Foundations of Basic Nursing

Third Edition

DEDICATIONS

Lois White:
To my beloved husband, John, who is on his last great adventure and learning experience.

Gena Duncan:
To my husband, who gives me unconditional love and brings balance, calmness, and excitement to my life.
To Lois White, who modeled the role of an author and committed much of her life to this textbook.
To Wendy Baumle, for her hard work and dedication in developing this textbook. Thanks.
To future nurses who are caring and competent.

Wendy Baumle:
This book is dedicated to my beloved family—Patrick, Taylor, Madeline, Blair, Connor, Janet, and Robert—for their love and support, to Juliet Steiner for inspiring me and for making a difference in my life, to Gena Duncan for her guidance and friendship, and to my friends, colleagues, and students for their support and valuable insight into today's nursing education.

Foundations of Basic Nursing

Third Edition

Lois White, RN, PhD
Former Chairperson and Professor Department of Vocational Nurse Education, Del Mar College, Corpus Christi, Texas

Gena Duncan, RN, MSEd, MSN
Former Associate Professor of Nursing, Ivy Tech Community College, Fort Wayne, Indiana

Wendy Baumle, RN, MSN
James A. Rhodes State College, School of Nursing, Lima, Ohio

CENGAGE Learning™
Australia • Brazil • Japan • Korea • Mexico • Singapore • Spain • United Kingdom • United States

DELMAR
CENGAGE Learning™

Foundations of Basic Nursing, Third Edition
Lois White, RN, PhD, Gena Duncan, RN, MSEd, MSN, and Wendy Baumle, RN, MSN

Vice President, Career and Professional Editorial: Dave Garza

Director of Learning Solutions: Matt Kane

Executive Editor: Steven Helba

Managing Editor: Marah Bellegarde

Senior Product Manager: Juliet Steiner

Editorial Assistant: Meghan E. Orvis

Vice President, Career and Professional Marketing: Jennifer Ann Baker

Marketing Director: Wendy Mapstone

Senior Marketing Manager: Michele McTighe

Marketing Coordinator: Scott Chrysler

Production Director: Carolyn Miller

Production Manager: Andrew Crouth

Senior Content Project Manager: James Zayicek

Senior Art Director: Jack Pendleton

Technology Project Manager: Mary Colleen Liburdi

Production Technology Analyst: Patricia Allen

Production Technology Analyst: Ben Knapp

Library of Congress Control Number: 2009929886
ISBN-13: 978-1-428-31774-1
ISBN-10: 1-428-31774-0

Delmar
5 Maxwell Drive
Clifton Park, NY 12065-2919
USA

Cengage Learning is a leading provider of customized learning solutions with office locations around the globe, including Singapore, the United Kingdom, Australia, Mexico, Brazil, and Japan. Locate your local office at: **international.cengage.com/region**

Cengage Learning products are represented in Canada by Nelson Education, Ltd.

To learn more about Delmar, visit **www.cengage.com/delmar**

Purchase any of our products at your local college store or at our preferred online store **www.CengageBrain.com**

Printed in the United States of America
2 3 4 5 6 7 12 11 10

CONTENTS

CHAPTER 4: LEGAL AND ETHICAL RESPONSIBILITIES / 62

UNIT 2

The Health Care Environment / 89

CHAPTER 5: THE HEALTH CARE DELIVERY SYSTEM / 90

CHAPTER 6: ARENAS OF CARE / 105

UNIT 3

Communication / 121

CHAPTER 7: COMMUNICATION / 122

CHAPTER 8: CLIENT TEACHING / 143

CHAPTER 11: CULTURAL CONSIDERATIONS / 229

CHAPTER 12: STRESS, ADAPTATION, AND ANXIETY / 257

CHAPTER 13: END-OF-LIFE CARE / 273

CHAPTER 20: SAFETY / HYGIENE / 416

UNIT 6
Infection Control / 439

CHAPTER 21: INFECTION CONTROL/ASEPSIS / 440

CHAPTER 25: MEDICATION ADMINISTRATION AND IV THERAPY / 515

CHAPTER 26: ASSESSMENT / 552

CHAPTER 27: PAIN MANAGEMENT / 573

CHAPTER 28: DIAGNOSTIC TESTS / 601

UNIT 8

Nursing Procedures / 657

CHAPTER 29: BASIC PROCEDURES / 658

CONTRIBUTORS

Joy E. Ache-Reed, RN, MS
Assistant Professor of Nursing
Indiana Wesleyan University
Marion, Indiana
Chapter 11, Cultural Considerations

Susan L. Bredemeyer, RN, MS
Former Assistant Professor
University of Saint Francis
Fort Wayne, Indiana
Chapter 26, Assessment

Ali Brown, RN, MSN
Assistant Professor
College of Nursing
University of Tennessee
Knoxville, Tennessee
Chapter 9, Nursing Process/ Documentation/Informatics

Donna J. Burleson, RN, MS
Chair of Nursing Department
Cisco Junior College
Abilene, Texas
Chapter 1, Student Nurse Skills for Success

Anne H. Cary, RN, PhD, MPH, A-CCC
Professor and Coordinator, PhD in Nursing Program
College of Nursing and Health Sciences
George Mason University
Fairfax, Virginia
Chapter 3, Nursing History, Education, and Organizations

Judy Conlon
Chapter 20, Safety/Hygiene

Jan Corder, RN, DNS
School of Nursing
Northeast Louisiana University
Monroe, Louisiana
Chapter 9, Nursing Process/ Documentation/ Informatics

Julie Coy, RNC, MS
Pain Consultation Service
The Children's Hospital
Denver, Colorado
Chapter 19, Rest and Sleep
Chapter 27, Pain Management

Cheryl Erickson, RN, BSN, MA, FNP-BC
Associate Professor
University of Saint Francis
Fort Wayne, Indiana
Chapter 26, Assessment

Mary Ellen Zator Estes, RN, MSN, FNP, APRN-BC, NP-C
Family Nurse Practitioner in Internal Medicine
Fairfax, Virginia
and
Adjunct Faculty
School of Health Professions
Marymount University
Arlington, VA
Chapter 26, Assessment

Mary Frost, RN, BSN
Covington, Louisiana
Chapter 17, Complementary/ Alternative Therapies

Susan Halley, RN, MS, FNP
Geriatric Nurse Practitioner
Fort Wayne, Indiana
Chapter 4, Legal and Ethical Responsibilities

Lucille Joel, RN, EdD, FAAN
Professor
College of Nursing
Rutgers, The State University of New Jersey
Newark, New Jersey
Chapter 5, The Health Care Delivery System

Denise M. Jordan, RN, BSN, MA
Chair of Nursing Program
IT Technical Institute
Fort Wayne, Indiana
Chapter 4, Legal and Ethical Responsibilities

Mary E. A. Laskin, RN, CS, MN
Clinical Nurse Specialist
Surgical/Orthopedic Services
Kaiser Permanente
San Diego, California
Chapter 27, Pain Management

Judy Martin, RN, MS, JD
Nurse Attorney
Louisiana Department of Health and Hospitals
Health Standards Section
Baton Rouge, Louisiana
Chapter 4, Legal and Ethical Responsibilities

Kim Martz
Instructor
Department of Nursing
Boise State University Department of Nursing
Boise, Idaho
Chapter 16: Spirituality

Linda McCuistion, RN, PhD
Assistant Professor
School of Nursing
Our Lady of Holy Cross College
New Orleans, Louisiana
Chapter 9, Nursing Process/ Documentation/Informatics

Betty Miller
Staff Development Coordinator
Meadowcrest Hospital
Gretna, Louisiana
Chapter 13, End-of-Life Care

Barbara S. Moffett, RN, PhD
Associate Professor of Nursing
School of Nursing
Southeastern Louisiana University
Hammond, Louisiana
Chapter 9, Nursing Process/ Documentation/Informatics

Mary Anne Mordcin-McCarthy, RN, PhD
Associate Professor and Director of the Undergraduate Program
College of Nursing
University of Tennessee–Knoxville
Knoxville, Tennessee
Chapter 9, Nursing Process/ Documentation/Informatics

Barbara Morvant, RN, MN
Louisiana State Board of Nursing
Metairie, Louisiana
Chapter 4, Nursing History, Education, and Organizations

Joan Fritsch Needham, RNC, MS
Director of Education
DeKalb County Nursing Home
DeKalb, Illinois
Chapter 6, Arenas of Care
Chapter 13, End-of-Life Care

Rebecca Osterhaut
Chapter 2, Holistic Care

Brenda Owens, RN, PhD
Associate Professor
School of Nursing
Louisiana State University Medical Center
New Orleans, Louisiana
Chapter 25, Medication Administration and IV Therapy

Demetrius Porche, RN, CCRN, DNS
Associate Professor and Director
Bachelor of Science in Nursing Program
Nicholsa State University
and
Adjunct Assistant Professor
Tulane University
School of Public Health and Topical Medicine
New Orleans, Louisiana
Chapter 20, Safety/Hygiene
Chapter 21, Infection Control/Asepsis
Chapter 22, Standard Precautions and Isolation

Suzanne Riche, RN
Charity School of Nursing
Delgado Community College
New Orleans, Louisiana
Chapter 9, Nursing Process/ Documentation/Informatics

Maureen Straight, RN, BSN, MSEd
Regents College
Albany, New York
Chapter 1, Student Nurse Skills for Success

Susan Stranahan, RN, DPH, BCC
Chaplain, Shell Point Retirement Community
Fort Myers, Florida
Chapter 11, Cultural Considerations

Leonie Sutherland, RN, PhD
Assistant Professor
Department of Nursing
Boise State University
Boise, Idaho
Chapter 16: Spirituality

Patricia R. Teasley, RN, MSN, APRN, BC
Central Texas College
Killeen, Texas
Chapter 23: Bioterrorism

John M. White, PhD
Former Chairperson, Professor
Biology Department
Del Mar College
Corpus Christi, Texas
Chapter 24, Fluid, Electrolyte, and Acid-Base Balance

Rothlyn Zahourek, RN, CS, MS
Certified Clinical Nurse Specialist
Amherst, Massachusetts
Chapter 17, Complementary/ Alternative Therapies

PROCEDURE CONTRIBUTORS

Gaylene Bouska Altman, RN, PhD
Director, Learning Lab
Faculty, School of Nursing
University of Washington
Seattle, Washington

Sharon Aronovitch, RN, PhD, CETN
Regents College
Albany, New York

Dale D. Barb, MHS, PT
Academic Coordinator of Clinical Education
Department of Physical Therapy
Wichita State University
Wichita, Kansas

Theresa A. Barenz, RN, MN

Susan Weiss Behrend, RN, MSN
Fox Chase Cancer Center
Philadelphia, Pennsylvania

Patricia Buchsel, RN, MSN, FAAN
Clinical Instructor
School of Nursing
University of Washington
Seattle, Washington

Bethaney Campbell, RN, MN, OCN
University of Washington Medical Center
Seattle, Washington

Curt Campbell
Integrated Health Services of Seattle
Seattle, Washington

Jung-Chen (Kristina) Chang, RN, MN, PhD
University of Washington
School of Nursing
Seattle, Washington

Eileen M. Collins, MN, ARNP, CNOR
University of Washington
School of Nursing
Seattle, Washington

Cheryl L. Cooke, RN, MN
Student Services Coordinator
University of Washington
School of Nursing
Seattle, Washington

Valerie Coxon, RN, PhD
Affiliate Assistant Professor
University of Washington
School of Nursing
Seattle, Washington
and
Chief Executive Officer
NRSPACE Software, Inc.
Bellevue, Washington

Gayle C. Crawford, RN, BSN,
Staff Nurse
University of Washington Medical Center
Seattle, Washington

Eleonor U. de la Pena, RN, BS
Northwest Asthma and Allergy Center
Seattle, Washington

Tom Ewing, RN, BSN
Hematology-Oncology
University of Washington Medical Center
Seattle, Washington

Amy Fryberger, RN, MN, ONC

Karrin Johnson, RN
Health Care Project Manager
NRSPACE Software, Inc.
Bellevue, Washington

Kimberly Sue Kahn, RN, MSN, FNP-C, CS, AOCN
University of Virginia
Portsmouth, Virginia

Catherine H. Kelley, RN, MSN, OCN
Chimeric Therapies, Inc.
Palatine, Illinois

Carla A. Bouska Lee, PhD, ARNP, FAAN
Clarkston College
Omaha, Nebraska

Kathryn Lilleby, RN
Clinical Research Nurse
Fred Hutchinson Cancer Research Center
Seattle, Washington

Joan M. Mack, RN, MSN, CS
Nebraska Medical Center
Omaha, Nebraska

Marianne Frances Moore, RN, MSN
Clarkson Hospital
Omaha, Nebraska

Susan Randolph, RN, MSN,CS
Manager, Transplant Services
Coram Healthcare
Parkersburg, West Virginia

Susan Rives, RN, BSN, OCN
CARE Center Coordinator
Martha Jefferson Hospital
Charlottesville, Virginia

Barbara Sigler, RN, MNEd, CORLN
Technical Publications Editor
Oncology Nursing Press, Inc.
Formerly: Clinical Nurse Specialist in Otolaryngology—Head and Neck Surgery
University of Pittsburgh Medical Center
Pittsburgh, Pennsylvania

Pam Talley, MN, PhD
University of Washington
School of Nursing
Seattle, Washington

Hsin-Yi (Jean) Tang, RN, MS, PhD
University of Washington
School of Nursing
Seattle, Washington

Robi Thomas, MS, RN, AOCN
Clinical Nurse Specialist for Oncology and the Pain Center
St. Mary's Mercy Medical Center
Grand Rapids, Michigan

Chandra VanPaepeghem, RN, BSN
University of Washington Medical Center
Seattle, Washington

REVIEWERS

Charlene Bell, RN, MSN, NCSN
Instructor
Associate Degree Nursing Program
Southwest Texas Junior College
Uvalde, Texas

Donna Burleson, RN, MS
Chair of Nursing Department
Cisco Junior College
Abilene, Texas

Dotty Cales, RN
Instructor
North Coast Medical Training Academy
Kent, Ohio

Carolyn Du, BSN, MSN, NP, CDe
Director of Education
Pacific College
Costa Mesa, California

Janice Eilerman, RN, MSN
Nursing Instructor
James A. Rhodes State College
Lima, OH

Jennifer Einhorn, RN, MS
Nursing Instructor
Chamberlain College of Nursing
Addison, Illinois

Patricia Fennessy, RN, MSN
Education Consultant
Connecticut Technical High School System
Middletown, Connecticut

Helena L. Jermalovic, RN, MSN
Assistant Professor
University of Alaska
Anchorage, Alaska

Lee Klopfenstein, MD, CMD
Family Physician
Long Term Care Medical Director
Van Wert, Ohio

Sharon Knarr, RN
Clinical Instructor
LPN Program
Northcoast Medical Training Academy
Kent, Ohio

Christine Levandowski, RN, BSN, MSN
Director of Nursing
Baker College
Auburn Hills, Michigan

Wendy Maleki, RN, MS
Director
Vocational Nursing Program
American Career College
Ontario, California

Deborah McMahan, MD
Health Commissioner of Fort Wayne-Allen County Department of Health
Fort Wayne, Indiana

Katherine C. Pellerin, RN, BS, MS
Department Head LPN Program
Norwich Technical High School
Norwich, Connecticut

Jennifer Ponto, RN, BSN
Faculty
Vocational Nursing Program
South Plains College
Levelland, Texas

Cheryl Pratt, RN, MA, CNAA
Regional Dean of Nursing
Rasmussen College
Mankato, Minnesota

Cherie R. Rebar, RN, MSN, MBA, FNP
Chair, Associate Professor, Nursing Program
Kettering College of Medical Arts
Kettering, Ohio

Patricia Schrull, RN, MSN, MBA, MEd, CNE
Director, Practical Nursing Program
Lorain County Community College
Elyria, Ohio

Laura Spinelli
Keiser Career College
Miami Lakes, Florida

Frances S. Stoner, RN, BSN, PHN
Instructor, NCLEX Coordinator
American Career College
Anaheim, California

Tina Terpening
Associate Nursing Faculty
University of Phoenix, Southern California Campus

Lori Theodore, RN, BSN
Orlando Tech
Orlando, Florida

Kimberly Valich, RN, MSN
Nursing Faculty, Department Chairperson
South Suburban College
South Holland, Illinois

Sarah Elizabeth Youth Whitaker, DNS, RN
Nursing Program Director
Computer Career Center
El Paso, Texas

Shawn White, RN, BSN
Clinical Coordinator, Nursing Instructor
Griffin Technical College
Griffin, Georgia

Christina R. Wilson, RN, BAN, PHN
Faculty, Practical Nursing Program
Anoka Technical College
Anoka, Minnesota

MARKET REVIEWERS AND CLASS TEST PARTICIPANTS

Deborah Ain
Nursing Professor
College of Southern Nevada
Las Vegas, Nevada

Mary Ann Ambrose, MSN, FNP
Program Director
Cuesta Community College Vocational Nursing Program
Paso Robles, California

Jennie Applegate, RN, BSN
Practical Nursing Instructor
Keiser Career College
Greenacres, Florida

Charlotte A. Armstrong, RN, BSN
Instructor
Northcoast Medical Training Academy
Kent, Ohio

Camille Baldwin
High Tech Central
Fort Myers, Florida

Priscilla Burks, RN, BSN
Practical Nursing Instructor
Hinds Community College
Pearl, Mississippi

Virginia Chacon
Colorado Technical University
Pueblo, Colorado

Sherri Comfort, RN
Practical Nursing Instructor Department Chair
Holmes Community College
Goodman, Mississippi

Brandy Coward, BNS, MA
Director of Nursing
Angeles Institute
Lakewood, California

Scott Coward, RN
Campus Director
Angeles Institute
Lakewood, California

Jennifer Decker
Clinical Instructor
College of Eastern Utah
Price, Utah

C. Kay Devereux
Professor
Department Chair, Vocational Nurse Education
Tyler Junior College
Tyler, Texas

Carolyn Du, BSN, MSN, NP, CDe
Director of Education
Pacific College
Costa Mesa, California

Laura R. Durbin, RN, BSN, CHPN
Instructor
West Kentucky Community and Technical College
Paducah, Kentucky

Robin Ellis, BSN, MS
Nursing Faculty
Provo College
Provo, Utah

Suzanne D. Fox, RN
Practical Nursing Instructor
Arkansas State University Technical Center
Marked Tree, Arkansas

Judie Fritz, RN, MSN
Instructor
Keiser Career College
Miami Lakes, Florida

Edith Gerdes, RN, MSN, BHCA
Associate Professor of Nursing
Ivy Tech Community College
South Bend, Indiana

Juanita Hamilton-Gonzalez
Professor
Coordinator—Practical Nursing Program
City University of New York–Medgar Evers
Brooklyn, New York

Jane Harper
Assistant Professor
Southeast Kentucky Community & Technical College
Pineville, Kentucky

Angie Headley
Nursing Instructor
Swainsboro Technical College
Swainsboro, Georgia

Lillie Hill
Clinical Coordinator/Instructor
Practical Nursing
Durham Technical Community College
Durham, North Carolina

Michelle Hopper
Sanford-Brown College
St. Peters, Missouri

Karla Huntsman, RN, MSN
Instructor
Nursing Program
AmeriTech College
Draper, Utah

Connie M. Hyde, RN, BSN
Practical Nursing Instructor
Louisiana Technical College
Lafayette, Louisiana

Kimball Johnson, RN, MS
Nursing Professor
College of Eastern Utah
Price, Utah

Sandy Kamhoot, BSN
Faculty
Santa Fe College
Gainesville, Florida

Juanita Kaness, MSN, RN, CRNP
Nursing Program Coordinator
Lehigh Carbon Community College
Schnecksville, Pennsylvania

Mary E. Kilbourn-Huey, MSN
Assistant Professor
Maysville Community and Technical College
Maysville, Kentucky

Gloria D. Kline, RN
Practical Nursing Instructor
Hinds Community College
Vicksburg, Mississippi

Christine Levandowski, RN, BSN, MSN
Director of Nursing
Baker College
Auburn Hills, Michigan

Mary Luckett, RN, MS
Professor Vocational Nursing
Level 1 Coordinator
Houston Community College
Coleman College for Health Sciences
Houston, Texas

Wendy Maleki, RN, MS
Director
Vocational Nursing Program
American Career College
Ontario, California

Luzviminda A. Malihan
Assistant Professor
Hostos Community College
Bronx, New York

Vanessa Norwood McGregor, RN, BSN, MBA
Practical Nursing Instructor
West Kentucky Community and Technical College
Paducah, Kentucky

Kristie Oles, RN, MSN
Practical Nursing Chair
Brown Mackie College
North Canton, Ohio

Beverly Pacas
Department Head/Instructor
Practical Nursing
Louisiana Technical College
Baton Rouge, Louisiana

Debra Perry, RN, MSN
Instructor
Lorain County Community College
Elyria, Ohio

Cheryl Pratt
Regional Dean of Nursing
Rasmussen College
Mankato, Minnesota

Charlotte Prewitt, RN, BSN
Practical Nursing Instructor
Meridian Technology Center
Stillwater, Oklahoma

Stephanie Price
Faculty, Practical Nursing
Holmes Community College
Goodman, Mississippi

Patricia Schrull, RN, MSN, MBA, M.Ed., CNE
Director, Practical Nursing Program
Lorain County Community College
Elyria, Ohio

Margi J. Schutlz, RN, MSN, Ph.D.
Director, Nursing Division
GateWay Community College
Phoenix, Arizona

Sherie A. Shupe, RN, MSN
Director of Nursing
Computer Career Center
Las Cruces, New Mexico

Sherri Smith, RN
Chairwoman
Arkansas State University Technical Center
Jonesboro, Arkansas

Cheryl Smith, RN, BSN
Practical Nursing Instructor
Colorado Technical University
North Kansas City, Missouri

Laura Spinelli
Keiser Career College
Miami Lakes, Florida

Jennifer Teerlink, RN, MSN
Nursing Faculty
Provo College
Provo, Utah

Dana L. Trowell, RN, BSN
LPN Program Director
Dalton State College
Dalton, Georgia

Racheal Vargas, LVN
Clinical Liaison
Medical Assisting/Vocational Nursing
Lake College
Reading, California

Sarah Elizabeth Youth Whitaker, DNS, RN
Nursing Program Director
Computer Career Center
El Paso, Texas

Shawn White, RN, BSN
Clinical Coordinator, Nursing Instructor
Griffin Technical College
Griffin, Georgia

Sharon Wilson
Program Director/Instructor, Practical Nursing
Durham Technical Community College
Durham, North Carolina

Vladmir Yarosh, LVN, BS
Program Coordinator—Vocational Nurse Program
Gurnick Academy of Medical Arts
San Mateo, California

DiAnn Zimmerman
Director, Instructor
Dakota County Technical College
Rosemount, Minnesota

PREFACE

Foundations of Basic Nursing, third edition, is designed for the beginning semester of a practical/vocational nursing program. It includes information on student nurse skills for success, microbiology, infection control (Standard Precautions), growth and development, legal and ethical issues, communication, documentation, nursing process, client teaching, cultural aspects, complementary/alternative therapies, wellness concepts, stress/anxiety, end-of-life care, rest/sleep, safety/hygiene, nutrition, fluid/electrolyte/acid-base balance, medication administration, IV therapy, assessment, pain management, diagnostic tests, and nursing procedures. There is a strong emphasis on life span development, older adult needs, and professional adjustments. Chapters on bioterrorism, spirituality, and self-concept enhance the student's learning of current nursing issues. Together with *Foundations of Adult Health Nursing,* third edition, and *Foundations of Maternal & Pediatric Nursing,* third edition, both also by White, Duncan, and Baumle, the books cover an entire curriculum for a practical/vocational nursing program.

Although a systems approach is presented, the concept of holistic care is fundamental to this text. Throughout the book, boxes highlight special topics regarding critical thinking questions, memory tricks, life span development, client teaching, cultural considerations, professional tips, community/home health care, safety, and infection control. Pharmacology basics, medication administration, and diagnostic testing are presented. The concept of critical thinking, presented in the first chapter, lays the foundation for the entire nursing process, presented in great detail and incorporating current NANDA diagnoses and NIC/NOC references. The student is provided with opportunities to demonstrate knowledge and develop critical thinking skills by completing Case Studies included in many of the chapters. Concept Maps and Concept Care Maps challenge the student to incorporate the interrelatedness of nursing concepts in preparation for clinical practice. The student has the opportunity to assess knowledge and critical thinking of essential nursing concepts by answering NCLEX®-style review questions at the end of each chapter.

Health care settings are changing, multifaceted, challenging, and rewarding. Critical thinking and sound nursing judgments are essential in the present health care environment. Practical/Vocational nursing students confront and adapt to changes in technology, information, and resources by building a solid foundation of accurate, essential information. A firm knowledge base also allows nurses to meet the changing needs of clients. This text was written to equip the LPN/VN with current knowledge, basic problem-solving and critical thinking skills to successfully pass the NCLEX®-PN exam and meet the demanding challenges of today's health care.

ORGANIZATION

Foundations of Basic Nursing, third edition, consists of 31 chapters grouped into 8 units.

- **Unit 1:** FOUNDATIONS—discusses student nurse skills for success (including critical thinking, time management, study skills, and life organizing skills); holistic care; nursing history, education, and organizations; and legal and ethical responsibilities.
- **Unit 2:** THE HEALTH CARE ENVIRONMENT—describes the health care delivery system and arenas of care, focusing on the various settings in which practical/vocational nurses practice.
- **Unit 3:** COMMUNICATION—addresses the process of communication, how communication is used in the nurse/client relationship; generational differences; and technical and legal aspects of documentation. Each component of the nursing process is explained in a clear, concise manner. Electronic medical records and technological information is incorporated throughout the chapters. The client teaching process is presented as a major nursing intervention for clients throughout the life span.
- **Unit 4:** DEVELOPMENTAL AND PSYCHOSOCIAL CONCERNS—describes the growth and development changes throughout the life span; cultural aspects and

considerations; stress, adaptation, and anxiety; grief and end-of-life care.

- **Unit 5:** HEALTH PROMOTION—addresses self-concept, spirituality, and complementary/alternative therapies. Wellness concepts, basic nutrition, rest and sleep, and safety/hygiene are presented as methods of promoting health.
- **Unit 6:** INFECTION CONTROL—presents the chain of infection, describes various types of pathogenic microorganism, presents the concepts of asepsis and aseptic technique along with Standard Precautions and isolation measures, and discusses issues regarding bioterrorism.
- **Unit 7:** FUNDAMENTAL NURSING CARE—discusses fluid, electrolyte and acid-base balance. Medication administration and IV therapy are presented in nursing process format. Also included are legal considerations, dose equivalents, and dosage calculations. Assessment is covered in great detail, including head-to-toe physical assessment, nursing history, and functional assessment. Pain management is detailed in causes of pain, transmission and perception, assessment methods, and nursing interventions for pain relief. Nursing care for a client encountering diagnostic tests is thoroughly covered. The most commonly-ordered diagnostic tests are presented in tables that provide the normal results and nursing considerations.
- **Unit 8:** NURSING PROCEDURES—basic, intermediate, and advanced procedures follow the nursing process format and are presented in step-by-step fashion. Rationale is given for each step, and figures add to the clarity of the procedures.

FEATURES

Each chapter includes a variety of learning aids designed to help the reader further a basic understanding of key concepts. Each chapter opens with a **Making the Connection** box that guides the reader to other key chapters related to the current chapter. This highlights the integration of the text material. Procedures used for the care of clients with medical/surgical disorders are identified as appropriate. **Learning Objectives** are presented at the beginning of each chapter as well. These help students focus their study and use their time efficiently. A listing of **Key Terms** is provided to identify the terms the student should know or learn for a better understanding of the subject matter. These are bolded and defined at first use in the chapter.

The content of each chapter is presented in nursing process format. Where appropriate, a **Sample Nursing Care Plan** is provided in the chapter. These serve as models for students to refer to as they create their own care plans based on case studies. **Case Studies** are presented at the conclusion of most chapters. These call for students to draw upon their knowledge base and synthesize information to develop their own solutions to realistic cases. **Nursing Diagnoses, Planning/Outcomes, and Interventions** are presented in a convenient table format for quick reference. **Concept Maps** and **Concept Care Maps** are visual pictures of interrelated concepts as they relate to nursing.

A bulleted **Summary** list and multiple-choice **NCLEX®-style Review Questions** at the end of each chapter assist the student in remembering and using the material presented. **References/Suggested Readings** allow the student to find the source of the material presented and also to find additional information concerning topics covered. **Resources** are also listed and provide names and internet addresses of organizations specializing in a specific area of health care.

Boxes used throughout the text emphasize key points and provide specific types of information. The boxes are:

- **Critical Thinking**: encourages the student to use the knowledge gained to think critically about a situation.
- **Memory Trick**: provides an easy-to-remember saying or mnemonic to assist the student in remembering important information presented.
- **Life Span Considerations**: provides information related to the care of specific age groups during the life span.
- **Client Teaching**: identifies specific items that the client should know related to the various disorders.
- **Cultural Considerations**: shares beliefs, manners, and ways of providing care, communication, and relationships of various cultural and ethnic groups as a way to provide holistic care.
- **Professional Tip**: offers tips and technical hints for the nurse to ensure quality care.
- **Safety:** emphasizes the importance of and ways to maintain safe care.
- **Community/Home Health Care**: describes factors to consider when providing care in the community or in a client's home, and adaptation in care that may be necessary.
- **Drug Icon**: highlights pharmacological treatments and interventions that may be appropriate for certain conditions and disorders.
- **Collaborative Care**: mentions members of the care team and their roles in providing comprehensive care to clients.
- **Infection Control**: indicates reminders of methods to prevent the spread of infections.

The back matter includes a **Glossary of Terms**. The appendices include **NANDA Nursing Diagnoses**; **Recommended Childhood, Adolescent, and Adult Immunization Schedules**; **Abbreviations, Acronyms** and **Symbols**; and **English/Spanish Words and Phrases**. **Standard Precautions** are found on the inside back cover.

NEW TO THIS EDITION

Added 3 new chapters:

- **Chapter 15**, *Self-Concept*, presents a global understanding of the dimensions, formation, and factors affecting self-concept to facilitate client coping and promote overall physical and mental wellness.
- **Chapter 16**, *Spirituality*, provides understanding of the basic human need for spirituality and prepares the nurse to integrate the spiritual aspect of each client into the care provided.
- **Chapter 23**, *Bioterrorism*, discusses the major agents of bioterrorism, protective measures prior to and following a terrorist attack, and delineates the roles of the nurse, various levels of government, and each person in the event of a terrorist attack.

Extensively updated chapters:

- **Chapter 13**, ***End-of-Life Care*** includes sections on fluids and nutrition, palliative care and hospice care, and pain management
- **Chapter 27**, ***Pain Management***, features an improved section on patient controlled analgesia (PCA) and oral patient controlled analgesia, medication on demand (MOD®); a discussion of gate control theory of pain; and a presentation of the Joint Commission standards for pain management and the World Health Organization's (WHO) pain management guidelines.

Updated content within chapters:

- Additional coverage of learning disabilities
- Information on preparing for exams and test-taking tips
- Includes coverage of Scientology beliefs in the Cultural Considerations chapter
- Follows the federal government's new recommended food pyramid, MyPyramid
- Updates to the Assessment chapter include assessing client using complementary/alternative therapy and assessment of edema
- Thorough updating of the basic, intermediate, and advanced procedure chapters with new photos for the visual learner
- Thorough updating of the Diagnostic Tests chapter with the addition of new current diagnostic testing procedures
- Added older adult content to the Life Span Development chapter and emphasized geriatric content in Life Span Considerations boxes

Other additions:

- Added case studies to all chapters as appropriate; case studies offer a mixture of critical thinking and nursing process questions
- Added Concept Maps to several chapters so the student can link facts with real life clinical practice
- Added Concept Care Maps to chapters as appropriate for visual picture of the nursing process
- Increased number of challenging and applicable critical thinking questions
- Cultural considerations updated and cultural content included throughout the text
- Added Adult Immunization Schedule along with Childhood and Adolescent Immunization Schedules
- Added current NANDA diagnoses according to NANDA-International (2009) *Nursing Diagnoses, 2009-2011 Edition: Definitions and Classification (NANDA Nursing Diagnosis)*.
- Added new NCLEX®-style review questions at the end of chapters to help students challenge their understanding of content while gaining practice with this important question style.
- Added memory tricks for ease of student recall of pertinent information.
- Numerous new photos and illustrations for improved presentation of concepts.
- New, free, StudyWARE™ CD-ROM provides interactive games, animations, videos, heart and lung sounds, and much more to augment the learning experience and support mastery of concepts.

EXTENSIVE TEACHING/ LEARNING PACKAGE

The complete supplements package for *Foundations of Basic Nursing*, third edition was developed to achieve two goals:

1. To assist students in learning the information and procedures presented in the text.
2. To assist instructors in planning and implementing their programs for the most efficient use of time and other resources.

INSTRUCTOR RESOURCES

Foundations of Nursing Instructor's Resource, fourth edition

ISBN-10: 1-428-31780-5
ISBN-13: 978-1-428-31780-2

The Instructor's Resource has four components to assist the instructor and enhance classroom activities and discussion.

Instructor's Guide

- **Instructional Approaches**: Ideas and concepts to help educators manage different presentation methods. Suggestions for approaching topics with rich discussion topics and lecture ideas are provided.
- **Student Learning Activities:** Ideas for activities such as classroom discussions, role play, and individual assignments designed to encourage student critical thinking as they engage with the concepts presented in the text.
- **Resources:** Additional books, videos, and resources for use in developing and implementing your curriculum.
- **Web Activities:** Suggestions for student learning experiences online, including specific websites and accompanying activities.
- **Suggested Responses to the Case Study:** Case studies located throughout the core book challenge student critical thinking with questions about nursing care. Suggested responses are included.
- **Answers to Review Questions:** Answers and rationales for all end-of-chapter NCLEX®-style questions are provided.

Computerized Testbank

- Includes a rich bank of questions that test students on retention and application of material in the text.
- Many questions are now presented in NCLEX® style, with each question providing the answer and rationale, as well as cognitive levels.
- Allows the instructor to mix questions from each of the didactic chapters to customize tests.

Instructor Slides Created in PowerPoint

- A robust offering of instructor slides created in PowerPoint outlines the concepts from text in order to assist the instructor with lectures.
- Ideas presented stimulate discussion and critical thinking.

Image Library

A searchable Image Library of more than 800 illustrations and photographs that can be incorporated into lectures, class materials, or electronic presentations.

Student Resources

Foundations of Basic Nursing Study Guide

ISBN-10: 1-428-31783-X
ISBN-13: 978-1-4283-1783-3

A valuable companion to the core book, this student resource provides additional review on all 61 chapters of *Foundations of Nursing* with Key Term matching review questions, Abbreviation Review Exercises, Self-Assessment Questions, and other review exercises and activities. Answers to questions are provided at the back of the book, making this an excellent resource for self-study and review.

Foundations of Basic Nursing Skills Checklist

ISBN-10: 1-428-31784-8
ISBN-13: 978-1-428-31784-0

This excellent resource helps students evaluate their comprehension and execution of all the basic, intermediate and advanced procedures covered in the core book.

Foundations of Nursing Online Companion

ISBN-10: 1-428-31779-1
ISBN-13: 978-1-428-31779-6

The Online Companion gives you online access to all the components in the Instructor's Resource as well as additional tools to reinforce the content in each chapter and enhance classroom teaching. Multimedia animations, additional chapters, and resources related to workplace transition are just some of the many resources found on this robust site.

CL eBook to Accompany Foundations of Basic Nursing, third edition

printed access code ISBN-10: 1-435-48790-7
printed access code ISBN-13: 978-1-435-48790-1
instant access code ISBN-10: 1-435-48789-3
instant access code ISBN-13: 978-1-435-48789-5

Foundations of Nursing WebTutor Advantage on Blackboard

ISBN-10: 1-428-31781-3
ISBN-13: 978-1-428-31781-9

Foundations of Nursing WebTutor Advantage on WebCT

ISBN-10: 1-428-31782-1
ISBN-13: 978-1-428-31782-6

- A complete online environment that supplements the course provided in both Blackboard and WebCT format.
- Includes chapter overviews, chapter outlines, and competencies.
- Useful classroom management tools include chats and calendars, as well as instructor resources such as the instructor slides created in PowerPoint.
- Multimedia offering includes video clips and 3D animations.

ABOUT THE AUTHORS

Lois Elain Wacker White earned a diploma in nursing from Memorial Hospital School of Nursing, Springfield, Illinois; an Associate degree in Science from Del Mar College, Corpus Christi, Texas; a Bachelor of Science in Nursing from Texas A & I University—Corpus Christi, Corpus Christi, Texas; a Master of Science in Education from Corpus Christi State University, Corpus Christi, Texas; and a Doctor of Philosophy degree in education administration—community college from the University of Texas, Austin, Texas.

She has taught at Del Mar College, Corpus Christi, Texas, in both the Associate Degree Nursing program and the Vocational Nursing program. For 14 years, she was also chairperson of the Department of Vocational Nurse Education. Dr. White has taught fundamentals of nursing, mental health/mental illness, medical-surgical nursing, and maternal/pediatric nursing. Her professional career has also included 15 years of clinical practice.

Dr. White has served on the Nursing Education Advisory Committee of the Board of Nurse Examiners for the State of Texas and the Board of Vocational Nurse Examiners, which developed competencies expected of graduates for each level of nursing.

Gena Duncan has worked as an RN for 36 years in the clinical, community health, and educational arenas. This has equipped Mrs. Duncan with a wide range of nursing experiences and varied skills to meet the educational needs of today's students. She has a MSEd and MSN.

During her professional career, Mrs. Duncan served as a staff nurse, an assistant head nurse of a medical-surgical unit, a continuing education instructor, an associate professor in an LPN program, and director of an Associate degree nursing program. She has taught LPN, ADN, BSN, and MSN nursing students. As a faculty member she taught many nursing courses and served on a statewide curriculum committee for a state college. As director of an Associate degree nursing program, she was instrumental in starting and obtaining state board approval of an LPN-RN nursing program.

Her master's research thesis was entitled, An Investigation of Learning Styles of Practical and Baccalaureate Students. The results of the study are published in the *Journal of Nursing Education*. She has coauthored two textbooks, a medical-surgical textbook, and a transitions text for LPN to RN students. She has been an active member of Sigma Theta Tau.

Wendy Baumle is currently a nursing instructor at James A. Rhodes State College in Ohio. She has spent 19 years as a clinician, educator, school district health coordinator, and academician. Mrs. Baumle has taught fundamentals of nursing, medical-surgical nursing, pediatrics, obstetrics, pharmacology, anatomy and physiology, and ethics in health care in practical nursing and associate nursing degree programs. She has previously taught at Lutheran College, Fort Wayne, Indiana, at Northwest State Community College, Archbold, Ohio, and at James. A. Rhodes State College in Lima, Ohio. Mrs. Baumle earned her Bachelor of Science degree in Nursing from The University of Toledo, Toledo, Ohio and her Master's degree in Nursing from The Medical College of Ohio, Toledo, Ohio. Mrs. Baumle is a member of a number of professional nursing organizations, including Sigma Theta Tau, the American Nurses Association, the National League for Nursing, and the Ohio Nurses Association.

ACKNOWLEDGMENTS

Many people must work together to produce any textbook, but a comprehensive book such as this requires even more people with various areas of expertise. We would like to thank the contributors for their time and effort to share their knowledge gained through years of experience in both the clinical and academic settings. Nancy Emke, clinical nurse oncology specialist at Parkview Health Comprehensive Cancer Center, contributed content to Chapter 2, Holistic Care.

To the reviewers, we thank you for your time spent critically reading the manuscript, expertise, and valuable suggestions that have added to this text.

We would like to acknowledge and sincerely thank the entire team at Delmar Cengage Learning who has worked to make this textbook a reality. Juliet Steiner, senior product manager, receives a special thank you. She has kept us on track and provided guidance with humor, enthusiasm, sensitivity, and expertise. We extend a special thank you to Steve Helba, executive editor, for his vision for this text, calm demeanor, and patience. Other members on the team—Marah Bellegarde, managing editor, James Zayicek, senior content product manager, Jack Pendleton, senior art director, and Meghan Orvis, editorial assistant, have all worked diligently for the completion of this textbook. Thank you to all.

HOW TO USE THIS TEXT

This text is designed with you, the reader, in mind. Special elements and feature boxes appear throughout the text to guide you in reading and to assist you in learning the material. Following are suggestions for how you can use these features to increase your understanding and mastery of the content.

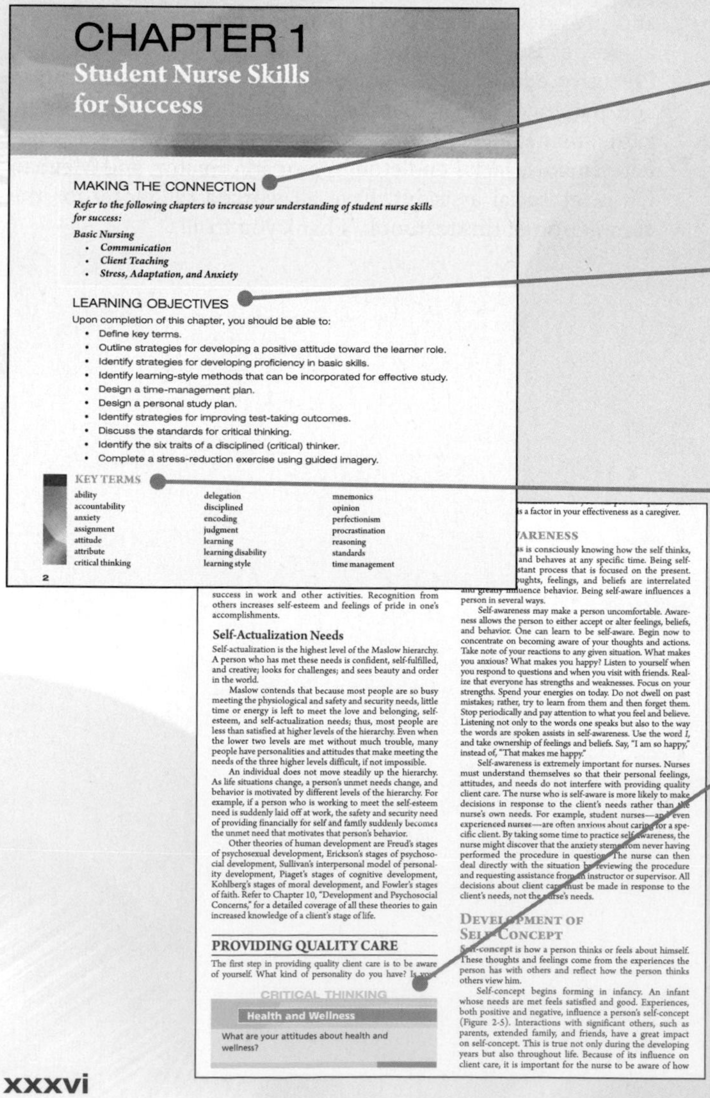

CHAPTER 1

Student Nurse Skills for Success

MAKING THE CONNECTION

Refer to the following chapters to increase your understanding of student nurse skills for success:

Basic Nursing

- *Communication*
- *Client Teaching*
- *Stress, Adaptation, and Anxiety*

LEARNING OBJECTIVES

Upon completion of this chapter, you should be able to:

- Define key terms.
- Outline strategies for developing a positive attitude toward the learner role.
- Identify strategies for developing proficiency in basic skills.
- Identify learning-style methods that can be incorporated for effective study.
- Design a time-management plan.
- Design a personal study plan.
- Identify strategies for improving test-taking outcomes.
- Discuss the standards for critical thinking.
- Identify the six traits of a disciplined (critical) thinker.
- Complete a stress-reduction exercise using guided imagery.

KEY TERMS

ability	delegation	mnemonics
accountability	disciplined	opinion
anxiety	encoding	perfectionism
assignment	judgment	procrastination
attitude	learning	reasoning
attribute	learning disability	standards
critical thinking	learning style	time management

2

success in work and other activities. Recognition from others increases self-esteem and feelings of pride in one's accomplishments.

Self-Actualization Needs

Self-actualization is the highest level of the Maslow hierarchy. A person who has met these needs is confident, self-fulfilled, and creative; looks for challenges; and sees beauty and order in the world.

Maslow contends that because most people are so busy meeting the physiological and safety and security needs, little time or energy is left to meet the love and belonging, self-esteem, and self-actualization needs; thus, most people are less than satisfied at higher levels of the hierarchy. Even when the lower two levels are met without much trouble, many people have personalities and attitudes that make meeting the needs of the three higher levels difficult, if not impossible.

An individual does not move steadily up the hierarchy. As life situations change, a person's unmet needs change, and behavior is motivated by different levels of the hierarchy. For example, if a person who is working to meet the self-esteem need is suddenly laid off at work, the safety and security need of providing financially for self and family suddenly becomes the unmet need that motivates that person's behavior.

Other theories of human development are Freud's stages of psychosexual development, Erickson's stages of psychosocial development, Sullivan's interpersonal model of personality development, Piaget's stages of cognitive development, Kohlberg's stages of moral development, and Fowler's stages of faith. Refer to Chapter 10, "Development and Psychosocial Concerns," for a detailed coverage of all these theories to gain increased knowledge of a client's stage of life.

PROVIDING QUALITY CARE

The first step in providing quality client care is to be aware of yourself. What kind of personality do you have? Is your

CRITICAL THINKING

Health and Wellness

What are your attitudes about health and wellness?

…is a factor in your effectiveness as a caregiver.

…ARENESS

…s is consciously knowing how the self thinks, … and behaves at any specific time. Being self-… stant process that is focused on the present. …oughts, feelings, and beliefs are interrelated and greatly influence behavior. Being self-aware influences a person in several ways.

Self-awareness may make a person uncomfortable. Awareness allows the person to either accept or alter feelings, beliefs, and behavior. One can learn to be self-aware. Begin now to concentrate on becoming aware of your thoughts and actions. Take note of your reactions to any given situation. What makes you anxious? What makes you happy? Listen to yourself when you respond to questions and when you visit with friends. Realize that everyone has strengths and weaknesses. Focus on your strengths. Spend your energies on today. Do not dwell on past mistakes; rather, try to learn from them and then forget them. Stop periodically and pay attention to what you feel and believe. Listening not only to the words one speaks but also to the way the words are spoken assists in self-awareness. Use the word *I*, and take ownership of feelings and beliefs. Say, "I am so happy," instead of, "That makes me happy."

Self-awareness is extremely important for nurses. Nurses must understand themselves so that their personal feelings, attitudes, and needs do not interfere with providing quality client care. The nurse who is self-aware is more likely to make decisions in response to the client's needs rather than the nurse's own needs. For example, student nurses—and even experienced nurses—are often anxious about caring for a specific client. By taking some time to practice self-awareness, the nurse might discover that the anxiety stems from never having performed the procedure in question. The nurse can then deal directly with the situation by reviewing the procedure and requesting assistance from an instructor or supervisor. All decisions about client care must be made in response to the client's needs, not the nurse's needs.

DEVELOPMENT OF SELF-CONCEPT

Self-concept is how a person thinks or feels about himself. These thoughts and feelings come from the experiences the person has with others and reflect how the person thinks others view him.

Self-concept begins forming in infancy. An infant whose needs are met feels satisfied and good. Experiences, both positive and negative, influence a person's self-concept (Figure 2-5). Interactions with significant others, such as parents, extended family, and friends, have a great impact on self-concept. This is true not only during the developing years but also throughout life. Because of its influence on client care, it is important for the nurse to be aware of how

MAKING THE CONNECTION

Read these boxes before beginning a chapter to link material across the holistic care continuum and to tie new content to the material you have already encountered.

LEARNING OBJECTIVES

Read the chapter objectives before reading the chapter to set the stage for learning. Revisit the objectives when preparing for an exam to see which entries you can respond to with "yes, I can do that."

KEY TERMS

Review this list before reading the chapter to familiarize yourself with the new terms and to revisit those terms you already know to link them to the content in the new chapter.

CRITICAL THINKING

Visit these boxes after reading the entire chapter to check your understanding of the concepts presented.

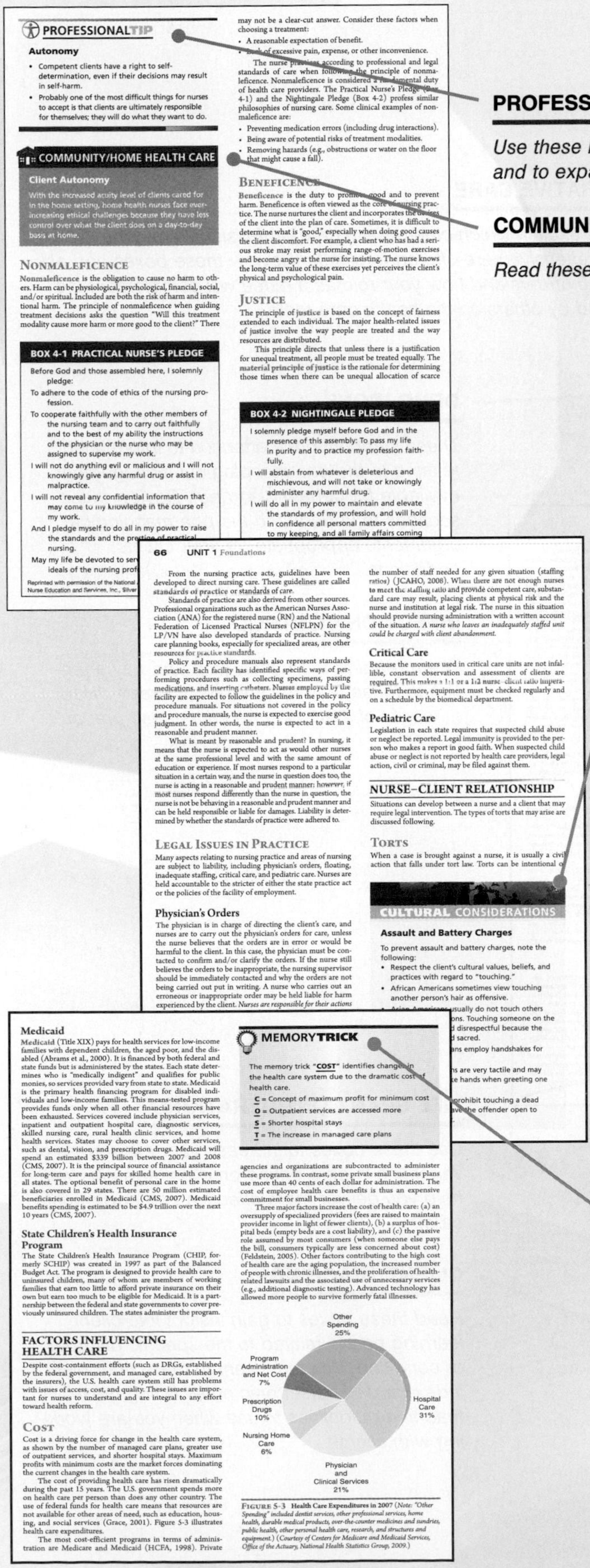

PROFESSIONAL TIP

Use these boxes to increase your professional competence and confidence, and to expand your knowledge base.

COMMUNITY/HOME HEALTH CARE

Read these boxes before making a home visit to a client with a given disorder.

CULTURAL CONSIDERATIONS

Test your sensitivity to cultural and ethnic diversity by scanning these boxes and using the guidelines and suggestions in your practice. You may also want to ask yourself what biases or preconceptions you have about different cultural practices before reading a chapter and then read these boxes for information that may help you be more sensitive in your nursing care and approach to clients.

MEMORY TRICK

Use the mnemonic devices provided in the new Memory Trick feature to help you remember the correct steps or proper order of information when working with clients.

HOW TO USE THIS TEXT (Continued)

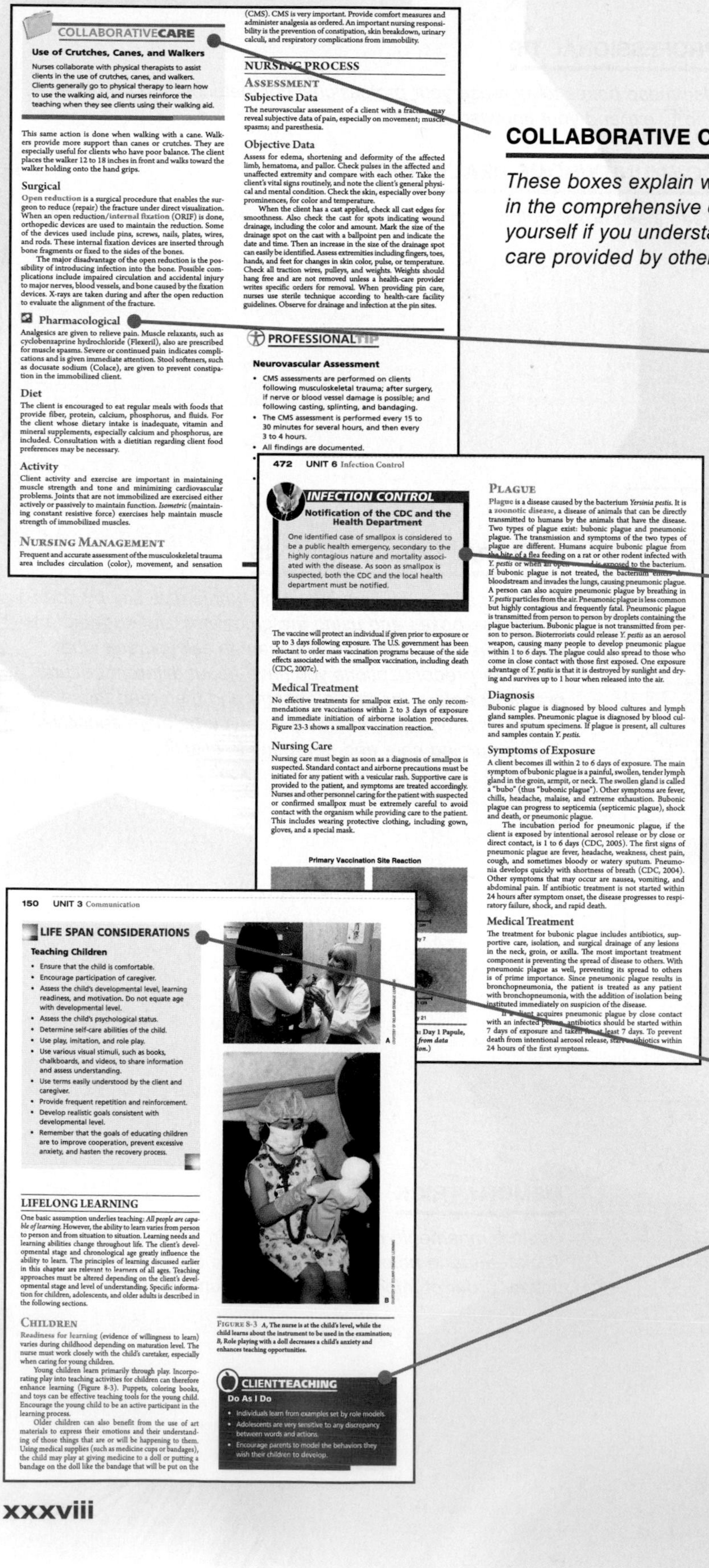

COLLABORATIVE CARE

Use of Crutches, Canes, and Walkers

Nurses collaborate with physical therapists to assist clients in the use of crutches, canes, and walkers. Clients generally go to physical therapy to learn how to use the walking aid, and nurses reinforce the teaching when they see clients using their walking aid.

This same action is done when walking with a cane. Walkers provide more support than canes or crutches. They are especially useful for clients who have poor balance. The client places the walker 12 to 18 inches in front and walks toward the walker holding onto the hand grips.

Surgical

Open reduction is a surgical procedure that enables the surgeon to reduce (repair) the fracture under direct visualization. When an open reduction/**internal fixation** (ORIF) is done, orthopedic devices are used to maintain the reduction. Some of the devices used include pins, screws, nails, plates, wires, and rods. These internal fixation devices are inserted through bone fragments or fixed to the sides of the bones.

The major disadvantage of the open reduction is the possibility of introducing infection into the bone. Possible complications include impaired circulation and accidental injury to major nerves, blood vessels, and bone caused by the fixation devices. X-rays are taken during and after the open reduction to evaluate the alignment of the fracture.

Pharmacological

Analgesics are given to relieve pain. Muscle relaxants, such as cyclobenzaprine hydrochloride (Flexeril), also are prescribed for muscle spasms. Severe or continued pain indicates complications and is given immediate attention. Stool softeners, such as docusate sodium (Colace), are given to prevent constipation in the immobilized client.

Diet

The client is encouraged to eat regular meals with foods that provide fiber, protein, calcium, phosphorus, and fluids. For the client whose dietary intake is inadequate, vitamin and mineral supplements, especially calcium and phosphorus, are included. Consultation with a dietitian regarding client food preferences may be necessary.

Activity

Client activity and exercise are important in maintaining muscle strength and tone and minimizing cardiovascular problems. Joints that are not immobilized are exercised either actively or passively to maintain function. *Isometric* (maintaining constant resistive force) exercises help maintain muscle strength of immobilized muscles.

NURSING MANAGEMENT

Frequent and accurate assessment of the musculoskeletal trauma area includes circulation (color), movement, and sensation (CMS). CMS is very important. Provide comfort measures and administer analgesia as ordered. An important nursing responsibility is the prevention of constipation, skin breakdown, urinary calculi, and respiratory complications from immobility.

NURSING PROCESS

ASSESSMENT

Subjective Data

The neurovascular assessment of a client with a fracture may reveal subjective data of pain, especially on movement; muscle spasms; and paresthesia.

Objective Data

Assess for edema, shortening and deformity of the affected limb, hematoma, and pallor. Check pulses in the affected and unaffected extremity and compare with each other. Take the client's vital signs routinely, and note the client's general physical and mental condition. Check the skin, especially over bony prominences, for color and temperature.

When the client has a cast applied, check all cast edges for smoothness. Also check the cast for spots indicating wound drainage, including the color and amount. Mark the size of the drainage spot on the cast with a ballpoint pen and indicate the date and time. Then an increase in the size of the drainage spot can easily be identified. Assess extremities including fingers, toes, hands, and feet for changes in skin color, pulse, or temperature. Check all traction wires, pulleys, and weights. Weights should hang free and are not removed unless a health-care provider writes specific orders for removal. When providing pin care, nurses use sterile technique according to health-care facility guidelines. Observe for drainage and infection at the pin sites.

PROFESSIONALTIP

Neurovascular Assessment

- CMS assessments are performed on clients following musculoskeletal trauma; after surgery, if nerve or blood vessel damage is possible; and following casting, splinting, and bandaging.
- The CMS assessment is performed every 15 to 30 minutes for several hours, and then every 3 to 4 hours.
- All findings are documented.

472 UNIT 6 Infection Control

INFECTION CONTROL

Notification of the CDC and the Health Department

One identified case of smallpox is considered to be a public health emergency, secondary to the highly contagious nature and mortality associated with the disease. As soon as smallpox is suspected, both the CDC and the local health department must be notified.

The vaccine will protect an individual if given prior to exposure or up to 3 days following exposure. The U.S. government has been reluctant to order mass vaccination programs because of the side effects associated with the smallpox vaccination, including death (CDC, 2007c).

Medical Treatment

No effective treatments for smallpox exist. The only recommendations are vaccinations within 2 to 3 days of exposure and immediate initiation of airborne isolation procedures. Figure 23-3 shows a smallpox vaccination reaction.

Nursing Care

Nursing care must begin as soon as a diagnosis of smallpox is suspected. Standard contact and airborne precautions must be initiated for any patient with a vesicular rash. Supportive care is provided to the patient, and symptoms are treated accordingly. Nurses and other personnel caring for the patient with suspected or confirmed smallpox must be extremely careful to avoid contact with the organism while providing care to the patient. This includes wearing protective clothing, including gown, gloves, and a special mask.

Primary Vaccination Site Reaction

PLAGUE

Plague is a disease caused by the bacterium *Yersinia pestis*. It is a **zoonotic disease**, a disease of animals that can be directly transmitted to humans by the animals that have the disease. Two types of plague exist: bubonic plague and pneumonic plague. The transmission and symptoms of the two types of plague are different. Humans acquire bubonic plague from the bite of a flea feeding on a rat or other rodent infected with *Y. pestis* or when an open wound is exposed to the bacterium. If bubonic plague is not treated, the bacterium enters the bloodstream and invades the lungs, causing pneumonic plague. A person can also acquire pneumonic plague by breathing in *Y. pestis* particles from the air. Pneumonic plague is less common but highly contagious and frequently fatal. Pneumonic plague is transmitted from person to person by droplets containing the plague bacterium. Bubonic plague is not transmitted from person to person. Bioterrorists could release *Y. pestis* as an aerosol weapon, causing many people to develop pneumonic plague within 1 to 6 days. The plague could also spread to those who come in close contact with those first exposed. One exposure advantage of *Y. pestis* is that it is destroyed by sunlight and drying and survives up to 1 hour when released into the air.

Diagnosis

Bubonic plague is diagnosed by blood cultures and lymph gland samples. Pneumonic plague is diagnosed by blood cultures and sputum specimens. If plague is present, all cultures and samples contain *Y. pestis*.

Symptoms of Exposure

A client becomes ill within 2 to 6 days of exposure. The main symptom of bubonic plague is a painful, swollen, tender lymph gland in the groin, armpit, or neck. The swollen gland is called a "bubo" (thus "bubonic plague"). Other symptoms are fever, chills, headache, malaise, and extreme exhaustion. Bubonic plague can progress to septicemia (septicemic plague), shock and death, or pneumonic plague.

The incubation period for pneumonic plague, if the client is exposed by intentional aerosol release or by close or direct contact, is 1 to 6 days (CDC, 2005). The first signs of pneumonic plague are fever, headache, weakness, chest pain, cough, and sometimes bloody or watery sputum. Pneumonia develops quickly with shortness of breath (CDC, 2004). Other symptoms that may occur are nausea, vomiting, and abdominal pain. If antibiotic treatment is not started within 24 hours after symptom onset, the disease progresses to respiratory failure, shock, and rapid death.

Medical Treatment

The treatment for bubonic plague includes antibiotics, supportive care, isolation, and surgical drainage of any lesions in the neck, groin, or axilla. The most important treatment component is preventing the spread of disease to others. With pneumonic plague as well, preventing its spread to others is of prime importance. Since pneumonic plague results in bronchopneumonia, the patient is treated as any patient with bronchopneumonia, with the addition of isolation being instituted immediately on suspicion of the disease.

If a client acquires pneumonic plague by close contact with an infected person, antibiotics should be started within 7 days of exposure and taken for at least 7 days. To prevent death from intentional aerosol release, start antibiotics within 24 hours of the first symptoms.

150 UNIT 3 Communication

LIFE SPAN CONSIDERATIONS

Teaching Children

- Ensure that the child is comfortable.
- Encourage participation of caregiver.
- Assess the child's developmental level, learning readiness, and motivation. Do not equate age with developmental level.
- Assess the child's psychological status.
- Determine self-care abilities of the child.
- Use play, imitation, and role play.
- Use various visual stimuli, such as books, chalkboards, and videos, to share information and assess understanding.
- Use terms easily understood by the client and caregiver.
- Provide frequent repetition and reinforcement.
- Develop realistic goals consistent with developmental level.
- Remember that the goals of educating children are to improve cooperation, prevent excessive anxiety, and hasten the recovery process.

LIFELONG LEARNING

One basic assumption underlies teaching: *All people are capable of learning*. However, the ability to learn varies from person to person and from situation to situation. Learning needs and learning abilities change throughout life. The client's developmental stage and chronological age greatly influence the ability to learn. The principles of learning discussed earlier in this chapter are relevant to learners of all ages. Teaching approaches must be altered depending on the client's developmental stage and level of understanding. Specific information for children, adolescents, and older adults is described in the following sections.

CHILDREN

Readiness for learning (evidence of willingness to learn) varies during childhood depending on maturation level. The nurse must work closely with the child's caretaker, especially when caring for young children.

Young children learn primarily through play. Incorporating play into teaching activities for children can therefore enhance learning (Figure 8-3). Puppets, coloring books, and toys can be effective teaching tools for the young child. Encourage the young child to be an active participant in the learning process.

Older children can also benefit from the use of art materials to express their emotions and their understanding of those things that are or will be happening to them. Using medical supplies (such as medicine cups or bandages), the child may play at giving medicine to a doll or putting a bandage on the doll like the bandage that will be put on the

FIGURE 8-3 *A*, The nurse is at the child's level, while the child learns about the instrument to be used in the examination; *B*, Role playing with a doll decreases a child's anxiety and enhances teaching opportunities.

CLIENTTEACHING

Do As I Do

- Individuals learn from examples set by role models.
- Adolescents are very sensitive to any discrepancy between words and actions.
- Encourage parents to model the behaviors they wish their children to develop.

COLLABORATIVE CARE

These boxes explain which other health care professionals may be involved in the comprehensive care offered to clients. Review these boxes and ask yourself if you understand how your role as a nurse will complement the care provided by others on the health care team.

DRUG ICONS

These symbols draw attention to information relating to the pharmacological management available for certain disorders. Review these sections to understand the pharmacological treatments appropriate for your clients' conditions.

INFECTION CONTROL

When reading a chapter, stop and pay attention to these features and ask yourself, "Had I thought of that? Do I practice these precautions?"

LIFE SPAN CONSIDERATIONS

Use these boxes to increase your awareness of variations in care based on client age; this will help you deliver more effective and appropriate care.

CLIENT TEACHING

Read these boxes to gain insight into client learning needs related to the specific disorder or condition. You may want to make your own index cards or electronic notes listing these teaching guidelines to use when you are working with clients.

HOW TO USE THIS TEXT (Continued)

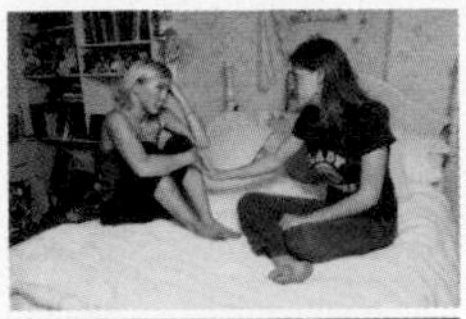

FIGURE 15-5 Support from friends promotes a healthy self-concept during adolescence.

comments and reactions from their peers can cause them to participate in substance abuse, inappropriate sexual behavior, and eating disorders as an attempt to fit in. Adolescents struggling with how to deal with anxiety and depression due to these expectations may use self-injury (self-mutilation) as a method of coping or even attempt suicide.

The development of a healthy self-concept for the adolescent often lies in parental involvement and support. As the adolescent becomes more independent, the parents may need to adapt and change their parenting style. While adolescents may begin to attain more independence, they still require the love, support, and involvement of their family and friends (Figure 15-5).

ADULTHOOD

The natural process of aging will lead to significant cha... in a person's self-concept. Over the course of a lifetim... adult will experience changes in one's roles, body, and i... tity. Young adults strive to develop relationships, careers... often a family. Older adults attempt to define themselv... their accomplishments. Major life events in adulthood... continuously shape a person's self-concept, such as obta... a college degree, getting a job, marriage, divorce, losing a... retirement, and the death of a significant other. How the ... vidual views and copes with these changes will determin... influence and impact they have on the person's self-con...

FACTORS AFFECTING SELF-CONCEPT

Self-concept can be affected by an individual's life ex... ences, heredity and culture, stress and coping, health st... and developmental stage. The nurse needs to evaluate ea... these factors and the influence each has on the client's ach... ment of a healthy self-concept (Figure 15-6).

LIFE EXPERIENCES

Life experiences, including success and failure, will dev... and influence a person's self-concept. Experiences in w... the individual has accomplished a goal and achieved su... will positively reinforce the development of a healthy... concept. Difficult experiences and/or failures can negat... impact a person's self-concept unless they have establ...

SAFETY

A mental health professional needs to be consulted immediately when self-injury, suicide, or eating disorders are suspected or committed.

Self-injury: Self-injury involves intentional self-inflicted tissue damage, such as cutting, burning, skin picking, or pulling one's hair out. This disorder occurs in either sex and in any religion or race and is not limited by education, age, or social status. Statistics are difficult to obtain because of the secretive nature of this disorder (Cleveland Clinic, 2005). Search online at http://www.clevelandclinic.org for more information.

Suicide: Suicide is the third-leading cause of death in clients aged 10 to 24. Boys, Native Americans/Alaskan Natives, and Hispanic youth have the highest rates of suicide. Approximately 32,000 suicides (one every 16 minutes) are committed in the United States each year (CDC, 2008b). Search online at http://www.cdc.gov for more information.

Eating disorders: Anorexia nervosa, bulimia, and binge eating are the three most common eating disorders. Anorexia nervosa and bulimia can lead to life-threatening conditions, resulting in permanent damage to major organs of the body. Statistics are difficult to obtain because of the secretive nature of these disorders (CDC, 2009).

SAFETY

Pause while reading to consider these elements and quiz yourself: "Do I take steps such as these to ensure my own and the client's safety? Do I follow these guidelines in every practice encounter?"

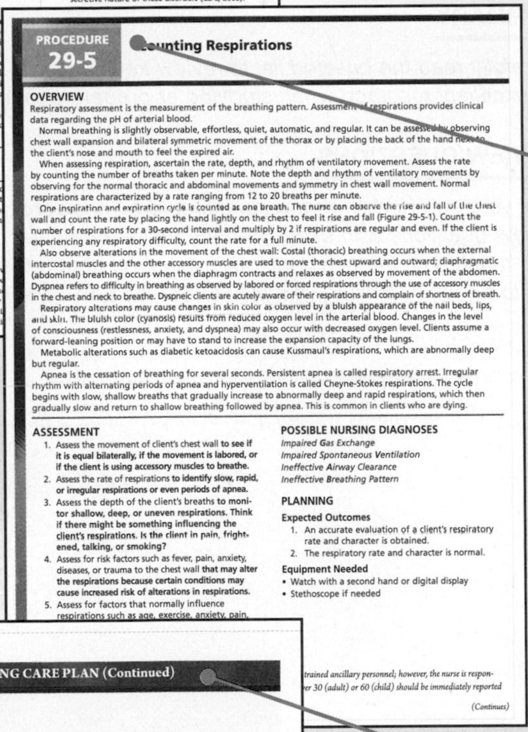

PROCEDURE 29-5 Counting Respirations

OVERVIEW

Respiratory assessment is the measurement of the breathing pattern. Assessment of respirations provides clinical data regarding the pH of arterial blood.

Normal breathing is slightly observable, effortless, quiet, automatic, and regular. It can be assessed by observing chest wall expansion and bilateral symmetric movement of the thorax or by placing the back of the hand next to the client's nose and mouth to feel the expired air.

When assessing respiration, ascertain the rate, depth, and rhythm of ventilatory movement. Assess the rate by counting the number of breaths taken per minute. Note the depth and rhythm of ventilatory movements by observing for the normal thoracic and abdominal movements and symmetry in chest wall movement. Normal respirations are characterized by a rate ranging from 12 to 20 breaths per minute.

One inspiration and expiration cycle is counted as one breath. The nurse can observe the rise and fall of the chest wall and count the rate by placing the hand lightly on the chest to feel it rise and fall (Figure 29-5-1). Count the number of respirations for a 30-second interval and multiply by 2 if respirations are regular and even. If the client is experiencing any respiratory difficulty, count the rate for a full minute.

Also observe alterations in the movement of the chest wall: Costal (thoracic) breathing occurs when the external intercostal muscles and the other accessory muscles are used to move the chest upward and outward; diaphragmatic (abdominal) breathing occurs when the diaphragm contracts and relaxes as observed by movement of the abdomen. Dyspnea refers to difficulty in breathing as observed by labored or forced respirations through the use of accessory muscles in the chest and neck to breathe. Dyspneic clients are acutely aware of their respirations and complain of shortness of breath.

Respiratory alterations may cause changes in skin color as observed by a bluish appearance of the nail beds, lips, and skin. The bluish color (cyanosis) results from reduced oxygen level in the arterial blood. Changes in the level of consciousness (restlessness, anxiety, and dyspnea) may also occur with decreased oxygen level. Clients assume a forward-leaning position or may have to stand to increase the expansion capacity of the lungs.

Metabolic alterations such as diabetic ketoacidosis can cause Kussmaul's respirations, which are abnormally deep but regular.

Apnea is the cessation of breathing for several seconds. Persistent apnea is called respiratory arrest. Irregular rhythm with alternating periods of apnea and hyperventilation is called Cheyne-Stokes respirations. The cycle begins with slow, shallow breaths that gradually increase to abnormally deep and rapid respirations, which then gradually slow and return to shallow breathing followed by apnea. This is common in clients who are dying.

ASSESSMENT

1. Assess the movement of client's chest wall **to see if it is equal bilaterally, if the movement is labored, or if the client is using accessory muscles to breathe.**
2. Assess the rate of respirations **to identify slow, rapid, or irregular respirations or even periods of apnea.**
3. Assess the depth of the client's breaths **to monitor shallow, deep, or uneven respirations. Think if there might be something influencing the client's respirations. Is the client in pain, frightened, talking, or smoking?**
4. Assess for risk factors such as fever, pain, anxiety, diseases, or trauma to the chest wall **that may alter the respirations because certain conditions may cause increased risk of alterations in respirations.**
5. Assess for factors that normally influence respirations such as age, exercise, anxiety, pain, ...

POSSIBLE NURSING DIAGNOSES

Impaired Gas Exchange
Impaired Spontaneous Ventilation
Ineffective Airway Clearance
Ineffective Breathing Pattern

PLANNING

Expected Outcomes

1. An accurate evaluation of a client's respiratory rate and character is obtained.
2. The respiratory rate and character is normal.

Equipment Needed

- Watch with a second hand or digital display
- Stethoscope if needed

...trained ancillary personnel; however, the nurse is respon-... ...er 30 (adult) or 60 (child) should be immediately reported

(Continues)

PROCEDURES

Reference the procedures as you read the chapters. Study the techniques, review the figures, and be prepared for your clinical days with questions of clarification for your instructor.

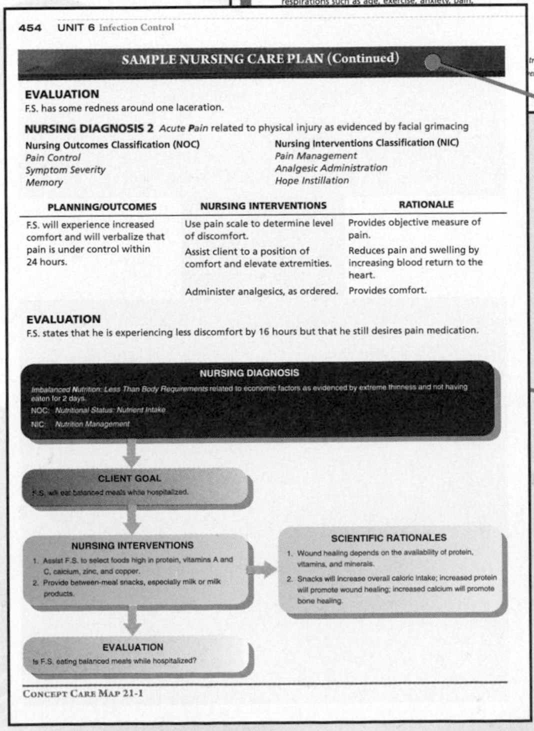

454 UNIT 6 Infection Control

SAMPLE NURSING CARE PLAN (Continued)

EVALUATION

F.S. has some redness around one laceration.

NURSING DIAGNOSIS 2 *Acute Pain* related to physical injury as evidenced by facial grimacing

Nursing Outcomes Classification (NOC)	Nursing Interventions Classification (NIC)
Pain Control	*Pain Management*
Symptom Severity	*Analgesic Administration*
Memory	*Hope Instillation*

PLANNING/OUTCOMES	NURSING INTERVENTIONS	RATIONALE
F.S. will experience increased comfort and will verbalize that pain is under control within 24 hours.	Use pain scale to determine level of discomfort.	Provides objective measure of pain.
	Assist client to a position of comfort and elevate extremities.	Reduces pain and swelling by increasing blood return to the heart.
	Administer analgesics, as ordered.	Provides comfort.

EVALUATION

F.S. states that he is experiencing less discomfort by 16 hours but that he still desires pain medication.

NURSING DIAGNOSIS

Imbalanced Nutrition: Less Than Body Requirements related to economic factors as evidenced by extreme thinness and not having eaten for 2 days.

NOC: *Nutritional Status: Nutrient Intake*

NIC: *Nutrition Management*

CLIENT GOAL

F.S. will eat balanced meals while hospitalized.

NURSING INTERVENTIONS

1. Assist F.S. to select foods high in protein, vitamins A and C, calcium, zinc, and copper.
2. Provide between-meal snacks, especially milk or milk products.

SCIENTIFIC RATIONALES

1. Wound healing depends on the availability of protein, vitamins, and minerals.
2. Snacks will increase overall caloric intake; increased protein will promote wound healing; increased calcium will promote bone healing.

EVALUATION

Is F.S. eating balanced meals while hospitalized?

CONCEPT CARE MAP 21-1

SAMPLE NURSING CARE PLAN

Use this feature to test your understanding and application of the content presented. Ask yourself "Would I have come up with the same nursing diagnoses? Are these the interventions that I would have proposed? What other interventions would be appropriate?"

CONCEPT CARE MAPS

Review these graphical tools to help incorporate the interrelatedness of nursing concepts in preparation for clinical practice.

HOW TO USE THIS TEXT (Continued)

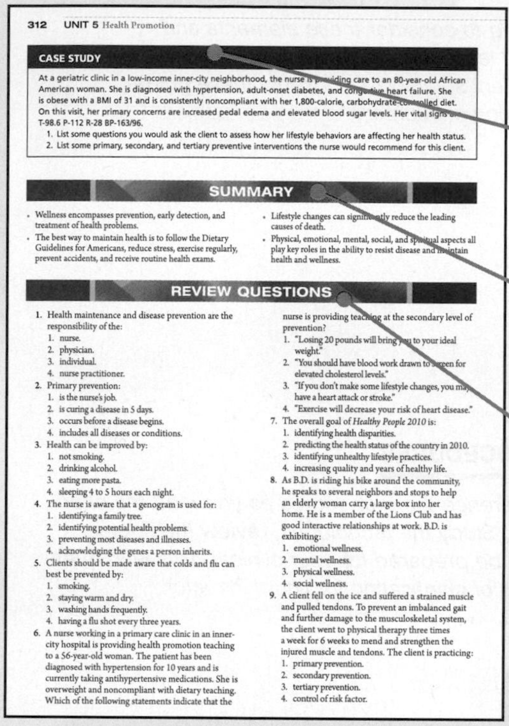

312 UNIT 5 Health Promotion

CASE STUDY

At a geriatric clinic in a low-income inner-city neighborhood, the nurse is providing care to an 80-year-old African American woman. She is diagnosed with hypertension, adult-onset diabetes, and congestive heart failure. She is obese with a BMI of 31 and is consistently noncompliant with her 1,800-calorie, carbohydrate-controlled diet. On this visit, her primary concerns are increased pedal edema and elevated blood sugar levels. Her vital signs are T-98.6 P-112 R-28 BP-163/96.

1. List some questions you would ask the client to assess how her lifestyle behaviors are affecting her health status.
2. List some primary, secondary, and tertiary preventive interventions the nurse would recommend for this client.

SUMMARY

- Wellness encompasses prevention, early detection, and treatment of health problems.
- The best way to maintain health is to follow the Dietary Guidelines for Americans, reduce stress, exercise regularly, prevent accidents, and receive routine health exams.
- Lifestyle changes can significantly reduce the leading causes of death.
- Physical, emotional, mental, social, and spiritual aspects all play key roles in the ability to resist disease and maintain health and wellness.

REVIEW QUESTIONS

1. Health maintenance and disease prevention are the responsibility of the:
   1. nurse.
   2. physician.
   3. individual.
   4. nurse practitioner.
2. Primary prevention:
   1. is the nurse's job.
   2. is curing a disease in 5 days.
   3. occurs before a disease begins.
   4. includes all diseases or conditions.
3. Health can be improved by:
   1. not smoking.
   2. drinking alcohol.
   3. eating more pasta.
   4. sleeping 4 to 5 hours each night.
4. The nurse is aware that a genogram is used for:
   1. identifying a family tree.
   2. identifying potential health problems.
   3. preventing most diseases and illnesses.
   4. acknowledging the genes a person inherits.
5. Clients should be made aware that colds and flu can best be prevented by:
   1. smoking.
   2. staying warm and dry.
   3. washing hands frequently.
   4. having a flu shot every three years.
6. A nurse working in a primary care clinic in an inner-city hospital is providing health promotion teaching to a 56-year-old woman. The patient has been diagnosed with hypertension for 10 years and is currently taking antihypertensive medications. She is overweight and noncompliant with dietary teaching. Which of the following statements indicate that the nurse is providing teaching at the secondary level of prevention?
   1. "Losing 20 pounds will bring you to your ideal weight."
   2. "You should have blood work drawn to screen for elevated cholesterol levels."
   3. "If you don't make some lifestyle changes, you may have a heart attack or stroke."
   4. "Exercise will decrease your risk of heart disease."
7. The overall goal of *Healthy People 2010* is:
   1. identifying health disparities.
   2. predicting the health status of the country in 2010.
   3. identifying unhealthy lifestyle practices.
   4. increasing quality and years of healthy life.
8. As B.D. is riding his bike around the community, he speaks to several neighbors and stops to help an elderly woman carry a large box into her home. He is a member of the Lions Club and has good interactive relationships at work. B.D. is exhibiting:
   1. emotional wellness.
   2. mental wellness.
   3. physical wellness.
   4. social wellness.
9. A client fell on the ice and suffered a strained muscle and pulled tendons. To prevent an imbalanced gait and further damage to the musculoskeletal system, the client went to physical therapy three times a week for 6 weeks to mend and strengthen the injured muscle and tendons. The client is practicing:
   1. primary prevention.
   2. secondary prevention.
   3. tertiary prevention.
   4. control of risk factor.

CASE STUDY

Read over these boxes within the text. Draw on the knowledge you have gained and synthesize information to develop your own educated responses to the case study challenges.

SUMMARY

Carefully read the bulleted list to review key concepts discussed. This is an excellent resource when studying or preparing for exams.

REVIEW QUESTIONS

Test your knowledge and understanding by answering the NCLEX®-style review questions with each chapter. These are an excellent way to test your mastery of the concepts covered in the chapter, and a good opportunity to become familiar with answering NCLEX®-style review questions.

HOW TO USE STUDYWARE™ TO ACCOMPANY FOUNDATION OF BASIC NURSING, THIRD EDITION

Minimum System Requirements

- Operating systems: Microsoft Windows XP w/SP 2, Windows Vista w/ SP 1, Windows 7
- Processor: Minimum required by Operating System
- Memory: Minimum required by Operating System
- Hard Drive Space: 500 MB
- Screen resolution: 1024 x 768 pixels
- CD-ROM drive
- Sound card & listening device required for audio features
- Flash Player 10. The Adobe Flash Player is free, and can be downloaded from http://www.adobe.com/products/flashplayer/

Setup Instructions

1. Insert disc into CD-ROM drive. The StudyWare™ installation program should start automatically. If it does not, go to step 2.
2. From My Computer, double-click the icon for the CD drive.
3. Double-click the *setup.exe* file to start the program.

Technical Support

Telephone: 1-800-648-7450
8:30 A.M.-6:30 P.M. Eastern Time
E-mail: delmar.help@cengage.com

GETTING STARTED

The StudyWARE™ software helps you learn terms and concepts in *Foundations of Basic Nursing,* third edition. As you study each chapter in the text, be sure to explore the activities in the corresponding chapter in the software. Use StudyWARE™ as your own private tutor to help you learn the material in your *Foundations of Basic Nursing,* third edition textbook.

Getting started is easy! Install the software by following the installation instructions provided above. When you open the software, enter your first and last name so the software can store your quiz results. Then choose a chapter or section from the menu to take a quiz or explore media and activities.

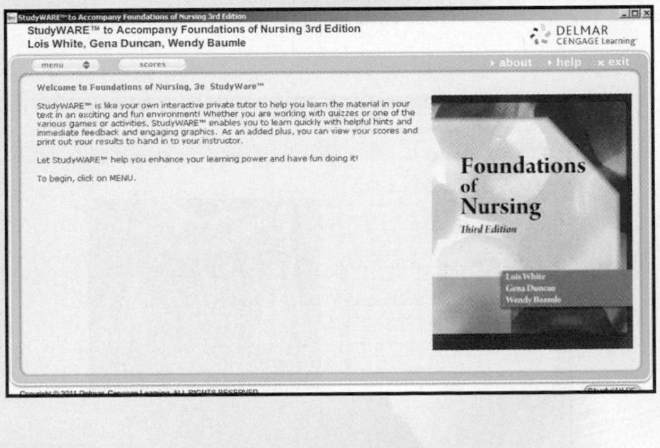

HOW TO USE STUDYWARE™ (Continued)

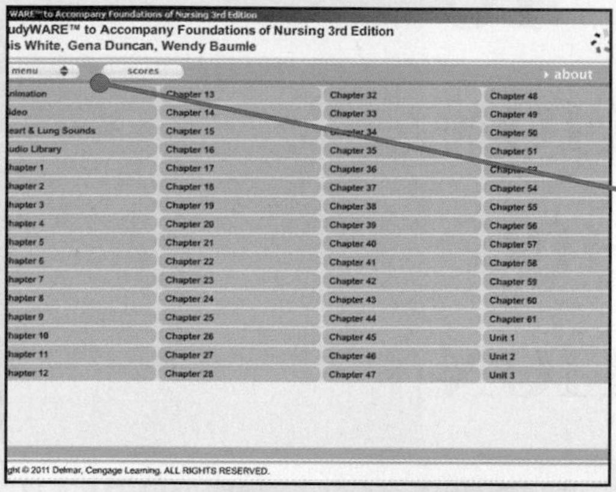

MENU

You can access the menu from wherever you are in the program. The Menu includes Animations, Video, Heart & Lung Sounds, Chapter activities for all didactic chapters, and NCLEX®-Style Quizzes for each major unit. You can also access your scores from the button to the right of the main menu button.

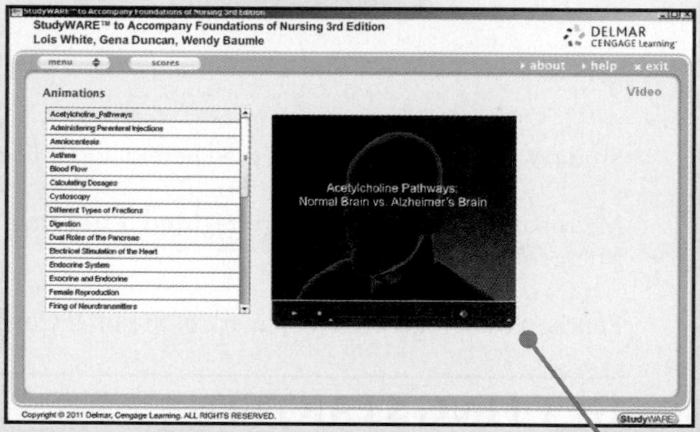

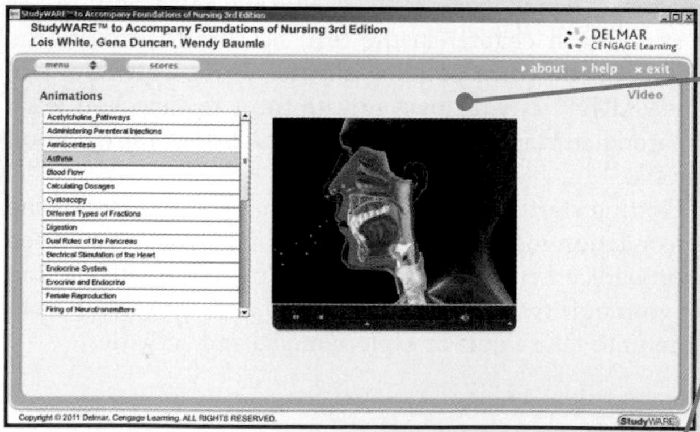

ANIMATION

This section on your StudyWARE™ CD-ROM provides 35 multimedia animations of biological, anatomical, and pharmacological processes. These animations visually explain some of the more difficult concepts and are an engaging resource to support your understanding.

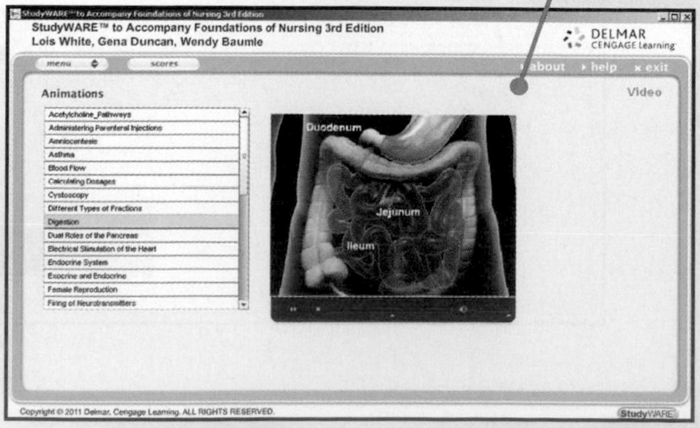

HOW TO USE STUDYWARE™ (Continued)

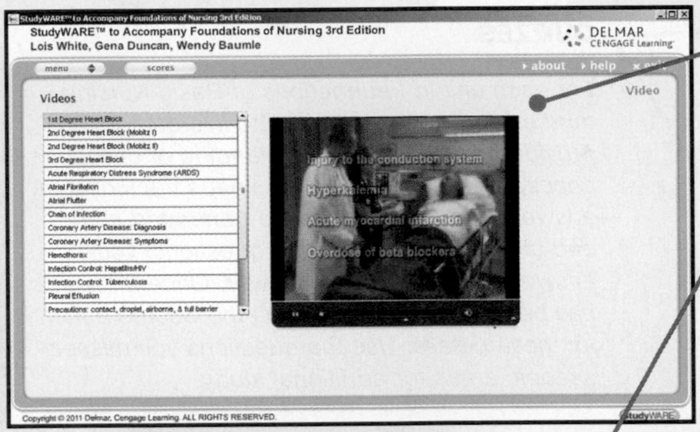

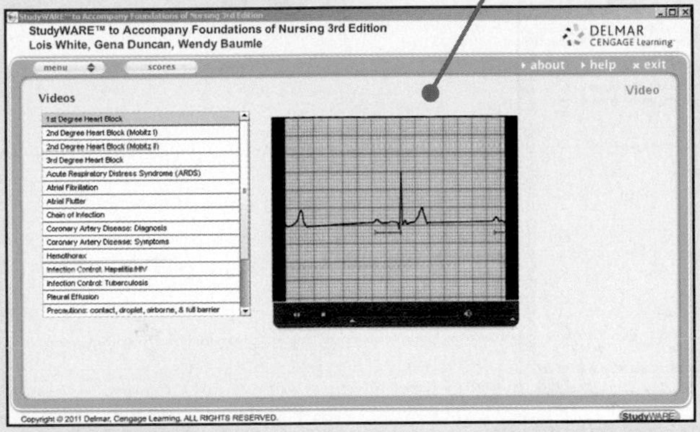

VIDEO

A selection of 20 high quality video clips on topics ranging from infection control to the cardiovascular and respiratory systems has been provided. Click on the clip you would like to view, then click on the play button on the media viewer in the center of the screen. These video clips, many of which were developed by Concept Media, are a wonderful resource to help visualize difficult processes and skills.

HEART & LUNG SOUNDS

This searchable multimedia program provides a comprehensive library of audio files for different heart and lung sounds that will be encountered by nurses. Sounds can be viewed according to category or specific sounds can be found by using the alphabetical term search function. In addition to hearing the sounds, related information about etiology and auscultation is provided.

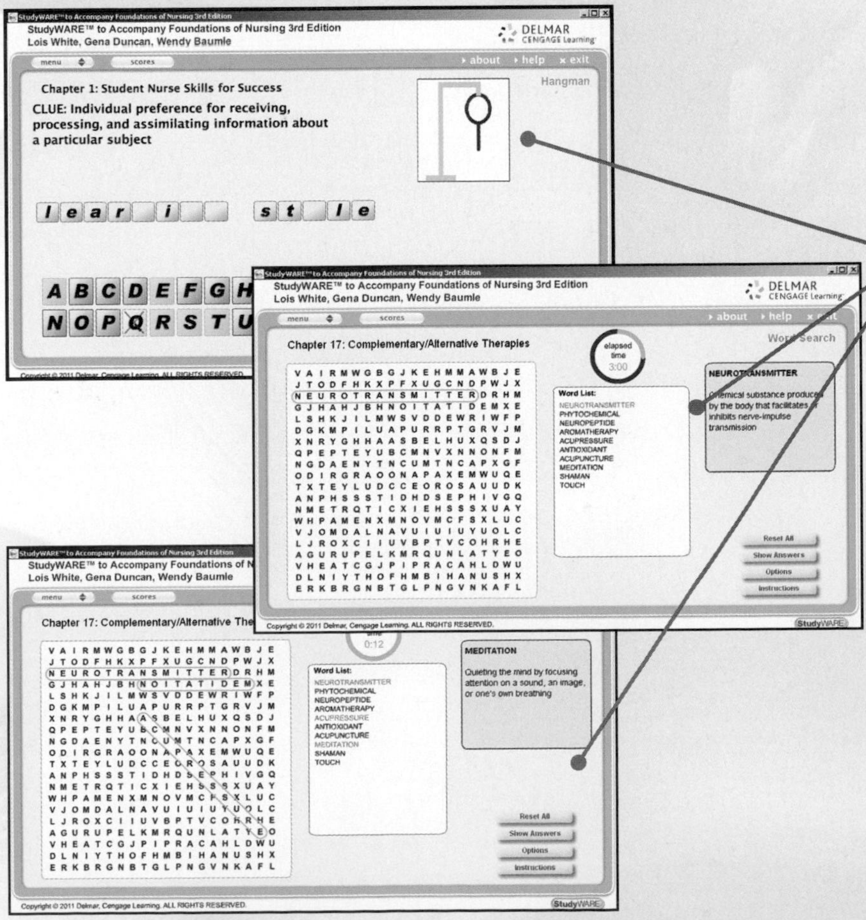

CHAPTER ACTIVITIES

For each chapter from Foundations of Basic Nursing, third edition, that contains glossary terms, games and activities are provided to help you master the terminology in a fun and interesting way. Concentration is a memory game that asks you to flip cards to match definitions with their terms. Flash Cards allow you to test your knowledge of a term by reading the term, thinking about the definition, then checking the actual definition. Hangman follows the traditional hangman game format and can be played by one or two players, challenging you to fill in the blanks for a term before the puzzle is completed. Crossword Puzzles provide definitions of key terms as clues so you can fill in the appropriate term and clear the board.

HOW TO USE STUDYWARE™ (Continued)

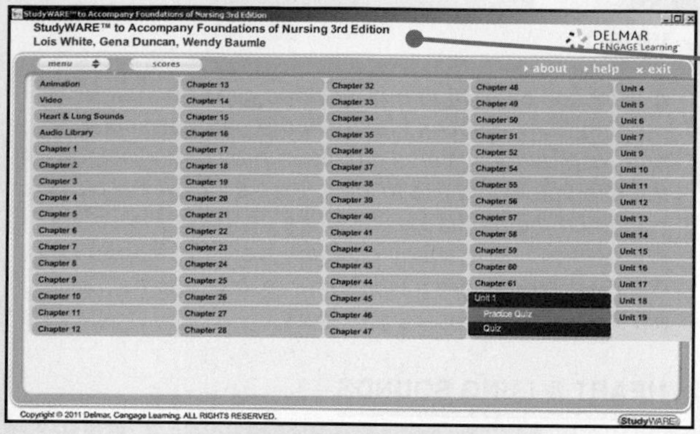

QUIZZES

For each unit in Foundations of Basic Nursing, third edition, both practice and live quizzes are provided to test your understanding of critical concepts. The quiz program keeps track of your answers and a report can be generated at the end of the quiz outlining the questions, your answer, and the correct answer. Once the quiz has been completed, click on the Scores button for these details. Use the questions you missed as topic areas for additional study.

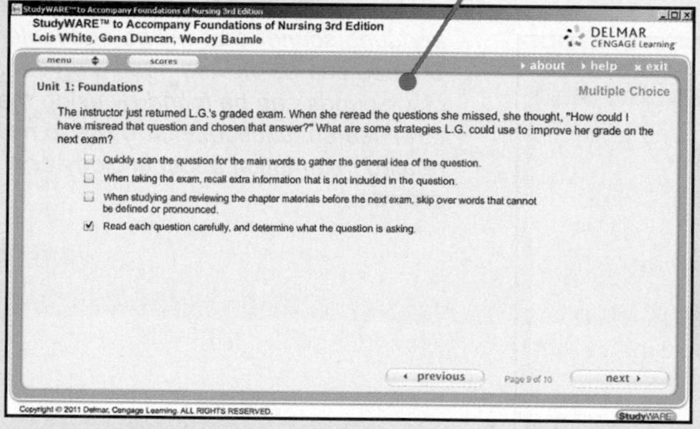

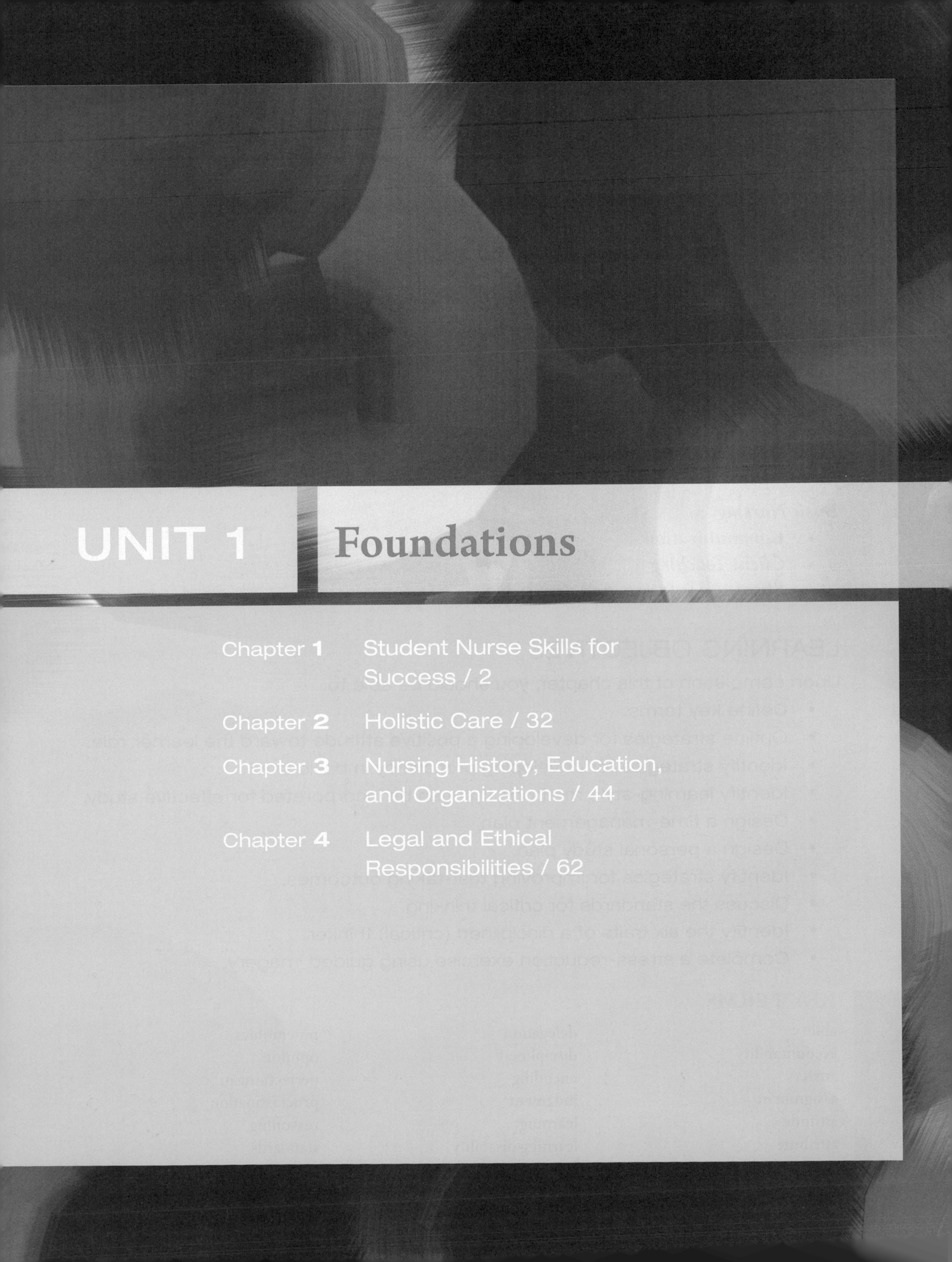

UNIT 1 Foundations

CHAPTER 1
Student Nurse Skills for Success

MAKING THE CONNECTION

Refer to the following chapters to increase your understanding of student nurse skills for success:

Basic Nursing

- ***Communication***
- ***Client Teaching***
- ***Stress, Adaptation, and Anxiety***

LEARNING OBJECTIVES

Upon completion of this chapter, you should be able to:

- Define key terms.
- Outline strategies for developing a positive attitude toward the learner role.
- Identify strategies for developing proficiency in basic skills.
- Identify learning-style methods that can be incorporated for effective study.
- Design a time-management plan.
- Design a personal study plan.
- Identify strategies for improving test-taking outcomes.
- Discuss the standards for critical thinking.
- Identify the six traits of a disciplined (critical) thinker.
- Complete a stress-reduction exercise using guided imagery.

KEY TERMS

ability
accountability
anxiety
assignment
attitude
attribute
critical thinking
delegation
disciplined
encoding
judgment
learning
learning disability
learning style
mnemonics
opinion
perfectionism
procrastination
reasoning
standards
time management

INTRODUCTION

Welcome to practical/vocational nursing. You have chosen one of life's rewarding careers. The next few months of your life will be challenging, exhilarating, frustrating, and full of new experiences. When you consider the difficulty of the nursing program's admission process, being a member of this nursing class is no small achievement. The fact that you have survived the admissions process demonstrates that you are capable of overcoming the challenges that lie ahead. Balancing family, community, and school responsibilities will require self-discipline.

LEARNING

Learning is defined as the act or process of acquiring knowledge and/or skill in a particular subject. An individual never stops learning. This is especially true in the field of nursing and health care. The amount of information within the health care domain has expanded exponentially in just the past several years. Consider, for example, the advances in drug therapies, complementary/alternative therapies, and genetics. By graduation, some of the information learned in the beginning of the program will have been displaced by new information and discoveries. We are living in the information age and have constant access to thousands of pieces of information through various media, including television and the Internet. Knowledge is never static. Learning also is not static but, rather, is a lifelong process.

Individuals seek knowledge to effect some type of change. As a student, you are seeking knowledge to learn skills and to prepare yourself for a career in nursing. Referring to yourself as a learner implies that you are an active participant in the learning process, as opposed to a passive recipient of information. You bring to this new adventure yourself, your past experiences, your abilities, and your motivation to master the knowledge necessary to reach your goals. You have already learned much in your lifetime and are ready to continue the process. It is important that you take some time to think about the competencies needed for the role of learner. It is equally important to realize that *you* are in charge of developing the competencies that will enable you to learn.

The learning you are seeking will afford you the knowledge and skills necessary to become a nurse and, thus, to demonstrate your ability to competently provide care to clients who seek your professional talents. Nursing education is different from many other college majors in the turnaround time allowed for learning. Few other disciplines require the student to apply on Thursday that which was acquired on Monday. Nursing students must acquire a greater depth of understanding in a shorter amount of time; to achieve this, basic learning processes will need to be well developed.

This chapter addresses *how* you learn rather than *what* you learn. It focuses on competencies necessary to master the learning process: attitude, basic skills, learning style, time management, study strategies, critical thinking, and test-taking strategies. Assessing which habits you already practice and which ones you have yet to incorporate, internalize, and utilize will assist you in improving your process of learning. As you do so, your potential for attaining your goals will increase.

> **PROFESSIONALTIP**
>
> **Learning**
>
> The key to your success is not how you are taught but how you decide to learn.

DEVELOP A POSITIVE ATTITUDE

Attitude is defined as a manner, feeling, or position toward a person or thing. In order to effect change in your behavior, you must first develop a positive attitude about the experience you are about to begin. You are in charge of setting yourself up for success. This is your opportunity to acquire the knowledge and skills that will make it possible for you to reach the goal of becoming a licensed practical/vocational nurse. Start by developing a positive attitude toward yourself as a person and a learner as well as a genuine desire to learn. To maintain this attitude late at night when you are struggling over the names of the latest drugs and writing client assessments, you must be convinced that you have the capability to complete your task, that some intrinsic factor will be able to support you in the pursuit of your goal. This positive self-attitude sustains the question "Why am I doing this?" Among the strategies you can practice to help you build a positive attitude are the following:

- Create positive self-images and visualize yourself attaining your goals.
- Recognize your abilities.
- Identify realistic expectations.

CREATE POSITIVE SELF-IMAGES

To create a positive self-image, you must know those attributes that are unique to you. An **attribute** is a characteristic, either positive or negative, that belongs to you. For instance, some positive attributes that are typical to nurses include caring and compassion. Attributes are sometimes referred to as strengths and weaknesses. Whatever you call them, you must actively engage in listing and recalling these qualities about yourself. Divide a paper into two columns, with one headed positive and the other negative. List as many words describing your attributes as you can.

Which side has more entries? Did you start with the negative list? It is unfortunate that sometimes we can recall the negatives faster than the positives. We often speak about ourselves in negative terms, which creates negative self-images. For example, you may recall thinking some of the following: "I wish I were thinner . . . ," "I hope I can do this, I'm not very good at math." Neither of these statements draws a positive image of the speaker. You may need to lose 10 pounds or improve your math skills, but these are not the total measure of your attributes. If they are the only qualities you recall, they might become the overall image you see of yourself. Regardless of where you started, you must concentrate on the positive side of the chart. You must actively recall your positive side at least as often as you recount the things that could be improved.

Begin to speak of yourself in positive terms and accept compliments from yourself! When an assignment is particularly difficult, you can refocus from "I hope I can do this. I have never been good at math" to "I can read and follow the chapter instructions on how to complete the problems." This simple restatement can sometimes make the difference between success or failure at attempts to acquire new knowledge.

The list does not have to stop at just the words you write today. Continue to practice and do periodic self-assessments. You will add more and more words to the positive side and begin to complement yourself more often. When things go awry, you will be able to draw on these positive attributes and know that you have these strengths.

Recognize Your Abilities

Recognizing your abilities is also an attitude builder. **Ability** can be defined as competence in an activity. An ability is something you can learn; competency is proficiency in a task. Your degree of competence as a nurse will depend on such factors as prior exposure, motivation, how often and with whom you practice, expectations of those things that you should be doing, and a willingness to laugh at attempts and learn from mistakes.

You have abilities and skills that you perform well. To acquire these skills took courage, discipline, and hard work. Recalling these abilities and the ways you developed competency in them not only adds to your positive self-image, but also showcases your strengths. Begin by making a four-column chart with the headings "I am really good at . . ."; "Skills I currently have to be 'really good' . . ."; "I avoid doing . . ."; and "Skills I need to be 'really good'. . ." In the second column, list the skills you presently have to be "really good." In the third column, write the things you tend to avoid doing. Finally, in the fourth column, list the skills you need to acquire to be "really good" at the tasks you "avoid doing" (refer to Table 1-1).

For example, perhaps you wrote, "I am really good at cooking." Some skills you could have written are the following:

- *Arithmetic:* You must have an understanding of fractions and the relationships of parts to the whole.
- *Reading:* You must comprehend the words in the recipe in order to follow all the steps.
- *Prioritizing:* You must know with what items to start in order to have all of the food ready at the same time.
- *Risk taking:* You may worry about whether your guests will like your dish, but you persist, confident in your ability to turn the raw ingredients into a delicious meal.

Now look at the third column. Maybe you wrote math. Mathematics is an ability you must develop in order to safely administer medications to your clients. If you view this skill only as something to avoid, you begin with a negative attitude toward an ability you will need. You are creating a negative image of yourself completing this task. Instead, look to your past experiences for your strengths; you may realize that you already possess much of the mathematical knowledge you need to correctly compute medication dosages. Realizing this puts a positive slant on this ability.

Now you must develop mathematical competency. Begin by listing the skills needed to perform mathematical operations. You must pay attention to details, understand the way parts relate to the whole, and have solid skills in arithmetic (addition, subtraction, division, and multiplication). Mathematics requires you to choose appropriate formulas to solve a variety of real-world problems. For example, to give the correct dose of medication to your client, you must know the correct formula to use for the calculation. This is a real-world problem for which you must both choose the correct formula and understand it. You must then accurately perform the arithmetic operations.

Identify Realistic Expectations

As mentioned earlier, developing a positive self-image is of primary importance to learning. Your expectations regarding how you will perform in the role as a learner affects your attitude toward both yourself and learning. You have an expectation about the way you will progress through the nursing program. Ideally, you will attend all classes, pass all exams, and graduate. Further, your current life responsibilities will cooperate with and support this plan. You will likely, however, encounter at least some obstacles. When you hit that first "speed bump" to your plan, your ability to look at the reality of your expectations will be important in regaining a positive focus. Consider the following example:

> G. is a 25-year-old female enrolled full time in a nursing program for the fall. She did well in high school and has already attended a college part time prior to this program. G. expects that she will get grades in the B and A range, as she did in prior course work. She works full time and has a 4-year-old daughter. When the class schedule is published, the times conflict with one of the days that she works. This will cause her to be 20 minutes late to work on that day. She has not shared with her employer that she is attending school. She has child care for her daughter, but the need to arrive at the clinical site at 7 A.M. means that she must rearrange her child care and that she will be 30 minutes late for clinical on Fridays. She does not tell her instructors of her time constraints for child care. She has always needed quiet time for study and is a morning person. G. finds her reading assignments take twice as long as she had planned. With all her other responsibilities, her only time for study is after her daughter goes to bed. She has a family that lives close by, but she does not like to burden them with

TABLE 1-1 Recognizing Your Abilities

"I AM REALLY GOOD AT . . ."	SKILLS I HAVE TO BE "REALLY GOOD . . ."	"I AVOID DOING . . ."	SKILLS I NEED TO BE "REALLY GOOD. . ."
Cooking	Arithmetic	Math	Attention to details
	Reading		Understanding the way parts relate to the whole
	Prioritizing		Solid skills in addition, subtraction, division, and multiplication
	Risk taking		

baby-sitting. She has always found a way to do things on her own in the past.

G. is a capable person, but her expectation of being able to control all the various facets of her life in perfect harmony is unrealistic. Maintaining a positive attitude while in the midst of the stress of completing all the tasks at hand is difficult, if not impossible, and the plan is often abandoned. In G.'s case, abandoning the plan may mean abandoning her plans for school. G.'s reality is that she cannot increase her time commitment by 30 hours of school work and keep everything else she does at the same level. She must set priorities with regard to the demands on her time, and she must identify realistic expectations for those things that she can accomplish.

When everything on your "to do" list cannot be completed, change the way you approach the list and realign your expectations. One way to do this is to ask for help. Asking for help is not a weakness, it is a success strategy. The most successful people are typically those who know when to ask for help and who have devised a plan to structure that help. In the previous example, G. needs to remove some of the stress related to work, child care, and school commitments by informing her employer and instructors of her situation and asking for their help in guiding her to manage the many demands. Help may mean something as simple as talking to the employer about coming in 20 minutes late and working 20 minutes longer and asking a family member to take her daughter to the child care place on Fridays.

If you do not set realistic expectations for yourself, you may fall victim to a positive attitude's biggest enemy, perfectionism. **Perfectionism** is an overwhelming expectation of being able to get everything done in a flawless manner. This is a setup for failure because it is a standard no one can achieve. Table 1-2 suggests some behaviors of perfectionists versus those of pursuers of excellence. Which list describes you most accurately? Remember to strive to be as realistic with your expectations as possible; be patient with yourself and ask for help when needed.

DEVELOP YOUR BASIC SKILLS

Reading, arithmetic and mathematics, writing, listening, and speaking are skills basic for success in academics and life. When you consider the importance of these basic skills, you must have a strong foundation in them to advance your knowledge beyond the level of memorization to comprehension and

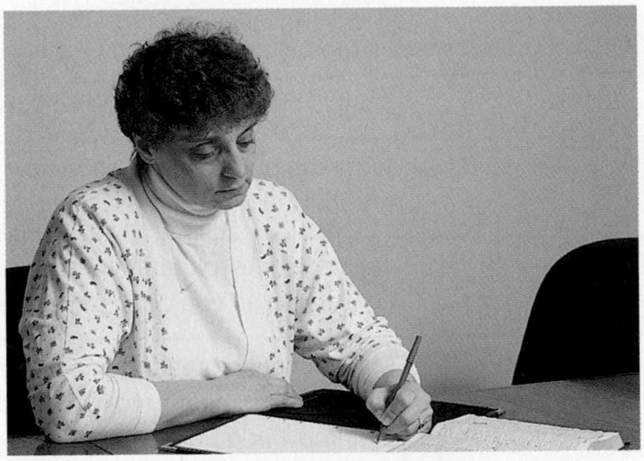

FIGURE 1-1 Keep a notebook of new terms to expand your vocabulary. Review your notebook and try to use the words in practice daily.

application. If you are struggling with these basic skills, you will have difficulty advancing. Developing these skills is basic to the habits of successful learners.

READING

A large percentage of your program is in written format. To study effectively, you must be highly adept in the basic skill of reading. To be competent in reading, you must be able to locate, understand, and interpret written information; determine the main idea or essential message; find the meanings for unknown or technical words; and judge the accuracy and plausibility of the writers.

Strategies to effectively improve your reading skills include vocabulary building, comprehension, and reading level. Your basic skill of reading encompasses vocabulary building, which includes the skill of identification and understanding of both English and medical terminology. Investing in quality medical and English dictionaries is a good step to understanding both these languages. When reading assignments, take the time to look up the words you do not know (Figure 1-1).

The primary reason for building a strong medical vocabulary is that words are the tools for thinking about and understanding your world, and you are entering the new world of nursing: You must therefore take the time to learn its language. Developing the habit of vocabulary building takes time initially, but as you persist in practicing this skill, your comprehension of the material will increase.

TABLE 1-2 Behaviors of Perfectionists and Pursuers of Excellence

PERFECTIONISTS	PURSUERS OF EXCELLENCE
Reach for impossible goals	Enjoy meeting high standards within reach
Value themselves for what they do	Value themselves for who they are
Get depressed and give up	Experience disappointment but keep going
Are devastated by failure	Learn from failure
Remember mistakes and dwell on them	Correct mistakes, then learn from them
Can only live with being number one	Are pleased with knowing they did their best
Hate criticism	Welcome criticism
Have to win to maintain high self-esteem	Do not have to win to maintain high self-esteem

Table 1-3 Strategies to Improve Comprehension

Reread	Do this after reading one section of the text or even after one paragraph.
Define new words	Write the definitions of each new word in new words the margin of your text and then reread the paragraph. Use a small notebook to build your own glossary. Make your own flashcards for further study.
Visualize	Create mental pictures of the material you are reading. You may even want to draw a simple stick figure, and as you continue to read, adjust the picture.
Research	Many times the reason you are unable to comprehend the material presented is that you have insufficient background in the subject. A solution may be to consult another text that is specific to that knowledge base. Use a dictionary, anatomy and physiology text, general subject text (like a psychology text), or a nursing journal to increase your background knowledge in a subject area (Meltzer & Marcus-Palau, 1997).
Summarize	Use your own words to "tell" yourself what you just read and how this connects to what you are going to be doing. Ask yourself, "Why might I need to know this material?"

Comprehension goes beyond rote memorization. One sign of true comprehension is the ability to summarize the writer's message. When you summarize, state the material in your own words. Unless you understand the words you have read, you will not be able to advance your level of knowledge from rote memorization to comprehension. When you are actively reading your nursing textbook and you realize that you are not understanding what you have read, you may find it helpful to use one, some, or all of the five strategies outlined in Table 1-3.

Reading level is another element of your reading skills. Reading level is not related to what you can understand but, rather, refers to the length of the words and the sentences used in a text to explain, describe, and convey information. It does not have anything to do with your intelligence, but it has a great deal to do with the length of time it takes you to read.

Arithmetic and Mathematics

A skill in which you must develop competency is arithmetic and mathematics. To be competent in this skill, you must be able to perform basic computations using whole numbers, percentages, fractions, and decimals, and choose the appropriate formula to use. You will be responsible for correctly calculating dosages and safely administering medications to your clients. You must be able to recognize whether your calculations are correct and logical. In nursing, your mastery of mathematical basic skills cannot be overemphasized. According to a research study, approximately 7,000 deaths annually are due to medication errors (Sakowski et al. 2005). Hughes and Edgerton (2005) state:

> The most common calculations involve fractions, percentages, decimals, and ratios. In mathematical tests, new interns and nurses have been found to have poor mathematical skills. . . . The inability to calculate the correct therapeutic volume of a drug dose accounts for the majority of pediatric medication errors. Research has found that the major problems behind many of these miscalculations are associated with an inability to conceptualize the right calculation to be performed and understand the mathematical process leading to the solution. . . . Misplacement of the decimal point is a common dosing error than can lead to a tenfold error in overdosing or underdosing. . . . Some errors of this type have been linked to performance on calculation tests because those who perform poorly on such tests are more likely to make a mistake in practice, especially when fatigued or distracted. (p. 81)

Give yourself a reality check on your competency in mathematics and commit to improving those areas where you are weakest. You may want to investigate a resource such as the learning services center at your school, enlist the assistance of a tutor, or use a programmed-learning text to refresh your skills. There are also numerous texts written to assist nursing students in developing these essential skills. Consider also using computer-assisted instruction (CAI) programs or self-paced study modules to hone your math skills. Whatever means you use, an honest assessment of your competency in mathematics and a commitment to improvement is essential to your practice in the nursing profession.

Writing

In your role as a student and as a professional, you will need writing skills. To be competent in writing, you must be able to communicate thoughts and information clearly and completely using proper grammar, spelling, and punctuation. Contrary to popular opinion, the influx of the computer into health care has not removed the need for this skill. You will be writing client assessments, transfer summaries, discharge summaries, and client-teaching plans. The skill of writing can be practiced and improved.

Listening

The old saying "I know you can hear me, but are you listening?" can be applied to all of us. You must be listening, understanding, and processing information, as opposed to just hearing, when you are in class, as well as when you begin working with clients. To be competent in listening you must receive, interpret, and respond to verbal messages and other cues such as body language while attempting to both comprehend the information and evaluate the speaker. You may need to polish up on ways that you can improve listening and evaluation skills to make the most of your class time. Listening effectively can make efficient use of the class period to increase your comprehension of the content.

Among the many strategies that can be used to improve listening skills are the following:

- *Be interested in the subject.* Make a connection with the reason you are going to this lecture. What is the connection between the information and your need for the information? Have you read the material and come with questions about the subject?
- *Be open to the information.* When you hear a topic and immediately react with your instinct, you often miss the point and some aspect of the presentation you had not considered before. Listening does not automatically mean you will change your mind on topics, but it will allow you to evaluate and incorporate those aspects that are beneficial to you.
- *Focus on the message, not the messenger.* The speaker may not be a member of a theatrical company that entertains you. The speaker's role is to impart information. You can concentrate on the information that you need to know and apply it properly.
- *Concentrate on the information.* Be attentive to the lecture. If you find yourself falling asleep, do muscle flexes or breathe deeply to try to stay alert and aware. Imagine test questions that might be asked on the information.
- *Evaluate the information.* Not every word is critical. Relate the information to what you know, where you may use it, and whether you agree with what is said. If you have difficulty with what is being said, use the next strategy to maintain your concentration.
- *Write down questions as you listen.* This allows you to follow the speaker to the end, and many of your questions may have been answered. If not, you have them written down and can refer later to the list. This promotes concentration on the information presented. You will not be distracted trying to remember questions you wanted to ask.

SPEAKING

You have entered one of the most "speaking"-oriented professions. You will communicate daily with clients, their families, instructors, peers, ancillary staff members, and the multiple members of the health care team. To be competent in speaking, organize your ideas and communicate them using verbal language in a tone, style, and level of complexity appropriate to the listener.

Many students will not ask questions during a lecture specifically because they believe themselves incapable of speaking clearly and identifying exactly the information they need. There is a saying, "There is no stupid question"; believe it. Develop the confidence to speak up when you have a question. There are potential serious consequences to your clients if you fail to clarify a medical order or question a procedure that is unclear.

The following strategies may help when you want to ask a question:

- *Understand why you are asking the question.* Instead of saying, "I don't understand," say, "I was with you on the physiology of the kidney until you reached the Bowman's capsule. Can you connect this particular part of the kidney with osmosis for me?" This puts you and the speaker in a positive light; you have not attacked the speaker's explanation, and you acknowledge your skill in listening. You are communicating what you need and asking the speaker to help by connecting the two concepts for you.
- *Know when to ask the question.* Writing down those topics on which you need further information may help you decide the correct time to ask a question. If the instructor begins by saying, "Today we will be speaking about pharmacokinetics," and you do not understand the word, stopping her before she has a chance to define the word may not be the most effective strategy. If instead you write down, "What does pharmacokinetics mean?" and listen for the meaning of that word in the context of the lecture, you will most likely hear clues as to the word's meaning. The instructor will use other words, such as *absorption, distribution, metabolism,* and *excretion* to describe what happens to a drug as it goes through the body. When an appropriate time in the presentation comes, review those things that have been said and clarify: "So, Prof. Z., am I correct when I say that pharmacokinetics has to do with the movement of drugs through all the systems of the body?" You will get your answer, and your instructor will know from your question that you have been listening.

Speak clearly and articulate your needs as you attend classes; listen to your instructors; listen to your clients; and transmit information to instructors, colleagues, support staff, doctors, and allied health care team members. Practice both the skills of listening and speaking equally and keep asking questions.

DEVELOP YOUR LEARNING STYLE

The term **learning style** refers to the ways you best receive, process, and assimilate information (knowledge) about a

PROFESSIONALTIP

Speaking

Thorough preparation is an important strategy for speaking. Formulating multiple examples is one way of increasing your comfort level with the given information. For example, if you are asked to explain the way the pancreas produces insulin, you might draw the organ and indicate where the islets of Langerhans are. Or you may use a lock and key to explain the way insulin works to open the channels for glucose to enter the cells. You may trace a cracker as it travels through the body from teeth to cells and indicate just where and when insulin is utilized. Regardless of the specifics, creating multiple examples will assist you in thoroughly learning a topic and creating a feeling of comfort about your knowledge of the subject.

particular subject. In your life as a student, you have probably had both of the following experiences:

You attend class with Professor A for Course 100. The professor arranges the room casually in small groupings and breaks up class time to alternate short lectures with small-group work. There is time for a hands-on demonstration of the principle along with actual work-related items used as examples. Professor A allows for student–teacher interchange of ideas and gives credence to experiences of the students during the class discussions. You leave the class exhilarated and with ideas, aware that this content connects with your desired outcome. You plan a review of the notes with a fellow student you met in your class group. You continue to prepare throughout the course and prior to the final, on which you get a B.

The next day you attend Course 200 with Professor B. The room is arranged in rows. Professor B puts up the class outline on the overhead, lectures for 40 minutes, then allows 10 minutes at the end for questions. If you hand him a written question, he will answer it during the next class. You dread his boring presentation and wish that Professor B was more like Professor A. You really do not know anyone in the class with whom to study, you cannot understand the text, and your grades are in the low C to D range. You know you need this class for your major. You try to do your part, but you just cannot "get into it."

PROFESSIONALTIP

Learning Disabilities

According to the National Center for Learning Disabilities (2008), 15 million children, adolescents, and adults have some form of learning disability. **Learning disability** is a generic term that refers to a heterogeneous group of disorders manifested as significant difficulties in the acquisition and use of listening, speaking, reading, writing, reasoning, or mathematical abilities.

Having a learning disability will not prohibit your success; you must, however, understand your different abilities. Find out the types of accommodations that will enhance your learning capabilities, and ask for those things that you need. Accommodations in postsecondary programs are mandated by the federal government; however, the onus to disclose, provide documentation, and request accommodations is on the student. Accommodations are determined on a case-by-case basis. Reasonable accommodations in the classroom may be as simple as having the instructor wear a microphone, being able to use a tape recorder or note taker, or requesting textbook tapes. In the clinical area, all reasonable accommodations are made within the confines of client safety and essential skills needed to participate in a nursing program. A quiet work area and ear protectors provide quiet for students who are hypersensitive to background noise. Using a computer for writing assignments, note taking in class, and studying may assist students who have difficulty writing. Getting a tutor who is skilled at working with students with learning disabilities is another intervention to consider.

Whatever you suspect your needs to be, getting professional testing to ascertain whether you have a disability and to determine any specific accommodations you need is crucial. Seek the assistance of your instructors, student service personnel, learning center personnel, or call the special education coordinator at the nearest high school. These resources will help you locate an accredited testing agency to provide you with further resources and documentation.

Think about Professor A, who presents information in a variety of methods—short lecture, small group, hands-on demonstration. As a student, you can grasp the information from whichever method appeals to you. You come away feeling connected to the subject and your classmates and want to continue learning about the subject. You are rewarded for your efforts through the academic grade system.

Now consider Professor B, who knows just as much about the subject as does Professor A but who presents it using only one method—lecture. Lecture is not your preferred learning style, and your ability to clarify your understanding through questions is limited by the class format. Your outcomes on tests are less rewarding, and you begin to avoid putting time into studying the subject all together. You end up thinking that you really do not do well in that subject and consider changing your major.

The difference in the outcomes of the two examples lies in the perceived role of the learner. In these examples, the student relied heavily on the *teacher's* ability to present material in the student's preferred learning style. Remember, *you* are in charge of your learning. Teacher presentations vary in ways that may not appeal to your primary learning style, but you can still learn the information. You must take charge of developing your abilities, increasing your awareness of your preferred learning styles, and implementing some simple strategies to enhance those styles. As you increase your skills in your preferred methods and strengthen those in your weaker ones, your outcomes will change.

Classification of Learning Styles

Learning styles are cognitive (mental) functions. They refer to the ways you perceive, remember, think, and solve problems: Their focus is *how* you learn as opposed to *what* you learn. Your preference for one style over another can be argued to be both genetic and developmental. Regardless, your awareness of the ways you best learn will affect your learning outcomes.

Learning styles are classified in many different ways. One classification method focuses on the route by which students best perceive and remember information: visual, auditory, or kinesthetic. These divisions are not mutually exclusive; we possess all three, and we use all of them to acquire information. Visual learners make up approximately 65% of the population, auditory learners approximately 30%, and kinesthetic learners approximately 5% (Mind Tools, 2008).

Visual learners think in pictures. No matter how information is obtained (reading, hearing, or seeing), it is stored as visual images. This person says "I see" or "I get the picture." Auditory learners relate best to the spoken word and prefer class discussion and oral presentations. This person says "That sounds right" or "I hear you." Kinesthetic learners process and remember information well if they touch, imitate, and practice what they are studying. All of us have the capacity to learn in all three modes. You naturally gravitate to one over the others based on which style has led to your greatest learning successes.

Another way to classify learning styles is according to brain-hemisphere dominance. The left hemisphere of the brain is associated with analytical activities, such as logic, structure, speech, reasoning, numbers, verbal expression, verification of data, and analysis of parts of the whole. The right side is associated with creativity and synthesizing parts to form a whole idea. The right side is also considered the more emotional side and links to insight, intuition, daydreams, visualization, music, rhythm, and color visualization.

We need both sides of the brain to function and learn. Numerous studies demonstrated that individuals with left-brain dominance are primarily auditory learners and those with right-brain dominance are primarily visual. Additional studies show that right-brain–dominant learners process, recall, and retain more from information presented in computer-assisted instructional programs, whereas left-brain–dominant learners derive more success from a lecture format. To overlook or use one style to the exclusion of the other is using only part of your overall potential learning ability.

Strategies for Learning

You can determine your preferred learning style by going to one of the following Web sites, doing a search for learning-style test, and taking the test (www.Vmentor.com; www.mindtools.com; and www.vark-learn.com). You can also check the Web site resources at the end of the chapter for more learning-style information. By determining your preferred learning style, you will adopt strategies to enhance that style when you study. You want to effectively move the required information into long-term memory and increase your knowledge level from memorization to comprehension and, finally, to application. To accomplish this you must know which strategies work with which learning styles. Refer to Table 1-4 and note all the strategies listed that you consistently use in your study routine. Start with the style you previously ascertained to be your preferred learning style.

Are there strategies listed under your preferred style that you currently do not use? To enhance your acquisition of material, begin to incorporate these into your study plan. Are there strategies listed under any of the other styles that you could use when the material you are learning is especially difficult for you?

One way to incorporate more than one learning style into your study program is to employ a CAI program. Many texts now come with an accompanying disk designed to enhance learning style. Such disks may contain the total text along with testing materials, exercises that accompany the text, and/or resource material for the text. For example, several medical terminology packages come as program-instruction texts with disks and provide audio pronunciation in the computer programs. The student can read the text, manipulate the information on the computer, and hear the correct pronunciation.

When faced with a particularly difficult passage or concept, incorporate more than one style and one strategy to process the information. The more action you put into your learning methods, the more effective your time and outcomes will be. **Mnemonics**, words or phrases used to aid memory, may help. For example, ABC reminds you of airway, breathing, and circulation. You will find several examples of mnemonics to illustrate concepts in Memory Trick boxes throughout the text.

DEVELOP A TIME-MANAGEMENT PLAN

Somewhere in your decision-making process to go to school, you decided you would have the time to do so. You now must make that a reality by actively engaging in a time-management plan. **Time management** is a system to help meet goals through problem solving. Practicing time-management strategies will not eliminate the need to perform tasks you do not like, but it will make doing so more manageable. Active application of time-management strategies will make a difference in what you can accomplish in the time you have.

Strategies for time management include the following:

- Analyzing your time commitments
- Knowing yourself
- Clarifying your goals
- Setting priorities and identifying one or two valued goals to achieve
- Disciplining yourself to adhere to the plan through changes and until the goal is reached

Table 1-4 Sample Learning Strategies

VISUAL LEARNER	AUDITORY LEARNER	KINESTHETIC LEARNER
Takes notes in class	Reads aloud	Takes notes and rewrites them to condense
Writes notes in margin of books	Reads into a tape recorder and plays it back to self	Expresses self with hands, even while reading
Looks for reference books with pictures, graphs, and charts	Discusses ideas about class content with others	Handles visual aids during class
Draws own illustrations	Requests explanations of illustrations	Requests to do a demonstration

Analyze Time Commitments

To analyze your time commitments, start by listing them. Provide yourself with both a big-picture plan and a daily plan. Creating a year-at-a-glance calendar that lists all of your important time commitments can provide a quick illustration of the way the months ahead will be used. Start by putting in your graduation date in red capital letters. This will give you an instant visual reminder of your current goal. Next, using a pencil, insert all important dates, including holidays, birthdays, work, and organizational obligations. Remember to also include activities for those in your household that will require your participation, such as carpooling, special school programs, after-school activities, and child care. Use your academic program calendar as the source for the dates that classes, as well as vacations, begin and end, financial aid forms and tuition payments are due, and the like. Use your individual class schedules as the sources for dates of exams, special review or clinical days, field trips, or any other time commitments you must meet in order to complete the courses. This exercise will give you a big-picture view of your time commitments and will also point out any conflicts.

Conflicts are not impossible obstacles. Knowing about them in advance will allow you to take steps now to prioritize and reschedule. When prioritizing, think about delegating some tasks to other people. Do not always solve a conflict by removing those tasks you enjoy or that will renew you. Taking care of yourself during this time is very important. Never give up the time you need to refresh and renew, even if it is just a hot bath, a brisk 15-minute walk, or a dinner out with family and friends. Place yourself near the top of the priority list to complete your goal.

Each learner's big-picture map will differ. The challenge is to mesh your map with your other relationships and keep yourself toward the top of the list. One strategy is to prominently display your big-picture calendar in an area where all of the members of your household can see it—including and especially you. Everyone will then have the opportunity to see that he is on the list and that he contributes to helping you reach your goal.

The next step is daily planning. Using a week-at-a-glance planner helps illustrate more concrete expectations of those things you plan to do and the amount of time you actually have (Figure 1-2). You should include time to sleep, eat, drive, work, attend class, and study.

You may find that you must rearrange your schedule. This does not mean continuing to do all of the things you have listed but just on different days; rather, it means choosing two valued goals on which to work. *One goal must be to be a learner. The other will be unique to you.* This does not mean that you replace all other goals with these two valued goals. Rather, it means that these goals must take precedence when choosing ways to use your time. If you choose child care and learner as your most valued goals, you could refine them even further to complement each other. For example, you may opt to keep driving the carpool but negotiate to drive every morning because doing so will afford you 2 hours to study prior to class. You may then have to make child care arrangements for after school, which might mean asking your neighbor or contracting with an after-school program. You may also have to set aside 1 hour each evening to get everything laid out for the next day, a task you might ask someone else in the household to do each night so that you can gain an extra hour of study time. That extra hour, in turn, might mean that you dedicate Saturdays for nothing but family commitments. Regardless of the way you choose to solve such problems, the solutions must be designed to help you reach your goals.

Know Yourself

To develop your system, you must know yourself. You must be honest with yourself about your work habits and preferences. Consider the time of day when you are at your intellectual best. Is it early in the morning, or do you come alive at 10 P.M.? You must be able to focus and concentrate when you are studying. Deciding you are going to carpool in the morning to get to school early to study will not be effective if you cannot concentrate until after noon. If this is the case, it would be better to do the more mechanical and less intellectually demanding tasks, such as the shopping or laundry, in the 2 hours before class. Are you a person who is more left-brain oriented (logical, orderly, structured, and plays by the rules)? Then writing out lists of tasks and crossing them off may be your time-management strategy to stay on track. Perhaps you are a more right-brain personality (creative, resists rules, has own sense of time)? Scheduling your task within a specific time frame that has a time-sensitive goal/reward at the end may assist you to use your available time more effectively.

	Monday	Tuesday	Wednesday	Thursday	Friday	Saturday	Sunday
7 AM	Work	Carpool	Carpool	Carpool	Clinical	House	
9 AM	Work	Class	Class	Class		House	Sunday school
11 AM	Work	Class	Class	Class		Chores	Church
1 PM	Work	Class	Class	Class			
3 PM	Work				Work	Work	
5 PM	Carpool Dinner				Work	Work	
7 PM	Study	Study	Study	Study	Work	Work	

COURTESY OF DELMAR CENGAGE LEARNING

Figure 1-2 Week-at-a-Glance Calendar

PROFESSIONALTIP

Time Wasters

Are you a time waster? We all sometimes behave in ways that sabotage the best of plans. Following are some examples of time wasters along with some strategies for helping you reclaim those wasted hours.

1. *Clutter:* Wisdom holds that you can save 1 hour each day by just clearing your work area of clutter and keeping it clean. This time can be put to good use in the form of study. Organize your study area so that when you arrive it is ready for work and take a few minutes at the end of your session to prepare your area for the next session.
2. *Interruptions:* Intrusions into your study or work hours (from either people or things) can be real time wasters. Try the following:
   - Learn to say "no." You do not have to agree to every request. Learn to pick your involvements carefully and according to those that are most important to you reaching your goals.
   - Put your answering machine on, and turn the phone's ringer off. Delegate a time to listen and respond to messages after studying.
   - Open your mail over the garbage can. Respond, delegate, or throw it out.
   - Organize your papers. For instance, have a folder for each child's paper/notes. Keep your class notebooks, your calendar, and phone lists in one three-ring binder so you have all your essentials together.
3. *Procrastination:* This refers to intentionally putting off or delaying something that should be done. **Procrastination** is a time waster because it does not afford effective use of time. Time management is not necessarily finishing everything at one sitting, but, rather, scheduling time to return to the task until you complete it; whereas procrastination is intentionally delaying the task without good cause or a plan to complete it in a time-efficient manner. Breaking the task down into manageable segments and rewards will encourage you to return to it again and again until it is complete.
4. *Perfectionism:* Very often we do not stick to a plan because it does not give us results immediately or does not give the results we expected. Perfectionism affects your time-management plan by prohibiting you from accepting anything less than perfection; it also damages your positive attitude of yourself by setting unrealistic expectations. Focus on your positive accomplishments, look for ways to improve, accept your failures, and build on your experiences.

Clarify Goals

Without setting goals, we cannot know whether we are making any progress. Goals are like grocery lists. Think about when you go to the store without a list. You may purchase many items, but when you get home you often discover that you did not get all the things you needed. If the next time you go to the store you make a list, you will likely get all the items you want.

Just like the grocery list, goals must be written down. They must be based on reality and broken down into manageable parts. Say your goal is to provide study time each week that will allow you to be successful in each unit exam of your program. This time will comprise the time you need to prepare and review material, prepare for clinical assignments, view information in the library, and practice new skills in the lab. As a rule, you will need 1 to 2 hours of study time for each hour you spend in class. If you are in class 12 hours per week, you will thus need to find 24 more hours to study; and if you are in clinical 6 hours 3 days per week for a total of 18 hours, you will need to fit in 36 hours of study. As a rough estimate, this would mean 12 class hours plus 24 study hours plus 18 clinical hours plus 36 preparation hours for a total of 90 hours per week (30 class hours plus 60 study hours) for the ideal study week and 30 hours (class attendance only) for a week without any study. So now you know what amount of time you are aiming for. You can now take this goal of 60 study hours per week and compare it to your written schedule and calendar to determine how to best arrange the demands on your time in order to meet your goals.

Set Priorities

Another part of setting goals is prioritizing tasks into general categories. Look at your daily calendar and list the general categories. Some examples might be as follows:

- Work
- Study
- Personal (eating, sleeping)
- Household chores (shopping, budget)
- Transportation (self, others)
- Supervising children
- Decision making (planning, outside organizational responsibility, time for self, time for spouse, friends, and children)

Next, rank these general categories in order of priority, keeping in mind that not everything is a primary priority. If you uncover conflicts, try to further clarify which items take top priority.

Another way to prioritize is to group tasks according to the time frame in which you wish them to be accomplished. To do this, divide a sheet of paper into three parts. Label the first part column A, the second, column B, and the third, column C. Under column A, write "I must work on these tasks now." This list includes your priority tasks that need immediate attention. Under column B, write "I can do these after A is done." Under

A	B	C
I must work on these tasks now	I can do these after A is done	I can delay, eliminate, or delegate until after B is done
school/study	supervise children	organization
child care		shopping
self-care		
work		

FIGURE 1-3 **Prioritizing Tasks**

column C, write "I can delay, eliminate, or delegate these until after B is done" (Figure 1-3).

If you placed your entire list under column A, go back to your original two goals—one of which includes your new role as learner—and rethink your list. You must prioritize your activities in order to reach your goal. You cannot be all things at all times to all people. You also must know how to work smarter, not longer or harder, to remain focused on the priority task.

Discipline Yourself

The hardest strategy to commit to may be discipline of self. The idea that you must actively engage in using the plan sounds simple. In practice, the plan will not always work. When this happens, you may be tempted to abandon the plan instead of changing it. If the plan is not working, you must ascertain the reasons. Maybe you lack resources, have not scheduled enough time, or need to revisit and reevaluate your goals. Build time to plan into your weekly schedule. If you really want to use a time-management system, your ability to go back to the plan and revise it is very important.

DEVELOP A STUDY STRATEGY

Developing a study plan involves more than just buying a textbook and reading it. Several strategies that will assist you to study more efficiently and effectively follow.

Set Up the Environment

Where and when you study are as important as how. The fact that you assign a specific behavior to your study space will set you up for success. The space should fit your style. Do you like everything organized in neat spaces, or do you just need it near you? What type of lighting, seating, or noise level will assist or detract from your concentration? Consider your preferred learning style when setting up your study space. If you are a kinesthetic learner, you may want to put motion into your space by, for instance, using a treadmill in your study plan. You may want to spend a percentage of your study time sitting to read and take notes and then switch to walking or running on the treadmill to recite and reflect on the material. You will be increasing comprehension and making connections, all while walking 2 miles! Regardless of the way you arrange your space, take into consideration the type of learner you are and your biological and personality preferences.

Gather Your Resources

Your resources should all be easily accessible from your study space. In some homes, the kitchen table serves as the study space. If your study space serves more than one function, as would the kitchen table, consider keeping your study resources in a milk crate or box, so they are portable yet readily at hand when needed.

Gathering your resources is your start to building a library of textbooks, which will serve you throughout your program. These resources become a reference library for you when you study. Some general resources to keep on hand include the following:

- A recent edition of an unabridged dictionary
- A medical dictionary
- An anatomy and physiology text

Additional resources you will need as you progress through your program may include texts on pharmacology, nutrition, and the nursing process. Depending on your personal knowledge base, you may need further resources in the foundation sciences—biology, psychology, and sociology. These areas serve as the knowledge base for your future profession.

Keeping your learning style in mind, consider purchasing accompanying workbooks or other study aids that come with the text and research CAI or videotapes available in your nursing program library. Using varied and multiple resources enhances your knowledge base and will increase your comprehension of the content. You must go beyond memorization, beyond amassing facts, to comprehension of this knowledge base in order to answer the questions on the exams. Keep in mind that you are studying for the program examination, the National Council Licensure Examination (NCLEX-PN®), and, ultimately, to apply your knowledge base to provide safe, effective care to your clients.

Remember to use journals as resources. The articles and related client situations can assist you in understanding the application of content to the clinical area. Your ultimate goal is to apply your content information to client care. Consider getting a subscription to your nursing journal, *Journal of Practical*

Nursing or *Practical Nursing Journal*. Nursing organizations such as the National Federation of Licensed Practical Nursing or the National Association for Practical Nurse Education and Service are also valuable resources, and many have Web sites that you can visit.

Whatever resources you ultimately choose, gathering them and having your resources readily at hand are simple strategies that will make the time you have allotted for study more efficient and effective.

Minimize Interruptions

Interruptions to your study time decrease the actual time you can focus on the material and affect your concentration. Interruptions may also become your procrastination "triggers." If you allow your study time to be constantly interrupted, you will soon be doing something other than studying. At the very least, these interruptions minimize your efficient use of time. When you plan your time to study, do not set yourself up for interruptions. Look realistically at your time schedule and do not schedule your study time around the household's naturally busy times of the day—typically mornings, mealtimes, early evenings, and bedtimes.

This is where you put the strategies listed in the section on time management to work. If you have set aside a time and a space for study, make it known that you are not to be interrupted unless there is an emergency. Hang a sign on the door that reads, "Think before you knock." Studying in 1- or 1½-hour blocks is also a way to cut down on interruptions. This is a reasonable time period for you to put the world on hold in order to accomplish your task.

Get to Know the Textbook

Your textbook is not intended to be read like the latest mystery novel, from beginning to end in one sitting. It has directions on the way to use it (introduction, preface) and built-in references (glossary, appendix, summary questions). It is arranged in sections, each dealing with a major topic, and then subdivided into the parts (chapters) that make up the sum of that topic. Getting to know your textbook and its resources and the author's approach to writing may constitute the first part of your study plan. Having this information gives you some insight into the way the material has been grouped and connected.

Another author may have written the book in totally stand-alone chapters and may encourage students to review the table of contents and start anywhere they feel they need to. Self-instruction modules or texts in math often give students instructions to first take all of the post-tests in the chapters and, as long as a certain score is reached, to go on. This is a means of giving students credit for knowledge already learned and facilitating recall of knowledge in preparation for new learning.

Take a look at various parts of this text. How is the information organized? What built-in references can assist you? Consider the cues given about the way to use this text to help you organize the big picture.

Set Up the Study Plan

Each time you enter your study space, your study plan should be with you. You should have a plan or a specific goal for that time. Each time you enter the space, bring a positive attitude toward reaching that goal. Your nursing course outline will drive your study plan. You will have a certain amount of material to cover in a specific time span. You first must know those things that are expected of you. Your course outline, curriculum, and instructors will give you this information.

As an example, consider a unit on vital signs, which is assigned to be completed in 1 week. The components of the unit include understanding the theory base about vital signs as well as learning the psychomotor skills involved in actually measuring these indicators. You are expected to acquire the knowledge by reading the chapter in the text, attending the lecture and demonstration, and practicing in the lab. You will be tested on your ability to apply your knowledge through a pencil-and-paper test and a redemonstration of your psychomotor skills. Now that you know the information you must cover, the sources of the information, and the way you will be tested, you can map out a study plan. Consider the following steps:

1. *Preview the material to be studied.* Your assigned reading from the text on the content of the unit may be contained in one chapter or may span several chapters. Always preview the assigned chapter(s). Often, the student reads only the pages assigned, thinking that this is the most efficient way to study. By not spending the 5 or 10 minutes to preview the entire chapter, the connections between the content may be lost. Previewing can be done very quickly by scanning the chapter headings, art, and tables.
2. *Consider the chapter heading.* The material about vital signs may be contained in a chapter labeled "Baseline Assessment" or "Measurement of Baseline Values" or "Physiologic Functions of the Body." All of these give you a cue as to what you are about to study.
3. *Read the objectives for the chapter.* The objectives list those things you should be able to do when you are finished learning the content of the chapter.
4. *Scan the vocabulary section and the end-of-chapter summary and questions.* Read the key terms and the summary and questions at the chapter's end. Doing so gives you an overview of the scope of the reading you will need to do and should take no more than 5 to 10 minutes.
5. *Set up your questions.* Beginning at the chapter objectives, write down those things you already know, questions about those things you must learn for each objective, and some additional resources that you think you should check. For example, in a chapter about vital signs, the initial page may look like the one in Figure 1-4. Jot down your current knowledge and your questions. The resources note relates to the reasons you are trying to learn this material. Connecting the material to your role in the profession is most important. You are now ready to read the chapter critically for the answers to your questions. You may uncover more and have more questions at the end; but you have a plan and can move on to the next step.
6. *Read and take notes.* Answer your questions and check your vocabulary knowledge as you read.
7. *Reread when necessary.* Remember your basic skills and concentration.

The Measurement of Vital Signs

At the completion of this chapter, you should be able to:

1. Describe the physiologic mechanisms controlling temperature, pulse, respiration, and blood pressure.

   Temp = ?, Pulse = heart, Respiration = lungs, Blood pressure = arteries need to find out about temp.

2. Identify the normal range for vital sign measurements.

   For adults? Children?

3. Select the appropriate equipment used to take vital signs.

   Thermometer, stethoscope, blood pressure cuff

4. Demonstrate the correct psychomotor technique used in measuring vital signs.

   I do this in the lab/get procedure from book or instructor? Ask in class.

5. Document the normal findings of the measurement of blood pressure.

   Temp = 98.6, p = 60–80, bp = 120/80; I need to know this to be able to tell if the client is normal or having trouble.

COURTESY OF DELMAR CENGAGE LEARNING

FIGURE 1-4 Start with the chapter objectives and devise questions and answers to determine the things you know and the things you need to give more attention.

8. *Reflect on the connections you can make between the material and client care.* Identify the reasons the information is important and the way you will use it.
9. *Recite or create your individual style cues.* This is where you will put your individual unique learning styles to work. Make up songs. Create mnemonics. Design flash cards for items that must be memorized. Try to create a logical connection when recalling information.
10. *Review or summarize the information.* Answer the objectives. Use your own words to answer your initial questions. Do you have more questions? Must you consult a second resource to answer them?
11. *End the session with a critical thinking question.* What would the client look like if his temperature were 103°F? What other body systems would be affected? What nursing measures might I use to support the client with this level temperature (e.g., monitor the client's fluid intake and output because the body would be losing fluid as a result of the thermoregulation [sweating and evaporation that would reduce the temperature]), and why? Write these questions down in your notes. You will soon have a collection of "client scenarios" that you will be able to build on as you increase your knowledge base.

The preceding 11 study plan steps require skill in five areas: reading, rereading, reflecting, reciting, and review. With each step, you are engaging in the process of encoding the material. **Encoding** is thought of as actually laying down tracks in the areas of your brain. Each time you read, reread, reflect, recite, and review, you increase the depth of the tract, and your ability to recall and utilize the information increases. You move the information from short-term to long-term memory, and you increase your level of knowledge. The more senses and action you put into your study plan, the more you are able to utilize the information.

You move your level of knowledge from the memorization of a group of facts to the comprehension of the facts in a logical, organized fashion that allows you to apply the information to the client's situation to whom you will provide care. Each time you sit down to study, make your goal the application of knowledge to the client's condition. You can preview, question, and quickly outline the major points in the chapters before class. Listen to the lecture and take notes. Approach new material with the read, reread, reflect, recite, and review steps before moving on to the next topic.

PROFESSIONAL TIP

Mnemonics

Create your own mnemonics to group the steps of a procedure. A mnemonic is simply a method for helping your association and recall; it consists of a memorable word or phrase created from the letters of the list of items you are trying to recall. For example, to remember all of the areas to include when assessing a client to whom a cast has been applied (pulse, circulation, sensation, movement, and temperature), you might make up a silly sentence to help you remember, such as "***P***aul ***C***an ***S***hine ***M***y ***T***uba." This type of statement will help you group these facts together (pulse, circulation, sensation, movement, temperature) and assist you in recalling them. You could sing this also. Do whatever you can to be active in moving material from short-term to long-term memory.

NOTE TAKING

Note taking is an action that connects you to the content of written material or a lecture presentation and will assist you in identifying the main ideas and their connection to the overall topic.

PROFESSIONAL TIP

Attending Class

In general, the best strategies for getting the most from classes are to:

- Get to class on time.
- Get a front row seat.
- Listen attentively with a pencil in your hand and take notes.

Keep materials for each of your classes or topics in a separate three-ring binder. Take notes on loose-leaf paper and write on one side only because this allows you to arrange your preview notes and lecture notes chronologically. You can also insert handouts from the class in the appropriate order as you receive them. Using this method, you can also review notes against additional information you have from other resources to assist you when it is time to review for the examinations.

When you are taking notes from the text, read with a pencil in your hand to put yourself in the action mode. You will thus be ready to receive and process information. You may also take notes from text readings on your computer, which facilitates editing and rearranging material.

Before class, preview your chapter material and divide your paper, leaving a 3-inch border on the left side. From the assigned reading, identify the main topic to be covered, list the main section and the subheadings, and summarize the information in the left column. Then write your questions in this column. This prepares you for more active participation in the lecture; use the right column to take notes from the lecture.

Regardless of the way you choose to take notes, note taking while you study sets you up for connecting with the content. It positions you as an active participant in the learning process, and any time you increase your active participation in the learning process, you increase your learning.

When taking notes in class, listen attentively, lean forward, and concentrate on the information the speaker is imparting (Figure 1-5). Take notes on the following:

- The topic, as stated by the speaker; write it on the top of the page
- The main ideas and the details that support the topic
- The most important points, based on the speaker's organization and emphasis
- Other students' questions and the responses from the speaker, which are often the very questions you had

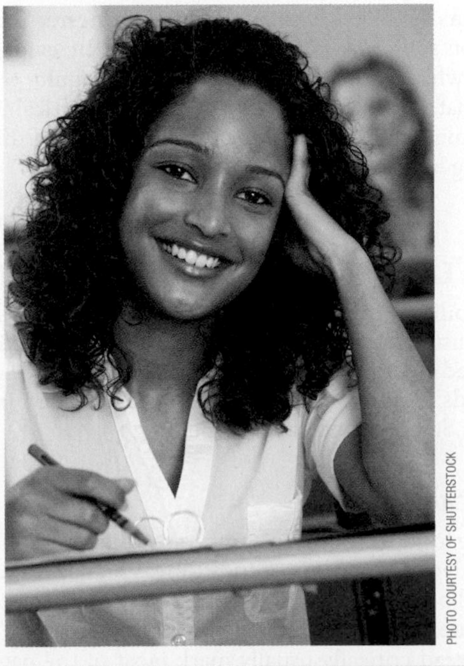

FIGURE 1-5 Note taking is an important component of increasing your comprehension of the material.

Look for visual and auditory cues from the speaker, for example, if the speaker says, "This is important," or writes steps on the board. Do not form an opinion of what is being said until you have heard the entire lecture. As stated earlier, a good strategy is to write your questions as you think of them. They may be answered by the time the lecture is over.

The purpose of note taking during a lecture is not to create a transcript of the information imparted but, rather, to record what you understand. The combination of attending lecture, listening, and note taking can provide you with much knowledge that you will not have to learn elsewhere. Previewing the material to be covered further contributes to this dynamic. When taking notes, consider the following guidelines to make your note taking efficient and effective:

- Do not take notes with the intent of writing them over. This is a waste of time, and, contrary to what you may expect, it does not improve recall.
- If your handwriting is sloppy, print or use a laptop computer.
- Condense the amount of actual writing you do by using symbols and abbreviations and leaving out everything but necessary words. For instance, instead of writing "If the client's blood pressure reading is greater than 140 systolic and 90 diastolic, . . ." write "If BP >140/90. . . ."
- Write definitions and mathematical formulas exactly as you heard them in lecture.
- In mathematics and science lab courses, write the process step by step exactly as explained. Indicate which formulas are used with which problems, for example:

  "Use ratio/proportion for word problems."
- Pick an abbreviation system and stick to it.
- Review the notes as soon as possible after class. Many studies have demonstrated that even a brief review of notes after class increases retention of the material by 50%.

PREPARE FOR EXAMS

The final plus of having a study plan is the ability to review for exams. Reviewing for exams is not studying all of the material over from the beginning. You will already have studied the subject matter you are going to cover on the exam; now, you are reviewing and recalling it through a series of exercises designed to increase your comprehension and facilitate application. Some nursing examinations are written at the comprehension or recall level. The NCLEX-PN® is written at the application level. On the NCLEX-PN® exam you will not see many questions about naming where the pulse points are (comprehension, recall). You will instead find questions about which of the pulse points of the body are most appropriate for assessing an infant (application). Making decisions about which fact or groups of principles you have learned will be the basis for most nursing examination questions.

Depending on the curriculum, you may have examinations every week or every month, a weekly quiz, a midterm, and a final. Regardless, you will know the schedule, and you must set aside review time for preparation. If you are to have weekly quizzes, you must build a time for review into your daily study plan. One way to do so is to set aside the last 30 minutes of each study session for review. Take each objective of your course outline and, without looking at your notes or text, turn them into questions and then answer them. If you are weak in one area, refer to your notes and devise a technique for recall, such as the use of flash cards, rhythms, mnemonics, pictures, or graphic drawings. Work through each of the objectives for the content that is covered.

If your examinations are by unit, you must divide the material up over the time you will need to cover it, leaving at least 2 days for review and recall before the examination. Each of these review sessions will also serve as preparation for both your final examination and the NCLEX-PN®. As you are successful in each of your examinations and continue to see further connections in your clinical application, your depth as well as breadth of content mastery will increase.

Participate in Test Reviews

Test reviews vary from one instructor or class to another but are a great way to review your level of knowledge and ability to succeed within a class and the nursing profession. As nurses, our final evaluation and rite-of-passage for nursing practices is the NCLEX-PN® exam. It is a computerized multiple-choice exam, and it is only by successfully passing the exam that a nurse begins a nursing career. So it is imperative that nursing students learn to successfully take exams. A test review is a great way to identify common mistakes or patterns of mistakes on exams. Some students learn that they frequently change from the right answer to a wrong answer. Others eliminate all but two answers and then struggle choosing the right one. Changing these patterns could make the difference between succeeding and failing in nursing school (DePew, 2008).

Learn from Mistakes

Some nursing student's mistakes might be failing an exam, skipping class, or choosing not to complete an assignment. The ability to learn from one's mistakes provides an opportunity to turn failure into success. A challenge after each exam might be to understand each missed question so that if a student sees those question concepts again, he would understand the concept and get that question correct. If pertinent information is missed from class because of an absence, then next time it is important to contact the instructor and peers to ensure that no information covered or provided in class is omitted. A mistake might occur in the clinical setting, and the clinical instructor offers time to review and relearn the skill. Mistakes are opportunities to learn and grow and are important not to repeat, since a nurse's mistakes could impact another human life. Taking time to learn from one's mistakes will lead to success in nursing care and nursing practice (DePew, 2008).

Talk with Instructors

Many people are available to discuss experiences and concerns with a nursing student. Some of these people are instructors, advisors, and peers. It is important to remember the value in talking with peers. Share with each other what is working and what is not working in class. Explore ideas that might help or hinder success in the class and nursing school.

If you feel you are not achieving the desired results and you are unable to identify ways to correct a class problem, ask to meet with the instructor. Instructors are often available before and after a class, or have specific office hours available to discuss student concerns. Instructors are great resources for explaining or clarifying class specific information and details. They also hold the key to what has worked for former students and assignments in the past. Collaboration between student and faculty is a very important part of a student's success when accompanied by a trusting relationship (Sayles, Shelton & Powell, 2003). Remember these resources when evaluating and modifying for success in nursing school. These tips help identify the resources needed to succeed (DePew, 2008).

PRACTICE CRITICAL THINKING

Most of this chapter thus far has been devoted to presenting strategies for the effective and efficient acquisition of knowledge. Your ultimate goal is to be able to use this knowledge to provide safe client care. To do so, you must go beyond the initial stage of simply acquiring information. In delivering nursing care, facts alone do not constitute a sufficient knowledge base for making sound decisions about client care. You must internalize these facts and be able to use them when presented with new situations.

In considering which actions you may need to take in a new situation, you must consider past experience and principles of care, postulate possible outcomes from a variety of interventions, and seek additional information from colleagues, clients, and resource materials. This process is called critical thinking, and it is what you will be expected to do with the knowledge you are acquiring.

The first step is to develop an understanding of **critical thinking**. A comprehensive definition is the **disciplined** (taught by instruction and exercise) intellectual process of applying skillful **reasoning** (use of the elements of thought to solve a problem or settle a question), imposing intellectual **standards** (a level or degree of quality), and self-reflective thinking as a guide to a belief or an action (Heaslip, 1994; Paul, 1995).

Many students find the process of becoming responsible for their own thinking painful. You, along with many other students, may be uncomfortable when asked to defend your **opinions** (subjective beliefs) and **judgments** (conclusions based on sound reasoning and supported by evidence) or to decide what is important. Probably you would prefer to be told what you need to know. Because practical/vocational nurses must make many decisions in the care of their clients, knowing how to make good decisions is essential.

Skills of Critical Thinking

Your abilities in the four basic skills of critical reading, critical listening, critical writing, and critical speaking can be measured by how well you achieve the universal intellectual standards (UIS). These standards are discussed in the next section: Standards of Critical Thinking.

Critical Reading

Reading for the meaning of concepts is basic to the acquisition of knowledge from books. Study time is reduced, and information will be retained, leading to better results on tests. Use of a highlighter to mark the main ideas is often helpful. Those who do not read critically usually mark most of the page. Form a study group to compare the main ideas marked in the assigned material. When reviewing tests, note when misreading or misinterpretation was the cause of your incorrect answer. Make a conscious effort to identify your weaknesses.

As you prepare your assignments, have a dialogue with yourself:

- Before beginning to read, preview the material and ask yourself: What is it about; how is it related to what I already know; how it is organized; and are other resources required?
- As you are reading, ask yourself: Does it make sense; are all terms familiar or should I look them up; how is this related to what I already know; and can I summarize this section?
- After reading, ask yourself: Do I understand the main points; can I outline the main points; how will I use or apply this information; does something need to be clarified; and what questions are likely to be on the exam?

Critical Listening

Communication skills, especially listening skills, are greatly emphasized in the nursing curriculum. Many students do not have effective listening skills. Many persons have developed the habit of tuning in only occasionally to what is said, resulting in lost communication. Improve your listening skills by restating the points made in a discussion with another student and ask that student to give feedback about how accurately you have restated her position. As you listen, focus on what the speaker is saying, listen for key points, and make a note of anything that seems confusing to you (Figure 1-6).

Critical listening requires a conscious commitment to focus on the topic of discussion. Recognize things that distract your attention. Attempting to take word-for-word notes, daydreaming, and focusing on the mannerisms or appearance of the speaker are common distractors. A good thinker is not afraid to identify weaknesses and strengths in order to improve.

Critical Speaking

Disciplined speaking is perhaps the most neglected skill. Examples of clear, logical, and accurate spoken communication are seldom heard. Oral communication is usually more spontaneous than written communication and must be carefully presented. Ambiguous statements are misleading, and personal biases influence what the other person hears. Small

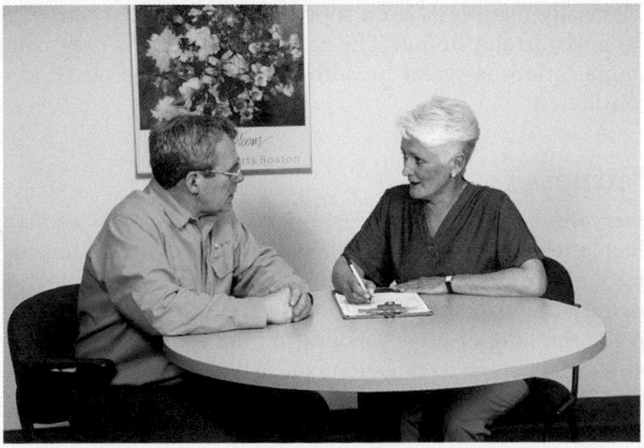

COURTESY OF DELMAR CENGAGE LEARNING

FIGURE 1-6 Effective listening skills are essential to all client interactions.

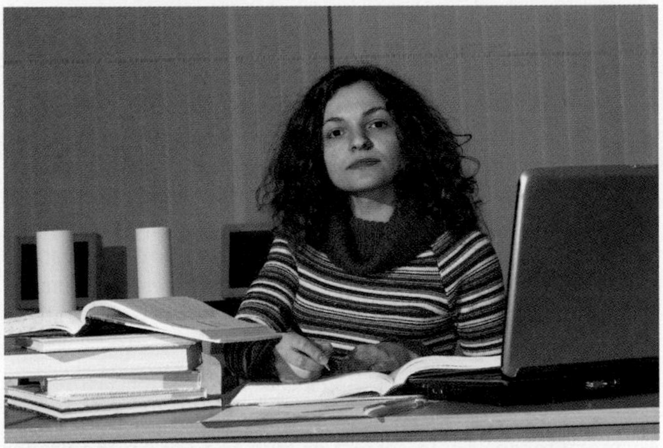

PHOTO COURTESY OF SHUTTERSTOCK

FIGURE 1-7 Effective writing skills are integral to critical thinking.

group practice followed by feedback from the listeners can help a student assess and improve speaking skills.

Critical Writing

Basic to good thinking skills is the ability to state one's thoughts coherently, clearly, and concisely. Many students arrive at college unable to write well. The quality of thinking is improved by the discipline required to write well. Many students feel that writing is too revealing and are afraid to write down their thoughts. Writing is important for the improvement of thinking because it can be reviewed using the standards for critical thinking to evaluate the quality of the thinking reflected in the writing (Figure 1-7). The standards for critical thinking are discussed next.

Standards for Critical Thinking

Critical thinking relies on the use of intellectual standards for checking the quality of thinking (Elder & Paul, 2008). The first requirement is to become familiar with the Universal Intellectual Standards developed at The Center for Critical Thinking. These are used in this discussion because they provide a valid and reliable measure for the quality of thinking. Whether you are reading, listening, writing, answering test questions, or speaking, the standards of clarity, accuracy, precision, relevance, consistency, logic, depth, breadth, and fairness should be applied.

Clarity

Fundamental to quality thinking is the ability to think clearly. Clarity of thought means placing facts and ideas into a logical and coherent framework. The standard is the degree to which others can understand your position. Pay particular attention to the exact meaning of words. There will be many new terms and concepts in your nursing curriculum. Practice the proper use of these terms and apply concepts appropriately to improve clarity of thought and increased retention of content.

Think about the word *clarity*. There are several shades of meaning in the dictionary. Look up the word for yourself and decide which definition applies to the use of clarity in describing a standard for critical thinking.

Think about expressions you use frequently. Would someone from another part of the country understand them? The term *this evening* is common in some parts of the country. When would you expect someone who told you that she would visit "this evening?" In some places, the person might arrive in the early afternoon; in other places, at night. When speaking to clients, families, and other health team members, be sure that the words used clearly express the intended message. Do not assume that you understand a term; take time to verify the meaning. When a statement is unclear, it cannot be determined whether it is accurate or relevant.

Accuracy

Accuracy means being correct or true and within the proper parameters. The need for accurate calculation of a drug dose or accurate measurement of blood pressure can readily be understood. In the same way, the collection and interpretation of data must be accurate. Being accurate implies the use of some measuring instrument. Accuracy in thinking may be hard to conceptualize. When a person uses the term *hypertension* to mean someone who is anxious and very active instead of the actual meaning, an elevation of blood pressure above the accepted normal maximum, the standard of accuracy is not met. Students can improve their accuracy in thinking by writing new information in their own words and asking another student to interpret what was written. Inaccurate information will become evident.

Accurate documentation of client care is essential to quality care. There are degrees of accuracy. For example, you might measure a client's temperature using a thermometer that can measure to the 0.01 degree, but this degree of accuracy is not necessary. On the other hand, when figuring a pediatric dosage, a difference of 0.01 is very important. A challenge to you is to learn the degree of accuracy required in given nursing situations.

Precision

Sometimes, students learn enough about a subject to be "in the ballpark" but not enough to hit a home run. The result is a general idea about a fact or idea, but not enough understanding to apply it. Precise thinking means that there is enough detail and specificity for a concept or word to be clearly understood in terms of its relationship to other concepts or words.

Relevance

Relevance refers to information connected to the issue as opposed to information that is not. Students may get sidetracked from the purpose of an exercise by failing to limit their discussion to the issue at hand. Their responses are not relevant. When studying, ask yourself how a particular concept is relevant to client care. It is also important to be able to recognize when sufficient relevant information is not available.

Consistency

Consistency is the appropriate use of principles and concepts. For instance, a particular nursing diagnosis based on specified indicators should be used when those indicators are present and never used when the indicators are not present.

Knowing the basic actions of epinephrine enables the nurse to predict client responses to the administration of the drug. It also helps the nurse understand that the client will have the same response when an increased secretion of epinephrine is released by the client's adrenal medulla.

Logic

Thinking brings a variety of thoughts together in some order. Logic asks the question "Does this make sense?" Symptoms exhibited by clients can usually be understood based on knowledge of normal physiology and those changes produced by the client's disease or condition. For example, a client with a gallstone blocking the common bile duct is concerned because his stool is very light gray in color. Bile is the substance that colors the stool brown, so it follows that if there is no bile, the stool will not be brown. These two items make sense in combination.

When calculating a medication dosage, the standard of logic is extremely important. If the calculation answer is to give the client 200 pills of a certain medication, this is not logical; it does not make sense. Most likely, there is a missing decimal point, with the correct answer being two pills.

Depth

Students are often tempted to rely on the specific learning objectives as an indicator of which material they must master. This may result in a superficial understanding of the material. The ability to recognize the depth to explore concepts and ideas can be learned. Students should ask themselves, "What are the most significant factors; and what are the complexities in this situation; and what other problems may be involved?" These questions will guide the student to see other aspects that also need to be explored for a thorough understanding. Your instructor and the learning aids within your textbook are useful guides for identifying relevant information and the appropriate depth of knowledge required to make good clinical decisions.

Breadth

Breadth of thinking entails considering another point of view and asking if there is another way to look at the question or problem. Consider a pregnant woman, with a 6-year-old son, who has been told she must stay in bed because of complications. The problem is broader than just the complication of the pregnancy. Who will care for the son, take him to school? Who will do the cooking, cleaning, laundry? Is this financially feasible? Can a mother or friend help out? Can the husband stay home? The narrow problem of a pregnancy complication has great breadth when the entire situation is considered.

Fairness

Everyone has a set of beliefs, opinions, and points of view. People tend to believe that what they think is true. Improving the quality of your thinking depends on your ability to identify the biases in your thinking and those biases present in the thinking of others. Following the standard of fairness will lead a person to question conclusions based on personal bias. When a nurse who responds to pain in a stoic manner assesses a person who responds to pain emotionally, the nurse may allow personal values to influence the assessment, with the result that the nurse provides inadequate pain relief for the client.

Reasoning and Problem Solving

Although reasoning involves thinking, all thinking is not reasoning. Thinking is occurring when a person daydreams, jumps to conclusions, or decides to listen to music. However, these activities cannot be called reasoning. In order to effectively use reasoning, to figure things out, or to problem-solve, the student must become familiar with the components of reasoning. These components are purpose, the question at issue, assumptions, point of view, data and information, concepts, inferences and conclusions, and implications and consequences.

Purpose

All reasoning is directed toward some specific purpose. This is one aspect where reasoning is different from daydreaming. For the nursing student, the purpose of reasoning is to use the information learned in class to effectively solve client care problems.

The Question at Issue

The purpose of the reasoning process is to figure something out, answer a question, or solve some problem. This problem or question must be clearly stated. At the beginning of a study period, state clearly the problems presented by this particular material. Good clinical judgment begins with a clear statement of problems presented by each client.

Assumptions

Assumptions are ideas or things that are taken for granted. They are accepted as being true without examination. Assumptions may be helpful in problem solving, but recognize them for what they are. An example of an assumption is that nursing makes a difference in the outcome of a client's illness. This is a necessary assumption for nurses to make in order to engage in problem-solving related to client care needs.

Assumptions that have proven reliable can help in decision making, while faulty assumptions may cause you to draw faulty conclusions and may lead to inadequate problem-solving. Learn to recognize your own assumptions and those of others. Never be afraid to challenge your own assumptions or to ask others to clarify the assumptions they are using.

Point of View

Each person reasons from his own point of view, which is influenced by previous experience, available information, the quality of thinking already acquired, and many other factors. All together these factors give each person a unique perspective and a unique way of thinking. Seek other points of view and evaluate their strengths and weaknesses. Each person sees things differently. An individual's point of view will determine what facts and information will be noticed, the importance given to the information, and even the acceptable solutions to the problem. Identify your own point of view and its limitations and acknowledge the right of others to have their own points of view (Figure 1-8).

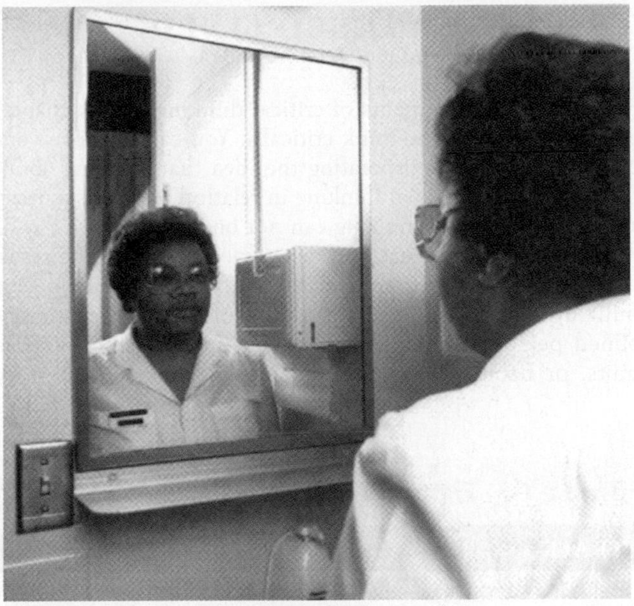

FIGURE 1-8 To be effective problem-solvers and critical thinkers, nurses must first take a good look at their own point of view.

Data and Information

Data and information are the basic materials of reasoning. Be sure that all information and data are clear, accurate, and relevant to the question or problem at issue. Search for information that not only supports your position but also refutes it. Make conclusions supported by the data you have collected.

Concepts

Identify concepts needed to explore the problem and the implications of each. The concepts (such as asepsis, pain, adaptation, and so on) important to nursing care must be part of the evidence supporting a nursing judgment.

Inferences and Conclusions

Reasoning requires interpretation of facts and information. The interpretation must be justified by the relevant facts. It must be supported by the data and information. Many times, students state opinions as judgments or inferences. This happens when inferences are based on assumptions and personal preferences rather than on the information.

Properly drawing judgments or inferences is basic to thinking well. For example, when the body's temperature goes above 98.6 degrees, the body's metabolic rate increases. Increased metabolism requires more oxygen for the tissues. More oxygen can be delivered to the tissues by increasing the heart rate. From these facts, it is inferred that an elevated body temperature results in an increased heart rate.

The product of reasoning is a conclusion regarding the problem. It is the answer to the question that began the process. The conclusion must be logical.

Implications and Consequences

The reasoning process usually produces more than one solution. Now it is necessary to examine the implications of each solution by thinking about the ease with which a solution can be applied, the ability of a person to carry out the required actions, or the risks involved. Look for both positive and negative consequences.

Consequences can result from action or inaction. It may not be possible to predict all consequences, but the possible outcomes should be examined as completely as possible.

Traits of a Disciplined Thinker

Reading the requirements of critical thinking in this chapter will not make anyone think critically. You can improve your own thinking by incorporating the idea that thinking about the quality of your own thinking in relation to UIS is a desirable goal. Improved thinking can not be acquired in a day or two. It takes time, effort, and disciplined practice. The result is well worth it, however. Consistent efforts to improve your thinking can result in the acquisition of the traits of a disciplined person (Center for Critical Thinking, 2008). These traits, or habitual ways of thinking, can be recognized by others and enable a person to compete successfully in the high-tech world (Table 1-5).

Critical Thinking and the Nursing Process

A nursing education program is intended to help students develop the logic of nursing. In other words, you will learn to think like a nurse. The method nurses have adopted to implement the practice of nursing is called the nursing process. The nursing process applies the problem-solving process to the practice of nursing and requires critical thinking. When you find the relationship between the content of the textbooks

Table 1-5 Traits of a Disciplined Thinker

TRAIT	DESCRIPTION
Faith in reason	Confident that interests of humankind are best served by giving free play to reason Values reasoning in self and others Has faith that people can learn to think for themselves, think coherently and logically, and come to reasonable conclusions
Intellectual humility	Aware of how much he does not know Sensitive to bias, prejudice, and limitations of own viewpoint Willing to examine beliefs and conclusions based on new evidence Respects thoughts and ideas of others Continually learning and improving own thinking
Intellectual courage	Addresses ideas, beliefs, or viewpoints causing strong negative emotions that have not received a serious hearing Recognizes that ideas considered dangerous are sometimes jusitified Willing to take unpopular positions based on reasoning
Intellectual integrity	Is true to own thinking Consistent in intellectual standards applied and does not change to suit circumstances or personal bias Admits discrepancies and inconsistencies in own thoughts and actions Practices what he advocates for others
Intellectual perseverance	Uses intellectual insights and truths despite difficulties and frustrations Pursues question or problem until conclusion is reached Adheres to rational principles Willing to struggle with confusion and unsettled questions over an extended time period to achieve deeper meaning
Intellectual empathy	Imaginatively puts self in place of others to genuinely understand them Able to reconstruct accurately the viewpoints and reasoning of others Remembers past occasions when he was wrong despite intense conviction of being right
Fair-mindedness	Considers all viewpoints Adheres to intellectual standards Is impartial

and the logic of nursing, the study of nursing will be an exciting and challenging process. Using the nursing process will improve the quality of your thinking, and using reasoning will enhance your use of the nursing process.

DEVELOP TEST-TAKING SKILLS

Testing is not studying; however, the skills you need for testing are similar to those needed for studying. The task involved in taking a test is not to pass it; to pass the test is the *outcome*. You cannot achieve the outcome if you do not perform the task. The task is to read the question, understand what the question is asking, and make a decision about a correct response.

To hone your test-taking behaviors, you must first perform a personal analysis with regard to your attitudes, preparation methods, and behaviors related to a testing situation. Only after you have identified these variables can you initiate strategies to improve your outcomes.

Attitude and Expectations

If you are like most students, you may feel quite anxious about taking a test. You may think of each test as the final chance to show your worth. Or you may consider receiving less than an A on an examination as being the same as failing. Neither of these is a reasonable expectation for testing. Testing is a useful tool for both measuring your level of knowledge and showing what you still need to learn. Have you ever considered that receiving a grade of C on an examination usually indicates that you know 75% of all of the knowledge that was tested? And the knowledge on any given test does not represent all the knowledge you possess. Your attitude toward testing is very important if you are to improve your outcome. Maintain a reasonable expectation about both the purpose of the test and the meaning of your grade. This is often a key factor in improving your test performance.

Preparation

In analyzing your preparation for test taking, you must critically examine your study habits. Review the section in this chapter on study strategies and consider whether you are on task when it comes to your study habits. There may be some areas where you can improve. If you know of an area of weakness, make a conscious effort to develop this part of your preparation. Be reasonable in your expectations and do not expect to see results overnight. Building your study habits takes time and persistence. Persevere and your outcome on tests will improve.

Next, consider the way you review for an examination. Do you cram the night before, or are you consistently planning for questions in your study plan and adding time for review of material before the examination? One strategy is to use the technique of note mapping to help you organize the material into manageable parts. (See the Professional Tip: Note Mapping.) Taking each part and developing a more detailed one-page outline that you can take with you to review for 15 to 20 minutes at a time is another method to try. Another suggestion is to change your study place and times. Instead of 1-hour sessions, break your review sessions into 30-minute recall sessions. You must draw an imaginary line between studying and reviewing. Studying is the learning of new knowledge; reviewing comprises recall, organization, and summary of information.

Do not study only just before the test. This is a poor technique. Approaching preparation in this manner serves only to put a few facts into short-term memory. Better to spend the time before the examination relaxing with a good book or good friends or at the spa or gym. You must be confident and rested and come to the testing area with that good feeling that results from doing something you like.

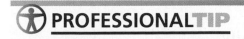

PROFESSIONALTIP

The 30-Second Vacation

For those of you who need an "anxiety buster," consider a "30-second vacation." The 30-second vacation is based on a guided imagery technique that is used often in the client care arena. This technique takes practice. Start by doing the following:

Sit in a comfortable spot where you will not be disturbed, close your eyes, and think of an event or a place that evokes a feeling of calmness (not necessarily happiness). This is an event or place that made you feel like everything was right with the world and with you. It can be from any time in your life.

It may take some time to settle on the right event or place. Relax and take a few minutes now and think.

Once you have it, don't tell anyone! This is your secret place, your place of peace, and when you go there, no one can find you.

Once you have selected this event or place, start to give it "life." To do this, you must begin to recall this event or place regularly. Practice doing so at the beginning of your study sessions, when you are stuck in traffic, when you are at the dentist, when you have something difficult to do, at the beginning of your test-taking exercises, or at the beginning of your real tests.

Each time you recall your event or place, give it more "life." Recall the time of day, the setting, the colors of that day. Was it raining, was it sunny, was it snowing? If it was raining, was it a summer rain or an autumn rain? Recall what you were wearing and what colors you had on. Were you alone or with others? Were you eating something? What did the food smell like?

Consider the rest you get the night before the examination. Physical stamina is needed for concentration. If you cram for a test by "pulling an all-nighter," you are setting yourself up for possible errors on the examination. Be reasonable, revisit your study plan, and get adequate rest.

Next, consider whether you have enough energy to take the test. You can eat what you want, but eat. The cells of the brain require glucose to function; this glucose is supplied in the calories you consume. Try not to increase caffeine intake immediately before a test because doing so may make you jittery.

Finally, ask yourself whether surrounding yourself with positive people helps keep you focused, or whether talking to students before a test only makes you more anxious. If the latter is the case, you should arrive with just enough time to walk into the testing room and you should not speak to anyone.

Minimize Anxiety

Anxiety is the physiologic response of the autonomic nervous system to a perceived stressful situation. As the situation becomes more stressful, the body's response increases. This affects the ability to process information and make rational choices. People are often not good at identifying what they are feeling and are often unaware of the degree to which stress affects the ability to take tests.

Develop a plan to deal with anxiety. Anxiety about performance is always present. Past experience with testing often contributes to the development of test anxiety. If the expectation regarding performance on a test is not mirrored in the grade we receive, our confidence in our ability is shaken, and we approach the whole experience with more and more anxiety.

To deal with anxiety, consciously develop an activity to counter the feeling that anxiety evokes. Some people listen to music, pace, or do deep breathing to combat feelings of stress and anxiety. All of these are good strategies, even if all of them cannot be done *while you are actually taking the test.*

Improve Test-Taking Skills

How do you improve your test-taking skills? You practice, practice, practice and analyze, analyze, analyze. Consider the following:

> *Treat every wrong answer as a treasure. Examine it and discover the secret of why you got it wrong.*

This is the only way to know which errors you are making. Always request to review your examinations, and track your incorrect responses using the analysis worksheet presented in Figure 1-9. Initially, when you review your tests, do not concern yourself with the content of the questions. Simply write the number of the question in the row that indicates the reason you got that question incorrect. You will also notice that there is a heavy black line before the last row of the worksheet. The first four rows represent what are known as *mechanical errors;* these can be eliminated by developing positive habits and revising current practices. You will notice after three or four quizzes that a pattern starts to emerge. Imagine that you just took a 100-question test and received a score of 60/100. You then use the worksheet to categorize your incorrect responses.

Of the 40 incorrect answers you provided, you see that 10 of them fell in "did not read carefully," 2 in "did not know the vocabulary," 7 in "inferred additional data," 4 in "identified priorities incorrectly," and 7 in "did not know the material." If you could eliminate the bad habits that resulted in the first 23 errors, this would improve your test score immediately. Your grade would be 83/100. More important, tests would truly represent only what you did not know, not areas where bad habits resulted in poor test scores.

After you have identified your error patterns, you can work on developing the counterhabits that will eliminate them. Work first on the one that is the most glaring.

Test Question Analysis Worksheet

Reason for Incorrect Response	Test 1 Date	Test 2 Date
Did not read carefully (missed details, missed key words)		
Did not know the vocabulary (medical terminology, English vocabulary)		
Inferred additional data (made assumptions, "read into the question")		
Identified priorities incorrectly (placed events in wrong order)		
Did not know the material		
Marked the correct answer and then changed it (changed answer instead of going with first choice)		

FIGURE 1-9 Test Question Analysis Worksheet

Read Carefully

Reading carefully is a test-taking behavior that must be practiced. The section on study strategies noted the value of scanning in looking for important words when you read. When you are reading a test question, however, you must *never* scan. Many students choose incorrect responses because they miss key words, scan the question for familiar terms, infer what the question is, or misinterpret words they read too quickly. Incorrect responses resulting from any of these actions represent poor reading habits rather than a substandard knowledge base. The following exercise will help improve your reading habits.

Exercise for Improving Your Literal Reading Skills

You will need:

- A timer (stove)
- An NCLEX-PN® review text or any comparable question and answer book. It is important that you have the answers and the rationales for each answer in a review text.
- Two sheets of paper: one to take the test on and one to make your analysis worksheet
- Pencil or pen
- Dictionary

PROFESSIONALTIP

Note Mapping

Note mapping is taking conventional notes and organizing them into a picture that allows one to see connections and links between ideas and concepts. A note map is similar to the concept maps within this text. When a note map is developed, one thinks through complex problems, fuses together the information, summarizes the content, and displays the information in a way that is easy to recall. More of the brain is engaged in assimilating and connecting the facts, so one can easily recall information because one can easily recall the shape and structure of the note map. The advantage of note mapping over conventional notes is that one can see the informational links and recall the basic facts within the notes. All the pages of notes are fit onto one page, so the note map is easy to carry and study in spare minutes. Here is an example of a note map for the section you are reading, "Develop Test-Taking Skills."

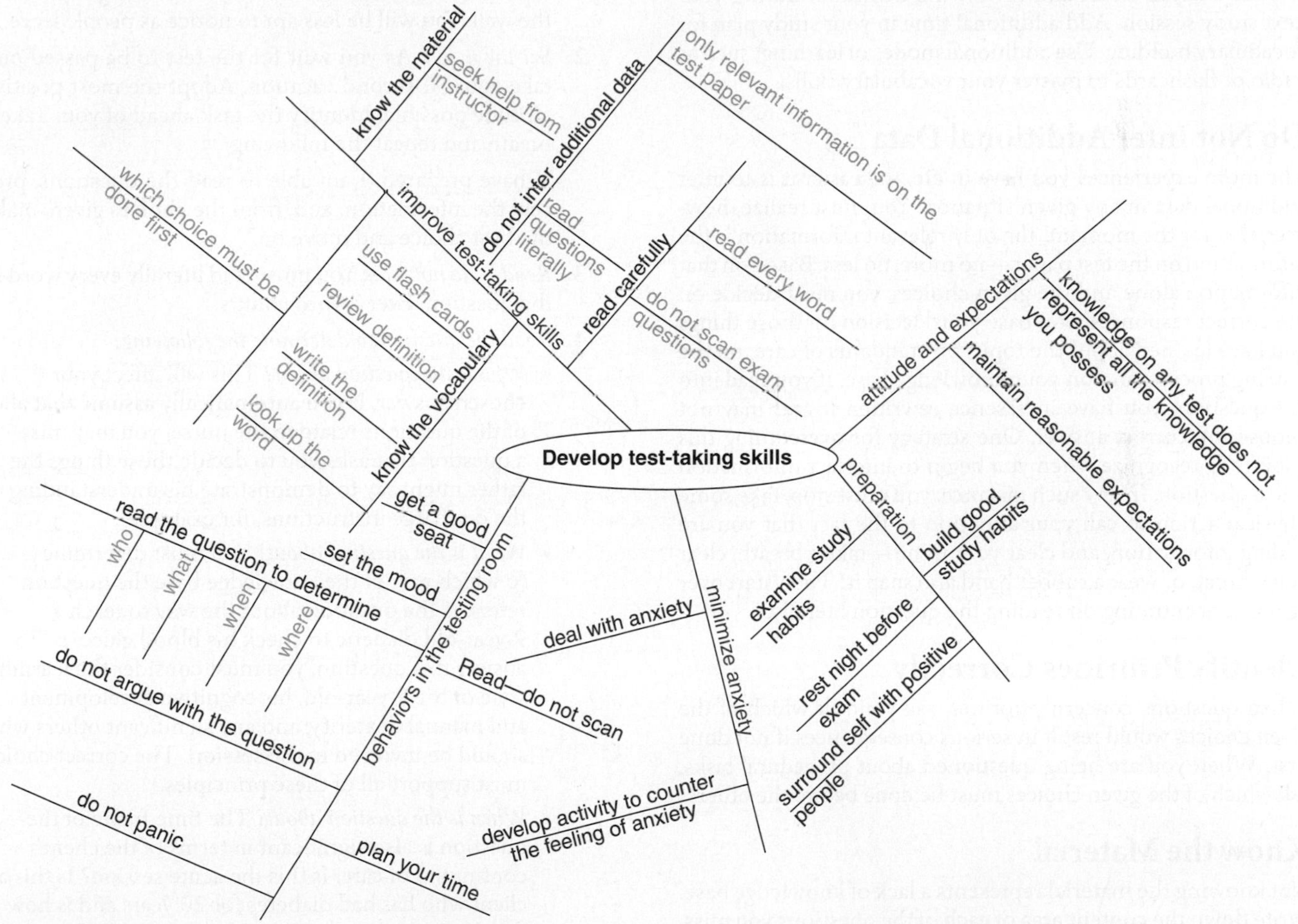

1. Pick a time and a place where there will be no interruptions for 20 minutes. You may neither speak to anyone nor get up to use any other resources. You are taking a test.
2. Randomly pick a page of the review book and choose five questions from that page. It does not matter whether you have studied the content in your program.
3. Set the timer for 5 minutes.
4. Start the test. Read each question out loud.
   a. If you read "over" a word, stop reading, make a mark next to that word, and begin again from the beginning.
   b. If you mispronounce a word, stop reading, make a mark next to that word, and begin again from the beginning.
   c. If you do not know the meaning of a word (English or medical), stop and look it up.
5. At the end of the question, restate what is being asked of you.
6. Read the choices, connect each to the question, and choose the most correct answer.
7. When the timer goes off, score your questions.
8. Analyze why you got questions correct or incorrect. You can use the test question analysis worksheet and your personal critical thinking skills to analyze the answers.

9. Repeat this exercise with five different questions three or four times a week.

The object of this exercise is not to finish all the questions, nor is it even to get all the answers right. Rather, the object is to consciously practice reading every word literally. Each time you do this exercise, you must treat it as a test—no food, no talking, no music, no interruptions. You must associate this type of reading with taking a test so that each time you take a test, this literal reading habit is instinctual.

Know the Vocabulary

If vocabulary is your weak area, there is only one thing to do-learn the vocabulary. Look up the word (English and medical) in the appropriate dictionary, write the definition on the back of your analysis sheet and review the definition during your next study session. Add additional time in your study plan for vocabulary building. Use additional modes of learning, such as audio or flashcards to master your vocabulary skills.

Do Not Infer Additional Data

The more experiences you have in life, the easier it is to infer additional data in any given situation. You must realize, however, that for the moment, the only relevant information is the information on the test paper—no more, no less. Based on that information alone and the given choices, you must decide on the correct responses. You base your decision on those things you have learned about the topic, on standards of care, on the nursing process, and on your knowledge base. If you read into the question, you have in essence rewritten it and may not choose the correct answer. One strategy for overcoming this habit is to recognize when you begin to interject information into a question. In any such instance, you must stop, take some physical action to call your attention to the fact that you are adding information, and clear your mind—take a breath, clear your throat, or wear a rubber band and snap it! Then start over again, concentrating on reading the question literally.

Identify Priorities Correctly

When questions concern priorities, ask yourself which of the given choices would result in serious consequences if not done first. When you are being questioned about procedural tasks, ask which of the given choices must be done before the others.

Know the Material

Not knowing the material represents a lack of knowledge base. Write down the content area of each of the questions you miss, then go back and review the concept or facts in question. If the same content areas are problematic over several tests, seek additional assistance from your instructor. You need clarification regarding your understanding of both the information and the questions.

Go with the First Answer

Have you ever found yourself reading a test question and then eliminating all but two choices? Finally you choose one of the answers. You start to go to the next question but then second-guess yourself and change the answer. When the exam is returned, you find your first choice was the correct answer.

Generally, a student's first choice is correct. Unless you have the thought, "Oh, my goodness, why did I choose that answer?" do not change the answer. That thought indicates you recalled or found information that made the second choice incorrect. Unless you know the answer is definitely wrong, go with your first intuition. Often the first choice is correct.

Behaviors in the Testing Room

Setting yourself up in the testing room for a positive experience can make a difference in your outcome. Be sure to practice the following behaviors:

1. *Get a good seat.* Unless your seat is assigned, sit in an area that is quiet and, has good light, and where you can "zone in" on the test and "zone out" the rest of the room. If you are a student who gets anxious when you are the last one left in the room, pick a seat in the front row and farthest from the door and turn your seat slightly toward the wall. You will be less apt to notice as people leave.
2. *Set the mood.* As you wait for the test to be passed out, take your 30-second vacation. Adopt the most positive attitude possible. Identify the task ahead of you. Take a breath and repeat the following:

   "I have prepared. I am able to read the questions, process the information, and, from the choices given, make the best choice and move on."
3. *Read—do not scan.* You must read literally every word in the question. Every word counts!
4. *Read the question to determine the following:*
   - *Who is the question about?* This will affect your chosen answer. If you automatically assume that all of the questions relate to the nurse, you may miss a question that asks you to decide those things the father might say to demonstrate his understanding of the discharge instructions, for example.
   - *What is the question about?* You must determine to which part of the knowledge base the question refers. Is the question about the way to teach a 9-year-old diabetic to check his blood glucose? To answer this question, you must consider the learning style of the 9-year-old, his cognitive development and manual dexterity, and any significant others who should be involved in the session. The correct choice must support all of these principles.
   - *When is the question about?* The time frame of the question is also significant in terms of the client's continuum of care. Is this the acute session? Is this a client who has had diabetes for 20 years and is now developing pulmonary vascular disease? Is this a new mother with her first child or a new mother with her fifth? Are you in the assessment phase of the nursing process, are you in the planning stage, or are you evaluating the effects of a treatment or a drug?
   - *Where is the question about?* The focus of the nurse in the acute care institution is different from that of the nurse in the community clinic. This will affect your choice.
5. *Do not argue with the question.* Whether you agree with the question is irrelevant. The task is to read the question, put your mind to the question and, given the choices offered, make your choice based on principles and the application of your knowledge base.
6. *Plan your time.* Do not spend an inordinate amount of time on one question. There are some things you will

not know, and if you spend so much time on one question, you can sabotage your success on others. You can come back to any question, but you must be able to clear your mind of this question before moving on to tackle another. This is a good place for a 30-second vacation to put you back on task! If you cannot let a question go, you will be unable to concentrate on the next few questions and, very likely, will get several questions in a row incorrect. It is best to read, choose, and move on. Going back may work for paper-and-pencil tests during the nursing program, but the NCLEX-PN®, which you will take on computer for licensure upon completion of the nursing program, does not allow going back. Each question must be answered in the order presented.

7. *Do not panic.* When you come to a question that you cannot immediately answer, do not panic. Use your 30-second vacation to counter your anxiety and facilitate your ability to process. Recite again, "I have prepared, I am able to read, process, choose, and move on." (See Memory Trick.) Remember, the answer is on the paper.

YOUR PROGRAM IS ALMOST COMPLETED

Additional skills for success are required when you leave the protection of your nursing program. These include scope of practice/competence, tasks of the unlicensed assistive personnel (UAP), delegation, prioritizing care, and the nursing team.

MEMORY TRICK

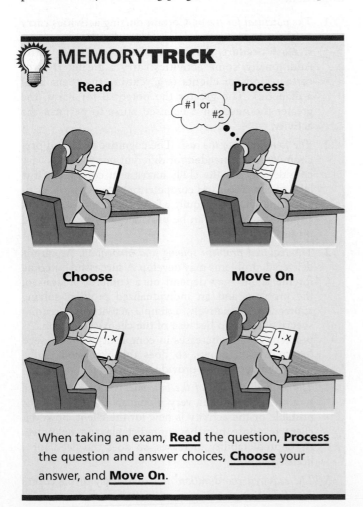

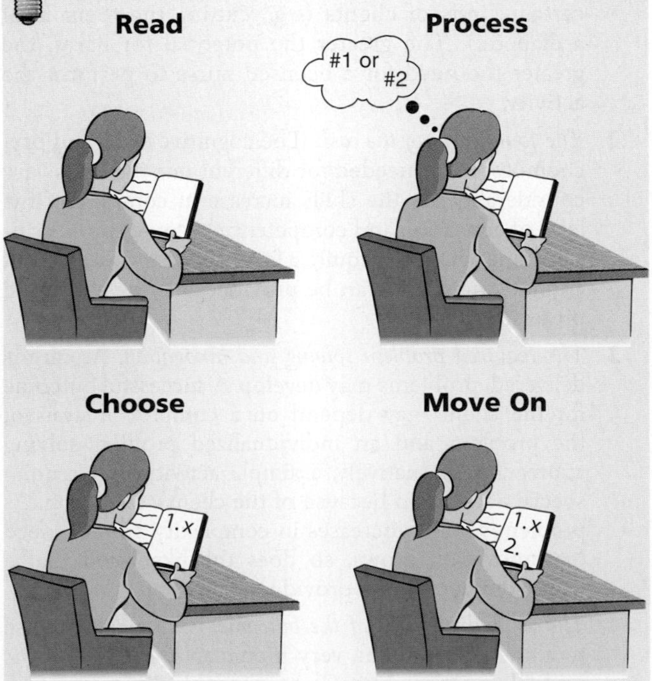

When taking an exam, **Read** the question, **Process** the question and answer choices, **Choose** your answer, and **Move On**.

PROFESSIONAL TIP

LP/VN Services

Any time nursing services are provided by an LP/VN, the supervising RN must be on the premises or immediately available by telephone. Being available by an answering machine or service does not fall within the definition of "immediately available." The amount of supervision is a function of the setting. In home health care or long-term care settings, it is common practice for the supervising RN to be available by telephone rather than on the premises.

SCOPE OF PRACTICE/ COMPETENCE

Registered nurses (RNs) and licensed practical/vocational nurses (LP/VNs) are individually licensed. Although some overlap exists in the scopes of practice of the LP/VN and the RN, there are also some significant differences. LP/VNs are dependent practitioners, meaning that an RN, doctor, dentist, or some other health care provider must supervise them. Most often the supervisor is an RN.

In addition to a scope of practice, LP/VNs and RNs have scopes of competence. Within the scope of practice, there are tasks and responsibilities the individual may or may not be competent to implement. For example, it is within the scope of practice for the LP/VN to perform phlebotomy, but this task does not fall within the scope of competence of every LP/VN. The scope of competence expands as new skills are acquired, but all skills must fall within the scope of practice.

LP/VNs are qualified to care for clients with common illnesses and to provide basic and preventive nursing procedures. LP/VNs can participate in data collection, planning, implementation, and evaluation of nursing care in all settings. In most states, some specific activities are considered beyond the scope of practice of the LP/VN. These activities, with some variances by state, include the following:

- Client assessments (can collect data but not perform physical assessments)
- Independent development of the nursing care plan
- Triage, case management, or mental health counseling
- Intravenous chemotherapy
- Administration of blood and blood products
- Administration of initial doses of any intravenous medication
- Any procedures involving central lines

TASKS OF THE UAP

Unlicensed assistive personnel do not have a scope of practice. A task that falls within the protected scope of practice of any licensed profession (including registered nursing and licensed practical/vocational nursing) *cannot* be performed by a UAP. These personnel can perform only those health-related activities for which they have been determined competent to perform. These activities include the following:

- Activities of daily living (feeding, grooming, toileting, ambulating, dressing)
- Vital signs
- Venipuncture
- Glucometer use
- Mouth care and oral suctioning
- Care of hair, skin, and nails
- Electrocardiogram measurements
- Applying clean dressings without assessment
- Nonnursing functions (clerical work, transport, cleaning)

DUTY DELEGATION

Delegation is the process of transferring to a competent individual the authority to perform a select task in a select situation. State provisions for the delegation of nursing tasks vary. Some states allow for the delegation of nursing tasks by an RN to both LP/VNs and UAP. In some states, LP/VNs may delegate certain nursing tasks to other LP/VNs or to UAP. Other states restrict delegation to licensed personnel only. It is *most* important to know what is allowed in your state. The National Council of State Boards of Nursing (NCSBN) Web site keeps a current listing of the address, telephone number, and Web site for each state board of nursing at www.ncsbn.org.

The licensed nurse retains accountability for the delegation. **Accountability** is defined as responsibility for actions and inactions performed by oneself or others. **Assignment**, another term frequently used to describe the transfer of activities from one person to another, involves the downward or lateral transfer of both responsibility and accountability for an activity.

At least one state differentiates between *delegating* nursing tasks to licensed nurses and *assigning* tasks to UAP. In New York, a nurse is not legally responsible for the process or outcome of care delegated to another licensed nurse. The nurse does remain responsible for tasks assigned to UAP, however. As an LP/VN, you are responsible for the decisions you make to delegate or assign tasks. Your knowledge of the client, activity, and worker will help you make sound decisions.

In most settings, RNs decide which nursing activities can be delegated or assigned to other licensed nurses (RNs or LP/VNs) and to UAP. Registered nurses and LP/VNs must consider five factors when making the decision to delegate or assign duties:

1. *The potential for harm.* Certain nursing activities carry a risk for harming the client. Generally, the more invasive a procedure, the greater the potential for harm. Additionally, some activities carry a greater risk for certain kinds of clients (e.g., cutting the toenails of a diabetic). The greater the potential for harm, the greater the need for a licensed nurse to perform the activity.
2. *The complexity of the task.* The cognitive skills and psychomotor skills needed for different nursing tasks vary considerably. As the skills increase in complexity, the level of education and competence becomes more critical. Some activities require a level of nursing assessment and judgment that can be provided only by a licensed professional.
3. *The required problem solving and innovation.* As care is delivered, problems may develop. A successful outcome for the client may depend on a complex analysis of the problem and an individualized problem-solving approach. Alternatively, a simple activity may require special adaptation because of the client's condition. As problem solving increases in complexity and the need for innovation grows, so does the likelihood that a licensed nurse should provide the care.
4. *The unpredictability of the outcome.* A client's response to an activity may be very predictable. If the client is unstable or the activity is new for the client, however, client response may be unpredictable and unknown. As unpredictability increases, so does the need for a licensed nurse.
5. *The required coordination and consistency of the client's care.* Effective planning, coordination, and evaluation of

PROFESSIONALTIP

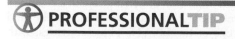

LP/VN Supervision

As defined in the Nursing Practice Acts, or in the state nursing board's rules and regulations, an LP/VN works under the direction of an RN, physician, or dentist. These are the professionals who directly supervise the LP/VN. In some states, the language of the law indicates that "other health care providers" can supervise the LP/VN. The question is, who are the other health care providers? In your state, do you follow orders written by a physician's assistant? A nurse practitioner? A physical therapist? The answers vary by state. It is critical that you know who can direct your nursing activities.

PROFESSIONALTIP

Unlicensed Personnel

Much controversy surrounds the role of UAP. Concerns have been raised that unlicensed personnel are functioning as de facto licensed nurses in violation of Nursing Practice Acts. Further, serious questions exist about the cost savings and quality of care in light of increased reliance on UAP and a corresponding reduction in licensed nurses. Understanding the role and limitations of UAP is critical.

client care requires the nurse to have direct client contact. The more stable the client and the more common the medical diagnosis, the more care can generally be delegated to support personnel. The need for a licensed nurse increases as the required coordination needed to deliver quality care increases.

The five rights of delegation provide further direction in making appropriate decisions about delegation. They are as follows:

1. *Right task:* The nurse must determine whether the task should be delegated for a specific client.
2. *Right circumstance:* Factors to consider include the client setting, availability of resources, client's condition, and other considerations.
3. *Right person:* The nurse must ask the question, "Is the right person delegating the right task to the right person to be performed on the right client?"
4. *Right direction/communication:* A clear, concise description of the task should be conveyed, including all expectations for accomplishing the task.
5. *Right supervision:* Appropriate monitoring, implementation, evaluation, and feedback must be provided.

Registered nurses are frequently responsible for delegating care and assigning clients to the other nursing staff. In some settings, however, LP/VNs make these decisions. LP/VNs should use the same guidelines to make decisions regarding delegating an activity to another LP/VN or assigning the task to UAP.

Prioritizing Care

Establishing priorities requires an understanding of the importance of different problems to the nurse, the client, the family, and other health care providers. For example, a client may be impatient to bathe because family is scheduled to visit. The nurse, however, does not want to remove the client's dressing for a bath until the physician has been able to examine the wound. Providing quality care while balancing such competing demands and ensuring completion of all tasks is challenging.

Information obtained during the change-of-shift report is needed to appropriately establish priorities. This information can be useful in creating a worksheet identifying a list of tasks and target times for accomplishing these tasks. The time allotted for activities varies based on the condition of the client, the availability of support personnel, the availability of supplies, and a number of other factors. The effective use of time is important whether caring for one client, caring for a group of clients, or supervising the activities of others providing care.

Although it is useful to get an overview of the day's activities, the clinical setting can change quickly and frequently. This is especially true in acute care settings. The nurse must be flexible and continually evaluate and reorder the priorities of care.

Given the same assignment, nurses will not necessarily establish the priorities of care in exactly the same way. If working closely with an RN, you should determine the priorities as she views them. When supervising UAP, you must be clear about your priorities and expectations. Among the factors that can be examined when establishing priorities are the following:

- *Safety:* You should ascertain whether a safety situation must be addressed immediately. A client experiencing a cardiac arrest, a fall, an insulin reaction, and other situations presenting an imminent threat must be tended to first.
- *Timing:* Medications, tests, and vital signs are frequently ordered at specific times. Often, there is very little flexibility in shifting the times. In hospitals, medications, for example, must be given within a specified time frame, usually half an hour before or after the established time.
- *Interdependence of events:* You must ascertain whether some activity must occur before another activity can take place. For example, a fasting blood sugar must be completed before the client receives either insulin or food; blood is drawn a specified time after the medication is given to ascertain the peak level of gentamyacin.
- *Client requests:* Quality care depends on meeting client needs. Some events—showers, bed changings, enema administration, and so on—can be scheduled after consulting with the client regarding personal preferences.
- *Availability of help:* If two people are needed to turn a client, ambulate a client, or provide other care, coordination of the health care team is essential for effective utilization of time. Ascertain which activities require assistance, then consult with coworkers about their availability.
- *Client's status:* Clients vary in the extent to which they can participate in their care. This factor influences the order of executing tasks and the length of time a task takes. A semi-independent client can be performing a task (e.g., bathing) with minimal assistance while the nurse attends to some other need.
- *Availability of resources:* If six clients are supposed to get out of bed and sit in chairs, and only two chairs are available, the clients clearly cannot get out of bed at the same time. Geri-chairs, wheelchairs, and other equipment are sometimes limited. Additionally, tasks may need to be delayed because supplies must be obtained from central supply.

Effectively organizing and establishing priorities with regard to care takes practice. Obtaining answers to certain questions when looking back at the day's events can help you hone this skill: Did you lack information that would have helped you prioritize more effectively? Did you fail to or inaccurately consider the client's status, the availability of help, or other factors? Did you establish priorities and set a schedule without getting client input? Did you fail to coordinate with coworkers? You will learn from experience. Both client and nurse feel the positive benefits of a day that flowed smoothly.

The Nursing Team

Within the nursing staff are different team members. Nursing staff includes nursing UAP, certified nurse assistants (CNAs), LP/VNs, RNs, and nurse practitioners (NPs). The roles, levels of education, skills, levels of independence, and lengths of education vary considerably (Figure 1-10). Familiarizing yourself with the roles of other nursing staff will help ensure that your practice conforms to the scope of practice as outlined by law.

Nursing UAP can have a number of different titles including UAP, patient care technician, clinical technician, and nursing assistant. These persons provide hands-on care to clients in addition to performing other duties. None of

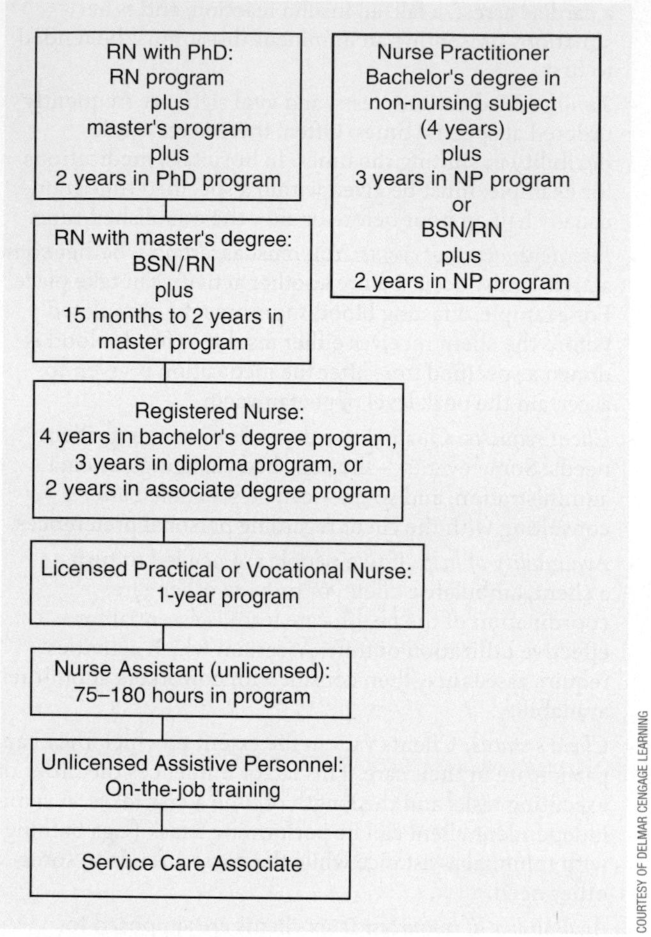

FIGURE 1-10 Workplace Hierarchy

these personnel has a license to practice. Rather, training is provided by the employer and may last from 2 to 10 weeks. The tasks they are expected to perform are designated by the employer.

A CNA is also unlicensed. In contrast to other UAP, however, the curriculum and length of training to become a CNA are prescribed. As part of health care reforms in the long-term care setting, the primary employment setting of CNAs, a set curriculum of a minimum of 100 hours duration must be completed to be certified.

LP/VNs work very closely with registered nurses. The LP/VN attends a 1-year program and must pass the NCLEX-PN®. The RN is educated in a 3-year hospital-diploma program, a 2-year college associate-degree program, or a 4-year college baccalaureate program and must pass the NCLEX-RN®.

An NP is an RN who has obtained additional education (usually a master's degree) and is certified by the state. The role of the NP typically includes diagnosis and treatment of commonly occurring medical conditions. Outpatient clinics frequently employ NPs. Increasingly, they are also found working in hospitals, long-term care facilities, and rehabilitation centers.

FROM STUDENT TO LP/VN

You have completed the LP/VN educational program. Through formal education and clinical supervision, you have studied and learned the skills necessary to become competent in providing client care. Now you are ready to graduate and begin your career as a nurse.

Your first task as a graduate practical nurse is to take and pass the NCLEX-PN® and obtain your nursing license. After you have obtained your license, you can begin the search for a job. The effort required in the period of time between the job search and employment can be considered a job in and of itself. There are many tasks to complete and skills to master to land your first job as an LP/VN.

EXAMINATION AND LICENSURE

In some states, you can begin work as a graduate LP/VN. A graduate LP/VN has completed the educational requirements and either is waiting to take the NCLEX-PN® or to receive test results and a license. Check with your state board of nursing to learn both the requirements for a temporary license to practice nursing as a graduate LP/VN and any restrictions put on your practice while working under this status. For most students, however, the time after graduation is used to prepare for the licensure exam.

The NCLEX-PN®

The examination that all practical/vocational nurses must pass in order to be licensed is the NCLEX-PN®. The NCLEX® tests the skills and knowledge required for entry-level practice. The state boards use the results of this examination to determine whether a license will be issued to the graduate. Figure 1-11 lists the steps each graduate must follow in order to take the examination. The NCLEX® tests knowledge of client needs such as physiologic and psychological needs, safety, and health promotion, as well as the nursing process, including data collection, planning, and implementation. The test is administered via a computer using a method called

1. The candidate applies for licensure in the state or territory in which he wishes to be licensed and meets their eligibility requirements.
2. Candidate gets an NCLEX® Examination Candidate Bulletin from the board of nursing, National Council of State Boards of Nursing (www.ncsbn.org), or on the NCLEX® Candidate website (www.vue.com/nclex).
3. The candidate receives registration confirmation from Pearson VUE.
4. The board of nursing with which you desire licensure sends eligibility to take the examination.
5. Pearson VUE sends an Authorization to Test (ATT) to the candidate.
6. After receiving the ATT, an appointment to test can be made through the Web (www.pearsonvue.com/nclex) or by telephone to Pearson VUE.
7. On the appointed day, the candidate takes the test at a Pearson Professional Center. The candidate presents an approved form of identification and the ATT at the testing center.
8. Test results from the board of nursing to which you applied are sent within one month of taking the examination.

COURTESY OF DELMAR CENGAGE LEARNING

FIGURE 1-11 NCLEX® Examination Process (Data from NCSBN, 2008c)

computerized adaptive testing (CAT), wherein the computer selects the test questions as you take the examination. You must answer all of the questions as they are presented to you, and you may not skip questions. Most of the questions are four-option multiple choice in format.

In April 2003, alternate item formats were added to the NCLEX®. These alternate item formats include multiple choice requiring more than one response, fill-in-the-blank (must be spelled correctly), and identifying an area on a picture or graphic. The answers will be either correct or incorrect; no partial credit will be given (National Council of State Boards of Nursing [NCSBN], 2007).

All LP/VN candidates answer a minimum of 85 questions and a maximum of 205 questions during the maximum 5-hour testing period (NCSBN, 2008b). The results are mailed to the candidate by the state board 1 month or less after the examination. Candidates may retake the examination; however, the National Council requires a wait of at least 91 days between testings. Your state board may have other policies related to retaking the exam.

Your License

After you have successfully passed the NCLEX®, you will be issued your nursing license from your state board. It is your responsibility to maintain your license according to your state's standards and inform your state board of any changes in name, address, and employment. Once licensed, you are ready to practice.

SUMMARY

- Developing a positive attitude enhances your learning experience.
- Strategies for developing a positive attitude include creating a positive self-image, recognizing your abilities, and identifying realistic expectations for meeting those goals.
- Competency in the basic skills of reading, arithmetic and mathematics, writing, listening, and speaking is necessary.
- It is important to build your vocabulary and comprehension of medical terminology to better enable you to meet your clients' learning needs.
- Identifying your preference for a particular learning style will help you identify the strategies you need to be a successful student.
- Organizing your study space and decreasing interruptions will increase your efficiency and facilitate your sticking to your study plan.
- Several methods can be used to take notes. Note taking in lectures and from your text is a strategy to help you retain the information presented.
- Critical thinking is the ability to apply your knowledge base.
- Critical thinking is a disciplined way of thinking that the nursing student can begin to develop. The effective use of the nursing process depends on the ability to think well.
- Four basic intellectual skills are essential to quality thinking: critical reading, critical listening, critical writing, and critical speaking.
- Reasoning is the process of applying critical thinking to some problem to find an answer or to figure something out. Therefore, reasoning has a purpose.
- When students begin to be aware of their own thinking and begin to assume responsibility for it, they will begin to use their own logic to discover the logic of nursing. The result will be better learning and the ability to make high-quality decisions related to client care.
- Consistent attention to improving the quality of thinking will produce the traits of an educated person.
- Developing a strategy to minimize anxiety when taking tests will improve your performance.
- To successfully complete a test, read each question thoroughly, do not infer additional information, and identify priorities.

REVIEW QUESTIONS

1. The sign of true comprehension of material is:
   1. the ability to repeat a paragraph word for word.
   2. memorization of the material.
   3. the ability to recite the material.
   4. the ability to summarize the material using your own words.
2. If you suspect you have a learning disability, it is important that you:
   1. ignore it; you will be able to work around it on your own.
   2. be tested to determine the assistance you will need to compensate for the disability.
   3. keep it to yourself; you will not be able to pass the program if you tell anyone about it.
   4. use it as an excuse to put less work into the program.
3. The best way to study is to:
   1. read only the assigned material.
   2. take notes in the lecture only.
   3. read, reread, reflect, recite, and review.
   4. read and attend lectures.
4. The best way to deal with any anxiety you may experience during a test is:
   1. jogging.
   2. listening to music.
   3. practicing deep breathing and imagery.
   4. asking for more time to take the test.

5. The person who has the ability to separate needed information from information not needed at the present time is practicing the standard for critical thinking called:
   1. logic.
   2. relevance.
   3. adequacy.
   4. significance.
6. To improve test-taking skills, one should: (Select all that apply.)
   1. quickly scan the question and answers and choose a response.
   2. connect each choice to the question to determine correctness.
   3. write definitions of unfamiliar words and study them prior to the exam.
   4. relate to life experiences and weave them into the answers.
   5. when determining priorities decide what choice would have the most serious consequences if not done first.
   6. not waste time reviewing the wrong answers on an exam.
7. The best strategy to decrease test anxiety is to:
   1. sit by the door so I can see all the students leave after taking their exam.
   2. postpone reviewing test content until the night before the exam.
   3. take a 30-second vacation right before the exam.
   4. use self-talk such as, "This is only one of the four exams in this course."
8. The instructor just returned L.G.'s graded exam. When she rereads the questions she missed, she thought, "How could I have misread that question and chosen that answer?" What is a strategy L.G. could use to improve her grade on the next exam?
   1. Stay up late the night before the next exam reviewing her notes.
   2. When she takes the exam, recall extra information that is not included in the question.
   3. Skip over words that she cannot define or pronounce as she reads the chapter.
   4. Read each question carefully and determine what the question is asking.
9. On the first clinical day, the nurse asks P.W., a new student nurse, to give P.L., the client in room 423, her medication because she is so busy. What right of delegation is the nurse violating?
   1. Right task
   2. Right circumstance
   3. Right person
   4. Right direction/communication
10. Note mapping is
    1. strategically placing class notes in visible places throughout the house.
    2. cramming the night before the final exam.
    3. putting class notes on flash cards to review in spare minutes.
    4. organizing notes into a picture to see connections and links between concepts.

REFERENCES/SUGGESTED READINGS

American Nurses Association. (2008). Unlicensed assistive personnel. Retrieved August 19, 2008, from http://www.nursingworld.org/MainMenuCategories/HealthcareandPolicyIssues/ANA Position

Browne, M., & Keeley, S. (2006). *Asking the right questions: A guide to critical thinking* (8th ed.). Upper Saddle River, NJ: Prentice Hall College Division.

Center for Critical Thinking. (2008). Valuable intellectual traits. Retrieved August 21, 2008, from http://www.criticalthinking.org/page.cfm?PageID=528&CategoryID=68

Center for New Discoveries in Learning, Inc. (2007). Personal Learning Style Inventory. Retrieved August 21, 2008, from http://www.howtolearn.com/lsinventory_student.html

Chaffee, J. (2006). *Thinking critically* (8th ed.). Boston: Houghton Mifflin College.

Chopra, D. (1997, May–June). How can I keep up? *Natural Health*, 208.

DePew, R. (2008). Successfully mastering medical-surgical content. Manuscript submitted for publication.

Duncan, G., & DePew, R. (2011). *Transitioning from LPN/VN to RN: Moving ahead in your career.* Clifton Park, NY: Delmar Cengage Learning.

Elder, L., & Paul, R. (2008). Universal intellectual standards. Retrieved August 18, 2008, from http://www.criticalthinking.org/articles/universal-intellectual-standards.cfm

Ham, K. (2001). *From LPN to RN—Bridges for role transitions.* Philadelphia: W. B. Saunders.

Heaslip, P. (1994, November). Defining critical thinking. *Dialogue: A Critical Thinking Newsletter for Nurses*, 3.

Higbee, K. (2001). *Your memory: How it works and how to improve it* (2nd ed.) Indianapolis, IN: Macmillan.

Holkeboer, R., & Walker, L. (2003). *Right from the start: Taking charge of you college success* (4th ed.). Belmont, CA: Wadsworth.

Hughes, R., & Edgerton, E. (2005). Reducing pediatric medication errors: Children are especially at risk for medications errors. *American Journal of Nursing*, 105(5), 79–84.

Korchek, N., & Sides, M. (1998). *Successful test-taking: Learning strategies for nurses* (3rd ed.). Philadelphia: Lippincott Williams & Wilkins.

Lesar, T. (1998). Errors in the use of medication dosage equations. *Archives of Pediatric Adolescent Medicine*, 152(4), 340–344.

Martin, C. (2002). The theory of critical thinking of nursing. *Nursing Education Perspectives*, 23(5), 243–247.

Meltzer, M., & Marcus-Palau, S. (1997). *Learning strategies in nursing: Reading, studying and test taking* (2nd ed.). Philadelphia: W. B. Saunders Company.

Mind mapping. (2008). Retrieved October 27, 2008, from http://www.achieve-goal-setting-success.com/mind-mapping.html

Mind Tools. (2008). Mind maps a powerful approach to note taking related variants: Spray diagrams, spider diagrams, spidograms, spidergrams and mindmaps. Buzan Organization. Retrieved October 31, 2008, from http://www.mindtools.com/pages/article/newISS01.htm

Mind Tools. (2008, August 15). Use of Mnemonics. Retrieved August 15, 2008, from http://www.mindtools.com/mnemlstylo.htm

National Center for Learning Disabilities, Inc. (NCLD) January 24, 1999 [Online]. Available. http://www.ncid.org

National Center for Learning Disabilities. (2008, August 18). Retrieved August 18, 2008, from http://www.guidestar.org/pqShowGsReport.do?partner+justgive&npoId=67112

National Council of State Boards of Nursing (NCSBN). (2007) Fast facts about alternative item formats and the NCLEX examinations. Retrieved August 21, 2008, from https://www.ncsbn.org/01_08_04_Alt_Itm.pdf

National Council of State Boards of Nursing (2008a). The NCLEX process. Retrieved August 20, 2008, from https://www.ncsbn.org/NCLEX_Process_public.ppp

National Council of State Boards of Nursing (2008b). 2008 NCLEX examination candidate bulletin. Retrieved August 20, 2009, from https://www.ncsbn.org/2008_NCLEX_Candidate_Bulletin.pdf

National Council of State Boards of Nursing (2008c). The eight steps of the NCLEX examination process. Retrieved August 20, 2008, from https://www.ncsbn.org/Eight_Steps_of_NCLEX.pdf

Nosich, G. (2008) *Learning to think things through: A guide to critical thinking across the curriculum* (3rd ed.). Upper Saddle River, NJ: Prentice Hall.

Nugent, P., & Vitale, B. (2000). *Test taking techniques for beginning nursing students* (3rd ed.). Philadelphia: F. A. Davis.

Paul, R. (1995) *Critical Thinking: How to Prepare Students for a Rapidly Changing World* (3rd ed.). Dillon Beach, CA: Foundation for Critical Thinking, http://www.criticalthinking.org/resources/books/how-to-prepare-students.cfm

Paul, R., & Elder, L. (2002). *Critical thinking: Tools for taking charge of your professional and personal life* (2nd ed.). Upper Saddle Rive, NJ: Prentice Hall.

Rubenfeld, M., & Scheffer, B. (1998). *Critical thinking in nursing: An interactive approach* (2nd ed.). Philadelphia: Lippincott Williams & Wilkins.

Sakowski, J., Leonard, T., Colburn, S., Michaelsen, B., Schiro, T., Schneider, J., & Newman, J. (2005). *Using a bar-coded medication administration system to prevent medication errors.* American Society of Health-System Pharmacists, 62(24), 2619–2625.

Saucier, B., Stevens, K., & Williams, G. (2000). Critical thinking outcomes of computer-assisted instruction versus written nursing process. *Nursing and Health Care Perspectives*, 21(5), 240–246.

Sayles, S., Shelton, D., & Powell, H. (2003). Predictors of success in nursing education. *ABNF Journal*, 14(6), 116–120.

Schank, R. (2000). *Dynamic memory revisited* (2nd ed.). Cambridge, UK: Cambridge University Press.

Scriven, M., & Paul, R. (2008) Defining Critical Thinking. Retrieved August 21, 2008, from http://www.criticalthinking.org/page.cfm?CategoryID=51

Sheehan, J. (2001). Delegating to UAPs—A practical guide. *RN*, 64(11), 65–66.

Smith, G., Davis, P., & Dennerll, J. T. (1999). *Medical terminology: A programmed systems approach* (8th ed.). Clifton Park, NY: Delmar Cengage Learning.

VARK: A guide to learning styles. (2006). Learning style quiz. Retrieved August 20, 2008, from http://vark-learn.com/english/index.asp

VMentor. (2006). Identifying your learning style strategies to help you be a better student. Retrieved August 20, 2008, from http://www.Vmentor.com/docs/learning_styles_module.pdf

Walter, T., Knudsvig, G., & Smith, E. (2002). *Critical thinking: Building the basics*, (2nd ed.). Belmont, CA: Wadsworth.

RESOURCES

Center for Critical Thinking at Sonoma State University, http://www.criticalthinking.org

Indentifying Your Learning Style Strategies to Help www.vmentor.com

Insight Assessment, http://www.calpress.com

LD Resources, http://www.ldresources.org/

Mind Tools, http://www.mindtools.com

National Association for Practical Nurse Education and Service, Inc., www.napnes.org/

National Center for Learning Disabilities, Inc., www.ncld.org

Socratic Arts, http://socraticarts.com

Vark a Guide to Learning Styles, http://www.vark-learn.com/

CHAPTER 2
Holistic Care

MAKING THE CONNECTION

Refer to the following chapters to increase your understanding of holistic care:

Basic Nursing

- ***Legal and Ethical Responsibilities***
- ***Life Span Development***
- ***Cultural Considerations***
- ***Stress, Adaptation, and Anxiety***
- ***Self-Concept***
- ***Spirituality***
- ***Complementary/Alternative Therapies***
- ***Basic Nutrition***
- ***Safety/Hygiene***
- ***Standard Precautions and Isolation***
- ***Fluid, Electrolyte, and Acid-Base Balance***

Basic Procedures

- ***Hand Hygiene***
- ***Proper Body Mechanics***

LEARNING OBJECTIVES

Upon completion of this chapter, you should be able to:

- Define key terms.
- Define health as it relates to the whole person.
- List and discuss the five aspects of total wellness.
- List and discuss Maslow's Hierarchy of Needs.
- Describe self-awareness and why it is important to nurses.
- Describe self-concept.
- Discuss the concept of personal responsibility for one's own illness.
- Discover personal attitudes about health and illness and take responsibility for personal well-being.
- Identify the components of a healthy lifestyle.

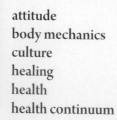

KEY TERMS

attitude
body mechanics
culture
healing
health
health continuum
holistic
homeostasis
intellectual wellness
Maslow's Hierarchy of Needs
physical wellness
psychological wellness
self-awareness
self-concept
sociocultural wellness
spiritual wellness
spirituality
wellness

INTRODUCTION

As a nurse, you will be a professional caregiver. Your intimate contact with clients allows you the opportunity not only to provide physical and emotional support but also to teach ways to take an active role in maintaining health.

You may have contact with hundreds of clients, each needing specialized treatment and care. The care you provide will vary from routine to critical to emergency. You will be part of a multidisciplinary team of caregivers that includes registered nurses, physicians, nursing assistants, physical therapists, respiratory therapists, laboratory technicians, dietitians, and social workers. All caregivers work together to promote and maintain client health.

Because the caregiver's goal is promoting and maintaining health, understanding the concept of health is paramount. Health is "the condition of being sound in body, mind, or spirit" (*Merriam-Webster Online Dictionary*, 2008).

INTERRELATED CONCEPTS OF HEALTH

In 1948, the World Health Organization (WHO) was founded. The WHO, which functions as an arm of the United Nations, places particular emphasis on combating communicable diseases, educating health care workers, and improving the health of all people of the world. The WHO defines **health** as follows: "Health is a state of complete physical, mental, and social well-being and not merely the absence of disease or infirmity" (WHO, 1974).

Many people believe that health or wellness is only the absence of disease. Health, in holistic terms, is more than the absence of disease. It is a state of well-being on a physical, emotional, and spiritual level while having a sense of fulfilling one's mission in life (Telstar Innovations, Inc., 2000). In its truest form, health refers to the total well-being of the whole person.

Holistic is a term derived from the Greek word *holos*, meaning "whole." Holistic health views the physical, intellectual, sociocultural, psychological, and spiritual aspects of a person's life as an integrated whole. These five aspects cannot be separated or isolated; anything that affects one aspect of a person's life also affects the other aspects. The environment within which a person lives and the manner whereby the person interacts with that environment are also considerations. Figure 2-1 illustrates the holistic perspective.

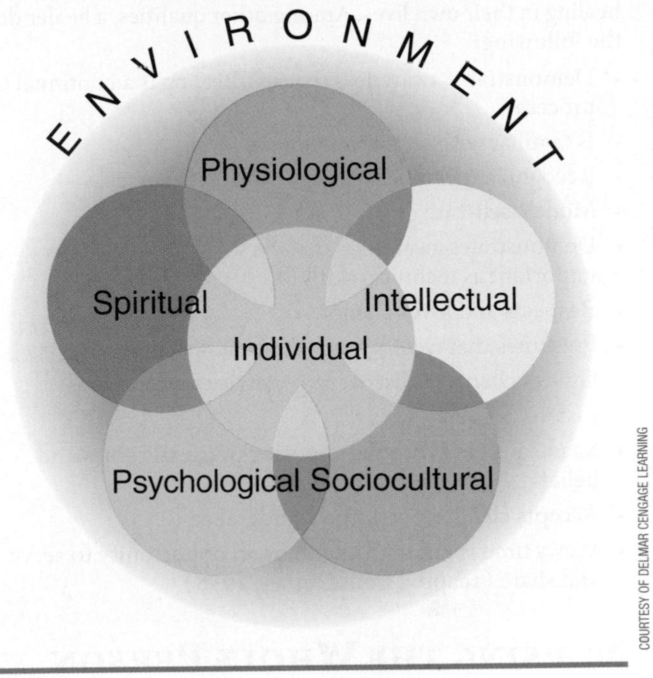

FIGURE 2-1 Holistic View of an Individual

Healing means to be or become whole (Quinn, 2005). It is a state of harmony or balance in the body, mind, and spirit connection. **Homeostasis** is the balance or stability that the body strives to achieve among these aspects of a person's life by continuous adaptation.

The goal of holistic nursing is the "enhancement of healing the whole person from birth to death" (American Holistic Nurses Association [AHNA], 2004). Nurses must understand the integration of these aspects of a person's life in order to help clients through healing processes. Healing is often different from curing. Although curing a disease may or may not be possible, healing is always possible. A major component of healing is caring. Thus, the goal in holistic care is to heal.

HOLISTIC CARE

The AHNA is the professional nursing organization dedicated to the promotion of holism and healing. It supports the belief that health involves the harmonious balance of body, mind, emotions, and spirit within an ever-changing environment. The AHNA serves as a bridge between the conventional medical model and complementary and alternative healing practices. The AHNA supports an integrative model, which involves integration of both complementary and alternative modalities and conventional therapies, enabling the client to benefit from all available therapies. The National Institutes of Health (NIH) established the National Center for Complementary and Alternative Medicine to investigate holistic modalities. The NIH defines holistic care as care that "considers the whole person, including physical, mental, emotional, and spiritual aspects." The final goal of investigating holistic modalities is to allow the validated therapies to be further integrated into general client care.

Success in using holistic modalities in client care requires an awareness of a fundamental principle of holism: The nurse *facilitates* the client in attaining the best state for healing to occur. Among the holistic modalities most frequently used in nursing are the following:

- Biofeedback
- Exercise and movement
- Goal setting
- Humor and laughter
- Imagery
- Journaling
- Massage
- Play therapy
- Prayer
- Therapeutic touch

Nurses must be open to new ideas and must not allow holistic modalities to become just another technology. According to the AHNA, the holistic nurse is "an instrument of healing and a facilitator in the healing process (AHNA, 2004). Nurses develop personal healing qualities and become more aware of healing in their own lives. Among other qualities, a healer does the following:

- Demonstrates awareness that self-healing is a continual process
- Is familiar with self-development
- Recognizes personal strengths and weaknesses
- Models self-care
- Demonstrates awareness that personal presence is as important as technical skills
- Respects and loves clients
- Presumes that clients know the best life choices
- Guides clients in discovering creative options
- Listens actively
- Shares insights without imposing personal values and beliefs
- Accepts client input without judgment
- Views time spent with clients as an opportunity to serve and share (adapted from Dossey, 1998)

Nursing the Whole Person

Nursing the whole person, or holistic health care, is a comprehensive approach to health care. It considers physical, intellectual, sociocultural, psychological, and spiritual aspects; the response to illness; and the effect of illness on a person's ability to meet self-care needs. Also taken into account is the individual's responsibility for personal well-being. Teaching preventive care is always a focus.

Nurses work with people throughout life to promote wellness and prevent illness (Figure 2-2). The highest level of wellness should be the goal of each nurse and every client.

Wellness

Wellness is a responsibility, a choice, a lifestyle design that helps maintain the highest potential for personal health (Hill & Howlett, 2005). The **health continuum** is a way to visualize the range of an individual's health, from highest health potential to death (Figure 2-3).

An individual's place on the continuum may change daily or even hourly depending on what is happening to that individual. Constant effort is required to balance all aspects of life and to maintain the highest level of health. A person at the highest level of wellness is one who demonstrates good physical self-care, emotional well-being, creative expression, and positive relationships with others.

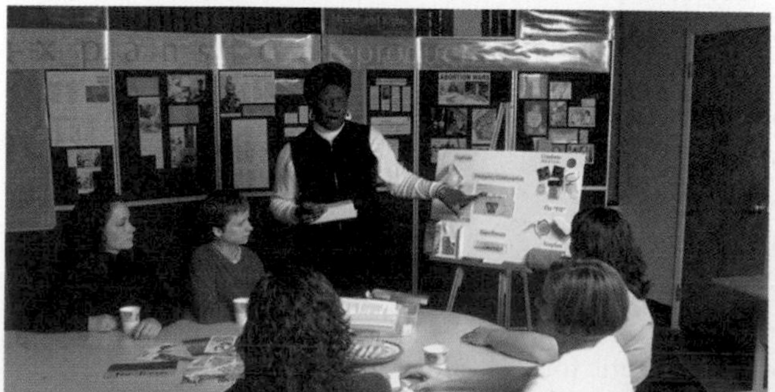

COURTESY OF DELMAR CENGAGE LEARNING

FIGURE 2-2 Nurses work with clients of all age-groups to encourage health and wellness.

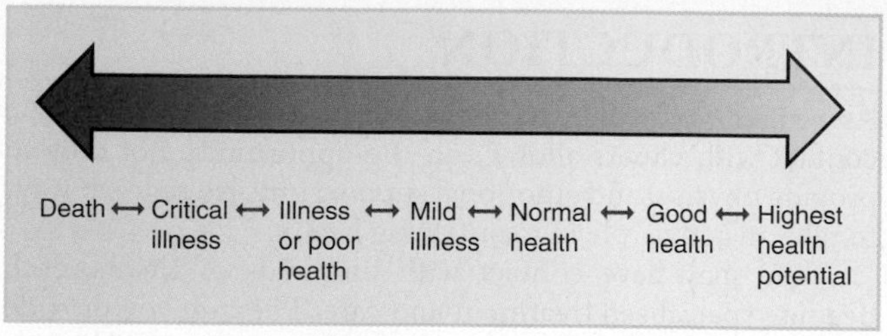

COURTESY OF DELMAR CENGAGE LEARNING

FIGURE 2-3 Health Continuum

Wellness incorporates physical, intellectual, sociocultural, psychological, and spiritual wellness. To provide holistic care, all aspects of the individual's wellness must be addressed.

Maslow's Hierarchy of Needs

Abraham Maslow developed a theory of behavioral motivation based on needs. This theory is often referred to as **Maslow's Hierarchy of Needs**. There are five levels in this hierarchy. The basic physiological needs must be met to maintain life. The rest of the needs are related to quality of life. They are safety and security, love and belonging, self-esteem, and self-actualization. The needs of the lower levels must be met before a person is motivated to meet the needs of the next higher level (Figure 2-4).

Many nursing programs use Maslow's Hierarchy of Needs as a basis for planning the care of clients. This ensures that basic physiological needs as well as the other needs are assessed and addressed in individualized care plans.

Physiological Needs

Although Maslow (1987) did not specifically identify the physiological needs, they are generally accepted to be the needs of oxygen, water, food, elimination, rest (sleep)/activity (exercise), and sex. With the exception of sex, all of these needs must be met for the life of the individual to be maintained. Satisfying the sexual need, while not necessary for individual survival, is necessary for survival of the human race. The basic physiological needs must be met before higher-level needs become motivators of behavior. For example, a person who is truly hungry is motivated by that need, and behavior is focused on getting food.

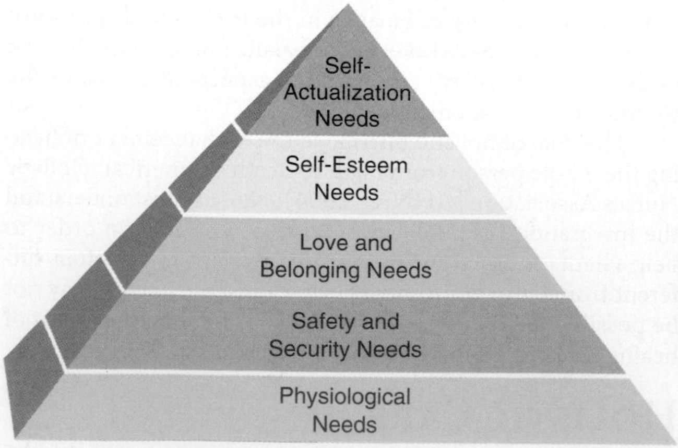

COURTESY OF DELMAR CENGAGE LEARNING

FIGURE 2-4 Maslow's Hierarchy of Needs

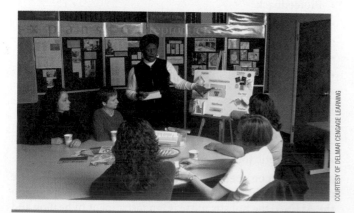

Safety and Security Needs

The next level, safety, encompasses the needs for shelter, stability, security, physical safety, and freedom from undue anxiety. Safety needs include both physical and emotional aspects. Illness is often a threat to safety because the stability of life is disrupted.

Love and Belonging Needs

The third level of the hierarchy, love and belonging, incorporates not only giving but also receiving affection. Having friends and participating with others in groups and organizations are two ways to meet these needs. Meeting these needs is extremely important for mental health.

Self-Esteem Needs

The needs of the self-esteem level are met by achieving success in work and other activities. Recognition from others increases self-esteem and feelings of pride in one's accomplishments.

Self-Actualization Needs

Self-actualization is the highest level of the Maslow hierarchy. A person who has met these needs is confident, self-fulfilled, and creative; looks for challenges; and sees beauty and order in the world.

Maslow contends that because most people are so busy meeting the physiological and safety and security needs, little time or energy is left to meet the love and belonging, self-esteem, and self-actualization needs; thus, most people are less than satisfied at higher levels of the hierarchy. Even when the lower two levels are met without much trouble, many people have personalities and attitudes that make meeting the needs of the three higher levels difficult, if not impossible.

An individual does not move steadily up the hierarchy. As life situations change, a person's unmet needs change, and behavior is motivated by different levels of the hierarchy. For example, if a person who is working to meet the self-esteem need is suddenly laid off at work, the safety and security need of providing financially for self and family suddenly becomes the unmet need that motivates that person's behavior.

Other theories of human development are Freud's stages of psychosexual development, Erickson's stages of psychosocial development, Sullivan's interpersonal model of personality development, Piaget's stages of cognitive development, Kohlberg's stages of moral development, and Fowler's stages of faith. Refer to Chapter 10, "Development and Psychosocial Concerns," for a detailed coverage of all these theories to gain increased knowledge of a client's stage of life.

PROVIDING QUALITY CARE

The first step in providing quality client care is to be aware of yourself. What kind of personality do you have? Is your self-concept positive, or do you have self-doubts and lack self-confidence? What are your beliefs and attitudes? Knowing the answers to such questions will help you in your role as caregiver.

The next step is taking care of your own needs (see the preceding section on Maslow's Hierarchy of Needs). When you attend to the needs in your own life, you are then free to concentrate on caring for others. Your example of self-care inspires clients to have confidence that you will provide quality care. Thus, self-care is a factor in your effectiveness as a caregiver.

> **CRITICAL THINKING**
>
> **Health and Wellness**
>
> What are your attitudes about health and wellness?

SELF-AWARENESS

Self-awareness is consciously knowing how the self thinks, feels, believes, and behaves at any specific time. Being self-aware is a constant process that is focused on the present. A person's thoughts, feelings, and beliefs are interrelated and greatly influence behavior. Being self-aware influences a person in several ways.

Self-awareness may make a person uncomfortable. Awareness allows the person to either accept or alter feelings, beliefs, and behavior. One can learn to be self-aware. Begin now to concentrate on becoming aware of your thoughts and actions. Take note of your reactions to any given situation. What makes you anxious? What makes you happy? Listen to yourself when you respond to questions and when you visit with friends. Realize that everyone has strengths and weaknesses. Focus on your strengths. Spend your energies on today. Do not dwell on past mistakes; rather, try to learn from them and then forget them. Stop periodically and pay attention to what you feel and believe. Listening not only to the words one speaks but also to the way the words are spoken assists in self-awareness. Use the word *I*, and take ownership of feelings and beliefs. Say, "I am so happy," instead of, "That makes me happy."

Self-awareness is extremely important for nurses. Nurses must understand themselves so that their personal feelings, attitudes, and needs do not interfere with providing quality client care. The nurse who is self-aware is more likely to make decisions in response to the client's needs rather than the nurse's own needs. For example, student nurses—and even experienced nurses—are often anxious about caring for a specific client. By taking some time to practice self-awareness, the nurse might discover that the anxiety stems from never having performed the procedure in question. The nurse can then deal directly with the situation by reviewing the procedure and requesting assistance from an instructor or supervisor. All decisions about client care must be made in response to the client's needs, not the nurse's needs.

DEVELOPMENT OF SELF-CONCEPT

Self-concept is how a person thinks or feels about himself. These thoughts and feelings come from the experiences the person has with others and reflect how the person thinks others view him.

Self-concept begins forming in infancy. An infant whose needs are met feels satisfied and good. Experiences, both positive and negative, influence a person's self-concept (Figure 2-5). Interactions with significant others, such as parents, extended family, and friends, have a great impact on self-concept. This is true not only during the developing years but also throughout life. Because of its influence on client care, it is important for the nurse to be aware of how

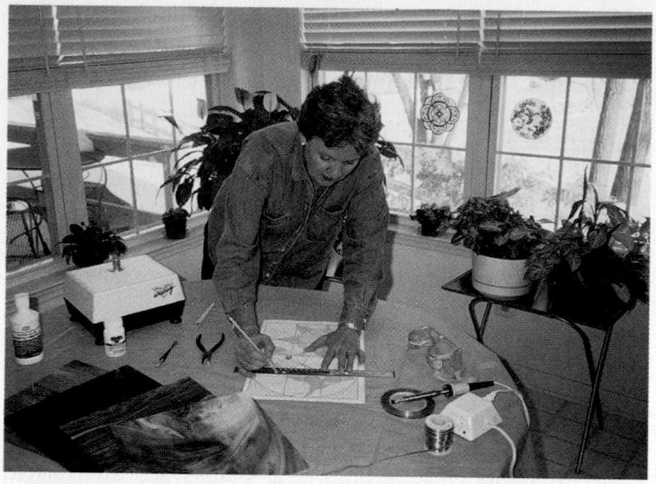

FIGURE 2-5 Self-concept and self-esteem can be enhanced by learning new skills.

her own self-concept has developed. Self-concept develops through feedback from others. The nurse is responsible for providing feedback that will not negatively affect the client's self-concept.

An individual who is constantly ignored or who receives messages such as "Don't bother me," "Can't you do anything right?" or "You don't have any sense" may very well begin to view himself in these terms, with the likely result being a negative self-concept. On the other hand, a person who is shown caring and who hears messages such as "Let me help you in a minute," "Let's try it this way," or "Have you thought about . . . ?" will move toward a positive self-concept.

SELF-CARE AS A PREREQUISITE TO CLIENT CARE

The most effective means to teach wellness is by positive example. By first practicing good health habits as a nursing student, you will become, by example, an important factor in your clients' overall well-being and good health. Remind yourself and your clients that health is a personal choice and that each person has control over his or her own wellness.

You will be helping clients recognize how their own actions can prevent many of the conditions that cause illness. Choosing to exercise regularly, to eat a balanced diet, to eat breakfast each day, to control fat content, and to select from the basic food groups are good rules for wellness. Choosing to not smoke, to practice moderation in the use of alcohol, to avoid all nontherapeutic drugs, and to practice safe sex can help prevent many of the conditions that cause disease and death.

While emphasizing health promotion and client education, the nurse must also encourage and respect the client's responsibility for wellness. This respect allows the client to become an active partner in, rather than a passive recipient of, health care. It is not enough to tell a client *what* can be done to improve health; the nurse must also be prepared to explain *why*. If a client understands the reason behind an action, the likelihood of compliance increases.

Just as you are aware of yourself as a whole person with many components, help your clients see themselves and their health care as more than physical health. Help clients understand how physical, intellectual, sociocultural, psychological, and spiritual health are all related and can lead to an overall sense of well-being. This is the full meaning of holistic care.

PHYSICAL WELLNESS

Physical wellness refers to a healthy body that functions at an optimal level. To achieve physical wellness, a person must practice good grooming; use proper body mechanics; have good posture; refrain from smoking and the use of drugs and alcohol; and have adequate nutrition, sleep, rest, relaxation, and exercise.

Grooming

The nurse communicates a message of health and well-being by being clean and neatly dressed (Figure 2-6). A daily bath or shower and the use of a deodorant form the basis of good grooming. Hair should be clean, combed, and neatly styled. Perfume should not be worn because some clients may have allergies, and it may be offensive to other clients. Frequent brushing, regular dental checkups, and avoiding refined sugars helps control dental caries.

While important for client safety, good hand hygiene is also crucial to the nurse's wellness. Antiseptic hand lotion can be used to prevent cracked, dry skin. Fingernails should be kept short because long nails not only harbor dirt and microorganisms but also can scratch clients.

Standard Precautions have been established by the Centers for Disease Control and Prevention in Atlanta, Georgia. These precautions are designed to protect all health care workers and their clients from the transmission of communicable disease. Good hand hygiene is an integral part of Standard Precautions. As soon as you have been taught the skill of hand hygiene, practice it. Make it a part of your daily life. Encourage your clients to establish good hand hygiene habits.

Jewelry, which can harbor bacteria, and excessive makeup are both inappropriate for the nurse in uniform. Clothing should be clean and free of stains and wrinkles. Clients will have confidence in the nurse who maintains a professional appearance and who practices good hygiene.

Body Mechanics

Wellness involves more than just good grooming practices. It also requires proper **body mechanics** (i.e., using the body in the safest and most efficient way to move or lift objects). The use of proper body mechanics is very important because many

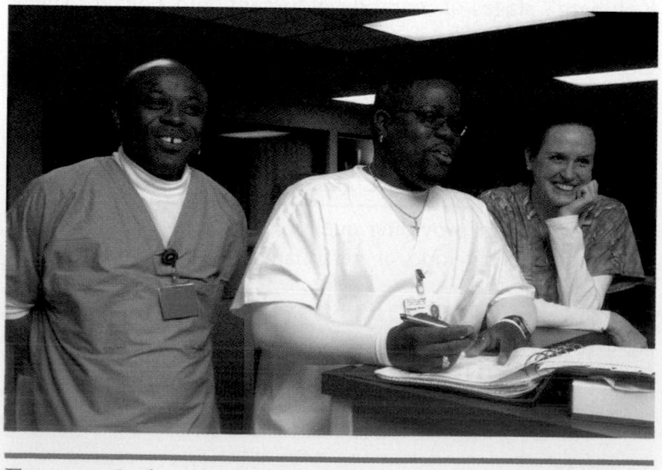

FIGURE 2-6 Holistically healthy nurses' positive attitudes are contagious.

of the skills and tasks you will perform as a nurse involve lifting or moving clients or objects. Bending, lifting, or stooping can cause injury if done incorrectly. One of the first skills you will study involves the practice of proper body mechanics to prevent physical disability, including safe methods for bending, lifting, and moving.

Posture

Good posture is the basis for proper body mechanics. Good posture means the ability to carry oneself well and in correct body alignment. Posture can also send messages about a person. A person who stands with feet spread apart and with hands on hips, for example, may be perceived as aggressive or authoritative, whereas one who holds the arms tightly folded over the chest may be viewed as closed minded.

Observe those around you as they communicate with others. Notice the differences in posture. Does the person who stands in good alignment, with shoulders back and head up, convey self-confidence and capability? Does the individual whose shoulders are drooped and head bowed convey depression, sadness, or lack of self-confidence?

As you continue your studies and begin client care, you will realize that clients appreciate having nurses who appear confident in their own abilities and decision making. When you are with clients, you must be particularly careful of the way you stand. Remember that your posture sends messages about your attitude and feelings. The client should feel that you are confident, caring, relaxed, and willing to listen.

Smoking

Smoking contributes to many health hazards and illnesses. It may also be personally offensive to clients. The odor of smoke on clothing or the breath (halitosis) may precipitate allergic reactions or lead to a feeling of nausea in some clients. Most health care facilities have strict rules about smoking. Many facilities are "smoke free." The nurse should never smoke in a client's room. Furthermore, great care should be taken to ensure that no offensive tobacco odors remain if the nurse uses or is in close proximity to tobacco products. In each situation, every effort should be made to enforce all safety rules for clients and visitors. "No smoking" signs should be posted and strictly enforced when oxygen is in use.

Drugs and Alcohol

A frightening trend in the United States is the increasing rate of alcohol and drug abuse. Drug abuse has become so widespread within the health professions that impaired caregiver programs have been implemented. Many states now provide access to treatment for the impaired nurse through the state board of nursing. Drug abuse can begin very insidiously when a nurse says to herself, "I'll borrow a pill just this once for my headache." The second time is easier, and the downward spiral begins.

A nurse should never give or make a drug available to anyone without the written order of a physician or other person who can legally prescribe medications, such as a nurse practitioner. Approximately 10% of nurses have a substance abuse problem (Dunn, 2005). If you believe that a colleague is abusing drugs, you have an obligation to let your supervisor know so that the colleague can receive help through the impaired nurse program in your state. If you become addicted, you have a duty to your clients, your peers, and yourself to accept help through a recovery program.

Nutrition

Nursing is emotionally, mentally, and physically demanding. Nurses must be able to think clearly and work efficiently. A balanced diet, including fruits and vegetables, whole grains and cereals, milk and milk products, and meats or other protein foods, is required for optimal body function.

Nursing students may be tempted to skip meals, omit breakfast, eat snacks, and follow fad diets. This is never a wise practice. While you are in school, your success depends on your functioning at your best. Skipping meals, especially breakfast, leaves a person tired, weak, and hungry. It is impossible to think efficiently when hungry. Remember Maslow's Hierarchy of Needs: The need for food must be satisfied before you will be motivated to meet the need to learn or to study.

Always eat a balanced breakfast. Pastries and coffee, although satisfying in the moment, elevate the blood sugar level only for a short while before the level plummets. This reaction leaves a person drained, irritable, and hungrier than before. Try to avoid snacking on junk foods, which contain empty calories, or those having very little nutritional value. Instead, plan to eat fruit or high-protein snacks.

Plan a routine for mealtimes and stick to it. Doing so helps prevent the urge to binge on unhealthy snacks. Also, drink plenty of water. Water is the body's most important nutrient (Figure 2-7). A human being can survive for weeks without food but only for a few days without water. By weight, approximately 60% of the adult body is water. In order to maintain proper fluid balance and to facilitate the elimination of body wastes, it is necessary to drink plenty of fluids.

LIFE SPAN CONSIDERATIONS

Nutrition

- Children's appetites vary with their growth spurts and growth plateaus.
- Healthy eating habits should be established during childhood.
- The amount of food eaten generally declines in the elderly person.
- Proper food choices are more important than quantity for the elderly person.

CLIENT TEACHING

Tips on Maintaining Proper Nutrition

- Read product labels.
- Avoid foods high in fat, sugar, and salt.
- Work to maintain or attain your ideal weight.
- If you drink alcohol, do so in moderation.
- Always eat breakfast.
- Make between-meal snacks healthy, such as raw fruits and vegetables.

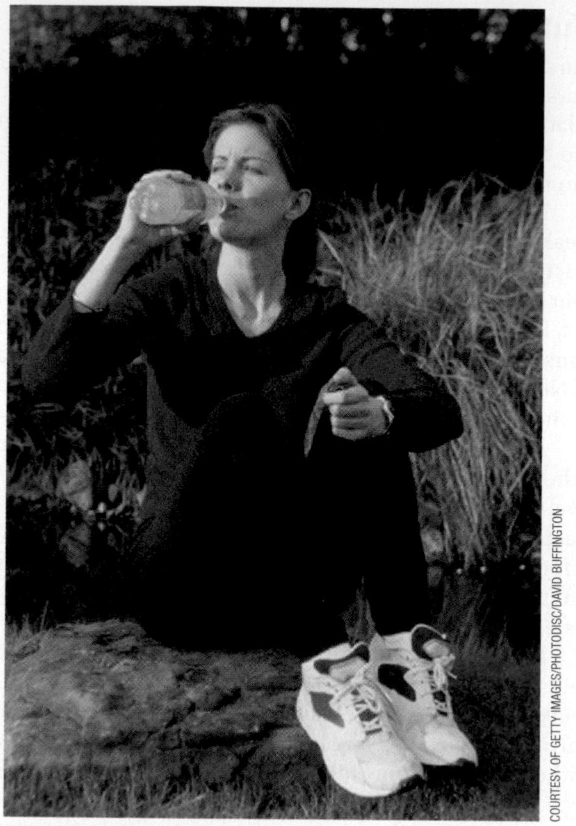
COURTESY OF GETTY IMAGES/PHOTODISC/DAVID BUFFINGTON

FIGURE 2-7 **Drinking plenty of water is an important element of proper nutrition.**

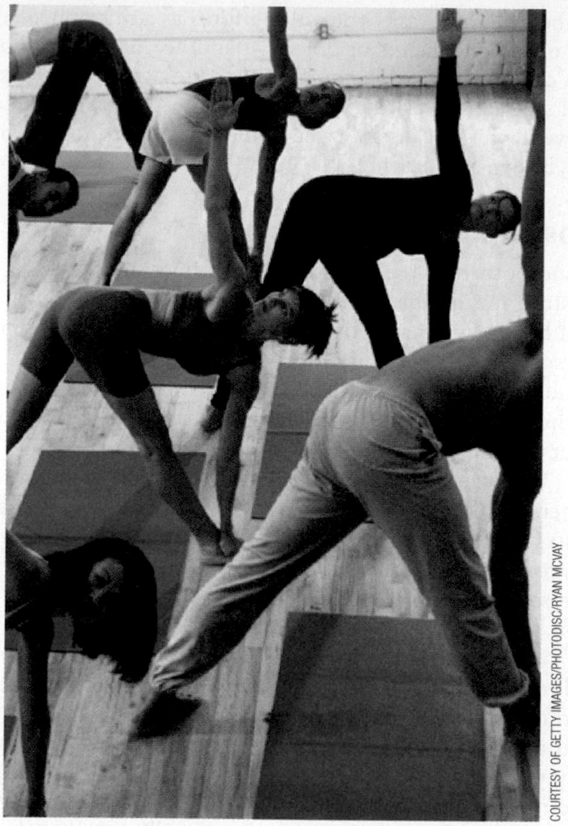
COURTESY OF GETTY IMAGES/PHOTODISC/RYAN MCVAY

FIGURE 2-8 **Exercise is an essential ingredient for wellness because it improves physiological functioning and increases ability to concentrate.**

Most authorities agree that the average adult needs six to eight (8-ounce) glasses of water each day. It is important to maintain a balance in the diet for optimal wellness.

Sleep, Rest, Relaxation, and Exercise

Wellness implies more than eating balanced meals, avoiding harmful substances, and practicing good grooming. Wellness also means taking time to enjoy yourself. It means making time for sleep, rest, relaxation, and exercise.

Sleep is time for the body to replenish its energy reserves and to heal itself. The amount of time needed may vary with the individual or even with the day. One person may need 8 hours of sleep after a heavy workday but need only 6 hours after a less strenuous day. An infant, of course, needs more sleep than does a young adult. Sleep is necessary to allow the body's organs to function at their most minimal levels. This period of rejuvenation for the body is necessary for total wellness.

Rest, meaning conscious freedom from activity and worry, is just as important as sleep. Rest is a time of inner quiet and physical inactivity. Only when a person is relaxed and at inner peace can that person rest.

Relaxation means doing something for the fun of it. That which is relaxing to one person may not be relaxing to another. Examples of relaxation activities include reading a novel, reading to children, playing cards or other games, fishing, painting, or sewing or other handwork.

Many experts agree that the best rest follows planned exercise. During exercise, heart rate and breathing increase, circulation improves, and muscles stretch. Exercise is also a time to free the mind of anxiety-producing thoughts. Sometimes after a day's work, a brisk walk frees the mind and allows the body to relax in preparation for rest.

Whichever form of exercise, rest, and relaxation is best for you, make time for it in each day (see Figure 2-8). Rest and relaxation as well as regular sleep and exercise are essential ingredients for wellness and result in reduced fatigue and irritability and possibly increased resistance to colds, flu, and serious infections. Furthermore, the capacity to concentrate increases, which should make a significant difference in your studies.

INTELLECTUAL WELLNESS

Intellectual wellness is the ability to function as an independent person capable of making sound decisions. Such decisions are based on the individual's needs but at the same time take into account the needs of others. Clear thinking, problem-solving skills, good judgment, and the desire to continually learn are all qualities found in the person who is intellectually well.

Nursing requires making many decisions, some of which may mean life or death to the client. The nurse must have intellectual wellness to make the best decisions possible with regard to client care.

SOCIOCULTURAL WELLNESS

Sociocultural wellness is the ability to appreciate the needs of others and to care about one's environment and the inhabitants of it. As a nurse, you will care for clients of all ages and races who speak different languages and come from various cultural groups. Each client's **culture** (behavior, customs, and beliefs of the family, extended family, tribe, nation, and society) influences the way that person views wellness and responds to illness.

It is important that the nurse understand that while everyone's basic needs are the same, the ways that those needs are met may vary based on the client's culture. Today's population is working, playing, and contributing to society for more years than ever before. People are more health conscious, better educated, and more involved in making health choices than perhaps any previous generation. Nurses should encourage such involvement and work to dispel discrimination by accepting each person as an individual.

Psychological Wellness

Psychological wellness encompasses the enjoyment of creativity, the satisfaction of the basic need to love and be loved, the understanding of emotions, and the ability to maintain control over emotions. Emotions are an integral part of the balance sought in life and are important factors in the way a person relates to others. They are measures of inner thoughts and feelings and are apparent in actions or behaviors.

Wellness requires that individuals recognize emotions and control their reactions in various situations. By controlling their emotions, nurses help create a therapeutic environment within which to help clients.

Another aspect of emotional wellness is a positive attitude. An **attitude** is a feeling about people, places, or things that is evident in the way one behaves. It can be positive or negative. Many books and hundreds of studies have described the role that a positive attitude plays in helping conquer illness. Many authorities believe that having a positive attitude is at least as important as having the best treatment for an illness.

Nursing requires that you see the best in people during the worst of times. In order to survive and function well, the nurse needs to see life as a challenge and as a gift to cherish and enjoy.

Because a positive attitude is so important when caring for your clients, it is vital that you share yours with them. An attitude can become a habit. If you repeatedly think positively, soon you will unconsciously find yourself seeing the positive aspects in any given situation. For example, you may find yourself at work when the usual number of staff does not show up. You can say to yourself at the beginning of your shift, "There is no way I will ever finish my work on time," or you can tell yourself, "This is the perfect opportunity to get organized early and work together as a team." Either way, you will have the same number of staff members. But whereas having a negative attitude will increase your chances of being miserable and unsuccessful, having a positive attitude will help the day go smoother and increase the likelihood of your coworkers being cheerful and willing to help.

Having a positive attitude will also help you in your studies. It will help open your mind and will spill into your daily life, making life more enjoyable.

Spiritual Wellness

Spiritual wellness manifests as inner strength and peace. **Spirituality** is a broad concept incorporating more than a client's religious affiliation. It encompasses the beliefs that a person has that give meaning and purpose to their existence (Fitchett, 2002). It encompasses values, purpose, caring, love, honesty, wisdom, and imagination (Roberts, 2005), and it may also reflect a belief in the existence of a higher power or guiding spirit outside of the client's self (Burkhardt & Jacobson, 2005). Spirituality manifests as meaningful work, creative expression, familiar rituals, and religious practices (Wright, 1998). It involves finding meaning in everything, including life, illness, and death. Spiritual needs include love, meaning in life, forgiveness, and hope. The human spiritual dimension is a major healing force. It can mean the difference between life and death and wellness and illness (Dossey, Keegan, & Guzzetta, 2004).

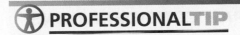

PROFESSIONAL TIP

Self-Nurturing

- Develop activities that recharge the body, mind, and spirit.
- Make time for fun. Any activity that brings happiness or joy is beneficial.
- Schedule a few minutes each day to do at least one fun thing.

CULTURAL CONSIDERATIONS

Sociocultural Wellness

Nurses and nursing students come from various cultural backgrounds and are thus excellent resources for you to learn about cultural variations.

CLIENT TEACHING

Tips for Wellness

Encourage clients to adopt the following tips for wellness:

- Eat healthy meals and healthy snacks.
- Eat breakfast.
- Do not use tobacco products.
- Exercise regularly.
- Do not use drugs.
- Do not drink alcoholic beverages or drink only in moderation.
- Focus on one problem at a time.
- Get enough sleep every night.
- Practice having a positive attitude.
- Think before speaking.
- Make a list of goals for each day.

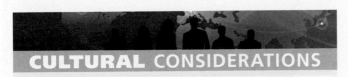

LIFE SPAN CONSIDERATIONS

Older Adult's Spiritual Wellness

As the older adult experiences life and all the challenges that are presented, spirituality is evolving. Spiritual needs and expressions of spirituality may change. The older adult may find new meaning to life. On the other hand, if confronted with many age-related changes and losses that seem insurmountable, the older adult may believe that there is no longer any meaning to life and that life is not worth living. The older adult may experience closeness to a higher power that has never been previously experienced. Older adults may become angry at a higher power because of all the losses they have endured. Age-related changes may have resulted in the older adult becoming bitter about "the golden years." A realistic goal to assist the older adult in achieving a spiritual sense of harmony is to encourage the person to discuss her feelings about spirituality (Brill & Anderson, 2003).

Florence Nightingale spoke boldly about the importance of the spiritual aspect of client care. Dossey and Dossey (1998) state that the richness of a person's interactions with others correlates with positive health outcomes and that practice of any religion correlates with greater health and increased longevity.

CRITICAL THINKING

Personal Well-Being

What are you doing or what can you do to take responsibility for your well-being?

Nurses are not asked to take over the role of spiritual counselors. Clark (2004) proposes that nurses ask simple, open-ended questions, such as asking the client to tell a story about the struggles in his journey to wholeness. The nurse encourages the client to explain what spirituality means to him. The nurse asks the client if he has thoughts about the purpose and meaning of his life and if he could share it. In addition, the nurse assesses if the client has ever felt "lost in life" and, if so, if anything has helped him find his way or if he is still feeling lost.

Because nurses play a key role in helping clients find hope and meaning in life, it is important that nurses understand spirituality. For many, religious practices are an expression of their spirituality. An important function for the nurse is to respect the religious beliefs of clients, provide clients with privacy to practice those beliefs, and make spiritual guidance available through the client's minister, priest, rabbi, or other representative, when requested.

NURTURE YOURSELF

The worthy and challenging profession of nursing requires unselfish caring for others. Those who select nursing as a

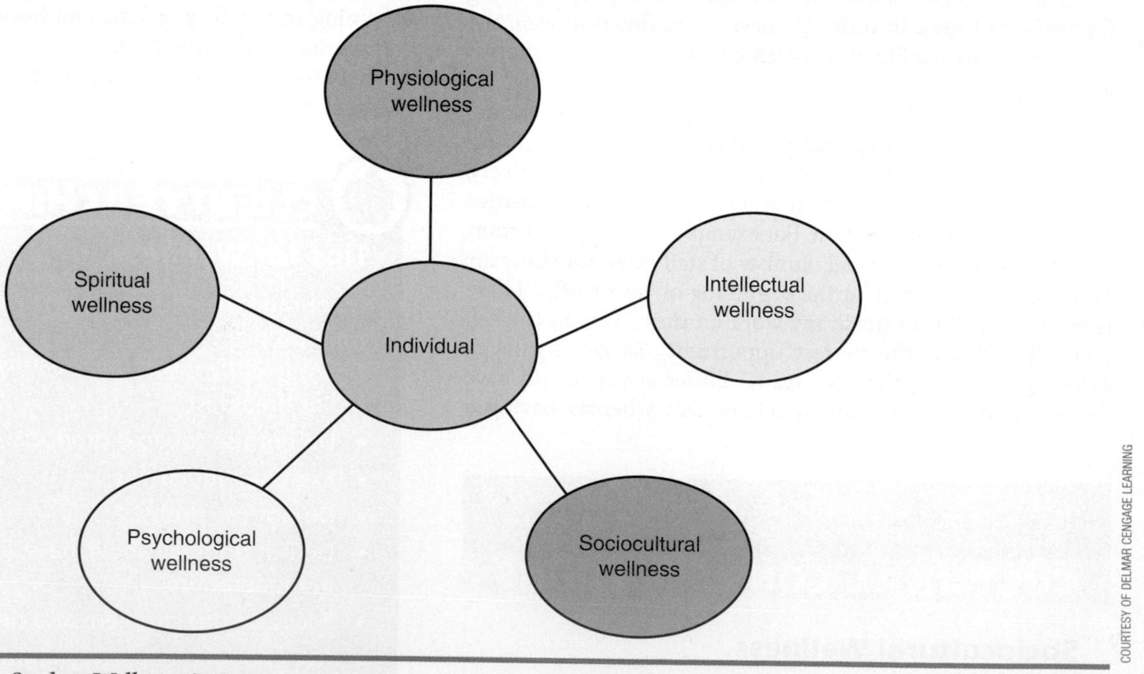

CONCEPT MAP 2-1 Student Wellness Activity

1. Read the chapter content for physiological, intellectual, sociocultural, psychological, and spiritual wellness.
2. Inside each wellness balloon, list areas of wellness that apply to the designated wellness category.
3. Highlight the listed areas where you are "whole" or "well."
4. How can you take responsibility to improve the areas that are not highlighted?

career generally want to make a difference in people's lives. The demands of clients, employers, and coworkers can cause stress for the nurse. The nurse's personal life may also be a source of stress. Many caregivers do not know how to care for themselves. Those who do not nurture themselves will suffer stress symptoms and illnesses (American Holistic Health Association, 2007).

Persons who are well physically, intellectually, sociocul-turally, psychologically, and spiritually lead productive, creative lives. They are better able to meet life's challenges and to control their stressors. For nurses, wellness means practicing wellness habits daily. Nurses are excellent role models when they are holistically healthy individuals.

CASE STUDY

H.B. is a 52-year-old woman who presents to the nurse practitioner with a 3-week history of right-sided abdominal pain. The pain first started infrequently at night, but H.B. has noticed that it is now happening during the daytime, and that the frequency has increased. H.B. states that the pain occurs a few hours after eating but is not associated with eating any particular types of food. She rates the pain as a 7 to 8 on a 0 to 10 scale. She is not having pain at the time of her appointment with the nurse practitioner.

H.B. is perimenopausal—experiencing "mild" hot flashes and periodic episodes of "feeling very edgy and not herself"—and she describes her menstrual cycles as being "normal" for her. She had a right oophorectomy for a benign cyst 20 years ago. She is allergic to ragweed, for which she takes Rhinecort and Singular.

As H.B. describes her pain, she becomes tearful and admits that this is the last thing that she needs. She admits to being fearful of what this pain could indicate. She states that she is "overwhelmed" by all the demands that she has going on with her life. She "doesn't have time for herself" to do the things that she enjoys.

When asked about her life struggles, H.B. admits that she has had a "rough" time. She married into an abusive relationship. She divorced at a young age, and despite having two small children at the time, she went to college and earned a degree in food science management. She is very active in her church and finds this to be a source of support. She admits that she has had to decrease her involvement over the past few years. She admits that she is just "living day to day . . . just trying to survive."

H.B. is a single mother with two teenage daughters. The youngest is having difficulties adjusting to middle school and is having behavior problems. H.B. has elderly parents who live nearby. They have multiple health problems, and H.B. is worried about their ability to live independently. H.B. is employed as a manager of a restaurant, often working 12-hour days and taking calls on the weekend.

The following questions will guide your development of a nursing care plan for the case study.

1. Assess H.B.'s physical, intellectual, sociocultural, psychological, and spiritual wellness.
2. Review your assessment and develop a plan written as a measurable goal of how H.B. could become "whole."
3. What are some steps (interventions) H.B. could take to improve her wholeness?
4. According to the plan and interventions you developed, how would you know if H.B. is becoming "well" or "whole"?

SUMMARY

- Wellness includes physical, intellectual, sociocultural, psychological, and spiritual health.
- The keys to wellness are prevention and education.
- Each individual learns to accept responsibility for his or her own wellness.
- The most effective means to reinforce teachings of wellness is by positive example.
- There are five levels in Maslow's Hierarchy of Needs: physiological, safety and security, love and belonging, self-esteem, and self-actualization.
- Self-awareness is important for nurses so their own needs do not interfere with providing quality client care.
- Nurses should get to know themselves by becoming aware of their thoughts, actions, and reactions to situations.
- Good posture is necessary for personal and client safety.
- Dental health is necessary for overall wellness and professionalism.
- Wellness tips include exercising regularly, getting enough sleep, and finding a quiet time each day for relaxing.
- A positive attitude is helpful in looking for the best in everyone.
- All nurses should learn to laugh at themselves and enjoy life's little pleasures.

REVIEW QUESTIONS

1. Rest is defined as:
   1. sleeping.
   2. physical inactivity.
   3. playing games with family or friends.
   4. conscious freedom from activity and worry.
2. What responsibility does the nurse have who believes a colleague is abusing drugs?
   1. Report it to the supervisor.
   2. Ignore it; it is not the nurse's concern.
   3. Tell the colleague to stop or the nurse will call the police.
   4. Assist the nurse to receive help through the local drug treatment program.
3. What can be the result when breakfast is omitted?
   1. The person loses weight faster.
   2. The person is left tired, weak, and hungry.
   3. The person eats more at the noon and evening meals.
   4. The person's mind is sharper, and study time is more productive.
4. Positive or negative feelings about people, places, or things are called:
   1. culture.
   2. empathy.
   3. symptoms.
   4. attitudes.
5. The aspects of total wellness are:
   1. rest, exercise, and good grooming.
   2. physical, psychological, spiritual, intellectual, and sociocultural.
   3. self-awareness; rest; balanced, nutritious diet; good grooming; dental care.
   4. physiological; safety and security; love and belonging; self-esteem; self-actualization.
6. The goal of holistic nursing is:
   1. curing the client of disease.
   2. assessing, planning, intervening, and evaluating the client.
   3. assisting the client to heal.
   4. collaborating with the client.
7. Spirituality includes: (Select all that apply.)
   1. the client's religious affiliation.
   2. beliefs that give meaning and purpose to life.
   3. values such as honesty, wisdom, and caring.
   4. a belief in the existence of a higher power.
   5. feeling "lost in life."
   6. telling a story of sustaining hope during a struggle toward wholeness.
8. A nurse desires a healthy lifestyle. What activities will contribute to her healthy lifestyle? (Select all that apply.)
   1. Choosing foods low in fat and high in vitamins, minerals, and nutrients for her and her family.
   2. The nurse refuses to forgive a colleague for a statement that hurt her deeply.
   3. The nurse sees working overtime once a week and having to rearrange daycare for her children as a challenge and opportunity.
   4. The nurse takes a class on the values and beliefs of other cultures.
   5. The nurse works all the overtime she can and averages 4 to 5 hours of sleep per night.
   6. The nurse stands in good alignment with her shoulders back and head up.
9. Holistic assessments consist of the following:
   1. physiologic, psychological, and spiritual aspects.
   2. psychological and physiological aspects.
   3. spiritual, social, psychological, and physiological aspects.
   4. environmental, social, spiritual, psychological, and physiological aspects.
10. A nurse establishes a therapeutic relationship by: (Select all that apply.)
    1. focusing on the client and her family.
    2. imposing personal values and beliefs on the client.
    3. establishing a foundation of trust with the client.
    4. actively listening and caring.
    5. collaboratively working with the client as an active partner.
    6. assessing the client's past and current relationships.

REFERENCES/SUGGESTED READINGS

American Holistic Nurses Association. (1994). AHNA philosophy. *Journal of Holistic Nursing, 12*(3), 350–351.

American Holistic Nurses Association. (2004) Standards of holistic practice. Retrieved April 10, 2007, from http://www.ahna.org

American Holistic Health Association. (2007). Wellness from within: The first step. Retrieved April 10, 2007, from http://www.ahha.org

Brill, C., & Anderson, M. (2003). Common clinical problems: Psychological. In M. A. Anderson (Ed.), *Caring for older adults holistically* (pp. 212–231). Philadelphia: F. A. Davis.

Burkhardt, M., & Jacobson, M. G. (2005). Spirituality and health. In B. Dossey, D. Guzzetta, & L. Keegan (Eds.), *Holistic nursing: A handbook for practice* (pp. 135–172). Sudbury, MA: Jones and Bartlett.

Cerrato, P. (1998a). Spirituality and healing. *RN, 61*(2), 49–50.

Cerrato, P. (1998b). Understanding the mind/body link. *RN, 61*(1), 28–31.

Clark, C. (2004). *The holistic nursing approach to chronic diseases.* New York: Springer Publishing.

Diluzio, J., & Spillane, E. (2002). Holistic nursing: Is it right for you? *RN, 65*(8), 32–35.

Dossey, B. (1997). *Core curriculum for holistic nursing.* Gaithersburg, MD: Aspen.

Dossey, B. (1998). Holistic modalities and healing moments. *American Journal of Nursing, 98*(6), 44–47.

Dossey, B. (2000). *Florence Nightingale: Mystic, visionary, healer*. Springhouse, PA: Springhouse.

Dossey, B., & Dossey, L. (1998). Attending to holistic care. *American Journal of Nursing, 98*(8), 35–38.

Dossey, B., Keegan, L., & Guzzetta, C. (2004). *Holistic nursing: A handbook for practice* (4th ed.). Sudbury, MA: Jones and Bartlett.

Dunn, D. (2005). *Substance abuse among nurses—Defining the issue* (PMID: 16370231). Wayne, NJ: St. Joseph's Wayne Hospital. Retrieved February 1, 2009, from http://www.ncbi.nlm.nih.gov/pubmed/16370231?ordinalpos=1&itool=EntrezSystem2.PEntr

Dyer, E. (1998, April 6). Faith and healing. *Corpus Christi Caller-Times*.

Edlin, G. (2004). *Health and wellness* (8th ed.). Sudbury, MA: Jones and Bartlett.

Fitchett, G. (2002). *Assessing spiritual needs: A guide for caregiver*. Lima, OH: Academic Renewal Press.

Frisch, N., Dossey, B., Guzzetta, C., Fristh, N., & Quinn, J. (2000). *AHNA standards of holistic nursing practice: Guidelines for caring and healing*. Gaithersburg, MD: Aspen.

Hill, S., & Howlett, H. (2005). Success in practical nursing: Personal and vocational issues (5th ed.). Philadelphia: W. B. Saunders.

Hughs, C. (1997). Prayer and healing: A case study. *Journal of Holistic Nursing, 15*(3), 318.

Ivker, R. (2002). Comparing holistic and conventional medicine. Retrieved August 28, 2008, from http://ahha.org/articles/ivker.htm

Jerome, A., & Ferraro-McDuffie, A. (1992). Nurse self-awareness in therapeutic relationships. *Pediatric Nursing, 18*(2), 153–156.

Kahn, S., & Saulo, M. (1995). *Healing yourself*. Clifton Park, NY: Delmar Cengage Learning.

Kurzen, C. (2000). *Contemporary practical/vocational nursing* (4th ed.). Philadelphia: Lippincott Williams & Wilkins.

Maslow, A. (1987). *Motivation and personality* (3rd ed.). New York: HarperCollins.

Merriam-Webster Online Dictionary. (2008). Health. Retrieved August 28, 2008, from http://www.merriam-webster.com/dictionary/health

National Institutes of Health. (2000). Complementary and alternative medicine at the NIH. Available: http://nccam.nih.gov/nccam/ne/newsletter/spring2000

Quinn, J. (2005). Transpersonal human caring and healing. In B. Dossey, D. Guzzetta, & L. Keegan (Eds.), *Holistic nursing: A handbook for practice* (pp. 39–54). Sudbury, MA: Jones and Bartlett.

Rivera-Andino, J., & Lopez, L. (2000). When culture complicates care, *RN, 63*(7), 47–49.

Roberts, D., Taylor, S., Bodell, W., Gostick, G. Silkstone, J., Smith, L., Phippen, A., Lyons, B., Denny, D., Norris, A., & McDonald, H. (2005). Development of a holistic admission assessment: An integrated care pathway for the hospice setting. *International Journal of Palliative Nursing*, 11, 322–332.

Selye, H. (1978). *The stress of life* (2nd ed.). New York: McGraw-Hill.

Taber's Cyclopedic Medical Dictionary (20th ed.). (2005). Philadelphia: F. A. Davis.

Telstar Innovations, Inc. (2000). Retrieved April 8, 2007, from http://www.findhealer.com

Walter, S. (1999). Holistic health. Available: http://ahha.org/rosen.htm

Waughfield, C. (2002). *Mental health concepts* (5th ed.). Clifton Park, NY: Delmar Cengage Learning.

World Health Organization. (1974). *Chronicle of WHO*. Geneva: Organization Interim Commission.

Wright, K. (1998). Professional, ethical, and legal implications for spiritual care in nursing. *Image: Journal of Nursing Scholarship, 30*(1)81–83.

RESOURCES

American Holistic Health Association, http://ahha.org

American Holistic Nurses' Association, http://www.ahna.org

National Center for Complementary and Alternative Medicine (NCCAM), http://nccam.nih.gov

Nurse Healers—Professional Associates International, Inc., http://www.therapeutic-touch.org

CHAPTER 3
Nursing History, Education, and Organizations

MAKING THE CONNECTION

Refer to the following chapters to increase your understanding of nursing history, education, and organizations:

Basic Nursing

- ***Legal and Ethical Responsibilities***

LEARNING OBJECTIVES

Upon completion of this chapter, you should be able to:

- Define key terms.
- Define nursing as an art and a science.
- Identify major historical and social events that have shaped current nursing practice.
- Describe Florence Nightingale's impact on current nursing practice.
- Discuss the contributions of early nursing leaders in the United States.
- Discuss the impact of selected landmark reports on nursing education and practice.
- Define the role of the RN.
- Define the role of the LP/VN.
- Describe select nursing organizations and their purposes and functions.
- Differentiate between program approval and program accreditation.

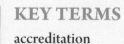

KEY TERMS

accreditation
autonomy
clinical
didactic
empowerment
health maintenance organizations (HMOs)
morbidity
mortality
nursing
primary care providers
primary health care
staff development

INTRODUCTION

Nursing is the art and science of promoting, restoring, and maintaining the health of clients founded on a knowledge base supported by evidence-based theory. Nursing has developed into a scientific profession resulting in change from mystical beliefs to sophisticated technology and caring. Nursing uses caring behaviors, critical thinking skills, and scientific knowledge.

Nursing focuses on the client's *response* to illness rather than on the illness. Nursing promotes health and assists clients move to a higher level of wellness, including assistance during a terminal illness with the maintenance of comfort and dignity during the final stage of life.

In this chapter, the development of nursing is traced through its rich history and the social forces that affected it. Nursing education and nursing organizations are also discussed.

HISTORICAL OVERVIEW

A basic knowledge about the history of nursing is necessary to understand what nursing is today. The study of nursing history helps the nurse better understand the issues of **autonomy** (being self-directed), unity within the profession, education, supply and demand, salary, and current practice. Learning from the role models of history, nurses can increase their capacity to make positive changes in the present and set goals for the future.

The major reason for studying history is to learn from the past. By applying the lessons learned from history, nurses will continue to be a vital force in the health care system.

By studying nursing history, nurses learn how the profession has advanced from its beginnings. The process of enabling others to do for themselves is called **empowerment**. Today, magnet hospitals encourage the autonomy of nurses (Summers, 2008). When nurses are empowered, they are autonomous. Historically, it has been difficult for nurses to achieve autonomy.

Empowerment and autonomy are necessary for nursing to bring about positive changes in health care today. Personal power comes to individuals who are clear about what they want from life and who see their work as essential to the contributions they wish to make.

EVOLUTION OF NURSING

Nursing has evolved alongside human civilization. Although it is not possible to present a complete history of nursing and health care within the scope of this text, it is necessary for all nurses to have some understanding of their profession's heritage and of those pioneers who led the way on the path to modern nursing. Table 3-1 is a chronological listing of events in the evolution of nursing.

Early Civilizations

Nursing dates back to 4000 B.C. to the primitive societies where mother–nurses worked with priests. The use of wet nurses in Babylonia and Assyria is recorded in 2000 B.C.

Ancient Greece

Temples to honor Hygiea, the goddess of health, were built by the ancient Greeks. These temples, religious institutions governed by priests, were more like health spas than hospitals. Priestesses (who were not nurses) attended to those visiting the temples. Nursing was done by women in the homes.

Hippocrates, a Greek physician born in 460 B.C., is considered the father of medicine. He used a system of physical assessment, observation, and record keeping in his care of the sick. Hippocrates wrote about many aspects of medicine, including anatomy, physiology, pathology, diagnosis, prognosis, mental illness, gynecology, obstetrics, surgery, client-centered care, bedside observation, hygiene, and professional ethics. Case histories that he wrote are still used as examples today. His emphasis on the importance of caring for the client laid a foundation for nursing. The Hippocratic Oath, taken by physicians today, is based on his principles.

Roman Empire

The first hospitals were established in the Eastern Roman Empire (Byzantine Empire). Fabiola, disciple of St. Jerome, was responsible for introducing hospitals in the West. These were primarily religious and charitable institutions sheltered in monasteries and convents. The caregivers who volunteered their time to nurse the sick had no formal training in therapeutic modalities.

Middle Ages

Hospitals in large Byzantine cities of the medieval era were staffed primarily by paid male assistants and male nurses. This was not true in the rural parts of the Eastern Roman Empire and in the West, where nursing was viewed as a natural nurturing job for women.

In Western Europe, medical practices remained basically unchanged until the 11th and 12th centuries. At that time, formal medical education for physicians was required in a university setting, but other caregivers were not required to receive any formal education.

Renaissance

Interest in the arts and sciences emerged during the Renaissance (A.D. 1400–1550). This was also the time of many geographic explorations by Europeans, which resulted in the expansion of the world.

Universities were established because of a renewed interest in science, but there were no formal nursing schools. Social status and customs encouraged women to stay at home and attend to the traditional role of nurturer/caregiver.

Industrial Revolution

The Industrial Revolution led to a proliferation of factories, where conditions for the workers were deplorable. Grueling work, long hours, and unsafe conditions prevailed in the workplace, and the health of laborers received little attention.

The Royal College of Surgeons in London and other medical schools were founded in 1800. Male barbers in France also functioned as surgeons by performing leeching, giving enemas, and extracting teeth.

It was still considered unseemly in the mid-1800s for women to be nurses, even though some hospitals (almshouses) relied on women to bathe the poor, make beds, and scrub floors. Most nursing care was still performed in the home by female relatives of the ill.

TABLE 3-1 Historical Events Influencing the Evolution of Nursing

DATE	EVENT
4000 B.C.	Primitive societies
2000 B.C.	Babylonia and Assyria
800–600 B.C.	Health religions of India
700 B.C.	Greece: source of modern medical science
460 B.C.	Hippocrates
3 B.C.	Ireland: pre-Christian nursing
A.D. 390	Fabiola: first hospital founded
390–407	Early Christianity, deaconesses
711	Field hospital with nursing, Spain
1096–1291	Military Nursing Orders (Knights Hospitalers of St. John in Jerusalem)
1100	Ambulatory clinics, Spain (Muslims)
1440	First Chairs of Medicine, Oxford and Cambridge
1500–1752	Deterioration of hospitals and nursing, "dark ages of nursing"
1633	Founded: Daughters of Charity
1820	Florence Nightingale born
1836	Kaiserswerth, Lutheran Order of Deaconesses reestablished
1841	Founded: Nursing Sisters of the Holy Cross
1848	Women's Rights Convention, Seneca Falls, New York
1854–1856	Crimean War
1859	Nightingale's *Notes on Nursing* published in England
1860	Founded: first Nightingale School of Nursing, St. Thomas Hospital, London
1861–1865	Civil War, United States
1861	Dorothea Dix appointed Superintendent of the Female Nurses of the Army
1871	Founded: New York State Training School for Nurses, Brooklyn Maternity, Brooklyn, New York
1872	New England Hospital for Women's one-year program for nurses yields America's first educated nurse, Linda Richards
1873	Founded: first three Nightingale schools in United States: Bellevue Hospital School of Nursing (New York City), Connecticut Training School (New Haven, CT), and Boston Training School (Boston, MA)
1881	Founded: American Red Cross, by Clara Barton
1892	Founded: Ballard School at YWCA Brooklyn, NY; first practical nursing school
1893	Founded: American Society of Superintendents of Training Schools for Nurses
1899	Founded: International Council of Nurses (ICN)
1900	*American Journal of Nursing* (*AJN*) established
1903	New York: efforts fail to pass a nurse licensing law
	North Carolina: first state nurse registration law passes
	Founded: Army Nurse Corps
1907	Thompson Practical Nursing School in Brattleboro, VT established
1910	Flexner report
1911	Founded: American Nurses Association (ANA), formerly the Associated Alumnae
1912	Founded: National League of Nursing Education, formerly the Superintendents' Society
1914	Mississippi is first state to license practical nurses
1917	Smith-Hughes Act passes (provided federal funds for practical nursing programs in vocational schools)
1918	Household Nursing Association School of Attendant Nursing in Boston, MA, established
1920s	First prepaid medical plan established, Pacific Northwest Hospitals offer a prepaid plan Baylor Plan (prototype of Blue Cross) established
1921	Women get the right to vote
1923	Goldmark Report: Nursing and Nursing Education in the United States
1935	Social Security Act passes
1941	Founded: Association of Practical Nursing Schools
1942	Association of Practical Nursing Schools becomes National Association of Practical Nurse Education (NAPNE)
	Practical nursing curriculum planned and advocated across United States

TABLE 3-1 Historical Events Influencing the Evolution of Nursing (Continued)

DATE	EVENT
1944	U.S. Department of Vocational Education commissions intensive study to differentiate tasks of the practical nurse
1945	New York only state to have mandatory licensure law for practical nurses
1948	Brown Report: Future of Nursing
1949	Founded: National Federation of Licensed Practical Nurses (NFLPN)
1952	National League of Nursing Education changes name to National League for Nursing (NLN)
1955	Practical nursing established under (Title III) Health Amendment Act
	All states pass licensure laws affecting practical/vocational nursing
1959	National Association of Practical Nurse Education (NAPNE) changes name to National Association for Practical Nurse Education and Service (NAPNES)
1960s	Established: Medicare and Medicaid
1961	National League for Nursing establishes a Council for Practical Nursing Programs
	Surgeon General's Consultant Group
1965	First nurse practitioner program, pediatric
	ANA position paper on entry into practice
1966	Educational opportunity grants for nurses
1970	Secretary's commission to study extended roles for nurses
1973	Health Maintenance Organization Act
1977	Rural Health Clinic Service Act
1979	U.S. Surgeon General Report *Healthy People*
1980	Omnibus Budget Reconciliation Act (OBRA)
1980	National Commission on Nursing
1982	Budget cut to Health Maintenance Organization Act
	Tax Equity Fiscal Responsibility Act (TEFRA)
1983	Institute of Medicine Committee on Nursing and Nursing Education study
1987	Secretary's Commission on Nursing
1990s	Health care reform
1991	U.S. Department of Health and Human Services *Healthy People 2000*
1996	Certification Examination for Practical and Vocational Nurses in Long-term Care
1997	Established: NLN Accrediting Commission (NLNAC)
2000	U.S. Department of Health and Human Services *Healthy People 2010*
2002	Nurse Reinvestment Act of 2002 (PL 107-205)

RELIGIOUS INFLUENCES

Religion had a strong influence on the development of nursing beginning in India in 800–600 B.C. The religious influence prospered in Greece and Ireland in 3 B.C. with male nurse–priests.

Theodor Fleidner, a pastor in Kaiserswerth, Germany in 1836, revived the Lutheran Order of Deaconesses to care for the sick in a hospital he had founded. He established the first real school of nursing to educate the deaconesses in the care of the sick. These deaconesses of Kaiserswerth became famous because they were the only ones formally educated in nursing. Pastor Fleidner had a profound influence on nursing through Florence Nightingale, who received her nursing education at the Kaiserswerth Institute.

Religious orders were established by the Catholic Church to care for the sick and poor. Only nurses who functioned within a religious order were approved by society. The need for nurses in the mid-19th century and changing social conditions set the stage for Florence Nightingale's reforms.

The order of the Nursing Sisters of the Holy Cross was founded in LeMans, France, by Father Bassil Moreau in 1841. Also in 1841, four sisters were brought to Notre Dame in South Bend, Indiana, by a Father Sorin. These sisters established St. Mary's Academy in Bertrand, Michigan, in 1844. In 1855, the school was moved to Notre Dame and became known as Saint Mary's College, which later had a strong influence on the emerging role of women (Wall, 1993).

FLORENCE NIGHTINGALE

The founder of modern nursing is Florence Nightingale (1820–1910), who grew up in a wealthy, upper-class family in England. Unlike other young women of her era, Nightingale was educated in Greek, Latin, mathematics, history, and philosophy. She always had an interest in relieving suffering and caring for the sick, but social mores of her time made it impossible for her to consider caring for others because she was not a member of a religious order. After receiving encouragement from a family visitor, Dr. Samuel Gridley Howe, however, she became a nurse over the objections of society and her family.

On completion of a 3-month course of study at Kaiserswerth Institute, Nightingale worked to reform health care.

CRITICAL THINKING

Florence Nightingale's Characteristics

Florence Nightingale has been described as being strong-minded and assertive. In what ways would it be helpful for you to develop such characteristics?

Britain's war in the Crimea presented her with the opportunity to volunteer with 38 other nurses to serve in the battle-site hospital (Figure 3-1). The physicians in charge assigned the nurses to nonclient care duties. Florence Nightingale persisted in advocating cleanliness, good nutrition, and fresh air. When battle casualties mounted, the nurses had a chance to prove their worth. They worked around the clock, caring for the wounded and carrying oil lamps to light their way in the darkness. The symbol of the oil lamp is still used today in nursing and is the reason Florence Nightingale is called the "Lady with the Lamp." The implementation of her principles in the areas of nursing practice and environmental modifications resulted in reduced **morbidity** (illness) and **mortality** (death) rates during the war.

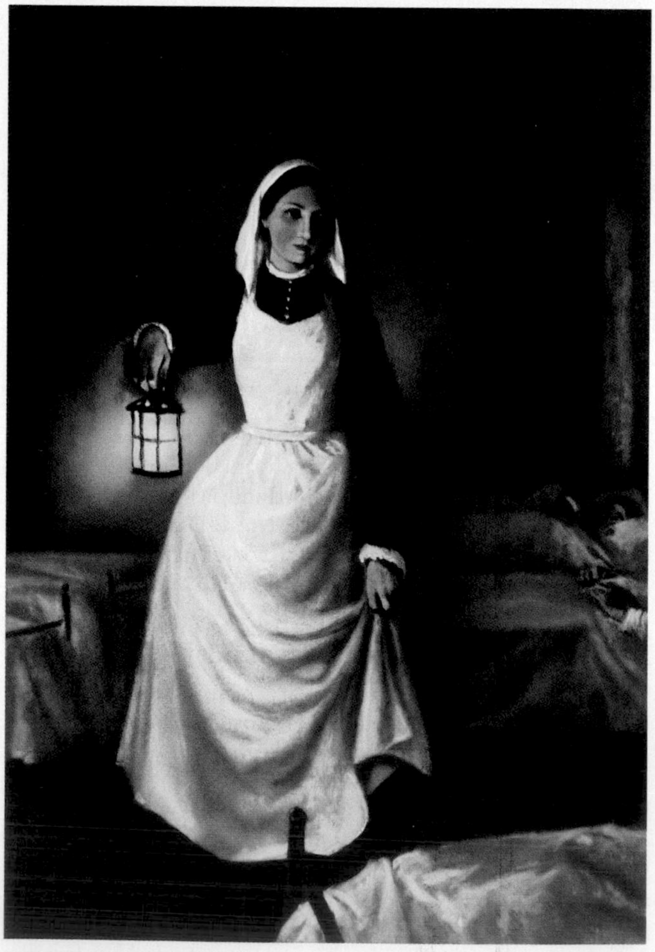

FIGURE 3-1 **Florence Nightingale in the Crimea** (*Reprinted with permission from Bettmann/Corbis.*)

Nightingale worked to further develop the public's awareness of the need for educated nurses and forged the future of nursing education as a result of her experiences in educating nurses to care for British soldiers. At St. Thomas' Hospital in London, she established the Nightingale Training School of Nurses. This was the first school for nurses providing both theory-based knowledge and clinical experience. She fundamentally changed both the public's perception of nursing and the method for educating nurses. Some of Nightingale's unique beliefs about nursing and nursing education were the need for the following:

- A holistic framework inclusive of illness and health
- A theoretical basis for nursing practice
- A liberal education as a foundation of nursing practice
- An environment that promotes healing
- A body of nursing knowledge distinct from medical knowledge (Macrae, 1995)

She introduced many other concepts that are still used today, although they were unique in her day. Specifically, Nightingale recommended (a) a systematic method of assessing clients, (b) individualized care based on the client's needs and preferences, and (c) confidentiality.

Recognizing the influence of environmental factors on health, she recommended that clean surroundings, fresh air, and light would improve the quality of care (Nightingale, 1969). She believed that nurses should be formally educated and function as client advocates (Selanders, 1994). She is credited with being the originator of modern nursing because many of these beliefs and concepts are still advocated in nursing schools today.

The Civil War and Nursing

During the Civil War (1861–1865), America's need for nurses increased dramatically. The Sisters of the Holy Cross were the first to respond to the need for nurses, with 12 sisters caring for wounded soldiers. By the end of the war, 80 sisters had cared for soldiers in Illinois, Missouri, Kentucky, and Tennessee (Wall, 1993).

Nursing care was also provided by the Sisters of Mercy, Daughters of Charity, Dominican Sisters, and the Franciscan Sisters of the Poor. These sisters, although influenced by the roles assigned to women during the 19th century, were willing to take risks when human rights were threatened (Wall, 1993). Other women also volunteered to care for the soldiers of both the Union and the Confederate armies. These women implemented sanitary conditions in field hospitals and performed various other duties.

Dorothea Dix (1802–1887) was the first woman ever appointed to an administrative position by the federal government when she was made superintendent of the female nurses of the army in 1861. Her recruitment efforts procured more than 2,000 women to care for the sick in the Union army. Following the Civil War, she concentrated on reforming the treatment of the mentally ill (Mohr, 2005).

Clara Barton (1821–1912), who volunteered her nursing services during the Civil War, organized the Red Cross in the United States in 1881.

Blanche E. Oberle was a World War I Red Cross Army Nurse. According to Oberle, nurses were not allowed to take blood pressures in 1918. Only a physician could take a client's blood pressure. However, registered nurses mixed sterile water into powdered medications that was injected into clients.

Men in Nursing

Males impacted nursing even though their involvement is overshadowed by female nurses. During the Middle Ages, men provided nursing care in the military and religious and lay orders, including the Knights Hospitalers, the Teutonic Knights, the Tertiaries, the Knights of St. Lazarus, and the Hospital Brothers of St. Anthony. St. Camillus was from this era and he originated the red cross symbol that is still used today and developed the first ambulance service (Kauffman, 1978). Male nurses served on both sides during the Civil War, but female nurses received more recognition as Union volunteers. The Confederate army had 30 men per regiment who were designated to care for the wounded (Pokorny, 1992). Male nursing schools—Mills School for Nursing and St. Vincent's Hospital School for Men—were started in 1888 in New York (Wilson et al., 2009). Male nurses served on a U.S. Navy hospital ship, the U.S.S. *Solace*, during the Spanish-American War (Navsource.com, 2007). Today, men are a vital component in the nursing profession.

The Women's Movement

The beginnings of social unrest started in 1848 with the Women's Rights Convention in Seneca Falls, New York. Women were not considered equal to men, women did not have the right to vote, and society did not value education for women. With suffrage, the rights of women and the nursing profession were advanced. More women were being accepted into colleges and universities by the mid-1900s, but there were only a few university-based nursing programs available.

Nursing Pioneers and Leaders

The contributions of many outstanding nurses through the years made nursing what it is today. Nursing pioneers and leaders established public health nursing, rural health care services, and advanced nursing education.

Linda Richards

In 1873, Linda Richards (1841–1930) was awarded the first diploma from an American school educating nurses. She established numerous hospital-based schools for nurses and introduced the practice of keeping nurses' notes and physicians' orders as part of medical records. She also instituted the practice of nurses' wearing uniforms. While working as the first superintendent of nurses at Massachusetts General Hospital, she showed that educated nurses gave better care than nurses without formal nursing education.

Mary Mahoney

Mary Mahoney (1845–1926) was America's first African American professional nurse (Figure 3-2). She was a noted nursing leader who encouraged respect for cultural diversity. Today, the American Nurses Association (ANA) bestows the Mary Mahoney Award to recognize individuals who have made significant contributions toward improving relationships among the various cultural groups.

Adelaide Nutting

As a nursing educator, historian, and scholar, Adelaide Nutting (1858–1947) actively campaigned for the university

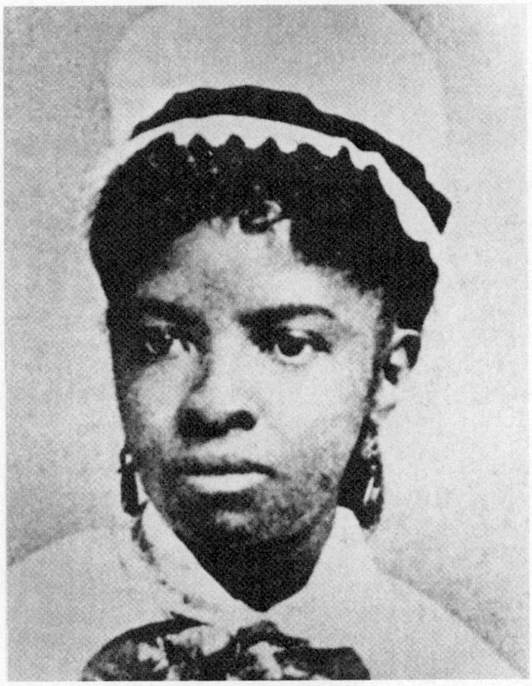

FIGURE 3-2 Mary Mahoney (*Photo courtesy of the American Nurses Association.*)

education of nurses. She was the first nurse appointed as a university professor.

Lavinia Dock

Another influential leader in nursing education, Lavinia Dock (1858–1956) graduated from Bellevue Training School for Nurses in 1886. She worked at the Henry Street Settlement House in New York City, caring for the indigent. Dock wrote one of the first nursing textbooks, *Materia Medica for Nurses*. Also, she was the first editor of the *American Journal of Nursing* (*AJN*) and wrote many other books.

Isabel Hampton Robb

Isabel Hampton Robb (1860–1910) was the founder of the Superintendents' Society in 1893 and the Nurses' Associated Alumnae of the United States and Canada in 1896. She knew it was important for nurses to participate in professional organizations and to work for unity across the profession on important issues. She worked to establish both the ANA and the National League of Nursing Education, the predecessor of the National League for Nursing (NLN). As an early supporter of the rights of nursing students, she urged that there be shorter working hours and stressed the role of the nursing student as a learner instead of an employee.

Lillian Wald

Lillian Wald (1867–1940) spent her life providing nursing care to poor people. She founded public health nursing with the establishment of the Henry Street Settlement Service in 1893 (Figure 3-3) in New York City (Silverstein, 1994). Wald was the first community health nurse and also established a school of nursing. As a tireless reformer, she worked to:

- Improve housing conditions in tenement districts
- Establish education for the mentally challenged

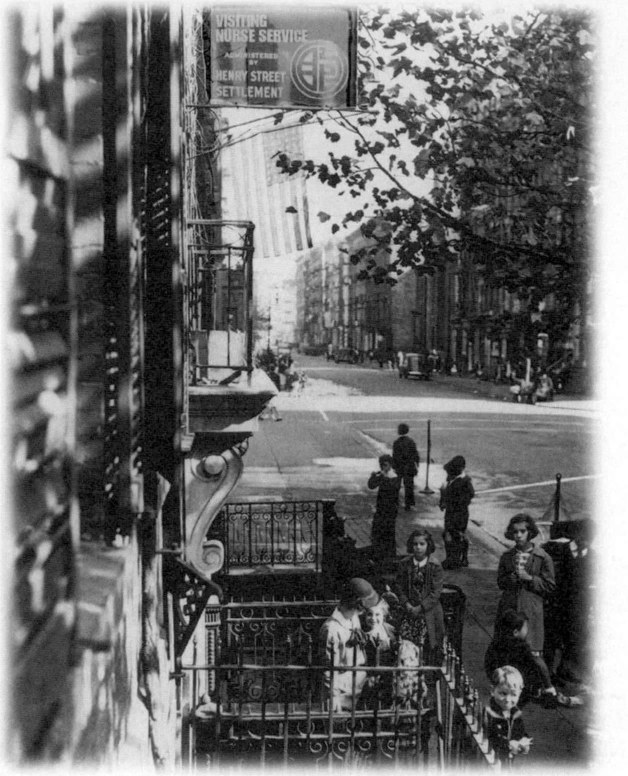

FIGURE 3-3 Nurses at the Henry Street Settlement in New York City (*Photo courtesy of Visiting Nurses Service of New York.*)

- Pass more lenient immigration regulations
- Initiate change of child labor laws and founded the Children's Bureau of the U.S. Department of Labor

Mary Breckenridge

In 1925, Mary Breckenridge (1881–1965) introduced a decentralized system of delivering health care to rural America. This system for providing primary nursing care services in the Kentucky Appalachian Mountains, called the Frontier Nursing Service, lowered the childbirth mortality rate in Leslie County, Kentucky, from the highest in the nation to below the national average.

Mamie Hale

The Arkansas Health Department hired Mamie Hale (1911–1968?) in 1942 to upgrade the educational programs for midwives. A graduate of Tuskegee School of Nurse-Midwifery, she gained the support of public health nurses, granny midwives, and obstetricians. Through education, she decreased illiteracy and superstition among those functioning as midwives. Hale's efforts improved mortality rates for both infants and mothers (Bell, 1993).

PRACTICAL NURSING PIONEER SCHOOLS

Women who cared for others but who had no formal education often called themselves "practical nurses." Formal education for practical nursing began in the 1890s. The first schools were the Ballard School, the Thompson Practical Nursing School, and the Household Nursing Association School of Attendant Nursing.

Ballard School

In 1892, the Ballard School, funded by Lucinda Ballard, was opened in New York City by the YWCA. It offered several courses for women, one of which was practical nursing. The 3-month course in simple nursing care focused on the care of infants, children, elders, and disabled persons in their own homes. The course included cooking, nutrition, basic science, and basic nursing procedures. When the YWCA was reorganized in 1949, the school closed.

Thompson Practical Nursing School

Thomas Thompson of Brattleboro, Vermont, left money in his will to help women who were making shirts for the army and were receiving only $1 per dozen. His executor, Richard Bradley, saw the need for nursing service and, in 1907, established a practical nursing school in Brattleboro. It is still operating today and is accredited by the NLN.

Household Nursing School

In 1918, a group of women in Boston were concerned about providing nursing care for people who were sick at home. After talking with Richard Bradley, they opened the Household Nursing Association School of Attendant Nursing. The name was later changed to the Shepard-Gill School of Practical Nursing. It closed in 1984.

NURSING IN THE TWENTIETH CENTURY

The beginning of the twentieth century brought about changes that have greatly influenced contemporary nursing. Several landmark reports about medical and nursing education, early insurance plans, the establishment of visiting nurse associations and their use of protocols, and health care initiatives are discussed next.

Flexner Report

In 1910, Abraham Flexner, supported by a Carnegie grant, visited the 155 medical schools in the United States and Canada. The goal of the resulting Flexner report, which was based on his findings, was to impose accountability for medical education. Flexner's study resulted in the closure of inadequate medical schools, consolidation of schools with limited resources, creation of nonprofit status for remaining schools, and establishment of medical education in university settings that was based on standards and strong economic resources.

Seeing the value and impact of the Flexner report on medical education, Adelaide Nutting, together with colleagues from the Superintendents' Society, presented a proposal to the Carnegie Foundation in 1911 to study nursing education. That study was never done.

In 1906, Richard Olding Beard established a 3-year diploma school of nursing at the University of Minnesota under the College of Medicine.

Early Insurance Plans

At the turn of the twentieth century, the concepts of third-party payments and prepaid health insurance were instituted. Third-party payment is the payment by someone other than the recipient of health care (usually an insurance company) for the health care services provided. Prepaid medical plans were started in lumber and mining camps of the Pacific Northwest, where employers contracted for medical services, for which they paid a monthly fee. As the first president of the National Organization for Public Health Nursing, Lillian Wald suggested that a national health insurance plan be established.

Visiting Nurses Associations

In 1901, Lillian Wald suggested that Metropolitan Life Insurance Company enter into an agreement with the Henry Street Settlement to provide visiting nursing services to its policyholders. One form of managed care began as Wald worked with Metropolitan to expand the services of the Henry Street Settlement to other cities.

Nurses providing care in the home had experienced greater autonomy of practice than did hospital-based nurses (Figure 3-4). This led to discord among physicians regarding the scope of medical practice versus the scope of nursing practice. Some physicians encouraged nurses to do whatever was necessary to care for the sick at home, whereas other physicians believed nurses were going to take over their practice.

In 1912, the Chicago Visiting Nurse Association developed a list of standing orders for nurses to follow when providing home care. When the nurse did not have specific orders from a physician, these orders were to direct the nursing care of clients. This established the groundwork for nursing protocols.

Blue Cross and Blue Shield

The main impetus for the growth of insurance plans was the Depression. The philosophy in the United States of health care for all further contributed to the growth of insurance plans. In 1920, American hospitals offered a prepaid hospital plan, which became the prototype for Blue Cross.

The American Hospital Association laid the groundwork for an insurance company to provide benefits to subscribers when hospitalized. This eventually became Blue Cross. The American Medical Association developed Blue Shield to provide subscribers reimbursement for medical services.

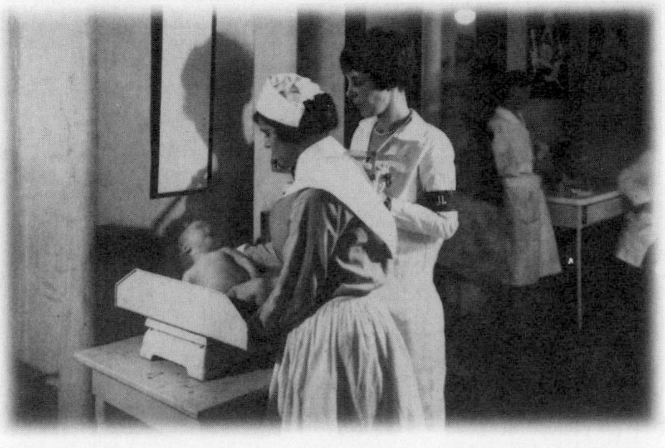

FIGURE 3-4 A baby being weighed by a student nurse and a Junior League volunteer in 1929. *(Photo courtesy of Touro Infirmary Archives, New Orleans, LA.)*

The federal government became involved in health care delivery in 1935 when the Social Security Act was passed. It provided for benefits for elderly persons, child welfare, and federal funding for educating health care personnel, among other things. During World War II, the U.S. government extended the benefits of military personnel to include their dependents and health care for veterans.

Landmark Reports in Nursing Education

Several reports were issued concerning nursing education and practice during the first half of the twentieth century. Three reports that had a profound impact on nursing education are the Goldmark, the Brown, and the Institute of Research and Service in Nursing Education.

Goldmark Report

In 1918, Adelaide Nutting approached the Rockefeller Foundation for support of nursing education reform. They provided funding, and, in 1919, the Committee for the Study of Nursing Education was established to investigate the education of public health nurses. A social worker, Josephine Goldmark, served as the secretary to the committee and developed the method of collecting data and the analysis for a small sampling of the 1,800 schools of nursing then in existence.

The Goldmark report, titled *Nursing and Nursing Education in the United States*, was published in 1923. Goldmark identified that the major weakness of the hospital-based education programs was that the needs of the institution (service delivery) were put before the needs of the student (education). The apprenticeship form of education along with nursing tradition put the needs of the client before the learning needs of the student.

Limited resources, low admission standards, poorly educated instructors, lack of supervision, and failure to correlate clinical practice with theory were identified by the study as major inadequacies in nursing education. The report concluded that nursing education should take place in the university setting if nursing was to be on equal footing with other disciplines.

Brown Report

In 1948, the social anthropologist Esther Lucille Brown published *Nursing for the Future and Nursing Reconsidered: A Study for Change*. The Brown report, published 26 years after the Goldmark report, identified many of the same problems in hospital nursing education, including the fact that nursing students were still being used for service by the hospitals, resources were inadequate, and authoritarianism still prevailed.

Brown understood that the proper intellectual climate for educating professional nurses would be the university setting. Visionary nurse educators were securing libraries, laboratories, and clinical facilities as necessary learning resources. Nurse leaders were implementing professional endeavors such as research and publication.

Institute of Research and Service in Nursing Education Report

The 1950s addressed different aspects of nursing. After World War II, a deficit in the supply of nurses coincided with an increased demand for nursing services. Hospitals were closed as a result of the nursing shortage. Other factors contributing to the scarce supply of nurses were the long hours combined with a heavy workload, low esteem of nursing as a profession, and low salaries.

The Institute of Research and Service in Nursing Education Report resulted in the establishment of practical nursing under Title III of the Health Amendment Act of 1955. There was a proliferation of practical nursing schools in the United States following this report.

Other Health Care Initiatives

In the 1960s, health care services were provided to the elderly and the indigent populations through the federal programs of Medicare and Medicaid.

The Nurse Training Act was passed in 1964 to provide federal funds to expand the enrollment in schools of nursing. Federal funds were made available to construct nursing schools and provide student loans and scholarships to nursing students.

The Health Maintenance Organization Act of 1973 provided an alternative to the private health insurance industry. **Health maintenance organizations (HMOs)** are prepaid health plans that provide primary health care services for a preset fee and focus on cost-effective treatment methods. **Primary health care** refers to the client's point of entry into the health care system and includes assessment, diagnosis, treatment, coordination of care, education, preventive services, and surveillance.

In 1977, the National Commission for Manpower Study resulted in amendments to Title XVIII of the Social Security Act, which provided payment for rural health clinic services. Anne Zimmerman, former president of the ANA, had the bill amended to substitute the term **primary care providers** (health care providers whom a client sees first for health care) for *physician extenders*, which allowed nurse practitioners to be paid directly for their services. This represented the first time that nurses could be directly reimbursed for care they rendered.

Costs and Quality Controls

During the 1970s, the rapid escalation of health care expenditures made the cost-control systems of various federal health programs inadequate. The 1982 Tax Equity Fiscal Responsibility Act (TEFRA) was passed in response to the $287 billion spent on health care in 1981. At the same time that the federal government was trying to control costs with TEFRA and prospective payment legislation, concern was also growing regarding the quality of health care.

Although business and industry embraced quality control systems in the 1940s and 1950s, the health care industry failed to see the need for such controls until the 1980s. The Joint Commission on Accreditation of Healthcare Organizations (formerly JCAHO, now the Joint Commission) in the late 1980s emphasized monitoring for quality of outcomes rather than process. This changed the system from a static quality assurance system to a dynamic quality improvement program. The Joint Commission (2008) views quality of care as an ongoing process that continuously looks for ways to improve the care provided.

CRITICAL THINKING
Learning from Experience

By studying nursing history, we gain a better understanding of autonomy, professionalism, advancements in nursing education, and nursing care. Think of some lessons you have learned from the past. Can you identify some life experiences that taught you something? List two things you learned from these experiences or situations.

Health Care Reform

With an ever-increasing number (over 60 million) of Americans being uninsured or underinsured, health care access and costs became a major focus of attention in the 1990s (Edelman & Mandle, 2002). Children are especially at risk for having their health care neglected, with one in five children in the United States being uninsured (Baker, 1994).

Nursing as a profession has made great strides in affecting federal and state health care legislation (Figure 3-5). Hospitals are moving away from the controlling, bureaucratic entities they once were and instead are more often being characterized by an environment of shared governance where nurses have a voice in both clinical and administrative decision making. Nurses now serve as case managers and collaborate with physicians and other health care providers. Advocates are working to obtain prescriptive privileges for all advanced practitioners.

Nurses are seeking to improve their scientific knowledge and client outcomes by developing evidence-based practice. Evidence-based practice is "the integration of best research evidence with clinical expertise, and patient values" (Sackett, Straus, Richardson, Rosenberg, & Haynes, 2000, p. 1). Evidence-based practice ensures best practice and best client outcomes.

NURSING EDUCATION

Educational programs that prepare graduates to take a licensing examination must be approved by a state board of nursing.

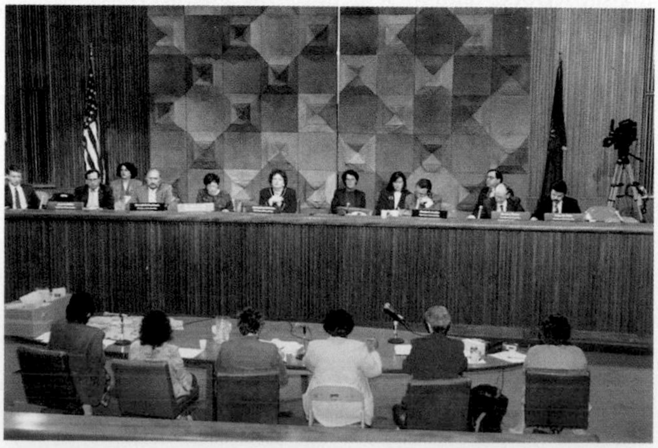

FIGURE 3-5 Nurses making a presentation before a state legislature. (*Photo courtesy of the New York State Nurses Association.*)

These boards approve entry-level programs to ensure the safe practice of nursing by setting minimum educational requirements and guaranteeing that graduates of the program are eligible candidates to take a licensing examination. Candidates in the United States must pass the National Council Licensure Examination (NCLEX®) before a state board of nursing will issue a license to practice nursing.

Types of Programs

There are two types of entry-level nursing programs available in the United States: licensed practical or vocational nurse (LPN or LVN) and registered nurse (RN). An entry-level educational program is one that prepares graduates to take a licensing examination. Graduates of licensed practical/vocational programs take the NCLEX® for practical nurses (NCLEX-PN®), and graduates of registered nurse programs take the NCLEX® for registered nurses (NCLEX-RN®).

Postgraduate programs prepare nurses to practice in various roles as advanced-practice registered nurses (APRNs). Statutory provisions for APRNs vary from state to state.

Licensed Practical/Vocational Nursing

Licensed practical nurses (LPNs) or licensed vocational nurses (LVNs, as they are called in Texas and California) work under the supervision of an RN or other licensed provider such as a physician or dentist. The LP/VN, like the RN, was first educated in hospitals. The Smith Hughes Act passed by Congress in 1917 gave impetus to the formation of vocational school–based practical nursing programs. In 2006, there were 11,172 students enrolled in practical nursing programs in the United States (National League for Nursing Accreditation Commission [NLNAC], 2008). In 2006, 8,047 new graduates entered the nursing workforce from practical nursing programs (NLNAC, 2008).

Programs are state approved and in some cases also have accreditation by the NLN. **Accreditation** is a process by which a voluntary, nongovernmental agency or organization appraises and grants accredited status to institutions and/or programs or services that meet predetermined structure, process, and outcome criteria. These educational programs are generally 1 year in length and provide both **didactic** (systematic presentation of information) and **clinical** (observing and caring for living clients) experience. The education is focused on basic nursing skills and direct client care. Although most clinical experience is in hospitals, long-term care facilities, physicians' offices, home health agencies, and ambulatory care facilities are also used.

Admission generally requires a high school diploma or General Education Development (GED) certificate. Schools may require a preentrance examination that assesses such skills as math, reading, and writing.

Once licensed, the LP/VN is prepared to work in structured settings such as hospitals, long-term care, home health, medical offices, and ambulatory care facilities. Just as the RN has been delegated duties previously considered the domain of the physician, the LP/VN has been assigned duties once considered the domain of the RN. Many hospitals offer programs that provide levels of advancement for the LP/VN.

The National Federation of Licensed Practical Nurses has written standards of nursing practice for the LP/VN. They are listed in Table 3-2.

Registered Nursing

Registered nurses are graduates of state-approved and, in many cases, NLN-accredited programs. They are prepared for entry into practice in one of three ways: hospital diploma programs, associate degree nursing programs, or baccalaureate degree nursing programs.

Diploma Program Diploma nursing programs are offered by hospitals and are typically 3 years in length. Most are now affiliated with colleges or universities that grant college credit for select courses. Graduates of these programs receive a diploma from the hospital rather than a college degree.

Program content historically prepared the graduate in basic nursing skills particularly suitable for hospitalized clients. Now, however, most diploma schools also use community-based settings such as physicians' offices, visiting nurse services, clinics, and health departments for clinical experiences.

Although prominent in the early history of nursing education, the number of diploma nursing programs in the United States has decreased. In 2006, 4% of all entry-level nursing programs in the United States were diploma programs with 11,266 students enrolled (ANA, 2008a; NLNAC, 2008). In 2006, 3,600 graduates or 8% of all new graduates eligible to enter the nursing workforce came from diploma programs (NLN, 2008a; NLNAC, 2008).

Associate Degree Program Associate degree programs are offered through community colleges and are typically 2 years in length. They may also be offered as an option at 4-year degree-granting universities. The graduate receives an associate degree in nursing (ADN). In 2006, 58.9% of all entry-level nursing programs in the United States were ADN programs with 139,008 students enrolled (ANA, 2008a; NLNAC, 2008). In 2006, 49,878 or 59% of all new graduates eligible to enter the nursing workforce came from ADN programs (NLN, 2008a; NLNAC, 2008). Traditionally, program content reflects basic skill preparation and emphasizes clinical practice in the hospital setting. Because of a decreasing use of hospital beds, however, students are now likely to spend a higher number of clinical hours in community-based institutions (e.g., ambulatory settings, clinics, or schools).

Baccalaureate Degree Program Baccalaureate degree programs are offered through colleges and universities and are typically 4 years in length. The graduate receives a bachelor of science in nursing (BSN). These programs emphasize a broader preparation for practice, not only in hospital settings but also for autonomous and collaborative practice. In 2006, 38% of all entry-level nursing programs in the United States were baccalaureate programs with 52,481 students enrolled (ANA, 2008a; NLNAC, 2008). In 2006, 14,233 graduates or 38% of all new graduates eligible to enter the nursing workforce came from baccalaureate programs (NLN, 2008a; NLNAC, 2008).

Continuing Education and Staff Development

Once a nurse is in practice, both continuing education and staff development are used to maintain the needed knowledge and skills for continuing practice.

Nurses are responsible for their own continuing education. Continuing education offers both personal and professional growth to the nurse and constitutes an essential dimension of

TABLE 3-2 Nursing Practice Standards for the Licensed Practical/Vocational Nurse

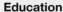

Education

The licensed practical/vocational nurse:

1. Shall complete a formal education program in practical nursing approved by the appropriate nursing authority in a state.
2. Shall successfully pass the National Council Licensure Examination for Practical Nurses.
3. Shall participate in initial orientation within the employing institution.

Legal/Ethical Status

The licensed practical/vocational nurse:

1. Shall hold a current license to practice nursing as an LP/VN in accordance with the law of the state wherein employed.
2. Shall know the scope of nursing practice authorized by the Nursing Practice Act in the state wherein employed.
3. Shall have a personal commitment to fulfill the legal responsibilities inherent in good nursing practice.
4. Shall take responsible actions in situations wherein there is unprofessional conduct by a peer or other health care provider.
5. Shall recognize and commit to meet the ethical and moral obligations of the practice of nursing.
6. Shall not accept or perform professional responsibilities that the individual knows (s)he is not competent to perform.

Practice

The licensed practical/vocational nurse:

1. Shall accept assigned responsibilities as an accountable member of the health care team.
2. Shall function within the limits of educational preparation and experience, as related to the assigned duties.
3. Shall function with other members of the health care team in promoting and maintaining health, preventing disease and disability, caring for and rehabilitating individuals who are experiencing an altered health state, and contributing to the ultimate quality of life until death.
4. Shall know and utilize the nursing process in planning, implementing, and evaluating health services and nursing care for the individual patient or group.
   a. Planning: The planning of nursing includes:
      1) assessment/data collection of health status of the individual patient, the family, and community groups
      2) reporting information gained from assessment/data collection
      3) the identification of health goals
   b. Implementation: The plan for nursing care is put into practice to achieve the stated goals and includes:
      1) Observing, recording, and reporting significant changes that require intervention or different goals
      2) Applying nursing knowledge and skills to promote and maintain health, to prevent disease and disability, and to optimize functional capabilities of an individual patient
      3) Assisting the patient and family with activities of daily living and encouraging self-care as appropriate
      4) Carrying out therapeutic regimens and protocols prescribed by an RN, physician, or other persons authorized by state law
   c. Evaluation: The plan for nursing care and its implementations are evaluated to measure the progress toward the stated goals and will include appropriate persons and/or groups to determine:
      1) The relevancy of current goals in relation to the progress of the individual patient
      2) The involvement of the recipients of care in the evaluation process
      3) The quality of the nursing action in the implementation of the plan
      4) A reordering of priorities or new goal setting in the care plan
5. Shall participate in peer review and other evaluation processes.
6. Shall participate in the development of policies concerning the health and nursing needs of society and in the roles and functions of the LP/VN.

Continuing Education

The licensed practical/vocational nurse:

1. Shall be responsible for maintaining the highest possible level of professional competence at all times.
2. Shall periodically reassess career goals and select continuing education activities that will help to achieve these goals.
3. Shall take advantage of continuing education opportunities that will lead to personal growth and professional development.
4. Shall seek and participate in continuing education activities that are approved for credit by appropriate organizations, such as the NFLPN.

Specialized Nursing Practice

The licensed practical/vocational nurse:

1. Shall have had at least one year's experience in nursing at the staff level.
2. Shall present personal qualifications that are indicative of potential abilities for practice in the chosen specialized nursing area.
3. Shall present evidence of completion of a program or course that is approved by an appropriate agency to provide the knowledge and skills necessary for effective nursing services in the specialized field.
4. Shall meet all of the standards of practice as set forth in this document.

(Reprinted with permission of the National Federation of Licensed Practical Nurses, Inc.)

lifelong learning. In some states, license renewal depends on acquiring continuing education units (CEUs) according to the board of nursing's rules. Lifelong learning is essential to career development and competency achievement in nursing practice.

Staff development generally occurs in the setting of employment and is described as the delivery of instruction to assist nurses to achieve the goals of the employer. It is guided by the accreditation standards of the Joint Commission and ANA's *Standards for Nursing Staff Development* (ANA, 1990).

Orientation is an important organizational tool for both recruitment and retention. The sessions typically occur at the beginning of employment and whenever positions or roles change. The sessions include information unique to the institution of employment, such as philosophy, goals, policies and procedures, role expectations, facilities, resources and special services, and assessment and development of competency with equipment and supplies used in the work setting.

In-service education occurs after orientation and throughout employment. It supports the nurse in acquiring, maintaining, and increasing skills to fulfill assigned responsibilities.

The American Nurses Credentialing Center (ANCC) is an international credentialing program that certifies registered nurses and advanced-practice nurses in specialty practice areas. The ANCC certification exams validate a "nurse's skills, knowledge, and abilities" (ANCC, 2009, p. 1). NAPNES provides certification for LPNs in long-term care that covers not only geriatrics but also chronic illnesses for all age-groups (NAPNES, 2009). For more information on certification for LPNs go to www.napnes.org and search for "Certifications for LPN/LVNs."

Trends in Nursing Education

Trends in nursing education reflect issues in nursing, nursing education, delivery of care, and the public's health. At the heart of many of these trends are two fundamental issues: competency development and delivery of care.

Competency Development

The debate about multiple education levels for entry into nursing practice will continue. Demonstration of basic competency by all entry-level graduates regardless of education is likely to gain great support from nursing. It allows for not only consensus about the outcome (competency) but also diversity (innovation) about the process. Many changes in nursing education are being stimulated by competency development.

Delivery of Care

The demand for nursing care will continue to be driven by a larger aging population that uses long-term care and home health services. Other changes will include expansion of primary and preventive care to focus on health promotion and wellness; an increased use of ambulatory care services because they are less expensive; increased complexity of health care delivery, which requires well-educated nurses; and increased demand to provide health services such as prenatal care, well-child clinics, adolescent clinics, and neighbor care clinics to underserved populations (such as inner-city residents).

Managed care arrangements are the delivery systems of the future. They emphasize wellness, health promotion, and disease prevention. More and more factors contributing to disease point to health behaviors as preventive interventions. The Healthy People 2010 goals, focus areas, and leading health indicators can be found on the Web at www.health.gov.

NURSING ORGANIZATIONS

Nursing organizations exist for LP/VNs and RNs. Some organizations also welcome as members those who are interested in nursing but who are not nurses. There are also many specialty nursing organizations.

All nurses are encouraged to maintain membership in a nursing organization. The organizations represent the nurses to the public; to legislative bodies, both state and national; to federal agencies; and to all health care facilities. Through these organizations, nurses' concerns about workplace issues are addressed, high standards of practice are fostered, ethics codes are established, continuing education programs are certified and provided, and nurses' general welfare is protected. It is a professional opportunity to be a participating member of a nursing organization. It is an option to present a strong unified voice regarding nursing issues. Table 3-3 provides pertinent information about selected nursing organizations.

National League for Nursing

The original organization, established in 1893, was named the American Society of Superintendents of Training Schools for Nurses. The last name change, National League for Nursing, was made in 1952. Because of the growth of practical/vocational nursing programs, the NLN established a Department of Practical Nursing Programs (now called Council of Practical Nursing Programs [CPNP]) in 1961. The NLN offers accreditation services to all nursing programs through an independent subsidiary called the National League for Nursing Accrediting Commission (NLNAC) (NLN, 2008b).

National Association of Practical Nurse Education and Service

Originally called the Association of Practical Nurse Schools, this organization was dedicated exclusively to practical nursing. The multidisciplinary membership planned the first standard curriculum for practical nursing. In 1959, the name was changed to the National Association of Practical Nurse Education and Service (NAPNES, 1998).

PROFESSIONAL TIP

Professional Memberships

Every nurse is encouraged to be involved in a nursing organization. Membership means more political clout for passing legislation to improve health care for all citizens and to improve the profession of nursing.

Nursing students have an opportunity to stay abreast of current issues and meet with local nursing leaders to discuss health care reform, alternative health care delivery models, and other issues. Then as graduates, they can share this information with both the public and legislators.

TABLE 3-3 Selected Nursing Organizations

ORGANIZATION	DESCRIPTION
National League for Nursing (NLN)	Established: 1893 as The American Society of Superintendents of Training Schools for Nurses. 1952 name changed to National League for Nursing. Purpose: To advance quality nursing education that prepares the nursing workforce to meet the needs of diverse populations in an ever-changing health care environment Activities: • Accredit (through voluntary participation from schools) nursing education programs • Conduct surveys to collect data on education programs • Provide continuing-education programs • Offer testing services, including: Achievement tests for use in nursing schools Preadmission testing for potential nursing students Membership: • Open to any individual (nurse or nonnurse) or agency interested in improving nursing services or nursing education Publications: • *Nursing Education Perspectives* • *The Scope and Practice for Academic Nurse Educators©* • *National Study of Faculty Role Satisfaction©* • *The NLN Report* • *NLN Member Update* • *Professional Development Bulletin* • *Nursing Education Policy*
National Association for Practical Nurse Education and Service, Inc. (NAPNES)	Established: 1941 Purpose: To improve the quality, education, and recognition of nursing schools and LP/VNs in the United States Activities: • Provide workshops, seminars, and continuing-education programs • Evaluate and certify continuing-education programs of others • Provide individual student professional liability insurance program • Inform legislatures and public on LP/VN issues • Authorize those who pass the Certification Examination for Practical and Vocational Nurses in Long-term Care (CEPN-LTC)™ to use the initials *CLTC* Membership: • LP/VNs • RNs, physicians, and caregivers in all fields • Practical/vocational nursing students Publications: • *Journal of Practical Nursing* • *NAPNES Forum*
National Federation of Licensed Practical Nurses, Inc. (NFLPN)	Established: 1949 Purpose: • Provide leadership for LP/VNs • Foster high standards of practical/vocational nursing education and practice • Encourage continuing education • Achieve recognition for LP/VNs • Advocate effective utilization of LP/VNs • Interpret role and function of LP/VNs • Represent practical/vocational nursing • Serve as central source of information on practical/vocational nursing education and practice Activities: • Promote continuing education of LP/VNs; evaluate programs for CEU credit • Offer IV and gerontology certification

TABLE 3-3 Selected Nursing Organizations (Continued)

ORGANIZATION	DESCRIPTION
	• Establish principles of ethics • Offer members an opportunity to participate in activities of the organization • Keep members informed on matters of interest and concern • Offer members best type of low-cost insurance • Represent and speak for LP/VNs in Congress • Encourage fellowship among LP/VNs • Develop mutual understanding and good will among members, other allied health groups, and the general public Membership: • Three-tier concept of local, state, and national enrollment • LP/VNs • Practical/vocational nursing students • Affiliate (person who has an interest in the work of NFLPN but is neither an LP/VN nor an LP/VN student) Publication: • *Practical Nursing Journal*
American Nurses Association (ANA)	Established: 1911 Purpose: To work for the improvement of health standards and availability of health care service for all people, foster high standards for nursing, stimulate and promote the professional development of nurses, and advance their economic and general welfare. Activities: • Establish standards for nursing practice • Establish a professional code of ethics • Develop educational standards • Promote nursing research • Oversee a credentialing system • Influence legislation affecting health care • Protect the economic and general welfare of registered nurses • Assist with the professional development of nurses (i.e., by providing continuing education programs) Membership: • Registered nurses only • Federation of state nurses' associations • Individual, by joining respective state nurses' association Publications: • *American Nurse Today* • *The American Nurse*
National Council of State Boards of Nursing, Inc. (NCSBN)	Established: 1978 Purpose: Provide an organization through which boards of nursing act and counsel together on matters of common interest and concern affecting the public health, safety, and welfare, including the development of licensing examinations in nursing Activities: • Develop and administer licensure examinations for registered nurse and licensed practical/vocational nurse candidates • Conduct job analyses that provide data required to support the NCLEX® examinations and the test development process • Maintain a national disciplinary data bank • Monitor and analyze issues and trends in public policy, nursing practice, and nursing education that impact nursing regulation • Serve as the national clearinghouse of information on nursing regulation • Offer educational conferences and regional meetings

(Continues)

Table 3-3 Selected Nursing Organizations (Continued)

ORGANIZATION	DESCRIPTION
	Membership: • Boards of nursing in the 50 states, the District of Columbia, and four United States territories • No individual membership Publications: • *Education Issues* • *NCLEX-PN® Program Reports* • *NCLEX-RN® Program Reports* • *NCLEX-PN® Detailed Test Plan* • *NCLEX-RN® Detailed Test Plan*

Data from About ANA (online), by American Nurses Association, 2008a, http://www.nursingworld.org/FunctionalMenuCategories/AboutANA.aspx; History of NAPNES by National Association for Practical Nurse Education and Service, Inc., 1998, Silver Spring, MD: Author; About Us (online), by National Association for Practical Nurse Education and Service, 2008, http://www.napnes.org/about/index.html; About NFLPN (online), by National Federation of Licensed Practical Nurses, 2008, http://www.nflpn.org/about.html; Bylaws, by National League for Nursing, 1995, New York: Author; About the NLN (online), by National League for Nursing, 2008, http://www.nln.org/aboutnln/index.htm; About NCSBN (online), by National Council of State Boards of Nursing, Inc., 2008a, https://www.ncsbn.org/about.htm.

National Federation of Licensed Practical Nurses

The National Federation of Licensed Practical Nurses (NFLPN) was founded in 1949 by a group of LPNs who recognized that to gain status and recognition in the health field and to have a channel through which they could officially speak and act for themselves, they needed an organization of their own. Since 1991, affiliate membership (lacking the rights to vote and hold office) has been available to anyone who is interested in the work of NFLPN but who is neither a practicing LP/VN nor an LP/VN student. The NFLPN is the official organization for LP/VNs (NFLPN, 2008).

American Nurses Association

The ANA represents registered nurses through its constituent state organizations. The ANA fosters high standards of nursing practice, promotes the economic and general welfare of nurses in the workplace, projects a positive and realistic view of nursing, and lobbies Congress and regulatory agencies on health care issues affecting nurses and the public (ANA, 2008a).

National Council of State Boards of Nursing

The National Council of State Boards of Nursing (NCSBN) was established in 1978 to assist member boards, collectively and individually, to promote safe and effective nursing practice in the interest of protecting public health and welfare. They have developed the NCLEX-PN® and NCLEX-RN® to test the entry-level nursing competence of candidates for licensure as LP/VNs and RNs.

In 1996, they began administration of the first large-scale, national certification examination available to LP/VNs. It is named the Certification Examination for Practical and Vocational Nurses in Long-Term Care (CEPN-LTC™). Those who pass the examination are certified in long-term care and are authorized by NAPNES to use the initials CLTC to signify their new status (Washington State Department of Health: The Nursing Commission Newsletter, 1999).

CASE STUDY

C.J. is a new nursing student. One of his first assignments is to read a chapter on nursing history. C.J. thinks that history is boring and considers skipping the assignment. However, he desires to make good grades and is a dedicated nursing student, so he reads the chapter.

1. How will knowing nursing history affect C.J.'s view of nursing?
2. What is presently happening in nursing that will become part of the nursing history archives in 10 years?
3. What is presently happening in nursing or legislation that will change the face of nursing in 5 years?

SUMMARY

- Nursing is the art and science of assisting people in learning to care for themselves whenever possible and of caring for them when they are unable to meet their own needs.
- By studying nursing history, the nurse is better able to understand such issues as autonomy, unity within the profession, supply and demand, salary, education, and current practice and can thus promote the empowerment of nurses.
- Nursing's early history was heavily influenced by religious organizations and the need for nurses to care for soldiers during wartime.
- Florence Nightingale forged the future of nursing practice and education as a result of her experiences in educating nurses to care for soldiers.
- Early American leaders, professional organizations, and landmark reports of nursing determined the infrastructure of current nursing practice.
- Influential nursing leaders such as Lillian Wald, Isabel Hampton Robb, Adelaide Nutting, and Lavinia Dock were instrumental in the advancement of nursing education and practice.
- Other nursing leaders such as Mary Breckenridge, Mary Mahoney, and Linda Richards made important contributions to both nursing education and practice.
- In 1923, the Goldmark Report concluded that for nursing to be on equal footing with other disciplines, nursing education should occur in the university setting.
- The Brown Report (1948) addressed the need for nurses to demonstrate greater professional competence by moving nursing education to the university setting.
- Title III of the Health Amendment Act of 1955 resulted in the establishment of practical nursing.
- The Health Maintenance Organization Act of 1973 provided an alternative to the private health insurance industry.
- Types of programs that currently prepare nurses for entry-level practice are practical/vocational, diploma, associate degree, and baccalaureate degree.

REVIEW QUESTIONS

1. The founder of modern nursing is considered to be:
   1. Lillian Wald.
   2. Dorothea Dix.
   3. Florence Nightingale.
   4. The Nursing Sisters of the Holy Cross.
2. The first practical nursing school was:
   1. Ballard School.
   2. Thompson Practical Nursing School.
   3. Bellevue Training School for Nurses.
   4. Household Nursing Association School of Attendant Nursing.
3. Practical nursing was established under:
   1. Bureau of Medical Services, 1908.
   2. Health Maintenance Organization Act of 1973.
   3. Title III of the Health Amendment Act of 1955.
   4. Nursing and Nursing Education in the United States, 1923.
4. A nursing organization that accredits schools of nursing is:
   1. ANA.
   2. NLN.
   3. NFLPN.
   4. NAPNES.
5. The National Council of State Boards of Nursing began administering a national certification examination available to the LP/VN. It is for:
   1. licensure.
   2. acute care.
   3. accreditation.
   4. long-term care.
6. The science of nursing is evidenced by: (Select all that apply.)
   1. critical thinking skills.
   2. using scientific knowledge.
   3. caring behaviors.
   4. using evidence-based practice.
   5. providing comfort and dignity in death.
   6. evidence-based practice.
7. The official organization to speak and act for the LPN/VN is the:
   1. National Council of State Boards of Nursing.
   2. American Nurses Association.
   3. National League of Nursing.
   4. National Federation of Licensed Practical Nurses.
8. A nurse desires to join a nursing organization because such organizations: (Select all that apply.)
   1. protect the nurse's welfare.
   2. stress best standards of nursing practice.
   3. establish the nurse's code of conduct and practice.
   4. develop curricula for nursing education programs.
   5. oversee and discipline nursing misconduct.
   6. leave continuing education programs to hospitals.
9. Studying nursing history: (Select all that apply.)
   1. gives the nurse a sense of autonomy.
   2. encourages nurses to make a positive impact on present nursing events.
   3. serves only to give a view of previous nursing events.
   4. enhances the present view of current practice.
   5. has little relevance to current nursing practices.
   6. increases understanding of advances in nursing education.

10. Nursing as a science: (Select all that apply.)
    1. promotes restores, and maintains the health of clients.
    2. is founded on evidence-based research.
    3. uses nursing principles based on scientific theory.
    4. is demonstrated in skillful caring acts.
    5. is individualized care based on the client's needs and preferences.
    6. is the application of data collection (research) in client care.

REFERENCES/SUGGESTED READINGS

American Nurses Association. (1990). Standards for nursing staff development. Kansas City, MO: Author.

American Nurses Association. (2008a). About ANA. Retrieved September 29, 2008, from http://www.nursingworld.org/FunctionalMenuCategories/AboutANA.aspx

American Nurses Association. (2008b). About nursing. Retrieved September 29, 2008, from http:/www.nursingworld.org/MainMenuCategories/CertificationandAccreditaition/AboutN

American Nurses Association. (2008c). ANA bylaws. Retrieved September 29, 2008, from http://www.nursingworld.org/DocumentVault/MemberCenter/ANABylaws2006PDF.aspx

American Nurses Association. (2008d). ANA's statement of purpose. Retrieved September 29, 2008, from http://www.nursingworld.org/FunctionalMenuCategories/AboutANA/WhoWeAre/ANAsStatementofPurpose.aspx

American Nurses Association. (2009). What is nursing? Retrieved February 7, 2009, from http://www.nursingworld.org/EspeciallyForYou/StudentNurses/WhatisNursing.aspx

American Nurses Credentialing Center. (2009). About ANCC. Retrieved February 7, 2009, from http://www.nursecredentialing.org/FunctionalCategory/AboutANCC.aspx

Anglin, L. (2000). Historical perspectives: Influences of the past. In J. Zerwekh (Ed.), *Nursing today: Transitions and trends* (3rd ed.). Philadelphia: W. B. Saunders.

Baker, C. (1994). School health: Policy issues. *Nursing and Health Care, 15*(4), 178–184.

Bell, P. (1993). "Making do" with the midwife: Arkansas' Mamie O. Hale in the 1940s. *Nursing History Review*, 155–169.

Calhoun, J. (1993, March). The Nightingale pledge: A commitment that survives the passage of time. *Nursing and Health Care, 14*(3), 130–136.

Cushing, A. (1995, Summer). A historical note on the relationship between nursing and nursing history. *International History Nursing Journal, 1*(1), 57–60.

Department of Health and Human Services: Centers for Disease Control and Prevention. (2008). Health people 2010. Retrieved September 29, 2008, from http://www.cdc.gov/nchs

Dossey, B. (1995). Endnote: Florence Nightingale today. *Critical Care Nursing, 15*(4), 98.

Edelman, C., & Mandle, C. (2002). *Health promotion throughout the lifespan* (5th ed.). St. Louis, MO: Mosby.

Estabrooks, C. (1995). Lavinia Lloyd Dock: The Henry Street years. *Nursing History Review, 3*, 143–172.

Guide to Nursing Organizations. (2000). *Nursing2000, 30*(5), 54–56.

Humphreys, K. (2002). Guide to 2002 nursing organizations. *Nursing 2002, 32*(5), 46–48.

Joint Commission on the Accreditation of Healthcare Organizations. (2008). Principles respecting joint commission core performance measurement activities. Retrieved September 29, 2008, from http://www.jointcommission.org/NR/rdonlyres/A2C1C8AF-D879-41DD-A4DF-E6D9CCA21362/0/AttachAPMPrinciplesFinalWebVersion.pdf

Kauffman, C. (1978). *The ministry of healing*. New York: Seabury Press.

Macrae, J. (1995). Nightingale's spiritual philosophy and its significance for modern nursing. *Image: Journal of Nursing Scholarship, 27*(1), 8–10.

Mason, D., & Leavitt, J. (1995). The revolution in health care: What's your readiness quotient? *American Journal of Nursing, 95*(6), 50–54.

Mohr, W. (2005). *Psychiatric-mental health nursing* (6th ed.). Philadelphia: Lippincott Williams & Wilkins.

National Association for Practical Nurse Education and Service. (1998). *History of NAPNES*. Silver Spring, MD: Author.

National Association for Practical Nurse Education and Service. (2008). About us. Retrieved September 29, 2008, from http://www.napnes.org/about/index.html

National Association for Practical Nurse Education and Service. (2009). Certifications for LPN/LVNs. Retrieved February 7, 2009, from http://www.napnes.org/certifications.htm

National Council of State Boards of Nursing. (2008a). About NCSBN. Retrieved September 29, 2008, from https://www.ncsbn.org/about.htm

National Council of State Boards of Nursing. (2008b). What is NCLEX? Retrieved September 29, 2008, from https://www.ncsbn.org/1200.htm

National Federation of Licensed Practical Nurses. (2008). About NFLPN. Retrieved September 29, 2008, from http://www.nflpn.org/about.html

National League for Nursing. (1995). *Bylaws*. New York: Author.

National League for Nursing. (1998). Research Department Communication. New York: Author.

National League for Nursing. (2000, August 15). *Unofficial, unpublished data from 1998*. Research Department Communication.

National League for Nursing. (2008a). About the NLN. Retrieved September 29, 2008, from http://www.nln.org/aboutnln/index.htm

National League for Nursing. (2008b). Number of nursing school graduates—Including ethnic and racial minorities—On the rise. Retrieved September 29, 2008, from http://www.nln.org/newsreleases/data_release_03032008.htm

National League for Nursing Accrediting Commision. (2008). NLNAC 2008 report to constituents. Retrieved September 29, 2008, from http://www.nlnac.org/reports/2008.htm

Navsource.com. (2007). NavSource online: Service ship photo archive. Retrieved on February 9, 2009, from http://www.navsource.org/archives/09/12/1202.htm

Nightingale, F. (1969). *Notes on nursing: What it is and what it is not*. New York: Dover.

Ogren, K. (1994). The risk of not understanding nursing history. *Holistic Nursing Practice, 8*(2), 10.

Pokorny, M. (1992). An historical perspective of confederate nursing during the Civil War, 1861–1865. *Nursing Research, 41*(1), 29.

Sackett, D., Straus, S., Richardson, W., Rosenberg, W., & Haynes, R. (2000). *Evidence-based medicine: How to practice and teach EBM* (2nd ed.). Edinburgh: Churchill Livingstone.

Secretary's Commission on Nursing. (1988). *Final report*. Washington, DC: Department of Health and Human Services.

Selanders, L. (1994). *Florence Nightingale: An environmental adaptation theory*. Newbury Park, CA: Sage.

Silverstein, N. (1994). Lillian Wald at Henry Street, 1893–1895. In P. L. Chinn (Ed.), *Developing the discipline: Critical studies in nursing history and professional issues.* Gaithersburg, MD: Aspen.

Summers, S. (2008). What is magnet status and how's that whole thing going? Retrieved September 10, 2008, from http://www.nursingadvocacy.org/faq/magnet.html

U.S. Department of Health and Human Services. (1996). The registered nurse population. Washington, DC: Author.

Washington State Department of Health: The Nursing Commission Newsletter. (1999). Self directed care. Retrieved September 29, 2008, from https://fortress.wa.gov/doh/hpqa1/hps6/Nursing/documents/nwsltr_f99.pdf

Wall, B. (1993). Grace under pressure: The nursing sisters of the Holy Cross, 1861–1865. *Nursing History Review,* 71–88.

Wilson, Sprouse, D., Gause, G., Jr., Tallent, D., Ahlfield, R., Holbrook, B. (2009). The story of men in American nursing. Retrieved February 9, 2009, from http://www.geocities.com/Athens/Forum/6011/sld002.htm

Wolf, P. (2003). Guide to nursing organizations. *Nursing 2003, 33*(5), 50–52.

RESOURCES

American Association of the History of Nursing (AAHN), http://www.aahn.org

American Nurses Association (ANA), http://www.ana.org

National Association for Practical Nurse Education and Service (NAPNES), http://www.napnes.org

National Council of State Boards of Nursing (NCSBN), http://www.ncsbn.org

National Federation of Licensed Practical Nurses (NFLPN), http://www.nflpn.org

National League for Nursing (NLN), http://www.nln.org

National League for Nursing Accrediting Commission (NLNAC), http://www.nlnac.org

CHAPTER 4
Legal and Ethical Responsibilities

MAKING THE CONNECTION

Refer to the following chapters to increase your understanding of legal and ethical responsibilities:

Basic Nursing

- ***Student Nurse Skills for Success***
- ***Nursing Process/Documentation/ Informatics***
- ***Cultural Considerations***
- ***End-of-Life Care***
- ***Safety/Hygiene***

LEARNING OBJECTIVES

Upon completion of this chapter, you should be able to:

- Define key terms.
- Describe the difference between public law and civil law.
- State the purpose and identify various sources of standards of practice.
- Discuss the difference between intentional and unintentional torts.
- Discuss ways that informed consent impacts nursing practice.
- Discuss the concept of advance directives.
- Describe the purpose and correct utilization of an incident report.
- Discuss ways the nurse can reduce personal liability.
- Identify the benefits of having one's own malpractice insurance policy.
- List steps to be taken when suspecting a colleague of being impaired by drugs or alcohol.
- Describe the major ethical principles that have an impact on health care.
- Explain the link between ethics and values and the process involved in reconciling the potential conflicts between them.
- Relate the ethical code developed by the National Federation of Licensed Practical Nurses daily nursing practice.
- Identify the rights of the client as established by the American Hospital Association.
- Discuss the roles of the nurse as client advocate and whistle-blower in the delivery of ethical nursing care.

KEY TERMS

active euthanasia
administrative law
advance directive
assault
assisted suicide
autonomy
battery
beneficence
bioethics
civil law
client advocate
confidential
constitutional law
contract law
criminal law
defamation
deontology
durable power of attorney for health care (DPAHC)
ethical dilemma
ethical principles
ethical reasoning
ethics
euthanasia
expressed contract
false imprisonment
felony
fidelity
formal contract
fraud
Good Samaritan laws
impaired nurse
implied contract
incident report
informed consent
justice
law
liability
libel
living will
malpractice
material principle of justice
misdemeanor
negligence
nonmaleficence
nursing practice act
passive euthanasia
peer assistance programs
privacy
public law
restraint
slander
standards of practice
statutory law
teleology
tort
tort law
utility
value system
values
values clarification
veracity
whistle-blowing

INTRODUCTION

Nursing, which embodies a concern for the client in every aspect of life, encompasses a great responsibility—one that requires knowledge, skill, care, and commitment. As society and technology change, the issues affecting nursing practice also change. We continue to recognize the importance of the right to decide what is best for oneself, informed consent, and belief in the client's bill of rights; however, difficult issues, such as advance directives, do-not-resuscitate (DNR) orders, and impaired nurses, now must be faced by the nursing profession. The delivery of ethical health care is becoming an increasingly difficult and confusing issue in contemporary society. Nurses are committed to respecting their clients' rights in terms of providing health care and treatment. This desire to maintain clients' rights, however, often conflicts with professional duties and institutional policies. Nurses must thus learn to balance these potentially conflicting perspectives to achieve the primary objective—the care of the client. This chapter provides a general overview of many legal and ethical concepts that affect nursing.

BASIC LEGAL CONCEPTS

Because it is useful to have working definitions of some basic legal concepts before applying them to a health care setting, a discussion of pertinent legal concepts follows.

DEFINITION OF LAW

Laws are decisions about conduct that guide the interactions of people. Laws are necessary, binding, and enforceable so people can live and work together. When laws are broken, a penalty is incurred.

The word **law** is derived from an Anglo-Saxon term meaning "that which is laid down or fixed." The two types of law are **public law**, which deals with the individual's relationship to the state, and **civil law**, which deals with relationships among individuals.

SOURCES OF LAW

The four sources of public law at the federal and state levels are constitutional, statutory, administrative, and criminal. At the federal and state levels, the three sources of civil law are contracts, torts, and protective/reporting laws.

Public Law

Constitutional law, set forth in the U.S. and state constitutions, defines and limits the powers of government. **Statutory law** is enacted by legislative bodies. State boards and professional practice acts, such as nursing practice acts, are created and governed under statutory laws.

Administrative law (regulatory law) is developed by those persons appointed to governmental administrative agencies. These persons are entrusted with enforcing the statutory laws passed by the legislature. Administrative law gives state boards of nursing the power to make rules and regulations governing nursing as set forth in the nursing practice acts. In these administrative rules, nursing boards delineate the specific processes for educational programs, licensure, grounds for disciplinary proceedings, and the establishment of fees for services and for penalties rendered by the board.

Criminal law, the most common example of public law, addresses acts or offenses against the safety or welfare of

Table 4-1 Types of Public Law

TYPE	FEDERAL EXAMPLES	STATE EXAMPLES
Constitutional law	U.S. Constitution Civil Rights Act	State constitutions
Statutory law	None	Various state boards and professional practice acts
Administrative law	Social Security Act National Labor Relations Act	Rules and regulations of various state boards
Criminal law	Controlled Substance Act Homicide	Criminal codes (defining manslaughter, murder, criminal negligence, rape, illegal possession of drugs, fraud, theft, assault, and battery)

the public. Under criminal law, there are two types of crime: **felony** (a crime of a serious nature that is usually punishable by imprisonment at a state penitentiary or by death or a crime violating a federal statute that involves punishment of more than 1 year incarceration) and **misdemeanor** (offense less serious than a felony that may be punishable by a fine or a sentence to a local prison for less than 1 year). Table 4-1 outlines the types of public law.

Civil Law

Civil law addresses crimes against a person(s) in matters such as contracts, torts, and protective/reporting law (Table 4-2). Most cases of malpractice fall under the civil law of torts (Flight, 2004).

Contract law is the enforcement of agreements among private individuals. The three essential elements in a legal contract are:

- Promise(s) between two or more legally competent individuals that state what each individual must do or not do
- Mutual understanding of the terms and obligations the contract imposes on each individual
- Compensation for lawful actions performed

Contract terms may be agreed on in writing or orally; however, a **formal** (written) **contract** cannot be changed legally by an oral agreement. An **expressed contract** gives, in writing, the conditions and terms of the contract. An **implied**

Table 4-2 Types of Civil Law

TYPE	FEDERAL EXAMPLES	STATE EXAMPLES
Contract law	None	Business contracts with clients Employment contracts
Torts	Federal Torts Claims Act	State Torts Claims Act (allows claims against the state) Assault Battery Defamation (libel and slander) Fraud False imprisonment Invasion of privacy Negligence (common law claim) Malpractice statutes (professional liability)
Protective/reporting laws	Child Abuse Prevention and Treatment Act Privacy Act of 1974	Good Samaritan law Abuse statutes (domestic violence, child, elderly) Age of consent statutes (medical treatment, drugs, sexually transmitted disease) Americans with Disabilities Act Living will legislation Involuntary Hospitalization Act Abortion statute

PROFESSIONALTIP

Good Samaritan Laws

Good Samaritan laws vary in coverage from state to state and may be amended periodically by legislation. It is the responsibility of caregivers to know the law for their respective jurisdictions.

contract acknowledges a relationship between parties for services.

In accord with U.S. Contract Law, the nurse is legally required to:

- Follow the employer's policies and standards unless they conflict with state or federal law
- Complete the terms of contracted service with the employer
- Respect the rights and responsibilities of other health care providers, especially to promote continuity of client care

Along with these legal responsibilities, the nurse has a right to expect:

- Adequate and qualified assistance in providing care
- Reasonable and prudent conduct from the client
- Compensation from the employer for services rendered
- A safe work environment with the necessary resources to render services
- Prudent, reasonable conduct from other health care providers

A **tort** is a civil wrong committed by a person against another person or property (Zerwekh & Claborn, 2003). **Tort law** is the enforcement of duties and rights among individuals independent of contractual agreements.

The protective/reporting law may be considered criminal law, depending on classification by the state. Two examples of protective law are the Americans with Disabilities Act (ADA) and the Good Samaritan laws.

The ADA was passed by the U.S. Congress in 1990. It prohibits discrimination in employment, public services, and public accommodations on the basis of disability. The ADA defines a disability as a physical or mental impairment that substantially limits one or more of the major life activities.

All 50 states and the District of Columbia have enacted **Good Samaritan laws**, which protect health care providers by ensuring immunity from civil **liability** (obligation one has incurred or might incur through any act or failure to act).

The Good Samaritan law applies only in emergency situations, usually those outside the hospital setting. It stipulates that the health care worker must not be acting for an employer or receive compensation for care given. In most states, health care professionals are not required to stop at the scene of accidents. If they do stop, however, they are held to higher standards than is a layperson. Health care professionals are expected to use their specialized body of knowledge when providing care. They are expected to act as would most other professionals with the same background and education.

THE LAW AND NURSING PRACTICE

Nursing practice falls under both public law and civil law. In all states, nurses are bound by rules and regulations stipulated by the **nursing practice act** as determined by the legislature.

Public laws are designed to protect the public. When these laws are broken by a nurse, while either on or off duty, she can be punished by paying a fine, losing her license, or being incarcerated. For example, a nurse guilty of diverting drugs, which is a crime against the state, could lose her license to practice and could be sent to jail. There is a common misconception that this only applies to the nurse's work behavior or that marijuana is not included.

Civil laws deal with problems occurring between a nurse and a client. For example, if a nurse catheterizing a client perforates the bladder, the client has sustained injury. No law affecting the population as a whole has been broken, but the client may bring a civil suit against the nurse. The client may receive compensation for injuries, but the nurse receives no jail time.

Multistate nursing practice has become a pressing issue with telehealth, transporting of clients across state lines, and employment by staffing companies operating in several states (Ventura, 1999b). The National Council of State Boards of Nursing (NCSBN), in 1997, endorsed a model of nursing regulations for RNs and LP/VNs now called the Nurse Licensure Compact that allows nurses licensed in one of the compact states to practice in any of the compact states. Nurses are licensed in their state of residence. When necessary, disciplinary action may be taken by any of the compact states against a nurse, even when licensed by another compact state. The 15 states that have passed the legislation and have implemented this compact are Arizona, Arkansas, Delaware, Idaho, Iowa, Maine, Maryland, Mississippi, Nebraska, North Carolina, North Dakota, South Dakota, Texas, Utah, and Wisconsin. Three states—Indiana, New Jersey, and Tennessee—are writing their rules for implementation (NCSBN, 2002).

STANDARDS OF PRACTICE

State boards of nursing have the responsibility of regulating nursing practice and setting educational guidelines for the programs. They stipulate who may practice nursing in their respective states through licensure. The related criteria usually involve graduating from a state-approved program, passing the National Council Licensure Exam (NCLEX)®, and meeting certain legal and moral standards. The boards have authority to bring disciplinary action against a nurse for violation of its rules and regulations. Disciplinary action may include revocation or suspension of the nurse's license and/or a fine.

PROFESSIONALTIP

Nursing Practice Act

Nursing practice acts state those things that the nurse can and cannot do. The nurse is responsible to know the state practice act for any state that she practices in.

From the nursing practice acts, guidelines have been developed to direct nursing care. These guidelines are called **standards of practice** or standards of care.

Standards of practice are also derived from other sources. Professional organizations such as the American Nurses Association (ANA) for the registered nurse (RN) and the National Federation of Licensed Practical Nurses (NFLPN) for the LP/VN have also developed standards of practice. Nursing care planning books, especially for specialized areas, are other resources for practice standards.

Policy and procedure manuals also represent standards of practice. Each facility has identified specific ways of performing procedures such as collecting specimens, passing medications, and inserting catheters. Nurses employed by the facility are expected to follow the guidelines in the policy and procedure manuals. For situations not covered in the policy and procedure manuals, the nurse is expected to exercise good judgment. In other words, the nurse is expected to act in a reasonable and prudent manner.

What is meant by reasonable and prudent? In nursing, it means that the nurse is expected to act as would other nurses at the same professional level and with the same amount of education or experience. If most nurses respond to a particular situation in a certain way, and the nurse in question does too, the nurse is acting in a reasonable and prudent manner; however, if most nurses respond differently than the nurse in question, the nurse is not be behaving in a reasonable and prudent manner and can be held responsible or liable for damages. Liability is determined by whether the standards of practice were adhered to.

Legal Issues in Practice

Many aspects relating to nursing practice and areas of nursing are subject to liability, including physician's orders, floating, inadequate staffing, critical care, and pediatric care. Nurses are held accountable to the stricter of either the state practice act or the policies of the facility of employment.

Physician's Orders

The physician is in charge of directing the client's care, and nurses are to carry out the physician's orders for care, unless the nurse believes that the orders are in error or would be harmful to the client. In this case, the physician must be contacted to confirm and/or clarify the orders. If the nurse still believes the orders to be inappropriate, the nursing supervisor should be immediately contacted and why the orders are not being carried out put in writing. A nurse who carries out an erroneous or inappropriate order may be held liable for harm experienced by the client. *Nurses are responsible for their actions regardless of who told them to perform those actions.*

Floating

Nurses sometimes are asked to "float" to an unfamiliar nursing unit. The supervisor should be informed about a float nurse's lack of experience in caring for the type of clients on the new nursing unit. The nurse should be given an orientation to the new unit and will be held to the same standards of care as are the nurses who regularly work on that unit.

Inadequate Staffing

The Joint Commission on Accreditation of Healthcare Organizations (JCAHO) has established guidelines for determining the number of staff needed for any given situation (staffing ratios) (JCAHO, 2008). When there are not enough nurses to meet the staffing ratio and provide competent care, substandard care may result, placing clients at physical risk and the nurse and institution at legal risk. The nurse in this situation should provide nursing administration with a written account of the situation. *A nurse who leaves an inadequately staffed unit could be charged with client abandonment.*

Critical Care

Because the monitors used in critical care units are not infallible, constant observation and assessment of clients are required. This makes a 1:1 or a 1:2 nurse–client ratio imperative. Furthermore, equipment must be checked regularly and on a schedule by the biomedical department.

Pediatric Care

Legislation in each state requires that suspected child abuse or neglect be reported. Legal immunity is provided to the person who makes a report in good faith. When suspected child abuse or neglect is not reported by health care providers, legal action, civil or criminal, may be filed against them.

NURSE–CLIENT RELATIONSHIP

Situations can develop between a nurse and a client that may require legal intervention. The types of torts that may arise are discussed following.

Torts

When a case is brought against a nurse, it is usually a civil action that falls under tort law. Torts can be intentional or

CULTURAL CONSIDERATIONS

Assault and Battery Charges

To prevent assault and battery charges, note the following:

- Respect the client's cultural values, beliefs, and practices with regard to "touching."
- African Americans sometimes view touching another person's hair as offensive.
- Asian Americans usually do not touch others during conversations. Touching someone on the head is considered disrespectful because the head is considered sacred.
- European Americans employ handshakes for formal greetings.
- Hispanic Americans are very tactile and may embrace and shake hands when greeting one another.
- Native Americans prohibit touching a dead body. This may leave the offender open to charges of assault.

TABLE 4-3 Selected Torts: Definitions and Examples

TYPE OF TORT	DEFINITION	EXAMPLE
Intentional		
Assault	Threaten or attempt to touch another person.	Tells client he will be tied in bed if he tries to get out.
Battery	Unconsented touching.	A treatment is performed against the client's will.
False imprisonment	Unwarranted restriction of the freedom of an individual.	A client who is of sound mind and is not in danger of inflicting injury on self or another is restrained.
Quasi-intentional		
Invasion of privacy	All individuals have the right to privacy and may bring charges against any person who violates this right.	Information is disclosed about a client that is considered private or photographs taken without client consent.
Defamation (libel and slander)	Verbal (slander) or written (libel) remarks that may cause the loss of an individual's reputation.	A statement is made that could either ruin the client's reputation or cause the client to lose his or her job.
Unintentional		
Negligence	Failure to use such care as a reasonably prudent person would use under similar circumstances, which leads to harm.	Client's property is lost. A medication error occurs. A client is burned from the improper use of equipment. A change in the client's condition is not observed and/or reported. Inaccurate count of sponges in the operating room is taken.
Malpractice	Failure of a professional to use such care as a reasonably prudent member of the profession would use under similar circumstances, which leads to harm.	An inaccurate nursing diagnosis is made and the wrong treatment is implemented. Physician's orders are not followed. Physician's clearly erroneous order is not questioned.

unintentional (Table 4-3). The person who commits an intentional tort violates the civil rights of another individual knowingly and willfully. Examples of intentional torts are assault and battery, defamation (libel and slander), fraud, false imprisonment, and invasion of privacy. Unintentional torts are those actions that cause harm to the client resulting from carelessness or negligence by the nurse. If found liable, the nurse generally must pay monetary damages. Prison terms are rare.

Intentional Torts

Assault and battery, defamation, fraud, false imprisonment, and invasion of privacy are types of intentional torts.

Assault and Battery **Assault** and **battery** are in fact two separate terms. Assault is the threat to do something that may cause harm or be unpleasant to another person. Battery is the unauthorized or unwanted touching of one person by another.

The key elements in assault are fear and intimidation. The person assaulted must believe that the threat can and will be carried out; for example, a client confined to a wheelchair is told, "If you do not finish your meal, you are going to sit there all night." The client complies because he believes the health care worker will leave him to sit there. The client knows the worker is in a position to carry out this threat.

Consent is the key factor in battery. People have the right to be free of unwanted handling of their person. Striking a client, performing a procedure without the client's consent, and forcing a person to take medication he does not want are all battery. Any unwanted touching can be construed as battery.

Defamation **Defamation** is using words to harm or injure the personal or professional reputation of another person. If the words are written down, they constitute **libel**. If the information is communicated verbally to a third party, it constitutes **slander**.

Negative or derogatory comments that are untrue leave the nurse no defense against charges of defamation. If comments are true, the relevance of the information is important. The most common examples of this tort are giving out inaccurate or inappropriate information from the medical record; discussing clients, families, or visitors in public areas; or speaking negatively about coworkers (Zerwekh & Claborn, 2003).

Fraud **Fraud** is a wrong that results from a deliberate deception intended to produce unlawful gain. Common forms of fraud in health care include deceit in obtaining or attempting to obtain a nursing license and illegal billing.

False Imprisonment **False imprisonment** refers to making the client wrongfully believe that she cannot leave a place. Any means used to confine a client or to restrict movement can be considered a restraint and a form of false imprisonment. This includes threats, physical restraints such as wrist or vest restraints, locked doors, side rails, geriatric chairs, and psychotropic drugs. A common example of this tort is telling a client not to leave the hospital until the bill is paid (Zerwekh & Claborn, 2003).

A dilemma arises when a client decides to leave the health care facility and no discharge order has been written. If the health care problem has not been resolved, the nurse may feel that it is not in the best interest of the client to leave. A client of sound mind has the right to make this decision, regardless of what others think is best. Detaining the individual could bring charges of false imprisonment.

Documentation is very important in these situations, including the client's reasons for leaving the facility and any teaching or interventions related to the situation. Facility policy usually requires that the client sign a form indicating that he is leaving against medical advice (AMA), which releases the facility of any liability. If the client refuses to sign the AMA form, the client's refusal should be documented, and the nursing supervisor and the client's physician should be notified.

Any device used to restrict movement is called a **restraint**. To prevent possible charges of false imprisonment, carefully assess the situation and include the client or significant other in the care planning process. If it is decided that a restraint is needed, the purpose and use of the restraint should be explained, including how the restraint fits into the plan of care, the length of time the restraint may be necessary, and the expected outcome. Document the planning session in the client's medical record. Documentation must show that the client is toileted, receives food and water, and has position changes.

In acute care settings, restraints can generally be applied temporarily as a nursing measure for client safety; however, in most states, a physician's order must be immediately obtained. In long-term care settings, a physician's order is required before utilizing any restraints.

Invasion of Privacy **Privacy** includes the right to be left alone, to choose care based on personal beliefs, to govern body integrity, and to choose when and how sensitive information is shared. People are entitled to **confidential** (nondisclosure of information) health care. All information gathered from working with a client or from his medical records must be kept confidential. Therefore, a client's health status may not be discussed with a third party, unless either the client is present and has given verbal permission or permission has been obtained in writing. This does not apply to nurses discussing a client's health status with other health care workers involved in the care of the client.

Invasion of privacy occurs when a person's private affairs become public knowledge without the person's permission. Photographing a client without his consent is an invasion of privacy, as is failure to pull curtains to shield the client when performing personal or intimate care.

Discussing clients in public areas is a common mistake made by health care personnel. When talking in the cafeteria or in the elevator, it is difficult to know who may overhear what is said. The client's job or family situation may be compromised, depending on the nature of the information. For example, news of an abortion, positive HIV status, or venereal disease may be socially damaging. *Clients or their health care status should never be discussed in public areas or with anyone not directly involved in the care of the client.*

To protect the client's privacy, permission should be obtained before going through a client's belongings, doors should be kept closed and curtains pulled when providing personal care, and people not involved in the performance of a procedure should not be invited to watch unless the client has given permission. Clients cannot be photographed or videotaped without their permission, and a release form must be signed. Nursing students should never use a client's full name on care plans, case studies, or other assignments. Only initials should be used to protect the client's privacy in case the papers are lost. The client's chart and other materials should not be left lying around, allowing a client's private information to become public knowledge.

Since the time of Florence Nightingale, nurses have been practicing and advocating clients' basic right to privacy and confidentiality. Now there is a federal regulation covering these aspects. On April 14, 2003, the Health Insurance Portability and Accountability Act (HIPAA) privacy regulations went into effect. Protected health information (PHI) includes all health care information that can be traced to or identified with a specific individual (Ziel & Gentry, 2003).

The rules now protect how client health care information is stored and transferred and prescribe to whom it can be revealed. Also, clients are given the right to access their health care records, amend health care information, and obtain a list of who has seen their health care records (Frank-Stromborg & Ganschow, 2002; Trossman, 2003). Clients must be given a written notice by hospitals, physicians, pharmacies, and other covered entities of their privacy practices (Frank-Stromborg & Ganschow, 2002; Ziel & Gentry, 2003). When a state's law is more stringent than HIPAA regulations, the state's law will prevail.

Unintentional Torts

Negligence and malpractice are considered unintentional torts.

Negligence **Negligence** is a general term referring to negligent or careless acts on the part of an individual who is not exercising reasonable or prudent judgment. All nurses, including student nurses, are expected to use good judgment when providing client care. For example, side rails should not be left down on confused clients' beds, and puddles and spills should be cleaned up immediately to prevent falls rather than waiting for housekeeping. Any person, even without the specialized knowledge required for nursing, could make these judgments. When a nurse fails to protect a client in such a situation or in one requiring similar judgment, the nurse could be found negligent.

Malpractice Negligent acts on the part of a professional can be termed **malpractice**, or professional negligence. Malpractice relates to the conduct of a person while acting in a professional capacity.

Not meeting the standards of care, not doing what a reasonable and prudent nurse would do in similar circumstances, results in negligent or careless acts on the part of a nurse. A nurse can be charged with malpractice for acts committed or acts omitted. Failing to properly assess a client or act on the assessment information are examples of omission. Giving a client the wrong medication and improperly performing a procedure resulting in client injury are acts of commission.

Malpractice differs from negligence in that anyone can be accused of negligence; only professionals can be accused of malpractice. Several factors must hold true for a nurse to be found guilty of malpractice (professional negligence):

- The nurse owed a special duty to the client; that is, a nurse–client relationship existed.
- The nurse failed to meet the standards of care.
- The injury occurred as a direct result of the nurse's action or inaction.
- Damage such as physical or emotional pain, suffering, monetary losses, or medical expenses must be proved. If there is not damage, the plaintiff is not entitled to an award (Lee, 2000).

The prudent nurse is protected by adhering to facility policy and procedure and attempting to meet the standards of care at all times.

Legal Risk

Nurses today are more likely to have problems for violating statutes (i.e., laws and regulations) than to be sued for malpractice (Infante, 2000). Two common sources of statutory liability are federal antifraud laws and state reporting requirements. Statutory liability may lead to criminal charges rather than just civil penalties (Infante, 2000). The best protection against statutory liability is to learn about the federal and state laws and regulations that apply to the nurse's particular practice setting. A good resource is the facility's risk manager.

Federal Antifraud Laws

The federal government has:

- Expanded the list of activities that constitute fraud
- Imposed new criminal sanctions on violators
- Increased the budget for investigating and prosecuting these activities

Infante (2000) lists as examples of fraudulent activities the following:

- Billing for services either unnecessary or not provided
- Falsifying care plans
- Forging physician's signature
- Filing false cost reports
- Falsifying or omitting information about a client's condition to obtain reimbursement

State Reporting Requirements

Nurses are required to report cases of suspected child abuse or neglect in every state (Infante, 2000). Most states also require nurses to report cases of suspected elder abuse and neglect. Infante (2000) identifies some criminal acts that must be reported. Many states require that:

- Police are notified of known or suspected cases of rape
- Reports of gunshot or stab wounds are made

Some states require that clients who have taken narcotics or who have a blood alcohol level higher than the legal limit for driving be reported.

These laws are not only for the general public but also for health care providers. If a suspected abuser is a health care provider, many states require that the event be reported to the agency that licenses that professional. Also, many states require nurses to report *any* provider who acts unprofessionally or is incompetent (Infante, 2000).

Professional Discipline

More than 5,000 nurses (RNs and LP/VNs) are annually disciplined for professional misconduct in the United States (LaDuke, 2000). That is, the nurses are found to have violated existing laws or regulations that govern a nurse's practice. LaDuke (2000) suggests that a nurse:

- Should *immediately* seek representation by an attorney specializing in professional misconduct and discipline if under investigation
- Is not obligated to talk to *any* investigator without an attorney present
- Know and understand the applicable state nursing practice act and established standards of care
- Look closely at the disciplinary process and ask questions to promote understanding

Sanctions

Boards of nursing determine and issue sanctions for nurses found to have demonstrated professional misconduct. Monetary damages are not generally awarded to consumers. A sample of sanctions from which boards of nursing may choose includes:

- Warn, censure, or reprimand the licensees.
- Impose a fine.
- Place on probation or set a condition of licensure.
- Limit the license.
- Suspend the license.
- Revoke the license.
- Dismiss the complaint.

Disciplinary Data Banks

The NCSBN maintains a Disciplinary Data Bank (DDB), as do many other professional organizations. The purpose of these data banks is to facilitate the communication of information about unsafe practitioners. In 1990, Congress created the National Practitioner Data Bank (NPDB) to improve the quality of health care by encouraging the identification and discipline of health care professionals (mostly physicians and dentists) who engage in incompetent and unsafe behavior.

As part of the HIPAA of 1996, the Healthcare Integrity and Protection Data Bank (HIPDB) was implemented in 2000. This data bank collects and discloses certain final adverse actions taken against nurses at all levels of practice, other licensed practitioners, and unlicensed persons who provide health care services or are involved in the health insurance business. The Data Banks' Proactive Disclosure Service Prototype (PDS) went online in 2007. PDS offers health care providers and facilities the opportunity to query enrolled practitioners. Health care practitioners and facilities that subscribe to PDS receive notification within 24 hours of the Data Banks' receipt of a report on any of its enrolled practitioners. PDS saves time and money when compared to the traditional method of querying the Data Banks (Health Resources and Services Administration, 2008).

DOCUMENTATION

The source of information regarding the client's clinical history is the medical record, or the chart. The chart should accurately reflect diagnosis, treatment, testing, clinical course, nursing assessment, and intervention. According to the law, "If it was not charted, it was not done." When a chart ends up in court, this is the standard the jury applies in determining what happened and who is at fault.

Medications should not be charted before they are given. This constitutes a direct violation of the standards of practice for documentation and medication administration. The standard of practice is that medications are documented *after* they are administered. All client care, including treatments, is documented after being provided.

Documentation must be objective and accurate. The nurse should describe what is seen and done. Nurses' notes should reflect facts, not inferences or opinions, about the client. It is not enough to chart nursing assessment or identified problems; any actions taken, including nursing interventions and physician's orders implemented, must also be documented.

Entries must be neat, legible, spelled correctly, written clearly, and signed or initialed. It is illegal to change a chart.

INFORMED CONSENT

Informed consent refers to a competent client's ability to make health care decisions based on full disclosure of the benefits, risks, potential consequences of a recommended treatment plan, and alternate treatments, including no treatment, and the client's agreement to the treatment as indicated by the client's signing a consent form. This detailed explanation, provided by the physician, lets the client make intelligent decisions about treatment options. Consent to treatment also protects health care workers from unwarranted charges of battery (Figure 4-1) (Delaune & Ladner, 2006).

Nurses must obtain consent for nursing procedures. Each client, on admission, signs a general care consent form. The nurse is obligated to explain what is to be done to the client and to receive at least implied consent, as indicated by lack of objection on the part of the client. Individuals who are declared incompetent are assigned a guardian or someone who has power of attorney to make heath care decisions and give consent for treatment. The physician is responsible for obtaining consent for medical or surgical treatment. The discussion about the risks and benefits of treatment generally takes place when the nurse is not present, often in the physician's office. The client usually decides on the basis of the discussion whether to accept the treatment recommendation. Confusion arises, however, because nurses are often delegated the duty of collecting the signature on the informed consent form. *Student nurses should neither ask the client to sign a consent form nor witness a consent form.*

When a nurse has a client sign the informed consent form, the nurse is verifying the following three things:

1. The client's signature is authentic.
2. The client has the mental capacity to understand what was discussed with the physician.
3. The client was not coerced into signing the form.

The client should not sign the form if the client still has questions or if the nurse is unsure about the client's understanding. The nurse should document the client's lack of understanding and contact the physician. Further clarification must come from the physician.

Clients older than age 18 may give consent for their own health care. Parents or guardians give consent for minor children. In most states, minors who live on their own, are married, become pregnant, or require treatment for sexually transmitted infections, substance abuse, or mental illness may give consent for themselves.

Complex situations occur when minors refuse treatments to which parents have consented or parents refuse consent or treatment that has been deemed medically necessary for their minor children. The court has had to intervene in such cases. In situations such as these, the child may be made a ward of the court and decision making temporarily taken away from the parents. An example would be the child of Jehovah's Witnesses who needs a blood transfusion but whose parents refuse treatment on the basis of religious beliefs.

A typical consent form (Figure 4-2) is used to obtain client permission for the performance of invasive medical, surgical, or diagnostic procedures, such as surgery, cardiac

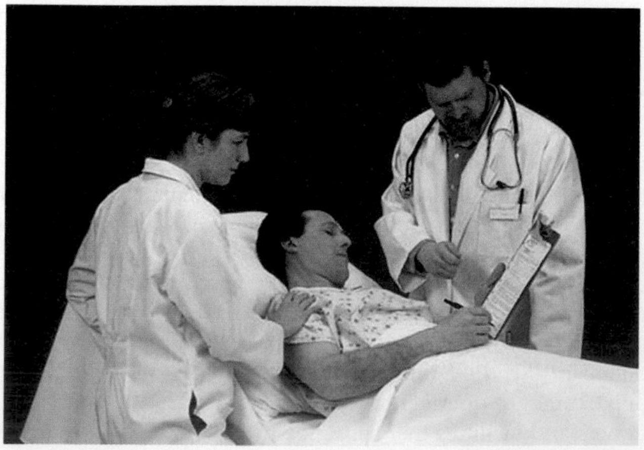

COURTESY OF DELMAR CENGAGE LEARNING

FIGURE 4-1 A nurse is witnessing the signing of a consent form after the physician has fully informed the client about the proposed treatment.

> **CLIENT TEACHING**
>
> **Informed Consent**
>
> Consent may be withdrawn, either verbally or in writing, at any time.

> **PROFESSIONAL TIP**
>
> **Consent in Emergencies**
>
> - Consent is implied when immediate action is necessary to save a life or to prevent permanent physical harm. Written consent is waived.
> - After the emergency is over, consent must be obtained for further care.

TO THE PATIENT: You have the right as a patient to be informed about your condition and the recommended surgical, medical, or diagnostic procedure to be used so that you may make the decision whether or not to undergo the procedure after knowing the risks and hazards involved. This disclosure is not meant to scare or alarm you, but is simply an effort to make you better informed so you may give or withhold your consent to the procedure. Any questions or concerns you may have with respect to the proposed procedure, its risks, complications, or benefits should be directed to your treating physician.

I (we) voluntarily request Dr. ______________________ as my physician, and such associates technical assistants and other health care providers as they may deem necessary to treat my condition, which has been explained to me as: ______________________

____

I (we) understand that the following surgical, medical, and/or diagnostic procedures are planned for me, and I (we) voluntarily consent and authorize these procedures: ______________________

____

I (we) understand that my physician may discover other or different conditions which require additional or different procedures than those planned. I (we) authorize my physician, and such associates, technical assistants, and other health care providers, to perform such procedures which are advisable in their professional judgment.

I (we) [DO] [DO NOT] consent to the use of blood and blood products as deemed necessary.

I (we) understand that no warrant or guarantee has been made to me as a result or cure.

Just as there may be risks and hazards in continuing my present condition without treatment, there are also risks and hazards related to the performance of the surgical, medical, and/or diagnostic procedures planned for me. I (we) realize that common to surgical, medical, and/or diagnostic procedures is the potential for infection, blood clots in veins and lungs, hemorrhage, allergic reactions, and even death. I (we) realize that the following risks and hazards may occur in connection with this particular procedure:

____

____

____

(Additional Consent Information On Back.)

INITIAL: ______________

CHRISTUS SPOHN HEALTH SYSTEM

DISCLOSURE AND CONSENT
MEDICAL AND SURGICAL PROCEDURES
PATIENT CARE SERVICES

2704980 NEW: 05/82
REVISED: 10/99

3025

I (we) understand that anesthesia involves additional risks and hazards, but I (we) request the use of anesthetics for the relief and protection from pain during the planned and additional procedures. I (we) realize the anesthesia may have to be changed, possibly without explanation to me (us).

I (we) understand that certain complications may result from the use of any anesthetic, including respiratory problems, drug reaction, paralysis, brain damage, or even death. Other risks and hazards which may result from the use of general anesthetics range from minor discomfort to injury to vocal cords, teeth, or eyes. I (we) understand that other risks and hazards resulting from spinal or epidural anesthetics include headache, chronic pain, remote possibility of nerve injury, hematoma, infection, septic and aseptic meningitis, nausea, vomiting, itching, and urinary retention.

I (we) consent to the photographing of the operations or procedures to be performed, including appropriate portions of the body, for medical, scientific, or educational purposes, provided my identity is not revealed by descriptive texts accompanying the picture.

I (we) consent to the disposition by hospital authorities of any tissues or parts which may be removed.

I (we) have been given the opportunity to ask questions about my conditions, alternative forms of anesthesia and treatment, risks of non-treatment, the procedures to be used, and the risks and hazards involved, and I (we) believe that I (we) have sufficient information to give this informed consent.

My physician has discussed the alternatives, risks and benefits, of the proposed procedures. I (we) certify that this form has been fully explained to me; that I (we) have read it or have had it read to me; that the blank spaces have been filled in, and that I (we) understand its contents.

____
PHYSICIAN'S SIGNATURE

DATE: ______________ TIME: ______________ A.M./P.M.

____
Witness (Signature of witness/print name of witness)

____
Patient/Other Legally Responsible Person
(Minor patient and parent/guardian signature)

FIGURE 4-2 Disclosure and Consent—Medical and Surgical Procedures (*Courtesy of CHRISTUS Spohn Health System, Corpus Christi, TX.*)

CRITICAL THINKING

Informed Consent

How would you address a situation in which a 17-year-old client is adamantly refusing to have surgery but the parents sign the consent form anyway?

catheterization, or HIV testing. Consent for procedures that are not invasive can be either given verbally or implied. Consent is implied when the client cooperates with the procedure offered. For example, if the orderly says, "Mr. Garza, I am here to take you for your hand x-ray," and Mr. Garza gets into the wheelchair, consent is implied by Mr. Garza's cooperation.

ADVANCE DIRECTIVES

An **advance directive** is a written instruction for health care, recognized under state law, related to the provision of care when the individual is incapacitated. Advance directives emphasize the client's right to self-determination. These instructions about health care preferences regarding life-sustaining measures may indicate who is to make health care decisions for the client if he becomes unable to do so for himself.

A client of sound mind has the right to make all health care decisions and even reverse previous decisions. When a situation arises and the person becomes incapable of making decisions, advance directives guide family members concerning those kinds of treatment that should or should not be allowed. Advance directives permit those involved in the decision-making process to know what the client prefers. Although these instructions are best put in writing, this is not always done. Sometimes, health care preferences are shared verbally with family members or friends. Verbal instructions can be interpreted differently by different people, creating difficulty for all involved—the physician, the health care facility, and the family. Thus, it is best to get this information in writing. When an advance directive indicates that the client does not wish to have cardiopulmonary resuscitation (CPR) performed in the event of cardiac arrest, the physician must write a DNR order, also referred to as a "No Code."

Health care facilities that receive Medicaid or Medicare monies are required to offer the opportunity to complete advance directives to all competent clients on admission. The client should be told about the availability and purpose of a living will and durable power of attorney for health care (discussed following). If desired, assistance in completing these documents is to be offered to the client. The medical record must show that the client was offered the opportunity to complete these documents, and documentation must indicate decisions made or not made at that time. Clients cannot be discriminated against for not signing an advance directive, nor can they be coerced into signing an advance directive.

PROFESSIONAL TIP

Consent in Special Situations

- If a client is unable to consent and the family is too far away, consent may be received over the telephone, according to agency policy. (Usually, two persons must hear the consent being given.)
- A client who has already received preoperative or preprocedure medication is not competent to sign a consent. When this situation arises, the surgery or procedure may have to be postponed.
- For blood transfusions, some facilities require that a denial form be signed if the client indicates *No* on the consent form.

CLIENT TEACHING

Advance Directives

- Advance directives should be discussed with the family and physician so that everyone understands the client's wishes and conflicts are less likely to occur at a later time.
- An advance directive may be changed by the client as long as the client is competent.

DURABLE POWER OF ATTORNEY FOR HEALTH CARE

A **durable power of attorney for health care (DPAHC)** is a legal document designating who may make health care decisions for a client when that client is no longer capable of decision making. This health care representative, appointed by the client, is expected to act in the best interests of the client. This appointment can be revoked any time the competent client chooses.

For example, if a client becomes comatose and the prognosis is poor, the health care representative having DPAHC can either give consent for certain types of treatment or withhold consent for treatment, even if the lack of treatment results in the client's death. Only when the client is no longer competent to make health care decisions is the DPAHC activated.

The person who has a regular power of attorney does not have the same authority about health care issues. The right to make health care decisions must be specified in the power of attorney agreement, or a DPAHC must be signed (Figure 4-3). A person who stands to benefit from the client's estate cannot be appointed health care representative.

CRITICAL THINKING

Advance Directives

You observe a coworker coercing a new nursing home resident into signing an advance directive. How would you handle this? What are the client's rights in this situation?

Part I. Durable Power of Attorney for Health Care

• If you do NOT wish to name an agent to make health care decisions for you, write your initials in the box [Initials]

This form has been prepared to comply with the "Durable Power of Attorney for Health Care Act" of Missouri.

It is suggested that only one Agent be named. However, if more than one Agent is named, anyone may act individually unless you specify otherwise.

1. Selection of agent. I appoint:
Name:__________
Address:__________
____
Telephone:__________
as my Agent.

2. Alternate Agents. Only an Agent named by me may act under this Durable Power of Attorney. If my Agent resigns or is not able or available to make health care decisions for me, or if an Agent named by me is divorced from me or is my spouse and legally separated from me, I appoint the person(s) named below (in the order named if more than one):

First Alternate Agent	Second Alternate Agent
Name:__________	Name:__________
Address:__________	Address:__________
Telephone:__________	Telephone:__________

This is a Durable Power of Attorney, and the authority of my Agent shall not terminate if I become disabled or incapacitated.

Part I. Durable Power of Attorney for Health Care (Continued)

3. Effective date and durability. This Durable Power of Attorney is effective when two physicians decide and certify that I am incapacitated and unable to make and communicate a health care decision.

• If you want ONE physician, instead of TWO, to decide whether you are incapacitated, write your initials in the box to the right. [Initials]

4. Agent's powers. I grant to my Agent full authority to:

A. Give consent to, prohibit, or withdraw any type of health care, medical care, treatment, or procedure, even if my death may result;

• If you wish to AUTHORIZE your Agent to direct a health care provider to withhold or withdraw artificially supplied nutrition and hydration (including tube feeding of food and water), write your initials in the box to the right. [Initials]

• If you DO NOT WISH TO AUTHORIZE your Agent to direct a health care provider to withhold or withdraw artificially supplied nutrition and hydration (including tube feeding of food and water), write your initials in the box to the right. [Initials]

B. Make all necessary arrangements for health care services on my behalf, and to hire and fire medical personnel responsible for my care;

C. Move me into or out of any health care facility (even if against medical advice) to obtain compliance with the decisions of my Agent; and

D. Take any other action necessary to do what I authorize here, including (but not limited to) granting any waiver or release from liability required by any health care provider, and taking any legal action at the expense of my estate to enforce this Durable Power of Attorney.

5. Agent's Financial Liability and Compensation. My Agent acting under this Durable Power of Attorney will incur no personal financial liability. My Agent shall not be entitled to compensation for services performed under this Durable Power of Attorney, but my Agent shall be entitled to reimbursement for all reasonable expenses incurred as a result of carrying out any provision hereof.

Part II. Health Care Directive

• If you DO NOT WISH to make a health care directive, write your initials in the box to the right, and go to Part III. [Initials]

I make this HEALTH CARE DIRECTIVE ("Directive") to exercise my right to determine the course of my health care and to provide clear and convincing proof of my wishes and instructions about my treatment.

If I am persistently unconscious or there is no reasonable expectation of my recovery from a seriously incapacitating or terminal illness or condition, I direct that all of the life-prolonging procedures which I have initialed below be withheld or withdrawn.

I want the following life-prolonging procedures to be withheld or withdrawn:

• artificially supplied nutrition and hydration (including tube feeding of food and water) .... [Initials]

• surgery or other invasive procedures.................. [Initials]
• heart-lung resuscitation (CPR) .... [Initials]
• antibiotic.................. [Initials]
• dialysis.................. [Initials]
• mechanical ventilator (respirator).................. [Initials]
• chemotherapy.................. [Initials]
• radiation therapy.................. [Initials]
• all other "life-prolonging" medical or surgical procedures that are merely intended to keep me alive without reasonable hope of improving my condition or curing my illness or injury.................. [Initials]

However, if my physician believes that any life-prolonging procedure may lead to significant recovery, I direct my physician to try the treatment for a reasonable period of time. If it does not improve my condition, I direct the treatment be withdrawn even if it shortens my life. I also direct that I be given medical treatment to relieve pain or to provide comfort, even if such treatment might shorten my life, suppress my appetite or my breathing, or be habit forming.

IF I HAVE NOT DESIGNATED AN AGENT IN THE DURABLE POWER OF ATTORNEY, THIS DOCUMENT IS MEANT TO BE IN FULL FORCE AND EFFECT AS MY HEALTH CARE DIRECTIVE.

Part III. General Provisions Included in the Directive and Durable Power of Attorney

YOU MUST SIGN THIS DOCUMENT IN THE PRESENCE OF TWO WITNESSES.
IN WITNESS WHEREOF, I have executed this document this______day of ______, year____.

____
Signature

Print name __________
Address __________

The person who signed this document is of sound mind and voluntarily signed this document in our presence. Each of the undersigned witnesses is at least eighteen years of age.

Signature__________	Signature__________
Print name __________	Print name __________
Address __________	Address __________

ONLY REQUIRED FOR PART I — DURABLE POWER OF ATTORNEY

STATE OF MISSOURI)
) as
)
______OF ______

On this ______day of ______, year______, before me personally appeared to me known to be the person described in and who executed the foregoing instrument and acknowledged that he/she executed the same as his/her free act and deed.

IN WITNESS WHEREOF, I have hereunto set my hand and affixed my official seal in the County of ______, State of Missouri, the day and year first above written.

____
Notary Public

My Commission Expires:

FIGURE 4-3 Durable Power of Attorney for Health Care and Health Care Directive (*Reprinted with permission of the Missouri Bar.*)

Living Will

A **living will** is a legal document that allows a person to state preferences about the use of life-sustaining measures in case she is unable to make her wishes known. These preferences can be expressed either with a living will or a Life-Prolonging Procedure Declaration. These documents allow the client to specify, in advance, those life-sustaining measures that are to be done or not done. Food, fluids, and comfort measures are generally continued, and the person is not abandoned; however, artificial means of sustaining life, such as ventilators or feeding tubes, are not to be used.

Although not all states currently recognize living wills, the client's requests should be given due weight when making health care decisions. The nurse must be knowledgeable about living will legislation in her state. A sample living will is shown in Figure 4-4.

A Life-Prolonging Procedure Declaration stating that the person wants all possible procedures done to delay the dying process, including the use of ventilators, is available in some places.

Sample Living Will

Declaration made this ____ day of __________, year______.
I, ________________________, willfully and voluntarily make known my desire that my dying not be artificially prolonged under the circumstances set forth below, and I do hereby declare:

If at any time I have a terminal condition and if my attending or treating physician and another consulting physician have determined that there is no medical probability of my recovery from such condition, I direct that life-prolonging procedures be withheld or withdrawn when the application of such procedures would serve only to prolong artificially the process of dying, and that I be permitted to die naturally with only the administration of medication or the performance of any medical procedure deemed necessary to provide me with comfort care or to alleviate pain.

It is my intention that this declaration be honored by my family and physician as the final expression of my legal right to refuse medical or surgical treatment and to accept the consequences for such refusal.

In the event that I have been determined to be unable to provide express and informed consent regarding the withholding, withdrawal, or continuation of life-prolonging procedures, I wish to designate, as my surrogate to carry out the provisions of this declaration:

Name: ________________
Address: ________________
________________ Zip Code: ________
Phone: ________________

I wish to designate the following person as my alternate surrogate, to carry out the provisions of this declaration should my surrogate be unwilling or unable to act on my behalf:

Name: ________________
Address: ________________
________________ Zip Code: ________
Phone: ________________

Additional instructions (optional):

I understand the full importance of this declaration, and I am emotionally and mentally competant to make this declaration.
Signed: ________________

Witness 1:
Signed: ________________
Address: ________________

Witness 2:
Signed: ________________
Address: ________________

FIGURE 4-4 Sample Living Will (*Reprinted by permission of Partnership for Caring, 1620 Eye Street NW, Suite 202, Washington, DC 20006.*)

INCIDENT REPORTS

An **incident report** is a risk management tool used to describe and report any unusual event that occurs to a client, visitor, or staff member. It is used by the facility to identify or track problem areas and to alert the legal department to possible lawsuits. An incident report is not a punitive device, although it is often perceived that it is.

Incident reports are completed to document such events as falls, medication errors, forgotten treatment, injuries—anything that happens out of the ordinary. An incident report may also be called a variance report or an occurrence report. The following three examples illustrate the types of occurrences that should be documented in an incident report.

- R.D. had blood drawn for various laboratory tests. It was later discovered that the laboratory work had been ordered on F.T., not R.D. The requisition had been stamped with the wrong name.
- C.S. was given Lasix 20 mg po at 9 A.M. When reviewing the physician's orders, the evening nurse discovered that Losec 20 mg had been ordered. C.S. received the wrong medication.
- M.C. was visiting her daughter, who had just given birth to the family's first grandchild. While walking down the hall, M.C. slipped and fell, injuring her right hip.

The previous examples are incidents or variances that occur in health care settings. For each situation, an incident report must be completed and channeled to the risk management department. Risk management convenes representatives from various departments, such as nursing administration, dietary services, environmental safety, and others, to review the incident reports. This group tries to identify those factors, if any, that contributed to the incident. Examples of questions asked include "Can the causal factors be eliminated or reduced?," "Does the possibility of a lawsuit exist as a result of the incident?" and "What can be done to prevent this incident from occurring again?"

Incident reports are filed by the person who was responsible for, who discovered, or who witnessed the incident. The report should state what was observed, as opposed to what is supposed. It should be concise and factual. In the third example given previously, if the nurse did not witness the actual fall, the correctly worded report would read, "M.C. found lying on floor outside room 222. Several puddles of liquid found under and around her; paper cup lying nearby." An incorrect, presumptuous, and potentially damaging report might read, "M.C. tripped and fell outside room 222. She slipped in a puddle of water." M.C. may have spilled the cup of water she was carrying during the fall; however, this second note implies that M.C. slipped in water that was already on the floor, thus implicating the facility.

Incident reports should include a description of the care given to the client or individual and the name of the physician who was notified. The incident should be charted in the client's medical record, but the incident report should not be referred to in any way. Although the incident report is not a part of the medical record, the details described in the medical record and in the incident report should be the same.

When completing an incident report, the nurse should be sure to include the date and time of the incident as well as assessments and interventions. The time that family members and physicians were notified should also be included. The nurse should refer to nursing administration policy and procedure regarding follow-up documentation.

LIABILITY INSURANCE

Many nurses assume the insurance provided by their employer is adequate and they do not need their own malpractice or liability insurance. This attitude may leave a nurse vulnerable both professionally and personally (LaDuke & Biondo, 2003).

Nurses assert they are knowledgeable and competent health care providers. Health care consumers hold nurses accountable for their actions, resulting in nurses being named as defendants in malpractice suits. Under the doctrine of *Respondeat Superior*, employers are responsible for the actions of their employees; however, if policy was violated and the employer has to pay damages, the employer has the right to sue the nurse to recover the loss. Also, this responsibility stops when the employee leaves work.

A professional liability policy provides the nurse with an attorney who will represent that nurse in court. The needs of an individual nurse will be secondary to an attorney representing the facility or a group of employees. The individual nurse is better represented in court by private counsel.

Friends and family members ask nurses for assistance and advice in health care matters. They seek this advice because of their experience and knowledge. Family members or friends might bring a law suit against the nurse later depending on the results of the advice. The nurse is accountable for the advice given even though no money was exchanged for information or services.

The nurse needs legal representation if the situation ends up in court, which is costly as are judgments against the nurse. The nurse is protected with a professional liability insurance policy that provides legal representation and pays the judgments.

Liability protection comes in two forms: the claims made policy and the occurrence policy. The claims made policy covers claims made while the policy is in effect. The nurse is not covered if a claim is made after the policy is terminated. An occurrence policy protects the nurse for events taking place during the active period of the policy even if a claim is filed after the policy is terminated. The occurrence policy seems to provide better protection for the nurse. Check if there is coverage for disciplinary claims (Sloan, 2002a).

Whether nurses should carry individual liability insurance is often debated. Some health care professionals and attorneys believe this practice encourages lawsuits. The benefits and cost of buying professional liability insurance must be compared against the loss of personal assets and cost of potential legal fees. When buying liability insurance the company's reputation should be investigated. Many nursing organizations offer group professional liability insurance. Sloan (2002a) suggests that nurses must assess their liability risk by considering their employment status (employee, independent contractor, or borrowed servant [agency nurse]); employer (well financed, having financial hardship, government); and area of specialty (ED, critical care, and obstetrics are considered high-risk settings).

IMPAIRED NURSE

A sensitive issue in nursing today is the impaired nurse. By definition, an **impaired nurse** is a nurse who is habitually intemperate or is addicted to the use of alcohol or habit-forming drugs. Although job performance may not be immediately compromised, substance abuse does eventually interfere with clinical judgment and performance. The chemical dependency rate among nurses is no higher than in the general population (Trinkoff et al., 2000).

In cases of impaired health care workers, the primary concern is client care. As a client advocate, the nurse cannot let loyalties to coworkers interfere with duty to the client. It is difficult reporting a coworker. No one wants to be a squealer. In many states, however, the board of nursing requires nurses to report impaired coworkers. Nurses suspected of being under the influence of drugs or alcohol must be reported to the proper authority at the place of employment. The second consideration is getting help for the impaired nurse and taking action to correct the problem.

When a coworker is suspected of diverting drugs or abusing alcohol, the nurse should:

1. Document the dates, times, and observed behavior. It is critical to be specific and descriptive of what was observed. For example:

   March 10, 2010. C.D. working 3–11 shift. Client A and Client B verbalized unrelieved postoperative pain. Documentation by C.D. stated both clients were comfortable after administration of Demerol 75 mg IM to each client. Narcotic count at shift change satisfactory.

   March 11, 2010. Client C and Client D verbalized unrelieved pain. Documentation by C.D. indicated both clients stated pain was relieved after administration of Demerol 100 mg IM. Narcotic count at shift change okay.

   March 12, 2010. Narcotic count listed 1 Demerol 100-mg syringe as broken and 1 Demerol 75-mg syringe as wasted, "client changed her mind." C.D. signed the narcotic sheet.

   or

   April 13, 2010. S.L. working the night shift. Strong odor of alcohol on his breath.

   April 14, 2010. S.L. observed walking with unsteady gait, speech is slurred, strong odor of alcohol on breath.

2. Report concerns to the supervisor and provide a copy of the documentation about the incidents. The supervisor is responsible for confronting the suspected employee. Intoxication requires immediate removal from the clinical area. In other situations, the supervisor will devise a plan before confronting the nurse.
3. Do not approach or confront the coworker yourself. The impaired coworker may become defensive and deny the problem or make threats. Also, once aware that someone is suspicious, the nurse may become more secretive, making detection less likely. Frequently, the nurse will leave one facility and go to another, repeating the same pattern.

Some employers offer an employee assistance program to rehabilitate the impaired nurse. In addition, most states have **peer assistance programs** (rehabilitation programs designed to provide an impaired nurse with referrals, professional and peer counseling support groups, and assistance and monitoring for reentry into nursing). These peer assistance programs operate under the guidance of the state nurses association in conjunction with the board of nursing. The goals of assistance programs are to protect the public from impaired nurses, provide the needed assistance to the impaired nurse, and assist the nurse to reenter nursing by monitoring the nurse's compliance. The peer counselor helps the impaired nurse develop a contract for treatment. Compliance is monitored, and confidentiality is ensured. Successful completion of the program allows the nurse to return to the practice setting.

Participation in these programs is optional. A nurse choosing not to cooperate, however, may be terminated, and the board of nursing may impose sanctions, including revoking the license to practice.

CONCEPT OF ETHICS

Ethics is the branch of philosophy concerned with determining right from wrong on the basis of knowledge rather than on opinions. Ethics deals with one's responsibilities (duties and obligations) as defined by logical argument. It is *not* a religious dogma. Ethics looks at human behavior—what people do in what circumstances. But ethics is *not* merely philosophical in nature; ethical persons put their beliefs into action.

HEALTH CARE AND ETHICS

Bioethics is the application of general ethical principles to health care. Every area of health care, including direct care of clients, utilization of staff, and allocation of finances is affected by ethics.

Ethics raises questions but does not provide easy answers. Ethical practice has more importance in health care today for several reasons. Some of these reasons are:

- An increase in technology. Advanced technology creates situations involving complicated issues, such as:
  - Newborns are surviving at earlier gestational ages, and many have serious health problems.
  - People are living much longer than ever before.
  - Organ transplants and use of bionic body parts are becoming more common.
- Changing of our society. Family structure is moving to more single-parent families and nonrelated groups living together as families.

TABLE 4-4 Overview of Ethical Principles

PRINCIPLE	EXPLANATION
Autonomy	Respect individual's right to self-determination; respect individual liberty
Nonmaleficence	Cause or do no harm to another
Beneficence	Do good to others and maintain a balance between benefits and harms
Justice	Distribute equitable potential benefits and risks
Veracity	Tell the truth
Fidelity	Do what one has promised

COURTESY OF DELMAR CENGAGE LEARNING

- Clients are more knowledgeable about their health and health care, resulting in a consumer-driven system.

ETHICAL PRINCIPLES

Ethical principles are widely accepted codes generally based on the humane aspects of society that direct or govern actions. Ethical decisions reflect what is best for the client and society. Table 4-4 summarizes the major ethical principles. Each principle is discussed in detail in the following paragraphs.

The nurse can become more systematic in solving ethical conflicts by using ethical principles. They can be used as guidelines in analyzing dilemmas and can serve as justification (rationale) for resolving ethical problems.

AUTONOMY

The principle of **autonomy** refers to the individual's right to choose and the individual's ability to act on that choice. Each person's individuality is respected. This respect is a dominant value in U.S. society.

Nurses must respect the client's right to decide and must protect those clients who are unable to decide for themselves. The ethical principle of autonomy respects the individual's right to self-determination for a competent person. The right to autonomy rests on the client's competency to decide; however, the legal definition of competency varies among states.

Informed consent is based on the client's right to make choices. Respecting autonomy means the nurse accepts client choices, even choices not in the client's best interests or choices that conflict with the nurse's values. Examples of autonomous client behavior that can hinder recovery or treatment include:

- Smoking after a diagnosis of emphysema or lung cancer
- Refusing to take medication
- Continuing to drink alcohol after being diagnosed with cirrhosis of the liver
- Refusing to receive a blood transfusion because of religious beliefs

PROFESSIONAL TIP

Autonomy

- Competent clients have a right to self-determination, even if their decisions may result in self-harm.
- Probably one of the most difficult things for nurses to accept is that clients are ultimately responsible for themselves; they will do what they want to do.

COMMUNITY/HOME HEALTH CARE

Client Autonomy

With the increased acuity level of clients cared for in the home setting, home health nurses face ever-increasing ethical challenges because they have less control over what the client does on a day-to-day basis at home.

NONMALEFICENCE

Nonmaleficence is the obligation to cause no harm to others. Harm can be physiological, psychological, financial, social, and/or spiritual. Included are both the risk of harm and intentional harm. The principle of nonmaleficence when guiding treatment decisions asks the question "Will this treatment modality cause more harm or more good to the client?" There may not be a clear-cut answer. Consider these factors when choosing a treatment:

- A reasonable expectation of benefit
- Lack of excessive pain, expense, or other inconvenience

The nurse practices according to professional and legal standards of care when following the principle of nonmaleficence. Nonmaleficence is considered a fundamental duty of health care providers. The Practical Nurse's Pledge (Box 4-1) and the Nightingale Pledge (Box 4-2) profess similar philosophies of nursing care. Some clinical examples of nonmaleficence are:

- Preventing medication errors (including drug interactions)
- Being aware of potential risks of treatment modalities
- Removing hazards (e.g., obstructions or water on the floor that might cause a fall)

BOX 4-1 PRACTICAL NURSE'S PLEDGE

Before God and those assembled here, I solemnly pledge:

To adhere to the code of ethics of the nursing profession.

To cooperate faithfully with the other members of the nursing team and to carry out faithfully and to the best of my ability the instructions of the physician or the nurse who may be assigned to supervise my work.

I will not do anything evil or malicious and I will not knowingly give any harmful drug or assist in malpractice.

I will not reveal any confidential information that may come to my knowledge in the course of my work.

And I pledge myself to do all in my power to raise the standards and the prestige of practical nursing.

May my life be devoted to service, and to the high ideals of the nursing profession.

Reprinted with permission of the National Association for Practical Nurse Education and Services, Inc., Silver Spring, MD.

BENEFICENCE

Beneficence is the duty to promote good and to prevent harm. Beneficence is often viewed as the core of nursing practice. The nurse nurtures the client and incorporates the desires of the client into the plan of care. Sometimes, it is difficult to determine what is "good," especially when doing good causes the client discomfort. For example, a client who has had a serious stroke may resist performing range-of-motion exercises and become angry at the nurse for insisting. The nurse knows the long-term value of these exercises yet perceives the client's physical and psychological pain.

JUSTICE

The principle of **justice** is based on the concept of fairness extended to each individual. The major health-related issues of justice involve the way people are treated and the way resources are distributed.

This principle directs that unless there is a justification for unequal treatment, all people must be treated equally. The **material principle of justice** is the rationale for determining those times when there can be unequal allocation of scarce

BOX 4-2 NIGHTINGALE PLEDGE

I solemnly pledge myself before God and in the presence of this assembly: To pass my life in purity and to practice my profession faithfully.

I will abstain from whatever is deleterious and mischievous, and will not take or knowingly administer any harmful drug.

I will do all in my power to maintain and elevate the standards of my profession, and will hold in confidence all personal matters committed to my keeping, and all family affairs coming to my knowledge in the practice of my profession.

With loyalty will I endeavor to aid the physician in his work, and devote myself to the welfare of those committed to my care.

resources. This concept specifies that resources may be allocated according to:

- Need
- Individual effort
- The individual's merit (ability)
- The individual's contribution to society

The Veterans Affairs (VA) Medical Centers are an example of the application of the material principle of justice (according to the individual's contribution to society). Only those who served their country by joining the military are eligible to receive health care through the VA in acute care, ambulatory, and psychiatric facilities.

VERACITY

Veracity means truthfulness (neither lying nor deceiving others). There are many forms of deception: intentional lying, partial disclosure of information, or nondisclosure of information. Veracity often is difficult to achieve. Telling the truth may not be hard, but deciding how much truth to tell may be very hard. Exceptions to truth-telling are sometimes upheld by the principle of nonmaleficence, when the truth does greater harm than good. The act of giving placebo medications is an example of when telling the truth does greater harm than good.

FIDELITY

Fidelity, which is the ethical foundation of nurse–client relationships, means faithfulness and keeping promises.

Clients have a right to expect nurses to act in their best interests. The nurse's function as a **client advocate** (a person who speaks up for or acts on behalf of the client) upholds the principle of fidelity. Fidelity is demonstrated when nurses:

- Share the client's wishes with other members of the health care team
- Keep their own personal values from influencing their advocacy for clients
- Support the client's decision, even if it conflicts with their own preferences

Within the nurse–client relationship, nurses are to be loyal to their responsibilities, maintain privacy, keep promises, and meet clients' reasonable expectations. Nurses also have a duty to be faithful to themselves. The nurse may question who is owed fidelity when conflict between commitments occurs. Remaining client centered may help clarify the question, but it may not resolve the conflict. For example, if the mother of a frightened teenage girl tried to pressure the nurse into revealing the results of the daughter's pregnancy test after the daughter had already requested that her mother not be told, although the nurse may believe that the mother has the girl's best interests at heart, the nurse must protect the client's right to privacy.

ETHICAL THEORIES

Ethical theories have been debated since the time of Plato and Aristotle. Ethical theories can be used to analyze ethical problems, but no theory by itself can provide the "correct" answer to any ethical conflict. Common ethical theories include teleology, deontology, situational theory, and caring-based theory.

CULTURAL CONSIDERATIONS

Smoke-Free Facilities

- Declaring health care facilities "smoke free" results in the most benefit and least harm for everyone.
- The minority group of smokers and the individual's right to smoke are ignored.

TELEOLOGY

Teleology is an ethical theory that states that the value of a situation is determined by its consequences. The criterion for determining the value of an action is the outcome of an action, not the action itself. An example would be immunizations—receiving an injection is not "good," but preventing the illness is.

A basic concept of teleology is the principle of **utility**, which states that an act must result in the greatest positive benefit for the greatest number of people involved. Thus, any act can be ethical if it delivers positive results. All alternatives are assessed for potential outcomes, both negative and positive. The action selected results in the most benefits and the least harm for all involved. Minority and individual rights may be ignored for the benefit of the masses.

DEONTOLOGY

Deontology is an ethical theory that considers the intrinsic significance of an act itself as the criterion for determination of good. A person must consider the motives of the individual performing the act, not the consequences of the act. For example, health care researchers might risk the well-being of a person participating in an experimental procedure for the sake of finding a drug that will save many people from suffering.

SITUATIONAL THEORY

The situational theory holds that there are no set norms, rules, or majority-focused results. Each situation must be considered individually, with an emphasis on the uniqueness of the situation and a respect for the person involved. Decisions made in one situation cannot be generalized to another situation (Pappas, 2000).

SAFETY

Immunizations

- The outcome of immunizations is the prevention of given illnesses in the individual and, thus, the prevention of the spread of those illnesses to the community.
- The greatest good for the greatest number of persons is achieved with immunizations.

Caring-Based Theory

Caring-based theory is founded on the idea that ethical decisions are not made based on principles but are made with respect to relationships, communication, caring, responsiveness, and a desire not to hurt others. Caring-based theory focuses on emotions, feelings, and attitudes. The ethical concept of caring is viewed by society as the core of the nurse's role (Daniels, Nosek, & Nicoll, 2007; Fry & Johnstone, 2002).

ETHICS AND VALUES

Ethics and values are closely related, both enlightening and complicating the nurse's balancing the ethical principles of the client with those of the health care profession. Nurses must understand their own values in order to practice ethically. **Values** influence the development of beliefs and attitudes rather than behaviors, although they often indirectly influence behaviors. A **value system** is an individual's collection of inner beliefs that guides the way the person acts and helps determine the choices the person makes in life. Although nearly nothing in life is value free, the impact of values on decisions and resultant behaviors is often not considered. Values are similar to the act of breathing; one does not think about them until a problem arises.

Nurses often care for clients whose value systems conflict with their own. For example, a client with a value system of "grin and bear it" may be insulted by a nurse's attempts to offer pain medications. In order to ascertain those things that are meaningful to the client, the nurse must have an understanding of the client's value system (Figure 4-5). Furthermore, nurses must be aware of their own values, especially when they conflict with the values of clients to prevent any personal values from influencing or interfering with client care.

Values Clarification

Values clarification is the process of analyzing one's own values to better understand those things that are truly important. Values clarification can increase nurses' self-awareness and help them better care for clients whose values differ from their own. Raths, Harmin, and Simon's (1978) classic work *Values and Teaching* explained their theory of values clarification and three-step process of valuing as follows:

- *Choosing:* Beliefs are chosen freely (without coercion).
- *Prizing:* The beliefs selected are cherished.
- *Acting:* The selected beliefs are demonstrated consistently through behavior.

Because values are individual and not universal, the nurse should not impose personal values on clients. Providing ethical nursing care is directly related to the nurse's values. For example, the nurse who strongly values the sanctity of life may experience an ethical conflict when caring for a terminally ill client who refuses treatment that might extend life for a short time.

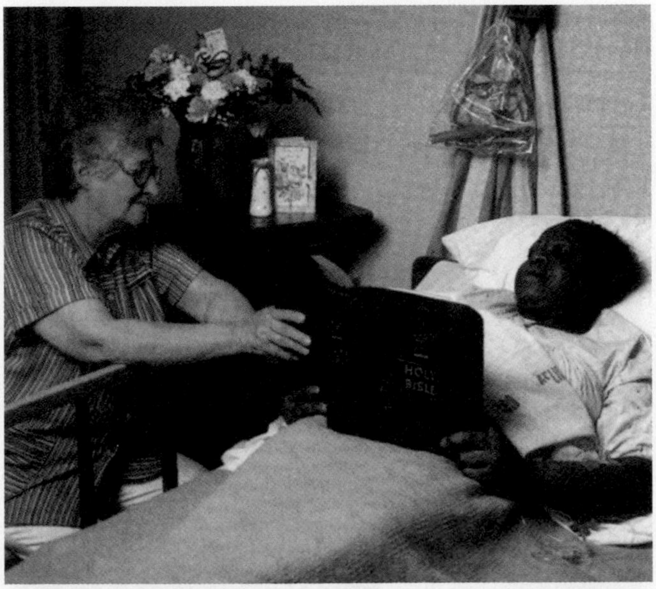

COURTESY OF DELMAR CENGAGE LEARNING

FIGURE 4-5 Clients' values determine those things that are meaningful to them.

PROFESSIONAL TIP

Values Clarification

It is the nurse's responsibility to make known to the supervisor any personal values that may influence or interfere with client care. For instance, a nurse who believes abortions should not be performed would find a conflict in working on a unit where abortions are performed. The nurse with this belief should make her values known to the employer before employment so that an assignment to that unit would not be made.

CODES OF ETHICS

Professions determine ethical behavior for their members. Several nursing organizations have developed codes as guidelines for ethical conduct. The Code for Licensed Practical/Vocational Nurses, developed by the National Federation of Licensed Practical Nurses, Inc. (NFLPN), is presented in Table 4-5. This code, providing motivation for establishing, maintaining, and elevating professional standards, was adopted by NFLPN in 1961 and revised in 1979 and in 1998. Each LP/VN entering the profession inherits the responsibility to adhere to the standards of ethical practice and conduct as set forth in this code.

A Code for Nurses was developed by both the International Council of Nurses (ICN) and the American Nurses Association (ANA) for the ethical conduct of registered nurses (See the ANA website for their code at http://www.nursingworld.org/ethics/chcode.htm). A code of ethics identifies broad principles for determining and evaluating nursing care but is not legally binding. Most state boards of nursing have authority to reprimand nurses for unprofessional conduct resulting from violation of the ethical code.

CLIENT RIGHTS

Culture defines rights and obligations. The dominant culture in the United States, however, holds the ethnocentric perspective that our rights and values are shared globally.

Table 4-5 The Code for Licensed Practical/Vocational Nurses

1. Know the scope of maximum utilization of the LP/VN as specified by the nursing practice act and function within this scope.
2. Safeguard the confidential information acquired from the source about the patient.
3. Provide healthcare to all patients regardless of race, creed, cultural background, disease, or lifestyle.
4. Uphold the highest standards in personal appearance, language, dress, and demeanor.
5. Stay informed about issues affecting the practice if nursing and delivery of health care and, where appropriate, participate in government and policy decision.
6. Accept the responsibility for safe nursing by keeping oneself mentally and physically fit and educationally prepared to practice.
7. Accept responsibility for membership in NFLPN and participate in its efforts to maintain the established standards of nursing practice and employment policies which lead to quality patient care.

From Nursing Practice Standards for the Licensed Practical/Vocational Nurse, by National Federation of Licensed Practical Nurses, Inc. (NFLPN), 2003, Garner, NC: Author. Copyright 2003 by Author. Reprinted with permission.

Clients have certain rights that apply regardless of the setting for delivery of care. These rights include, but are not limited to, the right to:

- Make decisions regarding their care (Figure 4-6)
- Be actively involved in the treatment process
- Be treated with dignity and respect

MEMORY**TRICK**

RIGHTS

An easy memory trick to use when learning about clients' rights is the acronym "**RIGHTS**." Clients have a right to:

R = Review their medical records

I = Inclusion in making decisions regarding their care

G = Give consent or decline to participate in treatment or care

H = Have an advanced directive

T = Treatment with respect and dignity

S = Sensitivity to their cultural, religious, age, gender, or other differences

COMMUNITY/HOME HEALTH CARE

The Client's Rights

The client's rights (Figure 4-8) should be respected regardless of the setting for delivery of care. For care delivered in the home environment, for instance, the home health care nurse should discuss the client's rights with the client during the initial assessment (Figure 4-7).

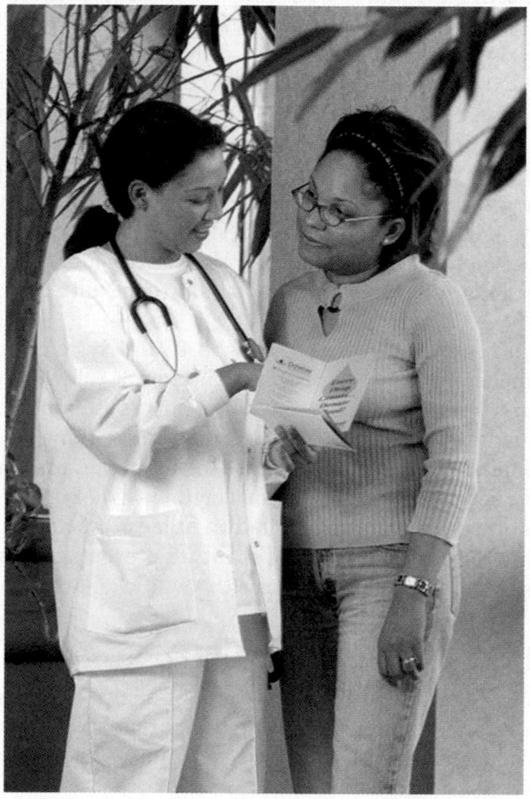

COURTESY OF DELMAR CENGAGE LEARNING

Figure 4-6 Clients have the right to information that will enable them to make decisions regarding their care.

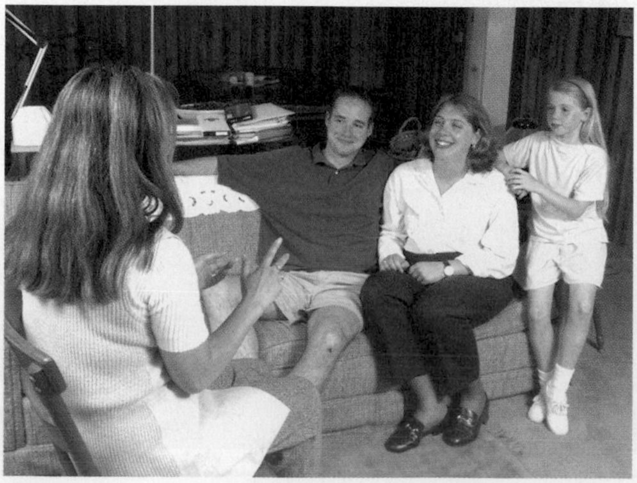

COURTESY OF DELMAR CENGAGE LEARNING

Figure 4-7 A home health nurse explains a client's rights.

Clients in short-term acute care agencies or extended care facilities are entitled to certain rights. The American Hospital Association (AHA) adopted *A Patient's Bill of Rights* in 1973. It identifies the rights and responsibilities of clients receiving care in hospitals. In 2003, this document was replaced by a brochure called *The Patient Care Partnership* (AHA, 2003) (Figure 4-8).

ETHICAL DILEMMAS

When two or more ideals or values are in conflict, there is an **ethical dilemma**. In an ethical dilemma, a choice is to be made between the conflicting ideals or values. Questions remain in some cases, even after the dilemma seems to have been settled. Areas where ethical dilemmas frequently occur are euthanasia, refusal of treatment, and scarcity of resources.

EUTHANASIA

The word *euthanasia* comes from the Greek word *euthanatos*, which literally means "good, or gentle, death." In current times, **euthanasia** refers to intentional action or lack of action that causes the merciful death of someone suffering from a terminal illness or incurable condition.

Active euthanasia refers to taking specific action to hasten a client's death, such as removing a client who is in a vegetative state from a respirator. **Passive euthanasia** is working with the client's dying process. An example is not putting in a feeding tube to provide nourishment when the client cannot or will no longer eat.

Assisted suicide is a form of active euthanasia where another person provides a client with the means to end his own life. Some nurses look on assisted suicide as violating ethical principles on which the practice of nursing is based, whereas other nurses see assisted suicide as an ethical dilemma. For example, in answer to the question "Does assisted suicide violate the principle of autonomy?" it might be argued that *refusing* to assist a suicide violates a client's autonomy.

Oregon and Washington allow physician-assisted suicide with laws that were adopted through ballot initiatives (Blesch, 2009). In 1997, Oregon enacted the *Death with Dignity Act*, which allows terminally-ill state residents to end their lives voluntarily by self-administration of a lethal medication that has been prescribed by a physician for that specific purpose (Oregon State Public Health, 2007). For more information regarding the *Death with Dignity Act*, visit *http://www.oregon.gov/DHS/ph/pas/faqs.shtml*. In November 2008, Washington state voters adopted physician-assisted dying in accordance with *Initiative 1000*. Washington Department of Health proposed rules similar to Oregon's in January 2009 that would govern *Initiative 1000* (O'Reilly, 2009a).

Montana is the third state that legalized physician-assisted suicide. In December 2008, a lower-court state judge ruled in the case *Baxter v. Montana* that terminally-ill clients have a constitutional right to physician-assistance in dying (O'Reilly, 2009b).

REFUSAL OF TREATMENT

The principle of autonomy is the basis of a client's right to refuse treatment. Only after treatment methods and their consequences have been explained can the client refuse treatment. The values of most health care providers are challenged when a client refuses treatment.

> Honoring the refusal of treatments that a patient does not desire, that are disproportionately burdensome to the patient, or that will not benefit the patient is ethically and legally permissible. (Curtin, 1995)

One possible ethical dilemma in this area relates to the use of ventilators for clients who would otherwise die. These clients continue to breathe as long as they are connected to the machine. What are the physical, emotional, psychological, and fiscal costs? What quality of life is prolonged by technology?

> **PROFESSIONALTIP**
>
> **Providing Ethical Care**
>
> - Find out about the client's wishes. Listen more than talk. (For example, it might be helpful to ask "If your heart stopped, would you want us to try to start it again?")
> - Assess the client's understanding of the illness and treatment options available.
> - Allow time for the client to explore values and to communicate.
> - Facilitate communication of the client's desires to family and other health care providers.

SCARCITY OF RESOURCES

The use of expensive services is being closely examined because of the emphasis on containing health care costs. For example, the length of a hospital stay and the number of office visits allowed for individual clients are already set by many third-party payers. The availability of goods (such as organs) contributes to a scarcity of resources.

Clients often wait extended periods to receive donated organs. Allocating scarce resources is a major ethical dilemma: Who should receive the benefit of such a scarce and precious resource as a living organ? How should the determination be made? Currently, organ recipient selection is based on objective criteria such as blood type, tissue type, size of the organ, medical urgency of the client, time on the waiting list, and distance between donor and recipient (Organ Procurement and Transplantation Network, 2009). Should only objective criteria be used in determining who receives a donated organ, or should moral judgments also be made?

ETHICAL DECISION MAKING

Ethical questions (dilemmas) are not easy to answer. **Ethical reasoning** is the process of examining the issue in a methodical manner. Ethical decisions should not be made based on emotions. Ethical decision making is used in situations where conflicts of rights and duties exist.

AMERICAN HOSPITAL ASSOCIATION PATIENT CARE PARTNERSHIP

The Patient Care Partnership: Understanding Expectations, Rights and Responsibilities

When you need hospital care, your doctor and the nurses and other professionals at our hospital are committed to working with you and your family to meet your health care needs. Our dedicated doctors and staff serve the community in all its ethnic, religious and economic diversity. Our goal is for your and your family to have the same care and attention we would want for our families and ourselves.

The sections explain some of the basics about how you can expect to be treated during your hospital stay. They also cover what we will need from you to care for you better. If you have questions at any time, please ask them. Unasked or unanswered questions can add to the stress of being in the hospital. Your comfort and confidence in your care are very important to us.

What to Expect During Your Hospital Stay

◎ **High quality hospital care.** Our first priority is to provide you the care you need, when you need it, with skill, compassion, and respect. Tell your caregivers if you have concerns about your care or if you have pain. You have the right to know the identity of doctors, nurses and others involved in your care, and you have the right to know when they are students, residents or other trainees.

◎ **A clean and safe environment.** Our hospital works hard to keep you safe. We use special policies and procedures to avoid mistakes in your care and keep you free from abuse or neglect. If anything unexpected and significant happens during your hospital stay, you will be told what happened, and any resulting changes in your care will be discussed with you.

◎ **Involvement in your care.** You and your doctor often make decisions about your care before you go to the hospital. Other times, especially in emergencies, those decisions are made during your hospital stay. When decision-making takes place, it should include:

- Discussing your medical condition and information about medically appropriate treatment choices. To make informed decisions with your doctor, you need to understand:
  - — The benefits and risks of each treatment.
  - — Whether your treatment is experimental or part of a research study.
  - — What you can reasonably expect from your treatment and any long-term effects it might have on your quality of life.
  - — What you and your family will need to do after you leave the hospital.
  - — The financial consequences of using uncovered services or out-of-network providers.

  Please tell your caregivers if you need more information about treatment choices.
- Discussing your treatment plan. When you enter the hospital, you sign a general consent to treatment. In some cases, such as surgery or experimental treatment, you may be asked to confirm in writing that you understand what is planned and agree to it. This process protects your right to consent to or refuse a treatment. Your doctor will explain the medical consequences of refusing recommended treatment. It also protects your right to decide if you want to participate in a research study.
- Getting information from you. Your caregivers need complete and correct information about your health and coverage so that they can make good decisions about your care. That includes:
  - — Past illnesses, surgeries or hospital stays.
  - — Past allergic reactions.
  - — Any medicines or dietary supplements (such as vitamins and herbs) that you are taking.
  - — Any network or admission requirements under your health plan.
- Understanding your health care goals and values. You may have health care goals and values or spiritual beliefs that are important to your well-being. They will be taken into account as much as possible throughout your hospital stay. Make sure your doctor, your family and your care team know your wishes.
- Understanding who should make decisions when you cannot. If you have signed a health care power of attorney stating who should speak for you if you become unable to make health care decisions for yourself, or a "living will" or "advance directive" that states your wishes about end-of-life care; give copies to your doctor, your family and your care team. If you or your family need help making difficult decisions, counselors, chaplains and others are available to help.

(Continues)

FIGURE 4-8 A Patient's Bill of Rights (*Reprinted with permission of the American Hospital Association, copyright 2003. All rights reserved.*)

AMERICAN HOSPITAL ASSOCIATION PATIENT CARE PARTNERSHIP (continued)

What to Expect During Your Hospital Stay (continued)

◎ **Protection of your privacy.** We respect the confidentiality of your relationship with your doctor and other caregivers, and the sensitive information about your health and health care that are part of that relationship. State and federal laws and hospital operating policies protect the privacy of your medical information. You will receive a Notice of Privacy Practices that describes the ways that we use, disclose and safeguard patient information and that explains how you can obtain a copy of information from our records about your care.

◎ **Preparing you and your family for when you leave the hospital.** Your doctor works with hospital staff and professionals in your community. You and your family also play an important role in your care. The success of your treatment often depends on your efforts to follow medication, diet and therapy plans. Your family may need to help care for you at home.

You can expect us to help you identify sources of follow-up care and to let you know if our hospital has a financial interest in any referrals. As long as you agree that we can share information about your care with them, we will coordinate our activities with your caregivers outside the hospital. You can also expect to receive information and, where possible, training about the self-care you will need when you go home.

◎ **Help with your bill and filing insurance claims.** Our staff will file claims for you with health care insurers or other programs such as Medicare and Medicaid. They also will help your doctor with needed documentation. Hospital bills and insurance coverage are often confusing. If you have questions about your bill, contact our business office. If you need help understanding your insurance coverage or health plan, start with your insurance company or health benefits manager. If you do not have health coverage, we will try to help you and your family find financial help or make other arrangements. We need your help with collecting needed information and other requirements to obtain coverage or assistance.

While you are here, you will receive more detailed notices about some of the rights you have as a hospital patient and how to exercise them. We are always interested in improving. If you have questions, comments, or concerns, please contact_____________________.

FIGURE 4-8 (*Continued*)

Kinsella (2001) identifies eight steps to guide ethical decision making:

1. Recognize the ethical dimension of the issue.
2. Identify the parties involved, their relationships to each other, and their rights and responsibilities.
3. Examine the values involved, what ideals or principles are at issue.
4. Compare benefits and burdens (positives and negatives) for each option.
5. Evaluate similar cases or ask colleagues about situations of ethical decision making.
6. Discuss, if possible, the issue with the relevant others.
7. Check legal and organizational policies so the decision meets legal, professional, and organizational standards.
8. Assess your comfort level with the decision, if uncomfortable reconsider.

CRITICAL THINKING

Ethical Decision

An 80-year-old woman is in a persistent vegetative state as a result of a cardiovascular accident. She has always talked about "someday" signing a living will requesting that heroic measures not be taken, but her family wants "everything to be done that can be done." Whose wishes should prevail? What ethical principles would come into play in this decision process?

NURSING AND ETHICS

Because nurses are accountable for protecting the interests and rights of the client, quality nursing practice involves making ethical decisions. Each practice setting has its own set of ethical concerns. Nurses must balance their ethical responsibilities to each client with their professional obligations.

ETHICS COMMITTEES

Providing ethical health care requires both dialogue among health care providers and self-examination by each care provider. Many health care agencies now recognize the need for a systematic manner for discussing ethical concerns (Figure 4-9). Multidisciplinary committees (also referred to as institutional ethics committees) constitute one arena for dialogue regarding ethical dilemmas. Ethics committees can serve as a forum for discussion of ethical issues and lead to policies and procedures for preventing and resolving dilemmas.

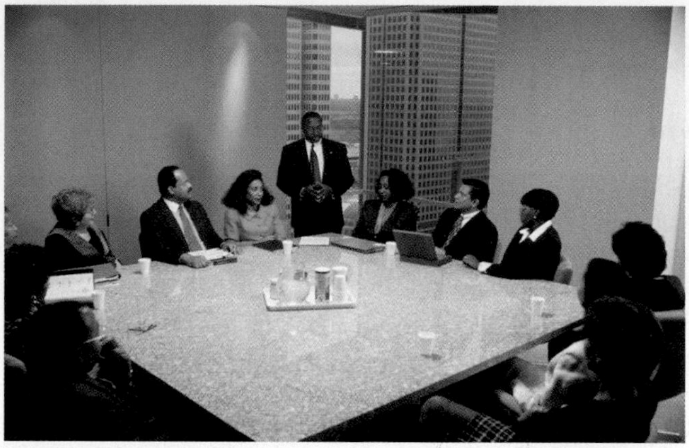
PHOTO COURTESY OF GETTY IMAGES/PHOTODISC

FIGURE 4-9 Ethics Committee Meeting

NURSE AS CLIENT ADVOCATE

The nurse's first step in acting as a client advocate is to develop a meaningful relationship with the client. The nurse is then able to make decisions with the client based on the strength of the relationship. The nurse's primary ethical responsibility is to protect clients' rights to make their own decisions.

NURSE AS WHISTLE-BLOWER

Whistle-blowing refers to calling public attention to the unethical, illegal, or incompetent actions of others. The ethical principles of veracity and nonmaleficence are the basis for whistle-blowing. Professionals are expected to monitor coworkers' abilities to perform their duties safely. Although nurses are expected to "blow the whistle" on incompetent health care providers, many are reluctant to do so because there are inherent risks in whistle-blowing. Haddad (1999) identifies some of the questions a person should consider before reporting unethical or incompetent behavior:

- Has the behavior in question created or is it likely to create serious harm?
- Have I gathered all appropriate information, and am I competent to judge this behavior?
- Do others confirm my information and judgment?
- Have all internal resources been exhausted to resolve the problem?
- Is it likely that past wrongdoing will be corrected or future damage prevented after the problem is reported?
- Is the harm created by whistle-blowing likely to be less than the harm done by the behavior in question?

The False Claims Act (FCA) encourages whistle-blowers to report evidence of fraud against the federal government (Sloan, 2002b).

Protection of privacy to whistle-blowers is provided by federal law and state laws (to varying degrees). The fear of reprisal and the inclination to protect one's coworkers may keep a nurse from fulfilling the ethical obligation to report substandard behaviors.

CASE STUDY

An alert and oriented 62-year-old client was diagnosed with colon cancer. Surgery was recommended, and she agreed to surgical excision of the tumor. Postoperatively, she experienced serious complications and remained in the surgical intensive care unit for 2 months. During that time, she experienced cardiac failure, temporary respiratory failure, and renal failure and required multiple surgical procedures.

One day she was asked to sign a consent form for surgical revision of her colostomy. She refused, stating that she could no longer tolerate any procedures and that she was ready to die a peaceful death. The nurse informed the resident of the client's decision. The resident called the attending physician, who ordered a stat dose of Valium 10 mg IM for the client. He then stopped by the nurses' desk and asked that the client be prepped for surgery.

1. Identify three elements needed to ensure informed consent.
2. Did this client give informed consent?
3. Identify which of the elements of informed consent were met or not met. Be sure to include your rationale.
4. What type of ethical dilemma does this case study present?
5. Which ethical principle pertains to this situation?
6. Explain the deontological view of this ethical dilemma.

SUMMARY

- Laws are rules that guide personal interaction. They are derived from several sources and can be classified as public or civil.
- Within most states, the nursing practice act indicates the scope of practice for nurses. Standards have been developed to guide nursing practice.
- The nurse must be familiar with client rights. Care must be taken not to falsely imprison a client or violate the client's right to privacy.
- The client's chart is a legal document and should accurately reflect client status and care. Entries should be neat and timely.

- Informed consent is more than just signing a form. It requires a competent client understanding the risks, benefits, and alternatives to treatment.
- Whether to purchase malpractice insurance is a personal decision, but having one's own policy provides both coverage off the job and individual legal counsel.
- Incident reports are a risk management tool. They are not meant to be used for punitive purposes.
- Advance directives are instructions about health care preferences. They both protect the rights of the client and guide the family through difficult decisions.
- Ethics examines human behavior—those things that people do under a given set of circumstances.
- There is a connection between acts that are legal and acts that are ethical. Nursing actions are to be both legal and ethical.
- Ethical decisions are based on principles such as autonomy, nonmaleficence, beneficence, justice, veracity, and fidelity.
- Because ethics and values are so closely associated, nurses must explore their own values in order to acknowledge the value systems of their clients.
- Ethical codes that have been developed by nursing organizations such as the NFLPN, the ICN, and the ANA establish guidelines for the ethical conduct of nurses with clients, coworkers, society, and the nursing profession.
- The Patient's Bill of Rights is designed to guarantee ethical care of clients.
- The roles of client advocate and whistle-blower enable nurses to protect their clients' rights and ensure the ethical and competent actions of their peers within the nursing profession.

REVIEW QUESTIONS

1. The nurse is providing care for a 25-year-old male client. His health is deteriorating, but he remains alert and oriented. His sister, an RN, asks to see his chart. What should the nurse do initially?
   1. Ask the client's permission.
   2. Ask the client's physician's permission.
   3. Deny her access to his chart.
   4. Provide her a private place to review the chart.
2. The nurse enters the room and tells the client that he has to take the medication, including an injection. The client refuses the medication, but the nurse continues to administer the medications. This action is an example of the intentional tort of:
   1. battery.
   2. invasion of privacy.
   3. libel.
   4. malpractice.
3. The nurse finds a client obnoxious and totally disapproves of the client's behavior. She writes on the chart that the client "is obnoxious and leads an immoral lifestyle, which has resulted in hospitalization." This is referred to as:
   1. assault.
   2. slander.
   3. libel.
   4. a supported statement.
4. Even though the nurse may obtain the client's signature on a form, obtaining informed consent for a medical treatment is the responsibility of the:
   1. client.
   2. physician.
   3. student nurse.
   4. supervising nurse.
5. Nurses would use the Code for Licensed Practical/ Vocational Nurses to: (Select all that apply.)
   1. solve an ethical dilemma.
   2. establish a guideline for ethical conduct.
   3. develop a nursing care plan.
   4. seek answers to a client care problem.
   5. understand the professional expectations of them.
   6. establish, maintain, and elevate professional standards.
6. The nurse is working the night shift with a colleague who has been his friend for several years. He discovers that his colleague is routing drugs regularly and is taking them herself. When confronted, the colleague tells the nurse that she needs the drugs to cope and that she cannot lose her job because she is a single parent of three young children. Which of the following is the most appropriate response by the nurse?
   1. "It will be alright. I can get help for you."
   2. "This must be a very difficult time for you. Would you like to talk about this?"
   3. "How long have you been doing this?"
   4. "This is illegal, and I must report this to the supervisor."
7. A nursing student is learning about client rights. Which of the following statements made by the student nurse indicates that further teaching is required?
   1. "My client can make her own decisions regarding her care."
   2. "I need to treat clients with dignity and respect."
   3. "I should do as much as possible for the client."
   4. "My client should be informed of the side effects of new medication."
8. A client is at risk for invasion of privacy when which of the following actions occur? (Select all that apply.)
   1. Photographing a client.
   2. Writing the client's allergies on the chart.
   3. Talking about the client during lunch break.
   4. Clarifying a physician's illegible written order.
   5. Closing the door to give an injection.
   6. E-mailing the client's HIV lab results.

9. Which of the following is an example of an ethical dilemma?
   1. A young couple seeking marriage counseling.
   2. A terminally ill client refusing treatment.
   3. A client signing an advanced directive.
   4. A client donating a kidney to his son.
10. A 17-year-old Jehovah's Witness is brought to the ED after passing out at the mall. It is determined that she is suffering from an ulcer that has perforated her stomach wall. The bleeding is severe, and she is in need of a blood transfusion to save her life. The client is refusing the blood transfusion. What is the most appropriate nursing intervention for this client?
    1. Administer the blood transfusion immediately.
    2. Contact the hospital's ethical advisory committee.
    3. Contact the client's parents.
    4. Follow the client's decision.

REFERENCES/SUGGESTED READINGS

American Hospital Association. 2003. The patient care partnership. Retrieved November 28, 2008, from http://www.aha.org/aha/issues/Communicating-With-Patients/pt-care-partnership.html

American Nurses Association. (2005). Code of ethics for nurses with interpretive statements. Retrieved November 28, 2008, from http://nursingworld.org/ethics/code/protected_nwcoe813.htm

Bandman, E., & Bandman, B. (2001). *Nursing ethics through the life span* (4th ed.). Norwalk, CT: Appleton-Lange.

Bemis, P. (2008). Nurses in the legal field. *RN, 71*(6), 20–21.

Blesch, G. (2009). Montana court hears arguments on physician-assisted death. Retrieved September 27, 2009 from http://www.modernhealthcare.com/article/20090902/REG/309029935

Brooke, P. (2003). How good a SAMARITAN should you be? *Nursing 2003, 33*(6), 46–47.

Burkhardt, M., & Nathaniel, A. (2008). *Ethics and issues in contemporary nursing* (3rd ed.). Clifton Park, NY: Delmar Cengage Learning.

Curtin, L. (1995). Nurses take a stand on assisted suicide. *Nursing Management, 26*(5), 71–76.

Daniels, R., Nosek, L., & Nicoll, L. (2007). *Contemporary medical-surgical nursing*. Clifton Park, NY: Delmar Cengage Learning.

Douglas, R., & Brown, H. (2002). Attitudes toward advance directives. *Journal of Nursing Scholarship, 34*(1), 61–65.

Flick, C. (2002). Organ donation: A delicate balance. *RN, 65*(12), 43–46.

Flight, M. (2004). *Law, liability, and ethics* (4th ed.). Clifton Park, NY: Delmar Cengage Learning.

Flores, J. (2002). What if you're named in a lawsuit? *RN, 65*(12), 65–68.

Frank-Stromborg, M., & Ganschow, J. (2002). How HIPAA will change your practice. *Nursing2002, 32*(9), 54–57.

Fry, S., & Johnstone, M. (2002). *International Council of Nurses Ethics in nursing practice: A guide to ethical decision-making*. Malden, MA: Blackwell.

Gebbie, K. (2001). Privacy: The patient's right. AJN, 101(6), 69–73.

Grace, P., & Hardt, E. H. (2008). Ethical issues: When a patient refuses assistance. *American Journal of Nursing, 108*(8), 36–38.

Haddad, A. (1999). Ethics in action. *RN, 62*(1), 23–26.

Health Resources and Services Administration. (2008). Practitioner data banks: National practitioner data bank. Retrieved November 28, 2008, from http://bhpr.hrsa.gov/dqa

Helm, A., & Kihm, N. (2001). Is professional liability insurance for you? *Nursing2001, 31*(1), 48–49.

Higginbotham, E. (2003). Does error 1 injury 5 negligence? *RN, 66*(5), 67–68.

Hill, S., & Howlett, H. (2001). *Success in practical nursing: Personal and vocational issues* (4th ed.). Philadelphia: W. B. Saunders.

Infante, M. (2000). Malpractice may not be your biggest legal risk. *RN, 63*(7), 67–73.

Joint Commission on Accreditation of Healthcare Organizations. (2008). Health care at the crossroads. Retrieved November 28, 2008, from http://www.jointcommission.org/NR/rdonlyres/5C138711-ED76-4D6F-909F-B06E0309F36D/0/health_care_at_the_crossroads.pdf

Kinsella, L. (2001). Truth telling in patient care: Resolving ethical issues. *Nursing2001, 31*(12), 52–55.

LaDuke, S. (2000). The effects of professional discipline on nurses. *American Journal of Nursing, 100*(6), 26–33.

LaDuke, S., & Biondo, T. (2003). Protect your future with personal liability insurance. *Nursing2003, 33*(2), 52–53.

Lee, N. (2000). Proving nursing negligence. *American Journal of Nursing, 100*(11), 55–56.

Maltz, A. (2001). Keeping pace with new patient privacy rules. *RN, 64*(9), 71–74.

McCurdy, D. (2008). Ethical spiritual care at the end of life. *American Journal of Nursing, 108*(5), 11.

Mock, K. (2001). Keep lawsuits at bay with compassionage care. *RN, 64*(5), 83–86.

National Council of State Boards of Nursing, Inc. (2000). NCSBN welcomes two more states to the nurse licensure compact. Available: http://www.ncsbn.org.public/nurselicensurecompact/nurselicensurecompact_index.htm

National Council of State Boards of Nursing, Inc. (2000). Why disciplinary databanks? Why the National Practitioner Data Bank (NPDB)? Available: http://www.ncsbn.org/files/publications/issues/vol171/ddb.171

National Council of State Boards of Nursing, Inc. (2002). What boards of nursing do . . . and what you can do. Available: http://www.ncsbn.org/public/regulation/boards_of_nursing.htm

Oregon State Public Health. (2007). FAQs about the Death With Dignity Act. Retrieved September 27, 2009 from http://www.oregon.gov/DHS/ph/pas/faqs.shtml

O'Reilly, K. (2009a). Montana judge rejects stay of physician-assisted suicide ruling. Retrieved September 27, 2009 from http://www.ama-assn.org/amednews/2009/01/26/prsd0129.htm

O'Reilly, K. (2009b). 5 people die under new Washington physician-assisted suicide law. Retrieved September 27, 2009 from http://www.ama-assn.org/amednews/2009/07/06/prsc0706.htm

Organ Procurement and Transplantation Network. (2009). Donor matching system. Retrieved June 21, 2009 from http://optn.transplant.hrsa.gov/about/transplantation/matchingProcess.asp

Pappas, A. (2000). Ethical issues. In J. Zerwekh & J. Claborn (Eds.), *Nursing today: Transitions and trends* (3rd ed.). Philadelphia: W. B. Saunders.

Raths, L., Harmin, M., & Simon, S. (1978). *Values and teaching* (2nd ed.). Columbus, OH: Merrill.

Roman, L. (2007). How to stay out of legal water. *RN, 70*(1), 26–31.
Sloan, A. (2002a). Liability insurance: Is your coverage adequate? *RN, 65*(10), 69–72.
Sloan, A. (2002b). Whistleblowing: Proceed with caution. *RN, 65*(1), 67–70.
Sloan, A., & Vernarac, E. (2001). Impaired nurses: Reclaiming careers. *RN, 64*(2), 58–63.
Trinkoff, A., Zhou, Q., et al. (2000). Workplace access, negative proscriptions, job strain, and substance use in registered nurses. *Nursing Research, 49*(2), 83.
Trossman, S. (2003). Protecting patient information. *American Journal of Nursing, 103*(2), 65–68.
U.S. Department of Health and Human Services. (2001). National standards to protect the privacy of personal health information. Available: http://www.hhs.gov/acr/hipaa
Ventura, M. (1999a). Staffing issues. *RN, 62*(2), 26–30.
Ventura, M. (1999b). The great multistate licensure debate. *RN, 62*(5), 58–62.
Ventura, M. (1999c). When information must be revealed. *RN, 62*(6), 61.
White, L., & Duncan, G. (2002). *Medical surgical nursing: An integrated approach* (2nd ed.). Clifton Park, NY: Delmar Cengage Learning.
Zerwekh, J., & Claborn, J. C. (2003). *Nursing today: Transitions and trends* (4th ed). Philadelphia: W. B. Saunders.
Ziel, S., & Gentry, K. (2003). Ready? HIPAA's here. *RN, 66*(2), 67–70.

RESOURCES

Partnership for Caring,
http://www.partnershipforcaring.org

The Living Bank International,
http://www.livingbank.org

Living Wills, Films for the Humanities and Sciences,
http://ffh.films.com

National Association for Practical Nurse Education and Service, Inc. (NAPNES),
http://www.napnes.org

National Federation of Licensed Practical Nurses, Inc. (NFLPN), http://www.nflpn.org

United Network for Organ Sharing (UNOS),
http://www.unos.org

UNIT 2 The Health Care Environment

CHAPTER 5
The Health Care Delivery System

MAKING THE CONNECTION

Refer to the following chapters to increase your understanding of the health care delivery system:

Basic Nursing

- ***Legal and Ethical Responsibilities***
- ***Arenas of Care***
- ***Wellness Concepts***

LEARNING OBJECTIVES

Upon completion of this chapter, you should be able to:

- Define key terms.
- Describe the three levels of service in the U.S. health care delivery system.
- Identify the members of the health care team and their respective roles.
- Describe the differences among financial programs for health care services and reimbursement.
- Explain the factors that influence health care delivery.
- Identify the challenges to providing care.
- Describe nursing's role in meeting the challenges within the health care system.
- Discuss the emerging trends and issues for the health care delivery system.

KEY TERMS

capitated rates
comorbidity
exclusive provider organizations (EPOs)
fee-for-service
health care delivery system
health maintenance organizations (HMOs)
managed care
Medicaid
medical model
Medicare
Medigap insurance
preferred provider organizations (PPOs)
prescriptive authority
primary care
primary care provider
primary health care
prospective payment
secondary care
single-payer system
single point of entry
tertiary care

INTRODUCTION

A **health care delivery system** is a method for providing services to meet the health needs of individuals. The U.S. health care delivery system is experiencing dramatic change. The once economically thriving health care institutions now search for ways to survive. Health care providers seek cost-effective ways to deliver a larger range of services to consumers, who are demanding greater accessibility to quality affordable health care services. The increase in consumerism is fueled by the Internet, regulatory changes, the rising popularity of nontraditional therapies, and frustration of clients and their families feeling they have been mistreated by the system (Haugh, 1999).

Because nursing is a major component of the U.S. health care delivery system, nurses must understand the changes occurring within the system and nursing's role in shaping those changes. This chapter explores the levels of health care services available, the settings offering those services, and the members of the health care team. The economics of health care, the challenges within the health care delivery system, and nursing's role in meeting those challenges are also addressed.

LEVELS OF HEALTH CARE SERVICES

Health care services are classified into three levels: primary, secondary, and tertiary. Table 5-1 provides an overview of the levels of care. The trend is toward holistic care (i.e., care of the entire person, including physiological, psychological, social, intellectual, and spiritual aspects).

CRITICAL THINKING

Levels of Health Care

A nurse is providing care for a 72-year-old female client diagnosed with terminal breast cancer. Which level of health care service will the client utilize? What is the purpose of this level of care? What would be an appropriate goal for this client?

PRIMARY CARE

The major purposes of **primary care** are to promote wellness and prevent illness or disability. Care is coordinated by the office of the primary care provider, usually a family practice physician, pediatrician, internal medicine physician, or family nurse practitioner. The U.S. health care system traditionally focused on treating illness rather than promoting wellness. Now, however, the focus is on health-promoting behaviors such as regular exercise, reducing fat in the diet, monitoring cholesterol level, and managing stress. Direct wellness promotion activities toward the individual, the family, or the community.

Under the traditional **medical model**, our health care delivery system was not a *health* care system at all but rather an *illness* care system. Services were directed toward care after disease or disability developed rather than preventive aspects of care. Today, however, there is more of an emphasis on the holistic promotion of wellness and on the preventive aspects of care.

SECONDARY CARE

Services within the realm of **secondary care**—diagnosis and treatment—occur after the client exhibits symptoms of

TABLE 5-1 Levels of Health Care Services

TYPE OF CARE	DESCRIPTION	EXAMPLES
Primary	*Goal:* To decrease the risk to a client (individual or community) for disease or dysfunction *Explanation:* General health promotion Protection against specific illnesses	Teaching Lifestyle modification for health (e.g., smoking cessation, nutrition counseling) Referrals Immunization Routine screenings Promotion of a safe environment (e.g., sanitation, protection from toxic agents)
Secondary	*Goal:* To alleviate disease and prevent further disability *Explanation:* Early detection and intervention	Diagnostic testing Acute care Various therapies Surgery
Tertiary	*Goal:* To minimize effects and permanent disability associated with chronic or irreversible conditions *Explanation:* Restorative and rehabilitative activities to attain optimal level of functioning	Education and retraining Provision of direct care Environmental intervention (e.g., advising on necessity of wheelchair accessibility for a person who has experienced a cerebrovascular accident [stroke])

illness. Acute treatment centers (hospitals) still constitute the predominant site for the delivery of these health care services, but there is a growing movement to provide diagnostic and therapeutic services in locations that are more easily accessed by the population. These are often satellite care centers of a major hospital, where holistic care is promoted.

Tertiary Care

Restoring an individual to the state of health that existed before the development of an illness is the purpose of **tertiary** (rehabilitative) **care**. When a person is unable to regain previous functional abilities, the rehabilitation goal is to reach the optimal level of health possible. For example, a client regains partial use of an arm after experiencing a stroke. Restorative care is holistic in that the physiological, psychological, social, and spiritual aspects of the person are all addressed in the provision of care.

HEALTH CARE DELIVERY SYSTEM

The intricate U.S. health care delivery system involves many providers, consumers, settings, personnel, and services.

Providers/Consumers

Health care services in the United States are delivered by public (including official and voluntary), public/private, and private sectors. Consumers are the individuals who receive the health care services.

Public Sector

Tax monies fund public agencies, and these agencies are accountable to the public. Official (or governmental) agencies and voluntary agencies make up the public sector.

The U.S. Public Health Service (USPHS), the major agency that oversees the actual delivery of care services, is administered by the U.S. Department of Health and Human Services (USDHHS). Table 5-2 lists the USPHS agencies and their purposes. The Veterans Administration (VA), also financed by tax monies, has hospitals and clinics providing services to veterans of the armed services.

The states vary in the public health services provided. Generally, activities of local health departments are coordinated by a state department of health. Local services provide immunizations, maternal–child care, and control of infectious and chronic diseases.

Voluntary agencies also constitute an important part of the public sector of the health care delivery system. These not-for-profit agencies (e.g., the National Federation of Licensed Practical Nurses [NFLPN], the American Nurses Association [ANA], the National League for Nursing [NLN], and the American Medical Association [AMA]) can exert significant legislative influence. Other voluntary agencies, such as the American Diabetes Association and the American Heart Association, provide educational resources to health care providers and the general public. Voluntary agencies receive

Table 5-2 Agencies of the U.S. Public Health Service

AGENCY	PURPOSE
Health Resources and Services Administration (HRSA)	Furnish health-related information; control programs of health care for the homeless; people with human immunodeficiency virus (HIV) and acquired immunodeficiency syndrome (AIDS); rural health care; organ transplants; and employee occupational health
Food and Drug Administration (FDA)	Protect the public from unsafe drugs, food, and cosmetics
Centers for Disease Control and Prevention (CDC)	Study and control the transmission of communicable diseases
National Institutes of Health (NIH)	Conduct research and education about specific illnesses
Alcohol, Drug Abuse, and Mental Health Administration (ADAMHA)	Serve as clearinghouse for information on substance abuse and mental health issues
Agency for Toxic Substances and Disease Registry (ATSDR)	Keep registry of certain diseases Provide information on toxic agents Study mortality and morbidity on defined population groups
Indian Health Service (IHS)	Furnish health care services to Native Americans, including health promotion, nutrition, maternal–child health, disease prevention, alcoholism, suicide prevention, and substance abuse
Agency for Health Care Research and Quality (AHRQ)	Serve as main source of federal support for research related to quality of health care delivery

funds from individual contributions, membership dues, and corporate philanthropy.

Public/Private Sector

A blending of the public and private sectors in many areas of health care has gradually occurred following the inception of Medicare and the diagnosis-related groups (DRGs), discussed in an upcoming section. Federal regulations guide both the care provided to clients in private nonprofit and for-profit agencies by private physicians and the reimbursement to both the agencies and the physicians.

Private Sector

The private sector of the health care delivery system is composed mainly of independent health care agencies and providers who are reimbursed on a **fee-for-service** basis (the recipient directly pays the provider for services as they are provided). Fee-for-service clients may have private insurance or use their own financial resources to pay for the services.

SETTINGS

The various settings where health care is delivered include acute care hospitals, extended care facilities, outpatient settings, home health care agencies, schools, and hospice, which are discussed in Chapter 6, "Arenas of Care."

PERSONNEL AND SERVICES

Many personnel and services exist within the various health care settings. Large hospitals provide the greatest number of services. Other health care settings may provide some but not all of these same services. The service departments most commonly found in the various settings include nursing units, specialized client care units, diagnostic departments, therapy departments, and support services.

HEALTH CARE TEAM

Health care services are delivered by a multidisciplinary team (Figure 5-1). Table 5-3 lists the various health care team members, their educational requirements, and their roles. Nurses work daily with other team members, so they must understand the role of each team member.

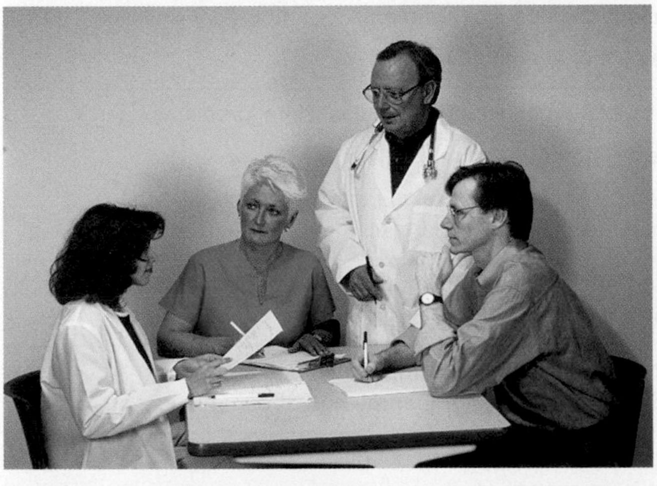

FIGURE 5-1 Members of the health care team work together for the benefit of the client.

Nurses have various roles when assisting clients to meet their needs. Table 5-4 identifies the most common nursing roles. Nurses function in independent, interdependent, and dependent roles. In the independent role, the nurse requires no direction or order from another health care professional (e.g., in deciding that a client's edematous arm should be elevated). In the interdependent role, the nurse works in collaboration with other health care professionals (e.g., in a client care conference where several members of the health care team together plan ways to meet the client's needs). In the dependent role, the nurse requires direction from a physician or dentist (e.g., medications must be ordered by a physician or dentist before a nurse may administer them to the client). The degree of autonomy nurses experience is related to client needs, nurse expertise, and practice setting.

HEALTH CARE ECONOMICS

Cost has been the primary motivation of the reform movement in health care. Control of costs has shifted from the health care providers to the insurers, with the result being increasing constraints on reimbursement. The predominant method of paying health care costs was for years fee for service, with little incentive for cost-effective delivery of care. All that is changing.

The U.S. health care system's financial base is composed of both public and private funding, resulting in administrative costs for health care reimbursement that are higher in this country than in countries with a **single-payer system** (a model wherein the government is the only entity to reimburse health care costs, such as in Canada). Despite the enormous expenditure of public funds, the United States has not found a way to provide health care coverage for all its citizens. Figure 5-2 shows the sources of the nation's health dollars in 2007.

PRIVATE INSURANCE

The private insurance model is the basis for the system of financing health care services in the United States. Private insurance companies constitute one of the largest sectors of the health care system. Payment rates to health care providers vary among insurance companies.

In the United States, insured individuals pay substantial monthly premiums for insurance coverage having high deductibles for health care services. For many, these costs may prove barriers to procuring necessary insurance coverage and health services. In addition, insurers will no longer pay for services that *they* deem unnecessary, effectively taking client care decisions out of the hands of physicians. The quality of care provided is now being monitored not only by providers (physicians) but also by third-party payers (insurance companies) and, ever increasingly, by consumers.

Medigap insurance to pay for costs not covered by Medicare is purchased from private insurance companies. As of 2006, an estimated 18% of Medicare beneficiaries were covered by a Medigap policy (Henry J. Kaiser Family Foundation, 2006). Nursing home care costs are covered 39% by private insurance, about 10% by Medicare, and 48% by Medicaid (CMS, 2002a). Long-term care insurance benefits vary greatly depending on the insurance company.

Table 5-3 Health Care Team Members

TEAM MEMBER	EDUCATION	FUNCTION/ROLE
Nurse (LP/VN, RN, and APRN)	LP/VN: 1 year RN: 2 to 4 year	Emphasize health (wellness) promotion Use a holistic approach to assist clients in coping with illness or disability by providing nursing care, health and health care education, and discharge planning Formulate nursing diagnoses to guide plan of care Address the needs of the client (individual, family, or community) Assist physician
	APRN (Advanced Practice Registered Nurse): 1 to 3 years post-RN	Functions may vary by state and specialization
Physician (medical doctor [MD])	8+ years	Formulate medical diagnoses and prescribe therapeutic modalities Perform medical and surgical procedures
Dentist (both doctor of dental surgery [DDS] and doctor of dental medicine [DMD])	8+ years	Diagnose and treat conditions affecting the mouth, teeth, and gums Perform preventive measures to promote dental health
Registered pharmacist (Rph)	5 to 6 years	Prepare and dispense drugs for therapeutic use May be involved in client education
Physician's assistant (PA)	2 years (plus a master's degree for PA licensure, required in many states)	Provide medical services under the supervision of a physician
Registered dietitian (RD)	4+ years	Plan diets to meet special needs of clients Promote health through nutrition education and counseling May supervise preparation of meals
Social worker (SW)	4 years	Assist clients with psychosocial problems (e.g., financial, housing, marital) Make referrals to other facilities and support groups May assist with discharge planning
Respiratory therapist (RT)	2 years	Provide various therapeutic treatments for respiratory illnesses Administer pulmonary function tests
Physical therapist (PT)	4 years	Work with clients experiencing musculoskeletal problems Assess client's strength and mobility Perform therapeutic measures (e.g., range of motion, massage, application of heat and cold) and teach new skills (e.g., crutch walking)
Occupational therapist (OT)	4 years	Work with clients who have functional impairment to teach skills for activities of daily living
Speech therapist	4 years	Assist clients who have speech impairments to speak understandably or to learn another method of communication
Chaplain	8 years	Assist clients in meeting spiritual needs Provide individual counseling and support to families Conduct religious services

TABLE 5-4 Nursing Roles

Caregiver: LP/VN and RN	Traditional and most essential role Function as nurturer Provide direct care Be supportive Demonstrate clinical proficiency Promote comfort of client
Teacher: LP/VN and RN	Provide information Serve as counselor Seek to empower clients in self-care Encourage compliance with prescribed therapy Promote healthy lifestyles Interpret information
Advocate: LP/VN and RN	Protect the client Provide explanations in client's language Act as change agent Support client's decision
Manager: LP/VN and RN	Make decisions Coordinate activities of others Allocate resources Evaluate care and personnel Serve as a leader Take initiative
Expert: RN	Advanced practice clinician Conduct research Teach in schools of nursing Develop theory Contribute to professional literature Provide testimony at governmental hearings and in court
Case manager: RN	Track client's progress through the health care system Coordinate care to ensure continuity
Team member: LP/VN and RN	Collaborate with others Use excellent communication skills

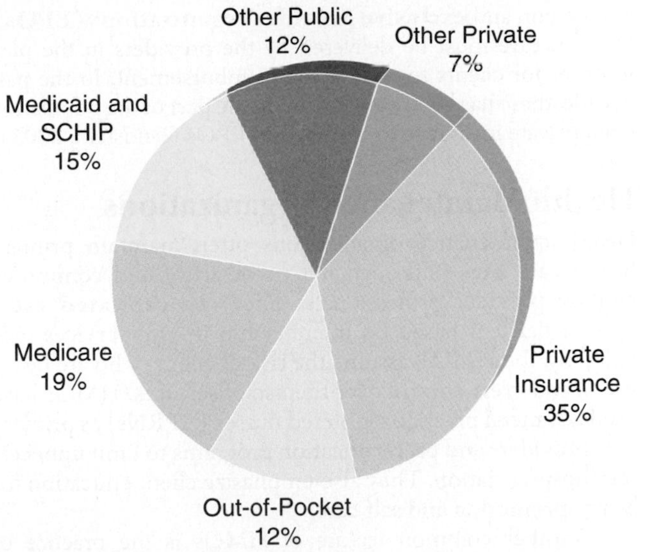

FIGURE 5-2 Source of the Nation's Health Dollar in 2007 *(Note: "Other Public" included workers' compensation, public health activity, Department of Defense, Department of Veterans Affairs, Indian Health Service, state and local hospital subsidies, and school health. "Other Private" includes industrial in-plant, privately funded construction, and nonpatient revenues, including philanthropy.) (Courtesy of Centers for Medicare and Medicaid Services, Office of the Actuary, National Health Statistics Group, 2009.)*

MANAGED CARE

Managed care is a system of providing and monitoring care wherein access, cost, and quality are controlled before or during delivery of services. Delivering services in the most cost-efficient manner possible is the goal of managed care. Managed care organizations combine financing and delivery of health care and try to control costs by monitoring delivery of services and restricting access to expensive procedures and providers.

Managed care was designed to provide coordinated services emphasizing prevention and primary care. The rationale behind managed care is to give consumers preventive services delivered by a **primary care provider** (a health care provider whom a client sees first for health care, typically a family practitioner, internist, or pediatrician). The primary care provider is responsible for managing or coordinating all care of a client when illness makes referrals necessary. This approach is supposed to result in less expensive interventions.

Although managed care has existed for years, only within the past 20 years has it enjoyed national prominence. In 1973 the Health Maintenance Organization Act implemented two mandates. First, federal grants and loans were made available to **health maintenance organizations (HMOs)** (prepaid health plans that provide primary health care services for a preset fee and that focus on cost-effective treatment measures) that complied with strict federal regulations instead of the less restrictive state requirements. Second, large employers were required to provide employees with an HMO option for health care coverage. From the beginning, HMOs have been a viable alternative to the traditional fee-for-service system.

Managed care is not a place but, rather, an organizational structure with several variations. One such variation is the HMO, which is both provider and insurer. Other variations are **preferred provider organizations (PPOs)**, wherein members must use providers within the system in order to obtain full reimbursement but may use other providers for lesser reimbursement, and **exclusive provider organizations (EPOs)**, wherein care must be delivered by the providers in the plan in order for clients to receive any reimbursement. In the past decade, there has been a great shift on the part of the population from private insurance to HMOs and PPOs (Feldstein, 2005).

Health Maintenance Organizations

Health maintenance organizations often maintain primary health care sites (although not necessarily) and commonly employ provider professionals. They use **capitated rates** (preset flat fees based on membership in, not services provided by, the HMO), assume the risk of clients who are heavy users, and exert control over the use of services. HMOs have used advanced practice registered nurses (APRNs) as primary care providers and precertification programs to limit unnecessary hospitalization. They also emphasize client education for health promotion and self-care.

Another common feature of HMOs is the practice of **single point of entry** (entry into the health care system through a point designated by the plan), through which primary care is delivered. **Primary health care** is the client's point of entry into the health care system and includes assessment, diagnosis, treatment, coordination of care, education, preventive services, and surveillance. It covers all the services provided by a family practitioner (nurse or physician) in an ambulatory setting. Primary care providers (PCPs) are "gatekeepers" to the health care system by deciding which, if any, referrals to specialists are needed by the client. HMOs purposely limit direct access to specialists to reduce costs. Managed care plans assume much of the risk of providing health care and, therefore, encourage wise use by both providers and consumers. In 1976, there were 175 HMOs in the United States; by 2002 there were 650 (Centers for Education and Research on Therapeutics [CERTS], 2003).

Preferred Provider Organizations

The most common managed care systems are PPOs. A PPO is a contractual relationship between providers, hospitals, insurers, employers, and third-party payers forming a network wherein providers negotiate with group purchasers to provide health services for a specific population at a preset cost (Feldstein, 2005). Care received within the network is associated with the highest reimbursement; care received outside the network is associated with lower reimbursement, with the client paying the difference. Preferred provider organizations have been very popular in the United States. In fact, the number of PPOs has increased from fewer than 10 in 1981 to more than 670 PPOs and over 55 PPO chains in 2008 (First Mark, 2008).

Exclusive Provider Organizations

Exclusive provider organizations create a network of providers (such as physicians and hospitals) and offer the incentive of consumer services for little or no copayment if the network providers are used exclusively. If a member receives treatment outside the network, no benefit is paid. For instance, a member who becomes ill and receives treatment while visiting relatives in another state would receive no benefits for the treatment.

FEDERAL GOVERNMENT PLANS

With the advent of Medicare and Medicaid in 1965, the federal government became a third-party payer for health care services. The Health Care Financing Administration (HCFA) is a federal agency that regulates Medicare, Medicaid, and Children's Health Insurance Program (CHIP) expenditures.

With the ultimate goal of curtailing spending for hospitalized Medicare recipients, the federal government created DRGs to categorize the average cost of care for each diagnosis. A prospective payment system was then created based on the DRGs. **Prospective payment** is a predetermined rate paid for each episode of hospitalization based on the client's age and principal diagnosis and on the presence or absence of surgery and **comorbidity** (simultaneous existence of more than one disease process in an individual). Hospitals are reimbursed the predetermined amount regardless of the actual cost of providing services to the client. The prospective payment system, originally designed for Medicare, has been adopted by other agencies and insurance companies.

Medicare

In 1965, **Medicare** (Title XVIII) was signed into law as an amendment to the Social Security Act. It was originally intended to protect those older than 65 years from excessive health care costs. In 1972, Medicare was modified to also cover permanently disabled individuals and those with end-stage renal disease. The federal government through the Centers for Medicare and Medicaid Services (CMS) administers Medicare. Medicare Part A covers inpatient hospital care, home health care, and hospice care. It may pay for care in a skilled nursing facility, but there are many restrictions, and coverage criteria changes frequently. Medicare Part B partially covers costs for physician services, outpatient rehabilitation, and certain services and supplies not covered by Part A. Limited skilled care and rehabilitation services in certified long-term care facilities may be paid if the client and the services provided meet specific criteria. Intermittent visits for skilled health care by a registered nurse may be reimbursed to certified home health care agencies. In 2006, the total expenditures for Medicare were $408.3 billion (U.S. Social Security Administration, 2007).

PROFESSIONALTIP

Impact of Prospective Payment System and DRGs

- Decreased length of client stay in hospitals
- More emphasis on preventive care
- Increased concern about consumer's (client's) response to care
- Increased number of critically ill clients in hospitals
- Clients sicker upon discharge from hospital
- Increase in outpatient care
- Client and family more responsible for care
- Greater need for home health care
- Mergers or closures of hospitals because of inordinate competition

Medicaid

Medicaid (Title XIX) pays for health services for low-income families with dependent children, the aged poor, and the disabled (Abrams et al., 2000). It is financed by both federal and state funds but is administered by the states. Each state determines who is "medically indigent" and qualifies for public monies, so services provided vary from state to state. Medicaid is the primary health financing program for disabled individuals and low-income families. This means-tested program provides funds only when all other financial resources have been exhausted. Services covered include physician services, inpatient and outpatient hospital care, diagnostic services, skilled nursing care, rural health clinic services, and home health services. States may choose to cover other services, such as dental, vision, and prescription drugs. Medicaid will spend an estimated $339 billion between 2007 and 2008 (CMS, 2007). It is the principal source of financial assistance for long-term care and pays for skilled home health care in all states. The optional benefit of personal care in the home is also covered in 29 states. There are 50 million estimated beneficiaries enrolled in Medicaid (CMS, 2007). Medicaid benefits spending is estimated to be $4.9 trillion over the next 10 years (CMS, 2007).

State Children's Health Insurance Program

The State Children's Health Insurance Program (CHIP, formerly SCHIP) was created in 1997 as part of the Balanced Budget Act. The program is designed to provide health care to uninsured children, many of whom are members of working families that earn too little to afford private insurance on their own but earn too much to be eligible for Medicaid. It is a partnership between the federal and state governments to cover previously uninsured children. The states administer the program.

FACTORS INFLUENCING HEALTH CARE

Despite cost-containment efforts (such as DRGs, established by the federal government, and managed care, established by the insurers), the U.S. health care system still has problems with issues of access, cost, and quality. These issues are important for nurses to understand and are integral to any effort toward health reform.

Cost

Cost is a driving force for change in the health care system, as shown by the number of managed care plans, greater use of outpatient services, and shorter hospital stays. Maximum profits with minimum costs are the market forces dominating the current changes in the health care system.

The cost of providing health care has risen dramatically during the past 15 years. The U.S. government spends more on health care per person than does any other country. The use of federal funds for health care means that resources are not available for other areas of need, such as education, housing, and social services (Grace, 2001). Figure 5-3 illustrates health care expenditures.

The most cost-efficient programs in terms of administration are Medicare and Medicaid (HCFA, 1998). Private agencies and organizations are subcontracted to administer these programs. In contrast, some private small business plans use more than 40 cents of each dollar for administration. The cost of employee health care benefits is thus an expensive commitment for small businesses.

Three major factors increase the cost of health care: (a) an oversupply of specialized providers (fees are raised to maintain provider income in light of fewer clients), (b) a surplus of hospital beds (empty beds are a cost liability), and (c) the passive role assumed by most consumers (when someone else pays the bill, consumers typically are less concerned about cost) (Feldstein, 2005). Other factors contributing to the high cost of health care are the aging population, the increased number of people with chronic illnesses, and the proliferation of health-related lawsuits and the associated use of unnecessary services (e.g., additional diagnostic testing). Advanced technology has allowed more people to survive formerly fatal illnesses.

MEMORY**TRICK**

The memory trick "**COST**" identifies changes in the health care system due to the dramatic cost of health care:

- **C** = Concept of maximum profit for minimum cost
- **O** = Outpatient services are accessed more
- **S** = Shorter hospital stays
- **T** = The increase in managed care plans

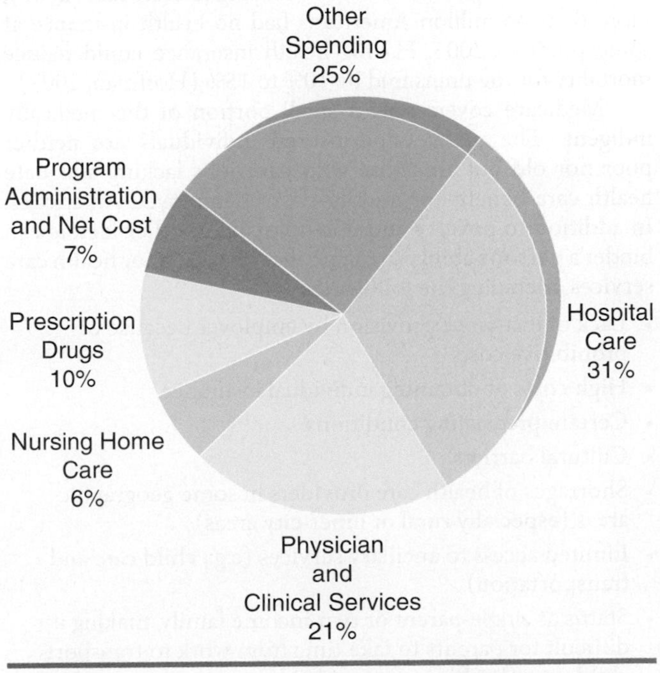

FIGURE 5-3 Health Care Expenditures in 2007 (*Note: "Other Spending" included dentist services, other professional services, home health, durable medical products, over-the-counter medicines and sundries, public health, other personal health care, research, and structures and equipment.*) (*Courtesy of Centers for Medicare and Medicaid Services, Office of the Actuary, National Health Statistics Group, 2009.*)

CULTURAL CONSIDERATIONS

Barriers to Health Care Services

Certain cultural beliefs and values may prevent individuals from seeking health care. These may include the following:

- Belief in divine healing
- Refusal of care on holy days
- Belief that the individual taking the ill person to a health care facility is responsible for the ill person for the rest of that person's life after recovery
- Belief that illness is a result of sins committed in previous life
- View of prayer as a tool for deliverance from illness
- Belief that illness is God's punishment

ACCESS

Related to the issue of cost is that of access to health care services, which carries serious implications for the functioning of the health care system. Health care for many people is crisis oriented and fragmented because of the high costs. Numerous people in the United States are unable to gain access to health care services because of inadequate or no insurance; thus, illness among these people may progress to an acute stage before intervention is sought. Their access is typically through emergency departments during acute illnesses. Emergency room and acute care services are very expensive compared to prevention and early intervention. According to Hoffman (2007), more than 46 million Americans had no health insurance at some point in 2005. Having health insurance could reduce mortality for the uninsured by 10% to 15% (Hoffman, 2007).

Medicare covers only a small portion of the medically indigent. The many underinsured individuals are neither poor nor old but are those who have jobs lacking adequate health care benefits or middle-class unemployed Americans. In addition to poverty and unemployment, other factors can hinder a person's ability to obtain insurance and/or health care services, including the following:

- Lack of insurance provision by employer because of prohibitive costs
- High costs of obtaining individual insurance
- Certain preexisting conditions
- Cultural barriers
- Shortages of health care providers in some geographic areas (especially rural or inner-city areas)
- Limited access to ancillary services (e.g., child care and transportation)
- Status as single-parent or two-income family, making it difficult for parents to take time from work to transport children to health care providers

QUALITY

Lee, Soffel, and Luft (1997) report that 30% to 40% of diagnostic and medical procedures performed in this country are unnecessary. This inappropriate use of resources can be traced to several factors, including:

- The litigious environment and resultant tendency toward defensive practice (e.g., ordering all possible tests instead of only those that the provider deems truly necessary)
- The widely held American belief that more is better
- Lack of access to and continuity of services and the subsequent misuse of acute care services

Quality may be sacrificed in an attempt to provide universal access to services in a cost-effective manner. For example, hospitals that reduce the number of nurses (downsizing) risk endangering quality. Safety and quality are often compromised by inappropriately substituting unqualified personnel for LP/VNs and RNs in direct client care. The quality of care in hospitals decreases with cross training of staff, greater use of unlicensed personnel, and reduction of full-time positions for nurses.

CHALLENGES WITHIN THE HEALTH CARE SYSTEM

The major challenges facing the U.S. health care delivery system, which also impact the control of costs, include the public's disillusionment with providers, consumers' and providers' loss of control over health care decisions, changing practice settings, decreased use of hospitals, vulnerable populations, and ethical issues.

DISILLUSIONMENT WITH PROVIDERS

Greed and waste have been identified as major problems of the U.S. health care system (Maraldo, 2001). The cause of these problems is irrelevant to the public. Reform success means starting with public expectations of eliminating the greed of providers and the waste in the health care system. Furthermore, people in the United States have become suspicious of health care providers. The high level of esteem in which medicine has traditionally been held has eroded over the past few years. Consumers, increasingly tired of paying the high cost of care, are questioning medical practices and fees (Zerwekh & Claborn, 2008); however, the public is not as disillusioned with nurses. As reported in the *American Journal of Nursing* (*AJN*), a November 1999 Gallup poll reported that almost three-quarters of those surveyed rated the honesty and ethics of nurses as "high" or "very high" (Health Care News, 2000). Nursing received higher ratings than any other profession, including other health care professionals. *Nurse Week* and Sigma Theta Tau International commissioned another survey. It revealed that 92% of the public trusts health information provided by registered nurses.

CRITICAL THINKING

Perception of Nurses

What factors do you think have contributed to a positive perception of nurses? A negative perception? What can you do specifically to promote positive images of nursing to the public?

Positive Perception of Nurses

Nurses are viewed as part of the solution, not the problem. If nurses were allowed to use their skills, the public believes they would significantly enhance quality and reduce costs. One survey (ANA, 1993) asked consumers about receptivity to nurses' having expanded responsibilities. Respondents supported *prescriptive authority* (legal recognition of the ability to prescribe medications) for RNs and endorsed the role of nurses in performing physical examinations and managing minor acute illnesses. Nurses should expand their focus on holistic care and spend as much time as possible on prevention of illness and wellness issues.

Loss of Control

Consumers express feeling terrorized by the health care delivery system. They feel they have lost personal control over their health care. Many stay in their current jobs because of their health care benefits or give up employment mobility out of fear of being denied a new policy because of preexisting conditions.

Providers feel they have lost control over the care they provide to their clients. Increasingly, the insurance companies or the managed care organizations decide which care can and cannot be provided to the client.

Changing Practice Settings

Most nurses practice in hospitals and will continue to do so in the future. The increasing presence of severely ill clients requires that nurses who work in hospitals possess technical expertise, critical thinking skills, and interpersonal competence. Outside the hospital setting, there is an ever-increasing need for nurses in different areas of practice. Home health services, in particular, will need to continue expanding in order to meet the growing needs of the steadily increasing elderly population. Social and political changes are affecting nurses by creating the need for expanded services and settings. More nurses will be needed in the future because:

- The increasing elderly population requires more health care services.
- Admissions to nursing homes is increasing.
- The number of homeless individuals is increasing rapidly.

Reforms may displace some nurses from their current jobs. The demand for greater access to health care services will create many more jobs. More nurses will be needed for primary care, extended care, home care, and public health.

Decreased Hospital Use

In the early 20th century, hospital focus was providing care to those who had no caregivers in the family or community. These early institutions provided care, not cure (Grace, 2001). In the mid-1940s the focus of hospitals changed because of technology and the 1946 Hill–Burton Act, which funded the renovation and construction of hospitals. This resulted in sizable oversupply of hospital beds. To keep the hospital beds occupied, everyone was put in the hospital, for everything from a complete physical examination to specific diagnostic testing to acute care or surgery, and health care costs escalated.

The demand for hospital beds steadily increased from 1945 to 1982. After 1982, there was a steady decline in hospital admissions and the average length of stay (Grace, 2001). In 1995, there were 23.7% fewer inpatient days than in 1985 (Feldstein, 2005). Many small hospitals have closed because they could no longer compete with the large hospitals.

Hospitals are still the center of the U.S. health care system. They employ a majority of health care workers. Fewer clients are in hospitals today because of earlier discharge and the large number of procedures performed in outpatient settings. Clients hospitalized today need more nursing care because of their complex needs and severity of illness. Additional factors that have contributed to the decreased hospital population include:

- Greater availability of outpatient facilities and services
- Advances in technology
- Expectations/demands of third-party payers

The changes in reimbursement practices resulted in hospital restructuring (also referred to as redesigning and reengineering). Examples include mergers with larger institutions; development of integrated systems that provide a full range of services focusing on continuity of care, such as preadmission, outpatient, acute inpatient, long-term inpatient, and home care; and the substitution of multiskilled workers for nurses.

Vulnerable Populations

Meeting the health care needs of underserved populations is especially challenging. Groups that may be unable to gain access to health care services include children, the elderly, people with AIDS, rural residents, and the homeless and others living in poverty. Increasing poverty strains hospitals because Medicaid can no longer meet the needs of the medically indigent.

Our current health care system neglects the overall needs of children who are more likely than adults to be uninsured or underinsured. Children who are covered by health insurance have a greater degree of well-being.

Many parents have their children immunized only when the children are ready to start school because immunization is a requirement for entry into the public school system. Preventive health care emphasizing early immunization should be encouraged and made available to children of all ages.

Rural areas have fewer health care providers and facilities than urban areas. Many people in rural areas have no health insurance because they tend to be self-employed or work for small businesses.

The Centers for Disease Control and Prevention (CDC) estimated that in 2006, 1,106,400 persons in the United States were living with an HIV infection (CDC, 2008). It is estimated that at least 56,300 persons were newly infected with HIV in 2006 (CDC, 2008). It is spreading most rapidly among women, children, and intravenous drug users and their sexual partners. Additional funding is necessary, and outpatient care

> **COMMUNITY/HOME HEALTH CARE**
>
> **Cost of Home Health Care**
>
> - Since the advent of Medicare and Medicaid, home health care has grown rapidly. Because it is much less costly to provide home care, clients are sent home to recuperate.
> - Expenditures for health care in the home are greatly increasing.

LIFE SPAN CONSIDERATIONS

Health Care for Children

- Approximately one-third of the 71,731,000 children younger than age 18 who live in poverty are younger than 6 years of age (U.S. Census Bureau, 2002).
- There are 9 million uninsured children in the United States (Agency for Healthcare Research and Quality [AHRQ], 2008).
- An estimated 2.3 million children with insured parents are uninsured (AHRQ, 2008).
- Six out of 10 parents whose children may qualify for Medicaid or State Children's Health Insurance Program (SCHIP) do not believe these programs apply to them (RWJF, 2001).
- Belief that their children do not qualify is highest in households where both parents work or when annual income is $25,000 or more (Robert Wood Johnson Foundation, 2001).
- By 1996, 90% or more of toddlers had received the most critical doses of vaccines for children by age 2 (CDC, 2002b).
- Nine percent fewer poor children complete the full series of immunizations (National Academies, 2002).
- Each day 11,000 babies are born who will need immunizations (National Academies, 2002).
- Federal funds supporting the immunization network are shrinking (CDC, 2002b).

settings (such as home care, hospices, and clinics) must be expanded to care for those affected.

The homeless and others living in poverty are often mobile, having no permanent address. They may not know which services are available to them or how to access the system except through inner-city hospitals. This creates a significant financial burden on these health care agencies. Illegal aliens, because of fears of being arrested and deported, may enter emergency departments under false identities and in acute distress, receive treatment, and then disappear.

ETHICAL ISSUES

The United States is struggling with the ethical issue of cost containment versus compassionate care. According to Hicks and Boles (1997), no country can provide all citizens with every health care service they need or desire. The U.S. health care delivery system has a dilemma of needs being greater than available resources. Difficult choices must be made to determine which needs are met and which remain unmet.

The national mentality, reflected in the expectation that everything must be done to save a dying person, has created an enormous drain on health care resources. There will be much debate about the ethics of decisions made about how scarce resources are to be allocated. Nurses must strongly advocate for just and ethical distribution of resources.

NURSING'S RESPONSE TO HEALTH CARE CHALLENGES

The United States will continue to seek ways to reform health care. There will be increasing implications for nursing. Some nurses feel threatened, but others are excited about changing the health care system into something better. The nursing profession responded to these challenges by proposing a plan for reform.

NURSING'S AGENDA FOR HEALTH CARE REFORM

In 1991, in response to high cost, limited access, and eroding quality affecting the U.S. health care system, the nursing community wrote a public policy agenda that was endorsed by more than 70 organizations. *Nursing's Agenda for Health Care Reform* (ANA, 1991) provides a framework for health care policy changes and establishes a legislative program through which to implement these changes. A major aspect of the proposal is that health care services be delivered in familiar, easily accessible, and consumer-friendly environments. Another essential aspect is that consumers are empowered in the area of self-care. The health care system continues to be costly and fragmented with unequal distribution of services (ANA, 2009). The *ANA's Health Care Agenda 2005* represents the ANA's commitment to the principle that all Americans are entitled to quality, accessible, and affordable health care services. ANA's updated *Health System Reform Agenda* (ANA, 2009) continues to represent ANA's role as a leading advocate for health care reform in the current national health care debate. For more information on ANA's health care agenda and reform, visit the ANA's website at *http://nursingworld.org/default.aspx*.

STANDARDIZATION OF CARE

A move toward standardization of care is another approach to the challenges of the health care delivery system. The Agency for Health Care Policy and Research (AHCPR) was established in December 1990 with the specific charge of reaching consensus within the medical/ health care community about the diagnosis and treatment of certain illnesses and diseases. The AHCPR aspires to identify standards of diagnosis and treatment for high-volume, expensive disease conditions to which the health care community can be held. Currently, 18

LIFE SPAN CONSIDERATIONS

Rural Elders

Health care barriers experienced by elderly persons living in rural areas include the following:

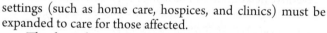

- Lower Medicare reimbursement rates for rural hospitals than for urban hospitals contributed to the closure of some rural hospitals
- Fewer health care providers available
- Greater travel distances to obtain services

AHCPR-published guidelines are available to the public and should be integral to nursing practice.

ADVANCED PRACTICE

Advanced-practice nursing developed as nursing became more complex and specialized. Nurse practitioners (NPs), clinical nurse specialists (CNSs), certified nurse midwives (CNMs), and other advanced practice registered nurses (APRNs) have provided primary health care services to individuals since the late 1960s. Many of these individuals would have had inadequate or no access to services (Boyd, Lowes, Guglielmo, & Slomski, 2000). The APRN has advanced skills and in-depth knowledge in specific areas of practice. Although there are differences among various advanced-practice roles, all APRNs are experts who work with clients to promote health and prevent disease.

Advanced-practice nurses are moving toward independent practice. Advanced-practice nurses prescribe less expensive diagnostic tests, have client visits comparable in length to that of physicians, and charge less for services because of the lower cost of professional liability insurance (Boyd et al., 2000). The single biggest obstacle to APRN practice is that most people are unaware of what APRNs can offer.

Currently, all states award APRNs some type of prescriptive authority (Pearson, 2000). In 10 states, this authority is complete and unrestricted and includes all classes of drugs (Pearson, 2000). According to the American Academy of Nurse Practitioners (2007), in 2007 there were approximately 120,000 NPs with an estimated 6,000 new graduates each year from 325 colleges and universities in the United States.

PUBLIC VS. PRIVATE PROGRAMS

The competition between the public and private sectors has encouraged quality and progress. Each setting has benefits as well as obstacles for health care recipients.

Public dollars are needed to help the poor and those who have no health care benefits through the workplace. To prevent the health care system from becoming a two-tiered process based on personal resources, both the poor and nonpoor and the privileged and nonprivileged should be enrolled in the same programs. Minimal national standards should be set, but local planning and implementation should be promoted.

The U.S. philosophy of states' rights is an obstacle to having national standards. Some consistency in the cost of services from coast to coast is needed with some local adjustments allowed.

CRITICAL THINKING

Health Care System

Even with the advantages of technology, biomedical research, and state-of-the-art clinical equipment and facilities, many consider the U.S. health care system to be in crisis. From your perspective, is the health care system in a state of strength or weakness? Explain your response.

LIFE SPAN CONSIDERATIONS

Meeting the Needs of Homeless Elderly Clients

The Health Resources and Services Administration (2003) listed recommendations from providers who serve elderly people who are homeless to assist in meeting their health care needs.

- Provide homeless elderly persons with a comprehensive multiservice center all under one roof
- Bring together the skills of different providers to provide comprehensive assessment and evaluation
- Develop health care resources for homeless persons 55 to 64 years old who are not eligible for benefits such as Medicare
- Provide outreach services to elderly persons who may be living alone, homeless, or living in a shelter who are at risk for depression and other health problems

PUBLIC HEALTH

In the past decade, public health has visibly deteriorated. Immunizations, environmental concerns (conditions that may affect health), prenatal care, and analysis of the prevailing disease patterns in a community are included in public health services. Current public health problems include:

- Prevalence of overweight population
- Emergence of drug-resistant strains of tuberculosis and other infections
- Presence of toxic environmental conditions

COMMUNITY HEALTH

Prevention and primary care are the focus of community-based care. Nursing has a rich legacy of contributing community aid, as demonstrated by the work of pioneers such as Mary Breckenridge and Lillian Wald.

ISSUES AND TRENDS

As various trends appear, the delivery of health care services will continue to change. The challenge is to improve the nation's delivery of health care services by preserving nursing integrity. Nursing must be involved from the beginning of any change. Factors that will continue to shape reform of the health care delivery system include:

- Aging of the U.S. population
- Increasing population diversity
- More single-parent families and children living in poverty
- Growth of outpatient care and a greater demand for primary care providers
- Technological advances resulting in more services in outpatient settings (including the home)

- More states using managed care to provide the medically indigent with services
- Incentives for those participating in preventive activities
- Federal funds for health care provider education requiring service to underserved populations and areas
- Managed care dominating service delivery
- Focus on quality improvement

CASE STUDY

A 45-year-old male client is diagnosed with lung cancer. In the past month, he has lost his job and his health insurance. He shares with you his concerns regarding his lack of income and insurance and his worries about providing for his wife and two young children.

1. What health care options are available for him? For his family?
2. What health care services could he be eligible to receive? His family?
3. As his nurse, what are your roles in providing care for him?
4. What level of care does he need?

SUMMARY

- The three levels of health care services are classified as primary, secondary, and tertiary.
- Health care services are financed and delivered by the public (official, voluntary, and nonprofit agencies), public/private, and private sectors.
- The health care team is composed of nurses, nurse practitioners, physicians, physician's assistants, pharmacists, dentists, dietitians, social workers, various therapists, and chaplains.
- Managed care organizations seek to control health care costs by monitoring the delivery of services and restricting access to costly procedures and providers.
- The primary federal government insurance plans are Medicare, which provides health care coverage for elderly persons and disabled persons; Medicaid, which is administered with the states to provide health care services for the poor; and CHIP, which provides health care to uninsured children.
- To achieve equity for all Americans, health care reform must address the three critical issues of cost, access, and quality of health care services.
- The challenges that the health care delivery system must overcome are the public's disillusionment with providers, provider and consumer loss of control over health care decisions, the decreased use of hospitals, the change in practice settings, ethical issues, and the health care needs of vulnerable populations.
- The Agency of Health Care Policy and Research aims to identify therapeutic standards to which the health care community can be held.
- A primary goal of the nursing profession is to provide health care services emphasizing prevention and primary health care, which will help reduce costs and increase the quality of health care.

REVIEW QUESTIONS

1. A nursing student is taught about the three levels of health care service in the United States. Which of the following statements made by the nursing student indicates that further teaching is needed?
   1. "A health care delivery system is a method for providing services to meet the health needs of individuals."
   2. "An example of primary care is when a parent takes her 6-month-old infant to the health department for immunizations."
   3. "Secondary care is when a client regains partial use of an arm after experiencing a stroke."
   4. "A client who is utilizing rehabilitation services is participating in tertiary care."
2. Which of the following is not considered a major challenge facing the U.S. health care delivery system?
   1. Changing practice settings.
   2. Ethical issues.
   3. Vulnerable populations.
   4. Health care teams.
3. As various issues and trends appear in health care, which of the following are factors that will shape the reform of the health care delivery system? (Select all that apply.)
   1. Aging of the U.S. population.
   2. More single-parent families.
   3. Fewer children living in poverty.
   4. Decreasing population diversity.
   5. Focus on quality improvement.
   6. Fewer states using managed care.

4. When a nurse tracks a client's progress through the health care system, this role is known as:
   1. caregiver.
   2. expert.
   3. case manager.
   4. team member.
5. A 64-year-old client asks the nurse, "What is the difference between Medicare and Medicaid?" The most appropriate response by the nurse is:
   1. "Medicare was originally intended to protect those older than 65 years from excessive health care costs, and Medicaid pays for health services for low-income families with dependent children, the aged poor, and the disabled."
   2. "Medicare covers the cost for low-income families with dependent children, and Medicaid pays for those older than 65 years of age."
   3. "Medicare is the primary health financing program for disabled individuals and low-income families, and Medicaid was modified to cover permanently disabled individuals and those with end-stage renal disease."
   4. "Medicare is for individuals that are over the age of 65, and Medicaid is for the wealthy that can afford it."
6. The major agency that oversees the actual delivery of care services is:
   1. U.S. Public Health Service.
   2. Medicare.
   3. American Medical Association.
   4. National Institutes of Health.
7. Factors that hinder a person's ability to obtain insurance and/or health care services include which of the following? (Select all that apply.)
   1. Certain preexisting conditions.
   2. Cultural barriers.
   3. High costs of obtaining individual insurance.
   4. Multiple surgical procedures.
   5. Upper-middle-class status.
   6. Shortages of health care providers.
8. As the homeless elderly population is increasing in numbers, the United States is facing the challenge of caring for this group of individuals. The best intervention to assist these individuals is:
   1. provide homeless elderly persons with a comprehensive multiservice center all under one roof.
   2. develop health care resources for homeless elderly persons who are not eligible for benefits such as Medicare.
   3. identify therapeutic standards to which the health care community is held.
   4. restrict access to costly procedures and providers.
9. A single working mother with three young children earns too little to afford private insurance and too much to be eligible for Medicaid. The nurse knows that which of the following is the best option for the client's children?
   1. Enroll the family in Medicare.
   2. Contact the States Children's Health Insurance Program (CHIP).
   3. Contact the local health department.
   4. Register for the Low-Income State Family Insurance Program.
10. A newly diagnosed diabetic client is being discharged home later today. The most important role for the nurse at this time is:
    1. teacher.
    2. advocate.
    3. caregiver.
    4. team member.

REFERENCES/SUGGESTED READINGS

Abrams, W. B., Beers, M. H., & Berkow, R. (Eds.). (2000). *The Merck manual of geriatrics* (3rd ed.). Whitehouse Station, NJ: Merck Research Laboratories.

Agency for Healthcare Research and Quality. (2008). More than 2 million children with uninsured parents are uninsured; most are low to middle income. Retrieved November 11, 2008, from http://www.ahrq.gov/news/press/pr2008/childuninspr.htm

American Academy of Nurse Practitioners. (2007). Why choose a nurse practitioner as your healthcare provider? Retrieved November 15, 2008, from http://www.npfinder.com/faq.pdf

American Nurses Association. (1991). *Nursing's agenda for health care reform*. Kansas City, MO: Author.

American Nurses Association. (1993, September). *Consumers willing to see a nurse for routine "doctoring" according to Gallup poll* [news release]. Washington, DC: Author.

American Nurses Association. (1995). Managed care: Challenges and opportunities for nursing. *Nursing facts* (Item PR-27). Washington, DC: Author.

American Nurses Association. (2009). Health system reform agenda. Retrieved September 27, 2009 from http://nursingworld.org/MainMenuCategories/HealthcareandPolicyIssues/HealthSystemReform/Agenda.aspx

Boyd, L., Lowes, R., Guglielmo, W., & Slomski, A. (2000). Advanced practice nursing today. *RN, 63*(9), 57–62.

Centers for Disease Control and Prevention. (2002). IOM Report—Calling the shots: Immunization finance policies and practice. Available: www.cdc.gov/nip/registry/ss/irc-2001p24.pps

Centers for Disease Control and Prevention. (2006). HIV/AIDS surveillance report: Cases of HIV infection and AIDS in the United States and dependent areas. Retrieved on November 5, 2008, from http://www.cdc.gov/hiv/topics/surveillance/resources/factsheets/prevalence.htm

Centers for Education and Research on Therapeutics. (2003). Annual report. Available: http://certs/hhs/gov/aboutcerts/annualreports/year2/y2certs.pdf

Centers for Medicare and Medicaid Services (2000). The state of the Children's Health Insurance Program. Available: www.cms.hhs.gov/schip/wh0700.pdf

Centers for Medicare and Medicaid Services. (2002a). Program information, June 2002, ed. Available www.cms.hhs.gov/chart/series/sec1.pdf

Centers for Medicare and Medicaid Services. (2002b). Program information, June 2002, ed. Available: www.cms.hhs.gov/chart/series/sec2.pdf

Centers for Medicare and Medicaid Services. (2007). Medicaid spending projected to rise much faster than the economy: Cumulative spending on Medicaid benefits projected to reach $ 4.9 trillion over 10 years. Retrieved November 11, 2008, from http://www.cms.hhs.gov/apps/media/press/release.asp?Counter=3311&intNumPerPage=10&checkDate=&checkKey=&srchType=1&numDays=350

Dochterman, J., & Grace, H. K. (Eds.). (2001). Current issues in nursing (6th ed.). St. Louis, MO: Mosby.

Feldstein, P. J. (2005). *Health care economics* (6th ed.). Clifton Park, NY: Delmar Cengage Learning.

First Mark. (2008). Preferred provider organizations list. Available: http://www.firstmark.com/fmkcat/ppo.htm

Grace, H. K. (2001). Can medical costs be contained? In J. Dochterman & H. K. Grace (Eds.), *Current issues in nursing* (6th ed.). St. Louis, MO: Mosby.

Grace, H. K., & Brock, R. M. (2001). Solving the health care dilemma: What will work? In J. Dochterman & H. K. Grace (Eds.), *Current issues in nursing* (5th ed.). St. Louis, MO: Mosby.

Haugh, R. (1999). The new consumer. *Hospital Health Network, 73*(12), 30–34, 36.

Health Care Financing Administration. (1998). Medicare and Medicaid expenses, 1997. Available: http://www.hcfa. gov/pubforms/finance/97/ch2n1216.htm

Health Care Financing Administration. (2002). The nation's healthcare dollar: 2000. Available: http://www.hcfa.gov/stats/nhe-oact/tables/chart.htm

Health Care News. (2000). Maryland group shows universal coverage can work. *American Journal of Nursing, 100*(8), 20.

Health Resources and Services Administration. (2003). Homeless and elderly: Understanding the special health care needs of elderly persons who are homeless. Retrieved November 15, 2008, from http://bphc.hrsa.gov/policy/pal0303.htm

Henry J. Kaiser Family Foundation. (2006). Examining sources of coverage among Medicare beneficiaries: Supplemental insurance, Medicare advantage, and prescription drug coverage. Retrieved November 11, 2008, from http://www.kff.org/medicare/upload/7801.pdf

Hicks, L. L., & Boles, K. E. (1997). Why health economics? In C. Harrington & C. L. Estes (Eds.), *Health policy and nursing: Crisis and reform in the U.S. health care delivery system* (2nd ed.). Boston: Jones & Bartlett.

Hoffman, C. B. (2007). Simple truths about America's uninsured. *American Journal of Nursing, 107*(1), 40–47.

Lee, P. R., Soffel, D., & Luft, H. (1997). Costs and coverage: Pressures towards health care reform. In P. Lee, C. Estes, & N. Ramsay (Eds.), *The nation's health* (5th ed.). Boston: Jones & Bartlett.

Maraldo, P. J. (2001). Nursing's agenda for health care reform. In J. Dochterman & H. K. Grace (Eds.), *Current issues in nursing* (6th ed.). St. Louis, MO: Mosby.

National Academies. (2002). Strengthening America's vaccine safety net. Available: http://www.national-academies. org/includes/shots.htm

National Information Center on Health Services Research and Health Care Technology. (2008). The nation's health dollar: 2000. Retrieved November 11, 2008, from http://www.nlm.nih.gov/nichsr/edu/healthecon/02_he_07.html

News. (2000). High public esteem for nurses. *American Journal of Nursing, 100*(1), 26.

Pearson, L. J. (2000). Annual legislative update: How each state stands on legislative issues affecting advanced nursing practice. *Nurse Practitioner, 25*(1), 16.

Peck, S. P. (2001). Community nursing centers: Implications for health care reform. In J. Dochterman & H. K. Grace (Eds.), *Current issues in nursing* (6th ed.). St. Louis, MO: Mosby.

Robert Wood Johnson Foundation. (2001). About covering kids. Available: http://www.coveringkids.org/ about

Stafford, M., & Appleyard, J. (2001). Clinical nurse and nurse practitioners. In J. Dochterman & H. K. Grace (Eds.), *Current issues in nursing* (6th ed.). St. Louis, MO: Mosby.

U.S. Census Bureau. (2002). Poverty 2000. Available: http://www.census.gov/hhes/poverty/poverty00/tables00.html

U.S. Social Security Administration. (2007). Annual statistical supplement. Retrieved November 12, 2008, from http://www.ssa.gov/policy/docs/statcomps/supplement/2007/medicare.pdf

Vrabec, N. J. (1995). Implications of U.S. health care reform for the rural elderly. *Nursing Outlook, 43*(6), 260–265.

Zerwekh, J., & Claborn, J. C. (2008). *Nursing today: Transitions and trends* (5th ed.). Philadelphia: W. B. Saunders.

Zerwic, J. J., Simmons, B., & Zerwic, M. J. (2007). Helping hands health center: Chicago-area volunteers respond to the uninsured. *American Journal of Nursing, 107*(1), 48–50.

RESOURCES

American Academy of Ambulatory Care Nursing (AAACN), http://www.aaacn.org

American Nurses Association (ANA), http://www.nursingworld.org

National Federation of Licensed Practical Nurses (NFLPN), http://www.nflpn.org

CHAPTER 6
Arenas of Care

MAKING THE CONNECTION

Refer to the following chapters to increase your understanding of areas of care:

Basic Nursing

- ***Legal and Ethical Responsibilities***
- ***Cultural Considerations***
- ***End-of-Life Care***
- ***Assessment***
- ***Pain Management***

LEARNING OBJECTIVES

Upon completion of this chapter, you should be able to:

- Define key terms.
- List three reasons for the growth in nonacute care services.
- Distinguish among licensure, certification, and accreditation.
- Describe the role of the LP/VN as a member of the interdisciplinary health care team in various health care settings.
- Discuss the types of clients that would benefit from participation in a rehabilitation program.
- Identify the responsibilities of the LP/VN in acute care, rehabilitation, long-term care, home care, and hospice.
- List the various types of long-term care services.

KEY TERMS

accreditation
adult day care
assisted living
certification
hospice
licensure
long-term care facility
rehabilitation
respite care
subacute care

INTRODUCTION

The traditional arenas for providing care have been physicians' offices and acute care hospitals. Many nonacute arenas of health care are now available, including long-term care, outpatient settings, home health care, and hospice, with rehabilitation provided in any of these. Most of these facilities must be licensed and certified, and some have accreditation.

AGENCY LICENSURE, CERTIFICATION, AND ACCREDITATION

Several methods have been designed to ensure that the agency, facility, or service meets minimal standards of care. Three of the methods are agency licensure, certification, and accreditation.

LICENSURE

Licensure is a mandatory system of granting licenses according to specified standards and is regulated by each state. All health care facilities must be licensed. A designated agency (often the department of public health) is responsible for licensing health care facilities in each state. Annually each facility is visited by a team of surveyors to determine if the facility complies with the rules and regulations of the state. Any area of noncompliance results in severe sanctions and financial penalties for the institution. A limited amount of time is given to the facility to correct any deficiencies. The facility may lose its license to operate if residents' lives or well-being are threatened.

CERTIFICATION

Certification is a voluntary process that establishes and evaluates compliance with rules and regulations but is required for any provider who seeks reimbursement from government funds, Medicare, and Medicaid. Because government funding is regulated by the federal government, certification rules are generated by the federal government.

State agencies perform this function under contract with centers for Medicare and Medicaid services. In some states, the long-term care survey for licensure and certification is done concurrently. The states have generally adopted the federal regulations but in some cases exceed federal regulations. Facilities not complying with regulations are not granted certification, resulting in no reimbursement from Medicare or Medicaid.

ACCREDITATION

Accreditation is an additional confirmation of quality and generally indicates that the delivery of care and service is above minimum standards. Accreditation is a voluntary (not required by law) process. Standards are issued by accrediting organizations, whereas rules and regulations are issued by state/federal licensure and certification agencies. The Joint Commission (JCAHO) has long been accrediting hospitals and skilled nursing facilities. The Commission on Accreditation of Rehabilitation Facilities (CARF) has been accrediting comprehensive inpatient rehabilitation programs since 1966. Rehabilitation facilities may seek accreditation from both groups.

ACUTE CARE HOSPITAL

Large acute care hospitals provide the greatest number of services. Other health care settings may provide some but not all of these services. The service departments most commonly found in acute care hospitals include nursing units, specialized client care units, diagnostic departments, therapy departments, and support services.

NURSING UNITS

Nursing units are composed of client rooms, where most nursing care is provided. Units often serve one particular type of client, such as cardiac, orthopedic, diabetic, surgical, pediatric, or obstetric. The nurse responsible for the unit may be called by several different titles, such as unit coordinator, nurse manager, or head nurse. Registered nurses (RNs), licensed practical/vocational nurses (LP/VNs), and nursing assistants provide the nursing care.

SPECIALIZED CLIENT CARE UNITS

Specialized units provide nursing care for specific needs of the clients. The LP/VN may work in these areas depending on experience, education, the size and location of the hospital, and the number of RNs available. Examples of specialized units include the following:

- Emergency department (ED): Provides care to clients involved in all types of accidents and those confronted with medical emergencies such as heart attack or stroke
- Intensive care unit (ICU): Provides care to critically ill clients until they are stabilized and can be managed with routine nursing interventions on a regular nursing unit
- Coronary care unit (CCU): Provides care to clients who have had a heart attack or who have had heart surgery such as coronary artery bypass or valve replacement
- Mental health unit: Provides care to clients who are having difficulty with relationships, coping with everyday demands, or dealing with a crisis
- Psychiatric unit: Provides care to clients diagnosed as having mental illness
- Rehabilitation unit: Provides care to clients who must learn to regain the highest level of self-care possible following injury, accident, or illness
- Dialysis unit: Provides care to clients who need dialysis because of renal failure
- Hospice unit: Provides both care to clients who are dying and support to their families; may be a unit in a hospital or a freestanding unit
- Outpatient unit: Provides care to clients when admission to the hospital is unnecessary
- Home care: Provides care to clients in their homes when professional supervision and/or minimal care is required; has been added to many hospitals to provide continuity of care
- Client education unit: Provides teaching to clients, either individually or in groups, about specific client conditions or other health-related issues

SURGICAL UNITS

Care of the client just before, during, and after surgery is performed by the operating room (OR) and recovery room (RR) personnel. In addition to the main surgical unit, many hospitals also have a day surgery/ambulatory surgery unit. Clients come in a couple of hours before their scheduled surgeries and leave when recovered from the anesthesia. Total length of stay is shorter than 24 hours.

Diagnostic Departments

Diagnostic departments provide specialized tests that assist the physician in making a diagnosis.

Clinical Laboratory

Clinical laboratory personnel examine specimens of tissues, feces, and body fluids, such as blood, sputum, urine, amniotic fluid, and spinal fluid. Testing assesses values of normal components and of any abnormal components of these specimens.

Radiology (Nuclear Medicine)

X-ray studies are performed in the radiology department, along with positron emission tomography (PET) scans, computed tomography (CT) scans, mammography, ultrasound, arteriograms, venograms, echocardiograms, and magnetic resonance imaging (MRI).

Other Diagnostic Services

Other diagnostic services may include the following:

- Sleep center: Provides observation, testing, and monitoring of clients as they sleep to identify sleep-related problems
- Electroencephalography (EEG): Records brain waves and ascertains electrical activity in the brain
- Electrocardiogram (EKG): Records electrical activity in the heart
- Electromyogram (EMG): Records electrical activity in body muscles

Therapy Departments

The function of the various therapy departments is to provide specialized treatments and/or rehabilitation services to clients to improve functional level in a specific area. Most hospitals have respiratory therapy and physical therapy departments. Some large teaching hospitals also have occupational therapy and speech therapy departments.

Support Services

Support services meet various other needs in providing care to clients. Pharmacists mix and dispense medications to the various client care units. Nurses then administer the medications to the clients. Dietitians supervise food preparation for all clients. They specifically choose the foods and calculate the amounts for special diets and provide client teaching for those clients on special diets. Social workers help clients deal with psychosocial problems, providing assistance in areas such as housing, finances, and referrals to support groups. Chaplains provide individual counseling to clients and support to families and assist clients in meeting spiritual needs. The admission department handles the admission process by preparing necessary paperwork and ensuring that the ordered preadmission laboratory testing and x-rays are performed. The business office oversees insurance and financial affairs on client discharge from the health care agency. Medical records, also called health information systems, maintains and stores all medical records for every client cared for by the health care agency. Housekeeping and maintenance keep the physical facilities and equipment clean, in good repair, and in proper working order.

Role of the LP/VN

Depending on the geographical location within the nation and nursing shortages, LP/VNs may have limited opportunities in acute care hospitals because of the high acuity level of clients in these facilities. Generally, in an acute care facility, LP/VNs provide direct client care on the general nursing units. This may include assisting with personal hygiene and ambulation, checking vital signs, and administering medications and IV therapy. LP/VNs perform client assessments and work with RNs to formulate nursing diagnoses and write plans of care. Each state has a scope of practice for the LP/VN. It is the LP/VN's responsibility to know the scope of practice for the state in which he or she is practicing. In some states, an LP/VN performs a partial assessment while another state allows full assessments. The Nurse Practice Act distinguishes between assessment data collection and assessment of the data. Generally, the LP/VN collects data, and then an RN assesses the data and determines the course of client care with the LP/VN's input (JCAHO, 2001). After some years of experience and additional education in specific areas, LP/VNs may work in specialized client care units, such as ICU, CCU, dialysis, and home care, as previously described.

Clients are transferred to rehabilitation centers and subacute facilities because of the short stays within an acute care facility. Some hospitals incorporate subacute units within the acute care facilities. Many LP/VNs are hired in rehabilitation centers and subacute facilities.

LONG-TERM CARE

Long-term care refers to the various services provided to individuals having an ongoing need for health care. Traditionally, long-term care has meant a community-based nursing home licensed for skilled or intermediate care. The rights of residents of long-term care facilities are regulated by the Omnibus Budget Reconciliation Act (OBRA) of 1987 (Table 6-1). There is a great demand for this level of care, and there is also a market for other levels of long-term care. It is estimated that by 2030, more than 8 million seniors will be residing in nursing homes It is estimated that by 2050, the older adult population will more than double to 87 million persons (Hollinger-Smith, 2005). Currently, 1.6 million persons live in 17,000 nursing homes. Of those residents, 90% are older than age 65, with almost half older than age 85 (Info USA & U.S. Department of State, 2008).

The growing population of elderly persons has caused tremendous changes in health care delivery. Various housing options are now part of the package of services available. The least restrictive level of care, appropriate for the client's needs, is generally the most cost effective. The Joint Commission has established standards for pain assessment and treatment in long-term care facilities (JCAHO, 2004; JCAHO, 2007).

TABLE 6-1 Residents' Rights—Long-Term Care

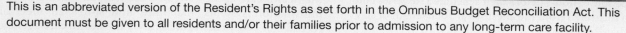

This is an abbreviated version of the Resident's Rights as set forth in the Omnibus Budget Reconciliation Act. This document must be given to all residents and/or their families prior to admission to any long-term care facility.

1. **The resident has the right to free choice, including the right to:**
   - choose an attending physician
   - full advance information about changes in care or treatment
   - participate in the assessment and care planning process
   - self-administration of medications
   - consent to participate in experimental research
2. **The resident has the right to freedom from abuse and restraints, including freedom from:**
   - physical, sexual, mental abuse
   - corporal punishment and involuntary seclusion
   - physical and chemical restraints
3. **The resident has the right to privacy including privacy for:**
   - treatment and nursing care
   - receiving/sending mail
   - telephone calls
   - visitors
4. **The resident has the right to confidentiality of personal and clinical records.**
5. **The resident has the right to accommodation of needs including:**
   - choices about life
   - receiving assistance in maintaining independence
6. **The resident has the right to voice grievances.**
7. **The resident has the right to organize and participate in family and resident groups.**
8. **The resident has the right to participate in social, religious, and community activities including the right to:**
   - vote
   - keep religious items in the room
   - attend religious services
9. **The resident has the right to examine survey results and correction plans.**
10. **The resident has the right to manage personal funds.**
11. **The resident has the right to information about eligibility for Medicare/Medicaid funds.**
12. **The resident has the right to file complaints about abuse, neglect, or misappropriation of property.**
13. **The resident has the right to information about advocacy groups.**
14. **The resident has the right to immediate and unlimited access to family or relatives.**
15. **The resident has the right to share a room with the spouse if they are both residents in the same facility.**
16. **The resident has the right to perform or not perform work for the facility if it is medically appropriate for the resident to work.**
17. **The resident has the right to remain in the facility except in certain circumstances.**
18. **The resident has the right to personal possessions.**
19. **The resident has the right to notification of change in condition.**

(As determined by Omnibus Budget Reconciliation Act [OBRA] of 1987)

LONG-TERM CARE FACILITIES

A **long-term care facility** may be licensed for either intermediate care or skilled nursing care. Long-term care facilities provide services to individuals who have continuing health care needs but are not acutely ill yet cannot function independently at home. Intermediate care facilities (ICFs) may be certified for Medicaid funding but are not certified for reimbursement from Medicare. Skilled nursing facilities (SNFs) are eligible to be certified by both Medicare and Medicaid, but not all facilities choose to do so. These facilities were formerly called rest homes, nursing homes, or convalescent centers. An *extended care facility* (ECF) is any facility that provides care for a long period of time and could refer to either an intermediate or a skilled facility. Every facility that receives government funds from any source is required by law to comply with OBRA regulations. It is estimated that 60% of persons over age 65 will need long-term care at some time in their lives (Info USA & U.S. Department of State, 2008).

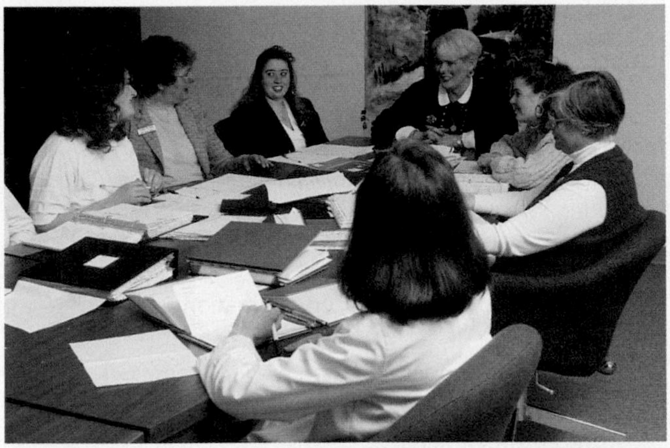

FIGURE 6-1 **An interdisciplinary team plans a client's care with the client's family as part of the team.**

Today's restorative philosophy of care directs the interdisciplinary team, which emphasizes assisting the client (usually called resident) to attain and maintain the highest level of physical, mental, and psychosocial function. The approach is holistic with family members part of the care team (see Figure 6-1).

Many facilities have special units for the care of residents with specific problems, such as Alzheimer's, diabetes, and respiratory disorders.

SUBACUTE CARE

Subacute care is a concept designed to provide services for clients who are out of the acute stage of their illnesses but who still require ongoing treatments, skilled nursing, and monitoring. The clients have complex medical needs. It is intended to fill the gap between the acute care hospital and the traditional long-term care facility (Cheek, Tumlinson, & Blum, 2005).

Subacute care facilities are usually part of a freestanding long-term care facility. Services may include intensive rehabilitation therapies, postsurgical services, wound and pain management, care for clients with acquired immunodeficiency syndrome (AIDS), oncology care, peritoneal dialysis, ventilator care, intravenous therapy, nutritional support, and cardiac monitoring. Many subacute care units specialize in one or two of these areas. Clients stay from 20 to 30 days. Thorough discharge planning with client teaching are essential components to the plan of care.

CONTINUING CARE RETIREMENT COMMUNITIES

Continuing Care Retirement Communities (CCRCs) are designed to provide continuous care as the individual's health care needs change. Such levels are the following:

- Independent living apartments on the premises with housekeeping services and meals provided.
- **Assisted living**—a combination of housing and services for those who need help with ADLs.
- Full care—short-term for persons recovering from a temporary disorder or permanent for long-term illnesses such as Alzheimer's disease; the CCRC health care facility may be licensed as either intermediate or skilled.

Usually, a fee is charged on entry and then a monthly fee. The client must show proof of adequate financial resources for acceptance into the system. The residents are secure knowing that they will receive care for the rest of their lives. Most CCRCs want individuals to enter the system when they can live independently in the apartments. The CCRC health care facility may be certified for Medicaid for clients who exhaust their financial resources; it may also be certified for Medicare for clients qualified to receive such services. Neither Medicaid nor Medicare will pay for the independent living or assisted living areas of a CCRC.

ASSISTED LIVING

Assisted living provides housing and services for those who require assistance with activities of daily living (ADLs). No nursing care is provided. These persons cannot live alone but do not need 24-hour care. The individual's independence and freedom of choice are maintained. This care may be available in a freestanding facility or as part of a long-term care facility or CCRC as previously described. The monthly fee covers meals, rent, utilities, housekeeping services, assistance with ADLs, health promotion, medication management, exercise programs, and transportation (Assisted Living Federation of America [ALFA], 2008a).

There are an estimated 20,000 assisted living residences in the United States with more than a million residents (ALFA, 2008a). The typical resident is a female (single or widowed) in her 80s (ALFA, 2008a). Assisted living residences are licensed by the state. The average cost is $3,241 per month and is paid mainly from personal funds (AFLA, 2008b). Some residents have financial assistant programs that aid with the cost. The Department of Veterans Affairs assists with assisted living costs for veterans and their widows if the veteran served in wartime.

ADULT DAY CARE

Adult day care centers may be freestanding, located in a private home or as a separate part of a long-term care facility. It is a protective setting for adults who are unable to stay alone but who do not need 24-hour care. A variety of services are provided. The centers are usually open 5 days a week and serve two or three meals. The daily or hourly fee does not include meals. Services may be comprehensive offering nursing care and some rehabilitation or limited to socialization. Working persons whose spouse or parent living with them cannot be left alone often use these services. Fifty-two percent of day care clients have some degree of cognitive impairment (National Adult Day Services Association, 2008).

RESPITE CARE

Respite care may be offered by long-term care facilities, adult day care centers, or private homes. It provides a break to caregivers for a few hours a week, for an occasional weekend, or for longer vacations. Supervision, meals, and planned activities are included.

FOSTER CARE

Foster homes for individuals unable to live independently yet who do not require care in a health care facility are being investigated in some states. These homes are similar to the foster home concept for children.

Role of the LP/VN

Long-term care facilities probably offer more career opportunities for the LP/VN than any other type of health care described in this chapter. Small facilities may use the LP/VN as supervisor during the evening or night shift according to the LP/VN scope of practice within the state. The LP/VN might have charge of one unit with an RN as house supervisor in larger facilities. The nurse needs good assessment skills and the ability to make nursing judgments based on assessment findings. The LP/VN may also be expected to coordinate and supervise the work of nursing assistants. LP/VNs may take the Certification Examination for Practical and Vocational Nurses in Long-Term Care (CEPN-LTC™ given by the National Council of State Boards of Nursing (NCSBN). Those who pass the examination are certified in long-term care and may use the initials "CLTC" to signify their certification.

OUTPATIENT CARE

Outpatient care includes services provided without actually admitting the client to a health care facility. Same-day surgery (in and out within 24 hours) may be found as a unit in an acute care hospital or as a freestanding facility. Various clinics and treatment centers offer diagnostic testing, chemotherapy, physical therapy, and other services.

Role of the LP/VN

The major role of LP/VNs is preparing the client for the treatment or procedure, checking vital signs, answering questions, and doing discharge teaching. They may also assist with the test or procedure.

HOME HEALTH CARE

Home care is the fastest-growing segment of health care and encompasses many services delivered to persons in their homes. Clients may receive IV therapy, chemotherapy, ventilator care, and parenteral nutrition at home. Nurse specialists often care for complicated cases involving wounds, diabetes, and respiratory or cardiac problems.

Medicare-certified agencies (7,747 in 1999) provide intermittent care to persons meeting the criteria for care (National Association for Home Care and Hospice (NAHC), 2008a). A registered nurse calls on the client a certain specified number of times each week to assess the client's condition, deliver skilled nursing care, and supervise the work of LP/VNs and unlicensed workers. Nursing assistants give personal care, check vital signs, and do positioning, transfers, and passive range-of-motion exercises. In addition, the agency may provide therapists and social workers to serve their clients, also on an intermittent basis. These services are time limited by Medicare and are not reimbursable if the client does not require skilled care.

The home health agency may provide homemaker services for light housekeeping tasks, companion services, transportation for outpatient care, and pain management. The home health nurse must be aware of the availability of respite care for family members needing a break from the rigors of caregiving and may need to encourage them to do so. Client rights and responsibilities are listed in Table 6-2.

Table 6-2 Client Rights and Responsibilities—Home Care

Clients receiving home health care services or their families possess basic rights and responsibilities. These include:

The right to:

1. be treated with dignity, consideration, and respect.
2. have their property treated with respect.
3. receive a timely response from the agency to requests for service.
4. be fully informed on admission of the care and treatment that will be provided, how much it will cost, and how payment will be handled.
5. know in advance if they will be responsible for any payment.
6. be informed in advance of any changes in care.
7. receive care from professionally trained personnel, to know their names and responsibilities.
8. participate in planning care.
9. refuse treatment and to be told the consequences of this action.
10. expect confidentiality of all information.
11. be informed of anticipated termination of service.
12. be referred elsewhere if denied services solely based on ability to pay.
13. know how to make a complaint or recommend a change in agency policies and services.

The responsibility to:

1. remain under a doctor's care while receiving services.
2. provide the agency with a complete health history.
3. provide the agency all requested insurance and financial information.
4. sign the required consents and releases for insurance billing.
5. participate in care by asking questions, expressing concerns, stating whether information is not understood.
6. provide a safe home environment in which care is given.
7. cooperate with the doctor, the staff, and other caregivers.
8. accept consequences for any refusal of treatment.
9. abide by agency policies that restrict duties the staff may perform.
10. advise agency administration of any dissatisfaction or problems with care.

PROFESSIONALTIP

Sharps Injuries in the Home

- A recent study found that 34.9% of home health care nurses had a sharps injury during their career. In analyzing the data from 2001–2007, no safety sharp was used in 65% of the sharp injury incidences (Quinn et al., 2008).
- OSHA cannot regulate private homes.
- Home health employers are responsible for meeting OSHA requirements that are not site specific, including sharps with built-in injury protection.

Role of the LP/VN

The role of the LP/VN in home care is expanding, with 56,610 LP/VNs working in home health care. Also, there are 126,453 RNs, 458,685 home care aids, 21,196 physical therapists, 12,564 social workers, and 6,272 occupational therapists working in home care (NAHC, 2008a). The LP/VN responsibilities vary among agencies. All nurses working in home care must have excellent assessment skills and a keen ability to identify actual and potential problems. Working with the family may be a greater challenge than meeting client needs. A major responsibility for the home health nurse is teaching the client and family. Clients with chronic health problems have ongoing needs after home health care is discontinued. They and their family caregivers must be taught the following:

The disease process

- Complications that may occur
- How to prevent complications
- Signs and symptoms of complications
- How to reduce risk factors, such as dietary adaptations and exercise programs

Medications

- Actions of medications
- Special administration guidelines, such as timing related to meals
- Side effects

Special skills

- Drawing up and administering insulin or other injectables
- Using a blood glucose monitor
- Changing dressings
- Monitoring vital signs
- Using special client care equipment, adaptive devices, and assistive devices

Documentation and communication

- How to keep records for nurse or physician visit, for example, blood glucose, blood pressure, and weight
- How and when to contact the home health nurse
- How and when to contact the physician
- How and when to contact emergency services

HOSPICE

Hospice is humane, compassionate care provided to clients who can no longer benefit from curative treatment and have 6 months or less to live. The special care is designed to provide sensitive support, allowing clients to be alert and pain free and have other symptoms managed so that the last days are spent with dignity and quality of life at home or in a homelike setting. This is sometimes referred to as palliative care.

The first hospice in the United States began in 1974. Today, there are 3,257 Medicare participating hospices, and in 2006, there were a total of 4,500 hospice programs. In 2006, 964,614 Medicare clients and their families received hospice services (Hospice Foundation of America [HFA], 2008).

The primary physician must refer the client to hospice. Care and support are provided to both client and family by a team consisting of the physician, nurses, counselors, therapists, social worker, aides, and volunteers. The team regards dying as a normal process and does nothing to hasten or postpone death. Relief of pain and other distressing symptoms is provided. The client is supported to live as actively as possible until death. The family is supported to help them cope during the client's illness and in their bereavement after the client's death. Health care workers may also need support because the task of caring for the dying is often quite stressful but can be fulfilling because most of the time the care encompasses all aspects of pure nursing care.

Benefits for hospice are included in most private health care insurance, HMOs, and managed care; Medicare; and in 43 states plus the District of Columbia by Medicaid. Forty-four states have licensure laws for hospice programs. Some programs are certified voluntarily by Medicare and accredited by the JCAHO or Community Health Accreditation Program (CHAP) (HFA, 2008).

Other health care environments include schools, community nursing centers, adult day care centers/programs, rural primary care hospitals, and industrial clinics. Table 6-3 describes arenas of care, services provided, and the nurse's role.

PROFESSIONALTIP

Hospice Settings

Hospice care may be implemented in a variety of settings: the client's home, a special area of hospitals or nursing homes, or freestanding inpatient facilities. Most clients receive care at home. In 2006, approximately 36% of all deaths in the United States were given care by hospice personnel (National Hospice and Palliative Care Organization, 2007).

CRITICAL THINKING

Working in Various Facilities

What are the pros and cons related to working for an acute care hospital, home health agency, hospice, or long-term care facility?

TABLE 6-3 Health Care Arenas

ARENA	SERVICES PROVIDED	NURSE'S ROLE
Acute care hospital	Diagnosis and treatment of illnesses (chronic and acute) Acute inpatient services Diagnostic procedures Surgical interventions Ambulatory care services Critical (intensive) care Rehabilitative care	Provide ongoing assessment Caregiver and educator Maintain client safety Coordinate care and collaborate with other health care providers Initiate discharge planning
Extended-care (long-term care) facilities (e.g., nursing homes, skilled nursing facilities)	Intermediate and long-term care for people who have chronic illnesses and are unable to care for themselves Restorative and rehabilitative care until client is ready for discharge home	Plan and coordinate care Provide care directed toward meeting basic needs (e.g., nutrition, hydration, comfort, elimination) Administer medications, treatments, and other therapeutic modalities Provide teaching and counseling
Outpatient (clinics, physician's offices, ambulatory treatment centers)	Treatment of illness (acute and chronic) Diagnostic testing Select surgical procedures	*Traditional role:* Prepare client for examination Check vital signs Assist with diagnostic tests *Expanded role:* Perform physical (or mental status) examination Provide teaching and counseling In some settings, advanced practice registered nurses (APRNs) act as primary care providers
Home health care agencies	Wide range of services, including curative and rehabilitative	Provide skilled nursing care Coordinate health-promotion activities (e.g., education)
Hospice	Care of individuals who have terminal illnesses Improve the quality of life until death	Promote comfort measures Provide pain control Support grieving families Educate family/client
Schools (school-based clinics [SBCs])	Federally funded to provide physical and mental health services in middle and high schools	Coordinate health-promotion and disease prevention activities Provide health education Treat minor illnesses
Community nursing centers	Direct access to professional services	Promote health and wellness Treat client's responses to health problems
Adult daycare centers/ programs	Maintain safety for clients Provide social experiences Monitor health	Provide safe environment Encourage socialization Health assessment and promotion
Rural primary care hospitals (RPCHs)	Stabilize clients until they are physiologically able to be transferred to more skilled facilities	Perform assessments and provide emergency care
Industrial clinics	Maintain safety and health of workers	Conduct ongoing screenings Provide preventive services (e.g., tuberculosis testing) Coordinate health-promotion activities Provide education for safety Provide urgent care as needed Maintain health records

REHABILITATION

Rehabilitation is the process of helping individuals reach their optimal level of physical, mental, and psychosocial functioning. This is accomplished by modifying the effects of the disability, preventing complications, and increasing independence. The individual's self-esteem is increased, thus improving the quality of life. Rehabilitation works to increase the client's ability to complete the basic ADLs and the instrumental activities of daily living (IADLs). ADLs include grooming and hygiene, dressing, eating, mobility, and toileting. IADLs include higher-level tasks such as using the telephone, household and money management, and driving a car. The goal is to teach clients to manage their own care when there is limited potential for regaining total independence.

THE INTERDISCIPLINARY HEALTH CARE TEAM

An interdisciplinary health care team (IHCT) is the essential component to the rehabilitation process. Client and family are the focus and are encouraged to participate in the planning of care. The client determines the amount of family participation. The professional members of the team are selected based on the needs of the client. The physician, rehabilitation nurses, social workers, dietitians, physical and occupational therapists, a speech-language pathologist, recreational therapists, and mental health professionals are usually required to provide services (see Figure 6-2).

Each discipline completes an assessment and shares this information at the care planning conference so that a consensus among members (including the client and family) can be reached. This avoids both duplication of services and fragmented care. A holistic approach is used so that the client's physical, mental, and psychosocial needs are identified.

FUNCTIONAL ASSESSMENT AND EVALUATION FOR REHABILITATION

Clients who need rehabilitation are screened before admission to a program. Assessments are completed by health care professionals whose services may be required by the client. The purpose of screening is to select the best setting for services. Criteria for admission to a program usually require that the client be the following:

- Medically stable
- Able to learn
- Able to sit supported for at least 1 hour per day and to actively participate in the program

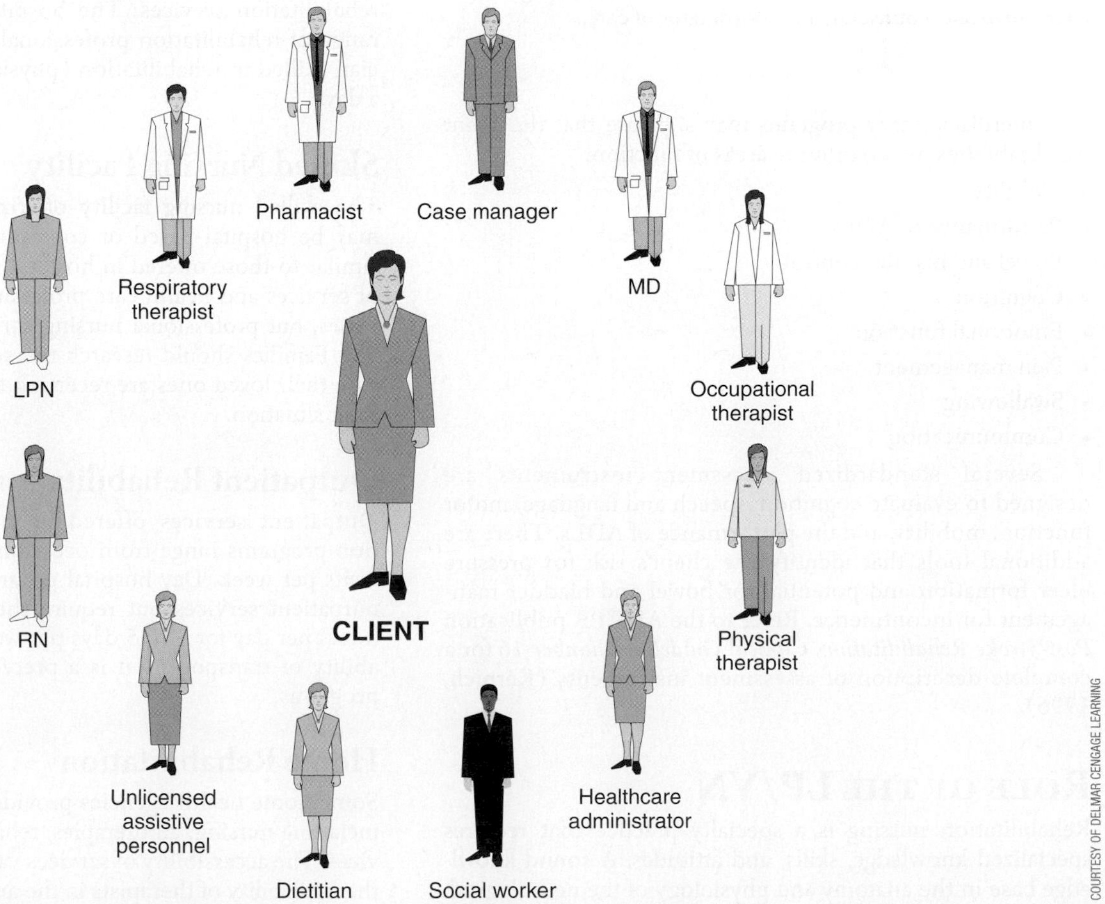

FIGURE 6-2 The Interdisciplinary Health Care Team

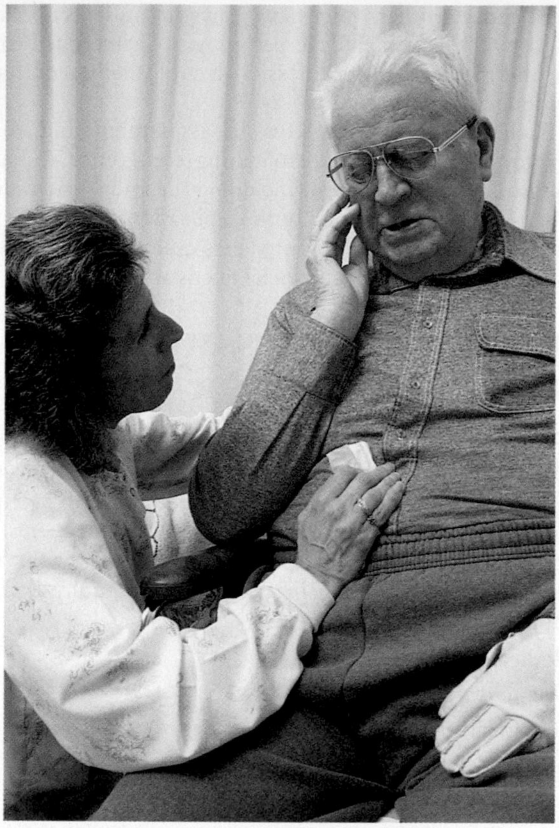

FIGURE 6-3 The role of a rehabilitative nurse is caregiver, client advocate, counselor, and coordinator of care.

Interdisciplinary programs may stipulate that the client has disabilities in two or more areas of function:

- Mobility
- Performance of ADLs
- Bowel and bladder control
- Cognition
- Emotional function
- Pain management
- Swallowing
- Communication

Several standardized assessment instruments are designed to evaluate cognition, speech and language, motor function, mobility, and the performance of ADLs. There are additional tools that identify the client's risk for pressure ulcer formation and potential for bowel and bladder management for incontinence. Refer to the AHCPR publication *Post-Stroke Rehabilitation, Clinical Guideline Number 16* for a complete description of assessment instruments (Kernich, 1996).

ROLE OF THE LP/VN

Rehabilitation nursing is a specialty practice that requires specialized knowledge, skills, and attitudes. A sound knowledge base in the anatomy and physiology of the neurological, musculoskeletal, gastrointestinal, and urological systems is a prerequisite. The nurse must have excellent clinical skills in the areas of therapeutic positioning, range-of-motion exercises, transfers, ambulation, and ADLs. The nurse is responsible for planning measures to prevent complications, such as impaired skin integrity and contractures, and to implement interventions for dysphagia, incontinence, and other identified problems.

The nurse, as a member of the interdisciplinary team, may function as caregiver, client advocate, counselor, and coordinator of care (see Figure 6-3). The nurse needs to understand the roles and responsibilities of each discipline and how to relate to each discipline.

REHABILITATION SETTINGS

Rehabilitation takes place in a variety of settings. It begins during the acute stage of illness when the client's medical condition stabilizes. Rehabilitative services are often needed after discharge from acute care, necessitating transfer to a hospital inpatient program, an outpatient rehabilitation program, a home rehabilitation program, or a skilled nursing facility. Entry into a rehabilitation program should reflect a consensus among the client, family or significant others, physician, and the rehabilitation program.

Hospital Inpatient Program

Hospitals may have a separate rehabilitation unit, or services may be available in a freestanding hospital specializing in rehabilitation services. The hospitals are staffed by a full range of rehabilitation professionals with RNs and a physician skilled in rehabilitation (physiatrist) available 24 hours a day.

Skilled Nursing Facility

The skilled nursing facility offering rehabilitation services may be hospital based or community based. Programs are similar to those offered in hospital settings, with a full range of services and health care professionals. Physician coverage varies, but professional nursing care is provided 24 hours a day. Families should research the services available to make sure their loved ones are receiving the best rehabilitation for their situation.

Outpatient Rehabilitation

Outpatient services offered by hospital-based rehabilitation programs range from occasional visits to three or four visits per week. Day hospital programs are another form of outpatient services but require the client to spend several hours per day for 3 to 5 days per week at the hospital. Availability of transportation is a prerequisite for all outpatient programs.

Home Rehabilitation

Some home health agencies provide a full scope of services, including nursing, all therapies, rehabilitation, and social services. The accessibility of services varies greatly depending on the availability of therapists in the area.

SAMPLE NURSING CARE PLAN

The Client Requiring Rehabilitation

M.J., 65 years old, was admitted to a skilled nursing facility following hospitalization for a right cerebral hemisphere stroke. He is unable to purposefully change position without assistance. His gag reflex is weakened, swallowing is delayed, and there is coughing after swallowing. M.J. has smoked for 50 years and is still doing so. Rehabilitation was initiated in the hospital. A feeding tube was put in place with the goal to assist M.J. to regain his swallowing ability so the tube can be removed. M.J. frequently expresses his discouragement with his dependency on the staff. He is married and lives in the community with his wife. M.J. had been retired for 1 year before the stroke. His wife, A.J., works full time. Two adult children live in other states. A.J. hopes that her husband will regain adequate mobility skills so she can eventually take him home.

NURSING DIAGNOSIS 1 *Impaired Physical **M**obility* related to musculoskeletal, neuromuscular, and sensoriperceptual impairments as evidenced by inability to purposefully change position of body without assistance

Nursing Outcomes Classification (NOC)
Ambulation: Walking
Body Positioning: Self-Initiated

Nursing Interventions Classification (NIC)
Exercise Therapy: Ambulation
Positioning

PLANNING/OUTCOMES	NURSING INTERVENTIONS	RATIONALE
M.J. will maintain current level of range of motion in all joints.	Change position at least every 2 hours. Do passive range-of-motion exercises twice a day on affected extremities.	Prevents contracture formation and pressure ulcers. Hemiplegic limbs are flaccid immediately after stroke and then become spastic.
M.J. will remain free of contractures.	Assist with active range-of-motion exercises on unaffected extremities. Teach to do self-range-of-motion exercises when condition permits.	Maintains joint mobility and prevents contracture formation, also increases strength and endurance.
M.J. will begin program of progressive mobilization.	Teach M.J. to move in bed: • Begin in supine position with the knees bent and feet flat in bed. • Raise the hips by pressing his heels down. • Stabilize the affected limb by nurse exerting pressure downward through the thigh just above the knee while assisting the client to lift the pelvis clear of the bed.	Increases the client's bed mobility. The recovery of a client with a stroke is dependent on the cooperative efforts of several interdisciplinary team members.
	Consult with physical therapist about program for progressive mobilization.	The physical therapist is an expert in mobility.

EVALUATION

Range of joint motion is preserved. No contractions noted. Progress in mobilization is achieved; movement in bed, transfers with 1 to 2 assists.

(Continues)

SAMPLE NURSING CARE PLAN (Continued)

NURSING DIAGNOSIS 2 *Impaired **S**wallowing* related to neuromuscular impairment as evidenced by weakened gag reflex, delayed swallowing, and coughing after swallowing

Nursing Outcomes Classification (NOC)
Swallowing Status

Nursing Interventions Classification (NIC)
Swallowing Therapy

PLANNING/OUTCOMES	NURSING INTERVENTIONS	RATIONALE
M.J. will swallow without aspirating.	Consult with speech-language pathologist regarding video-recorded fluoroscopy for swallowing evaluation.	Makes a definitive diagnosis of impaired swallowing and is the basis for intervention.
	Serve semisolid foods of medium consistency. Use a commercial thickener for liquids. Avoid milk, citrus juices, and water.	Requires less manipulation in the mouth and allows concentration on swallowing rather than chewing. Liquids are more manageable when thickened. Milk and citrus juices stimulate production of saliva.
	Allow rest period before eating. Position client at 60- to 90-degree angle before, during, and for 1 hour after eating.	Decreases risk of aspiration.
	Maintain head in midline with neck slightly flexed.	Facilitates the passage of food through the pharynx.
	Face M.J., avoid haste.	Allows feeder to evaluate the eating process.
	Minimize distractions, keep conversation minimal.	Focuses the client's attention on eating.
	Allow M.J. to see and smell food. Give verbal descriptions. Use regular metal teaspoon, give one-half teaspoon at a time.	Sensory cues promote awareness of eating.
	Place food on unaffected side of mouth. Teach to hold food in mouth, think about swallowing, and then swallow twice.	Buccal pocketing of food in the cheek on the affected side is common after a stroke.

EVALUATION

There are no signs of aspiration.

NURSING DIAGNOSIS 3 *Situational Low **S**elf-Esteem* related to the functional impairments of inability to move and delayed swallowing as evidenced by verbal expression of discouragement

Nursing Outcomes Classification (NOC)
Grief Resolution
Psychosocial Adjustment: Life Change

Nursing Interventions Classification (NIC)
Grief Work Facilitation
Coping Enhancement

SAMPLE NURSING CARE PLAN (Continued)

PLANNING/OUTCOMES	NURSING INTERVENTIONS	RATIONALE
M.J. will verbalize acceptance of self, situation, and lifestyle changes.	Assess for signs of severe or prolonged grieving.	May indicate need for counseling.
	Assess client's interactions with significant others.	Others may reinforce the concepts of helplessness and invalidism.
	Listen in nonjudgmental fashion to comments about situation.	Builds trust and encourages verbalization of thoughts.

EVALUATION

M.J. is progressing through all rehabilitation therapies and presents no signs of prolonged grieving.

SUMMARY

- There has been a significant increase in the growth of nonacute care settings.
- Medicare (federal funds) and Medicaid (state and federal funds) are major sources of health care payment, especially for the elderly and permanently disabled.
- Rehabilitation can be provided in a variety of settings.
- There is a need for the services and skills of the LP/VN in all health care services. Experience and additional education may be required for employment in special care settings.

REVIEW QUESTIONS

1. Subacute care is most often provided:
   1. in a step-down unit of the hospital.
   2. in a special care unit of a skilled care facility.
   3. for clients who are terminally ill.
   4. for clients who require life support.
2. Which of the following clients would be most likely to benefit from rehabilitation services?
   1. Mr. J, 64 years old, had a stroke, is responsive and stable.
   2. Mrs. B, 89 years old, has Alzheimer's disease in the fourth stage.
   3. Miss Z, 26 years old, is recovering from pneumonia.
   4. Mr. K, 56 years old, has terminal cancer of the lung.
3. As a member of the interdisciplinary health care team, the LP/VN must be able to:
   1. participate in the planning of client care.
   2. plan the appropriate diet for clients.
   3. teach the new amputee how to walk with a prosthesis.
   4. provide alternative methods of communication for the client with recent stroke.
4. In the home health care setting, it is essential that the LP/VN possess skills in:
   1. advanced intravenous therapy.
   2. respiratory therapy treatments.
   3. physical assessment.
   4. planning and providing speech therapy.
5. In a long-term care facility, the LP/VN may serve as the:
   1. charge nurse of a unit.
   2. physical therapist.
   3. clinical nurse specialist.
   4. social worker.
6. Agency certification: (Select all that apply.)
   1. is regulated by the state.
   2. is required for government reimbursement.
   3. rules are generated by federal government.
   4. establishes and evaluates compliance with rules and regulations.
   5. assures that delivery of care and service is above minimum standards.
   6. is a voluntary process.
7. Long-term care services include: (Select all that apply.)
   1. assisted living.
   2. acute care hospital.
   3. subacute care.
   4. hospice.
   5. outpatient care facility.
8. The nurse's roles, as a member of the interdisciplinary team, are: (Select all that apply.)
   1. instruct in ambulation techniques.
   2. provide care.
   3. evaluate home environment.
   4. order medications.
   5. advocate for the client.
   6. coordinate client care.

9. The goal of rehabilitation is to:
    1. improve quality of life.
    2. assist the client to reach optimal physical, mental, and psychosocial level.
    3. restore the client's activities of daily living only.
    4. regain total independence.
10. Nonacute arenas of health care includes a(n): (Select all that apply.)
    1. acute care hospital.
    2. school-based clinic.
    3. industrial clinic.
    4. adult day care center/program.
    5. skilled nursing home.
    6. home health care agency.

REFERENCES/SUGGESTED READINGS

American Association of Retired Persons. (1998). *A profile of older Americans*. Washington, DC: U.S. Department of Health and Human Services.

Assisted Living Federation of America (ALFA). (2003). What is assisted living? Retrieved September 13, 2008 from http://www.hospicefoundation.org/hospiceInfo/dearabby/default.asp

Assisted Living Federation of America. (2008a). About assisted living. Retrieved September 13, 2008, from http://www.alfa.org/i4a/pages/Index.cfm?pageid=3285

Assisted Living Federation of America. (2008b). As costs continue rising, assisted living remains the more affordable care choice. Retrieved September 13, 2008, from http://www.alfa.org/i4a/pages/Index.cfm?pageIC=4706

Assisted Living Info. (2003). What is assisted living? Retrieved on 5-17-09 at http://www.assistedlivinginfo.com/alserve.html

Barker, E. (1999). Life care planning. *RN, 62*(3), 58–61.

Boon, T. (1998). Don't forget the hospice option. *RN, 61*(2), 30–33.

Bral, E. (1998). Caring for adults with chronic cancer pain. *American Journal of Nursing, 98*(4), 26–32.

Bulecheck, G., Butcher, H., McCloskey, J., & Dochterman, J., eds. (2008). *Nursing Interventions Classification (NIC)* (5th ed.). St. Louis, MO: Mosby/Elsevier.

Cheek, M., Tumlinson, A., & Blum, J. (2005). American health keeping pace—Trends, options and opportunities in long term care. Retrieved September 12, 2008, from http://www.ahcancal.org/research_data/funding/Documents/Avalere_TrendsOptionsAndOpportunitiesInLTC.pdf

Feldkamp, J. (2002). The legal landscape of long-term care. *RN, 65*(4), 61–62.

Ferrell, B., & Coyle, N. (2002). An overview of palliative nursing care. *American Journal of Nursing, 102*(5), 26–31.

Ferrell, B., & Coyle, N. (Eds.). (2005). *Textbook of palliative nursing* (2nd ed.). Oxford: Oxford University Press.

Grove, N. (1997). Helping families select a nursing home. *RN, 60*(3), 37–40.

Haddad, A. (2003). When should you suggest hospice? *RN, 66*(5), 27–30.

Hollinger-Smith, L. (2005). Averting a care crisis. *Extended Care Product News, 98*(2), 18–23.

Hospice Foundation of America. (2008). What is hospice? Retrieved September 13, 2008, from http://www.hospicefoundation.org/hospiceInfo/dearabby/default.asp

Info USA & U.S. Department of State. (2008). What is long-term care? Retrieved September 12, 2008, from http://usinfo.state.gov/infousa/government/social/longtermcare.html

Joint Commission. (2001). LPN's performing assessment. Retrieved September 12, 2008, from http://www.jointcommission.org/AccreditationProgramams/Hospitals/Standards/FAQs/Provis

Joint Commission. (2004). Nutritional, functional, and pain assessments and screens. Retrieved September 12, 2008, from http://www.joint commission.org/AccreditationPrograms/Hospitals/Standards/FAQs/Provis

Joint Commission. (2007). Provision of care, treatment, and services. Retrieved September 12, 2008, from http://www.jointcommission.org/NR/rdpm;ures/D315C586-0D2B-4DB4-A9E4-FFC7681A55CC/0/LTC2008PCChapter.pdf

Kennison, M. (1999). A case study in care. *RN, 62*(1), 46–48.

Kernich, C. (1996). Post-stroke rehabilitation: Clinical practice guideline, number 16. *Journal of Neuroscience Nursing, 4,* 1–248.

Kovner, C., & Harrington, C. (2003). Nursing care in assisted living facilities. *American Journal of Nursing,* 102(1), 97–98.

Lattanzi-Licht, M. E. (1998). *The hospice choice: In pursuit of a peaceful death*. New York: Simon and Schuster/Fireside.

Loeb, J., & Pasero, C. (2000). JCAHO standards in long-term care. *American Journal of Nursing, 100*(5), 22–23.

Mitty, E. (2003). Assisted living and the role of nursing, *American Journal of Nursing, 103*(8), 32–43.

Moorhead, S., Johnson, J., & Mass, M. (2004). *Nursing Outcomes Classification (NOC)* (3rd ed.). St. Louis, MO: Mosby.

National Adult Day Services Association. (2008). Adult day services: Overview and facts. Retrieved September 13, 2008, from http://www.nadasa.org/adsfacts/default.asp

National Association for Home Care and Hospice. (2008a). Basic statistics about home care. Retrieved September 13, 2008, from http://www.nahc.org/home.html

National Association for Home Care and Hospice. (2008b). Hospice facts and statistics. Retrieved September 13, 2008, from http://www.nahc.org/facts

National Center for Assisted Living. (2006). Assisted living resident profile. Retrieved September 13, 2008, from http://www.ncal.org/about/resident.cfm

National Hospice and Palliative Care Organization. (2007). NHPCO facts and figures: Hospice care in America. Retrieved September 13, 2008, from http://www.nhpco.org/files/public/Statistics_Research/NHPCO_facts-and-figures_Nov2007.pdf

NewsHour. (2008). Today's nursing homes. Retrieved September 12, 2008, from http://www.pbs.org/newshour/health/nursinghomes

Puopolo, A. (1999). Gaining confidence to talk about end-of-life care. *Nursing99, 29*(7), 49–51.

Quinn, M., Markkanen, P., Galligan, C., Chalupka, S., Kim, H., Gore, R., et al. (2008). *Risk of sharps injuries and blood exposures among home health care workers* (182600). San Diego, CA: American Public Health Association.

Resnick, B., & Fleishell, A. (2002). Developing a restorative care program: A five-step approach that involves the resident. *American Journal of Nursing, 102*(7), 91–95.

Skokal, W. (2000). IV push at home? *RN, 63*(10), 26–29.

Ufema, J. (1999). Reflections on death and dying. *Nursing99, 29*(6), 56–59.

RESOURCES

American Association of Homes and Services for the Aging (AAHSA), http://www.aahsa.org

American Association of Retired Persons (AARP), http://www.aarp.org

American Health Care Association (AHCA), http://www.ahca.org

American Hospital Association (AHA), http://www.ahcanca.org

Assisted Living Federation of America (ALFA), http://www.alfa.org

Association of Rehabilitation Nurses (ARN), http://www.rehabnurse.org

Department of Health and Human Services (DHHS), http://www.hhs.gov

Home Healthcare Nurses Association (HHNA), http://www.hhna.org

Hospice Association of America (HAA), http://www.nahc.org/HAA

Hospice Education Institute, http://www.hospiceworld.org

Hospice Foundation of America (HFA), http://www.hospicefoundation.org

National Adult Day Services Association Inc. (NADSA), http://www.nadsa.org/ncoa

National Association for Home Care (NAHC), http://www.nahc.org

National Center for Assisted Living (NCAL), http://www.ncal.org

National Citizens' Coalition for Nursing Home Reform (NCCNHR), http://www.nccnhr.org

National Hospice and Palliative Care Organization (NHPCO), http://www.nhpco.org

National Rehabilitation Association, http://www.nationalrehab.org

National Rehabilitation Information Center (NARIC), http://www.naric.com

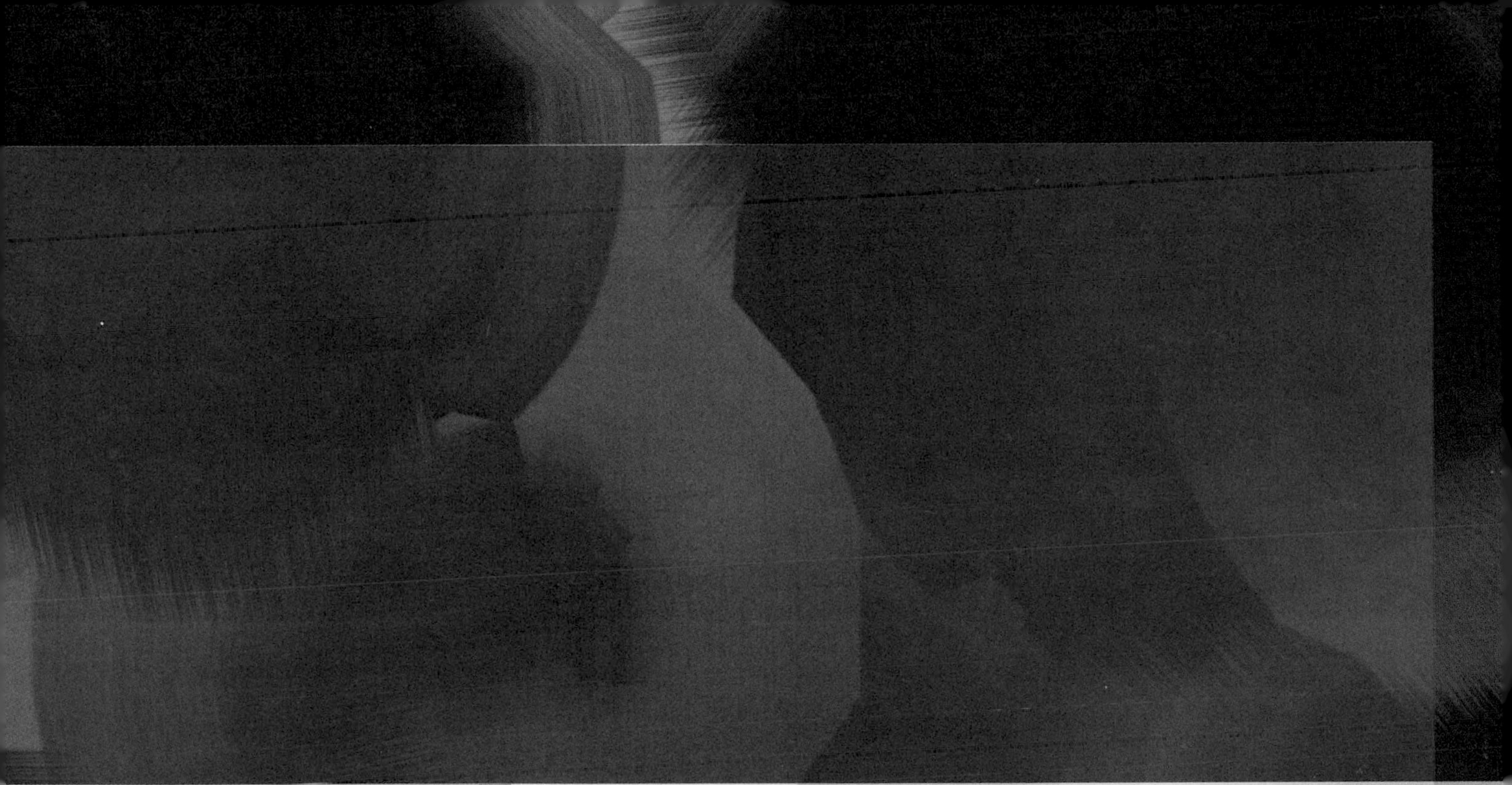

UNIT 3 Communication

CHAPTER 7
Communication

MAKING THE CONNECTION

Refer to the following chapters to increase your understanding of communication:

Basic Nursing

- ***Student Nurses Skills for Success***
- ***Legal and Ethical Responsibilities***
- ***Nursing Process/Documentation/Informatics***
- ***Cultural Considerations***
- ***End-of-Life Care***
- ***Self-Concept***
- ***Complementary/Alternative Therapies***
- ***Assessment***

LEARNING OBJECTIVES

Upon completion of this chapter, you should be able to:

- Define key terms.
- Discuss the process of communication and factors that influence it.
- Compare and contrast between verbal and nonverbal communication.
- Utilize therapeutic communication.
- Describe the psychosocial aspects of communication.
- Demonstrate proper telephone communication.
- Communicate effectively with clients and families.
- Communicate with special clients who are visually impaired, hearing impaired, speech impaired, unconscious, and non-English speaking.
- Communicate effectively with terminally ill clients and their families.
- Communicate effectively with other members of the health care team.

KEY TERMS

active listening
aphasia
communication
congruent
dysarthria
dysphasia
empathy
feedback
hearing
interpersonal communication
intrapersonal communication
listening
nonverbal communication
professional boundaries
proxemics
rapport
shift report
telehealth
telemedicine
telenursing
therapeutic communication
verbal communication

INTRODUCTION

Why study communication? Students in a nursing program have generally had a minimum of 17 years of communicating. Have you ever told another person a story and then heard the story repeated by someone else? Or have you ever played the game "telephone," where a message is whispered from one person to another and the last one states the message out loud? In both situations, when you hear the story or message again, it typically has changed from the original. When communicating with a client, family, or another member of the health care team, it is important that the message be sent and received accurately.

This chapter addresses the process of communication; methods of communicating, including verbal and nonverbal communication; and factors that influence communication, such as age, culture, education, language, attention, emotions, and surroundings. Techniques that promote effective (therapeutic) communication are also described, as are barriers to communication, and examples of both are presented. Also explored are psychosocial aspects of communication, such as style, gestures, meaning of time, meaning of space, cultural values, and political correctness, and their importance to the health care system. Finally, communication with the client, family, and health care team as well as self-communication is discussed.

PROCESS OF COMMUNICATION

Communication is the process by which information is exchanged between the sender and receiver. The six aspects of communication are sender, message, channel, receiver, feedback, and influences.

Sender

The person who has a thought, idea, or emotion to convey to another person is called the sender. Messages stem from a person's need to relate to others, to create meanings, and to understand various situations.

Message

The thought, idea, or emotion one person sends to another person is called the message. It is a stimulus produced by the sender and responded to by the receiver. A person's perception (the meaning that the individual assigns to any sensory input) can alter the message.

Channel

The person sending the message must decide how to send the message. The method by which a message may be transmitted is verbal or nonverbal (Table 7-1).

Receiver

The physiological component involves auditory, visual, and kinesthetic processes. The person's psychological processes may enhance or hinder the receiving of messages. For example, anxiety may cause an individual to experience alterations in **hearing** (act or power of perceiving sounds), vision, or feeling.

The cognitive element is the "thinking" part of receiving. It involves interpreting stimuli and converting them into meaning, as in **listening** (interpreting sounds heard and attaching meaning to them).

Feedback

Feedback is a response from the receiver that enables the sender to verify that the message received was the message sent. When these are not the same, more messages are sent and received until the receiver understands the message sent by the sender.

Table 7-1 Methods of Communication

SENDING	RECEIVING	DESCRIPTION	EXAMPLE
Verbal	Auditory		
Speaking	• Hearing	Receives auditory stimulus	Hears the client say, "My head hurts"
	• Listening	Interprets sounds heard and attaches meaning to them	Hears loud moaning in a client's room, and nurse checks if the client is in pain
Nonverbal or Verbal	Visual		
Writing	• Sight	Receives a visual stimulus	Sees reddened area on heels
Gestures	• Reading		Documents on client's record
Facial Expressions	• Observation	Interprets a visual stimulus by noting accompanying sounds	Makes note of moaning sounds when client turns to side and concludes that client has pain
Body Posture			
Eye Contact			
Physical Appearance	• Perception	Assigns meaning to a visual event	Decides client has pain when grimaces
Nonverbal	Kinesthetic		
Touch	• Procedure sensation	Performs nursing care	Gives the client a back rub
	• Caring sensation	Conveys emotional support	Places hand on client's shoulder

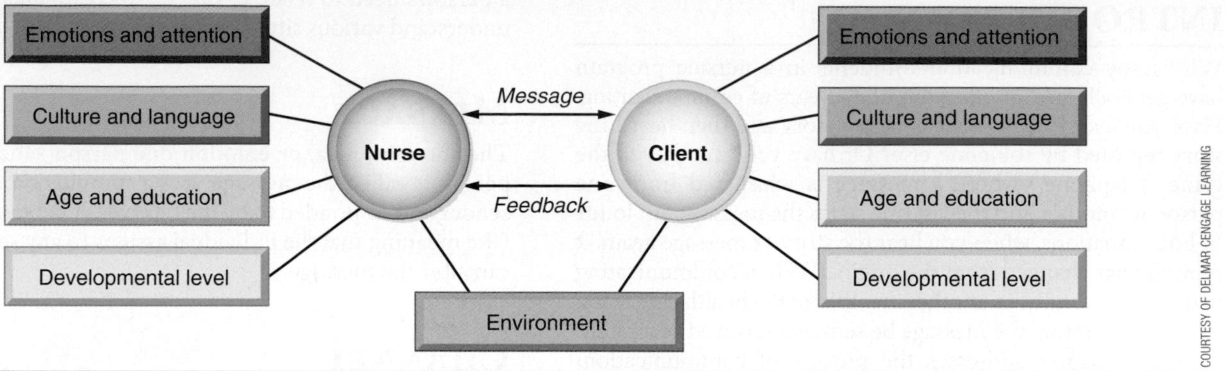

FIGURE 7-1 **Concept Map representing the communication process with influences identified.**

INFLUENCES

Culture, age, emotions, language, and attention influence both the sender and receiver as well as the situation within which they find themselves. All of these elements together are called a person's frame of reference. These influences sometimes help communication, and sometimes they hinder communication. Figure 7-1 shows the process of communication with the influences affecting both the sender and receiver.

METHODS OF COMMUNICATION

There are two methods of communicating: verbally and nonverbally. Which is better? The answer is neither, or, more accurately, it depends on what the sender is trying to communicate. Nonverbal aspects accompany virtually every spoken message. Since nonverbal communication is usually conveyed unconsciously by the sender, it is believed to be more honest than is verbal communication.

VERBAL COMMUNICATION

Verbal communication is the use of words, either spoken or written, to send a message. Methods of verbal communication include speaking, listening, writing, and reading.

Speaking/Listening

Speaking is usually thought of as verbal communication, but the receiver of a spoken message must listen. For communication to take place, both speaking and listening must occur. Have you ever spoken to someone in the same room with you and received a nonmeaningful, senseless response from that person or no response at all? The other person probably was only hearing words but not listening to the message.

Communication experts say that people speak at a rate of 125 to 150 words per minute (WPM) but hear at a rate of 400 to 800 WPM. This extra time allows for distractions. Listeners are generally distracted because they are not concentrating on what is being said. Listening is one of the most difficult skills to learn and execute well.

Intonation

Tone of voice has been estimated to convey 23% of the context of a message. When the same words are said in different tones of voice, they can have very different meanings. Tone of voice might be pleasant, sincere, sorrowful, sarcastic, joyful, or angry.

Writing/Reading

The other method of verbal communication is writing. The receiver of the written message reads the words. The reader must understand the words and then attach meaning to them. With a written message, there is generally no opportunity for immediate feedback. Therefore, great care should be taken to ensure clarity when composing a written message. A good example is charting. The physician may read the caregivers' notes after they have gone home, allowing no opportunity for immediate feedback. In such an instance, if the notes read that a client was "uncooperative," the physician would have little idea exactly what the caregiver meant. An entry of "refused to eat lunch, refused to get out of bed and sit in chair," however, is far more exact, illustrating the clarity in writing that is essential to good communication.

NONVERBAL COMMUNICATION

Nonverbal communication, or body language, is a method of sending a message without using speech or writing. Communication without words is done in many ways, including gestures, facial expressions, posture and gait, tone of voice, touch, eye contact, body position, and physical appearance.

Nonverbal communication, which is part learned behavior and part instinct, is generally unconscious. Feelings are believed to be most honestly expressed nonverbally because there is little conscious control over nonverbal communication.

Clients are particularly sensitive to nonverbal messages and seem to believe them. Nurses must therefore make every effort to be aware of the nonverbal messages they may be sending to clients. Consider, for example, the nursing skills that are not pleasant yet must be done. How would the client feel if the nurse had a facial expression of disgust or revulsion when emptying a bedpan?

Nurses must also be aware of and sensitive to the client's nonverbal messages. Many clients do not want to bother "busy" nurses, so they say they are fine or do not need anything when in fact they do. The perceptive nurse will observe nonverbal signs, such as clenched fists, stiff posture, or a frowning expression, and know that something is not right. The nurse would then proceed with further assessment to determine the reason the client is sending those nonverbal clues.

Gestures

Gestures are often referred to as "talking with hands." Gestures may be used to help clarify a verbal message, to emphasize an idea, to hold another's attention, or to relieve stress. Fingertapping, fidgeting, or ring twisting generally indicates tension, nervousness, or impatience. Shaking a fist indicates anger, whereas pointing may be used to clarify directions.

Facial Expressions

Although some people have very expressive faces, others do not. A big smile is easily interpreted as indicating happiness. Eyebrows can be very expressive, showing surprise, worry, thoughtfulness, or displeasure. The manner in which the forehead is wrinkled also sends a message.

Nurses must be very aware of their own facial expressions, especially when caring for a client under "unpleasant" conditions, such as when a client is vomiting or suffering from bowel incontinence. An expression of displeasure manifested as a "curled-up" nose or disgust is easily identified by the client. The client, often already embarrassed at requiring such care, will be reassured and comforted by a nurse's facial expression indicating caring, concern, and empathy.

Posture and Gait

Good posture, with the head held up, and a purposeful gait are usually interpreted as meaning self-confidence, competence, and a positive self-image. Stooped shoulders, a downward-held head, and a shuffling gait generally convey low self-esteem, depression, lack of confidence, or apathy.

Touch

Touch is a simple yet powerful form of nonverbal communication that even a newborn infant can understand. Touch can communicate caring, understanding, encouragement, warmth, reassurance, or affection. Of course, touch can also communicate anger, displeasure, or a lack or caring and understanding.

Many nursing tasks involve touching the client (i.e., bathing, dressing changes, ambulating). Touch, along with other nonverbal communication such as facial expression, posture, eye contact, and tone of voice, will convey the nurse's caring and acceptance. Most clients accept touch as an integral part of nursing care when it is done appropriately and professionally.

CULTURAL CONSIDERATIONS

Eye Contact

In some Asian cultures, it is considered rude or disrespectful to make direct eye contact.

Eye Contact

Eyes, it is said, mirror the soul. Have you ever seen joy, sadness, pain, or laughter in someone's eyes? It is very difficult to control these messages of the eyes.

Eye contact is generally interpreted as indicating interest and attention, whereas lack of eye contact is thought to indicate avoidance, disinterest, or discomfort.

Body Position

Body position is often a good indicator of a person's attitude. For example, crossed arms generally indicate withdrawal, although the person could just be cold. The nurse needs to be cautious not to misinterpret the client's body language. Open body positions, with the arms held freely at the sides, are usually taken to mean a receptive attitude.

Physical Appearance

A person's physical appearance says a great deal about that person. A clean, neat, appropriately dressed individual conveys a positive self-image, knowledge, and competence. A dirty, sloppy, or inappropriately dressed person conveys the message of "I don't care how I look," with the potential implication of "maybe I am not too knowledgeable or competent" or "I am sloppy in what I do."

It is very important for every nurse to be clean, neat, and professionally dressed. Clients and families understand the nonverbal message that appearance conveys. Appearance does influence communication.

INFLUENCES ON COMMUNICATION

Communication involves more than just sending and receiving verbal and nonverbal messages. How a person sends or receives a message is influenced by such factors as age, education, emotions, culture, and language. Attention to the message and the surroundings are other influences. These factors must be taken into account for accurate communication to take place.

AGE

Factors related to age affect communication. For instance, communicating with a child is different from communicating with an adult and depends on the child's age. Nonverbal communication, particularly touch, and facial expression can be understood by infants. Before learning to understand words, a child can interpret tone of voice and gestures. Preschool children respond well to communication involving toys or play situations. They should be allowed some choices, but no more than two alternatives should be offered. As the child's vocabulary increases, more verbal communication can take place.

Elderly persons may have some degree of hearing loss or a slowed response time. The nurse should face the elderly client when speaking and allow time for a response. The client should be addressed as "Mr." or "Ms." unless he or she asks to be called by his or her first name. These measures reflect respect to the individual from the caregiver.

Generational categories are determined by a person's age. By understanding the characteristics of the four main generations (traditional, baby boomers, Generation X, and Generation Y), communication between the nurse and the client, family members, coworkers, and others will be enhanced (Box 7-1).

Developmental Level

Age and developmental level do not necessarily go hand in hand. Individuals with mental retardation or developmental delays will communicate at their level of development, not at what is usually expected for their chronological age.

Education

Education is another strong influence on communication. Vocabulary generally increases as does the ability to discuss and understand concepts and abstract ideas.

Emotions

A person's emotional state greatly influences how messages are sent or received. Someone who is very anxious or upset, for example, may not hear what is said or may interpret the message differently than the sender intended. This same person typically speaks in an abrupt manner, loudly, and in harsh tones. The depressed person, on the other hand, typically says very little, speaking only one or two words or in very short sentences.

Box 7-1 CHARACTERISTICS OF THE FOUR MAIN GENERATIONS

Traditional
(1922–1945)
This generation is known for surviving the Great Depression, developing the space program, creating vaccines, developing suburbia, and pursuing equality through the civil rights movement.

Values
Respect authority and rules
Defined sense of right and wrong
Honor loyalty

Attributes
Disciplined
Detailed oriented
Dislike conflict
Learn from history to plan for the future

Work Style
Command-and-control leadership style
Prefer hierarchical organization
Uniformity and consistency

Medical
Chronic diseases common to the age group: chronic obstructive pulmonary disease, diabetes, osteoporosis, high blood pressure, and cardiovascular disease. Compliance to treatment depends on ability to afford medical care and medication. Least likely to seek mental health services (i.e., depression) because of embarrassment and the stigma attached to it.

Communication
Given this generation's respect for authority, communication needs to be respectful, direct, and in person or by phone. The client will most likely follow the health care provider's orders out completely and not question them.

Baby Boomers
(1946–1964)
This generation is known for the civil rights movement, the women's movement, an equal opportunity workplace, increased educational and financial opportunities, space exploration, and prosperity for many Americans.

Values
Health and wellness
Prosperity
Community involvement
Self-actualizing
Individual choice
Ownership

Attributes
Adaptive
Goal oriented
Positive attitude
Focus on individual choices and freedom

Work Style
Avoid conflict
Team building
Group decision making
Collaborative

Medical
Chronic diseases common to this age group include diabetes, high cholesterol, high blood pressure, and heart and lung disease. Cosmetic advancements have helped this generation try to delay the aging process. Lifestyle issues include obesity, certain forms of cancer (i.e., lung cancer from smoking), and liver problems from alcohol consumption. This generation feels an added stress by not only raising their own children but also caring for and managing the health care for their aging parents. This age group participates in self-improvement services and preventive health care.

Communication
Given this generation's respect for individual choice, the client will prefer to be a part of the decision-making process. This age group prefers to be called on the phone or to meet in person to discuss important topics. The client will expect to hear all of his or her health care options and for health care to be a collaborative effort.

(Continues)

Box 7-1 CHARACTERISTICS OF THE FOUR MAIN GENERATIONS (continued)

Generation X (Boomerang)
(1965–1980)
This was an era of emerging technology, autonomy, self-reliance, economic decline, and political and institutional issues, such as Watergate, Three Mile Island, and the Iranian hostage crisis. This is the first generation to be recognized as "latchkey" kids because of parents working and the rise in divorce.

Values
Autonomy
Feedback and recognition
Time with manager
Contribution

Attributes
Multitasking
Independence
Adaptability

Work Style
High-quality end results
Productivity
Free agent
Independent (Don't look over my shoulder)
Flexible work hours/job sharing appealing
Balance between work and life—work to live, not live to work
Sees self as marketable commodity
Technically competent
Ethnic diversity

Medical
Typically, this generation has waited to marry and begin having children at an older age than previous generations because of careers. Medical issues affecting this age group include pregnancy, smoking, depression, anxiety, and eating disorders.

Communication
Phone calls and e-mails are the preferred methods of communication for this age group. Given this generation's respect for independence and feedback, the client will prefer making his or her own health care decisions, obtaining second opinions, confidentiality, and prompt feedback from health care providers regarding health care (i.e., diagnostic testing results). This client will extensively research health issues on the Internet and bring the findings with him or her to physician appointments.

Generation Y (Millennial)
(1980–1995)
This was the era of technology; self-expression; being a team player; the Columbine High School shootings; the attacks of September 11, 2001; "a village raising a child"; and "No Child Left Behind." This age group has been nurtured and protected by their parents and is now entering the workforce with expectations of wanting everything instantly because of parental upbringing and technology.

Values
Self-expression is more important than self-control
Marketing and branding self is important
Violence is an acceptable means of communication
Fear living a poor lifestyle
Respect must be earned; it is not freely granted based on age, authority, or title

Attributes
Adapt rapidly/create constantly
Crave change and challenge/exceptionally resilient
Committed and loyal when committed to an idea or cause
Accept others of diverse backgrounds easily and openly
Global in perspective

Work Style
Seek work in teams/virtual problem solving
Prefer flexible work hours and dress code
View their work as an expression of themselves, not a definition of themselves
Want to know how what they do fits into the big picture and need to understand how everything fits together
Exceptional at multitasking (need more than one activity happening at a time)
Feeling of entitlement/wanting everything instantly
Seek to balance work and lifestyle, with more focus on lifestyle

Medical
This age group is young with few medical issues. Common health care issues include motor vehicle accidents, pregnancy, depression, anxiety, asthma, acne, drug experimentation, and binge drinking. Visits to the emergency room are more common for this generation than making an appointment to see the family physician, as it provides more immediate care.

Communication
This generation prefers communication via technology including cell phone, texting, e-mail, pagers, blogging, skyping, Facebook, chat rooms, and Webcams. It is common for parents to be present with the client during a health care appointment.

Adapted from www.ValueOptions.com, 2009.

CULTURE

Each culture has its own standards of communication, especially with regard to nonverbal behavior. In the United States, for example, eye contact is considered a sign of openness and honesty. Those of Spanish heritage, however, believe eye contact to be disrespectful. Similarly, in many parts of Europe, a kiss on the cheek between two men is accepted. People from other parts of the world, however, may look suspiciously on this behavior.

Language

Language certainly influences communication. Speaking the same language assists people in understanding each other, although regional accents or dialects of a language can inhibit communication and understanding. When verbal communication comes to a standstill, nonverbal communication is often employed to assist. Any nurse who works in an area where there is a predominant second language should learn a few words or phrases in that language to help put clients at ease and to facilitate their understanding. Most health care facilities are required to have certified language interpreters for consultation.

Attention

The amount of attention each individual focuses on a given communication greatly affects the outcome. In selective listening, the receiver hears only what he wants or expects to hear. Pain or discomfort, physical or mental, may result in preoccupation, limiting the attention given to the communication.

Surroundings

Most people do not want to talk about the intimate details of their health care concerns in public (Figure 7-2). Thus, privacy should be provided. If the client occupies a room alone, the nurse should close the door; if the client shares a room, the nurse should take the client to a conference room or to another private place, if possible, to discuss personal information.

The nurse should respect the client's current "home" (e.g., the hospital room) as she would any person's home, knocking on the door before entering the room, not sitting on the bed without permission, and asking before moving any personal articles. These simple courtesies show respect for the client as a person. When the client feels respected, communication is enhanced.

CONGRUENCY OF MESSAGES

It is important that verbal and nonverbal communications are in agreement, or **congruent**. Saying, "I really appreciate what you just did," in a pleasant tone of voice while smiling is congruent and clear; saying the same words in a disgusted tone of voice while frowning is incongruent and, thus, potentially unclear. The receiver may not know whether the sender is genuinely pleased with what was done or is displeased and being sarcastic. Messages such as these can confuse the receiver, who then may require feedback in order to correctly interpret the message.

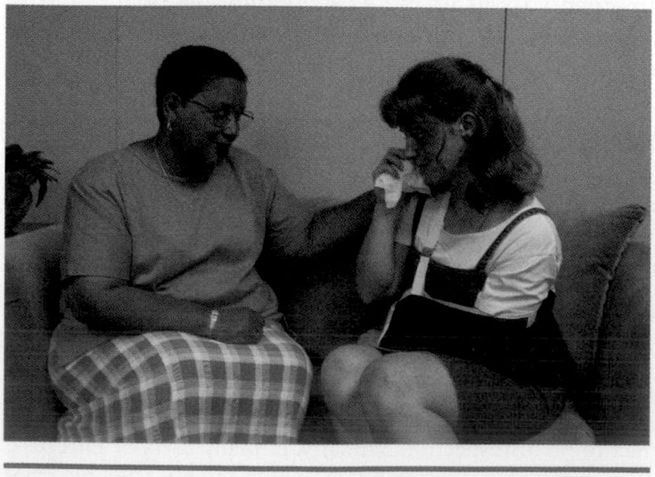

COURTESY OF DELMAR CENGAGE LEARNING

Figure 7-2 Provide privacy when discussing personal or intimate health concerns with clients.

It is important for the nurse to watch for congruency between verbal and nonverbal messages and to ask for clarification when incongruity exists.

LISTENING/OBSERVING

Listening and observing are two of the most valuable skills a nurse can have. These two skills are used to gather the subjective and objective data for the nursing assessment. Because the nursing diagnoses and nursing interventions are based on the assessment, it is imperative that the assessment be accurate.

The term **active listening** has been used to describe the behavior of listening and observing; it reflects the process of hearing spoken words and noting nonverbal behavior. It is listening for the meaning behind the words. This takes energy and concentration. To show undivided attention to the client, the nurse should be at eye level with the client, lean slightly forward toward the client, and make eye contact. In this position the nurse will be able to listen and observe more accurately. Responses from the nurse such as "go on," "yes," "tell me more," "mmhm," or "what else?" communicate that the nurse is really listening and encourage the client to continue.

PSYCHOSOCIAL ASPECTS OF COMMUNICATION

The psychosocial aspects of communication are important for nurses to understand and then apply when caring for individual clients. Consideration of these aspects makes communication more effective.

The psychosocial aspects of communication include gestures, style, meaning of space, meaning of time, cultural values, and political correctness. These aspects are based on individuality and culture and influence the nurse–client relationship.

Gestures

Gestures are movements of the body to reflect a thought, feeling, or attitude. Some gestures are known globally, such as applause to indicate approval. Some gestures, however, have entirely different meanings in various countries. The nurse must be sensitive to cultural variances and exercise good judgment when caring for clients of different backgrounds and heritages.

Style

Each person has a style of communication reflecting the personality and self-concept of that person. According to Jack (2000), there are three common types of style: passive, aggressive, and assertive. Remember that a person's style of communication is learned and has been reinforced over the years. Because communication style is learned, it can be changed.

PROFESSIONALTIP

When Clients Block Communication

In instances when clients block communication, keep the following things in mind:

- The client may not wish to discuss the topic introduced by the nurse or may not wish to talk at all. Everyone needs time alone to think.
- Accept and respect the client's desires to not communicate at a particular time.
- Let the client know that you are ready to listen whenever the client is ready to talk.

The stress, fear, and anxiety associated with being a client in the health care system may change a client's style to passive or aggressive.

Passive

The person using the passive style of communication is not able to share feelings or needs with others, has difficulty asking for help, does not stand up for himself, and is hurt and angry when others take advantage of him. This person has a weak, soft voice; uses apologetic words; makes little eye contact; and is often fidgety. The person with a passive style of communication will often go along with others without expressing a personal desire for an alternate plan of action. The client who is generally very compliant, asks for nothing, and gets little attention has a passive style of communication.

Aggressive

The person using the aggressive style of communication puts his own needs and feelings first. Communication is done in a haughty or angry manner. The voice is often demanding. This person works to control or manipulate others, shows no concern for anyone else's feelings, and has an attitude of superiority.

CULTURAL CONSIDERATIONS

Gestures

The meaning of gestures is not universal. For instance, in many places, a small circle made with the thumb and forefinger means "okay." This is not true in Japan and France, however, where this gesture means "money" and "zero," respectively. And in Brazil and Turkey, this gesture is a symbol for female genitalia and is considered an insult.

PROFESSIONALTIP

Being Assertive

"I" messages—I think . . . , I expect . . . , I feel . . . , I need . . .—are excellent ways to begin practicing assertive communication. Such messages indicate ownership of the thought, feeling, or need—a fact with which no one can argue.

Assertive

The assertive person stands up for himself without violating the basic rights of others. True feelings are expressed in an honest, direct manner, and others are not allowed to take advantage of him. The voice is firm and confident, and appropriate eye contact is made. Such a person also respects the rights, needs, and feelings of others; takes responsibility for the consequences of his actions; and behaves in a manner that enhances self-respect.

A person using the assertive style of communication effectively lets others know his thoughts, feelings, and needs. He also listens to and acknowledges the other person's thoughts, feelings, and needs. If the thoughts, feelings, or needs of the persons communicating are in conflict, a compromise acceptable to both can usually be worked out.

Meaning of Space

For many years Edward T. Hall (1959) studied **proxemics**, the study of space between people and its effect on interpersonal behavior. Hall says that like other animals, humans are territorial. Consider the following examples of human territoriality: People on a beach mark territory with a towel or blanket; space is marked in waiting rooms with a hat, jacket, luggage, or newspaper; and students in a classroom generally sit in the same place and expect others to respect that space.

How much space do you prefer between yourself and another person? This distance usually varies with the person and the situation. The distance at which one person is comfortable with another person is influenced by age, gender of those interacting, and cultural values. Hall (1959) categorizes these comfort zones as intimate, personal, social, and public space, defined as follows:

- Intimate—touch to 18 inches; usually limited to family and close friends; necessary when performing most nursing procedures
- Personal—18 inches to 4 feet; used with friends and coworkers; effective for many nurse–client interactions involving interviewing or data gathering
- Social—4 to 12 feet; preferred distance with casual acquaintances
- Public—12 feet or more; generally used with strangers in public places

Comfort zone distances vary from person to person. While some people are comfortable being very close to the person with whom they are interacting, others prefer a greater distance. Nurses should always be aware of the client's spatial comfort level (Figure 7-3).

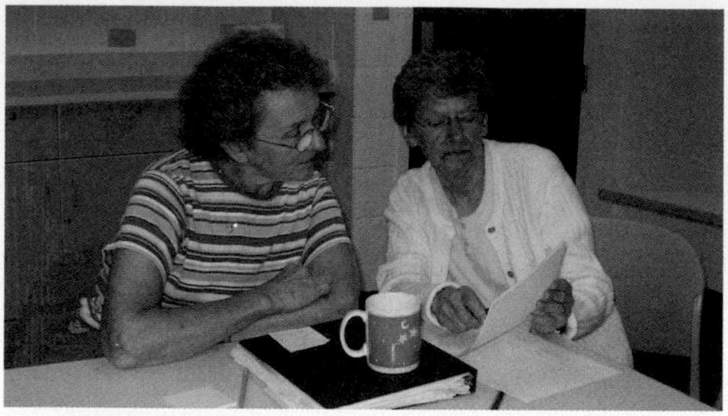

FIGURE 7-3 Personal space (18 inches to 4 feet) is used by friends and coworkers.

Much of nursing care involves touching the client, yet on admission the nurse and client generally do not know each other. The nurse must move from the client's public space to the client's intimate space in a very short span of time to provide care. When care is given competently and professionally, it helps the client feel more comfortable as the nurse occupies the client's intimate space.

Meaning of Time

In the United States, great emphasis is placed on schedules and being on time. Time is money. The clock is watched, so individuals know where they are to be every hour of the day and night. When scheduled appointments are kept, the person is considered to be dependable.

Some cultures do not have an instrument for telling time. They have other ways of perceiving and dividing time. Some cultures know a day has passed because the sun has risen, has set, and is rising again. Scheduling in these cultures often means "when we get around to it."

Cultural Values

It is important that the nurse be familiar with the cultural values of the people in the nurse's region of employment, especially when those values differ from the values of the dominant culture. For example, optimal health for all is the focus of the dominant U.S. culture. In some cultures, however, health is not a major concern, and little financial or political effort is dedicated to health. Likewise, individualism is stressed in our culture. In many other cultures, however, the social group, not the individual, is the primary focus.

As another example, consider that a number of cultural groups have learned to enjoy what they have and do not feel the need to keep working for some goal or material object. This contrasts with the dominant U.S. culture, where persons must work hard, achieve, and keep busy in order to be considered successful. Finally, in the dominant U.S. culture, cleanliness is closely related to optimal health and is a dominant value. Few cultural groups emphasize cleanliness in the way the U.S. culture does.

> **PROFESSIONALTIP**
>
> **Time Orientation**
>
> Be sensitive to the fact that clients of different cultural backgrounds may value time differently than you do. Do not jump to conclusions that the client who is always late is lazy or inconsiderate of schedules.

Political Correctness

Politically correct communication uses language that shows sensitivity to those who are different from oneself. It is intended to avoid the use of language that offends and to help eliminate prejudice. Terms that suggest inferior status for members of minority groups and terms that exclude older people, women, and those with handicaps are replaced by politically correct language. Prejudice and false ideas, which often lead to violence, are perpetuated by racist and bigoted language.

THERAPEUTIC COMMUNICATION

Therapeutic communication, sometimes called effective communication, is purposeful and goal directed, creating a beneficial outcome for the client. The focus of the conversation is the client, the client's problems, or the client's needs, not the problems or needs of the nurse.

Goals of Therapeutic Communication

Therapeutic communication has several goals or purposes. One or more of these goals guides each therapeutic communication between the nurse and client. The goals are to develop trust, obtain or provide information, show caring, and explore feelings.

Develop Trust

Clients and nurses are generally strangers when they first meet. The nurse then works to establish trust with each client. Examples of ways to build trust include answering questions honestly, responding to call lights promptly, and following through. When caring is shown, trust develops faster. Mutual trust established between client and nurse is termed **rapport**.

Obtain or Provide Information

The nurse obtains information from the client about general health and specific health problems. With this information, the nurse can make an accurate assessment and plan of care.

The nurse provides information to the client from admission to discharge, beginning with the orientation of a new client to the hospital policies and routines. Sharing of information continues throughout the hospital stay as the nurse explains procedures, treatments, and tests; teaches the client self-care; clarifies instruction from other health care workers; and answers client questions. The discharge instructions constitute the final stage of information provision.

Show Caring

Two ways to show caring are offering a drink of water without being asked or fluffing a pillow. Knocking on the room door

TABLE 7-2 Ways to Show Caring

ACTIVITY	STATEMENTS TO USE WITH ACTIVITY
Cover the client with a blanket.	"It feels chilly in here. Perhaps this blanket will help."
Assist the client to dress.	"I noticed you're having a little trouble getting your robe on. Perhaps I can help."
Serve a tray to the client.	"It's time to eat. I hope you're hungry because it really looks good."
Offer assistance.	"Here, let me help you. Perhaps together we can arrange these flowers."
Ask when leaving the room.	"Is there anything more I can do for you before I go?" or "I'm leaving now, but I'll be back in 20 minutes."
Move the client up in bed.	"You look so uncomfortable. Let me move you up in bed."
Make the client's bed.	"Now you have a nice fresh bed."
Regulate environmental temperature.	"It seems very warm in here. Perhaps if I turn the air conditioner up, it will help."
Turn the client in bed.	"Changing position really makes a difference, doesn't it?"
Straighten a pillow.	"Let me straighten your pillow for you."

before entering and taking time to always greet the client by name are additional ways to show caring.

Explore Feelings

After rapport is established, the nurse can encourage the client to explore feelings. Many clients are anxious about their illness. Some have anxiety about being in the hospital, and some fear the results of diagnostic tests. Some individuals will not admit they are anxious or fearful. The nurse is often able to help the client talk about feelings and reduce anxiety by using therapeutic communication techniques. Sometimes, only a clarifying statement is needed to alleviate fear or anxiety. Other times, fear and anxiety are reduced by allowing the client to talk.

BEHAVIORS/ATTITUDES TO ENHANCE COMMUNICATION

Behaviors and attitudes that enhance therapeutic communication include warmth, active listening, caring, genuineness, empathy, acceptance and respect, and self-disclosure.

Caring

Caring is an attitude that enhances communication as well as a goal of therapeutic communication. Caring is the basis of a nurse–client relationship and makes the client feel important. The client can easily identify a caring attitude. Table 7-2 gives some examples of ways to show caring.

MEMORY**TRICK**

SOLER

The nurse should use the memory trick **SOLER** when talking with a client:

- **S** = Sit upright
- **O** = Open arms
- **L** = Lean forward
- **E** = Eye contact
- **R** = Relax

Warmth

Warmth, expressed predominantly by nonverbal communication, makes the client feel relaxed, welcomed, and unjudged.

While touch is an important method to show warmth, it must be used appropriately. Society dictates the touching that is appropriate in various situations. Communication may be greatly enhanced by holding a client's hand or putting a hand on the shoulder. This touching provides a connection between the nurse and the client. Remember that touch may not always be welcomed by the client.

Active Listening

As implied, listening is an active process requiring energy and concentration. It involves listening to the spoken words as well as being attentive to the nonverbal messages.

Responses from the nurses indicate that the nurse is really listening to the client. It is important that the nurse concentrate on the interaction at hand and not become distracted by other thoughts (Figure 7-4).

Genuineness

Effective communication is genuine. The nurse must be honest about personal feelings. Sometimes it is appropriate to cry with a client.

Genuineness means being truthful and not attempting to answer a question when the answer is not known. After admitting not knowing, the nurse should offer to find the answer and then do so. Knowing that being genuine builds trust, the nurse must use good judgment about confronting a family member, client, or another health care worker or expressing negative thoughts.

Empathy

Empathy, the capacity to understand another person's feelings or perception of a situation, is an objective awareness of or a sensitivity to another person's feelings and thoughts. Although the nurse is not involved in the thoughts and feelings of the

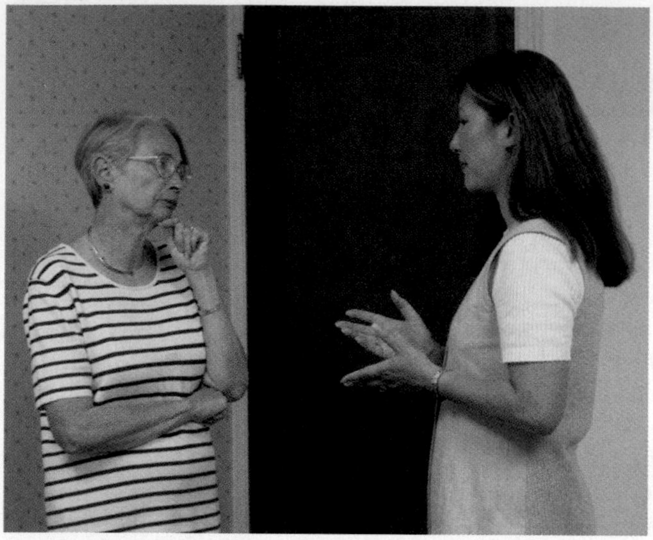

FIGURE 7-4 **Active listening, concentrating on the interaction with the client, enhances communication.**

client, through empathy the nurse is able to understand and accept the feelings and thoughts of the client. Sympathy is different from empathy. In sympathy, the nurse shares in the feelings and thoughts of the client. These feelings and thoughts are generally related to a loss.

Acceptance and Respect

Acceptance of clients as individuals with values and beliefs of their own is an attitude that enhances communication. Nurses must accept the fact that clients may have different values and beliefs. It is called being nonjudgmental when a client is accepted at face value.

Acceptance is shown by not expressing differing beliefs or values and by simply accepting the statements or complaints of clients. Clients then feel free to communicate and cooperate in their care.

After acceptance comes respect. In order to understand clients as unique individuals, they must be accepted in a nonjudgmental way. Acceptance and respect by the nurse lets clients know that they can be themselves and that they will still receive quality nursing care even though they have different values and beliefs than the nurse. Respect is shown when the nurse introduces herself and also addresses the client by name (preceded by "Mr.," "Mrs.," or "Ms.").

Self-Disclosure

Sharing something about yourself such as thoughts, expectations, feelings, or ideas is termed self-disclosure. It does not mean sharing personal problems. A nurse who shares something, such as personal future goals in nursing, is trusting the client with that knowledge. The client who feels trusted will trust the nurse, and therapeutic communication is augmented.

Techniques of Therapeutic Communication

Certain techniques promote therapeutic communication. These techniques should be learned and incorporated into the nurse's manner of communicating.

Clarifying/Validating

Clarifying or validating are used when the nurse is not sure of the meaning of a message. Clarifying is the technique used to understand verbal messages, such as the following:

"Do you mean . . . ?"

Validating is used to establish truth or accuracy. It is used for nonverbal as well as verbal messages. Examples are as follows:

"Are you saying that you did not get your medication today?"

"You are holding your side. Are you having pain there?"

Open-Ended Questions

Open-ended questions encourage clients to express their own thoughts and feelings. *How, when, where,* and *what* are words with which to begin an open-ended question. Open-ended questions cannot typically be answered with "yes" or "no" or with just one or two words, such as the following:

"How has this medication affected your vision?"

"What did the doctor tell you about going home?"

Open-Ended Statements

An open-ended statement calls for a response from the client. Because it is a statement and not a question, the client does not feel quizzed. Open-ended statements allow the client to determine the direction of the conversation, thus helping the client maintain a feeling of independence. Examples of open-ended statements are as follows:

"Tell me about your physical therapy today."

"You were telling me about . . ."

Reflecting

Reflecting is repeating all or part of a message back to the sender. Often, reflecting focuses on feelings and helps the sender "hear" the message from the receiver. This allows the sender a chance to clarify the message and shows that the listener is trying to understand the message. Reflecting can be a very useful technique if not overused. Examples include the following:

Client: "I'm really nervous about my surgery tomorrow. My friend got an infection after her surgery. I'm very frightened."

Nurse: "You are anxious about your surgery and afraid of getting an infection?"

Paraphrasing/Restating

Paraphrasing is restating the message in the receiver's own words. This lets the sender know how the receiver interpreted the message. Clarification can then be done if necessary. The sender is aware that the receiver is listening and trying to understand the message, as in the following:

Nurse: "You are afraid that you might have complications from your surgery?"

Summarizing

Summarizing is stating in a sentence or two the major points of a conversation to let the sender know what was heard.

The sender can then add more information or clarify what was originally heard. An example might be as follows:

"Let me see, we have discussed . . ."

Focusing

Keeping communication focused on the topic being discussed can sometimes be difficult. Clients may wander off to other topics, or the topic may shift to the nurse. It is important to keep the focus on the client and not the nurse. For example, the nurse could say the following:

"We can discuss that in a minute, right now I'd like to discuss . . ."

"A minute ago you mentioned that you'd had an upset stomach after taking your medication. Tell me more about that."

Silence

Silence is one of the most difficult but effective techniques to use. In the dominant U.S. culture, most people are uncomfortable with silence and feel the need to fill the gap by saying something. Silence can be a valuable therapeutic technique, allowing the client time to gather thoughts or check emotions. Silence also gives the nurse a chance to decide how best to continue the interaction. If the nurse employs behaviors to enhance communication during the silence, the client will often verbalize thoughts or feelings.

BARRIERS TO COMMUNICATION

Employing behaviors and attitudes to enhance communication will be of little use if the nurse also employs barriers to communication. Although the communication process is intense, it should not be threatening. The purpose in learning about things that block communication is to enable the nurse to identify them and avoid using them. Many mistakes can be corrected when identified. A simple "I'm sorry, I shouldn't have said that" will often take care of the situation. Practice helps sharpen communication skills. The most common barriers are discussed in the following sections.

PROFESSIONALTIP

Improve Communication Skills

Communication skills can be improved by the following:

- Minimizing distractions
- Making eye contact
- Listening
- Being patient
- Not interrupting
- Checking congruency of words spoken with non-verbal cues
- Using clear, easy-to-understand terminology and explaining medical terms when used
- Asking client to paraphrase important information

PROFESSIONALTIP

Therapeutic Communication

Practice the techniques of therapeutic communication with family, classmates, friends, and instructors. This may seem artificial and uncomfortable at first, but it will become easier with practice. If you begin using the techniques of therapeutic communication now, you will have incorporated them into your manner of communication by the time you begin clinical experience.

Closed Questions

Questions that can be answered with "yes" or "no" or with only one or two words are considered closed. After the one- or two-word answer, communication is usually ended; there is no other avenue for the communication to follow. This type of question is appropriate in certain circumstances, however, such as when taking a health history or in an emergency. Examples of closed questions are as follows:

"Is the pain gone?"

"Did you sleep well?"

Clichés

Clichés are overused, trite phrases that are almost meaningless. They are impersonal and often used when individuals are at a loss for anything better to say. They are used without thinking of the impact on the other person and often seem disrespectful of the client's individual circumstances. Examples include the following:

"Hang in there; tomorrow is another day."

"It could be worse."

False Reassurance

False reassurance about the outcome of a situation is often used in an effort to cheer up the client regardless of the facts. False reassurance can be especially traumatic to a terminally ill client who may be desperate to believe assurances even if they are not founded in reality. An example of false reassurance is as follows:

"Don't worry, I'm sure everything will be fine."

Judgmental Responses

Judgmental responses are based on the nurse's personal value system and imply right or wrong. Such responses allow no room for further discussion, such as the following:

"You shouldn't feel that way."

"You ought to do . . ."

Agreeing/Disagreeing or Approving/Disapproving

Whether the nurse is agreeing/approving or disagreeing/disapproving, offering an opinion implies that one belief is right and the other wrong. Clients are thus prevented from sharing their feelings and may feel pressured to express the same values and opinions as the nurse. One example is as follows:

"I wouldn't do it that way."

Giving Advice

Giving advice involves offering personal rather than professional opinion. When the nurse does this, the client's responsibility for making decisions is diminished. Furthermore, some clients may end up feeling unable to make their own choices and may therefore become more dependent on the nurse. One example might be the following:

"I think you should . . ."

Stereotyping

Stereotyping occurs when individual differences are ignored and a person is automatically put into a specific category because they have certain characteristics. Examples might be the following:

"Someone your age shouldn't worry about that."

"Boys aren't supposed to cry."

Belittling

Belittling conveys to a person that his thoughts or feelings really have no value, that it is silly to think or feel a certain way, or that he is no different from other individuals in similar circumstances. Examples include the following:

"Many people have it much worse."

"Yes, everyone feels like that."

Defending

Defending is a response to a feeling of being directly or indirectly threatened. The nurse may make statements in defense of self, another nurse, a doctor, or the health care facility. Defending implies that the client is not permitted to criticize or express feelings. This may be one of the most difficult communication barriers to overcome. No one likes to be criticized or to hear coworkers criticized. A natural first response is to defend why something was said, done, or not done. An example of defending is as follows:

"No one on this unit would say that."

Requesting an Explanation

It can be very intimidating for a client when a nurse asks for an explanation of behaviors, feelings, or thoughts. Often, the client does not know the "why." The usual results are increased anxiety, becoming defensive, and an end to communication. Examples are as follows:

"Why did you do that?"

"Why do you feel that way?"

Changing the Subject

An abrupt change of subject by the nurse generally indicates to the client that the nurse is uncomfortable or anxious about the topic under discussion. It often is used to avoid listening to a client's fear, distress, or problems and is interpreted by the client as a lack of interest:

Client: "I don't think I'll ever get well."

Nurse: "Isn't it a beautiful day?"

PROFESSIONAL BOUNDARIES

All communication with clients must take place within **professional boundaries** (the limits of the professional relationship that allow for a safe, therapeutic connection between the professional and the client). The nurse must abstain from obtaining personal gain at the expense of the client and refrain from inappropriate involvement in the client's personal relationships.

NURSE–CLIENT COMMUNICATION

One of the most important aspects of nursing care is communication. Good communication skills are essential whether the nurse is gathering admission information, taking a health history, teaching, or implementing care. **Interpersonal communication** is an exchange of information between the nurse and the client. This basic level of communication occurs between 2 or more people in a small group and is the most common form of communication in nursing.

Nurses have both an ethical and a moral responsibility to use any information gathered from the client in the client's best interest. Information that affects the health status or care of the client should be shared with other members of the health care team. All information concerning a client is confidential and should never be discussed in elevators, the cafeteria, the hallways, or other public places outside the health care facility.

Nurses' competence is often judged by their communication skills. Client satisfaction is increased by good communication, and increased client satisfaction leads to better compliance with the therapeutic regimen.

A key factor in the client's perception and evaluation of the health care services provided is communication.

Formal/Informal Communication

Formal communication is purposeful and is employed in a structured situation, such as information gathering on admission or scheduled teaching sessions (Figure 7-5). Specific items covered in a planned sequence provide more information in the shortest amount of time.

Informal communication does not follow a structured approach, although it often reveals information that is pertinent to the client's care. For instance, a client may comment that the tape holding her bandage in place is irritating to her skin. This would lead the nurse to assess the wound area and take action to correct the problem. This interaction, although not planned or structured, was nonetheless helpful in ensuring quality nursing care.

CRITICAL THINKING

Communication Barriers

Can you identify communication barriers you may have seen in the past? If so, list them and discuss ways to eliminate these communication barriers.

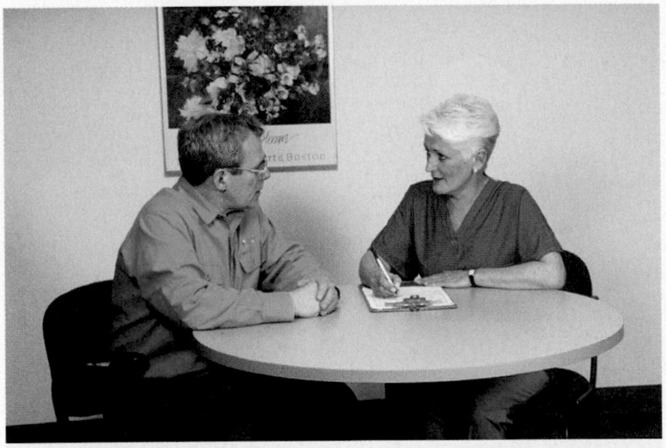

FIGURE 7-5 Formal Interaction, Admission Interview

SOCIAL COMMUNICATION

Everyday conversations with friends, family, and acquaintances are called social communication. Topics usually are those of interest to both parties and reflect the social relationship of the persons involved. Both people share information, feelings, and thoughts. Social communication provides a way to get acquainted with clients to learn about each other and to begin a nurse–client relationship.

Although social communication is not considered therapeutic communication, it is used in the nurse–client relationship. It is nonthreatening and puts the client at ease, allowing the nurse to get to know the client and what is important to the client. Social communication is often interpreted by clients as expressions of caring on the part of the nurse—that is, the nurse cares enough about the client to spend time communicating as a person rather than as a nurse.

INTERACTIONS

Nurse–client interactions and relationships progress through three phases. The purpose of the interaction dictates the amount of time spent on each phase.

Introduction Phase

The introduction phase of any interaction is usually fairly short. After greeting the client by name, the nurse should introduce himself and define his role. Then expectations of the interaction are clarified, and mutual goals are set. A good format might be as follows:

> "Good morning, Mrs. Ishdu. My name is Lorenzo Lopez. I am a student practical (vocational) nurse. I will be caring for you today and tomorrow. During this time, I will be teaching you some leg exercises that you will have to do after your surgery tomorrow."

Working Phase

The working phase generally constitutes the major portion of any interaction and is used to accomplish the goal or objective defined in the introduction. Feedback should always be asked for to ensure understanding on the part of the client. In the previously presented scenario, the client's demonstrating the leg exercises and verbalizing why the exercises are necessary would indicate understanding.

Termination Phase

The termination phase is the final phase of any interaction. Seldom do nurses have unlimited time to spend with one client, and there are several ways for the nurse to indicate the end of an interaction. The nurse may ask whether the client has any questions about the topic discussed. Summarizing the topic is another good way for the nurse to indicate closure.

FACTORS AFFECTING NURSE–CLIENT COMMUNICATION

As mentioned previously, factors such as age, education, emotions, culture, language, attention, and surroundings affect both parties in a communication. In nurse–client communications, additional factors relating to both the nurse and the client also come into play. The nurse must be sensitive to these factors and avoid personal biases in order to provide appropriate nursing care.

Nurse

Many factors pertaining to the nurse influence nurse–client communication. The nurse's state of health, home situation, workload, staff relations, and past experiences as a nurse can all impact the attitude, thinking, concentration, and emotions of the nurse. These all influence the way a nurse sends and receives messages. Self-awareness (an awareness of all these factors) is very important for the nurse when communicating.

Client

Factors related to the client that must be considered include social factors, religion, family situation, visual ability, hearing ability, speech ability, level of consciousness, language proficiency, and state of illness. The National Institute on Deafness and Other Communication Disorders (NIDCD, 2008) estimates that more than 46 million Americans suffer from a communication disorder and that approximately 36 million Americans have some degree of hearing loss (NIDCD, 2008a).

Hearing Ability If a hearing-impaired person is able to read, writing may be the easiest method of communication; however, many hearing-impaired persons have learned to speech read at least to some degree. This was formerly known as lip-read. Communicating with a client who is hearing impaired requires time and patience.

The client may experience frustration when communicating. Such frustration generally stems more from trying to understand others rather than from trying to be understood. Face the client and speak slowly and deliberately using slightly exaggerated word formation. Gesturing can also be very effective. Check to see whether the client has a hearing aid and, if so, encourage its use during the communication.

Speech Ability Dysphasia, the impairment of speech, and **aphasia**, the absence of speech, are most commonly seen as the result of a stroke, although both can result from a brain lesion. Other neurological diseases such as Parkinson's disease may also cause **dysphasia**. A dysfunction of the muscles used for speech is termed **dysarthria**, which makes a person's speech difficult, slow, and hard to understand. Dysphasia, aphasia, and dysarthria create communication problems.

LIFE SPAN CONSIDERATIONS

Communication

With Older Client

- Assess for sensory disturbances.
- Face the client when speaking.
- Have patience; response may be slow.
- Show respect and be considerate of the older client's personal dignity.

With Children

- Be at eye level with the child.
- Use vocabulary appropriate for the child's level of development.

CRITICAL THINKING

Communication and the Unconscious Client

Why should you communicate with an unconscious client?

How can you communicate with an unconscious client?

The person with dysphasia has difficulty putting thoughts and feelings into words and sending messages. It should be noted, however, that seldom does the person with dysphasia have difficulty receiving and interpreting messages; thus, explanations should be given before doing anything. If the client can write, paper and pencil can be used for communication. A picture board, word board, letter board, or computer may also be employed. A person with speech impairments may feel frustrated and helpless. Establishing some method of communication for the client provides hope and maintains self-esteem while minimizing or preventing feelings of depression, anger, and hostility.

Level of Consciousness True communication cannot be accomplished with unconscious or comatose clients. It should be remembered, however, that unconscious or comatose clients may be able to hear even though they cannot respond. Caregivers should speak to these clients just as they would to alert clients. Always greet the client by name, identify yourself, and explain why you are in the room (i.e., what you are going to do). Then let the client know when you are leaving and, if possible, when you will return. Although one sided, this interaction is critical to the client's care.

Language Proficiency The client's ability to communicate effectively through spoken language also influences the nurse–client interaction. Clients who do not speak English generally come from another culture. Learning about the other culture, especially about the values and beliefs, will help prevent the nurse from violating those values and beliefs.

A family member who speaks English could be used as an interpreter, as shown in Figure 7-6. When another health care

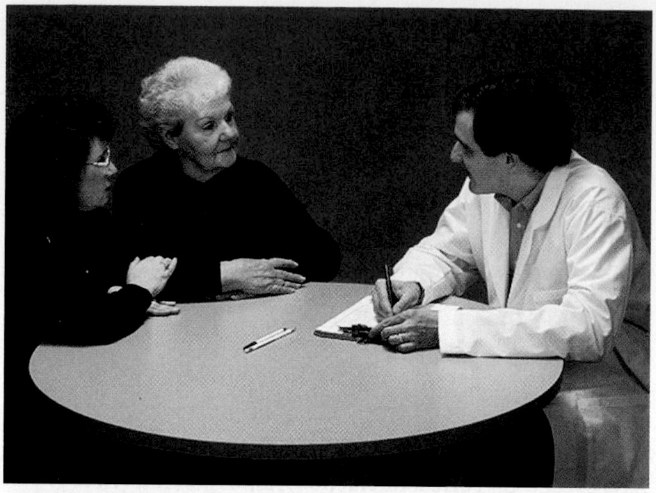

FIGURE 7-6 A family member interprets communication with a non–English-speaking client.

worker on the nursing unit speaks the same language as does the client, that person could also be used as an interpreter as long as it does not interfere with his or her work. Speak directly to the client whether an interpreter is present or not. Make eye contact with the client and speak slowly and clearly. Use simple words and avoid slang and medical jargon. The nurse may recommend a professional interpreter when obtaining informed consent.

Pictures or a two-language dictionary are often helpful. When another language is prevalent in the community, nurses should learn some phrases in that language to use in client assessment and care. *Remember, gestures, facial expressions, and other nonverbal communication send messages without the use of language.*

Social Factors Socially acceptable health concerns, such as having the gallbladder or appendix removed or having the flu, are easy to discuss. It may be more difficult to communicate with a woman who is having a breast removed. The symbolic meaning of the breast may make it difficult for the client to accept its removal and may influence how she relates to others. A person who is HIV positive or has another sexually transmitted infection may be very reluctant to discuss the illness.

Stage of Illness The stage of a client's illness may influence the client's desire to communicate with the nurse. Clients in the early stages of illness may be eager to learn all they can about the illness or may express anger and resentment at their current state of health.

Terminally ill clients may pose special challenges for the nurse. Most terminally ill clients know they are dying and are concerned about those whom they love. It is thus important for the nurse to have the client identify those persons the client considers to be "family." Family and nurses often struggle with effective communication techniques when speaking with one who is dying. Death is not a prime subject for discussion, as it is often considered a defeat by health care workers. *Remember that silence and listening are both part of communication and can relay caring, compassion, and acceptance.*

Whenever a client begins talking about death, the nurse must be willing to listen and take part in the conversation. Many times nurses hesitate to communicate with the terminally ill for fear they will say the wrong thing. The client who wishes to talk needs a good listener. Allow the client to guide

PROFESSIONALTIP

Caring for the Client Who Is Hearing Impaired

- Check to see whether the client wears a hearing aid. Be sure it is in working order and turned on.
- Make every effort to move the client to a setting with minimal background noise.
- Always face the client.
- Speak in a normal tone and at a normal pace.
- Determine whether the client uses sign language. If signing is used, enlist the assistance of an interpreter.
- Pay particular attention to nonverbal cues of the client and to your own nonverbal behavior.
- Provide a pen and paper to facilitate communication, if necessary.

the conversation. Listen and accept what the client says. Trying not to give advice may be very difficult to do.

The nurse and the family must work together to understand the ways that the terminally ill client communicates. It can take persistence and insight to identify and decipher some messages. "Listening" to the client's gestures and facial expressions helps facilitate understanding of messages.

Religion Communication can be difficult when religious beliefs conflict with those of the health care team. Members of some religions seek healing only through faith and not through conventional medical services, including not receiving blood transfusions. When a client has a minister, priest, or rabbi visit, privacy should be provided if at all possible.

Family Situation Illness often unites family members around the client, but communication between the family and client may be strained if the family has not been close to or supportive of the client before the illness. The nurse must be careful not to discuss aspects of the client's condition or treatment in front of family members. It is usually best to ask family members to step out of the room when any nursing care is being given. This maintains the client's right to privacy and confidentiality.

If the client asks for a specific person to remain in the room, it is usually allowed unless specifically contraindicated.

Visual Ability Communicating with clients who are visually impaired may not seem to be a challenge at first; however, because the nonverbal part of any message, such as facial expressions, gestures, and other body language, is not able to be observed, an important part of every message is lost to the client.

Generally, persons who are visually impaired speak only when spoken to. Their speech is often loud when they are not sure where the other person is. Silence makes them uncomfortable.

When orienting a new client who cannot see, the nurse must include an explanation of "hospital sounds." Describe the room in detail and guide the client around the room if possible. Always speak and identify yourself when entering the

PROFESSIONALTIP

Caring for the Client Who Is Visually Impaired

- Look directly at the client when speaking.
- Use a normal tone and volume of voice.
- Advise the client when you are entering or leaving the room.
- Orient the person to the immediate environment; use clock hours to indicate positions of items in relation to the client.
- Ask for permission before touching the client.

PROFESSIONALTIP

Objectivity

The nurse must remain objective and nonjudgmental when the client's idea of family is different from the nurse's idea of family.

CULTURAL CONSIDERATIONS

Family Interaction Patterns

- In some families, the male members make all the decisions.
- In some families, decisions are made jointly, with all members (or all adults) participating.
- In some families, unrelated persons such as godparents or special friends are involved in decision making.

room. Each step of a procedure as well as any touching should be described before it is initiated. To prevent startling a client, always inform the visually impaired client before touching.

COMMUNICATING WITH THE HEALTH CARE TEAM

Because providing care to clients is a team effort, effective communication is necessary. This communication between team members may be oral or written, individual, group, or on computer.

ORAL COMMUNICATION

Oral communication takes place among all health care team members. To provide continuity of care to the client, all persons who provide that care communicate orally concerning that care.

Nurse–Student Nurse

Student nurses communicate not only with their clinical instructor but with the staff nurses too. How well staff nurses interact with student nurses depends on the experiences the staff nurses have had with other student nurses and also on how the staff nurses were treated as students. Student nurses are present in the clinical facility for very specific learning experiences that are selected by the instructor and relate to classroom discussion. They will review client records, communicate with and care for their clients, and, when possible, observe others performing procedures. Depending on how far they have progressed through the nursing curriculum, students may be limited in their nursing activities. Communication between student nurses and staff nurses is essential because staff nurses are responsible for the care of clients even though clients are assigned to students. Usually, a helping relationship develops between staff nurses and nursing students.

Nurse–Nursing Assistant

The nurse is responsible for assigning duties to the nursing assistants. A relationship of trust and mutual respect is established by answering questions and providing reasons for specific activities requested.

Nursing assistants are often much more comfortable and confident in providing bedside care. Therefore, they can be of considerable assistance to the new graduate (whether an LP/VN or RN). They often have creative solutions to problems and should be included in planning care.

Nurse–Nurse

Nurse–nurse communications can be either peer–peer or superior–subordinate communication. Peer–peer communication takes place many times every day. When each nurse uses effective communication with peers as well as clients, the unit runs more efficiently, and client care will be more effective. Superior–subordinate communication often occurs when the superior discusses client care to be performed by the subordinate. The way this communication is handled affects both the attitude of the subordinate and the client care given.

Nurse–Physician

Nursing education and expertise have evolved over the years to a professional level. Nurses are responsible for their own actions even when under the direction of a physician. Nurses have a duty to secure physician clarification of any order that is illegible, that is unclear, or that violates hospital policy or procedure.

Nurses must communicate openly and honestly with physicians, demonstrating competence in assessments, nursing skills, provision of quality care, reporting change in client status, and accurate documentation.

Nurse–Other Health Professionals

Communicate with professionals in other departments on a peer-to-peer basis. The focus of communication should be clarification of goals for each client and ways to meet those goals. Top-quality care is provided to clients by listening to those in other departments and establishing mutual respect for each other's area of expertise.

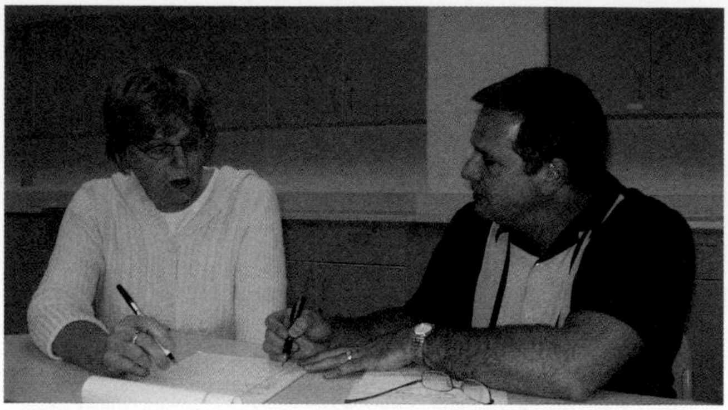

FIGURE 7-7 **Nurses work together to plan client care.**

Group Communication

Client care conferences may be scheduled whenever the need arises or on a regular basis. Some conferences may be only for the staff of a specific nursing unit; others may include some members of other departments. Only persons directly involved with client care should be invited (Figure 7-7).

The objectives of the conference are established by the conference leader, who makes all necessary arrangements. The meeting site should be a conference room or other private place. One person should record the discussion. When the conference is about a particular client, only facts are to be documented on the client's chart. When the topic is general and not related to any one client, only a record of the discussion is needed.

Telephone

When a student nurse takes a telephone call, the call should be answered with the name of the department or floor and the student's full name and position (i.e., student nurse). If a message is taken, the student nurse should write it down and read it back to the caller, asking for the caller's name and for the caller to spell out his or her name. The student nurse must never give out any information about clients.

SHIFT REPORT

Vital to continuity of client care is the **shift report** (report about each client between shifts). An oral report is the most common. The charge nurse of the outgoing shift may report to all members of the incoming shift or only to the incoming charge nurse who, in turn, shares the information with the appropriate caregivers on the incoming shift.

Sometimes, the report is put on a tape recorder for the next shift. This allows no chance for feedback, which can be a disadvantage.

Another method is a "walking report." The outgoing nurse reports to the oncoming nurse on each client as they walk from bed to bed. This way the client is included and aware of the information provided to the next shift.

The shift report about each client should be complete and concise no matter which method is used. The report should be focused on the clients and given in an orderly manner. This is not the time for social conversation.

WRITTEN COMMUNICATION

Most written communication relates to the client's chart. All aspects of a client's care are recorded on that client's chart.

PROFESSIONALTIP

Client Information for Shift Report

- Name, room and bed, age, sex
- Physician, diagnosis, admission date, any surgery
- Diagnostic tests (results if available) or treatments in past 24 hours
- General status, significant changes in condition
- Changed or new physician's orders
- Nursing diagnoses with nursing orders
- Evaluation of nursing interventions
- Last PRN medication given, IV fluids left hanging and amount given
- Any concerns about the client or family

Requisitions to x-ray or to physical or respiratory therapy and requests for laboratory services for a client are all forms of written communication. The reports resulting from these requests become part of the client's chart.

One type of written communication not pertaining to a specific client is the interdepartmental memo requesting equipment, supplies, maintenance, or housekeeping. Documents such as this are necessary to keep the nursing unit functioning efficiently and effectively.

ELECTRONIC COMMUNICATION

Computers are being used extensively in the business offices of health care agencies and have been so for years. The introduction of computers into the departments of direct client care has been slower, however. Nonetheless, in many places, computers are used by client care departments to send requisitions to other departments and to receive test results. Some hospital pharmacies use computer programs that show safe dosages and drug interactions. There are also programs to aid physicians in diagnosing and treating some conditions. Some acute care and long-term facilities have implemented full online documentation, including nursing notes, nursing care plans, and the medication administration record MAR.

Hing, Burt, and Woodwell (2007) studied the use of electronic medical records (EMR) by office-based physicians throughout the United States as well as plans to install new EMR systems or replace current systems within the next 3 years. Approximately 29% of physicians reported using full or partial EMR systems. This represents a 22% increase since 2005 and a 60% increase since 2001. With the expanding use of computers in health care and the corresponding potential for increased use, it is important for all health care workers to have some knowledge about computers.

Telehealth

According to Hutcherson (2001), **telehealth** is using telecommunication equipment and communication networks to transfer health care information between participants at different locations. It can be used in almost every area of health care.

Telenursing, an element of telehealth, permits nurses to provide care through a telecommunication system. The simplest form has been used for years—the telephone. **Telemedicine**, another element of telehealth, permits physicians to provide care through a telecommunication system. Recognized subspecialties include teledermatology, teleoncology, telepathology, and teleradiology.

Two issues related to telehealth that are especially important to nursing include licensure and standards of practice. The National Council of State Boards of Nursing (NCSBN) developed a plan for multistate licensure through legal agreement (interstate compacts) between a group of states. In these agreements, a nurse is licensed in one state but can practice nursing in any of the states in the compact. Before multistate licensure, nurses could participate in telenursing only within the state of their licensure. Practice standards for telenursing are in the process of being established. To assist nurses when providing telenursing care, the American Nurses Association (ANA) has developed some core principles for telehealth (ANA, 1999) and telehealth protocols (ANA, 2001).

The use of two-way video allows the client and health care provider to see, hear, and talk to each other. A stethoscope or otoscope (called peripherals) can be included in the hookup so that the sounds and visual images can be transmitted (Granade, 1997). This allows physician specialists in large medical centers to examine a client many miles away.

COMMUNITY/HOME HEALTH CARE

Use of Telenursing

- From the office, a home health nurse can watch a client at home change a dressing or self-administer insulin.
- During a video consult, a home health nurse might assist by manipulating the peripherals or actually performing a physical assessment.

PROFESSIONALTIP

Cell Phones in Health Care

According to C. Peter Waegermann, CEO, Medical Records Institute (Waegemann, 2007). "A healthcare revolution is on the horizon. The new capabilities of modern cell phones, smart phones, PDAs, and others . . . are creating new possibilities for healthcare." Physicians and nurses are using cell phones to load client information to be synchronized with the hospital's IT system at the end of the shift. Clients are downloading their medical records on their cell phones, PDAs, and so on to have on hand for easy retrieval in case of an emergency and to share with health care providers. Cell phones with e-mail capabilities can send images and diagnostic testing results to physicians as well as the client. The use of cell phones is an exciting development in the health care telecommunications industry.

Nurses should document all activities, assessment findings, information provided by the client, and any instructions given to the client. All data transmissions (e.g., telemetry printouts or videotapes) should be stored in the client's record. Most telemedicine laws require that existing confidentiality rules be maintained.

COMMUNICATING WITH YOURSELF

People talk to themselves every day whether they admit it or not. **Intrapersonal communication** is internal thoughts and discussion with oneself. This self-talk is what people say to themselves, thus influencing their personalities and how they interact with others. Self-talk may be positive or negative.

Positive Self-Talk

The practice of positive self-talk is key to positive self-concept. You can send positive thoughts to yourself about yourself, but, better yet, say the thoughts out loud. Thinking, saying, and hearing positive statements about oneself reinforces a positive self-concept. When you have had a difficult day, whether in the classroom or clinical area, remind yourself of your good attributes and accomplishments. Every day, tell yourself out loud what you learned or what good care you gave to your client(s).

The desire to succeed is reinforced by positive self-talk. When things are not going well and frustration sets in, memories of success can serve as positive influences.

Positive affirmation is a positive thought or idea on which a person consciously focuses to produce a desired result. Positive affirmation can be used to change negative inner messages to positive messages. For instance, say, "I know I can pass this test" instead of saying, "I don't know if I can pass this test." Of course, positive affirmation cannot be a substitute for studying and preparing for the test. Positive affirmation merely serves to modify your attitude about the test—or about any other situation.

Negative Self-Talk

Whenever you say to yourself, "I can't do . . . ," you are decreasing your self-concept with the negative self-talk. Negative self-talk may originate within you or may be a replay of things that others have said about you. Negative self-talk is self-destructive. Your self-image is lowered by your own criticism, and you begin to see yourself as a failure.

CASE STUDY

Self-Talk

A student nurse is sitting in a preconference meeting with her peers and clinical instructor preparing for the first day of clinical to begin. She begins to think to herself, "Oh, I'm so nervous. I can't do this. I am terrible at meeting and talking with people. How am I ever going to go into my client's room and introduce myself?"

1. This is an example of which type of self-talk? Explain.
2. List three positive thoughts or ideas that the student nurse could tell herself.
3. What other positive affirmations could the student nurse use to increase her self-concept?
4. What affect does negative self-talk have on a person's self-concept?

SUMMARY

- Communication is influenced by factors such as age, education, emotions, culture, language, attention, surroundings, and past experience.
- Nonverbal messages are generally more accurate in communicating a person's feelings.
- Verbal and nonverbal messages must be congruent for clear communication to take place.
- Techniques of therapeutic communication should be practiced and incorporated into the nurse's communication.
- Barriers to communication should be identified and avoided when communicating.
- People have four comfort zones of closeness: intimate, personal, social, and public.
- Therapeutic communication is purposeful and goal directed.
- Psychosocial aspects of communication may hinder or aid communication.
- Most nurse–client interactions should involve therapeutic communication.
- Nurse–client communication is influenced by both the client and the nurse.
- The nurse is many times a role model for the family in terms of communicating with the terminally ill client.
- Accurate communication among the health care team is necessary for continuity of client care.

REVIEW QUESTIONS

1. B.R. is in the bathroom with the door partially closed. A nurse enters his room and says, "You will not be able to eat or drink after supper because of tests tomorrow," and then leaves. Did communication take place?
   1. No, there was no feedback.
   2. No, there was no eye contact.
   3. Yes, Mr. George had to hear the message.
   4. Yes, there was a sender, receiver, and message.
2. Which of the following are all examples of verbal communication?
   1. Singing, dancing, smiling.
   2. Reading, writing, listening.
   3. Shaking hands, reading, grimacing.
   4. Whispering, making eye contact, answering.
3. When a client says, "I'm not sure how I'll handle all this," which response of the nurse represents clarification?
   1. "Handle all this?"
   2. "Well, you can ask your sister to help."
   3. "Oh, you'll be able to handle things. You're an intelligent person."
   4. "I'm not sure I understand what it is you're concerned about being able to handle."
4. A critically ill client denies there is anything wrong and talks constantly about going home. The nurse should:
   1. listen but say nothing.
   2. acknowledge the client's wishes and hopes.
   3. advise the client that it will be impossible to go home.
   4. assist the client in planning when to return home.
5. A client tells the nurse that she would rather die than have chemotherapy. The nurse should report this communication to:
   1. the physician only.
   2. all nurses on the unit.
   3. the physician and charge nurse.
   4. no one; it is a confidential communication.
6. The nurse is establishing a helping relationship with a new client on the unit. In addressing the client, the nurse should:
   1. gently touch the client on the shoulder right away.
   2. ask the client why he or she is in the hospital.
   3. call the client by his or her first name.
   4. knock before entering the client's room.
7. In using communication skills with clients, the nurse evaluates which response as being the most therapeutic?
   1. "Don't worry, I'm sure everything will be fine."
   2. "I noticed that you didn't take your medication this morning. Is something wrong?"
   3. "I think you should try the medication first before having surgery."
   4. "Why do you feel that way?"
8. The nurse asks the client, "What did the physician tell you about going home?" This is an example of:
   1. an open-ended question.
   2. a confrontational question.
   3. a closed question.
   4. a double-barreled question.
9. The client informs the nurse of her concerns that she might be experiencing depression due to her sad feelings, lack of energy, and daily episodes of crying. She states that she has thoroughly researched depression on the Internet and has brought the information to discuss with the physician. The client is most likely in which generation?
   1. Traditional.
   2. Baby boomer.
   3. Generation X.
   4. Generation Y.
10. The student nurse stated, "I think that Mr. Smith is showing improvement because his vital signs are stable today." This is an example of which type of communication?
    1. Passive.
    2. Assertive.
    3. Aggressive.
    4. Congruent.

REFERENCES/SUGGESTED READINGS

American Nurses Association. (1999). Core principles on telehealth. Retrieved September 3, 2008, from http://www.nursingworld.org

American Nurses Association. (2001). Developing telehealth protocols: A blueprint for success. Retrieved September 3, 2008, from http://www.nursingworld.org

Barry, P., & Farmer, S. (2000). *Mental health and mental illness* (7th ed.). Philadelphia: Lippincott Williams & Wilkins.

Bush, K. (2001). Do you really listen to patients? *RN, 64*(3), 35–37.

Calloway, S. D. (2001). Preventing communication breakdowns. *RN, 64*(1), 71–74.

Deering, C., & Jennings, D. (2002). Communicating with children and adolescents. *American Journal of Nursing, 102*(3), 34–41.

Estes, M. E. Z. (2010). *Health assessment and physical examination* (4th ed.), Clifton Park, NY: Delmar Cengage Learning.

Frisch, N. C, & Frisch, L. E. (2011). *Psychiatric Mental Health Nursing* (4th ed.). Clifton Park, NY: Delmar Cengage Learning.

Granade, P. (1997). The brave new world of telemedicine. *RN, 60*(7), 59–62.
Gravely, S. (2001). When your patient speaks Spanish—And you don't. *RN, 64*(5), 65–67.
Hall, Edward T. (1959). *The silent language*. New York: Doubleday.
Hing, E. S., Burt, C. W., & Woodwell, D. A. (2007). *Electronic medical record use by office-based physicians and their practice: United States, 2006*. Atlanta: Centers for Disease Control and Prevention.
Hutcherson, C. (2001, September 30). Legal considerations for nurses practicing in a telehealth setting. *Online Journal of Issues in Nursing, 6*(3), manuscript 3. Available: http://www.nursingworld.org/onjin/topic16/tpc16_3.htm
Kübler-Ross, E. (1969). *On death and dying*. New York: Macmillan.
Kübler-Ross, E. (1975). *Death: The final stage of growth*. Englewood Cliffs, NJ: Prentice Hall.
Kübler-Ross, E. (1978). *To live until we say good-bye*. Englewood Cliffs, NJ: Prentice Hall.
Lyon, B. (2000). Conquering dysfunctional anxiety: What you say to yourself matters. *Reflections on Nursing Leadership, 26*(4), 33–35.
Milliken, M. (2004). *Understanding human behavior* (7th ed.). Clifton Park, NY: Delmar Cengage Learning.
National Institute on Deafness and Other Communication Disorders. (2008). Mission. Retrieved September 3, 2008, from http://www.nidcd.nih.gov/about/learn/mission.asp
National Institute on Deafness and Other Communication Disorders. (2008a). Quick statistics. Retrieved September 3, 2008, from http://www.nidcd.nih.gov/health/statistics/quick.htm
North American Nursing Diagnosis Association International. (2010). *NANDA-I nursing diagnoses: Definitions and classification 2009-2011*. Ames, IA: Wiley-Blackwell.
Rochman, R. (2000). Are computerized patient records for you? *Nursing2000, 30*(10), 61–62.
Tamparo, C., & Lindh, W. (2007). *Therapeutic communications for health professionals* (3rd ed.). Clifton Park, NY: Delmar Cengage Learning.
Thomas, N., & Thompson, J. (2003). Tomorrow's nurses need your help today. *RN, 66*(6), 51–53.
Waegemann, C. P. (2007). The next big wave is m-health: Smart phones in healthcare. Retrieved September 3, 2008, from http://www.medrecinst.com/cellphone/articles.html
Waughfield, C. (2002). *Mental health concepts* (6th ed.). Clifton Park, NY: Delmar Cengage Learning.

RESOURCES

American Health Information Management Association, http://www.ahima.org
American Nurses Association, http://www.nursingworld.org
Health Resources and Services Administration, http://telehealth.hrsa.gov
Language Line Services, http://www.languageline.com
National Council of State Boards of Nursing, http://www.ncsbn.org
ValueOptions, http://www.valueoptions.com

CHAPTER 8
Client Teaching

MAKING THE CONNECTION

Refer to the following chapters to increase your understanding of client teaching:

Basic Nursing

- ***Legal and Ethical Responsibilities***
- ***Communication***
- ***Nursing Process/Documentation/ Informatics***
- ***Life Span Development***
- ***Cultural Considerations***
- ***Stress, Adaptation, and Anxiety***

LEARNING OBJECTIVES

Upon completion of this chapter, you should be able to:

- Define key terms.
- Explain the importance of client education in today's health care climate.
- Relate principles of adult education to client teaching.
- Identify common barriers to learning.
- Explain the ways that learning varies throughout the life span.
- Discuss the nurse's professional responsibilities related to teaching.
- Relate the teaching–learning process to the nursing process.
- Describe teaching strategies that make learning meaningful to clients.

KEY TERMS

affective domain
auditory learner
cognitive domain
formal teaching
informal teaching
kinesthetic learner
learning
learning plateau
learning style
motivation
psychomotor domain
readiness for learning
teaching
teaching–learning process
teaching strategies
visual learner

INTRODUCTION

Client education is an integral part of nursing care. The nurse is responsible to help the client identify learning needs and resources that will restore and maintain that client's optimal level of functioning. This chapter discusses the teaching–learning process, including barriers and responsibilities, and relates it to the nursing process.

THE TEACHING–LEARNING PROCESS

The **teaching–learning process** is a planned interaction that promotes behavioral change that is not a result of maturation or coincidence. **Teaching** is an active process wherein one individual shares information with another to facilitate learning and thereby promote behavioral changes. A teacher is someone who uses a variety of goal-directed activities to promote change by assisting the learner to absorb new information.

Learning is the process of assimilating information, resulting in behavior change. Knowledge is power. By sharing knowledge with clients, the nurse helps them achieve their maximum level of wellness. The teaching–learning process has the same basic steps as the nursing process: assessment, identification of learning needs (nursing diagnosis), planning, implementation of teaching strategies, and evaluation of learner progress and teaching efficacy. These steps are discussed in greater detail later in this chapter.

Edelman and Mandle (2002) describe the goal of health education as helping individuals achieve optimal states of health through their own actions. Often, deficient knowledge about the course of illness and/or self-care practices hinders the client's recovery or in practicing health-promoting behaviors. The nurse's role is to help bridge the gap between those things a client knows and those things a client needs to know to achieve optimal health.

Client teaching is done for a variety of reasons, including to:

- Promote wellness
- Prevent illness
- Restore health
- Facilitate coping abilities

Client education focuses on the client's ability to practice healthy behaviors. The client's ability to care for self is enhanced by effective education. Client education may:

- Improve quality of care
- Decrease length of hospital stays
- Decrease chance of hospital readmission
- Improve compliance with treatment regimens

These benefits are enhanced through nurses' continued active participation as client educators.

Formal teaching is planned and goal directed, but informal teaching can occur in any setting at any time.

Formal Teaching

Formal teaching takes place at a specific time, in a specific place, and on a specific topic. It is planned and goal directed (Figure 8-1). The teacher prepares the information and/or activities related to the topic. Formal teaching may take place in a class setting with several learners, or it may be performed one-on-one. For example, many health care facilities provide formal classes related to diabetes. The same basic information is necessary for all clients with diabetes.

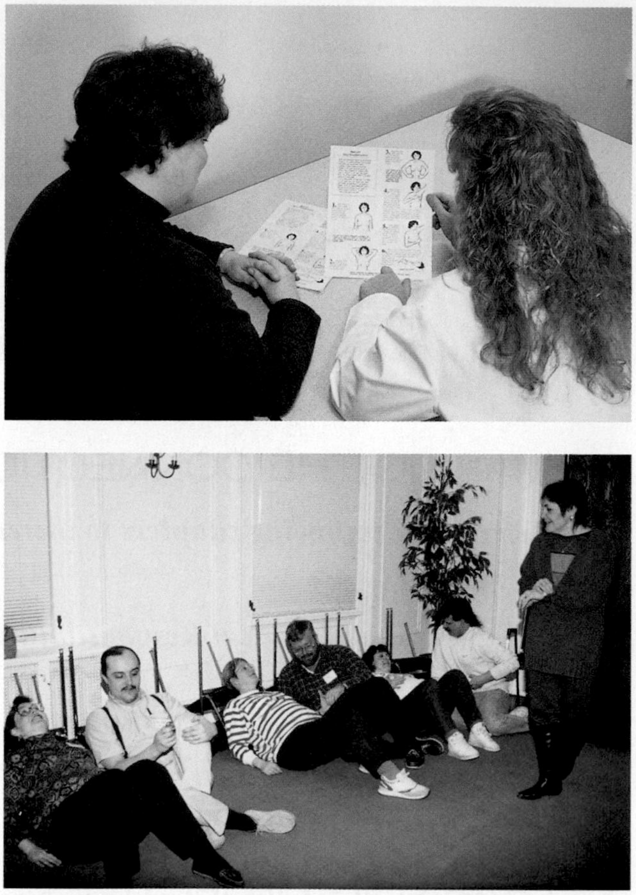

COURTESY OF DELMAR CENGAGE LEARNING

FIGURE 8-1 Nurses engage in formal teaching with both individual and groups clients. (*Bottom photo courtesy of Bellevue Woman's Hospital, Niskayuna, NY.*)

Informal Teaching

Informal teaching takes place any time, any place, whenever a learning need is identified. While providing nursing care, nurses have many opportunities for informal teaching, such as answering the clients' questions and explaining care being given to the client. Informal teaching may also occur in the midst of formal teaching. A comment or question from a learner in a formal setting may trigger some informal teaching in response. For example, during a class on diet for the diabetic client, a question about dietary cholesterol may be asked. The response would be considered informal teaching because it was not the planned topic.

An understanding of learning domains, learning principles, learning styles, learning barriers, and teaching methods is helpful. These topics are discussed as follows.

Learning Domains

In his classic work, Bloom (1977) identifies three areas or domains wherein learning occurs: the **cognitive domain**, which involves intellectual understanding; the **affective domain**, which involves attitudes, beliefs, and emotions; and the **psychomotor domain**, which involves the performance of motor skills. Information is processed in each domain.

TABLE 8-1 Learning Domains

DOMAIN	DEFINITION	EXAMPLE
Cognitive	Learning involving the acquisition of facts and data; used in decision making and problem solving	Client states the symptoms of possible complications
Affective	Learning involving attitude, emotion, and belief changing; used in making judgments	Client begins to accept the lifestyle changes required
Psychomotor	Learning involving gaining motor skills; used in physical application of knowledge	Client uses glucose monitor

TABLE 8-2 Teaching Strategies for the Learning Domains

COGNITIVE	AFFECTIVE	PSYCHOMOTOR
Lecture or discussion	Role playing	Demonstration
Audiovisual materials	Discussion group	Return demonstration
Printed materials	Support group	Audiovisual materials
Programmed instruction	Role modeling	Discovery
Computer-assisted learning	Printed materials	Skill repetition
Independent study	One-on-one counselling	Printed materials

From *Teaching the Client and Family*, by R. Smith, 2008, manuscript submitted for publication, adapted from *Community Based Nursing* (2nd ed.), by R. Hunt, 2001, Philadelphia: Lippincott.

Table 8-1 briefly outlines the three learning domains and provides clinical examples.

Nurses must be sensitive to all three learning domains when developing effective teaching plans and must use **teaching strategies**, or techniques to promote learning, that will tap into each of the domains. For instance, teaching a diabetic client how insulin works in the body falls within the cognitive domain; helping the same client learn how to use a glucose monitor falls within the psychomotor domain; and encouraging the client to view diabetes as only one aspect of the individual falls within the affective domain. Table 8-2 gives examples of teaching strategies for each learning domain.

LEARNING PRINCIPLES

Fundamental principles of learning can be used when teaching clients. Knowles, Holton, and Swanson (2005) cite four basic assumptions about adult learners, which are applicable to client education:

- *Assumption 1:* Personality develops in an orderly fashion from dependence to independence. *Nursing application:* Plan teaching–learning activities promoting client participation. This encourages independence and increases client control and self-care.
- *Assumption 2:* Learning readiness is affected by developmental stage and sociocultural factors. *Nursing application:* Conduct a psychosocial assessment before planning teaching–learning activities.
- *Assumption 3:* Previous learning experiences are a foundation for further learning. *Nursing application:* Perform a complete assessment to ascertain what the client already knows and build on that knowledge base.
- *Assumption 4:* Immediacy reinforces learning. *Nursing application:* Provide opportunities for immediate application of knowledge and skills and incorporate feedback as part of each nurse–client interaction.

Learning principles include relevance, motivation, readiness, maturation, reinforcement, participation, organization, and repetition.

Relevance

The material to be learned must be meaningful to the client, easily understood by the client, and related to previously learned information. Individuals must believe that they need to learn the information before learning can occur. If an individual sees the information as being personally valuable, the information is more likely to be learned. Because relevance is individually determined, the nurse must assess the personal meaning of learning for each client.

Motivation

One of the most critical indicators of the potential success of a teaching session is the client's motivation level. Redman (2006) describes **motivation** as forces acting on or within an organism that initiate, direct, and maintain behavior. Motivation is complex and constantly changing dependent on positive or negative influences in life (Smith, 2008). To maximize motivation, the nurse must keep the teaching–learning goals realistic by breaking the content down into small, achievable steps. For example, the cardiac client must see value in information about exercise, such as that the heart will be strengthened and the client will have more energy.

Readiness

The client should be able and willing to learn. Readiness is closely related to growth and development. For example, the

PROFESSIONALTIP

Checking Literacy

"Lscean uyro sdhna. Seu yver dloc rweat."

The preceding is what some clients see when given printed educational materials. Avoid making assumptions about client literacy. Check comprehension through return explanation of the written material.

client must have the requisite cognitive and psychomotor skills for learning a particular task, and the client must comprehend the information. One indicator of learning readiness is if clients ask questions; another is if clients become involved in learning activities, such as participating in return demonstration of a dressing change. Some indicators of lack of client readiness are anxiety, avoidance, denial, and lack of participation in discussion, demonstration, or self-care activities.

Maturation

The client should be developmentally able to learn and have requisite cognitive and psychomotor abilities. Assess the client for characteristics that will hinder or facilitate learning, such as developmental stage. Assess the client's developmental stage. Do not automatically assume that a 34-year-old client has mastered the developmental tasks of earlier stages.

Maturity level greatly influences the client's ability to learn information. Each developmental stage is characterized by unique skills and abilities affecting the response to various teaching tools. Developmental stage greatly determines the type of data taught, the method(s), the vocabulary, and the location of teaching. In addition to developmental stage, the nurse should also evaluate the client's cognitive skills, problem-solving abilities, and attention span.

Reinforcement

Feedback provided to the learner should be immediate and positive to reinforce the client's motivation and readiness to learn. For example, the client who is learning to apply a sterile dressing to an open wound should be told during the application of the dressing that it is being done correctly (if it is) and should be praised upon completion for learning so quickly (or whatever is appropriate). If some aspect of the dressing application is lacking, the nurse must maintain a positive approach in guiding the client to correctly perform the application.

Participation

The client's active involvement in the learning process promotes and enhances learning. Client involvement is relatively easy to monitor when a psychomotor skill is learned, as the client is actively involved in practicing a physical skill. Learning that takes place in the cognitive or affective domain is also most effective when active involvement of the client is encouraged. For example, the client who is on a low-fat diet can be involved in learning to self-regulate with regard to diet by reading labels of foods and planning menus of low-fat meals.

LIFE SPAN CONSIDERATIONS

Ability to Learn

Remember that age is not always synonymous with developmental level; observation of behavior provides the clearest picture of developmental level.

Organization

The material to be learned should incorporate previously learned information and be presented in sequence from simple to complex and from familiar to unfamiliar. Again using the example of the client learning about a low-fat diet, the nurse begins the teaching session by finding out what the client knows about the nutrient content of foods and then proceed by helping the client learn to read food labels, then plan a meal, and plan a menu for a day and a week, and so forth.

Repetition

Retention of material is reinforced with practice, repetition, and presentation of the same material in a variety of ways. The more often the learner hears or sees the material, the greater the chance of retention.

It is good to keep in mind that a **learning plateau**, or peak in the effectiveness of teaching and depth of learning, will occur in relation to the client's motivation, interest, and perception of relevance of the material. Frequent reinforcement of learning through immediate feedback and continual reassessment of effectiveness will enhance the value of the learning process for both the teacher and the learner. Making the information-acquisition process as user friendly as possible also increases satisfaction and success. This can be done by making learning as creative and interesting as possible and by adopting a flexible approach to allow the learning process to be dynamic.

CRITICAL THINKING

Learning

Will knowledge acquisition alone result in learning (behavioral change)? Why? Why not?

PROFESSIONALTIP

Beliefs about Learning

- Each individual has the capacity to learn, but learning ability varies.
- The pace of learning varies from person to person.
- Learning occurs throughout the life span.
- Learning occurs in formal and informal settings.
- Learning is an individualized process.
- Learning new information is based on previous knowledge and experiences.
- Motivation and readiness are necessary prerequisites for learning.
- Prompt feedback facilitates learning.

Learning Style

Each individual has a unique way of processing information. The manner whereby an individual takes in new information and processes the material is called **learning style**. Some people learn by processing information visually (**visual learner**), others by listening to the words (**auditory learner**), and others by experiencing the information or by touching, feeling, or doing (**kinesthetic learner**). According to Reed (2007), approximately 40% to 65% of students are visual learners, and 10% to 30% are kinesthetic learners. Use a variety of techniques, such as lecture, discussion, role play, modeling, games, return demonstration, imitation, problem solving, and question-and-answer sessions, to match various learning styles of clients. A good way to discover learning style is by asking the client, "What helps you learn?" or "What kinds of things do you enjoy doing?" Then teaching strategies can be matched to the client's learning style. Web sites with tools to determine an individual's learning style are listed in the "Resources" section at the end of the chapter. Table 8-3 gives suggestions for teaching–learning methods and study methods for each learning style. Students may use these to assist in personal study habits and when teaching clients.

Barriers to the Teaching–Learning Process

The giving and receiving of information does not, in and of itself, guarantee that learning will occur. Several barriers can impede the teaching–learning process. In a nursing

Table 8-3 Teaching–Learning Methods and Study Methods for Learning Styles

STYLE OF LEARNING	TEACHING–LEARNING METHODS	STUDY METHODS
Visual	Printed outline for student to follow PowerPoint slides Supplemental reading/articles Pictures/visual display (charts, graphs, diagrams) Demonstration with return demonstration Brainstorming with ideas written on whiteboard Short lecture with opportunity to try new methods Guided imagery Games	Workbooks Lab manuals Computer-aided instruction Assembly kits Videos Reading material
Auditory	Lecture Discussion Problem solving Question and answer Brainstorming Interactive video Guided imagery Verbally explain how to solve math problems Verbally explain any slides, charts, graphs, diagrams	Videos verbal explanation CDs Study with background music Read out loud
Kinesthetic	Role playing Modeling Games Demonstration/return demonstration Writing assignments Hold and play with pen or other object when reading or listening to lecture Take notes during lecture Field trips Experiential situations Short lecture with opportunity to try new methods	Workbooks Lab manuals, computer-aided instruction Assembly kits Hold and play with squeeze toys when reading

Adapted from "An Investigation of Learning Styles of Practical and Baccalaureate Nursing Students," by G. Duncan, 1996, *Journal of Nursing Education*, 35(1); "A New Definition for Individual: Implications for Learning and Teaching," by A. Gregorc and H. Ward, 1977, *NASSP Bulletin*; and Learning Your Way, by S. Reed, 2007, from www.presentations.com/msg/content_display/training/e3i7639605670451237f7bf2bea3bf8bad3.

CULTURAL CONSIDERATIONS

Overcoming Sociocultural Barriers

- Use pictures whenever possible.
- Provide written material in the appropriate language.
- Use a culturally sensitive interpreter or a family member who understands health care terminology.
- Avoid the use of clichés, jargon, or value-laden terms.
- Learn about the client's cultural norms.
- Be aware of your own values.
- Tailor teaching (information and questions) to the client's ability to read and write.
- Have the client verbalize his understanding from the teaching–learning session.

situation, the nurse, the client, or both may encounter one or more of these barriers. Learning barriers can be classified as either internal (psychological or physiological) or external (environmental or sociocultural). Examples of these barriers are listed in Table 8-4. To facilitate the learning process, the nurse must assess for the presence of learning barriers. Specific assessment information is presented later in this chapter.

Environmental Barriers

Both the nurse and client are subject to environmental barriers. As part of planning for a teaching session, the nurse ensures necessary privacy and minimizes interruptions and extraneous stimuli.

TABLE 8-4 Barriers to Learning

EXTERNAL BARRIERS	INTERNAL BARRIERS
Environmental • Lack of privacy • Extraneous stimuli • Interruptions	Psychological • Anxiety • Anger • Fear • Depression
Sociocultural • Language • Level of education • Values	Physiological • Pain • Oxygen deprivation • Fatigue • Hunger

Sociocultural Barriers

When language is a barrier to the teaching–learning process, several steps can be taken to ensure that learning takes place, such as using pictures, providing printed material in the appropriate language, or using an interpreter. Even when the nurse and client both speak the same language, a language barrier may exist when clichés, health care jargon, or value-laden terms are used. Furthermore, the meanings that the nurse and client attach to specific types of body language may differ depending on cultural influences. Nurses must be aware of their own value systems but focus client teaching within the client's value system. The client's level of education is kept in mind and words tailored to the client's educational level without "talking down" to the client.

Psychological Barriers

Nurses may be anxious about client teaching. Knowing the client's learning needs and adequate preparation related to content, environmental and sociocultural aspects, and developmental ability of the client alleviates some of this anxiety. What little anxiety is left will likely make the nurse more alert and sensitive.

Clients and families are often upset about the health situation. They may be anxious, angry, fearful, or depressed. In addition to the client's words, the nurse should pay attention to body language and behavior. If clients or family members are obviously angry, the nurse should acknowledge the anger by saying something like "You appear to be very angry about something. Tell me what you are feeling." Allowing clients and family members to express their emotions clears the air and allows learning to take place.

PROFESSIONALTIP

Overcoming Psychological Barriers

- Recognize your own emotions related to client teaching.
- Assess for psychological barriers to learning.
- Acknowledge the client's emotions but do not respond in kind.

PROFESSIONALTIP

Physiological Comfort and Learning

- Administer pain medication, as appropriate, before a teaching session to enable the client to concentrate on the information presented.
- Plan teaching sessions when the client is not fatigued, as might be the case after a physical therapy session, for example.
- Ensure that the client is in a comfortable position and does not have to go to the bathroom.

CRITICAL THINKING

Barriers to Learning

A 56-year-old male is admitted to the ER with epigastric discomfort, pain radiating from the chest down the right arm, weakness, pallor, diaphoresis, and shortness of breath. He is an executive with a large corporation and has a wife and two adolescent children. His wife is at his bedside and is very anxious and upset over his condition. He is also anxious and believes that he is having a heart attack. The client states that his father died of a massive heart attack at age 56. What barriers to learning would be affecting this client? How could the nurse's approach help overcome these barriers?

Physiological Barriers

The physiological situation affects the client's ability to learn. The client who is struggling to breathe, for example, is unable to pay attention to any teaching. A teaching session should be planned for a time when the client is rested and free from pain.

TEACHING METHODS

Many different teaching methods can be used depending on the client's learning need and the applicable learning domain.

Teaching Methods Applicable in the Cognitive Domain

Effective methods for promoting cognitive learning include discussion, formal lecture, question-and-answer sessions, role play, and games/computer activities.

Discussion Discussions may involve the nurse and one or several clients who need to learn the same information. Active participation in the discussion is promoted. Group discussions allow peer support.

Formal Lecture In formal lectures, the teacher presents the information to be learned, and learner participation is usually minimal.

Question-and-Answer Sessions Question-and-answer sessions can take two forms. In one, the client's concerns are addressed by the client asking the questions and the nurse providing answers. In the other, the nurse assists the client in applying the knowledge learned by asking the client questions that the client then answers (Figure 8-2).

Role Play Role play provides the client an opportunity to apply knowledge in a safe, controlled environment. In role play, the nurse and client each assume a certain role in order to play out different possible scenarios. For instance, the nurse teaching a client sex education information intended for an adolescent may have the client assume the role of parent, while the nurse assumes the role of the teenager. The two can then engage in practice discussion sessions to prepare the client for the actual parent–teen discussion.

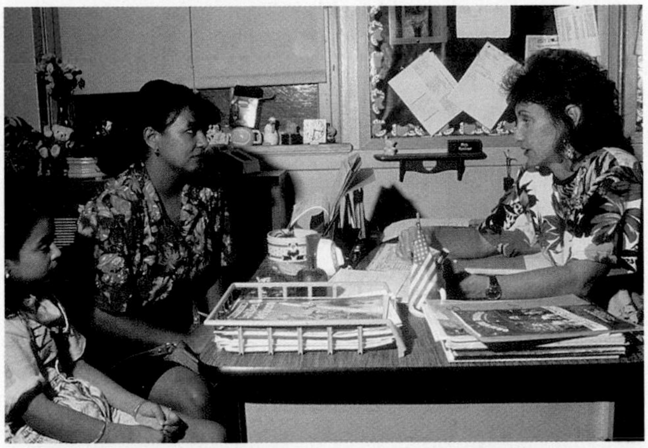

COURTESY OF DELMAR CENGAGE LEARNING

FIGURE 8-2 A Question-and-Answer Session with School Nurse, Mother, and Child

Games/Computer Activities Games and computer activities can be used to teach clients at a level that is appropriate for them. These methods allow the client to use the new information in various situations and to have fun while learning.

Teaching Methods Applicable in the Affective Domain

Role play and discussion are both effective methods for stimulating affective learning.

Role Play Role play allows expression of feelings, attitudes, and values in a safe, controlled environment. The client can try out different attitudes and values.

Discussion One-on-one discussion between nurse and client is effective for personal or sensitive topics related to values, feelings, attitudes, and emotions.

Teaching Methods Applicable in the Psychomotor Domain

Demonstration, supervised practice, and return demonstration assist the client to learn psychomotor skills.

Demonstration In demonstration, the nurse presents in a step-by-step manner the skill or procedure to be learned, explaining what is done and why. In this way, the client sees not only the equipment and the way it is used, but also the nurse's attitude and behaviors.

Supervised Practice In supervised practice, the client uses the equipment and performs the skill or procedure while the nurse watches. The nurse gives suggestions or corrects the client as the practice proceeds. Repetition can continue until the client feels confident in performing the skill or procedure.

Return Demonstration In return demonstration, the client performs the skill or procedure without any coaching from the nurse. Upon completion of the task, the nurse provides feedback and reinforcement to the client.

LIFE SPAN CONSIDERATIONS

Teaching Children

- Ensure that the child is comfortable.
- Encourage participation of caregiver.
- Assess the child's developmental level, learning readiness, and motivation. Do not equate age with developmental level.
- Assess the child's psychological status.
- Determine self-care abilities of the child.
- Use play, imitation, and role play.
- Use various visual stimuli, such as books, chalkboards, and videos, to share information and assess understanding.
- Use terms easily understood by the client and caregiver.
- Provide frequent repetition and reinforcement.
- Develop realistic goals consistent with developmental level.
- Remember that the goals of educating children are to improve cooperation, prevent excessive anxiety, and hasten the recovery process.

LIFELONG LEARNING

One basic assumption underlies teaching: *All people are capable of learning.* However, the ability to learn varies from person to person and from situation to situation. Learning needs and learning abilities change throughout life. The client's developmental stage and chronological age greatly influence the ability to learn. The principles of learning discussed earlier in this chapter are relevant to learners of all ages. Teaching approaches must be altered depending on the client's developmental stage and level of understanding. Specific information for children, adolescents, and older adults is described in the following sections.

CHILDREN

Readiness for learning (evidence of willingness to learn) varies during childhood depending on maturation level. The nurse must work closely with the child's caretaker, especially when caring for young children.

Young children learn primarily through play. Incorporating play into teaching activities for children can therefore enhance learning (Figure 8-3). Puppets, coloring books, and toys can be effective teaching tools for the young child. Encourage the young child to be an active participant in the learning process.

Older children can also benefit from the use of art materials to express their emotions and their understanding of those things that are or will be happening to them. Using medical supplies (such as medicine cups or bandages), the child may play at giving medicine to a doll or putting a bandage on the doll like the bandage that will be put on the

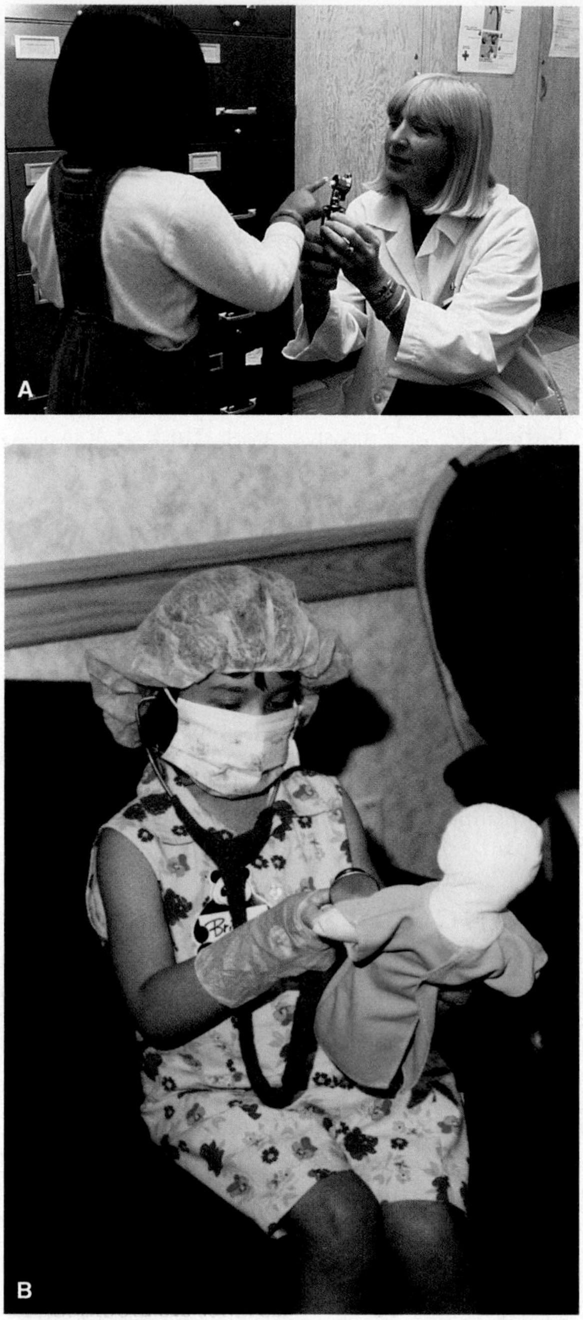

COURTESY OF DELMAR CENGAGE LEARNING

COURTESY OF DELMAR CENGAGE LEARNING

FIGURE 8-3 ***A,*** **The nurse is at the child's level, while the child learns about the instrument to be used in the examination;** ***B,*** **Role playing with a doll decreases a child's anxiety and enhances teaching opportunities.**

CLIENT TEACHING

Do As I Do

- Individuals learn from examples set by role models.
- Adolescents are very sensitive to any discrepancy between words and actions.
- Encourage parents to model the behaviors they wish their children to develop.

child. While the child is involved in play, the nurse is both teaching the child what to expect regarding treatment procedures and alleviating anxiety.

Adolescents

Individuals approaching adolescence are able to understand relationships between things. Usually, reading and comprehension ability have advanced, and the adolescent understands more complex information. Because one of the strongest influences on the adolescent is peer support, group meetings are often useful in teaching. The nurse can be a potent teacher as a role model.

Older Adults

Many physiological changes accompany aging. These changes cause some older adults to experience perceptual impairments in vision and hearing. The nurse assesses for these changes and adjusts teaching materials accordingly. For example, providing large-print written material and verifying that the client hears all instructions and directions are strategies helpful in teaching older clients.

PROFESSIONAL RESPONSIBILITIES OF TEACHING

The nurse empowers clients in their self-care abilities through teaching. Teaching provides information to clients about health-promoting behaviors, specific disease processes, and treatment methods. Although each state has its own definition of nursing practice, teaching is a required function of nurses in most states. Redman (2006) cites National League for Nursing documents dating back to 1918 as stating that "the nurse is essentially a teacher and an agent of health."

Providing client education is an expected role of all nurses. However, because of the nursing shortage and personal time constraints, some nurses are omitting the important responsibility of client teaching. If nurses give up their

LIFE SPAN CONSIDERATIONS

Teaching Adolescents

- Respect the adolescent.
- Boost their confidence by seeking their input and opinions on health care matters.
- Encourage exploration of their own feelings.
- Be sensitive to peer pressure.
- Help adolescents identify and build on their positive qualities.
- Use language that is clear yet appropriate to the health care setting.
- Encourage independent and informed decision making by engaging them in problem-solving activities.

LIFE SPAN CONSIDERATIONS

Teaching Older Adults

- Ensure that the client is comfortable. Fatigue, pain, a full bladder, or hunger can hinder learning.
- Assess the client's developmental level, motivation, and learning readiness.
- Assess the client for depression, anxiety, or denial, which can interfere with learning.
- Determine client's ability for self-care.
- Use words easily understood by the client.
- Avoid talking down to the client; a condescending, paternalistic manner hinders learning.
- Find the time of day when the client is most alert.
- Present material slowly using examples.
- Encourage client participation.
- Ask for feedback and listen actively.
- Provide feedback frequently.
- Assess for perceptual impairments and individualize teaching strategies accordingly:

For memory-impaired clients:

- Repeat material.
- Use different cues (spoken words, pictures, written materials, and symbols).

For visually impaired clients:

- Use large-print materials.
- Furnish a magnifying glass.
- Be sure prescription eyeglasses are worn.
- Arrange adequate lighting and reduce glare.

For hearing-impaired clients:

- Face the client when speaking.
- Use short sentences with words that are easily understood.
- Use gestures and demonstrate to reinforce verbal information.
- Eliminate distractions (activities or noises in the environment) as much as possible.

role as client educators to spend time performing additional tasks, nursing's worth to the health care system could greatly diminish. Client teaching requires the depth of information that only nurses possess; as such, it is one of the truly independent functions of nursing practice.

Client teaching is also required by several accrediting bodies, including the Joint Commission (2008). The American Hospital Association's *Patient Care Partnership* (2009) calls for the client's understanding of health status and treatment approaches. Only clients who are well informed can give informed consent. Nurses assess clients' level of understanding about treatment methods and correct any knowledge deficits. The nurse often serves as an interpreter for the client by explaining, clarifying, and referring.

Teaching supports behavioral changes that lead to positive adaptation by the client. Teaching decreases the fear of change by reducing anxiety and anticipation stresses.

Client teaching is an essential nursing function in every practice setting. All clients require information about disease prevention, growth and development, safety, first aid, nutrition, and hygiene. The hospitalized client needs information about his condition, the expected treatment, and the environment of the health care facility. By the time of discharge, clients must also have information about postdischarge care related to medications, dietary modifications, activity, complication prevention, and rehabilitation plans.

Clients recovering at home and their families also have significant learning needs. A primary role of the home health nurse is to teach the client about caring for himself at home. This often involves teaching family members ways to provide care (Figure 8-4) and information about their illness, accident, or injury. They should also be taught ways to achieve and maintain a maximum state of wellness. Accurate teaching plans for the home-based client and family are established by assessing many factors, such as:

Support system

- Individuals available to help give care
- Caregivers' knowledge about necessary care

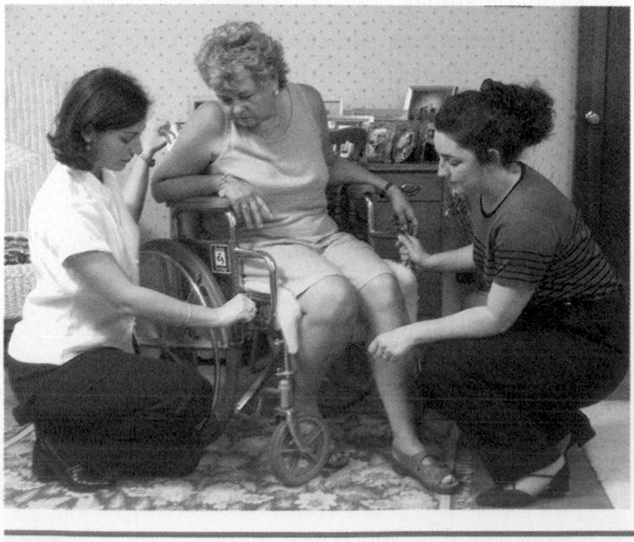

COURTESY OF DELMAR CENGAGE LEARNING

FIGURE 8-4 The nurse teaches a family member how to provide care.

COMMUNITY/HOME HEALTH CARE

Client Teaching Considerations

- Preparation of the client and family for home care begins at the time of hospital admission, not at the time of discharge.
- Discharge planning should consider current and potential learning needs of clients and caregivers.
- Teach about community resources.

Environmental

- Home accessibility
- Space to meet special needs of the client
- Need for and availability of equipment and supplies
- Need for assistance with self-care activities
- Need for information about environmental cleanliness related to health

Economic

- Ability to purchase medications, equipment, and supplies
- Available financial assistance

Community resources

- Area resources
- Awareness of and access to support services
- Respite availability for the family

SELF-AWARENESS

Several characteristics of nurses influence the outcome of the teaching–learning process. Nurse self-awareness with regard to the concepts discussed in the following sections is an all-important first step in teaching.

Knowledge Base

It is impossible for nurses to teach if they lack the knowledge or skills that are to be taught. Staying both current in knowledge and proficient in skills is the first step to maintaining efficacy and credibility as a teacher. Although it is impossible for one individual to be an expert in every area of nursing, knowing when to refer the client to others for teaching is an important critical-thinking skill.

Interpersonal Skills

Effective teaching is based on the nurse's ability to establish rapport with the client. The empathic nurse shows sensitivity to the client's needs and preferences. An atmosphere in which the client feels free to ask questions promotes learning. Activities that help establish an environment conducive to learning include:

- Showing genuine interest in the client
- Including the client in *every* step of the teaching–learning process
- Employing a nonjudgmental approach
- Communicating at the client's level of understanding

CRITICAL THINKING

Teaching Ethics

Is it ethical for a nurse to attempt to change a client's beliefs under the guise of teaching? Should a nurse "teach" a client the "right" attitude or belief?

PROFESSIONALTIP

Medical Jargon and Teaching

- Consider the language used by most nurses; think of the terms nurses take for granted. When a client is asked to "void," for example, does the client understand what is meant?
- These frequently used terms can easily be misunderstood by clients and families: *ambulate, defecate, dangle, NPO, vital signs,* and *contraindicated*.
- How can you communicate without using professional jargon?

Documentation

The standard is for nurses to document client education. From a legal perspective, if the nurse teaches a client but does not document it, the teaching never occurred. Documentation of teaching facilitates accurate communication to other health care colleagues and promotes continuity of care.

Many different approaches are used to document client teaching. Figure 8-5 is an example of a documentation form related to client teaching in an inpatient setting.

Because client education is a standard and essential component of nursing practice, each nurse must document the teaching interventions used and the client's response. Elements to be documented in all practice settings include:

- Content
- Teaching methods
- Learner(s) (e.g., client, family member, other caretaker)
- Client/family response to teaching activities

TEACHING–LEARNING AND THE NURSING PROCESS

The teaching–learning process and the nursing process are interdependent. Both are dynamic and comprise the same phases: assessment, diagnosis, planning, implementation, and evaluation.

Assessment

Primary (client) and secondary (family or significant other) sources are used by nurses to assess learning needs. Communication is the foundation of assessment related to learning. Factors to be considered include:

- Actual learning needs
- Potential learning needs
- Ability and readiness to learn
- Client strengths and limitations
- Previous experiences

Actual Learning Needs

Everyone who receives health care services has some need for learning. Client teaching may be indicated when a client:

- Asks for information to make decisions
- Requires new skills
- Desires to make lifestyle changes
- Is in an unfamiliar environment

The client's knowledge about the content to be taught must be evaluated. Previous knowledge can be used as a foundation for new concepts. The client's learning needs can be determined in a variety of ways, including:

- Asking the client directly
- Observing client behaviors
- Asking the client's family or significant others

The nurse first addresses the client's immediate need for knowledge. For example, preoperative clients are taught deep breathing exercises and leg exercises before surgery so that they are able to perform those exercises after surgery and thereby prevent potential complications. As soon as possible after surgery, begin teaching incision care so that the client is ready to care for the incision when discharged.

Potential Learning Needs

Potential learning needs are also assessed so that anticipatory planning can be done to prevent a relapse in the recovery process or to maintain wellness. Following are two scenarios with related potential learning needs noted:

- N.L. is pregnant for the first time. *Potential learning need:* Infant care
- T.A. has diabetes and has just been told that he must take insulin daily. *Potential learning need:* Self-administration of insulin

PROFESSIONALTIP

Learning Needs Assessment

Assess the client's learning needs by answering the following:

- Is the client uncertain about an upcoming procedure?
- Does the client know about medications, purposes, and side effects?
- Can the client describe necessary lifestyle modifications?
- Is the client able to correctly perform treatment procedures (e.g., colostomy irrigations, injections, blood glucose monitoring)?

Date/Time	Location of Pain	Pain Rating 0–10	Pharmacologic/ Nonpharmacologic	Mode of Administration	Source of Information	BP	P	R	Loc. / Side Effects	Safety	Time of Evaluation	Evaluation of Interventions/ Rating 0–10 Response/ Comments	Initials

PAIN SCALES: Mild = 0–3 Moderate = 3–7 Severe = 7–10

No Pain — Worst Pain

0 1 2 3 4 5 6 7 8 9 10

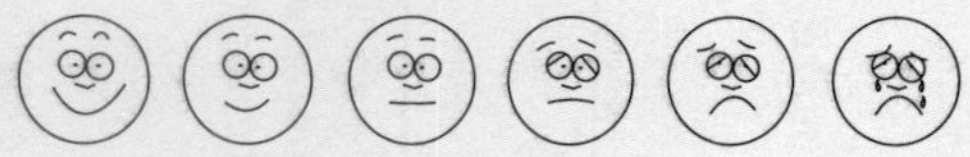

0 1 2 3 4 5 6 7 8 9 10

Initials	Signature

Pediatrics/Noncommunicative Clients (0–10)

A. Verbal/Vocal
0 = positive
1 = other complaint, whimper
2 = pain, crying
3 = screaming

B. Body Movements
0 = moves easily
1 = neutral shifting
2 = tense, flailing arms & legs

C. Facial
0 = smiling
1 = neutral
2 = frown, grimace
3 = clenched teeth

D. Touching (localizing pain)
0 = no touching
1 = reaching, patting
2 = grabbing

Source of Information:	Side Effects:	Safety:
1 = Patient	1 = Nausea/Vomiting	1 = Bed Low
2 = Child	2 = Resp. Depression	2 = Call bell in reach
3 = Parent	3 = Pruritis	3 = Side rails x2
4 = Nurse	4 = Urinary Retention	4 = Side rails x4
5 = Family	5 = Altered Mental Status	5 = Bed alert
6 = Other	6 = None	6 = Family/Sitter

Nonpharmacological Interventions
1 = Cold, 2 = Distractions, 3 = Environmental Control, 4 = Exercises, 5 = Heat, 6 = Imagery, 7 = Massage, 8 = Music, 9 = Positioning, 10 = Relaxation, 11 = TENS

Pediatrics
1 = Holding, 2 = Rocking, 3 = Pacifier, 4 = Security object

Mode of Administration
PCA, IV, IM, Epidural (EP), Transdermal (TD), SQ, PO, SL, Rectal (R), Nasal (N)

LEVEL OF CONSCIOUSNESS KEY (LOC)*
1. Alert, engages in conversation; purposefully travels with eyes, if mute.
2. Lethargic, drowsy, sedate – focuses on personal interchange – but unable to maintain focus.
3. Responds only to maximal stimulation (shaking). Response only a grunt or moan – not a clear sentence.
4. Coma – unable to respond at all.

4017

CHRISTUS SPOHN HEALTH SYSTEM

PAIN/EDUCATION/DIABETES
FLOW SHEET

2755824

NEW: 07/99.FM6

INITIAL EDUCATIONAL ASSESSMENT

EDUCATIONAL
Patient Family Learning Needs: (initial all that apply)
__Present Illness __Rehabilitation __Hypertension __Diabetes __Heart Disease __Cancer
__Incontinence __Medications __Diet __Skin Care __Post-Op Care __Home Equipment
__Community resources __Personal hygiene & grooming __*Other______

All "yes" answers require comment
Patient/Family Ability to Learn:
*Physical Limitations: ___No ___Yes *Cognitive Limitations: ___No ___Yes *Emotional Barriers: ___No ___Yes
*Language Barrier: ___No ___Yes *Primary Language Spoken ___English ___Spanish ___Other:______
Ability to read ___English ___Spanish ___Other ___None
Religious or cultural practices that may impact care of education ___No ___Yes
Financial implications of care choices. ___No ___Yes
COMMENTS: ______
Patient/Family Preferences for Learning: (initial all that apply)
___Video ___Demonstration ___1 to 1 instruction ___Handout material
___Other (please comment) ______
Patient/Family Readiness to Learn: ___Express readiness ___Express desire to delay learning (Comment) ______
Date:______ Time:______ Signature:______

KEYS:

Learner
Patient [P] Spouse [S]
Family [F] Other [O]
Demonstration [D]
Video [V]

Teaching Methods
Written Material [W] Video [V]
Demonstration [D] Explanation [E]

Limitations to Learning
None [1] Pain [2] Anxiety [3]
Physical Limitation [4]
Unable to Understand [5]
Disinterested [6]

Evaluation
States Understanding [S]
Reference (See CPG, Problem List Teaching Records) [Ref]
No Indication Learning Has Occurred [N]
Return Demonstration [R]
Needs ongoing instruction [O]

DATE	TIME	CONTENT	LEARNER	TEACHING METHODS	LIMITA-TIONS	EVALUA-TION	SIGNATURE/ DEPT.
		Discussion of disease process, diagnosis, or condition. (Specify) ______ ☐ Signs and Symptoms ☐ Risk Factors ☐ Treatment Modalities ☐ Follow-up Care ______					
		Pre Op Teaching/Preparation for diagnostic tests/ invasive procedure (Specify) ______					
		Post Op Teaching for invasive procedures (Specify) ______					
		Food/Drug interactions (list drugs) ______					
		Diet Education ______					
		Medication Use (List drugs) ______					
		Medical Equipment (List) ______ ☐ No Need Identified					
		Topic ______					
		Topic ______					
		Topic ______					

(Continues)

FIGURE 8-5 Documentation Form for Client Teaching: Inpatient Setting (*Courtesy of CHRISTUS Spohn Health System, Corpus Christi, TX.*)

DATE	TIME	CONTENT	LEARNER	TEACHING METHODS	LIMITA-TIONS	EVALUA-TION	SIGNATURE/ DEPT.
		Rehabilitation (Describe) PT ______ TR ______ OT ______ Speech ______					
		Special Treatments (Describe)					
		Community Resources (Specify) ______					
		Diabetes Teaching ☐ DM Medication ☐ Insulin Adm. Techniques ☐ Diet Guidelines ☐ Hypoglycemia–Sx., Tx, Prev. ☐ Foot Care ☐ Sick Day Guidelines Referred to OP Diabetes Class					
		Explanation of safety program, level precautions, and wristband					
		Topic: Pain Management Information Sheet					
		Topic ______					
		Topic ______					
		Topic ______					
		Topic ______					
		Topic ______					
		Topic ______					
		Topic ______					
		Topic ______					
		Topic ______					
		Topic ______					

Initial/Signatures
1.____ / ______ 8.____ / ______ 15.____ / ______
2.____ / ______ 9.____ / ______ 16.____ / ______
3.____ / ______ 10.____ / ______ 17.____ / ______
4.____ / ______ 11.____ / ______ 18.____ / ______
5.____ / ______ 12.____ / ______ 19.____ / ______
6.____ / ______ 13.____ / ______ 20.____ / ______
7.____ / ______ 14.____ / ______ 21.____ / ______

DIET: ______

INJECTION SITE:
RA – Right Arm
LA – Left Arm
RT – Right Thigh
LT – Left Thigh
RG – Right Gluteal
LG – Left Gluteal
RQ – Right Abdominal Quadrant
LQ – Left Abdominal Quadrant

For Documentation of Routine Blood Sugar Results i.e. BID, TID or AC and HS

DATE		AC Break-fast	AC Lunch	AC Dinner	AC HS Snack	2 AM	COMMENTS	DATE		AC Break-fast	AC Lunch	AC Dinner	AC HS Snack	2 AM	COMMENTS
	Bld Glu								Bld Glu						
	Meter #								Meter #						
	Insulin Admin.								Insulin Admin.						
	Bld Glu								Bld Glu						
	Meter #								Meter #						
	Insulin Admin.								Insulin Admin.						
	Bld Glu								Bld Glu						
	Meter #								Meter #						
	Insulin Admin.								Insulin Admin.						
	Bld Glu								Bld Glu						
	Meter #								Meter #						
	Insulin Admin.								Insulin Admin.						

Int.	#	Problem	Goal	Exp. Date of Resol.	Date Comp. Int.	Int.	#	Problem	Goal	Exp. Date of Resol.	Date Comp. Int.
		Alteration in Comfort	Comfort maintained					Impaired Skin Integrity	Regain Skin Integrity		
		Injury Potential	Safety Maintained					Pot. For Skin Impairment	Skin Integrity Maintained		
		Fever	Temp. within Normal Limits					Activity Intolerance	Maintain/Increase Activity		
		Anxiety/Fear	Reduced Anxiety/Fear					Impaired Mobility	Imp. Function/ Mobility		
		Knowledge Deficit	Increased Understanding					Self Care Deficit	Improve ADL's		
		Infection	Minimized/Absent Signs					Altered Thought Process	Reduced Disorientation		
		Body Image Disturbance	Acknowledge Change					Impaired Communication	Improve Communication		
		Fluid/Lyte Imbalance	Main. Fluid/Lyte Bal.					Constipation	Bowel Elim. With WNL		
		Impaired Gas Exchange	Main./Increase Gas Ex.					Diarrhea	Bowel Elim. With WNL		
		Ineffective Airway Clearance	Maintain Patient Airway					Incontinence	Maintain Bowel Integrity		
		Ineffective Breathing Pattern	Maintain Patient Airway					Impaired Swallowing/ Chewing	Optimal Nutrition Status		
		Altered Tissue Perfusion	Optimal Tissue Perfusion					Alteration in Nutrition	Optimal Nutrition Status		

Pain-Ed-Diabetes.FM6 09/16/99

FIGURE 8-5 *(Continued)*

CULTURAL CONSIDERATIONS

Learning and Culture

- Culture plays an important role in knowledge acquisition.
- Attitudes, which are derived from a cultural context, toward what is appropriate to learn and who should teach may require alterations in the nurse's approach.
- Sensitivity to cultural values affects every aspect of the teaching–learning process.

Ability and Readiness to Learn

Assess the client for factors that will hinder or facilitate learning. Age does not determine developmental level. Behavior provides the best indication of developmental level. The client's cognitive skills and attention span, along with developmental level, all indicate a client's ability to learn.

Readiness to learn is influenced by the client's ability to learn, the client's comfort, and the client's motivation (or lack of) to learn.

Client Strengths and Limitations

Identification of the client's strengths and limitations is the foundation for realistic expectations. Understanding the client's strengths and limitations allows the nurse to plan successful teaching–learning experiences. Determining a client's strengths assists the nurse to select appropriate teaching methods. For example, a client who has limited vision should not be given pamphlets or other reading material in small print from which to learn the intended information.

Previous Experiences

The client's knowledge base acquired from life experiences affects the client's attitude about learning and perception of the importance of the information to be learned. A client who has had several experiences of hospitalization will have both a basis of knowledge and feelings (positive and negative) about those experiences. Current attitudes about this hospitalization are influenced by prior hospital experiences.

NURSING DIAGNOSIS

Several nursing diagnoses are pertinent to the learning process. When lack of knowledge is the primary learning need, the diagnosis of *Deficient **K**nowledge (specify)* is applicable. For example:

- A client who is to use crutches for assisted ambulation may have the diagnosis of *Deficient **K**nowledge: Crutchwalking,* R/T lack of exposure AEB many questions and hesitancy to walk.
- A client who must give self-insulin and will be discharged soon may have a diagnosis of *Deficient **K**nowledge: Insulin Injection,* R/T lack of exposure AEB many questions.

*Deficient **K**nowledge* may also be a component of many other nursing diagnoses that encompass risk or impaired ability. For instance, *Risk for **C**onstipation* may relate to a client's compromised health status; this risk may be modified or reduced through certain dietary changes and client education. A client having a diagnosis of *Feeding **S**elf-Care Deficit* may need both assistance in cutting the food and opening containers related to present physical ability.

PLANNING

Learning does not just happen by chance—it is planned. An important part of planning is goal setting. The client and family or significant others be involved in setting goals. Specific learning goals include the following elements:

- Measurable behavioral change
- Time frame
- Methods and intervals for evaluation

Teaching–learning goals must be realistic (i.e., based on the abilities of the learner and the teacher).

Establishing teaching–learning goals involves setting priorities. One way to set priorities with regard to goals is to teach "need-to-know" content (that which is necessary for survival) before moving on to "nice-to-know" content. For example, Mrs. Stone, who is in her first trimester of pregnancy, must be taught guidelines for diet and exercise ("need-to-know" content); information about infant care ("nice-to-know" content at this time) can be given later in the pregnancy.

Planning involves considering the following:

- Why teach?
- What should be taught?
- How should teaching be done?
- Who should teach and who should be taught?
- When should teaching occur?
- Where should teaching occur?

Why Teach?

Client need is *why* teaching is done. The client may realize the need for knowledge about a given subject and ask for information or ask questions about the subject. The nurse recognizes the client's need for knowledge even when the client does not recognize that need. For example, the nurse recognizes that a preoperative client needs to know how to do deep breathing exercises and leg exercises after surgery. The nurse then plans teaching for that purpose.

What Is Taught?

Determination of *what* to teach is accomplished through comprehensive assessment. The content to be taught depends greatly on the client's knowledge base, current health status, and readiness to learn.

How Is Teaching Done?

Deciding *how* to teach involves deciding which teaching strategies are best for the content and the client's learning style and abilities. The effective teacher uses methods that capture the client's interest. Teaching methods are often influenced by the teaching location. For example, videos can often be used effectively in inpatient settings; however, the same information may need to be presented with flip charts or brochures in the home setting.

Who Teaches and Who Is Taught?

Planning includes deciding *who* will teach the client. The nurse is the coordinator of the health care team's teaching activities. Responsibility for a comprehensive teaching approach rests with the nurse. The teaching plan greatly affects continuity of care. The "who" part of planning also relates to who will be taught. The nurse must determine who in addition to the client (e.g., family members, significant others) will receive the teaching.

When Does Teaching Occur?

When to teach should be carefully considered. The nurse should recognize that every interaction with the client is an opportunity for teaching. When a client asks a question, it is an opportunity for teaching. These opportunities for teaching must be used. A client's motivation to learn is quickly destroyed when comments such as "Ask your doctor that" or "We'll talk about that later. Right now, take your medicine" are made. The best time for teaching is when the client is comfortable—physically and psychologically.

Where Does Teaching Occur?

Where teaching occurs must also be well planned. The location of teaching affects the quality of learning. Some factors to be considered in determining the location of teaching include privacy and equipment availability.

PROFESSIONALTIP

Guidelines for Effective Client Teaching

- Assess the client's needs and knowledge.
- Organize content from the simple to the complex, building on what the client already knows.
- Be creative.
- Ensure a comfortable environment.
- Maintain a flexible approach.
- Use a variety of teaching methods.
- Relate material to client's prior knowledge.
- Encourage the client's active participation.
- Reinforce learning frequently.
- Provide immediate feedback.
- Provide for immediate application of knowledge or skill.
- Emphasize oral instructions with the written word and pictures.
- Expect learning plateaus.

IMPLEMENTATION

Katz (1997) suggests several strategies to achieve successful client teaching, as outlined in the following sections.

Get and Keep the Client's Attention

Begin a teaching session by telling the client what will be taught and why it is important to the client. The client's interest is held by varying the tone of voice and using assorted teaching methods to present the material. Making the abstract concrete by using realistic examples from the client's experience also keeps the client's attention.

Stick to the Basics

Because the average adult remembers only five to seven points at a time, the nurse is specific about what the client is to learn. Simple, everyday language is used, and the most critical information presented first.

Use Time Wisely

The nurse incorporates teaching into client care by providing information during each nurse–client interaction. Involving the client's family and friends, allowing them to discuss the material with the client, is also helpful. The nurse considers supplementing teaching with written material for the client and/or family to read; this provides time for the learners to review the material and then ask questions to clarify understanding.

Reinforce Information

Repetition creates habits; the nurse takes advantage of this by reviewing the material with the client and serving as a role model. For example, when teaching a client a procedure, the nurse takes care to do it correctly each time and to avoid taking shortcuts. The nurse rewards the client by giving positive reinforcement such as a smile, a nod, or a few words of praise.

EVALUATION

Evaluation of teaching–learning is a twofold process:

1. Determining what the client has learned
2. Assessing the nurse's teaching effectiveness

Evaluation of Client's Learning

In performing the continual process of evaluating what the client has learned, the nurse determines whether a behavior

PROFESSIONALTIP

Evaluation of Learning

- Did the client meet the goals and objectives?
- Can the client demonstrate skills?
- Did the client's attitude change?
- Can the client cope better?
- Does the family understand how to help?

PROFESSIONALTIP

Evaluation of Teacher Effectiveness

- Were learning objectives stated in behavioral terms (i.e., easy to evaluate)?
- Was content presented clearly and at the client's level of comprehension?
- Did the nurse show interest in the client and in the material?
- Were a variety of teaching aids used?
- Were the teaching aids appropriate for the client and the content?
- Was the client encouraged to participate?
- Did the nurse give frequent feedback and allow for immediate return demonstration?
- Was the nurse supportive?

change has occurred, whether the behavior change is related to learning activities, whether further change is necessary, and whether continued behavior change will promote health. The following strategies are used to evaluate client learning:

- Asking questions
- Observation
- Return demonstration
- Written follow-up (e.g., questionnaires)

Evaluation of Teaching Effectiveness

A major purpose of evaluation is to assess the effectiveness of the teaching activities and to decide which modifications, if any, are necessary. If learning objectives are not met, teaching–learning activities are reassessed and modified. Goals that are measurable and specific facilitate evaluation. Evaluating teaching effectiveness is accomplished through:

- Feedback from the learner
- Feedback from colleagues
- Self-evaluation

CASE STUDY

The nurse admitted a 46-year-old male who has recently been diagnosed with stage II colon cancer. He has a wife and two school-age children and has just started his own construction company in the past year. The client is scheduled for a colon resection with a colostomy in 2 days. The nurse is assessing him and his wife for preoperative teaching. They are verbalizing a significant amount of distress and anxiety over the diagnosis and pending surgery.

1. What assessment data would you need to collect before initiating teaching?
2. What barriers would you expect to encounter in the teaching and learning process?
3. What would be two teaching goals for the session?
4. Identify two prioritized nursing diagnoses for this client?
5. Identify teaching strategies you might utilize in this teaching session?
6. How would you evaluate the teaching goals?

SUMMARY

- The teaching–learning process is a planned interaction that promotes behavioral change that is not a result of maturation or coincidence.
- Learning is the process of assimilating information that results in behavioral change.
- Three domains of learning are the cognitive (intellectual), the affective (emotional), and the psychomotor (motor skills).
- Learning readiness is affected by developmental and sociocultural factors.
- Elements of documenting client education include the content taught, the teaching methods used, the person(s) taught, and the response of the learners.
- Evaluation of the teaching–learning process involves: determining what the client has learned and assessing teacher efficacy.

REVIEW QUESTIONS

1. Bloom identified three areas wherein learning occurs: the psychomotor domain, the affective domain, and the:
   1. attitude domain.
   2. cognitive domain.
   3. emotional domain.
   4. knowledge domain.
2. A clinical example of psychomotor learning is when a client:
   1. changes the dressing on a leg ulcer.
   2. states an acceptance of a chronic illness.
   3. states the name and purpose of a medication.
   4. chooses to change the type of exercise performed.

3. When teaching a client, the nurse is aware that learning needs:
   1. change daily.
   2. are the same for everyone.
   3. change throughout the life span.
   4. change as teaching approaches are modified.
4. Nurses are required to provide teaching by:
   1. all state nursing practice acts.
   2. the National League for Nursing.
   3. the American Hospital Association.
   4. the Joint Commission.
5. Because age is not synonymous with developmental level, the nurse, when preparing to teach a client, must:
   1. teach everyone the same way.
   2. set the goals for the client.
   3. observe the client's behavior.
   4. ask the client about self-efficacy.
6. The nurse is providing discharge teaching to a 65-year-old male who is newly diagnosed with adult-onset diabetes. He is being discharged on an 1,800-calorie American Diabetes Association diet, oral hypoglycemic medications, and blood glucose checks four times a day using a glucometer. What learning domain is the nurse addressing when teaching the client how to perform blood glucose checks?
   1. Affective.
   2. Psychomotor.
   3. Cognitive.
   4. Social.
7. The nurse is teaching a 48-year-old female who was recently diagnosed with breast cancer. The nurse observes that she is an avid reader while in the hospital. What teaching strategies would be most effective in helping her understand her disease and the treatment process?
   1. Pamphlets, pictures, and written materials.
   2. Support group, discussion, and audiotapes.
   3. Videos, role modeling, and games.
   4. Examples, discovery, and explanation.
8. The nurse is caring for a 55-year-old Hispanic woman who was recently diagnosed with renal failure and placed on a protein-restricted diet. When the nurse enters the room, the client is observed eating shredded beef with refried beans that the family brought from home. Which of the following responses indicate that the nurse is aware of the client's dietary restrictions and is sensitive to her cultural needs?
   1. "I see your family brought in some home-cooked food. I'm glad you are able to enjoy this."
   2. "Those foods you are eating are all high in protein. You will not be able to eat them anymore."
   3. "The meal you are eating is too high in protein for your diet. Substituting beans and eating a smaller amount of meat in your tortilla would satisfy your diet restrictions."
   4. "The foods you are eating are too high in protein. I will have the dietitian bring you a list of acceptable foods for your diet."
9. The nurse is providing care to a 15-year-old female who is a newly diagnosed diabetic. When planning diabetic teaching for this client, what developmental considerations could guide the nurse's choice of teaching strategies?
   1. Adolescents respond well to authority figures, so the client will be very attentive to what the nurse says.
   2. The reading level of an adolescent may be low, so written materials are not used.
   3. Family involvement is not encouraged because as an adolescent she is striving for independence.
   4. Adolescents identify with their peer group and often respond well to peer-led support groups.
10. A 76-year-old female is discharged home from a subacute nursing facility. She has a history of osteoarthritis and underwent a right-knee replacement about 2 weeks ago. The teaching goal of the nurse at discharge is that the client will gradually increase weight bearing to the right knee to the point that she is able to support full weight bearing in 3 weeks. What client statement indicates that the teaching goal is met?
    1. "Until the pain improves, I will take it easy on my knee."
    2. "I can't wait to get home so I can walk without this walker."
    3. "I will increase the weight on my knee a little each day while continuing to use my walker."
    4. "Exercise is not helpful in my rehabilitation."

REFERENCES/SUGGESTED READINGS

American Hospital Association. (1998). A patient's bill of rights. Chicago: Author. Retrieved November 30, 2008, from http://www.patienttalk.info/AHA-Patient_Bill_of_Rights.htm

American Hospital Association. (2009). The patient care partnership. Retrieved June 18, 2009, from http://www.aha.org/aha/issues/Communicating-With-Patients/pt-care-partnership.html

Bandura, A. (1977). Social learning theory. Englewood Cliffs, NJ: Prentice Hall.

Beare, P., & Myers, J. (1998). *Principles and practice of adult health nursing* (3rd ed.). St. Louis, MO: Mosby.

Bloom, B. (1977). *Taxonomy of educational objectives: The classification of educational goals, handbook I: Cognitive domain.* New York: Longman.

Bruccoliere, T. (2000). How to make patient teaching stick. *RN, 63*(2), 34–38.

Clark, M. (2003). *Community health nursing: Caring for populations* (4th ed.). Upper Saddle River, NJ: Prentice Hall.

Doak, C., Doak, L., & Root, J. (1996). *Teaching patients with low literacy skills* (2nd ed.). Philadelphia: Lippincott Williams & Wilkins.

Duffy, B. (1997). Using creative teaching process with adult patients. *Home Healthcare Nurse, 15*(2), 102–108.

Duncan, G. (1996). An investigation of learning styles of practical and baccalaureate nursing students. *Journal of Nursing Education, 35*(1), 40–42.

Edelman, C., & Mandle, C. (2002). *Health promotion throughout the lifespan* (5th ed.). St. Louis, MO: Mosby.

Freda, M. (1997). Don't give it away. *MCN—The American Journal of Maternal/Child Nursing, 22*(6), 330.

Gregorc, A., & Ward, H. (1977). A new definitions for individual: Implications for learning and teaching. *NASSP Bulletin*, 20–26.

Hunt, R. (2001). *Community based nursing* (2nd ed.). Philadelphia: Lippincott.

Joint Commission. (2008). Healthcare organization survey activity guide. Retrieved November 30, 2008, from http://www.jointcommission.org/NR/rdonlyres/481CE5EA-D02C-46C3-AA5F-DF328FE13174/0/08_HCO_SAG_3.pdf

Joint Commission for Accreditation of Healthcare Organizations. (2002). *Accreditation manual*. Chicago: Author.

Jubeck, M. (1994). Teaching the elderly: A commonsense approach. *Nursing94, 24*(5), 70–71.

Katz, J. (1997). Back to basics: Providing effective patient teaching. *American Journal of Nursing, 97*(5), 33–36.

Knowles, M., Holton, E., & Swanson, R. (2005). *The adult learner: The definitive classic in adult education and human resource development* (6th ed.). St. Louis, MO: Elsevier Science and Technology Books.

Mayer, G., & Rushton, N. (2002). Writing easy-to-read teaching aids. *Nursing2002, 32*(3), 48–49.

Messner, R. (1997). Patient teaching tips from the horse's mouth. *RN, 60*(8), 29–31.

Meyers, D. (1998). *Client teaching guides for home health care* (2nd ed.). New York: Aspen.

Muma, R., Lyon, B., & Newman, T. (Eds.). (1996). *Patient education: A practical approach*. New York: McGraw-Hill.

Redman, B. (2006). *The practice of patient education: A case study approach* (10th ed.). St. Louis, MO: Elsevier Science.

Reed, S. (2007). Learning your way. Retrieved June 20, 2009, from http://www.presentations.com/msg/content_display/training/e3i7639605670451237f7bf2bea3bf8bad3

Ruholl, L. (2003). Tips for teaching the elderly. *RN, 66*(5), 48–52.

Seley, J. (1994). 10 strategies for successful patient teaching. *American Journal of Nursing, 94*(11), 63–65.

Smith, R. (2008). *Teaching the client and family*. Manuscript submitted for publication.

Sodeman, W., Jr., & Sodeman, T. (2005). *Instructions for geriatric patients* (3rd ed.). St. Louis, MO: Elsevier Health Sciences.

VARK a Guide to Learning Styles. (2009). Research and statistics. Retrieved June 20, 2009, from http://www.vark-learn.com/english/page.asp?p=research

Weissman, M., & Jasovsky, D. (1998). Discharge teaching for today's times. *RN, 61*(6), 38–40.

Winslow, E. (2001). Patient education materials: Can patients read them, or are they ending up in the trash? *American Journal of Nursing, 101*(10), 33–38.

RESOURCES

Center for Research on Learning and Teaching, http://www.crlt.umich.edu/index.php

Gregorc Associates, Inc., http://gregorc.com

The Learning Web, http://www.thelearningweb.net

VARK, http://www.vark-learn.com

CHAPTER 9
Nursing Process/ Documentation/Informatics

MAKING THE CONNECTION

Refer to the following chapters to increase your understanding of the nursing process:

Basic Nursing

- ***Holistic Care***
- ***Legal and Ethical Responsibilities***
- ***The Health Care Delivery System***
- ***Communication***
- ***Assessment***

LEARNING OBJECTIVES

Upon completion of this chapter, you should be able to:

- Define key terms.
- Explain the nursing process.
- Describe the components of assessment.
- Describe the three types of nursing diagnoses.
- Discuss planning and outcome identification.
- Discuss the types of skills that nurses must possess in order to perform the nursing interventions during the implementation step of the nursing process.
- Identify factors that may influence evaluation.
- Explain how critical thinking and problem solving are related to the nursing process.
- Use the nursing process to provide safe, effective client care.
- Discuss the purposes of documentation in health care.
- Explain the principles of effective documentation.
- Describe various methods of documentation.
- Identify various types of documentation records.
- Document client care accurately and completely.

KEY TERMS

actual nursing diagnosis
analysis
assessment
assessment model
charting by exception (CBE)
collaborative problems
comprehensive assessment
critical pathways
data clustering
defining characteristics
dependent nursing interventions
discharge planning
documentation
etiology
evaluation
expected outcome
focus charting
focused assessment
goal
health history
implementation
incident reports
independent nursing interventions
initial planning
interdependent nursing interventions
Kardex
long-term goal
medical diagnosis
narrative charting
nursing care plan
nursing diagnosis
nursing intervention
Nursing Interventions Classification (NIC)
Nursing Minimum Data Set (NMDS)
Nursing Outcomes Classification (NOC)
nursing process
objective data
ongoing assessment
ongoing planning
planning
point-of-care charting
primary source
Problem, Intervention, Evaluation (PIE) charting
problem-oriented medical record (POMR)
risk nursing diagnosis
secondary sources
short-term goal
SOAP
source-oriented charting
subjective data
synthesis
wellness nursing diagnosis

INTRODUCTION

The nursing process and documentation depend on each other for providing safe and effective client care. The nursing process lays out a plan of care that guides not only the care provided but also the accurate recording of that care. Documentation provides a legal record that all aspects of the nursing process were properly carried out and that professional standards of care, regulatory standards, and agency policies were met.

Every day, individuals process information and take steps that lead to goal attainment. For example, when a meal is prepared, the cook goes through a process of obtaining the food, then preparing the meal for the ultimate goal of eating good food. In deciding what to wear, an individual goes through a process of considering the weather for appropriate clothing, then choosing matching clothes for the goal of looking attractive in the chosen outfit. Nursing has a process, called the nursing process, that provides quality care to a client. There are several steps in the nursing process that a nurse takes to provide effective care.

This chapter first explains the nursing process in general and then each step individually. The legal aspects, methods, and forms for documenting are explained. Many examples are provided throughout the chapter.

NURSING PROCESS HISTORY

The first reference to nursing as a "process" was in a 1955 journal article by Lydia Hall, yet the term *nursing process* was not widely used until the late 1960s (Edelman & Mandle, 2002). Johnson (1959), Orlando (1961), and Wiedenbach (1963) referred to the nursing process as a series of three steps: assessment, planning, and evaluation. Yura and Walsh (1967) identified four steps in the nursing process:

1. Assessing
2. Planning
3. Implementing
4. Evaluating

The term *nursing diagnosis* was first used by Fry (1953). After the first meeting of the group now called NANDA-International in 1974, nursing diagnosis was added as a separate step in the nursing process. Now, the steps of the nursing process are:

1. Assessment
2. Diagnosis
3. Planning and outcome identification
4. Implementation
5. Evaluation

THE NURSING PROCESS

A **process** is a series of steps or acts that lead to accomplishing some goal or purpose. According to Bevis (1989), "processes have three characteristics: (1) inherent purpose, (2) internal organization, and (3) infinite creativity." These characteristics are found in the nursing process. The **nursing process** is a systematic method for providing care to clients. The purpose is to provide individualized, holistic, effective

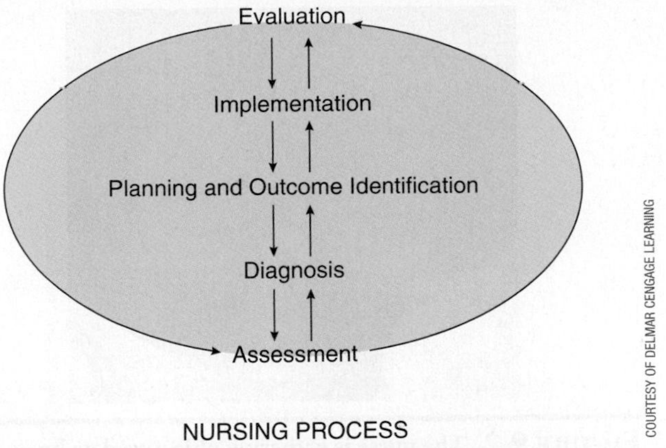

FIGURE 9-1 Five Components of the Nursing Process: Assessment, Diagnosis, Planning and Outcome Identification, Implementation, and Evaluation. The arrows going down represent revisions.

client care efficiently. Although the steps of the nursing process build on each other, they are not linear. Each step overlaps with the previous and subsequent steps (Figure 9-1).

The nursing process is dynamic and requires creativity in its application. The steps are the same for each client situation, but the correlation and results will be different. The nursing process is used with clients of all ages and in any care setting. It is also the organizing system for the National Council Licensure Examination for both practical/vocational nurses (NCLEX-PN®) and registered nurses (NCLEX-RN®).

Assessment

Assessment, the first step in the nursing process, includes systematic collection, verification, organization, interpretation, and documentation of data. The completeness and correctness of this data relate directly to the accuracy of the steps that follow. Assessment involves the following steps:

- Data collection from a variety of sources
- Data validation
- Data organization
- Data interpretation
- Data documentation

In some states, LPN/VNs do not perform complete assessments but collect data. For safe practice, LPN/VNs follow the Standards of Practice in their state of employment.

Purpose of Assessment

The purpose of assessment is to organize a database regarding a client's physical, psychosocial, and emotional health so that health-promoting behaviors and actual and/or potential health problems can be identified. The nurse ascertains the client's functional abilities, the absence or presence of dysfunction, normal activities of daily living, and lifestyle patterns through assessment. Identifying the client's strengths gives the nurse information about the abilities, behaviors, and skills the client can use during the treatment and recovery process. Assessment also provides an opportunity to form a therapeutic interpersonal relationship with the client. During assessment, the client can discuss health care concerns and goals with the nurse.

PROFESSIONALTIP

The Nursing Process

- The nursing process involves overlapping steps.
- The steps are explained one after the other for ease of understanding, but in actual practice, there may not be a definite beginning or ending to each step.
- Work in one step may begin before work in the preceding step is completed.

Types of Assessment

The information needed for assessment is usually determined by the health care setting and needs of the client. Three types of assessment are comprehensive, focused, and ongoing. A comprehensive assessment is most desirable when first determining a client's need for nursing care. Time limits or special circumstances may require an abbreviated data collection, as shown in a focused assessment. The assessment database can then be broadened through ongoing assessment.

Comprehensive Assessment A **comprehensive assessment** provides baseline client data including a complete health history and current needs assessment. It is usually completed upon admission to a health care agency. Changes in the client's health status can be measured against this database. It includes assessment of the client's physical and psychosocial health, perception of health, presence of health risk factors, and coping patterns.

Focused Assessment A **focused assessment** is limited to potential health care risks, a particular need, or health care concern. They are not as detailed as comprehensive assessments and are often used when short stays are anticipated (e.g., outpatient surgery centers and emergency departments), in specialty areas such as mental health settings, labor and delivery, or for screening for specific problems or risk factors (e.g., well-child clinics).

Ongoing Assessment When problems are identified during a comprehensive or focused assessment, follow-up is required. An **ongoing assessment** includes systematic monitoring of specific problems. This type of assessment broadens the database and allows the nurse to confirm the validity of data obtained during the initial assessment. Systematic monitoring allows the nurse to determine the client's response to nursing interventions and to identify any other problems.

Sources of Data

Although data are collected from a variety of sources, the client is considered the **primary source** of data (the major provider of information about a client). As much information as possible should be gathered from the client, using both interview techniques and physical examination skills. Sources of data other than the client are considered **secondary sources** and include family members, other health care providers, and medical records.

LIFE SPAN CONSIDERATIONS

Assessment and Interventions for Hearing Impairment

Approximately 30% of those over 65 have a hearing impairment. According to Wallhagen, Pettengill, and Whiteside (2006), studies show that hearing is not a routine assessment in older adults, even those in nursing homes. Some observational assessment techniques that may assist a nurse in determining hearing impairment are:

- Does the client cup her hand behind her ear?
- Does she tilt her head or lean into you as you speak?
- Is the volume higher than normal on the television?
- Does she misunderstand questions or respond inappropriately?

If you notice these signs in a client, use these interventions to improve communication and nursing care:

- State the client's name, pause, and then ask a question or make a statement.
- Speak in a normal tone and enunciate clearly without exaggerating lip movements.
- Keep your mouth visible to the client (e.g., avoid placing hand over mouth when speaking or turning face away from the client).
- Make sure the hearing aids are in place and that the batteries are correctly operating.
- Restate a phrase rather than repeat the same phrase.

Types of Data

Two types of information are collected through assessment: subjective and objective. **Subjective data** are data from the client's (sometimes family's) point of view and include perceptions, feelings, and concerns. The primary method of collecting subjective data (also called symptoms) is the interview. The **health history**, a review of the client's functional health patterns prior to the current contact with the health care agency, provides much of the subjective data.

Objective data (also called signs) are observable and measurable data that are obtained through both standard assessment techniques performed during the physical examination (Figure 9-2) and the results of laboratory and diagnostic testing. Table 9-1 provides examples of both subjective and objective data.

PROFESSIONALTIP

Clients Who Were Adopted

Remember that clients who were adopted will have varying degrees of knowledge about their biological parents. Sensitivity to this issue is critical in gaining client trust during the interview process.

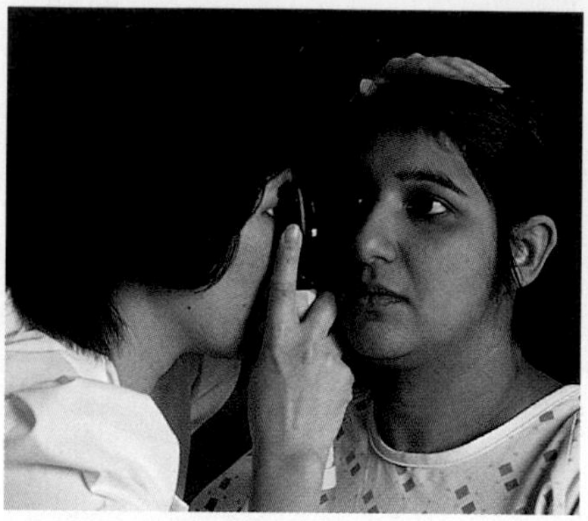

FIGURE 9-2 The nurse is gathering objective data by examining retinal structures.

Validating the Data

Objective data may add to or validate subjective data. Validation is a critical step that prevents misunderstandings, omissions, and incorrect inferences and conclusions (Figure 9-3). This process is particularly important if data sources are considered unreliable, such as when a client is confused or unable to communicate. If two sources provide conflicting data, further information or clarification must be sought. Findings should also be compared with norms, and grossly abnormal findings should be rechecked and confirmed.

Organizing the Data

Collected data must be organized so as to be useful to the health care professional collecting the data and to others involved in the client's care. After being organized into categories, the data are clustered into groups of related pieces. **Data clustering** is the process of putting data together in order to identify areas of the client's problems and strengths. Many health care agencies use an admission assessment format, which assists the nurse in collecting and organizing data.

An **assessment model** is a framework providing a systematic way to organize data. A few of the many assessment models available to nurses are described in the next sections.

TABLE 9-1 Types of Data

DATA

An African American male, age 79, comes to the emergency room because he cannot move his left arm. The client states, "It happened about an hour ago when my headache got worse. Now I am nauseated and dizzy."

The nurse takes his vital signs—T 99, P 100, R 28, BP 200/102—and observes that he cannot move his left arm and his face is flushed.

SUBJECTIVE	OBJECTIVE
Headache	T 99, P 100
Nausea	R 28, BP 200/102
Dizziness	Cannot move left arm
	Flushed face

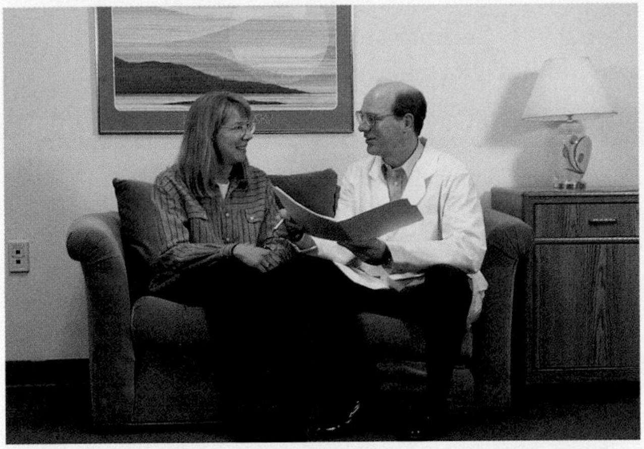

FIGURE 9-3 The nurse is validating information collected from the client during assessment.

Hierarchy of Needs Maslow's Hierarchy of Needs proposes that an individual's basic needs (physiological) must be met before higher-level needs can be met. An initial assessment of all physiological needs followed by assessment of the higher-level needs is necessary when using this model.

Body Systems Model The body systems model organizes data collection according to tissue and organ function in the various body systems (e.g., respiratory, cardiovascular, gastrointestinal). Physicians frequently use this model, so it is sometimes called the "medical model."

Functional Health Patterns Gordon's Functional Health Patterns (Gordon, 1998) provides a framework for data collection focusing on 11 functional health patterns. These functional health pattern areas cluster information about a client's habitual patterns and any recent changes to determine if the client's current response is functional or dysfunctional. For example, the elimination pattern is assessed for a client who now has diarrhea several times a week. Data collection would be focused on elimination habits, diet, and fluid intake before the diarrhea began and the effect of any changes on the client's functional ability and lifestyle. The 11 patterns are:

- Health perception/health management pattern
- Nutritional/metabolic pattern
- Elimination pattern
- Activity/exercise pattern
- Cognitive/perceptual pattern
- Sleep/rest pattern
- Self-perception/self-concept pattern
- Role/relationship pattern
- Sexuality/reproductive pattern
- Coping/stress-tolerance pattern
- Value/belief pattern (Gordon, 1998)

Theory of Self-Care Orem (2001) developed the theory of self-care based on a client's ability to perform self-care activities. Self-care, learned behavior with deliberate actions responding to need, includes activities an individual performs to maintain health. This theory focuses on the assessment of the client's ability to meet self-care needs and identifying existing self-care deficits. This theory is concerned primarily with illness states. The self-care essentials are:

- Maintenance of a sufficient intake of air
- Maintenance of a sufficient intake of water
- Maintenance of a sufficient intake of food
- Provision of care associated with elimination processes and excrements
- Maintenance of a balance between activity and rest
- Maintenance of a balance between solitude and social interaction
- Prevention of hazards to human life, human functioning, and human well-being
- Promotion of human functioning and development within social groups in accord with human potential, known human limitations, and the human desire to be normal (Orem, Taylor, and Renpenning, 2001)

Interpreting the Data

After data is collected, the nurse can begin developing impressions or inferences about the meaning of the data. Organizing data in clusters helps the nurse recognize patterns of response or behavior. When data are placed in clusters, the nurse can:

- Distinguish between relevant and irrelevant data.
- Determine whether and where there are gaps in the data.
- Identify patterns of cause and effect.

Documenting the Data

Assessment data must be recorded and some reported. The nurse must decide which data should be immediately reported to the head nurse and/or physician and which data can just be recorded. Data reflecting a significant change from the normal (e.g., BP 180/100, severe difficulty in breathing, or a high level of anxiety) would need to be reported as well as recorded. Data that need only be recorded include the fact that prescribed medication relieved a headache and that an abdominal dressing is dry and intact.

It is essential for accurate and complete recording of assessment data to communicate information to other health care team members. The basis for determining quality of care is documentation, which includes data to support identified problems.

DIAGNOSIS

The second step in the nursing process involves further **analysis** (breaking down the whole into parts that can be examined) and **synthesis** (putting data together in a new way) of the collected data. A list of nursing diagnoses is the result of this process. According to NANDA-International, a **nursing diagnosis**

> is a clinical judgment about individual, family, or community responses to actual or potential health problems/life processes. A nursing diagnosis provides the basis for selection of nursing interventions to achieve outcomes for which the nurse is accountable. (NANDA-I, 2010, p. 419)

The nursing diagnoses provide the basis for client care through the remaining steps. Clients have both medical and nursing diagnoses. Table 9-2 compares the two categories of diagnoses. It is important to have a clear understanding of the nature of a nursing diagnosis as compared to a **medical diagnosis** (clinical judgment by the physician that identifies or determines a specific disease, condition, or pathological state). Table 9-3 compares selected nursing and medical diagnoses.

TABLE 9-2 Comparison of Nursing and Medical Diagnoses

NURSING DIAGNOSIS	MEDICAL DIAGNOSIS
Recognizes situations that the nurse is licensed and qualified to treat	Recognizes conditions the physician is licensed and qualified to treat
Concentrates on the client's responses to health problems or life processes	Concentrates on injury, illness, or disease processes
Varies as the client's responses and/or health problems change	Stays the same until a cure is realized or client dies
Example: *Nausea* *Acute Pain* *Acute Pain* *Impaired Physical Mobility*	Example: Choleithiasis Exploratory surgery Cholecystectomy

The nurse uses critical-thinking and decision-making skills in developing nursing diagnoses. These skills are discussed later in the chapter. The LPN/VN's role in developing nursing diagnoses varies from state to state. For safe practice, the LPN/VN must be familiar with the Standards of Practice in the state of employment.

Components of a Nursing Diagnosis

The nursing diagnosis may be stated as a two-part statement or a three-part statement. The two-part statement is NANDA-International approved and used by most nurses because it is brief and precise. The three-part statement is often required of nursing students and is preferred by nurses who desire the diagnostic statement to include specific manifestations. Refer to the appendices for the list of NANDA-International approved nursing diagnoses.

Two-Part Statement The first part, the actual nursing diagnosis, is a problem statement or diagnostic label describing the client's response to an actual or risk health problem or a wellness condition.

PROFESSIONALTIP

Benefits of Nursing Diagnosis

- Nursing diagnosis is unique because it focuses on a client's *response* to a health problem rather than on the problem.
- Nursing diagnosis provides a way for effective communication.
- Holistic care is facilitated through the use of nursing diagnosis.

TABLE 9-3 Comparison of Select Nursing and Medical Diagnoses

NURSING DIAGNOSIS	MEDICAL DIAGNOSIS
Decreased Cardiac Output *Ineffective Breathing Pattern* *Risk for Imbalanced Fluid Volume*	Congestive heart
Impaired Physical Mobility	Ménière's disease
Death Anxiety	Lung cancer
Ineffective Airway Clearance *Ineffective Breathing Pattern* *Anxiety*	Chronic obstructive pulmonary disease

The second part is the **etiology**, the related cause or contributor to the problem, which is identified in the complete NANDA-International diagnosis description. The diagnostic label and etiology are linked by the term *related to* (R/T). Because the NANDA-International list of nursing diagnoses is constantly evolving, there may be times when no etiology is provided. In such cases, the nurse attempts to describe likely contributing factors to the client's condition. Examples of a two-part nursing diagnosis statement are *Disturbed **Body** Image* R/T loss of left lower extremity and ***Activity** Intolerance* R/T decreased oxygen-carrying capacity of cells.

Three-Part Statement In a three-part statement, the first two parts are the diagnostic label and the etiology. The third part consists of **defining characteristics** (collected data, also known as signs and symptoms, subjective and objective data, or clinical manifestations). The third part is joined to the first two parts with the connecting phrase *as evidenced by* (AEB). An example of a three-part nursing diagnosis statement is *Ineffective **Breathing** Pattern* R/T pain AEB respiratory rate less than 11 and use of accessory muscles. Table 9-4 provides other examples.

Types of Nursing Diagnoses

Analysis of the collected data leads the nurse to make a diagnosis in one of three categories:

- An **actual nursing diagnosis** indicates that a problem exists; it is composed of the diagnostic label, related factors, and signs and symptoms. An example of an actual diagnosis is *Situational Low **Self-Esteem*** R/T loss (first chair trumpet in band) AEB self-negating verbalization "I'm no good anymore."

PROFESSIONALTIP

Nursing Diagnosis

- The nursing diagnosis must evolve from the data, never the other way around.
- Never try to fit a client to a nursing diagnosis; select the appropriate diagnosis based on the data presented by the client. Failing to do this may result in errors in nursing diagnoses.

Table 9-4 Examples of Nursing Diagnoses Written as Two- and Three-Part Statements

TWO-PART STATEMENT	THREE-PART STATEMENT
*Toileting **S**elf-Care Deficit* R/T neuromuscular impairment	*Toileting **S**elf-Care Deficit* R/T neuromuscular impairment, right sided AEB inability to ambulate to the bathroom
*Impaired **S**wallowing* R/T mechanical obstruction	*Impaired **S**wallowing* R/T/mechanical obstruction AEB presence of tracheostomy tube
*Impaired **U**rinary Elimination* R/T urinary tract infection	*Impaired **U**rinary Elimination* R/T urinary tract infection AEB frequency and dysuria
*Impaired **M**emory* R/T fluid and electrolyte imbalance	*Impaired **M**emory* R/T fluid and electrolyte imbalance AEB inability to recall recent or past events
*Impaired **H**ome Maintenance* R/T individual/family member disease or injury	*Impaired **H**ome Maintenance* R/T individual/family member disease or injury AEB repeated lice infestations

- A **risk nursing diagnosis** (potential problem) indicates that a problem does not yet exist but that specific risk factors are present. A risk diagnosis begins with the phrase *Risk for* followed by the diagnostic label and a list of the risk factors. An example of a risk diagnosis is *Risk for Situational Low **S**elf-Esteem*; risk factors include unrealistic self-expectations AEB receiving "B" in two college courses while working full-time (expected "A").
- A **wellness nursing diagnosis** denotes the client's statement of a desire to attain a higher level of wellness in some area of function. It begins with the phrase *Readiness for Enhanced* followed by the diagnostic label. For example, a wife who has been caring for her husband who had a stroke two months ago asks the nurse about meeting with other wives who are/have been in a similar situation. The nurse would make a wellness diagnosis of *Readiness for Enhanced Family **C**oping.*

Examples of the three types of diagnoses are shown in Table 9-5.

After formulation, the nursing diagnoses is discussed with the client, but if this is not possible, the diagnoses is discussed with family members. The list of nursing diagnoses is recorded on the client's record, and the remainder of the client's care plan is completed. The list of nursing diagnoses is dynamic, changing as more data are collected and as client goals and responses to interventions are evaluated.

Table 9-5 Types of Nursing Diagnoses

TYPE	EXAMPLE
Actual diagnosis	*Perceived **C**onstipation* R/T faulty appraisal AEB expectation of passage of stool at same time every day
Risk diagnosis	*Risk for **A**spiration* R/T decreased cough and gag reflexes
Wellness diagnosis	*Readiness for Enhanced **S**piritual Well-Being*

Carpenito (2009) discusses situations in which nurses intervene in collaboration with other disciplines. She defines **collaborative problems** as "certain physiologic complications that nurses monitor to detect onset or changes in states. Nurses manage collaborative problems using physician-prescribed and nursing-prescribed interventions to minimize the complications of the events." She has identified 52 specific collaborative problems grouped under nine generic problem categories. For example, under the generic collaborative problem category of *Potential Complication (PC): Respiratory* are the specific collaborative problems of "PC: Hypoxemia, PC: Atelectasis/pneumonia, PC: Tracheobronchial Constriction, and PC: Pneumothorax."

The collaborative problem statement *always* begins with *Potential Complication* or PC. This differentiates it from a nursing diagnosis. A benefit of using collaborative problem statements is that they identify, and thus keep the nurses aware of, the potential complications a client may encounter. As in the previous example, the specific potential complication for a client with a respiratory problem would be listed on the care plan.

Planning and Outcome Identification

Planning and outcome identification are the third step of the nursing process and include both establishing guidelines for the proposed course of nursing action to resolve the nursing diagnoses and developing the client's plan of care. After the nursing diagnoses and the client's strengths have been identified, planning begins.

The planning occurs in three phases: initial, ongoing, and discharge. **Initial planning** involves development of a preliminary plan of care by the nurse who performs the admission assessment and gathers the comprehensive admission assessment data. Progressively shorter stays in the hospital make initial planning very important to ensure resolution of the problems. **Ongoing planning** updates the client's plan of care. New information about the client is collected and evaluated and revisions made to the plan of care. **Discharge planning** involves anticipation of and planning for the client's needs after discharge.

The planning phase involves several tasks:

- Prioritizing the nursing diagnoses
- Identifying and writing client-centered long- and short-term goals and outcomes (outcome identification)
- Identifying specific nursing interventions
- Recording the entire nursing care plan in the client's record

Prioritizing the Nursing Diagnoses

Prioritizing the nursing diagnoses involves deciding which diagnoses are the most important and require attention first. Maslow's hierarchy of needs is one of the most common methods of selecting priorities. After basic physiological needs (e.g., respiration, nutrition, temperature, hydration, and elimination) are met to some degree, the nurse can then consider needs on the next level of the hierarchy (e.g., safe environment, stable living condition, affection, and self-worth) and so on up the hierarchy until all the nursing diagnoses have been prioritized.

Alfaro-LeFevre (2008) suggests a three-level approach to prioritizing client problems (nursing diagnoses):

- **First-level priority problems (immediate):**
  Airway problems
  Breathing problems
  Signs (vital sign problems)
- **Second-level priority problems (immediate, after treatment for first-level problems is initiated):**
  Mental status change
  Acute pain
  Acute urinary elimination problems
  Untreated medical problems requiring immediate attention (e.g., a diabetic who has not had insulin)
  Abnormal lab values
  Risks of infection, safety, or security (for client or others)
- **Third-level priority problems:**
  Health problems that do not fit in the above categories

She also proposes that *sometimes* the priority order may change. For example, if acute pain causes breathing problems, managing the pain may have the higher priority; if abnormal lab values are life threatening, then they have a higher priority. Table 9-6 illustrates the prioritizing process.

TABLE 9-6 Prioritizing Nursing Diagnoses

NURSING DIAGNOSIS	PRIORITIZING METHOD	PRIORITY
*Decreased **C**ardiac Output* R/T altered heart rate rhythm	Maslow, physiologic	High
	Alfaro-LeFevre, cardiac/circulatory	High
***D**iarrhea* R/T travel	Maslow, physiologic	High
	Alfaro-LeFevre, untreated medical problem	Moderate
***R**elocation Stress Syndrome* R/T isolation from family/friends	Maslow, safety and security	Moderate
	Alfaro-LeFevre, risk to security	Moderate
*Disturbed **S**leep Pattern* R/T daytime activity pattern	Maslow, safety and security	Moderate
	Alfaro-LeFevre, other health problems	Low
*Ineffective **C**oping* R/T inadequate resources available	Maslow, self-esteem	Low
	Alfaro-LeFevre, other health problems	Low

COURTESY OF DELMAR CENGAGE LEARNING

Identifying Outcomes

Outcome identification includes establishing goals and expected outcomes, which together provide guidelines for individualized nursing interventions and establish evaluation criteria to measure the effectiveness of the nursing care plan.

Goals A **goal** is an aim, intent, or end. Goals are broad statements that describe the desired or intended change in the client's condition or behavior. Client-centered goals are established in collaboration with the client when possible. Goal statements refer to the diagnostic label (or problem statement) of the nursing diagnosis. Client-centered goals ensure that nursing care is individualized and focused on the client.

A **short-term goal** is a statement that profiles the desired resolution of the nursing diagnosis over a short period of time, usually a few hours or days (less than a week). It focuses on the etiology part of the nursing diagnosis. A **long-term goal** is a statement that profiles the desired resolution of the nursing diagnosis over a longer period of time, usually weeks or months. It focuses on the problem part of the nursing diagnosis. Table 9-7 provides examples of short-term and long-term goals.

Expected Outcomes After the goals have been established, the expected outcomes can be identified based on those goals. An **expected outcome** is a detailed, specific statement describing the methods to be used to achieve the goal. It includes direct nursing care, client teaching, and continuity of care. Outcomes must be measurable, realistic, and time limited. Several expected outcomes may be required for each goal (Table 9-8). Then nursing interventions are formulated to enable the client to reach the goals.

TABLE 9-7 Short- and Long-Term Goals

Nursing Diagnosis: *Disturbed **B**ody Image* R/T Surgery for Breast Cancer

Short-Term Goals (focus on etiology)	**Long-Term Goals** (focus on problem)
Will verbalize loss of breast	Will verbalize acceptance of change in physical self
Will identify negative feelings about body	
Will touch chest where breast was	

COURTESY OF DELMAR CENGAGE LEARNING

TABLE 9-8 Goal and Expected Outcomes

Nursing Diagnosis: *Impaired **U**rinary Elimination* R/T Urinary Tract Infection AEB Frequent Urination in Small Amounts	
GOAL	**EXPECTED OUTCOMES**
Client will have improved urinary elimination.	Client will take antibiotic as ordered.
	By next visit, client will identify three factors to prevent a urinary tract infection.
	In 2 days, client will have a plan to increase water intake.
	By next visit, client will be urinating at least 150 mL at 2-hour or longer intervals.
Nursing Diagnosis: ***P**owerlessness* R/T Illness-Related Regimen AEB Nonparticipation in Care or Decision Making When Opportunities Are Provided	
GOAL	**EXPECTED OUTCOMES**
Client will participate in care and decision making.	In 2 days, client will participate in one aspect of own care each day.
	Client will state preference in decision making situation within 1 week.

Identifying Specific Nursing Interventions

A **nursing intervention** is an action performed by the nurse that helps the client achieve the results specified by the goals and expected outcomes. Nursing interventions refer directly to the related factors or the risk factors in nursing diagnoses. Nursing interventions that reduce or remove the related factors and risk factors resolve or prevent the problem.

There may be a number of nursing interventions for each nursing diagnosis. Nursing interventions are stated in specific terms. Examples of nursing interventions are as follows:

- Assist client to turn, cough, and deep breathe q 2 h beginning at 0800, 4/15
- Teach cord care at 1000, 6/20
- Weigh client at 0700 each day

Interventions formulated for each diagnosis are recorded on the client's care plan. The list of interventions is also dynamic and may change as the nurse interacts with the client, assesses responses to interventions, and evaluates those responses.

CRITICAL THINKING

Goals and Outcomes

How are goals and outcomes different?

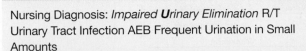

CRITICAL THINKING

Nursing Interventions

Differentiate among the three categories of nursing interventions: independent, interdependent, and dependent.

Categories of Nursing Interventions

Nursing interventions are classified into one of three categories: independent, interdependent, or dependent. **Independent nursing interventions** are initiated by the nurse and do not require direction or an order from another health care professional. Most states' nursing practice acts allow independent nursing interventions for activities such as daily living, health education, health promotion, and counseling. An example of an independent nursing intervention is elevating a client's edematous extremity.

Interdependent nursing interventions are implemented collaboratively by the nurse in conjunction with other health care professionals. For example, the nurse may assist a client to perform an exercise taught by the physical therapist.

Dependent nursing interventions require an order from a physician or another health care professional. Administration of a medication is an example of a dependent intervention. This intervention requires specific nursing knowledge and responsibilities, but it is not within the realm of legal practice for LP/VNs to prescribe medications. The nurse is responsible for knowing the classification, normal dosage, pharmacological action, contraindications, adverse effects, and nursing implications of the drug. Dependent nursing interventions must be governed by appropriate knowledge and judgment.

Recording the Nursing Care Plan

The **nursing care plan** is a written guide of strategies to implement to help the client achieve optimal health. Nursing care plans usually include components such as assessment, nursing diagnoses, goals and expected outcomes, and nursing interventions. The care plan is begun on the day of admission and is continually updated until discharge.

Care plans may be standardized, institutional, or computerized.

The standardized care plan is a printed guide for the care of clients with common needs. This care plan usually follows the nursing process format. It may be individualized by including handwritten notes for unusual problems.

Institutional nursing care plans are concise documents that become a part of the client's medical record after discharge. This care plan may simply include the nursing diagnoses, nursing interventions, and evaluation. Figure 9-4 provides an example of an institutional care plan.

Computers can generate both standardized and individualized nursing care plans. Appropriate diagnoses are selected from a menu, which lists possible goals and nursing interventions. Figure 9-5 is an example of a computerized nursing care plan.

IMPLEMENTATION

The fourth step in the nursing process is **implementation**, the performance of the nursing interventions identified during the planning phase. It also involves the delegation (process of transferring a select nursing task to a licensed individual who is

Nursing Diagnosis	Nursing Interventions	Evaluation
Ineffective Breastfeeding R/T deficient knowledge AEB inability to latch on to the maternal breast correctly	1. Teach various breastfeeding positions and techniques to encourage the infant. 2. Stay with mother during feeding and assist as needed.	1. Client tried the various positions and techniques. 2. Client able to assist infant to latch on to breast correctly.
Risk for Constipation R/T abdominal muscle weakness and hemorrhoids	1. Assess daily for bowel movement frequency and consistency. 2. Encourage more fluid and fiber intake.	1. Bowel movement daily, very firm consistency. 2. Asking for fruit between meals; drinking 8 oz water every 2 hours when awake.

FIGURE 9-4 Handwritten Institutional Care Plan

competent to perform that specific task) of some nursing interventions to staff members or assigning a specific nursing task to assistive (unlicensed) personnel capable of competently performing the task. The nurse is accountable for appropriate delegation and supervision of care provided by unlicensed personnel.

Requirements for Effective Implementation

Implementation involves many skills, including assessing the client's condition before, during, and after each nursing intervention. Positive responses add information to the database to use when evaluating the intervention. Negative responses must be dealt with immediately.

Psychomotor, interpersonal, and cognitive skills are also needed to perform the planned nursing interventions. Psychomotor skills are used when handling medical equipment and performing skills such as changing dressings, giving injections, and helping a client perform range-of-motion (ROM) exercises.

Interpersonal skills are used when collecting data, providing information in teaching sessions, and offering support in times of grief.

Cognitive skills enable the nurse to make appropriate observations, understand the rationale for the activities performed, ask appropriate questions, and make decisions about those things that need to be done. Critical thinking is an important element within the cognitive domain. It helps the nurse analyze data, organize observations, and apply prior knowledge and experiences to current client situations.

Orders for Nursing Interventions

Nursing interventions are written as orders in the care plan and may be initiated by nurses or physicians or from collaboration with other health care professionals. Interventions can be implemented on the basis of specific orders, standing orders, or protocols.

A **specific order** is an order written in a client's medical record by a physician or nursing care plan by the nurse especially for that individual client; it is not used for any other client.

A **protocol** is a series of standing orders or procedures that should be followed under certain specific conditions. It defines interventions that are permitted and circumstances under which the nurse can implement the measures. Health care agencies or individual physicians often use standing orders or protocols for preparing clients for diagnostic tests or for immediate interventions in life-threatening circumstances. Protocols prevent needlessly writing the same orders for different clients, saving valuable time.

Documenting and Reporting Interventions

The implementation step also involves documentation and reporting. Data to be recorded include the client's condition before the intervention, the specific intervention performed, the client's response to the intervention, and client outcomes. Documentation provides valuable communication among health care team members to ensure continuity of care and evaluate progress toward expected outcomes. Written documentation also provides data necessary for reimbursement.

Verbal communication between nurses generally occurs at the change of shift, when care responsibility changes. Nursing students must report relevant information to the nurse responsible for their clients when they leave the unit. Information that should be shared in the verbal report includes:

- Completed activities and those not completed
- Status of current relevant problems
- Assessment changes or abnormalities
- Results of treatments
- Diagnostic tests scheduled or completed (and results)

Both written and verbal communication must be objective, descriptive, and complete. It must include observations, not opinions and be stated or written to show an accurate picture of the client's condition. Communication of implementation activities is basic to client care and evaluation of progress toward goals.

EVALUATION

Evaluation, the fifth step in the nursing process, determines whether client goals have been met, partially met, or not met. When a goal is met, the nurse decides whether nursing interventions should stop or continue for the status to be maintained. When a goal is partially met or not met, the nurse reassesses the situation. The reasons the goal is not met and modifications to the plan of care are determined by more data collection. Reasons that goals are not met or are only partially met include:

- Initial assessment data were incomplete.
- Goals and expected outcomes were unrealistic.

Client Name: J. W. **Sex**: Female
Age: 77 **Temp:** 101.5 **BP:** 168/74 **Pulse:** 124 **O_2 Sat:** 89%

Client Health History

J.W. has smoked two to three packs of cigarettes a day for the past 60 years. She was diagnosed with COPD 4 years ago and has required supplemental oxygen at 2 L/min for the past 18 months. Her chief complaints are increasing dyspnea on exertion and a cough, which is sometimes productive, yielding thick, green-yellow sputum. She states, "I don't know why I'm coughing up this awful stuff."

Assessment Findings

Respiratory Rate 38
Sonorous and sibilant wheezes on expiration in the posterior lung fields with superimposed coarse crackles heard in the right posterior lower lung field.
Unable to ambulate to the bathroom or complete other ADLs because of dyspnea

Nursing Diagnosis: *Ineffective **B**reathing Pattern* R/T diseased lungs, infection, and increased secretions AEB severe dyspnea, elevated blood pressure, and increased pulse
Goal: J.W. will have an effective respiratory rate.
Outcomes: J.W. will:
1. Have a respiratory rate of 12–20 within 1 week.
2. Have clear lung sounds within 1 week.
3. Complete ADLs within 1 week.
4. Increase oral fluid intake to 2 L within 1 day.

Planning and Intervention

Intervention	Rationale
1. Assist client in assuming a high Fowler's position	Maximizes thoracic cavity space, decreases pressure from diaphragm and abdominal organs, facilitates use of accessory muscles
2. Provide humidified, low flow (2 L/min) oxygen, as ordered	Provides some supplemental oxygen to improve oxygenation and makes secretions less viscous
3. Administer bronchodilators, as ordered	Reduces bronchospasm and improves air flow
4. Administer IV fluids and increase oral fluids (2000–3000 mL/day as tolerated), as ordered	Improves hydration, decreases secretions
5. Administer expectorants, as ordered	Decreases secretions of previously ineffective cough
6. Administer antibiotics, as ordered	Eradicates respiratory infection or pneumonia and reduces secretions and end inflammation
7. Administer xanthines (aminophylline, theophylline), as ordered	Decreases smooth muscle spasm and edema of the mucosa
8. Administer non-narcotic cough suppressants, as ordered	Coughing can lead to fatigue. It is important for COPD clients to get adequate rest and not become fatigued with coughing

Evaluation:
Client's breathing is eupenic with a respiratory rate of 16
Client is able to cough up secretions
Client is able to ambulate to bathroom and complete ADLs
Client is drinking at least 2000 mL/day of water

Nursing Diagnosis: *Impaired **G**as Exchange* R/T lower airway (alveolar) wall destruction preventing adequate exchange of gases of respiration and airway obstruction (secretions) preventing adequate oxygenation AEB severe dyspnea, tachypnea, elevated blood pressure, increased pulse, and decreased oxygen saturation
Goal: J.W. will have improved gas exchange in her lungs.
Outcomes: J.W. will:
1. Have O_2 saturation of 95% within 1 week.
2. Have vital signs within normal ranges within 1 week.

Planning and Interventions

Intervention	Rationale
1. Assist client in assuming a high Fowler's position	Decreases the work of breathing (at least through crisis period)
2. Administer medications to loosen secretions, as ordered	Loosens secretions of previously ineffective cough
3. Provide humidified, low flow (2 L/min) oxygen, as ordered	Improves oxygenation, moistens thick secretions

Evaluation:
Client's O_2 saturation is 94%.
Client's vital signs are within normal ranges—T 98.6 P 80 R 20 BP 120/74.

FIGURE 9-5 Computer-Generated Nursing Care Plan

- Time frame was not adequate.
- Nursing interventions were not appropriate for the client or situation.

Evaluation is a fluid process that depends on all the other components of the nursing process. As shown in Figure 9-6, evaluation affects and is affected by the other four parts. Table 9-9 shows how evaluation is woven into every component of the nursing process. Ongoing evaluation is essential for the nursing process to be implemented appropriately. As Alfaro-LeFevre (2003) states,

> When we evaluate early, checking whether our information is accurate, complete, and up-to-date, we're able to make corrections *early*. We avoid making decisions based on outdated, inaccurate, or incomplete information. Early evaluation enhances our ability to act safely and effectively. It improves our *efficiency* by helping us stay focused on priorities and avoid wasting time continuing useless actions.

THE NURSING PROCESS AND CRITICAL THINKING

Many skills are necessary when nurses use the nursing process as a framework for providing client care. Critical thinking is one. Critical thinkers ask questions, identify assumptions,

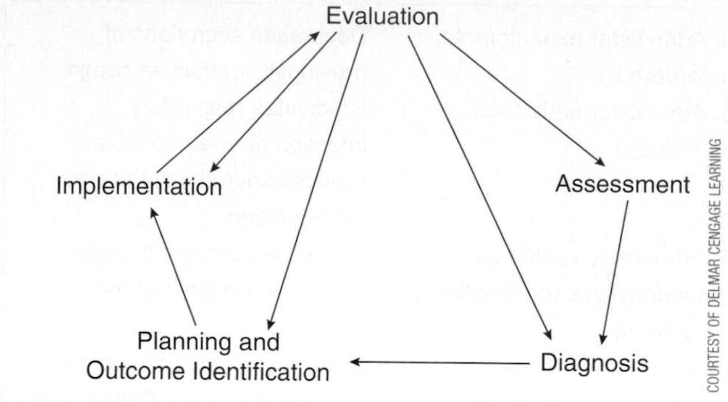

FIGURE 9-6 Relationship of Evaluation to the Other Components of the Nursing Process: Evaluation Impacts Every Component

evaluate evidence, examine alternatives, and seek to understand various points of view.

Critical thinking can be learned, just as other skills are learned. The skill of critical thinking is an especially vital tool for the nurse but is useful in all aspects of a person's life.

COMMUNITY/HOME HEALTH CARE

Effectiveness of Care

In the home, the nurse can use the following questions to evaluate client achievement of expected outcomes:

- Were the goals realistic for client abilities and the time frame?
- Did external variables (e.g., finances, housing problems, impaired family dynamics) prevent goal achievement?
- Did the family have resources (e.g., money, transportation) necessary to meet the goals?
- Was care appropriately coordinated with other providers?

Examples of questions the nurse, as critical thinker, might ask at each step in the nursing process are listed in Table 9-10.

TABLE 9-9 Interaction of Other Components of the Nursing Process with Evaluation

NURSING PROCESS COMPONENTS	EVALUATION QUESTIONS
Assessment	Are data relevant to client needs? Are data obtained appropriately? Are data collected from many, varied sources? Is a systematic, organized method used to collect data? Is data collection complete?
Diagnosis	Are diagnoses based on the data collected? Is each nursing diagnosis complete? Are nursing diagnoses client centered and relevant? Do nursing diagnoses guide planning and implementation of care? Are nursing diagnoses prioritized?
Planning and Outcome Identification	Are expected outcomes relevant to nursing diagnoses? Are outcomes realistic?
Implementation	Are resources (also team members) used effectively and efficiently? Are care plans documented? Is care plan revised according to the client's needs? Is plan of care followed by all team members? Are necessary resources available? Do nursing actions assist client in meeting expected outcomes? Are expected outcomes achieved? Does documentation reflect client status and responses to nursing interventions?

TABLE 9-10 Use of Critical Thinking with the Nursing Process

STEP OF NURSING PROCESS	SAMPLE CRITICAL THINKING QUESTIONS
Assessment	What data are necessary to prevent, anticipate, or detect health problems? What data are necessary to manage or eliminate a client's health problems? From what other sources can data be obtained? How does the client view his health situation? How efficient is care delivery? What assumptions or biases does the nurse have?
Diagnosis	How can the data be put together and analyzed? Are there any gaps in the data? What health problems can be identified? What are the underlying causes of risk factors for the health problems? What are the client's strengths and resources? Which satisfactory aspects of the client's health could be improved?
Planning and Outcome Identification	What are the specific desired outcomes for this client? What interventions will detect or prevent health problems? Which interventions will manage the client's health problems? What interventions will promote optimum wellness and independence for the client? How can the desired outcomes be achieved in a cost-effective, timely manner? Who is best qualified to carry out the interventions? How much does the client wish to be involved?
Implementation	How ready is the health care giver to perform the interventions? What are the critical steps of this intervention? How can the intervention be altered to meet this client's needs yet maintain principles of safety? How does the client respond during and after the intervention? What is to be documented to monitor the client's progress toward the goals and outcomes?
Evaluation	Were the specific desired goals and outcomes met? If all were met, can these goals and outcomes be eliminated? If not met, how should the plan be modified (revised)? If revision of the plan, goals, or outcomes is necessary, what ongoing, continuous assessments (data) are required? Were assumptions or biases missed that affected the interventions? What other nursing diagnosis(es) may be appropriate? What additional outcomes and interventions should be considered?

THE NURSING PROCESS AND DECISION MAKING

Every day, nurses make decisions. These decisions should be the best decisions possible based on reliable information, and made using critical thinking. Each step of the nursing process requires decisions.

Each decision, resulting from critical thought and reliable information, leads to appropriate nursing interventions for the client.

THE NURSING PROCESS AND HOLISTIC CARE

The broad base of nursing knowledge is derived from many fields, including natural science, social science, behavioral science, arts and humanities, and nursing science. With this broad knowledge base, the nurse interacts with the client in a holistic manner. Referral and collaboration among nurses and other health care professionals contribute to holistic achievement of client goals.

In some settings, the traditional nursing care plan formulated solely by nurses has been replaced by plans that are developed by a multidisciplinary team and referred to as critical pathways. Critical pathways are comprehensive, standard plans of care for specific conditions.

DOCUMENTATION

The methods of recording and reporting information relevant to client care have developed as a response to standards of practice, legal and regulatory standards, institutional standards and policies, and society's norms.

Recording and reporting are the major ways health care providers communicate. The client's medical record is a legal document of all activities regarding client care.

Documentation is any printed or written record of activities. In health care it should include:

- Changes in the client's condition
- The administration of tests, treatments, procedures, and client education, with the results of or client's response to them
- The client's response to an intervention
- The evaluation of expected outcomes
- Complaints from client or family

PURPOSES OF DOCUMENTATION

The two primary reasons for documentation are professional responsibility and accountability. The professional responsibility of all health care practitioners, documentation provides evidence of the practitioner's accountability to the client, the institution, the profession, and society. Other reasons are communication, legal and practice standards, education, reimbursement, research, and auditing.

Communication

Documentation is a communication method that confirms the care provided to the client and clearly outlines all important information regarding the client. Thorough documentation provides:

- Accurate data to plan care and ensure continuity of care
- Communication to health care team members involved in the client's care
- Evidence of things done to or for the client, the client's response, and revisions made in the plan of care
- Evidence of compliance with professional practice standards
- Evidence of compliance with accreditation criteria (e.g., those of the Joint Commission)
- A resource for reimbursement, education, and research and audit
- A written legal record to protect the client, institution, and practitioner

The client's medical record contains documents for recordkeeping. The type of documents that constitute the medical record in a given health care institution is determined by that institution. Table 9-11 outlines the content of the documents generally found in a client's record.

Practice and Legal Standards

Thoroughly documenting care in the medical record provides legal evidence that the care provided meets approved standards of care (Ferrel, 2007). *The medical record is a legal document, and in a lawsuit, it is the record that serves as the description of exactly what happened to a client.* In 80% to 85% of client care lawsuits, the determining factor in providing proof of

TABLE 9-11 Documents of the Client Medical Record

DOCUMENT	CONTENT
Face Sheet	*Demographic Data:* name, client's identifying number, address, telephone number, date of birth, place of birth, sex, race, marital status, religion, name and address of closest relative, social security number, admission date and hour, type of admission *Financial Data:* expected payer(s), insured's name and sex, client relationship to insured, employer's name and location, group name, insurance group number, insured's policy number *Clinical Data:* admitting diagnosis, admitting diagnosis-related group (DRG), client's advance directive (if has one) *Discharge Data* (to be entered by the physician on discharge of client): name of attending physician, discharge date and hour, principal diagnosis and other diagnoses, external cause of injury code, procedures and dates, operating physician(s), disposition of client
Medical History and Physical Examination	Client's description of chief complaint, present and past illnesses, personal and family histories, and review of systems as elicited by the physician, findings of physician's assessment of all body systems
Nursing Admission Assessment	Data from interview and physical assessment performed by the nurse
Prescriber's Orders	Physician's written or verbal orders to admit, to direct client's diagnostic and therapeutic course, and to discharge
Consultation Report	Findings of a physician whose opinion or advice is requested by another physician for evaluation and/or treatment of a client
Physician's Progress Notes	Provides a pertinent, chronologic report of the client's course in the hospital and reflects any changes in condition and response to treatment. May also contain notes by other members of the health care team (e.g., dietary or social service)
Laboratory Reports	Results from laboratory tests ordered by the physician
Radiology Reports	Radiologists interpretation of radiologic and fluoroscopic diagnostic services
Nuclear Medicine	Describes diagnostic studies and therapeutic procedures performed using radiopharmaceutical agents
Graphic Sheet	Various client parameters, most commonly: T, P, R, and BP. May also include weight, diet, I&O
Client Care Plan (Nursing Plan of Care)	Treatment plan including nursing diagnoses or problem list, client goals, nursing actions, and evaluation
Nurse's Progress Notes	Details care and treatments provided, client's response to care and treatments, achievement of expected outcomes that do not duplicate information on Flow Sheet (if used)

TABLE 9-11 Documents of the Client Medical Record (Continued)

DOCUMENT	CONTENT
Flow Sheet	All routine interventions that can be indicated by a check mark or other simple descriptor
Medication Administration Record (MAR)	Contains all medications administered orally, topically, by injection, inhalation, and infusion in one place; includes date, time, dosage, route of administration, and name of professional administering the drug. Routine, PRN, and single dose orders generally have separate sections
Consent Forms	*Admission:* gives the institution and physician permission to treat *Surgical:* explains the reason for and nature of the treatment, the risks, complications, alternate forms of treatment, no treatment, consequences of treatment or procedure. Sometimes surgical and anesthesia consents are separate so that responsibility is placed appropriately *Blood Transfusion:* gives specific permission to administer blood or blood products *Other:* procedure specific consent forms, participate in research project, photography
Client Education Record	Describes the nurse's teaching to the client, family, or other caregiver and the learner's response
Health Care Team Record	Used by respiratory, physical therapy, dietary when physician's progress are used only by physicians
Nursing Discharge Summary	Contains brief summary of care provided, medications, teaching, and other instructions (e.g., return appointment, referrals), discharge status, and mode of discharge
Discharge Plan and Summary	Review of events describing the client's illness, investigation (diagnostic studies), treatment, response, and condition at discharge. Instructions to the client and plans for follow-up care as included
Advance Directive	Both a living will and a durable power of attorney for health care are considered advance directives. Federal law requires that all clients be given written information about their rights so they can make decisions concerning medical care. An advance directive is not required to be in a client's medical record
Other Documents	These may or may not be in a client's medical record: Operative report, Anesthesia report, Pathology report, Transfusion record, Rehabilitation report, Critical pathway, Restraint record, and Autopsy report

significant events is the medical record (Iyer & Camp, 2005). The legal aspects of documentation require:

- Writing, legible and neat
- Spelling and grammar, properly used
- Authorized abbreviations
- Time-sequenced, and factual descriptive entries

State Nursing Practice Acts State nursing practice acts establish guidelines to ensure safe practice and to demonstrate accountability to society. The standards of care set forth in the practice acts are based on the nursing process components and require documentation as evidenced of compliance. Nurses must be familiar with the practice act of the states in which they work.

The Joint Commission The Joint Commission surveys health care facilities that voluntarily apply for accreditation to measure compliance with its standards for providing safe health care. Eligibility for Medicare, Medicaid, and private funding reimbursement depends on Joint Commission accreditation.

The Joint Commission requires documented evidence of an individualized plan of care (Joint Commission, 2008). The Joint Commission standards require:

- The involvement of the client or family in the development of the plan, which must be documented in the medical record
- Interdisciplinary planning and implementation of all aspects of care

The reviewers during an accreditation survey look for evidence of an organized and systematic method of monitoring and evaluating client care by checking documentation in medical records. Documenting the steps of the nursing process ensures compliance with the Joint Commission's plan of care requirements.

Confidentiality The client record is **confidential** and is to be read only by those health care providers directly involved in the care of that client. The record should not be left where just anyone has access to it. Keep it in its proper storage place when not being used.

Informed Consent Informed consent is a competent client's ability to make health care decisions based on full disclosure of the benefits, risks, and potential consequences of a recommended treatment plan and of alternative treatments, including no treatment, and the client's agreement to the treatment. Informed consent can be given either orally or in writing. A written informed consent document records the process of informed consent and is invaluable in the event of a lawsuit. The physician who will perform the procedure is responsible for obtaining the client's informed consent, but the nurse is often the one who actually has the client sign the form.

PROFESSIONALTIP

The Importance of Communication

Important assessment information needing immediate intervention should be documented and communicated orally to the other practitioners involved in the client's care. Time must direct decision making when critical information is obtained.

The nurse's signature as a witness on an informed consent form is vouching that the client or appropriate surrogate is the person signing and that the person signing is making an autonomous, noncoerced informed decision to have the procedure, treatment, or research completed. It is the nurse's responsibility to assess if the client is adequately informed, especially if the procedure has potential, serious consequences, and to advocate for the client to receive additional explanation as needed from the physician (Grace & McLaughlin, 2005; White, 2000).

Advance Directives An advance directive (i.e., living will and durable power of attorney for health care) is written instructions about an individual's health care preferences regarding life-sustaining measures to guide family members and health care professionals as to those treatment options that should or should not be considered when the individual is no longer able to decide. This allows competent clients to make end-of-life decisions and to choose the types of life-sustaining procedures they wish to be performed.

Reimbursement

The federal government requires peer review organizations (PROs) to monitor and evaluate the quality and appropriateness of care provided. Medical records are reviewed for documentation of intensity of services and severity of illness.

The diagnosis-related group (DRG) classification system changed the reimbursement process from a cost-per-case to a prospective payment system (PPS). With PPS, the medical record must have documentation supporting the DRG and the appropriateness of care. It also must show evidence of client and family education and discharge planning.

From the agency's perspective, when information in the medical record shows compliance with Medicare and Medicaid standards, reimbursement is maximized. Failure to document equipment or procedures used daily (e.g., feeding pump; daily weight, intake and output; intravenous therapy; drug additives) can result in reimbursement being denied.

PROFESSIONALTIP

Consent from Sedated Clients

Sedated clients should never be asked or allowed to sign an informed consent. If the client is not capable of understanding the nature of and risks associated with the procedure, the consent is invalid, and the nurse and institution are legally at risk. Either wait for the client to be competent and free of sedation (usually 4 hours after administration of medication that alters the level of consciousness) or have a legally acceptable family member sign.

COMMUNITY/HOME HEALTH CARE

Documentation

Home health agencies also keep client medical records. They must also comply with state and federal regulations affecting health care, documentation, and reimbursement.

Education

Health care students use the medical record as a tool to learn about disease processes, medical and nursing diagnoses, complications, and interventions. The results of laboratory and diagnostic testing and physical examinations provide valuable information about specific diagnoses and interventions.

Nursing students can enhance their critical-thinking skills by examining and analyzing the records of the health care team's plan of care, including the way the care plan was developed, implemented, and evaluated. All health care professionals including students must maintain confidentiality when reading any client's chart.

Research

The client's medical record is used by researchers to determine whether a client meets the research criteria for a study. Documentation can also indicate a need for research. For example, if documentation shows an increased rate of falls on certain nursing units, researchers can look for and study the variables associated with the increased fall rate.

Nursing Audit

A **nursing audit** is a method of evaluating the quality of care provided to clients. A nursing audit can focus on implementation of the nursing process, on client outcomes, or on both in order to evaluate the quality of care provided. The nursing audit is follow-up evaluation that not only evaluates the quality of care of an individual client but also provides an evaluation of overall care given in that health care facility. During a nursing audit, the evaluators look for documentation of all five components of the nursing process in the client records.

Each health care facility has an ongoing nursing audit committee to evaluate the quality of care given. The nursing audit committee reviews client records after discharge of the clients. They examine the records for data related to:

- Safety measures
- Treatment interventions and client responses to them
- Expected outcomes as basis for interventions
- Client teaching
- Discharge planning
- Adequate staffing

EFFECTIVE DOCUMENTATION PRINCIPLES

The health care facility (hospital, nursing home, home health agency), the setting within the facility (e.g., emergency room,

PROFESSIONALTIP

Follow the Nursing Process

Document according to the nursing process to ensure compliance with nursing practice acts and with reimbursement and accreditation criteria.

perioperative unit, medical-surgical unit), and the specific client population (e.g., obstetric, pediatric, geriatric) determine different documentation requirements. Even so, the documentation of the client care provided must reflect the nursing process. General documentation guidelines are listed in Table 9-12.

FOLLOW THE NURSING PROCESS

Nursing notes must be logical, focused, and relevant to care, and the outcomes must represent each phase in the nursing process.

TABLE 9-12 General Documentation Guidelines

- Ensure that you have the correct client record or chart and that the client's name and identifying information are on every page of the record.
- Document as soon as the client encounter is concluded to ensure accurate recall of data (follow agency guidelines on frequency of charting).
- Date and time each entry.
- Sign each entry with your full legal name and with your professional credentials, per your institutional policy.
- Do not leave space between entries.
- If an error is made while documenting, use a single line to cross out the error, then date, time, and sign the correction (follow institutional policy); avoid erasing, crossing out, or using correction fluid.
- Never change another person's entry, even if it is incorrect.
- The first entry of the shift should be made early (e.g., at 7:30 A.M. for the 7–3 shift, as opposed to 11:30 A.M. or 12 P.M.). Chart at least every 2 hours, or per institutional policy.
- Use quotation marks to indicate direct client responses (e.g., "I feel lousy").
- Document in chronological order; if chronological order is not used, state why.
- Write legibly.
- Use a permanent-ink pen (black is usually preferable because it photocopies well).
- Document in a complete but concise manner by using phrases and abbreviations as appropriate.
- Document all telephone calls that you make or receive that are related to a client's case.

Adapted from *Health Assessment & Physical Examination* (4th ed.), by M. Estes, Clifton Park, NY: Delmar Cengage Learning.

Nursing documentation based on the nursing process facilitates effective care because client needs can be traced from assessment, through identification of the problems to the care plan, implementation, and evaluation. A brief outline of the elements of the nursing process as they relate to documentation follows:

- *Assessment:* Assessment data related to an actual or potential health care need are summarized without duplication. With reassessment, any new findings or any changes in the client's condition (e.g., increased pain) are highlighted.
- *Nursing diagnosis:* NANDA-International terminology is used to identify the client's problem or need.
- *Planning and outcome identification:* The expected outcomes and goals of client care, as discussed with the client and communicated to members of the multidisciplinary team, should be documented on the care plan or critical pathway rather than in the progress notes.
- *Implementation:* After an intervention has been performed, observations, treatments, teaching, and related clinical judgments should be documented on the flow sheet and progress notes. Client teaching should include learning needs, teaching plan content, methods of teaching, who was taught, and the client's response.
- *Evaluation:* The effectiveness of the interventions in terms of the expected outcomes is evaluated and documented: progress toward goals; client response to tests, treatments, and nursing interventions; client and family response to teaching and significant events; and questions, statements, or complaints voiced by the client or family.
- *Revisions of planned care:* The reasons for the revisions along with the supporting evidence and client agreement are documented.

EFFECTIVE DOCUMENTATION ELEMENTS

If documenting on paper forms, the elements for effective documentation are:

- Document accurately, completely, and objectively including any errors that occurred
- Note date and time
- Use appropriate forms
- Identify the client
- Write in ink (Usually all charting is written with black ink, but each agency determines protocol.)
- Use standard abbreviations
- Spell correctly
- Write legibly
- Correct errors properly
- Write on every line
- Chart omissions
- Sign each entry

If documenting electronically, the guidelines are the same in documenting accurately, completely, and objectively. However, many of the issues of paper charting are completed automatically on an electronic health record, such as not needing to use ink to chart, writing legibly, and signing each entry. A nurse cannot obtain a client's electronic health record without logging on to the computer, which automatically signifies the writer, date, time, and entry.

NURSE'S PROGRESS RECORD

DATE	HOUR	PROGRESS NOTES
2/3/10	0815	Client verbalizes severe abdominal pain (8 on a 0-10 pain
		scale). Lying on Right side. States "I don't want to take a
		bath, and I don't want any breakfast". Abdomen distended.
		No bowel sounds asculated. Acute Pain R/T no flatus
		passed since surgery. ——— L. White, RN
2/3/10	0820	Administered Prostigmin Injection 0.5 mg (1 mL of 1:2000
		solution) given IM in Right gluteus maximus. Assisted to Left
		side (Sim's position). ——— L. White, RN
2/3/10	0900	Client states "I passed some gas, the pain is much less now,
		about a 4 (on 0-10 pain scale). ——— L. White, RN

FIGURE 9-7 Accurate, Complete, Objective Documentation

Accurate, Complete, and Objective

Record just the facts—exactly what you see, hear, and do. For example, "Two 4 × 4s completely soaked with yellow-green drainage in 20 minutes" is more accurate than "large amount of drainage." Never record opinions or assumptions. Chart relevant information relating to client care and reflecting the nursing process (Figure 9-7). *Remember, if it is not charted, it was not done.* It is difficult to prove in court that an aspect of client care was provided if it was not documented.

Document information promptly; the information is more likely to be accurate and complete. Important details may be forgotten if charting is left until the end of the shift, and those details may later become a legal issue. Chart medications immediately *after* administration. This prevents errors such as another nurse administering pain medication when the first dose was not charted.

Avoid subjective statements such as "client is uncooperative." Record the client's exact words using quotation marks, for example, *Client stated, "I don't want to take a bath, and I don't want any breakfast."*

Date and Time

Be sure each entry is dated and has a specific time. Especially note the exact time of sudden changes in a client's condition, nursing actions, and other significant events. Do not chart in blocks of time, such as 7 A.M. to 11 A.M. This is vague and sounds like the client has had no attention during that time frame.

When military time is used, there is no confusion between A.M. and P.M. entries. For this reason, many facilities use military time (Figure 9-8).

If documentation cannot be done in a timely manner, explain the delay. For example, "chart in x-ray with client." When an entry must be added after notes are completed, follow the facility's policy for recording a late entry. Generally, the practice is to enter the date and time and note "Late Entry."

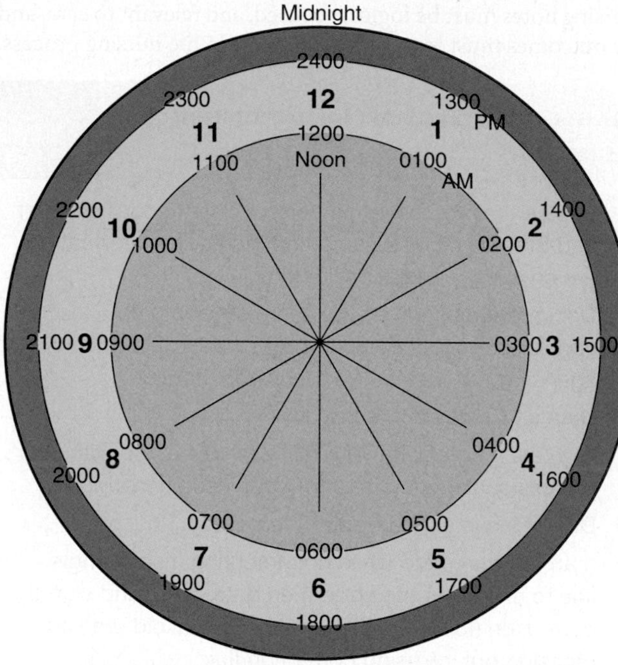

FIGURE 9-8 Military time uses a 24-hour clock.

This indicates that the entry is out of sequence. Then the date and time the entry should have been made is followed by the information to be recorded (Figure 9-9). A nurse charts a late entry on the electronic health record by changing the time notation as needed on all entries during her shift.

Use Appropriate Forms

Use the appropriate forms as required by the facility's policy manual. The forms used are not the same in every facility. Some facilities use flow sheets instead of progress notes.

NURSE'S PROGRESS RECORD

DATE	HOUR	PROGRESS NOTES
2/3/10	1100	Late Entry (2/3/10—0900) Client crying after talking to
		mother on the telephone. ——— L. White, RN

FIGURE 9-9 Recording a Late Entry

PROFESSIONALTIP

Abbreviations

Avoid abbreviations that can be misunderstood (Figure 9-10). For example, what does the abbreviation *Pt* mean? Does it refer to the patient, prothrombin time, physical therapy, or part time? Refer to your institution's approved abbreviations listing.

Identify the Client

Each page of the client's record should have the client's name on it. This aids in preventing confusion and helps ensure that information is charted on the correct record. Many facilities use the addressograph to stamp the client's name on each page. When charting electronically, make sure the correct client document is on the screen before making an entry.

Write in Ink

The client's record is a permanent document, and information should be charted in ink or printed out from a computer. Only black ink should be used because it will photocopy well. Felt-tipped pens are not to be used, especially on forms with carbons, because they do not hold up under pressure to make a clear copy. Also, they often bleed through the paper.

Use Standard Abbreviations

Each health care facility has a list of approved abbreviations and symbols for documenting information on its client records. This is to meet the Joint Commission standards and the regulations in many states. Such a list prevents confusion. The use of some abbreviations causes ambiguity that could be misleading and endanger a client's health (Figure 9-10). Appendix C lists commonly used abbreviations and terms that the Joint Commission officially lists as "Do not to use" terms.

Spell Correctly

Misspelled words on client records may be confusing and certainly convey a sense of unprofessionalism. They may generate questions about the quality of the care provided, increase the chance of liability, and produce a loss of the writer's credibility. When you are unsure of how to spell a word, *look it up*. Most units in a health care facility have a dictionary and other books to use as references. If these resources are not available and if spelling correctly is difficult, carry a small pocket dictionary and use it as needed.

Write Legibly

Legible handwriting is imperative for effective documentation. Sloppy writing hinders communication, and errors in client care can occur. Trying to decipher illegible writing wastes time. Illegible handwriting also creates a poor impression of the person who did the writing and damages that person's credibility. Print rather than use cursive writing; it is usually easier to read.

Correct Errors Properly

Promptly correct any error you make in documenting on a client's record. Know and follow your facility's policy for correcting errors. Generally, it is acceptable to draw a single line through the mistaken entry so that what was written can still be read. Above it carefully write "Mistaken Entry" followed by your initials and the date (Brooke, 2002; Dumpel, James, & Phillips, 1999; Pethtel, 2000). The original entry must still be readable. *NEVER scratch out, erase, or use correction fluid (white-out)* on a mistaken entry. Using these methods makes it look as if something is trying to be hidden. Be sure the mistaken entry is still readable (Figure 9-11).

Write on Every Line

Fill each line completely. Leave no blank lines or partially blank lines. Draw a line through the empty part of the line (see Figure 9-12). This prevents others from inserting information later that may change the meaning of the original documentation. On forms, when information requested does not apply to a particular client, write "NA" (not applicable) or draw a line through the space. This indicates that every item on the form has been addressed.

NURSE'S PROGRESS RECORD

DATE	TIME	ORDER
11/18/10	1400	Give MS 2 mg I.V. every 4 hours Dr. D. Ledbetter

Does the MS stand for morphine sulphate, or magnesium sulfate?

COURTESY OF DELMAR CENGAGE LEARNING

FIGURE 9-10 Misleading Abbreviation

NURSE'S PROGRESS RECORD

DATE	HOUR	PROGRESS NOTES
2/3/10	0600	Client verbalizes severe abdominal pain (8 on a 0–10 pain
		scale) when lying on ~~Left side~~ (Mistaken Entry LW 2/3/0) Right side.—L. White, RN

COURTESY OF DELMAR CENGAGE LEARNING

FIGURE 9-11 Mistaken Entry

NURSE'S PROGRESS RECORD

DATE	HOUR	PROGRESS NOTES
2/3/10	0900	Abdominal dressing not changed. Client in x-ray for a flat
		plate of the abdomen.——— L. White, RN

FIGURE 9-12 Charting an Omitted Part of the Care Plan

NURSE'S PROGRESS RECORD

DATE	HOUR	PROGRESS NOTES
2/3/10	1300	to assess client's knowledge of diabetes (Continued on next
		page)——— L. White, RN

NURSE'S PROGRESS RECORD

DATE	HOUR	PROGRESS NOTES
2/3/10	1300	(Continued from previous page) on the 3rd or 4th day
		post op——— L. White, RN

FIGURE 9-13 Entry Continues on Another Page

Chart Omissions

Charting is supposed to show implementation of the medical and nursing plans of care. Whenever a part of the plan is omitted, document the reason for the omission. For example, a treatment is not provided or medication is not administered because the client was in x-ray (Figure 9-12).

Sign Each Entry

Each entry on the nurse's notes (progress notes) is to be signed with your first name or initial, full last name, and professional licensure (i.e., LVN, LPN, RN). The signature should be at the end of the entry on the far right side. When there is not enough room on the last line of the documentation, draw a line from the last word to the end of the line and on the next line, leaving enough room to sign the entry at the far right.

For a long entry that will conclude on another page, record "(Continued on Next Page)" and sign your name. Begin the next page with "(Continued from Previous Page)", finish the entry, and sign your name (Figure 9-13).

Documenting a Medication Error

An incident report is required for all medication errors (discussed later). The medication given in error should be recorded on the Medication Administration Record (MAR) and in the nurse's progress notes. Remember, the purpose of the medical record is to report any care or treatment the client receives; this includes any errors made. Document in the nurse's notes the name and dosage of the medication, time it was given, client's response to the medication, time and name of the practitioner notified of the error, nursing interventions or medical treatment to counteract the error, and client's response to treatment. Do not mention that an incident report was completed.

Some health care facilities are now using a specific medication incident (variance) report for situations related to medications (Figure 9-14). This provides the facility with specific information to possibly change policies or procedures that will work to prevent medication incidents.

SYSTEMS OF DOCUMENTATION

Systems of recording and reporting data pertinent to client care have evolved primarily in response to demands that health care practitioners be held to societal norms, professional standards of practice, legal and regulatory standards, and institutional policies and standards. The documentation systems used today reflect specific needs and preferences of the many health care agencies.

Among the many systems used for documentation are the following:

- Narrative charting
- Source-oriented charting
- Problem-oriented charting
- PIE charting
- Focus charting
- Charting by exception
- Computerized documentation
- Critical pathways

Addressograph CHRISTUS Health *Addressograph*

QUALITY COMMITTEE
Medication Safety And Quality Report
Adverse Drug Event(Errors/Reactions)
Medical Record #:
Γ Male Γ Female
Name:

Address:

Medication Error: any preventable event that may cause or lead to inappropriate medication use or patient harm, including prescribing, order communication, product labeling, packaging, compounding, dispensing, distribution, administration and use. (adapted from USP); any variance from the established process.

Instructions: Person discovering event completes Sections 1 through 13 according to facility policy and procedure. Forward to manager for additional review and investigation. Manager or analyst completes sections 14 through 19.

Event Number: ________ **(# assigned by Risk Management)** **1. Diagnosis:**

2. FACILITY NAME ________ **3. Date of Occurrence:** ___/___/___ Time ___:___ AM PM

Check if event occurred on: □Holiday □Weekends

4. Event Type: Variance Occurred to: □ Patient(01) □ Other(OT)

5. Type/Event Indicator:

□ Adverse Drug Reaction	(70.10)	□ Monitoring Error	(70.60)	□ Wrong Rate	(77.10)
□ Deteriorated Drug Errors (dispensing expired drug)	(70.20)	□Clinical (lab, vital signs)	(70.61)	□Too Fast	(71.11)
□ Dose Omission	(70.30)	□Documented Allergy	(70.62)	□Too Slow	(71.12)
□ Improper Dose	(70.40)	□Drug-Disease Interaction	(70.63)	□ Wrong Route of Administration	(71.20)
□Extra Dose	(70.41)	□Drug-Drug Interaction	(70.64)	□ Wrong Strength/Concentration	(71.30)
□Frequency	(70.42)	□Drug-Food/ Interaction	(70.65)	□ Wrong Technique	(71.40)
□Resulting in Overdosage	(70.43)	□ Narcotic Discrepancy	(71.60)	□ Wrong Time	(71.50)
□Resulting in Under Dosage	(70.44)	□ Wrong Dosage Form	(70.70)	□ Other	(79.99)
□ IV Infiltration/Extravasation	(70.50)	□ Wrong Drug	(70.80)		
		□ Wrong Duration	(70.90)		
		□ Wrong Patient	(70.00)		

6. Setting of initial event:(Dept. or unit) **7. Setting where event discovered: (Dept or unit)**

8. Medication as Ordered: (Name, Dose, Route, Frequency) **9. Medication as Dispensed or Administered:**

10. DESCRIPTION OF EVENT:

11. Patient Outcome: (Errors or reactions with ** to left of description require physician notification and notification of Risk Management according to facility policy and procedure)

- □ No Error, but circumstances, policies or procedures that could lead to error (31.0)
- □ Error occurred but medication did not reach patient.(i.e. dispensing error, caught in pharmacy or on delivery to unit) (32.1)
- □ Error or reaction that reaches patient (32.2)
  - □ Medication reaches the patient but not administered (32.4)
  - □ ** Medication reaches the patient and is administered, no additional treatment, monitoring or intervention (32.3)
- □ ** Increased patient monitoring only(more frequent vital signs, laboratory tests ordered) (32.5)
- □ ** Treatment or intervention required(meds ordered, procedures required) (33.1)
- □ **Initial or prolonged hospitalization (33.2)
- □ ** Permanent patient harm (33.3)
- □ **Near-death event (e.g., anaphylaxis, cardiac arrest) (33.4)
- □ **Death (34.0)

12. Reported By: ________ **Date:** ___/___/___ **Time:** ___:___ AM PM **Risk Mgmt notified?** □Yes □No

13. Physician Notified □Yes □No **By:** ________ **Date:** ___/___/___ **Time:** ___:___ AM PM

THIS IS A COMMITTEE DOCUMENT & IS PRIVILEGED AND CONFIDENTIAL.

Sections 14 through 19 to be completed by Manager

14. Persons Involved (include name and phone, if appropriate, for purpose of followup or participation in possible root cause analysis)

Ordered Med: ________ □ Intern (A1) □ Resident(A2) □ Other Physician(A3) □ Nurse Practitioner/Advanced Practice (C1)

Prepared/Administered Med: ________ □ Registered Nurse(C2) □ Licensed Practical Nurse(C3) □Pharmacy Technician (E) □ Pharmacist (B) □ Other(H) ________

Dispensed Med ________ □ Pharmacist (B) □ Other(H) ________

15. System Breakdown Points: Were any of the following items identified during error investigation? Check all that apply

□ Administration not documented	(C1)	□ Location(adjacent medications)	(C27)
□ Allergy information not in chart	(C2)	□ Look alike/Sound alike product name/packaging	(C28)
□ Allergy information not on MAR/Karcex	(C3)	□ Look alike/Sound alike patient name	(C29)
□ Armband/name not checked	(C4)	□ MAR/Kardex incorrect, misleading or unclear	(C30)
□ Abbreviations	(C5)	□ Medication not available at scheduled admin time	(C31)
□ Automated dispensing device	(C6)	□ Medication stored in wrong drawer/location	(C32)
□ Calculation error in pharmacy	(C7)	□ Multiple orders for same medication	(C33)
□ Calculation error on nursing unit	(C8)	□ Order entry error (user error)	(C18)
□ Change of shift	(C9)	□ Order not sent to/received by pharmacy	(C34)
□ Computer system down	(C10)	□ Order overlooked/missed by pharmacy	(C35)
□ Computer system functionality	(C50)	□ Order overlooked/missed by nursing	(C36)
□ Decimal error(NOT Leading/Trailing Zeros)	(C11)	□ Order misinterpreted by pharmacy	(C37)
□ Delayed dose	(C12)	□ Order misinterpreted by nursing	(C49)
□ Documentation	(C17)	□ Order stamped/labeled for wrong patient	(C19)
□ Error in stocking/restocking/cart fill/floor stock etc	(C13)	□ Order unclear or ambiguous	(C38)
□ Handwriting	(C14)	□ Patient off unit	(C39)
□ Illegible fax or NCR order copy	(C15)	□ Patient with stated allergy to medication given	(C40)
□ Incomplete order	(C16)	□ Policy/procedure not followed	(C41)
□ Insufficient staff	(C20)	□ Prepared in patient care area	(C42)
□ Inexperienced staff	(C21)	□ Pump programmed incorrectly	(C43)
□ Fatigue or extended shift	(C22)	□ Pump/Equipment failure	(C44)
□ Lack of training	(C23)	□ Transfer patient /orders	(C45)
□ Leading/Trailing zeros	(C24)	□ Transcription error	(C46)
□ Labeling of drug incorrect or misleading	(C25)	□ Verbal order	(C47)
□ Lack of knowledge	(C26)	□ Other (Explain in section 16)	(C48)

16. Notes regarding investigation, action, recommendations for system improvement:

17. Nature of Injury: (Check all that apply)

□ Abscess (04)	□ Blood Disorder (62)	□ Hearing Disorder (39)	□ Respiratory Disorder/ Asphyxia/Choking (43)	□ Tissue Damage (61)
□ Amputation (06)	□ Circulatory Impairment (11)	□ Heart Attack (41)	□ Rupture (59)	□ Visual Impairment (40)
□ Anoxia (44)	□ Dermatitis/Skin Disorder(29)	□ Hematoma (51)	□ Seizure (22)	□ Other (99)
□ Blister (50)	□ Deterioration in Condition(14)	□ Infection (31)	□ Shock (Non-Electrical) (37)	
	□ Fever (24)	□ Inflammation (27)	□ Stroke (45)	□ No Injury Noted (48)
	□ Headache (52)	□ Phlebitis (19)		

18. Does this injury involve one of these outcomes... (Check only one)

□ Amputation (01)	□ Burn (04)	□ Loss of Hearing (13)	□ Residual Paralysis (18)
□ Birth Injury (02)	□ Events Resulting in Disability (06)	□ Loss of Eyesight (12)	□ Septicemia After Admission (19)
□ Brain Damage (03)	□ Kidney Failure (11)	□ Loss of Sensation (14)	□ Unexpected Death (20)

19. Manager Review: ________ Date:

20. Director/Administrator Review: ________ Date:

THIS IS A COMMITTEE DOCUMENT & IS PRIVILEGED AND CONFIDENTIAL.

FIGURE 9-14 Medication Incident Report (*Courtesy of CHRISTUS Spohn Hospital Shoreline, Corpus Christi, TX.*)

NURSE'S PROGRESS RECORD

DATE	HOUR	PROGRESS NOTES
2/3/10	1630	Client 6 hours post op; awakens easily, oriented x 3.
		Abdominal dressing dry and intact. Denies pain but stated he
		felt nauseated and immediately vomited 50 mL of clear fluid.
		Attempted to ambulate to bathroom with assistance, but felt
		dizzy. Assisted to lie down in bed. Voided 250 mL clear, yellow
		urine in urinal. Client encouraged to turn in bed, cough, and
		deep breathe.——————L. White, RN
2/3/10	1650	Continues to feel nauseated. Zofran 4 mg IV given
		——————L. White, RN
2/3/10	1730	States he is no longer nauseated. Remains pain free.
		Properly demonstrated coughing and deep breathing.——
		——————L. White, RN

FIGURE 9-15 Narrative Charting

NARRATIVE CHARTING

Narrative charting, the traditional method of nursing documentation, is a chronologic account written in paragraphs that describe client status, interventions and treatments, and the client's response to treatments. This was the only method for documenting care before the advent of flow sheets.

Narrative documentation is the most flexible of all systems and is usable in any clinical setting. The relationship between nursing interventions and client's responses is clearly shown (Figure 9-15).

However, subjectivity is a common problem. Client problems may be difficult to track because the same information may not be consistently documented. The client's progress may be difficult to identify. Narrative charting often fails to reflect the nursing process.

SOURCE-ORIENTED CHARTING

Source-oriented charting is a narrative recording by each member (source) of the health care team on separate documents. Each discipline uses a separate record, often resulting in fragmented care and time-consuming communication between disciplines.

PROBLEM-ORIENTED CHARTING

Problem-oriented medical record (POMR) employs a structured, logical format and focuses on the client's problem. There are four critical components of POMR:

- Database (assessment data)
- Problem list (client's problems numbered according to when identified)
- Initial plan (outline of goals, expected outcomes, and learning needs and further data, if needed)
- Progress notes (charting based on the **SOAP**, SOAPIE, or SOAPIER format)

The format in which progress notes are written includes SOAP, SOAPIE, or SOAPIER:

- S: subjective data (what the client or family states)
- O: objective data (what is observed/inspected)
- A: assessment (conclusion reached on the basis of data formulated as client problem or nursing diagnosis)
- P: plan (expected outcomes and actions to be taken)

SOAPIE and SOAPIER refer to formats that add the following:

- I: implementation
- E: evaluation
- R: revision

An entry need not be made for each component of SOAP(IER) at every documentation (Figure 9-16); however, each problem must have a complete note every 24 hours if unresolved or whenever the client's condition changes.

Continuity of care is shown when the plan of care and interventions performed are documented together. Figure 9-16 shows an example of SOAPIE charting. Some physicians use this format when writing progress notes.

PIE CHARTING

After the SOAP format gained popularity, the **Problem, Intervention, Evaluation (PIE) charting** system was developed to streamline documentation. The main parts of this system are an integrated plan of care, assessment flow sheets, and nurse's progress notes. Figure 9-17 shows an example of PIE charting.

FOCUS CHARTING

Focus charting is a documentation system using a column format to chart Data, Action, and Response (DAR) (Smith, 2000c) (Figure 9-18). Usually the focus is a nursing diagnosis, but it may also be:

- A sign or symptoms (e.g., abnormal vaginal bleeding)
- An acute change in the client's condition (e.g., sudden increase in blood pressure)
- A patient behavior (e.g., crying after talking on the phone)
- A treatment of procedure (e.g., dressing change with wound drainage)
- A special need (e.g., a discharge referral) (Smith, 2000a)

Focus charting reflects the stages of the nursing process. Data are the subjective and objective information describing

NURSE'S PROGRESS RECORD

DATE	HOUR	PROGRESS NOTES
2/3/10	0730	#1 Pain
		S: Client states "The pain in my hip is so bad."
		O: Client states pain is 9 (0–10 scale); skin warm, moist,
		pale. Lying stiffly in bed with fists clenched.
		A: Acute Pain, needs medication for relief
		P: Check orders for analgesia; check vital signs; if within
		normal limits give analgesia as ordered; then recheck in 30
		minutes for response. ——— L. White, RN
2/3/10	0740	#1 Pain
		O: BP 142/86, P 110, R 28
		I: meperidine 75 mg IM in right gluteus maximus. ——— L. White, RN
2/3/10	0810	#1 Pain
		S: Client states "The pain is better."
		O: Client states pain now 4 (0–10 scale); skin warm, dry,
		normal color. Lying relaxed in bed.
		A: Pain relieved
		P: Continue to monitor for pain
		E: Analgesic effective ——— L. White, RN
2/3/10	0810	#2 Anxiety
		S: Client states "I'm still worried about the surgery onmy
		hip."
		O: Client clutching sheet
		A: Anxiety R/T surgery the next day
		P: Encourage verbalization of concerns and feelings. Involve
		family in discussion of concerns, if client agreeable. ———
		——— L. White, RN

FIGURE 9-16 SOAPIE Charting

NURSE'S PROGRESS RECORD

DATE	HOUR	PROGRESS NOTES
2/3/10	0830	P #1: Disturbed Body Image R/T bilateral mastectomy ———
		I #1: Encourage verbalization of feelings and concerns and
		remain alert for client's comments about body changes;
		encourage looking at surgical site when ready ———
		E #1: Glanced at chest during dressing change. Continue
		encouraging client's involvement in dressing changes. ———
		——— L. White, RN
2/3/10	0830	P #2: Ineffective Breathing Pattern R/T musculoskeletal
		impairment following mastectomy ———
		I #2: Encourage use of incentive spirometer every 2 hours
		increasing level each day; assess breath sounds, rate, and
		quality of respirations every 4 hours; monitor O_2 saturation
		with pulse oximeter ———
		E #2: Using incentive spirometer every 2 hours when
		awake. Breath sounds normal, respirations 20 shallow, O_2
		saturation 93%. ——— L. White, RN

FIGURE 9-17 PIE Charting

NURSE'S PROGRESS RECORD

DATE	HOUR	FOCUS	PROGRESS NOTES
2/3/10	1300	Deficient	D: Client states that she does not
		Knowledge R/T	understand why she has to take three
		medications	medications. "I don't like to take pills."
			A: Reason for each medication explained,
			dosages, and side effects.——
			R: Client verbalizes action and side effects
			of her medications.——L. White, RN
2/3/10	1600	Abnormal	D: Client states that her period just
		vaginal bleeding	started and she is passing clots.
			A: One maxi pad saturated in 30 minutes.
			BP 110/68, P 100, R 20. No clotsseen.
			Status reported to Dr. Medoffer and
			orders received. IV started with 20 G
			catheter, 1000 mL normal saline hung at
			100 mL/h. Continue monitoring bleeding
			and vital signs. Dr. Medoffer will see
			client in 1 hour.
			R: Client states reason for IV.——
			——L. White, RN

FIGURE 9-18 Focus Charting

the focus. The data information corresponds to assessment in the nursing process. Action is the nursing interventions and mirrors the planning and implementation stages of the nursing process. Response is the client's response to the interventions reflecting the evaluation stage of the nursing process (Smith, 2000a). The column format of this system is used within the progress notes but is easily distinguished from other entries.

Charting by Exception

Charting by exception (CBE) is a documentation system using standardized protocols stating what the expected course of the illness is, and only significant findings (exceptions) are documented in a narrative form. It assumes that client care needs are routine and predictable and that the client's responses and outcomes are also routine and predictable.

The rule of thumb related to charting "if it is not charted, it was not done" is replaced in CBE by the presumption that unless documented otherwise, all standardized protocols have been met and no further documentation is needed. Time spent by nurses documenting client care may be reduced. Murphy (2003) states that when CBE is designed and implemented properly within a facility and when charting follows state or local requirements, CBE is not illegal. However, Guido (2001), states, "Charting by exception may make it impossible to show the attentiveness of the nursing staff to patients" and "may not assist nurses in being able to defend themselves, because even they cannot recreate what was done and not done" (p. 183).

Computerized Documentation

Health care facilities have been using computers for many years to order diagnostic tests and medications and to receive results of diagnostic tests. Using a totally computerized client record is slowly being adopted. In terms of both time and finances, it is a huge commitment for a facility to plan for and make the change to computerized client records.

Issues to be addressed when considering computerized client records include data standards, vocabularies, security, legal issues, and costs.

- Data standards—include length of fields, how dates and times are shown, and ASCII or binary data
- Vocabularies—the most commonly used are the combination of the NANDA-International nursing diagnoses, Nursing Interventions Classification (NIC) nursing interventions, and **Nursing Outcomes Classification (NOC)** nursing outcomes
- Security—includes privacy, confidentiality, who has access to which data, how errors are to be corrected, and protection against data loss
- Legal issues—electronic signatures
- Costs—include planning, hardware, software, and training for all users

Nursing information systems (NIS) are various software programs that allow nursing documentation in an electronic record. These systems generally follow the components of the nursing process. The NIS works in conjunction with the

CRITICAL THINKING

Systems for Charting

Why are there so many systems for charting? Of what value is each?

hospital information system (HIS). Each NIS can be customized to fit a facility's documentation forms.

Decision-support systems are available to alert nurses, physicians, and pharmacists of client drug incompatibility, appropriate antibiotics based on culture and antibiotic susceptibility results, and adverse drug reactions. Another decision-support system uses assessment data to suggest possible nursing diagnoses, goals and outcome criteria, and interventions from which the nurse selects those appropriate for a specific client. A medical spell check is also available.

Bedside computer terminals allow the nurse to immediately document client assessments, medications given, and interventions performed; the nurse can also check care plans and revise if necessary, check test results, and many other functions. Timeliness, completeness, and the quality of nursing documentation are improved.

Voice-activated systems are available in some facilities. The nurse speaks into a special telephone handset, and the words appear on the computer screen. These are generally located at a central place rather than at the bedside.

Besides reducing documentation time and increasing accuracy, computerized charting increases legibility, stores and retrieves information quickly and easily, helps link diverse sources of client information, and uses standardized terminology, thus improving communication among health care departments. Planners for health care, researchers, lawyers, and third-party payers can quickly and easily retrieve information for their respective jobs.

Problems with computerized charting may occur if used incorrectly, and client information may be mixed up. When security measures are neglected, client confidentiality may be compromised. Users (e.g., nurses, physicians) should never share computer ID numbers or passwords with anyone. Many systems keep a record of what each user has done in the system.

To prevent these problems, users must also remember to log off to prevent unauthorized access by others. Users should also follow facility protocol for correcting errors and keep monitors and print versions of client information where others cannot see the information.

Information is temporarily unavailable when the computer system is "down" either for routine servicing or an unexpected failure. Processing time may be slow during peak usage times when too few terminals are available.

Point-of-Care Charting

Point-of-care charting is a computerized documentation system allowing health care providers to have immediate access to client information. The system permits input and retrieval of client data at the bedside with a handheld portable computer. This is especially useful for nurses working in home health care.

The advantages of point-of-care charting are related to the computer system efficiency, through which the following can be achieved:

- Operating costs are controlled.
- Existing information systems are complemented.
- Redundant data entry is eliminated.
- The practitioner has more one-on-one time for client care.
- Crucial client information is available to all health care providers in a timely fashion.

Point-of-care charting enhances continuity of care by providing each health care practitioner with client data. It also fosters compliance with accreditation and regulatory standards.

Critical Pathway

A **critical pathway** (care map) is a comprehensive preprinted interdisciplinary standard plan of care reflecting the ideal course of treatment for the average client with a given diagnosis or procedure, especially those with relatively predictable outcomes. They are generally not written for extremely complex client situations with less predictable outcomes.

The overall goal for critical pathways is to improve the quality and efficiency of client care. The sequence and timing of interdisciplinary activities is established, including assessments, consultations, diagnostic tests, nutrition, medications, activities, treatments, therapeutics, education, and discharge planning. Although nursing diagnoses as such are not generally included in a critical pathway, a nurse may identify nursing diagnoses and interventions for a specific client.

Health care facilities develop their own critical pathways. An interdisciplinary team, including nurses, physicians, dietary, rehabilitative services, social services, and others when needed, develops the critical pathway through consensus about the management of the identified case situation. This is a time-consuming task, but once written, a critical pathway can be revised based on a review of the variances.

Goals not met or interventions not performed within the established time frame are called **variances**. The nurse documents on a variance form why a goal is not met or an intervention is not performed. Documentation becomes complicated when clients have more than two diagnoses or variations. Additional documentation forms are needed to complement the pathway.

FORMS FOR DOCUMENTATION

Forms for recording data include Kardex, flow sheets, nurse's progress notes, and discharge summaries. They are designed to facilitate record keeping and allow quick, easy access to information.

Kardex

A **Kardex** is a brief worksheet with basic client care information that traditionally is not part of the medical record. The Kardex is used as a reference throughout the shift and during change-of-shift reports. It comes in various sizes, shapes, and types, including computer-generated. The Kardex usually contains the following information:

- Client name, age, marital status, religious preference, physician, family contact with phone number
- Medical diagnoses: listed by priority
- Nursing diagnoses: listed by priority
- Allergies
- Medical orders: diet, medications, intravenous (IV) therapy, treatments, diagnostic tests and procedures (including dates and results), consultations, DNR (do-not-resuscitate) order (when appropriate)

COMMUNITY/HOME HEALTH CARE

Home Health Kardex

The home health Kardex also contains information related to family contacts, practitioners (physician), other services, and emergency referrals.

- Activities permitted: functional limitations, assistance needed in activities of daily living, and safety precautions

Some facilities are eliminating the Kardex in favor of keeping all data at fingertips on the computer.

Flow Sheets

Flow sheets, with vertical or horizontal columns for recording date, time, and assessment data and intervention information, make it easy to track the client's changes in condition. Special equipment used in client teaching and IV therapy are other parts of the flow sheet. These forms usually contain legends identifying the approved abbreviations for charting data because they have small spaces for recording (Figure 9-19). Flow sheets must be completely filled out because blank spaces imply that something was not recognized, attempted, or completed.

Because they decrease the redundancy of charting in the nurse's progress notes, flow sheets are used as supplements in many documentation systems. They do not, however, replace the progress notes. Nurses still must document observations, client responses and teaching, detailed interventions, and other significant data in the progress notes.

Nurse's Progress Notes

Nurse's progress notes are used to document the client's condition, problems, and complaints; interventions; the client's response to interventions; and achievement of outcomes. Documents falling under the general heading of nurse's progress notes includes nurse's notes, personal care flow sheets, MAR, teaching records, vital sign records, intake and output forms, and specialty forms (e.g., diabetic flow sheet or neurologic assessment form). Progress notes can be either narrative or incorporated into a standardized flow sheet (Figure 9-19) to complement SOAP(IE), PIE, focus charting, and other documentation systems.

Discharge Summary

The client's illness and course of care are highlighted in the discharge summary. A narrative discharge summary in the progress notes includes:

- Client status on admission and discharge
- A brief summary of the client's care
- Intervention and education outcomes
- Resolved problems and continuing care needs for unresolved problems, including referrals
- Client instructions about medications, diet, food-drug interactions, activity, treatments, follow-up, and other special needs

Many facilities have a form itemizing discharge and client instructions. The form has a duplicate copy for the client, with the original being placed in the medical record. Figure 9-20 is an example of this form.

DOCUMENTATION TRENDS

Computerized charting is one of the most widespread trends in nursing documentation; however, computerized nursing documentation can demonstrate the quality, effectiveness, and value of the services nurses provide only if standardized databases are developed that ensure accuracy and precision of the information. The need to define and develop standard terminology for nursing data, nursing diagnoses, nursing interventions, and nursing outcomes is continually evolving.

Nursing Minimum Data Set

In 1985, Werley and Lang convened an invitational working conference to identify the elements that should be included in a **Nursing Minimum Data Set (NMDS)** (elements that should be in clinical records and abstracted for studies on the effectiveness and costs of nursing care) (Werley & Lang, 1988). The three categories into which the 16 identified elements were grouped are:

1. *Demographics:* personal identification, date of birth, gender, race and ethnicity, and residence
2. *Service:* unique facility or service agency number, episode admission or encounter date, discharge or termination date, disposition of client, expected payer, unique health record number of client, and unique number of principal registered nurse provider
3. *Nursing care:* nursing diagnosis, nursing intervention, nursing outcome, and intensity of nursing care (Werley & Lang, 1988)

The development of standard terminology for the four nursing care categories: diagnoses, interventions, outcomes, and intensity is challenging. For example, automated information systems must be able to support cost-effective nursing practice with efficient, comprehensive documentation. The consistent use of a taxonomy promoting validity and reliability is basic to standardizing databases. The NMDS, however, does not specify for any of the four elements a taxonomy such as NANDA-International nursing diagnoses, Nursing Interventions Classification (NIC), Nursing Outcomes Classification (NOC), or acuity ratings. Nursing must find consensus in terminology so clinical data can be included in the nursing care elements of an NMDS.

Nursing Diagnoses

NANDA-International is recognized as the pioneer in diagnostic classification in nursing. The NANDA-International definition of a nursing diagnosis is: "A nursing diagnosis is a clinical judgment about individual, family, or community responses to actual or potential health problems or life processes" (NANDA-International, 2010). Currently, there are approximately 188 approved nursing diagnoses classified into 47 classes and 13 domains.

Many diagnostic labels (nursing diagnoses) now have new descriptors. The word *altered* has been removed and a more specific term used. This allows for more specific documentation and for the nursing diagnoses to be linked to NIC and NOC. The nursing diagnoses are now listed in alphabetical order by the diagnostic concept, not by the first word of the nursing diagnosis (NANDA-International, 2010). For example: *Excess **Fluid** Volume* is found under "fluid." The entire listing can be found in Appendix A.

Each diagnosis has a label, definition, major and minor defining characteristics, and related factors. The diagnoses identify client states which can then be used to select interventions that are intended to achieve the desired outcomes.

In 1992, the NANDA-International terms were accepted into the Unified Medical Language System (UMLS). The UMLS was begun in 1986 by the National Library of Medicine as a way to help health professionals and researchers retrieve and integrate electronic biomedical information from a variety of sources (National Library of Medicine, 2006).

Date:

Nutrition:	Hygiene:	7-3			3-11			11-7		
Diet ☐ NPO ☐	Bath ☐ Sitz ☐	self ☐ assist ☐ total			self ☐ assist ☐ total			self ☐ assist ☐ total		
Hyperal ☐ Tube Fed ☐	Shower ☐	refused ☐			refused ☐			refused ☐		
Breakfast: All ☐ >½ ☐ <½ ☐ 0 ☐	Oral Care	self ☐	assist ☐	Total	self ☐	assist ☐	Total	self ☐	assist ☐	Total
	Shave	self ☐	assist ☐	Total	self ☐	assist ☐	Total	self ☐	assist ☐	Total
	Peri Care	self ☐	assist ☐	Total	self ☐	assist ☐	Total	self ☐	assist ☐	Total
Lunch: All ☐ >½ ☐ <½ ☐ 0 ☐	Other:									
	Comments:									
Dinner: All ☐ >½ ☐ <½ ☐ 0 ☐										
Snacks: All ☐ >½ ☐ <½ ☐ 0 ☐										

Tube Feeding Residuals		Intake						Output			
Time	Amount	7-3	PO	IV	NG & Flush	Enteral	Other	Urine	Ng/Emesis	Stool	Drains
		7-3 Total									
Weight		3-11									
Today:											
Previous:											
Vital/Signs											

Time	T	P	R	B/P	P/S										
						3-11 Total									
						11-7									
						11-7 Total									
						24 / Total									

4010

CHRISTUS SPOHN HEALTH SYSTEM

FLOW SHEET - 24 HOUR RECORD
PATIENT CARE SERVICES

2705066

REV. 06/00

	Date:	7-3 Time:	3-11 Time:	11-7 Time:
Neuro	Normal: alert, oriented to time, place, person, follows command, speech clear	WNL: ☐ *	WNL: ☐ *	WNL: ☐ *
Respiratory	Normal: Regular, unlabored symmetrical respirations, no abnormal lung sounds	WNL: ☐ *	WNL: ☐ *	WNL: ☐ *
Cardiovascular	Normal: Heart rhythm regular, peripheral pulses easily palpable and strong bilaterally, no edema, capillary refill brisk	WNL: ☐ *	WNL: ☐ *	WNL: ☐ *
Musculo-Skeletal	Normal: Full ROM of All joints, no weakness, steady balance and gait, handgrips equal	WNL: ☐ *	WNL: ☐ *	WNL: ☐ *
Nutrition	Normal: Consumes greater than 1/2 of solid food meals	WNL: ☐ *	WNL: ☐ *	WNL: ☐ *
G.I.	Normal: Abdomen soft, bowel sounds present all 4 quadrants, no nausea/ vomiting, diarrhea/constipation Last BM:	WNL: ☐ *	WNL: ☐ *	WNL: ☐ *
G.U.	Normal: Voiding without difficulty, clear urine, no bladder distention	WNL: ☐ *	WNL: ☐ *	WNL: ☐ *
Skin	Normal: Skin warm, dry, intact, tugor elastic, oral cavity moist and intact Date of Last EZ Graph ______ Site: ______	WNL: ☐ *	WNL: ☐ *	WNL: ☐ *
Psychosocial	Normal: Thought processes logical, memory intact, behavior appropriate for situation	WNL: ☐ *	WNL: ☐ *	WNL: ☐ *
Incision	Normal: Incision clean, no redness, drainage Site: ______	WNL: ☐ *	WNL: ☐ *	WNL: ☐ *
Wound	Normal: Dry, no drainage no odor Site: ______	WNL: ☐ *	WNL: ☐ *	WNL: ☐ *

Safety Assessment

STATUS MENTAL/PHYSICAL

D E N
☐☐☐ (5) Confused/judgement impaired
☐☐☐ (5) Sensory impairment
☐☐☐ (5) Combative/aggressive
☐☐☐ (5) "Sundowners" syndrome
☐☐☐ (5) Noncompliance/uncooperative
☐☐☐ (5) Paralysis/amputee
☐☐☐ (5) Urgent/frequent elimination needs
☐☐☐ (10) Restraints in use
☐☐☐ (5) Weakness/debilitation/mobility impaired

MEDICATIONS

D E N
☐☐☐ (5) Diuretics
☐☐☐ (5) Laxatives/G.I. preps
☐☐☐ (3) Antihypertensives
☐☐☐ (3) Antiseizures
☐☐☐ (5) Sedative/hypnotics
☐☐☐ (3) Analgesics
☐☐☐ (3) Antipsychotics/ antidepressants

HISTORY

D E N
☐☐☐ (5) Age greater than 60
☐☐☐ (5) History of previous falls
☐☐☐ (3) From nursing home
☐☐☐ (3) Has had sitter/ companion at home

SAFETY LEVEL

D E N
☐☐☐ Level 1 (0-17)
☐☐☐ Level 2 (18-24)
☐☐☐ Level 3 (25 or greater)

TOTAL D ______ E ______ N ______

FIGURE 9-19 Assessment and Intervention Flow Sheet (*Courtesy of CHRISTUS Spohn Health System, Corpus Christi, TX.*)

(*Continues*)

EDUCATION REASSESSMENT

Have the Education needs of the patient changed in past 24 hours?	☐ Yes	☐ No
Is the patient scheduled for any new test or procedure today?	☐ Yes	☐ No
Explanation given?	☐ Yes	☐ No
Patient/significant other verbalizes understanding:	☐ Yes	☐ No

Patient desires/requires education on: ______________________________

____

Have Discharge Planning needs changed in past 24 hours? If yes, send consult to Social Services and document changes below.	☐ Yes	☐ No

ALL EDUCATION MUST BE DOCUMENTED ON THE MULTIDISCIPLINARY EDUCATION FORM

TIME	PROBLEM #	PROGRESS NOTES

TIME	PROBLEM #	PROGRESS NOTES

PLAN OF CARE VERIFICATION	______________ RN	______________ Time

IV SITE ASSESSMENT		7-3 Time:	3-11 Time:	11-7 Time:
Normal: IV Patent; No redness, drainage or edema	Site #1: Start Date:	WNL: ☐ *	WNL: ☐ *	WNL: ☐ *
# of IVAC's in use ___	Site #2: Start Date:	WNL: ☐ *	WNL: ☐ *	WNL: ☐ *

IV Site Care per hospital standard ☐ Time: *

IV Tubing Change per hospital standard ☐ Time: *

IV Start:	Time	Attempts	Site	Needle Size	S	U
					☐	☐
					☐	☐
Site prep per Standard ☐					☐	☐

INITIALS	SIGNATURE	INITIALS	SIGNATURE

FIGURE 9-19 *(Continued)*

Tulane
UNIVERSITY
Medical Center

COORDINATION OF DISCHARGE CARE

DISCHARGE ASSESSMENT

DESCRIPTION				COMMENT	DESCRIPTION				COMMENT	DESCRIPTION				COMMENT
LOC	NL	AB			respiration quality	NL	AB			Foley removed/voided	N	Y	NA	
pupils	NL	AB			lung auscultation	NL	AB			bladder habit problems	N	Y		
range of motion	NL	AB			heart sounds	NL	AB			sleep problems	N	Y	UTO	
extremity strength	NL	AB			telemetry removed	N	Y	NA		IV removed and intact	N	Y	NA	
appetite	NL	AB	UTO		peripheral pulses	NL	AB			break in skin integrity	N			
swallowing difficulty	N	Y	UTO		bowel sounds	NL	AB			discomfort/pain	N	Y	UTO	
feeds self	N	Y			bowel habit problems	N	Y		Date Last BM					

Signature RN Date Time

DISCHARGE MEDICATIONS

☐ None Medication	Dosage	Route	Schedule	Special Instructions (▼ medication instruction sheets given; food/drug interaction sheet given ▼)	RX given
				☐ ☐	
				☐ ☐	
				☐ ☐	
				☐ ☐	
				☐ ☐	
				☐ ☐	
				☐ ☐	
				☐ ☐	

HOME ROUTINE

Activity: ☐ As tolerated ☐ Restrictions ______

Diet: ☐ Regular ☐ Modified

Special Instructions: (document discharge sheet given to patient)

Social Services:

(SIGNATURE)

Physical Therapy ☐ Exercise Program ☐ Equipment

☐ Gait Instruction

(SIGNATURE)

Occupational Therapy:

(SIGNATURE)

Nutrition Care:

(SIGNATURE)

Other Services:

(SIGNATURE)

FOLLOW-UP CARE

Your MD is: To Contact Call: In An Emergency Call:

☐ No Appointment ☐ Appointment(s) made:

Name clinic/floor date/time phone #

Name clinic/floor date/time phone #

Appointment(s) not made:

Call phone # ext. for an appointment in days/weeks with MD

Call phone # ext. for an appointment in days/weeks with MD

I understand the above instructions.

Patient or Guardian's Signature Date Time of Discharge Nurse's Signature & Title

FIGURE 9-20 **Discharge Summary** *(Reprinted with permission of Tulane University Hospital & Clinic, New Orleans, LA.)*

Nursing Interventions Classification

The **Nursing Interventions Classification (NIC)** is a comprehensive standardized language for nursing interventions organized in a three-level taxonomy. This taxonomy sorts, labels, and describes interventions used by nurses for various diagnostic categories. Initiated by a research team (Iowa Intervention Project, 1993) at the University of Iowa in 1987, the three-level taxonomy now comprises 7 domains, 30 classes, and 542 interventions. The seven domains are:

1. Physiological: basic
2. Physiological: complex
3. Behavioral
4. Safety
5. Family
6. Health system
7. Community

A nursing intervention is any direct care treatment that a nurse performs using clinical judgment and knowledge to improve a client's outcomes (University of Iowa College of Nursing, 2008a). These treatments include nurse-initiated treatments resulting from nursing diagnoses, physician-initiated treatments resulting from medical diagnoses, and performance of the daily essential functions for the client who cannot do these. NIC interventions address physiological and psychological needs and include illness treatment, illness prevention, and health promotion.

Each nursing intervention has a label, a definition, a set of activities to carry out the interventions and a list of references. *Activities are not interventions and should not be identified as such in nursing information systems* (Bulecheck, Butcher, & Dochterman, 2008).

Although continuing to evolve, this classification system already provides assistance in choosing interventions based on nursing diagnoses or problems. The NIC interventions have been incorporated into health care data sets and the computerized client medical record. The NIC is included in the *National Library of Medicine's Metathesaurus,* one of four knowledge sources for the UMLS.

Nursing Outcomes Classification

An outcome is a measurable individual, family, or community state, behavior, or perception that is measured along a continuum and is responsive to nursing interventions (University of Iowa College of Nursing, 2008b).

The Iowa Outcomes Project being conducted at the University of Iowa has developed a taxonomy of client outcomes for nursing care, called **Nursing Outcomes Classification (NOC)**. This classification system now comprises 330 outcomes grouped into 31 classes and 7 domains (Moorhead, Johnson, & Maas, 2008). The seven domains are:

1. Functional health
2. Physiologic health
3. Psychosocial health
4. Health knowledge and behavior
5. Perceived health
6. Family health
7. Community health

Each NOC outcome has the outcome label, the outcome definition, a list of indicators for measurement, an outcome rating, identification of data source, a 5-point measurement scale, and a list of references (University of Iowa College of Nursing, 2008b). The NOC includes 311 individual, 10 family, and 9 community outcomes. The NOC is included in the *National Library of Medicine's Metathesaurus for a Unified Medical Language* (NIH: United States National Library of Medicine, 2009AA).

REPORTING

Reporting summarizes the current critical information pertinent to clinical decision making and continuity of care. Reporting, like recording, is based on the nursing process, standards of care, and legal and ethical principles. To verbally report in a well-organized efficient manner, the nurse should consider the following questions:

- What to say
- Why to say it
- How to say it

Another critical element of reporting is listening. Reports require everyone present to participate. When receiving a report, enhance listening skills by eliminating distractions, putting thoughts and concerns aside, concentrating on those things being said, and not anticipating the presenter's next statements. The reporting process is integral to promoting continuity of client care. Some facilities tape record the end-of-shift report. Summary reports, walking rounds, telephone reports and orders, and incident reports are all types of reporting.

Summary Reports

Information pertinent to the client's needs and identified by the nursing process is outlined in summary reports. Summary reports commonly occur either at the change of shift when new caregivers arrive or when the client is transferred to

PROFESSIONAL TIP

Information for Shift Report

1. Client name, room and bed, age, and gender
2. Physician, admission date and diagnosis, and any surgery
3. Diagnostic tests or treatments performed in the past 24 hours; results, if available
4. General status, any significant change in condition
5. New or changed physician's orders
6. Nursing diagnoses and suggested nursing orders
7. Evaluation of nursing interventions
8. Intravenous fluid amounts
9. Administration time of last PRN medication
10. Concerns about the client

another area. A summary report should include the following information in the order indicated:

1. Background data obtained from client interactions and assessment of the client's functional health patterns
2. Prioritized medical and nursing diagnoses
3. Identified client risks
4. Recent changes in condition or in treatments (e.g., new medications, elevated temperature)
5. Effective interventions or treatments of priority problems, inclusive of laboratory and diagnostic results (e.g., client's response to pain medication)
6. Progress toward expected outcomes
7. Adjustments in the plan of care
8. Client or family complaints

This logical and time-sequenced format follows the nursing process and thus provides structure and organization to the data. In order to provide continuity of care, the new caregiver must receive an accurate, concise report about those things that happened during the previous shift. Because client and family complaints usually generate questions and discussion, they should be addressed last.

Walking Rounds

Walking rounds can take the form of nursing rounds, instructor–student rounds, physician–nurse rounds, or multidisciplinary rounds. **Walking rounds** is when the members of the care team walk to each client's room and discuss progress and care with each other and with the client, as shown in Figure 9-21.

Nursing rounds are used most frequently by charge nurses as their method of report. The oncoming nurse is introduced to the client and the offgoing nurse discusses with the client and the oncoming nurse any changes in the plan of care. This is more time consuming than a summary report, but gives the nurses and the client time to evaluate the effectiveness of care together.

Nursing rounds are also used for teaching when the instructor introduces the client to the student and they discuss the client's care together. The student's observation, communication, and decision-making skills can also be assessed by the instructor.

Nurse–physician rounds involve the physician and either staff nurse or the charge nurse. These rounds usually occur daily and allow the nurse, the physician, and the client to evaluate the effectiveness of care.

Multidisciplinary rounds involving all disciplines occur less frequently than other types of rounds, primarily because it is difficult to schedule everyone. Multidisciplinary rounds are done most commonly to discuss discharge planning or to supplement case conferences.

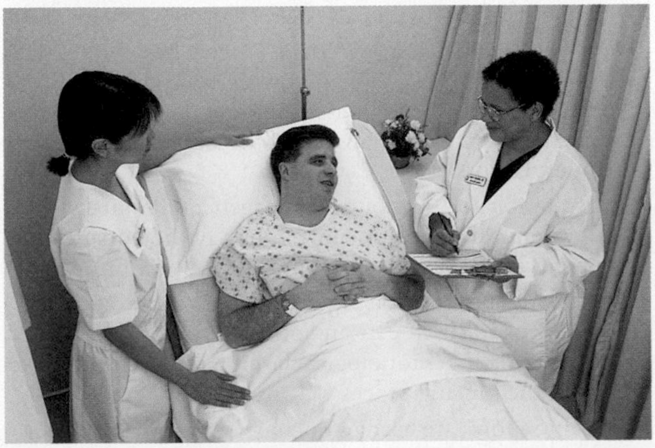

Figure 9-21 Nursing Rounds

Telephone Reports and Orders

Nurses are expected to exhibit courtesy and professionalism when using the telephone. When initiating a phone call, the nurse organizes the information to be reported or received. For example, the nurse:

- Ensures that all lab results are back; if they are not, identify those that are missing and telephone the lab or check the computer to ascertain whether the results are available. Spell the client's name and provide the client's medical record number when calling the lab to minimize the chances of receiving results for the wrong client. Write down the tests and the results.
- Has the client's assessment data available, especially any significant data related to abnormal results.
- Minimizes the chance of being interrupted during the call by informing the charge nurse or someone else at the nurses' station of the call.

State the reason for the call, for example, "I am calling Dr. Wojtal regarding the blood culture results for Mrs. Beacon." Be brief, listen carefully, and verify the test results and any orders received by repeating them back to the physician.

The date and time the phone call was placed, the client data reported by the nurse, the name of the person with whom the nurse spoke, and whether an order was obtained is recorded accurately in the client's record. Telephone orders are charted and the nurse's progress notes updated immediately after the call to prevent another caregiver from writing an entry before the telephone orders are written.

Figure 9-22 shows how to write a telephone order on the physician's order sheet: the entry is dated and timed; the order as given by the physician is recorded; the order is signed beginning with t.o. (telephone order); the physician's name is written; and the nurse's name is signed. If another nurse witnesses the phone order, that nurse's signature follows the first nurse's signature.

The physician must countersign the order within a time frame specified by the facility's policy. The use of fax machines and computers has decreased the need for lengthy or complicated telephone orders, saving time and minimizing errors. The physician is phoned to confirm the physician's identity as the initiator of the fax orders. The physician countersigns the fax orders according to agency policy.

PROFESSIONAL TIP

Documenting an Incident

The incident should be factually documented in the nurse's notes, but the notes should not say "incident report filed."

PHYSICIAN'S ORDER SHEET

DATE	HOUR	ORDERS
2/3/10	1420	Give Demerol 50 mg IM stat.
		T.O. Dr. Weng/L. White RN

COURTESY OF DELMAR CENGAGE LEARNING

FIGURE 9-22 Documenting a Telephone Order

INCIDENT REPORTS

Incident reports, also called occurrence reports or variance reports, document any unusual occurrence or accident in the facility. Incident reports are not a means of punishment, but ethical practice requires that an incident report be filed to protect the individual involved.

Incident reports are not only an internal device for the facility; they are required by federal, national, and state accrediting agencies. For legal reasons, nurses are often advised not to document the filing of an incident report in the nurse's notes.

An incident report serves two functions:

1. It informs the facility's administration of the incident and allows risk management personnel to consider ways to prevent similar occurrences in the future.
2. It alerts the facility's insurance company to a potential claim and the possible need for investigation.

Incident report forms vary from one facility to another, but the following information must be recorded on the report:

- The date, exact time, and place the nurse discovered the occurrence.
- The person(s) involved in the occurrence, including witnesses.
- The exact occurrences witnessed by the nurse (e.g., "Found the client sitting on the floor, client stated that . . . ," rather than "Client fell").
- The exact details and time sequence of what happened and the consequences for the persons involved.
- The nurse's actions to provide care and the results of the nurse's assessment for injuries and client complaints.
- The supervisor on duty who was notified and the time and name of the physician notified; if telephone orders were received from the physician, these should be documented as previously discussed and the orders implemented.
- Never record personal opinions, assumptions, judgments, or conclusions about what happened; point blame; or suggest ways to prevent similar occurrences. Forward the incident report to the designated person defined in the facility's policy.

Iyer and Camp (2005) suggest writing a brief, accurate description of the incident and keeping it at home. The description should include details of the incident and the names of the people who were involved. Because lawsuits may take several years until the case goes to court, personal notes will help accurate recall of the incident. The notes may be read by the plaintiff's attorney and should reflect the same elements as the incident report.

SUMMARY

- The nursing process composed of five steps: assessment, diagnosis, planning and outcome identification, implementation, and evaluation, is an organized way to plan and deliver nursing care.
- The nurse uses the assessment process to establish a database about the client, to form an interpersonal relationship with the client, and to provide the client with an opportunity to discuss health care concerns.
- The second step in the nursing process involves further analysis and synthesis of the data and results in a list of nursing diagnoses.
- Nursing diagnoses identify knowledge unique to nursing, improve communication among nurses and other health care professionals, and promote individualized client care.
- Planning and outcome identification, the third step in the nursing process, involves prioritizing nursing diagnoses, identifying and writing goals and client outcomes, developing nursing interventions, and recording the plan of care in the client's record.
- The implementation step of the nursing process is directed toward meeting client needs, resulting in health promotion, prevention of illness, illness management, or health restoration.
- Evaluation, the fifth step in the nursing process, measures the effectiveness of nursing interventions by the examination of the goals and expected outcomes, which provide direction for the plan of care and serve as standards against which the client's progress is measured.
- Critical-thinking, decision-making, and holistic skills are important in the nursing process.
- Documentation provides a system of written records that reflect client care provided on the basis of assessment data and the client's response to interventions.
- Nurses are responsible for assessing and documenting that the client has an understanding of the treatment prior to the intervention.
- Accreditation and reimbursement agencies require accurate and thorough documentation of the nursing care rendered and the client's response to interventions.
- Effective documentation requires clear, concise, accurate recording of all client care and other significant events in an organized and chronological fashion representing each phase of the nursing process.
- Incident reports are used to document any unusual occurrence in a health care facility.

REVIEW QUESTIONS

1. M. R. was admitted to the unit 2 hours ago. The following data are recorded on her chart. Which data are objective?
   1. Temperature 102°F.
   2. Nausea.
   3. Headache.
   4. Pain in abdomen.
2. The nursing care plan includes:
   1. collected documentation of all team members providing care for the client.
   2. physician orders, demographic data, and medication administration and rationales.
   3. client's nursing diagnoses, goals, expected outcomes, nursing interventions, and evaluation.
   4. client assessment data, medical treatment regimen and rationales, and diagnostic test results and significance.
3. Systematic documentation is critical because it:
   1. is done every hour.
   2. shows the care given by all health care providers.
   3. identifies the planning and implementation phases.
   4. presents in a logical fashion the care provided by nurses.
4. The person responsible for ensuring that the client understands the procedure or intervention and has signed the informed consent is the:
   1. nurse.
   2. physician.
   3. social worker.
   4. admission officer.
5. Documentation of the nursing care the client receives must:
   1. never have an error.
   2. be neatly spaced out.
   3. reflect the nursing process.
   4. be signed at the end of each shift.
6. A nurse is giving oxygen at 2 L/min per nasal cannula. What phase of the nursing process is the nurse's action an example?
   1. Assessment.
   2. Planning and Outcome Identification.
   3. Implementation.
   4. Evaluation.
7. A 78-year-old woman fell and broke three ribs with one of the ribs puncturing her lung. She arrives in the emergency room short of breath and anxious. She is on Plavix, so she has multiple bruises over her entire body with possible internal hemorrhaging. After the nurse assesses her, she finds she also is blind and hard of hearing and has difficulty empting her bladder. Of the listed symptoms, what is the priority problem that the nurse needs to address?
   1. Difficulty breathing.
   2. Internal hemorrhaging.
   3. Difficulty with urination.
   4. Blindness and difficulty hearing.
8. Of the following medical and nursing diagnoses, which ones are nursing diagnoses? (Select all that apply.)
   1. Chronic obstructive pulmonary disease.
   2. Congestive heart failure.
   3. Nausea.
   4. Acute pain.
   5. Ineffective breathing.
   6. Parkinson's disease.
9. During and after a nursing assessment, the nurse organizes data to identify areas of the client's problems and strengths. The charting form that assists the nurse to cluster data is:
   1. flow sheet.
   2. client care plan or nursing plan of care.
   3. assessment sheet following an assessment model.
   4. client education record.
10. What type of nursing diagnoses is the nursing diagnosis *Decreased* **C***ardiac Output* R/T altered heart rhythm AEB irregular pulse, cyanosis, weak pedal pulse, and weakness?
    1. Data cluster.
    2. Actual nursing diagnosis.
    3. Risk nursing diagnosis.
    4. Wellness nursing diagnosis.

REFERENCES/SUGGESTED READINGS

Alfaro-LeFevre, R. (2009). *Applying nursing process: A tool for critical thinking* (7th ed.). (5th ed.). Philadelphia: Lippincott Williams & Wilkins.

Alfaro-LeFevre, R. (2008). *Critical thinking and clinical judgment: A practical approach to outcome-focused thinking* (4th ed.). Philadelphia: W. B. Saunders.

American Nurses Association. (1991). *Standards of nursing practice.* Kansas City, MO: Author.

Bevis, E. (1989). *Curriculum building in nursing: A process* (3rd ed., Publication No. 15-2277). New York: National League for Nursing.

Beyea, L. (1996). *Critical pathways for collaborative nursing care.* Menlo Park, CA: Addison-Wesley Nursing.

Brooke, P. (2002). Legal questions: Documentation errors. *Nursing 2002, 32*(1), 67.

Bulecheck, G., Butcher, H., McCloskey, J., & Dochterman, J., eds. (2008). *Nursing Interventions Classification (NIC)* (5th ed.). St. Louis, MO: Mosby-Elsevier.

Calloway, S. (2001). Preventing communication breakdowns. *RN, 64*(1), 71–74.

Carpenito, L. (2009). *Nursing diagnosis: Application to clinical practice* (13th ed.). Philadelphia: Lippincott Williams & Wilkins.

Celia, L. (2002). Keep electronic records safe! *RN, 65*(6), 69–71.

Chaffee, M. (1999). A telehealth odyssey. *American Journal of Nursing, 99*(7), 26–32.

Charting Tips. (1999a). Documenting discharges and transfers in long-term care. *Nursing99, 29*(6), 17.

Charting Tips. (1999b). Easy as PIE. *Nursing99, 29*(4), 24.

Clark, M. (1998). Implementation of nursing standardized languages NANDA, NIC, and NOC. *Online Journal of Issues in Nursing 2*(2). Available: http://www.nursingworld.org

DeWitt, A. (2000). *Documentation: Legal principles of good charting, Penumbra Seminars LLC.* Available: http://www.respiratorycase-online.com/doc_handoutPDF

Dumpel, H., James, M., & Phillips, T. (1999). Charting by exception. *California Nurse,* June/July 1999, 9.Dykes, P., & Wheeler, K. (Eds.) (1997). *Planning, implementing, and evaluating critical pathways.* New York: Springer Publishing.

Edelman, C., & Mandle, C. (2002). *Health promotion throughout the lifespan* (5th ed.). St. Louis, MO: Mosby.

Estes, M. (2010). *Health assessment and physical examination* (4th ed.). Clifton Park, NY: Delmar Cengage Learning.

Ferrel, K. (2007). Documentation, part 2: The best evidence of care. *American Journal of Nursing, 107*(7), 61–64

Fry, V. (1953). The creative approach to nursing. *American Journal of Nursing, 53*(3), 301–302.

Gardner, P. (2002). *Nursing process in action.* Clifton Park, NY: Delmar Cengage Learning.

Gordon, M. (1998). Nursing nomenclature and classification system development. *Online Journal of Issues in Nursing.* Retrieved November 20, 2008, from http://www.nursingworld.org/MainMenuCategories/ANAMarketplace/ANAPeriodicals/OJIN/TableofContents/Vol31998/No2Sept1998/NomenclatureandClassification.aspx

Gordon, M. (2002). *Manual of nursing diagnoses* (10th ed.). St. Louis, MO: Mosby.

Grace, P., & McLaughlin, M. (2005). When consent isn't informed enough: What's the nurse's role when a patient has given consent but doesn't fully understand the risks? *American Journal of Nursing, 105*(4), 79–84.

Grane, N. (1995). Documenting a "harmless" medication error. *Nursing95, 25*(4), 80.

Gregory, K. (2000). Nurse the patient! *RN, 63*(9), 52–54.

Grulke, C. (1995). Seven ways to help a student nurse. *American Journal of Nursing, 96* (60), 24L.

Guido, G. (2001). *Legal and ethical issues in nursing* (3rd ed.). Upper Saddle River, NJ: Prentice Hall.

Heery, K. (2000). Straight talk about the patient interview. *Nursing2000, 30*(6), 66–67.

Humphrey, C. (1998). *Home care nursing handbook* (3rd ed.). Gaithersburg, MD: Aspen.

Iowa Interventions Project. (1993). The NIC taxonomy structure. *Image: Journal of Nursing Scholarship, 25*(3), 187–192.

Iyer, P., & Camp, N. (2005). *Nursing documentation: A nursing process approach* (4th ed.). Fleminiton, NJ: Medical League Support Services.

Johnson, D. (1959). A philosophy for nursing diagnosis. *Nursing Outlook, 7,* 198–200.

Johnson, M., & Maas, M. (1998). Implementing the nursing outcomes classification in a practice setting. *Outcomes Management for Nursing Practice, 2*(3), 99–104.

Johnson, M., Bulechek, G., Dochterman, J., Maas, M., & Moorhead, S. (2001). *Nursing diagnoses outcomes and interventions, NANDA, NOC and NIC linkages.* St. Louis, MO: Harcourt Health Sciences.

Joint Commission. (2008, November 10). Table of contents (standard PC.4.10). Retrieved November 17, 2008, from http://www.jointcommission.org/NR/rdonlyres/6530941D-98AD-4AC7-8944-9DSE1116E503/0/OBS_Standards_Sampler_2007_final.pdf

Joint Commission on Accreditation of Healthcare Organizations. (1998). *1998 Hospital accreditation standards.* Oakbrook Terrace, IL: Author.

Klenner, S. (2000). Mapping out a clinical pathway. *RN, 63*(6), 33–36.

LaDuke, S. (2000). Spotlight: What you really do with this powerful documentation tool. *Nursing2000, 30*(6), 68.

Malestic, S. (2003). A quick guide to verbal reports. *RN, 66*(2), 47–49.

McCloskey, J., & Bulechek, G. (1995). Validation and coding of the NIC taxonomy structure. *Image: Journal of Nursing Scholarship, 27*(1), 43–49.

McCloskey, J., & Maas, M. (1998). Interdisciplinary team: The nursing perspective is essential. *Nursing Outlook, 46*(4), 157–163.

McConnell, E. (1999). Charting with care. *Nursing99, 29*(10), 68.

Moorhead, S., Johnson, M., & Maas, M. (Eds.). (2008). *Nursing outcomes classification (NOC)* (4th ed.). St. Louis, MO: Mosby.

Murphy, E. (2003). Charting by exception—OR nursing law. *AORN Journal, 11.* Retrieved November 19, 2008, from http://findarticles.com/p/articles/mi_m0FSL/is_5_78/ai_111011830/print?tag=artBody;coll

National Institutes of Health (NIH): United States National Library of Medicine. (2009AA). Appendix to the License Agreement for Use of the UMLS® Metathesaurus. Retrieved July 29, 2009 from http://www.nlm.nih.gov/research/umls/metaa1.html

National Library of Medicine. (2006). Fact sheet: Unified medical language system®. Retrieved June 22, 2009, from http://www.nlm.nih.gov/pubs/factsheets/umls.html

North American Nursing Diagnosis Association International. (2010). *NANDA-I nursing diagnoses: Definitions and classification 2009–2011.* Ames, IA: Wiley-Blackwell.

Oermann, M., & Huber, D. (1999). Patient outcomes: A measure of nursing's value. *American Journal of Nursing, 99*(9), 40–47.

Olson-Chavarriaga, D. (2000). Informed consent: Do you know your role? *Nursing2000, 30*(5), 60–61.

Orem, D., Taylor, S., & Renpenning, K. (2001). *Nursing: Concepts of practice* (6th ed.). St. Louis, MO: Mosby.

Orlando, I. (1961). *The dynamic nurse–patient relationship.* New York: Putnam.

Pethtel, P. (2000). *Nursing documentation.* Available: http://garnet.indstate.edu/ppethtel/chartingforweb

Raymond, L. (2001). How to chart for peer review. *RN, 64*(6), 67–70.

Raymond, L. (2002). Documenting for the "PROs." *Nursing2002, 32*(3), 50–53.

Roberts, D. (2002). How to keep electronic health records private. *Nursing2002, 32*(10), 95.

Rochman, R. (2000). Are computerized patient records for you? *Nursing2000, 30*(10), 61–62.

Seaback, W. (2001). *Nursing process: Concepts and application.* Clifton Park, NY: Delmar Cengage Learning.

Sheehan, J. (2001). Delegating to UAPs—A practical guide. *RN, 64*(11), 65–66.

Smith, L. (2000a). Charting tips. Nursing2002. Retrieved November 18, 2008, from http://findarticles.com/p/articles/mi_qa3689/is_200005/ai_n8880050/print?tag+artBody;c

Smith, L. (2000b). How to use focus charting. *Nursing 2000, 30*(5), 76.

Smith, L. (2000c). Safe computer charting. *Nursing 2000, 30*(9), 85.

Smith, L. (2002). How to chart by exception. *Nursing 2002, 32*(9), 30.

Springhouse. (2005). *Charting made incredibly easy.* Springhouse, PA: Author.

Stewart, K. (2001). Charting tips: Documenting adverse incidents. *Nursing2001, 31*(3), 84.

Sullivan, G. (2000). Keep your charting on course. *RN, 63*(5), 75–79.

Thede, L. (2003). *Informatics and nursing: Opportunities and challenges* (2nd ed.). Philadelphia: Lippincott Williams & Wilkins.

Thompson, C. (1995, May). Writing better narrative notes. *Nursing95, 25*(5), 87.

Tucker, S., Canobbio, M., Paquette, E., & Willis, M. (2000). *Patient care standards: Collaborative planning and nursing interventions* (7th ed.). St. Louis, MO: Mosby.

United States National Library of Medicine. (2006). Fact sheet: Unified medical language system®. Retrieved June 22, 2009 from http://www.nlm.nih.gov/pubs/factsheets/umls.html

University of Iowa College of Nursing. (2008a). Nursing Interventions Classification (NIC): Overview of NIC. Retrieved November 19, 2008, from http://www.nursing.uiowa.edu/excellence/nursing_knowledge/clinical_effectiveness/nicoverview.htm

University of Iowa College of Nursing. (2008b). Nursing Outcomes Classification (NOC): Overview of NOC. Retrieved November 19, 2008, from http://www.nursing.uiowa.edu/excellence/nursing_knowledge/clinical_effectiveness/nocoverview.htm

Wallhagen, M., Pettengill, E., & Whiteside, M. (2006). Sensory impairment in older adults: Part 1: Hearing loss. *American Journal of Nursing, 106*(10), 40–48.

Werley, H., & Lang, N. (1988). The consensually derived nursing minimum data set: Elements and definitions. In H. H. Werley & N. M. Lang (Eds.), *Identification of the nursing minimum data set* (pp. 402–411). New York: Springer Publishing.

White, G. (2000). Informed consent. *American Journal of Nursing, 100*(9), 83.

Wiedenbach, E. (1963). The helping art of nursing. *American Journal of Nursing, 63*(11), 54–57.

Wilkinson, J. (2004). *Prentice Hall nursing diagnosis handbook: With NIC interventions and NOC outcomes* (8th ed.). Upper Saddle River, NJ: Prentice Hall.

Wilkinson, J. (2006). *Nursing process and critical thinking* (4th ed.). Upper Saddle River, NJ: Prentice Hall.

Yocum, R. (2002). Documenting for quality patient care. *Nursing2002, 32*(8), 58–63.

Yura, H., & Walsh, M. (1967). *The nursing process.* Washington, DC: Catholic University of America Press.

RESOURCES

American Health Information Management Association, http://www.ahima.org

American Nursing Informatics Association (ANIA), http://www.ania.org

Center for Nursing Classification, http://www.nursing.uiowa.edu

NANDA International, http://www.nanda.org

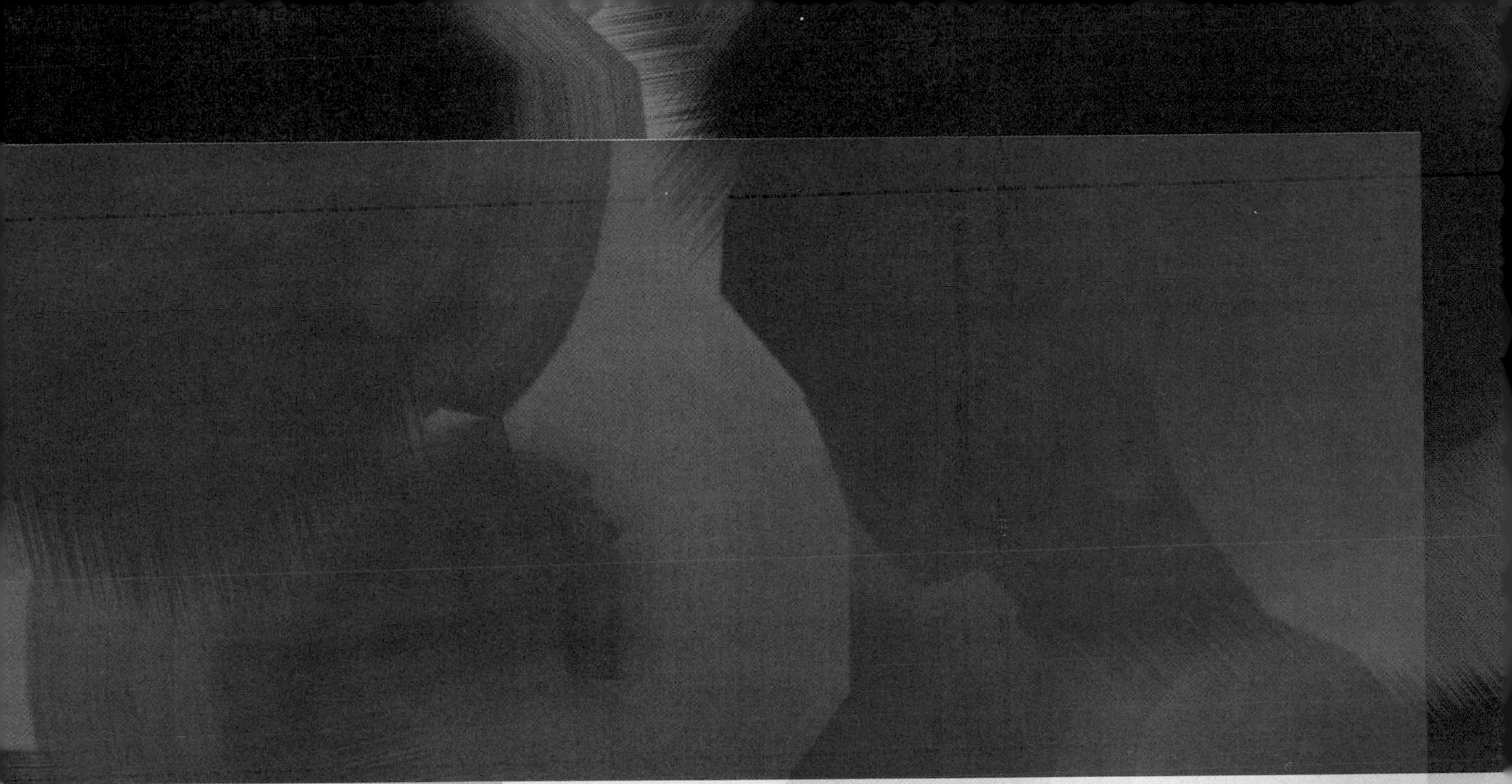

UNIT 4 Developmental and Psychosocial Concerns

CHAPTER 10
Life Span Development

MAKING THE CONNECTION

Refer to the following chapters to increase your understanding of the life span:

Basic Nursing

- ***Communication***
- ***End-of-Life Care***
- ***Self-Concept***
- ***Spirituality***
- ***Basic Nutrition***
- ***Safety/Hygiene***

LEARNING OBJECTIVES

Upon completion of this chapter, you should be able to:

- Define key terms.
- Discuss the basic concepts and principles of growth and development.
- Identify the factors influencing growth and development.
- Compare the major developmental theories.
- Discuss the importance of growth and development as a holistic framework for assessing and promoting health.
- Describe the important milestones for each developmental period.
- Discuss the specific nursing interventions relevant to each developmental stage.

KEY TERMS

accommodation
adaptation
adolescence
assimilation
bonding
critical period
development
developmental tasks
embryonic phase
fetal alcohol syndrome (FAS)
fetal phase
germinal phase
growth
infancy
learning
maturation
menarche
middle adulthood
moral maturity
neonatal stage
older adulthood
polypharmacy
preadolescence
prenatal stage
preschool stage
puberty
school-age stage
self-concept
spirituality
teratogenic substance
toddler stage
young adulthood

INTRODUCTION

Individuals constantly change from conception to death. Physical growth; emotional maturation; psychological, cognitive, and moral development; and spiritual growth occur throughout life. Progress through each developmental stage influences health status. Quality nursing practice depends on a thorough understanding of developmental concepts. This chapter presents the eleven life span stages.

BASIC CONCEPTS OF GROWTH AND DEVELOPMENT

Development occurs continuously through the life span. Adults continue to have transition periods during which growth and development occur.

Growth is the measurable changes in the physical size of the body and its parts. Examples of growth are the changes in height, weight, bone density, and dental structure. Growth patterns can be predicted even though growth is not a steady process. The rate varies from periods of rapid growth to periods of slower growth. Rapid growth is most common in the prenatal, infant, and adolescent stages.

Development is the behavioral changes in skills and functional abilities. Thus, developmental changes are not as easily measured. **Maturation,** the process of becoming fully grown and developed, applies to the individual's physiological and behavioral aspects. It depends on biological growth, behavioral changes, and **learning** (assimilation of information resulting in a behavior change). During each life span stage, certain goals (**developmental tasks**) must be accomplished. These developmental tasks are the foundation for future learning.

The time of most rapid growth or development in a stage of the life span is called the **critical period**. An individual is most vulnerable to stressors during a critical period.

Growth, development, maturation, and learning are interdependent processes. The individual must be mature enough to grasp the concepts and make required behavioral changes for learning to occur. Physical growth is essential for many types of learning; for example, a child must have the physical ability to reach the door knob before learning to open the door. Likewise, cognitive maturation precedes learning.

> **MEMORYTRICK**
>
> **GROWTH**
>
> G = Goals (developmental tasks) must be accomplished in each life span stage.
>
> R = Rapid growth occurs during the "critical period."
>
> O = Observe for changes in bone density and dental structure.
>
> W = Weight changes will occur throughout the life span stages.
>
> T = Time routine wellness checks throughout the life span to monitor growth.
>
> H = Height changes are expected during the process of aging.

PRINCIPLES OF GROWTH AND DEVELOPMENT

Individual abilities and talents contribute to each person's development as a unique entity. *The exact rate of development for any given individual cannot be predicted.* There are a few general principles relating to growth and development of all humans (Table 10-1).

The sequence of development is predictable, but performance of specific skills varies with each person. For example, not all infants roll over at the same age, but most roll over before they crawl.

FACTORS THAT INFLUENCE GROWTH AND DEVELOPMENT

Many factors such as heredity, health status, life experiences, and culture influence growth and development. A person's choices about health behaviors are also determined by these factors.

Heredity

Genetic information is passed from parents to children. An individual's genetic makeup determines not only physical characteristics such as skin color, facial features, hair texture, and body structure but also a predisposition to certain diseases (i.e., sickle cell anemia, Huntington's disease). Heredity is the genetic blueprint for an individual's growth and development. The role of heredity is complex and not yet fully understood.

Health Status

Individuals experiencing wellness progress through the life span as expected. Achievement of developmental milestones can be delayed by illness or disability. Individuals with a chronic condition may meet developmental milestones but later.

Life Experiences

The rate of growth and development can be influenced by life experiences. For example, a child whose family has few resources for food, shelter, and health care has a higher risk of lagging in physical and mental growth and development than a child whose family has plenty of resources.

Culture

Individuals are expected to master certain skills at each developmental period, but the age for mastery is determined partly by culture. For instance, some cultures expect mate selection at age 12 or 13, with the birth of a child soon after.

DIMENSIONS AND THEORIES OF HUMAN DEVELOPMENT

Nurses need to thoroughly understand growth and development so they can provide individualized care. Remember, *chronological age and developmental age are not the same.* An overview of the dimensions and major theories of human development follows.

TABLE 10-1 Principles of Growth and Development

PRINCIPLE	EXAMPLE
Growth and development are orderly and predictable, occurring from:	Everyone goes through the same processes.
• *cephalocaudal* (head to toe)	Head larger at birth in relation to body. Head controlled before crawling, and sitting occurs before walking.
• *proximodistal* (functions near midline develop before those distant)	Arm movements controlled before finger movements.
• *general to specific*	Sounds and noises made before words are spoken. Walking occurs before hopping or skipping.
Rate of growth and development:	Rapid growth in infancy and adolescence.
• is not consistent	Slower growth in school age and young adulthood.
• is individual	Slower-growing child will be smaller than others of the same age.
Each stage has specific characteristics.	Infants depend on others for survival. Adolescents search for their own identity.
Certain tasks must be accomplished in each stage.	Infants must develop trust so as adolescents they can establish individual identity.
Some stages are more critical than others.	First few weeks of pregnancy are critical for embryonic development.

CRITICAL THINKING

Heredity or Life Experiences

What is most important in determining a person's behavior: the person's genetic predisposition or the response of other people and socialization?

CULTURAL CONSIDERATIONS

Growth and Development

The time for mastery of such developmental tasks as speaking and toilet training is as dependent on cultural norms as it is on physiological development. In Japan, toilet training begins at a later age (Norimatsu, 2006). In 1990, 22% of mothers with an 18-month-old child had not started toilet training. In 2000, that percentage increased to 52%. Japanese consumers purchase approximately 5 million big-size diapers a month for recommended ages of 3 to 7 years (Connell, 2005).

PHYSIOLOGICAL DIMENSION

The physiological dimension of growth and development consists of physical size and functioning of the individual. It is influenced by the interaction of genetic predisposition, nutrition, the central nervous system (CNS), and the endocrine system.

PSYCHOSOCIAL DIMENSION

Growth and development's psychosocial dimension consists of feelings and interpersonal relationships. A positive **self-concept** (perception of one's self, including body image, self-esteem, and ideal self) is an important part of a person's happiness and success. Characteristics of an individual with a positive self-concept include:

- Self-confident
- Willing to take risks
- Able to accept criticism and not become defensive
- Able to adapt to stressors
- Has innovative problem-solving skills

People with a positive self-concept believe in themselves and set goals they can achieve. Achieving the goals reinforces their positive self-concept.

An individual with a negative or poor self-concept, on the other hand, is likely to have low self-esteem, a lack of confidence, and difficulty setting and achieving goals. A person with a positive self-concept is more likely to change unhealthy habits (such as smoking and sedentary lifestyle) to promote health than someone with a negative self-concept.

Various psychosocial theories have been put forth to explain the development of self-concept. A discussion of various theories of personality development follows.

Theorists

Two major theorists of personality development are Sigmund Freud and Erik Erikson. Freud's theory is called the psychosexual theory (Table 10-2). He identified sexuality (anything that gives bodily pleasure) as the underlying motivation for behavior. He believed that all behaviors have meaning and that repressed sexual problems in childhood cause problems later in life. Excessive gratification or excessive frustration at any stage, he thought, may cause a fixation (preoccupation with the pleasures of that stage).

Erikson (1968) theorized that psychosocial development proceeds throughout life. His theory is known as the psychosocial theory. Erikson believed that each stage has a task to be mastered. His eight developmental stages of life are described in Table 10-2.

Cognitive Dimension

The way a person thinks and understands the world shapes that person's perception, memory, attitude, action, and judgment and is the basis of cognitive theory. It develops as an individual progresses through life. Cognition is an adaptive process. Intelligent beings are able to change behavior in response to the demands of an ever-changing environment.

Jean Piaget (1963) studied the differences in children's thinking patterns at various ages and how they used intelligence to answer questions and solve problems. He theorized that children learn to think by playing.

Piaget (1963) lists four stages of intellectual development: sensorimotor, preoperational, concrete operations, and formal operations. Table 10-2 describes these stages. Each stage is characterized by the ways that the child interprets and uses the environment. There is great variation in age for each phase; ages are approximate.

Individuals learn by interacting with the environment using three processes: assimilation, accommodation, and adaptation. **Assimilation** is the process of taking in new experiences or information. **Accommodation** allows for adjustment of thinking to take in new information and increase understanding. **Adaptation** is the change resulting from assimilation and accommodation.

Moral Dimension

The moral dimension is a person's value system, which helps one differentiate right and wrong. Closely related to emotional and cognitive development is **moral maturity** (the ability to independently decide for oneself what is "right"). Lawrence Kohlberg (1977) described a framework for understanding how individuals decide on a moral code.

According to Kohlberg, there are six stages of moral development. Each stage is built on the previous stage and becomes the foundation for the next stage. Moral development evolves relative to cognitive development. Individuals who think at higher levels have the reasoning skills on which to base moral decisions. Table 10-2 provides an overview of Kohlberg's stages of moral development. Kohlberg indicates that individuals move through the six stages sequentially, but not everyone reaches stages five and six (Kohlberg, 1977).

Spiritual Dimension

The spiritual dimension is described as a sense of personal meaning. The term *spirit* is derived from the Latin word meaning breath, air, and wind. Thus, spirit refers to whatever gives life to a person. **Spirituality** refers to relationships with oneself, others, and a divine source or a higher power. It does not refer to a specific religion. Spirituality is developed throughout life.

The work of Erikson, Piaget, and Kohlberg all influenced Fowler's theory of spiritual development. Fowler's theory has a prestage and six distinct stages of faith development (Fowler, 1995). The sequence of stages remains the same, although the age at which individuals experience each stage varies. Table 10-3 outlines Fowler's theory.

Some clients seem to be unaware of their spiritual natures. The understanding of a client's spirituality is basic to nursing. Caring for the whole person is the distinguishing characteristic of a holistic nurse. Table 10-2 (shown on page 202) provides a summary of the ages and stages of the developmental theories.

HOLISTIC FRAMEWORK FOR NURSING

A basic concept of nursing is to provide care to the whole person. So it is essential for nurses to know growth and development concepts. Nursing interventions must be appropriate to each client's stage of development. Nursing's holistic perspective recognizes that an individual's development progresses throughout life. Progress, or lack thereof, in one dimension affects the other dimensions of development. Figure 10-1 shows the holistic nature of individuals.

Knowledge of growth and development is useful as a guideline for assessment. When developmental milestones are not met, prompt identification and comprehensive intervention is essential. For example:

- The infant who does not roll over, sit, or walk at expected times
- The adolescent girl who has not experienced menarche by the expected time
- The adult who fails to adjust to physiological changes

LIFE SPAN STAGES

Eleven developmental stages will be discussed: prenatal, neonatal, infancy, toddler, preschooler, school-age, preadolescent, adolescent, young adult, middle adult, and older adult. The indications of growth and development in the physiological, psychosocial, cognitive, moral, and spiritual dimensions are discussed for each stage, along with pertinent nursing implications.

Prenatal Stage

The **prenatal stage** (development beginning with conception and ending with birth) is a critical time in growth and

Table 10-2 Summary of Ages and Stages Developmental Theories

STAGE/AGE	PIAGET'S COGNITIVE STAGES	FREUD'S PSYCHOSEXUAL STAGES	ERIKSON'S PSYCHOSOCIAL STAGES	KOHLBERG'S MORAL STAGES
1. **Infancy** Birth to 1 year	**Sensorimotor** (birth to 2 years): Begins to acquire language, develops sense of cause and effect Task: Object permanence	**Oral:** Pleasure from exploration with mouth, tongue, and through sucking Task: Weaning	**Trust vs. Mistrust:** Establish a sense of trust Task: Trust Socializing agent: Mothering person Central process: Mutuality Ego quality: Hope	
2. **Toddler** 1 to 3 years	**Sensorimotor** continues **Preoperational** (2 to 7 years) begins: Use of representational thought (symbolism) and imagination Task: Use language and mental images to think and communicate	**Anal:** Control of elimination muscles Task: Toilet training	**Autonomy vs. Shame and Doubt:** Do things for self Task: Autonomy Socializing agent: Parents Central process: Imitation Ego quality: Self-control and willpower	**Preconventional Level:** (birth to 9 years) 1. **Morality Stage:** Avoid punishment by not breaking rules of authority figures
3. **Preschool** 3 to 6 years	**Preoperational** continues	**Phallic:** Attracted to opposite-sex parent Task: Resolve Oedipus/Electra complex	**Initiative vs. Guilt:** Iniate activities and moral responsibility Task: Initiative and moral responsibility Socializing agents: Parents Central process: Identification Ego quality: Direction, purpose, and conscience	2. **Individualism, Instrumental Purpose, and Exchange Stage:** "Right" is relative, follow rules when in own interest
4. **School Age** 6 to 12 years	**Preoperational** continues **Concrete Operations** (7 to 12 years) begins: Engage in inductive reasoning and concrete problem solving Task: Learn concepts of conservation and reversibility	**Latency:** Identify with same-sex parent Task: Identify with same-sex parent, and test and compare own capabilities with peer norms	**Industry vs. Inferiority:** Develop self-esteem, social and scholastic skills Task: Industry, self-assurance, self-esteem Socializing agents: Teachers and peers Central process: Education Ego quality: Competence	**Conventional Level:** (9 to 13 years) 3. **Mutual Expectations Relationships, and Confirmity to Moral Norms Stage:** Need to be "good" in own and others' eyes, believe in rules and regulations

5. Adolescence 12 to 18 years	**Formal Operations** (12 years to adulthood): Engage in abstract reasoning and analytical problem solving Task: Develop a workable philosophy of life	**Genital:** Develops sexual relationships Task: Establish meaningful relationship for lifelong pairing	**Identity vs. Role Confusion:** Seek sense of identity and values Task: Self-identity and concept Socializing agents: Society of peers Central process: Role experimentation and peer pressure Ego quality: Fidelity and devotion to others, personal and sociocultural values	**4. Social System and Conscience Stage:** Uphold laws because they are fixed social duties
6. Young Adult 18 to 30 years	**Formal Operations** continues		**Intimacy vs. Isolation:** Choose career and develop intimate relationships Task: Intimacy Socializing agent: Close friends, partners, lovers, spouse Central process: Mutuality among peers Ego quality: Intimate affiliation and love	**Postconventional Level:** (13+ years) **5. Social Contract or Utility and Individual Rights Stage:** Uphold laws in the interest of the greatest good for the greatest number; uphold laws that protect universal rights
7. Early Middle Age 30 to 50 years			**Generativity vs. Stagnation:** Become productive and establish a family (30 to 65 years) Task: Generativity Socializing agent: Spouse, partner, children, sociocultural norms Central process: Creativity and person-environment fit Ego quality: Productivity, perserverence, charity, and consideration	
8. Late Middle Age 50 to 70 years			**Generativity vs. Stagnation** continues	**6. Universal Ethical Principles Stage:** Support universal moral principles regardless of the price for doing so
9. Late Adult 70 years to death			**Ego Integrity vs. Despair:** Accept one's life (65 years to death) Task: Ego integrity Socializing agent: Significant others Central process: Introspection Ego quality: Wisdom	

Adapted from *Health Assessment and Physical Examination* (4th ed.), by M. E. Estes, 2010, Clifton Park, NY: Delmar Cengage Learning.

Table 10-3 Fowler: Stages of Faith

STAGE	AGE	CHARACTERISTICS
Prestage: *undifferentiated faith*	Infant	Trust, hope, and love compete with environmental inconsistencies or threats of abandonment.
Stage 1: *intuitive-projective faith*	Toddler and preschooler	Has no understanding of spiritual concepts but imitates parents' behaviors and attitudes about religion and spirituality.
Stage 2: *mythical-literal faith*	School-age child	Accepts existence of a deity. Religious and moral beliefs are symbolized by stories. Accepts concept of reciprocal fairness.
Stage 3: *synthetic-conventional faith*	Adolescent	Questions values and religious beliefs while attempting to form own identity.
Stage 4: *individuative-reflective faith*	Late adolescent and young adult	Assumes responsibility for own attitudes and beliefs.
Stage 5: *conjunctive faith*	Adult	Integrates other perspectives about faith into own definition of truth.
Stage 6: *universalizing faith*	Adult	Makes concepts of love and justice tangible.

Data from *Stages of Faith: The Psychology of Human Development and the Quest for Meaning*, by J. W. Fowler, 1995, New York: Harper & Row. Copyright 1995 by Harper & Row; *Psychiatric-Mental Health Nursing: Evidence-Based Concepts, Skills and Practices* (7th ed.), by W. Mohr, 2009, Philadelphia: Lippincott Williams & Wilkins. Copyright 2009 by Lippincott Williams & Wilkins.

development and consists of three phases: germinal, embryonic, and fetal. The **germinal phase** begins with conception and lasts approximately 10 to 14 days. Rapid cell division and implantation of the fertilized egg in the uterine wall delineates this stage. In this very early stage, the central nervous system (CNS) is already forming.

The **embryonic phase** (weeks 2 to 8 after conception) is marked by rapid differentiation of cells, development of the body systems, and growth. In this period, the embryo is most vulnerable for a spontaneous abortion (i.e., miscarriage).

The **fetal phase** (the intrauterine developmental period from 8 weeks to birth) is characterized by rapid growth and differentiation of body systems and parts.

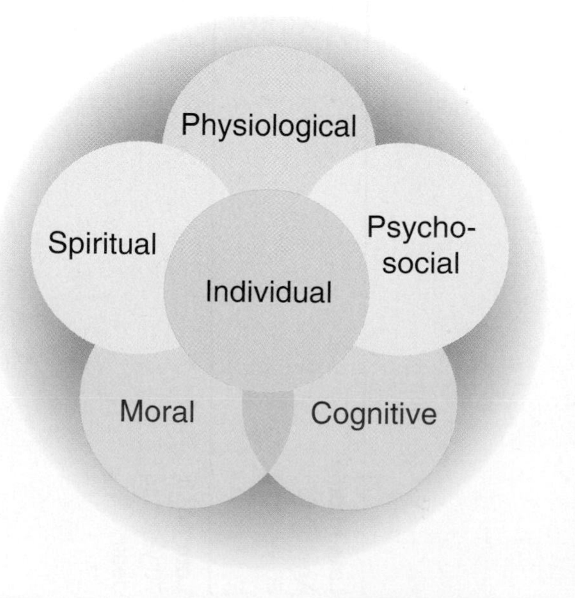

Figure 10-1 Holistic Nature of Individuals

Significance for Nursing

Early prenatal care is essential for a positive pregnancy outcome, with physical examinations and screenings throughout pregnancy.

Enhancing Wellness The primary environment affecting prenatal growth and development is the uterus.

The mother must provide a sufficient supply of nutrients. Women who consume an insufficient amount of protein during pregnancy have a high rate of preterm and low birth weight infants. Teaching must emphasize that vitamin supplements are not substitutes for adequate food intake. Other ways to promote prenatal health include:

- Screening (blood pressure, urine glucose, and albumin)
- Teaching (e.g., nutrition, self-care)
- Assisting economically disadvantaged clients to obtain prenatal care

Safety Concerns Any substances consumed by the mother affect the fetus, whether they are wholesome nutrients or deadly toxins. Cigarette toxic substances, including nicotine, cross the placenta and interfere with oxygen transport to the fetus. These toxins may result in fetal death, premature birth, retarded growth, and learning difficulties.

SAFETY

Use of Tobacco and Alcohol During Pregnancy

No cigarette smoking is advised during pregnancy. All pregnant women should abstain from drinking alcohol, because a "safe" amount of alcohol consumption has not been determined.

Alcohol use during pregnancy can result in **fetal alcohol syndrome (FAS),** a condition wherein fetal development is impaired, resulting in physical and intellectual problems. Alcohol consumption is most dangerous during the first 3 months of pregnancy, when the embryo's brain and other vital organs are developing. The effects of alcohol on the fetus are permanent. Fetal alcohol syndrome is considered to be the leading cause of mental retardation among infants, and the incidence continues to increase (Hockenberry & Wilson, 2007).

There are many other teratogenic substances in addition to nicotine and alcohol. A **teratogenic substance** is anything that crosses the placenta and impairs normal growth and development. The Food and Drug Administration (FDA) requires that all manufactured drugs list the potential for causing birth defects. Illegal drug use by pregnant women is a very serious threat to the unborn.

Neonatal Stage

The **neonatal stage** (the first 28 days of life following birth) is a time of major adjustment to extrauterine life. The neonate (newborn) focuses energy on achieving equilibrium by stabilizing major body systems. Table 10-4 outlines neonatal development.

The neonate's activities are reflexive, consisting mainly of sucking, crying, eliminating, and sleeping. Reflexes play a major role in the neonate's ability to survive. The neonate progresses developmentally from a mass of reflexes to behavior that is more purposeful.

Adjusting to the parental figure(s) is the major psychological task of neonates. **Bonding,** the attachment between parent and child, begins when the parent and neonate make initial eye contact. Parent–neonate bonding is the foundation for trust necessary when developing future interpersonal relationships.

Significance for Nursing

A thorough assessment of the neonate is performed immediately after delivery. The neonate's reflexes should be evaluated at the same time or when the neonate is physiologically stable.

Soon after birth, encourage the parents to cuddle the newborn, explain the neonate's interactive abilities, and encourage mutual eye contact between neonate and parents by showing parents how to hold the child in a position facing them.

Enhancing Wellness The most important nursing activity in promoting neonatal wellness is teaching. Other nursing interventions enhancing neonatal wellness are:

- Continually assess physiological status
- Provide a warm environment
- Monitor nutritional status
- Provide a clean environment; teach parents that neonates need a clean environment, not a sterile one
- Conduct screening tests; for example, the blood test for phenylketonuria (PKU)
- Promote *early* parent–neonate interaction

Safety Concerns Because neonates depend totally on others to meet their needs, safety is a primary concern. One important method to prevent neonatal accidents is to teach parents about using infant car seats. Under current federal law, neonates and infants must be secured in an approved infant car seat each time the child travels in a motor vehicle.

According to the World Health Organization (WHO, 2008a), the primary causes of neonatal deaths in the world are premature birth, low birth weight, and infections. Infections are a serious health risk to the neonate. Newborns should not be near anyone who has an infectious disease. It is essential that the neonate's skin integrity be maintained. Teach parents the importance of skin cleanliness. Diaper rash, a common skin problem for newborns and infants, is caused by the ammonia found in urine, which can burn and irritate the skin. In addition to changing wet diapers promptly, bathing and protective creams may be useful in preventing skin breakdown.

Infancy Stage

Infancy (development from the end of the first month to the end of the first year of life) is a period of continued adaptation,

CLIENT TEACHING

Pregnancy and Medications

Pregnant women should check labels of *all* medicines, especially over-the-counter, about potential effects on the fetus. Expectant mothers should question their practitioner about the safety of any drug taken during pregnancy.

CRITICAL THINKING

Changes in the Family

What are the typical changes that occur in a family after the birth of a new baby?

SAFETY

Car Seats

A neonate should never be sent home from the hospital in a car unless an infant seat is available for the trip.

Table 10-4 Neonatal Stage: Growth and Development

DIMENSION	CHARACTERISTICS	NURSING CONSIDERATIONS
Physiological	Heart takes over circulatory function from umbilical cord.	Accurately assess neonate's cardiovascular status.
	Gas exchange shifts from placenta to lungs.	Immediately after birth, hold the neonate's head lower than body to allow fluids that may block respiratory passages to drain.
	Respiratory reflexes are activated within seconds of birth.	Resuscitate immediately if spontaneous respirations do not occur.
	Neck and shoulder muscles are weak.	Support the neonate's head.
	Temperature-regulating mechanism is immature.	To conserve heat: • Dry neonate immediately after birth and place in a warmed bassinet and • Place a stockinette cap on neonate's head.
	Ossification (process of cartilage changing to bone) is incomplete.	Protect the anterior fontanel on neonate's skull.
	Visual acuity is poor, and visual focus is generally rigid.	Teach parents to be directly in front of the neonate (about 9–12 inches from child's face) when communicating.
Motor	Reflexes direct the majority of movement.	Teach parents to recognize neonate's protective reflexes.
	The full-term neonate has some limited ability to hold the head erect and is able to lift the head slightly when lying prone.	Support neonate's neck and head when lifting.
Psychosocial	Crying is the neonate's way of communicating. There is a reason for crying.	Teach parents about the dynamics of crying so that they neither label the neonate as "fussy" nor develop the misconception that they are inadequate caregivers.
	The bonding process begins shortly after birth.	Encourage parents to distinguish the various cries. Encourage parents to interact with the neonate during every contact (feeding, bathing, changing, cuddling).
Cognitive	Neonates learn through sensory experiences. Learning is enhanced in an environment providing stimuli without bombarding the neonate. Learning occurs by repeated exposure to stimuli.	Encourage parents to provide frequent sensory stimuli (touching, talking, looking the neonate in the eyes).

Data from *Health Assessment: A Nursing Approach* (3rd ed.), by J. Fuller and J. Schaller-Ayers, 2000, Philadelphia: Lippincott Williams & Wilkins. Copyright 2000 by Lippincott Williams & Wilkins; *Health Promotion Strategies through the Life Span* (8th ed.), by R. B. Murray and J. P. Zentner, 2008, Upper Saddle River, NJ: Prentice Hall. Copyright 2008 by Prentice Hall; *Wong's Nursing Care of Infants and Children* (8th ed.), by M. J. Hockenberry and D. Wilson, 2007, St. Louis, MO: Mosby Elsevier. Copyright 2007 by Mosby Elsevier.

CLIENT TEACHING

Parents and Newborn

Parents need information about:

- Basic newborn needs
- Nutrition
- Infection control (especially hand hygiene and hygienic diaper changing practices)
- Care of the umbilicus
- Incorporating the newborn into the family unit
- Growth and development milestones in order to provide appropriate stimulation and have realistic expectations for their newborn

with rapid physiological growth and psychosocial development (Figure 10-2). Table 10-5 provides an overview of infant development.

Significance for Nursing

The nurse providing care to an infant must focus on safety, prevention of infection, and teaching parents about incorporating the child into the family. It is essential for parents and other caregivers to know the developmental milestones. Nursing care involves providing information, support, and reassurance to the parents.

Enhancing Wellness Nurses enhance infant wellness by teaching growth and development concepts to parents. Knowing the behavior to expect at certain ages both guides and reas-

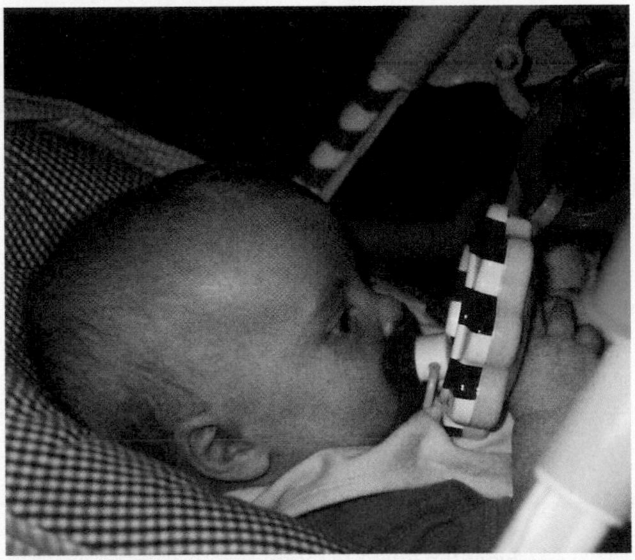

FIGURE 10-2 This infant is exploring his world and is developing in both the physiological and cognitive dimensions.

CULTURAL CONSIDERATIONS

Choice of Infant Feeding Method

There are some cultural sanctions against breastfeeding, and some cultures view bottle-feeding as a status symbol. The changing role of women in American society has impacted breastfeeding practices. Modern-day parenting practices discourage breastfeeding and influence women to not breastfeed for social reasons. Formula feeding in the United States has become a sign of affluence, sophistication, modernity, and freedom (Spangler, 2009). Be sensitive to the client's cultural background and norms when discussing infant feeding.

TABLE 10-5 Infancy Stage: Growth and Development

DIMENSIONS	CHARACTERISTICS	NURSING CONSIDERATIONS
Physiological	Physical growth is rapid. Birth weight usually triples by age 1 and length increases approximately 9 inches.	Teach parents the developmental norms.
	All body systems move toward maturation.	Encourage parents to have recommended "well-baby" checkups.
	Teeth eruption begins at 4–6 months.	
	Brain grows rapidly (reaching approximately half the adult size).	
	Eyes begin to focus.	Provide visual stimulation.
Motor	Physical maturation allows for development of motor skills.	Teach parents anticipated ages for various motor skills to develop.
	Primitive reflexes are replaced by movement that is more voluntary and goal directed.	
	Motor skills develop rapidly: • 6 months: rolls over voluntarily • 8–10 months: crawls • 8 months: sits alone	
	Grasping of objects, reflexive for the first 2–3 months, gradually becomes voluntary.	
Psychosocial	***Freud:*** oral stage	Encourage parents to provide toys and objects for sucking and teething.
	Seeks immediate gratification of needs.	
	Receives pleasure and comfort through mouth, lips, and tongue.	
	Erikson: trust vs. mistrust stage	Encourage parents to feed promptly and consistently (feed on demand rather than a fixed schedule).
	A sense of self begins to develop.	
	Responds to caregiver's voice.	Promote trust by providing warmth, diapering, and comforting.
	Separation anxiety develops at approximately 6 months.	

(Continues)

TABLE 10-5 Infancy Stage: Growth and Development (Continued)

DIMENSIONS	CHARACTERISTICS	NURSING CONSIDERATIONS
Cognitive	***Piaget:*** sensorimotor stage Infant learns by interacting with the environment.	Encourage parents to provide a variety of sensory stimuli: visual, sensory, auditory, and tactile (e.g., colorful mobiles; musical toys; soft, plush animals; rubbing, patting, and stroking of the infant's skin).
	Language development includes babbling, repetition, and imitation. 8–10 months says "mama" and "dada."	Encourage caregivers to talk to the infant and to name objects that are the focus of the infant's attention.
Moral	***Kohlberg:*** preconventional stage	Parents should start teaching (by role modeling) the difference between "right" and "wrong."
Spiritual	***Fowler:*** stage of undifferentiated faith	Encourage caregivers to model the values they want the infant to learn.

Data from *Health Promotion Strategies through the Life Span* (8th ed.), by R. B. Murray and J. P. Zentner, 2008, Upper Saddle River, NJ: Prentice Hall. Copyright 2008 by Prentice Hall; *Wong's Nursing Care of Infants and Children* (8th ed.), by M. J. Hockenberry and D. Wilson, 2007, St. Louis, MO: Mosby Elsevier. Copyright 2007 by Mosby Elsevier.

sures parents. Parents often need guidance about nutrition, protection from infection, and promotion of sleep.

An important factor enhancing infant wellness is providing adequate nutrients in a loving, consistent manner. Special formulas are available for infants who have PKU, are hypersensitive to protein, or experience fat malabsorption. Soy-based formulas are available for the infant who is lactose intolerant or allergic to regular formula. Infants who are formula fed usually have more subcutaneous fat. Whole cow's milk is not recommended for infants younger than 1 year of age. Human milk and commercially prepared formula are more easily digested.

Solid foods are usually introduced at 3 to 4 months of age. Rice cereal is the first solid food of choice because it causes the fewest allergic responses.

Infants are especially vulnerable to infections because the immune system is not fully matured.

Immunizations are important for infants. Nurses should advocate the administration of all recommended immunizations, which now include pneumococcal conjugate vaccine (PCV) to prevent invasive pneumococcal infections (WHO, 2008b), and should confirm those received by the infant. Refer to the appendices for a recommended schedule for immunizations.

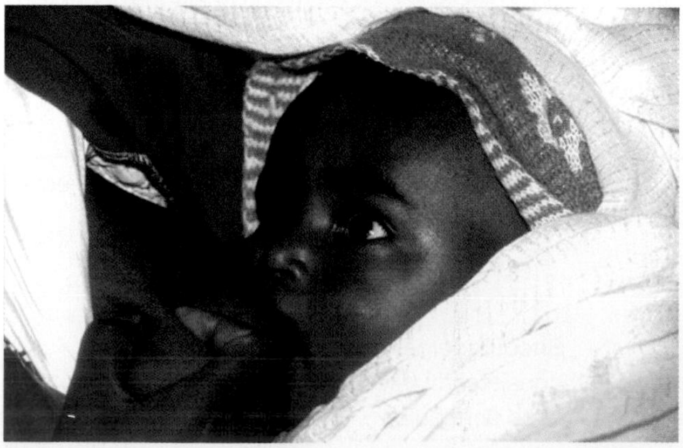

FIGURE 10-3 Breast milk is easily digested and the preferred nutrition for an infant in the first year of life. (*Courtesy of WHO/P. VIROT.*)

INFECTION CONTROL

Hand Hygiene and Infant Care

Hand hygiene is important to prevent the transmission of microorganisms. This is especially true when caring for infants, whose immune systems are still immature.

Information about normal sleep patterns of infants and how those patterns change with maturation is often needed by parents. To promote sleep, parents should:

- Provide a quiet room for the infant.
- Schedule feedings and other care activities during periods of wakefulness rather than drowsiness.
- Develop awareness to the unique sleep and rest periods of the infant.
- Provide comfort and security measures (e.g., rocking, singing).
- Establish routine times for sleep.

Safety Concerns Most infant injuries and deaths are related to motor vehicle accidents. The consistent and proper use of infant car seats is one of the most effective measures to ensure the infant's safety.

TODDLER STAGE

The **toddler stage** begins at 12 to 18 months of age, when a child begins to walk alone, and ends at approximately 3 years of age. The family promotes language development and teaches toileting skills. The child becomes more independent, and temper tantrums often result when attempts at autonomy

CLIENT TEACHING

Bottle-Feeding

- Assume a comfortable position and place the baby in a semireclining position, cradled close to your body.
- Never prop a bottle; choking may result.
- Use care if heating bottles. Do not warm bottles in the microwave; the hot liquid may burn the mouth and throat.
- Avoid using the bottle as a pacifier; this may result in tooth decay and may set the stage for overeating in the future.

are prevented. This stage is often called "the terrible twos." The toddler's frequent use of the word *no* is an expression of developing autonomy.

Nurses greatly influence the quality of parent–child interaction when teaching parents developmental concepts. This information helps parents have realistic expectations of the toddler's behavior. Using firm limits consistently applied helps the toddler learn and provides parameters for safe, socially acceptable behavior. Table 10-6 outlines the toddler's growth and development.

Significance for Nursing

Nurses working with toddlers must be sensitive that children this age are often anxious and fearful in the presence of strangers. Establishing rapport by playing with the child helps alleviate stranger anxiety.

Fear and anxiety can make a hospital experience a negative one. The major stressor is separation from the parents. The unfamiliar environment is also a stressor for the toddler. Nurses can help reduce stress by teaching both the child and parents about procedures. Anxiety is lessened through play.

Regular health examinations and immunizations are an essential part of health care for toddlers. Involve parents during examinations and immunizations. They can alleviate the toddler's stress by holding the child and talking calmly when the health care provider is present.

Enhancing Wellness Teaching involves both toddlers and their parents. Use play to establish an effective relationship with the child. Play is a valuable process for toddlers because it is the primary way they learn and socialize. When teaching, the nurse should be at the toddler's eye level and use words she can understand.

Respiratory infections are common health problems for toddlers. Parasitic diseases are also fairly common. Teach parents about preventive measures such as frequent hand washing with antibacterial soaps. The nurse should also verify which immunizations are needed.

As the rate of growth slows, nutritional needs change. Toddlers need fewer calories than do infants. The required amounts of protein and fluids (Hockenberry & Wilson, 2007) also decrease. Most toddlers become picky about the foods they will eat, so it may be difficult to provide enough calcium and iron. Toddlers should consume an average of 2 to 3 cups of milk per day to ensure adequate calcium intake. Drinking more than a quart of milk per day increases the risk of developing anemia, because the child will be "full" and may not eat other foods (Hockenberry & Wilson, 2007). Nurses can play a key role in nutritional counseling for toddlers.

CLIENT TEACHING

Preventing Infant Accidents

- To prevent vehicular accidents: Use infant seats and keep infants out of the paths of automobiles and other vehicles.
- To prevent burns: Keep infants away from open heaters, fireplaces, hot stoves, and matches.
- To protect from falls: Keep crib rails up at all times, never leave the infant lying unattended on furniture, and use protective gates and barriers to block stairways.
- To prevent drowning: Never leave the infant unattended near water (buckets, bathtubs, swimming pools).
- To prevent electrocution: Keep electrical cords out of the infant's reach and use plastic safety plugs to cover all electrical outlets.
- To prevent choking: Closely monitor the infant exploring the environment. During this oral phase, the infant tests out the environment and seeks pleasure through the mouth. Aspiration accidents are common, with infants choking on objects such as buttons and coins.

SAFETY

Aiding a Choking Infant

Never use the Heimlich maneuver on a choking infant. Instead, use alternating back blows and chest compressions to dislodge the object.

PROFESSIONAL TIP

Health Care for Toddlers

- Explain what is being done in a calm voice.
- Alleviate anxiety with play (e.g., demonstrate a procedure on a doll or teddy bear; allow the child to handle equipment, such as a stethoscope, before using it on the child).
- Provide simple, short directions.
- Comfort the child after a painful procedure.
- Encourage active participation of parents.

TABLE 10-6 Toddler Stage: Growth and Development

DIMENSIONS	CHARACTERISTICS	NURSING CONSIDERATIONS
Physiological	Overall rate of growth slows. By 24 months of age, weight is usually four times that at birth.	Instruct parents on need for vitamin D, calcium, and phosphorus.
	Brain grows rapidly.	
	Bones in extremities grow in length. Physiological readiness for bowel and bladder control develops.	Explain timing for toilet training and need for consistency and patience.
Motor	Learns to walk, run, climb stairs, jump, ride a tricycle, and throw a ball.	Have parents assess home environment for safety.
Psychosocial	*Freud:* anal stage	Have parents avoid overemphasis on toilet training.
	Receives pleasure from contraction and relaxation of sphincter muscles.	
	Erikson: autonomy vs. shame and doubt stage	Teach parents to encourage toddler's attempts at independence (e.g., trying to feed and dress self).
Cognitive	*Piaget:* preoperational stage	
	Can follow simple directions.	Instruct parents to give only one direction at a time.
	Thought processes are concrete.	
	Able to anticipate future events.	Use a calendar to show today's date and the number of days until a significant event.
	Child has short attention span.	
	Child comprehends self as a separate entity.	Teach caregivers importance of calling child by name.
	Language: At approximately 1 year of age, the child can make two-syllable sounds (e.g., ma-ma, da-da)	Have caregivers talk to child frequently but avoid "baby talk."
	By age 3, the child can form short sentences and has a vocabulary of approximately 900 words.	
Moral	*Kohlberg:* preconventional stage	Parents should be consistent in setting limits.
	Child learns to distinguish right from wrong.	Emphasize the significance of modeling desired behavior to the child.
Spiritual	*Fowler:* intuitive-projective stage of faith	Instruct parents to provide simple answers to questions related to religion, God, and church. Instruct on the importance of incorporating religious rituals and ceremonies into daily life.

Data from *Health Promotion Strategies through the Life Span* (8th ed.), by R. B. Murray and J. P. Zentner, 2008, Upper Saddle River, NJ: Prentice Hall. Copyright 2008 by Prentice Hall; *Wong's Nursing Care of Infants and Children* (8th ed.), by M. J. Hockenberry and D. Wilson, 2007, St. Louis, MO: Mosby Elsevier. Copyright 2007 by Mosby Elsevier.

Safety Concerns Accidents (especially those involving automobiles) are a frequent cause of disability and death among toddlers (Figure 10-4) (Edelman & Mandle, 2010). The information regarding use of car seats for neonates and infants also applies to toddlers.

Another common type of accident among toddlers involves toys. As children gain new skills (Figure 10-5), parents must reassess the safety of toys and the environments where the toddler might play.

With their increased mobility and curiosity, toddlers are especially prone to accidental poisoning. Parents should thus childproof the home and carefully observe the toddler.

SAFETY

Toys for Toddlers

Parents should check toys for:

- Age appropriateness
- Sharp pieces or corners
- Small parts that can be swallowed
- Poisonous paint (e.g., lead-based paint)
- Flammable or toxic materials
- Manner in which toys are used

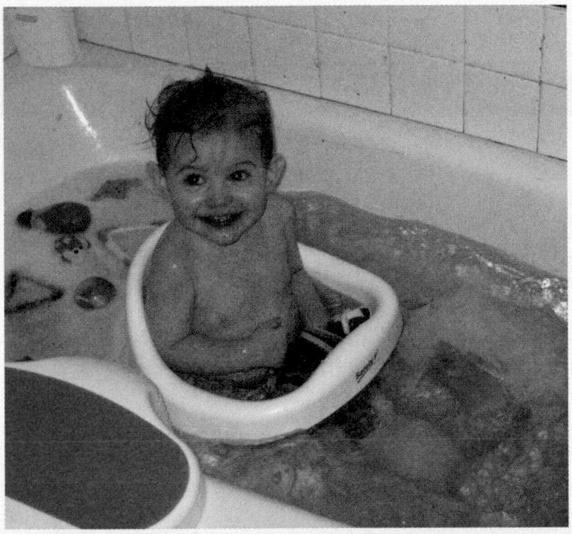

FIGURE 10-4 Parents should carefully observe toddlers and childproof their home to prevent accidents, as shown here with the use of a bath safety seat.

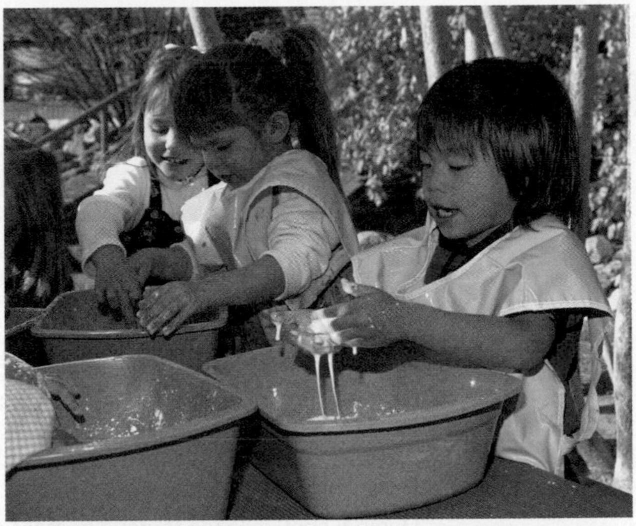

FIGURE 10-5 Parents must ensure that all materials a child plays with are safe, nontoxic, and nonflammable.

CLIENT TEACHING

Toddler Nutrition

- Avoid using food as a reward because doing so encourages overeating.
- Do not serve large helpings; it may overwhelm the child, possibly resulting in a refusal to eat.
- Expect sporadic eating patterns (eating a lot one day and very little the next, or enjoying one food for several days and then suddenly refusing to eat that food).
- Avoid power struggles related to meals. It is counterproductive to establishing healthy eating habits to force a child to eat.
- Establish a mealtime routine and follow it; toddlers like rituals.
- Provide nutritional snacks to meet dietary requirements.

CRITICAL THINKING

Male/Female Stereotypes

Our society labels certain characteristics as "masculine" or "feminine." How do you think these stereotypes influence the development of young boys and girls in our society?

PRESCHOOL STAGE

Development from ages 3 to 6 years is called the **preschool stage.** During this stage, physical growth slows, and psychosocial and cognitive development accelerate. Table 10-7 outlines preschool development in detail.

During this period, curiosity increases, and the child is better able to communicate. Parents should be taught that the child's frequent use of the word *why* is necessary for normal psychosocial and cognitive development.

The child's world continues to expand outside the immediate home environment. The preschooler uses play to both learn about and develop relationships.

Significance for Nursing

Play is a tool that can be used by nurses to help reduce fear and anxiety in the preschooler. Play helps preschoolers reduce tension, learn about the environment, and incorporate socially defined expectations for behavior (Figure 10-6).

Enhancing Wellness It is important to communicate at the child's level of comprehension yet not talk down to the child. Include the child in decisions and activities as much as possible. During the preschool years, the child begins showing an interest in health. To promote the development of lifelong health-promoting lifestyles, the astute nurse capitalizes on this by making health education fun. Immunizations are a major wellness intervention for preschoolers. At each checkup the nurse should verify that immunizations are up to date.

Safety Concerns Accidents are the leading cause of death among young children. Cognitive immaturity coupled with an eagerness to explore the environment lead to the preschooler's risk for accidents. Parents must understand the importance of teaching young children the meaning of the word *no*.

Common accidents among preschoolers include automobile accidents, falls, burns, animal bites, drowning, and ingestion of poisonous substances.

The nurse should emphasize parental education about protecting preschoolers from potential hazards. The safety practices learned as a preschooler will be lifelong. Accident prevention can be best taught through modeling. Parents who always buckle their seatbelts in a car protect themselves and teach their children an important accident prevention measure.

Table 10-7 Preschooler Stage: Growth and Development

DIMENSION	CHARACTERISTICS	NURSING CONSIDERATIONS
Physiological	Physical growth slows; average weight at age 5 years is 45 pounds. Head size approximates that of an adult. Deciduous teeth come in fully; these "baby teeth" start to fall out about age 6 and will be replaced by permanent teeth.	Eats a variety of foods and larger meals.
Motor	Fine motor skills develop (e.g., can skip, throw a ball overhand, use scissors, tie shoelaces).	Emphasize providing a safe environment for play and exploration. Praise attempted independent activities.
Psychosocial	*Freud:* phallic stage Oedipal conflict leads to development of superego (conscience). *Erikson:* initiative vs. guilt stage	Self-control is learned by interacting with others.
Cognitive	*Piaget:* preoperational stage Vocabulary over 2,000 words. Play more reality based. Increased ability to communicate, increases socialization with peers.	Tell parents that children of this age learn through frequent use of the word *why.*
Moral	*Kohlberg:* preconventional stage A conscience begins to develop. Fears wrongdoing, and seeks parental approval.	Encourage parents to teach the child basic values, ideally by modeling. Encourage parents to provide consistent praise and acceptance of child.
Spiritual	*Fowler:* intuitive-projective stage of faith Not yet able to understand spiritual concepts but imitates parent's behaviors.	Teaching by example is the best approach for a child of this age.

Data from *Health Promotion Strategies through the Life Span* (8th ed.), by R. B. Murray and J. P. Zentner, 2008, Upper Saddle River, NJ: Prentice Hall. Copyright 2008 by Prentice Hall; *Wong's Nursing Care of Infants and Children* (8th ed.), by M. J. Hockenberry and D. Wilson, 2007, St. Louis, MO: Mosby Elsevier. Copyright 2007 by Mosby Elsevier.

CLIENT TEACHING

Promoting Wellness

- Encourage healthy lifestyles (nonsedentary activities, nutritious meals).
- Teach children appropriate hygienic measures.
- Schedule regular checkups.
- Keep immunizations up to date.
- Schedule dental checkups and encourage daily brushing and flossing.
- Teach safety precautions.
- Establish sleep patterns.
- Report any symptoms of illness to the health care provider.

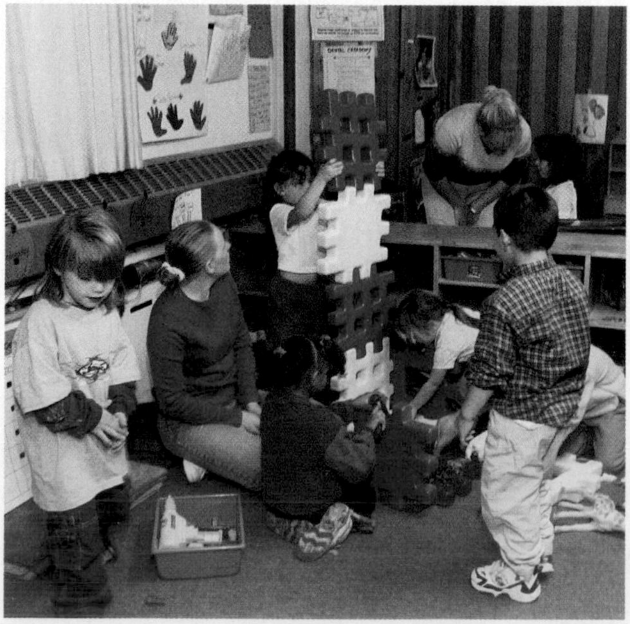

COURTESY OF DELMAR CENGAGE LEARNING

Figure 10-6 Play is an important vehicle for socialization among preschoolers.

School-Age Stage

During the **school-age stage** (development from the ages of 6 to 10 years), physical changes are slow, even, and continuous. Table 10-8 gives an overview of growth and development of the school-age child.

The world of a school-age child expands greatly. Participating in school activities, team sports, and play enlarges their social network. As they mature, play becomes more structured and less spontaneous. Communication increases, and an expanded vocabulary allows the expression of thoughts, needs, and feelings.

The school-age child's cognitive abilities expand, and academic, sporting, and social activities stimulate creativity.

Significance for Nursing

Common health problems among school-age children are minor illnesses such as upper respiratory infections and accidents. Teaching health promotion is a major role when caring for school-age children.

Enhancing Wellness Nurses can promote healthy lifestyles among children in schools. This is a cost-effective way to teach wellness behaviors.

Table 10-8 School-Age Stage: Growth and Development

DIMENSION	CHARACTERISTICS	NURSING CONSIDERATIONS
Physiological	Steady physical growth (approximately 3–6 pounds and 2–3 inches per year). Body has an overall slimmer shape. CNS maturation is nearly complete. By age 12, all permanent teeth (except second and third molars) are present.	Emphasize to parents the need for a balanced diet to sustain growth requirements. Need daily dental hygiene (brushing and flossing) and regularly scheduled visits to the dentist. Change toothbrush every 3 months.
Motor	Motor control continues to develop. Less dependent on parents for activities of daily living.	Encourage participation in physical activities. Praise independent activities.
Psychosocial	*Freud:* latency stage Same-gender companions are preferred. *Erikson:* industry vs. inferiority stage Develops initiative and high self-esteem as manifested in school and sports. Less dependent on family.	To develop a sense of confidence, encourage child to: • Participate in group and individual activities Encourage parents to praise child's efforts.
Cognitive	*Piaget:* concrete operations stage Ability to cooperate with others and to see other points of view leads to more meaningful communication. Reasoning now logical and rational. Abstract thinking is not fully developed. The concept of time develops: • Knows difference between past and present • Begins to learn to tell time Able to categorize, classify, and order objects. Relationships between objects seen.	Encourage group activities. Remember child's level of comprehension.
Moral	*Kohlberg:* conventional stage Understands what is unacceptable behavior but may need assistance to choose between right and wrong.	Encourage parents to provide consistent limits. Emphasize modeling appropriate behavior. Praise appropriate behavior.
Spiritual	*Fowler:* mythical-literal stage Accepts deity existence. Beliefs are symbolized through stories.	Encourage parents to discuss their beliefs. Stories reinforce understanding of spiritual concepts.

Data from *Health Promotion Strategies through the Life Span* (8th ed.), by R. B. Murray and J. P. Zentner, 2008, Upper Saddle River, NJ: Prentice Hall. Copyright 2008 by Prentice Hall; *Health Promotion throughout the Lifespan* (7th ed.), by C. L. Edelman and C. L. Mandle, 2010, St. Louis, MO: Mosby Elsevier. Copyright 2010 by Mosby Elsevier.

SAFETY

Accidents and Abductions

- Children must learn safety rules for riding toys (e.g., use of protective equipment, see Figure 10-7).
- Parents must frequently remind children of the danger of playing near traffic.
- Teach children to use caution with strangers because of the possibility of abduction.

Safety Concerns School-age children often experience accidents during play. Common injuries relate to the use of trampolines, skates, skateboards, and bicycles.

PREADOLESCENT STAGE

Preadolescence (development from the ages of 10 to 12 years) is marked by rapid physiological changes having psychological and social implications. The child begins to experience hormonal changes that will result in the onset of **puberty** (the emergence of secondary sex characteristics). Girls generally experience puberty at a younger age than do boys—approximately 9 to 10 years of age, as compared to 10 to 11 years of age for boys (Edelman & Mandle, 2010). Table 10-9 provides an overview of preadolescent development.

In girls, breast development begins between the ages of 10 and 11. The release of estrogen during puberty stimulates further breast development. **Menarche** (onset of the first menstrual period) occurs about 2 years after breast buds appear. The first menstrual periods are usually scant, irregular, and ovulation may or may not occur. The average age of menarche has declined over the past century in the United States and is now 12.8 years. This decline is probably caused by improved general health status (Hockenberry & Wilson, 2007).

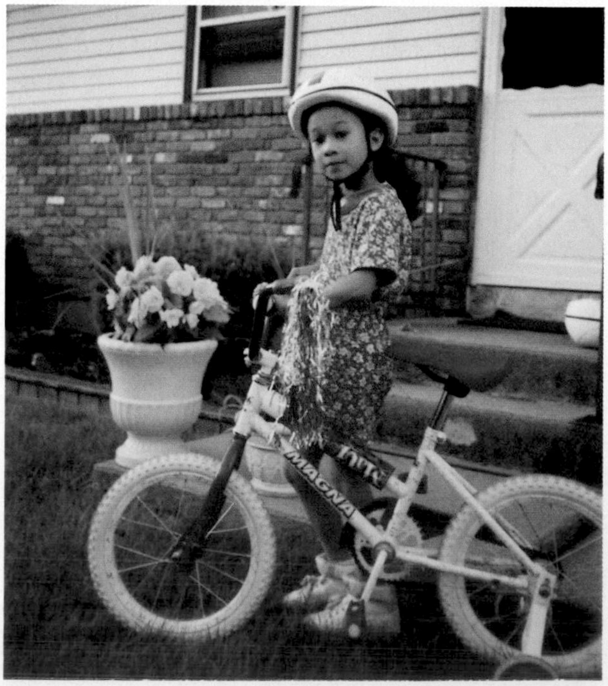

COURTESY OF DELMAR CENGAGE LEARNING

FIGURE 10-7 Safety equipment such as helmets helps protect school-age children from injury.

The menstrual cycle has physiological and psychological changes occurring monthly. A girl's cycle usually is established in a regular pattern after the first 6 to 12 months. Nurses must remember that some girls may receive incorrect or inadequate information regarding menstruation. Client teaching should emphasize the physiological changes, emotional changes, and personal hygiene.

In preadolescent boys, the first signs of puberty are:

- Testicles enlarge
- Penis enlarges
- Scrotum becomes redder and thins
- Pubic hair grows

Significance for Nursing

Sensitivity is essential in working with the preadolescent. To increase sensitivity, the nurse should use a nonjudgmental approach and attend to the preadolescent's body language.

Enhancing Wellness Information about nutrition, activity and rest, and physiological changes is needed by the preadolescent. This client should be taught about the dramatic growth spurt, the sexual changes, and the psychosocial changes that characterize this life stage (Figure 10-8). Preparing the preadolescent for upcoming changes promotes physical and emotional health. Confirm that immunizations are current.

Safety Concerns The preadolescent is at risk for injury during play and sports activities.

Other areas in which to promote safety are development of healthy lifestyle, substance abuse prevention, and sex education.

ADOLESCENT STAGE

Adolescence (development from the ages of 13 to 20 years) begins with the onset of puberty. The individual undergoes the transition from child to adult as many physiological changes and rapid growth occur. The rapid changes occurring are not only physical; many psychosocial adjustments must also be made. Friendships become very important (Figure 10-9). Establishing a sense of personal identity takes up a great amount of the adolescent's psychic energy. Questions such as "Who am I?" and "What is really important?" are common ones among adolescents.

Most adolescents are very concerned with their appearance. The importance of physical attractiveness may cause eating disorders, such as anorexia nervosa (self-imposed starvation that results in a 15% loss of body weight), bulimia nervosa (episodic binge-eating followed by purging), or obesity (weight that is 20% or more above ideal body weight).

PROFESSIONALTIP

Preadolescent–Nurse Relationship

To encourage the preadolescent to ask questions about health-related concerns, the nurse must establish a trusting relationship with the preadolescent.

TABLE 10-9 Preadolescent and Adolescent Stage: Growth and Development

DIMENSION	CHARACTERISTICS	NURSING CONSIDERATIONS
Physiological	*Physiological changes:* Physical growth accelerates and is accompanied by changes in body proportion. Extremities grow first, then trunk and hips.	Teach child and parents to expect growth spurts.
	Endocrine changes: Hypothalamus stimulates pituitary to secrete gonadotropins, causing reproductive maturity. Primary and secondary sex characteristics develop. Beginning of puberty is evidenced in girls by: • Breasts develop. • Pubic and axillary hair grows. • Menarche (onset of menses). • Height increases. Beginning of puberty is evidenced in boys by: • Genitals develop. • Facial, pubic, and axillary hair grows. • Ejaculations occur at night. • Height increases. • Voice deepens.	Provide information and support about sexual changes.
	Musculoskeletal changes: Bones ossify. Muscle mass and strength increase.	Encourage physical activities and adequate intake of calcium.
	Dental changes: Last four molars erupt.	Continue daily dental hygiene.
	Integumentary changes: Skin becomes thicker and tougher. Activation of sebaceous glands may lead to acne. Pubic hair appears.	Encourage sunscreen use and to avoid prolonged sunlight exposure. Support preadolescent experiencing acne.
Motor	Completely independent in performing self-care activities.	Encourage parents to allow some freedom of expression and choice.
Psychosocial	*Freud:* genital stage *Erikson:* identity vs. role diffusion stage The major task is to develop a sense of identity. A new body image develops. Intimacy with members of opposite gender is established.	Provide sex education.
	Primary support is the peer group. Often rebels against adult authority.	Educate parents that rebellion is a normal developmental experience.
Cognitive	*Piaget:* formal operations stage Approach to thinking is logical, organized, and consistent. Most adolescents think in terms of cause and effect. Sees self as exceptional, special, and unique, and views self as being immune to problems. Tends to be extremely idealistic. Egocentric (self-centered) thinking is common, as is a view of self as omnipotent.	False sense of immunity ("It can't happen to me" attitude) has an impact on health behaviors. Educate about safety in: • Sex practices • Driving practices (no driving with alcohol use)

(Continues)

TABLE 10-9 Preadolescent and Adolescent Stage: Growth and Development (Continued)

DIMENSION	CHARACTERISTICS	NURSING CONSIDERATIONS
Moral	*Kohlberg:* postconventional stage The adolescent tends to support the morality of law and order in determining right from wrong. Adolescents begin to question and discard the status quo and to choose different values. Moral maturity depends on the context of the situation and the relationship. Own moral reasoning may be overcome by peer pressure.	Teach parents that questioning of values is normal. Teach assertiveness skills preadolescent can use when communicating with peers.
Spiritual	*Fowler:* synthetic-conventional stage The adolescent questions values and beliefs.	Curiosity about other religious beliefs is normal.

Data from *Health Promotion throughout the Lifespan* (7th ed.), by C. L. Edelman and C. L. Mandle, 2010, St. Louis, MO: Mosby Elsevier. Copyright 2010 by Mosby Elsevier.

Significance for Nursing

Support the adolescent by providing information about the many bodily changes experienced during this developmental stage. Encourage adolescents to share health concerns with parents, but honor the adolescent's choice to keep sensitive information from parents. The confidentiality of the client as well as of those in a relationship with the client (sexual partners) must be protected.

Enhancing Wellness The adolescent's wellness is enhanced primarily through teaching. Areas to emphasize in health education for adolescents include nutrition, hygiene, developmental changes, sex education, and substance abuse prevention. Information is available from the American Academy of Pediatrics (AAP, 2008a).

Teaching adolescents about the physical changes they are undergoing is often done by school nurses.

Safety Concerns Unhealthy behaviors contribute to the three major causes of adolescent death: accidents, homicide, and suicide. The adolescent's risk for accidents increases because of:

- Impulsive behavior
- Feeling invulnerable to accidents
- Testing limits
- Rebelling

As a result, many adolescents engage in unhealthy behaviors such as smoking, consuming alcohol and other drugs, reckless driving, unprotected sexual activity, and violence.

Many adolescent health problems relate to sexual behaviors. For example, consider the following facts:

- The CDC estimates that approximately 19 million new sexually transmitted infections occur each year, almost half of them among young people ages 15 to 24. Young females aged 15 to 19 had the highest Chlamydia rate (CDC, 2007).
- Approximately one-third of girls in the United States get pregnant before age 20. In 2006, a total of 435,427 infants were born to mothers aged 15 to 19 years (CDC, 2008c).

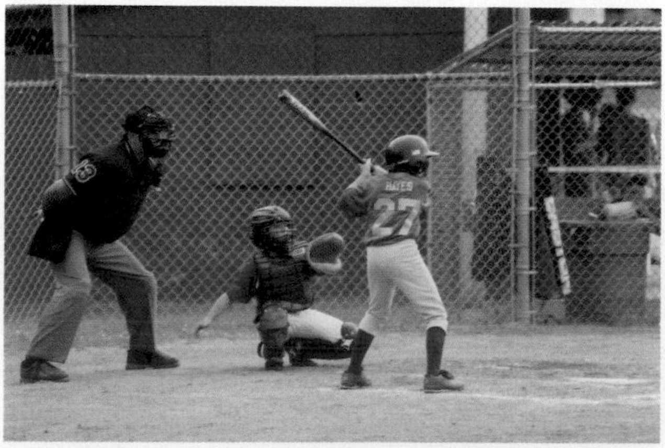

COURTESY OF DELMAR CENGAGE LEARNING

FIGURE 10-8 Preadolescence is a time of gender role discovery and increasing independence.

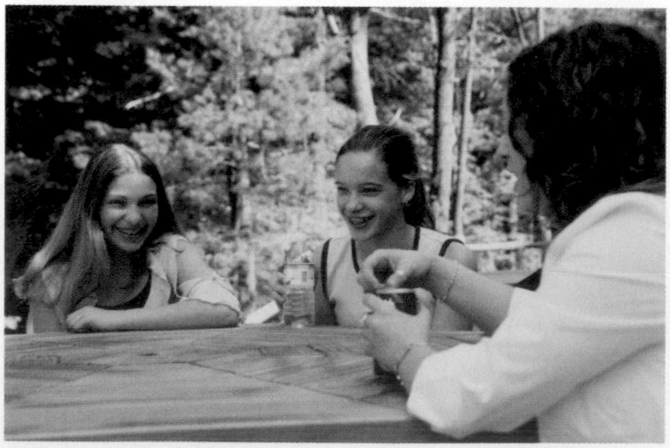

COURTESY OF DELMAR CENGAGE LEARNING

FIGURE 10-9 Adolescence is a time of developing peer group relationships.

PROFESSIONALTIP

Working with Adolescents

- Use a nonjudgmental attitude to establish rapport when working with adolescents.
- Treat every adolescent in a respectful, dignified manner.
- Avoid using a condescending attitude when communicating with the adolescent.
- To form a collaborative partnership, treat the adolescent as an active participant in health care.
- Answer all questions honestly.
- Be sensitive to nonverbal clues. Adolescents are often too embarrassed to initiate discussion.
- Remember that the peer group is of major importance to the adolescent; use group settings.
- Demonstrate acceptance of the adolescent even when limits must be established.
- Questioning adult authority is a normal part of adolescence. Do not personalize such behavior. Nurses who do so become defensive and lose their interpersonal effectiveness and credibility with adolescents.

Teen pregnancy has a great effect on families and communities. Social programs providing resources to meet the needs of pregnant adolescents are decreasing. Many pregnant teens become trapped in a cycle of school failure (or dropout), limited employment opportunities, and poverty.

The pregnant adolescent needs information, expert prenatal care, and a supportive environment. Teaching must emphasize preventing STIs because the pregnancy is evidence of high-risk (i.e., unprotected) sexual activity. According to the AAP (2007), 47.8% of youth (grades 9–12) have engaged in sexual intercourse, and 61.5% used a condom during their most recent sexual intercourse. Nurses teaching safe-sex practices must be sensitive to cultural influences on sexual activity.

A high risk of suicide is a major health problem during adolescence. The rate is higher among adolescent males than females. Suicide is often thought to be the only alternative to an overwhelming situation. Suicidal behavior can be traced to low self-esteem, lack of maturity, and resultant impulsive behaviors.

Assessment for suicide potential should always be direct questions about plans for harming or killing themselves. The following are signs of suicide risk in adolescents:

- Change in eating and sleeping habits
- Writing suicide notes
- Discussion of suicide
- Aggressive behavior
- Substance abuse
- Loss of interest in pleasurable activities
- Preoccupation with death
- Neglect of personal hygiene
- The giving away of treasured objects
- Marked personality change

SAFETY

Suicide Prevention

- Never leave the suicidal adolescent alone.
- The best deterrent to suicide is close observation.

- Verbal cues (e.g., "You won't have to worry about me much longer.")
- Fatigue, headache, stomachache
- Social withdrawal

When someone exhibits signs of suicide risk, contact a health care professional *immediately*. Most communities have a special suicide-prevention telephone line available.

Another significant health problem for many adolescents is substance abuse. A common maladaptive way to cope with the stressors of adolescence is using alcohol or other drugs.

Nurses can help adolescents make responsible, informed decisions before experimenting with drugs.

Young Adulthood Stage

Physical growth stabilizes during **young adulthood** (development from the ages of 21 years through approximately 40 years). The young adult still experiences physical and emotional changes, but at a slower rate than the adolescent. Table 10-10 outlines the development of young adults. This is a time of transition from adolescence to adulthood. According to Estes (2010), this time of separation and independence leads to new commitments and responsibilities in work, social, and family roles and relationships (Figure 10-10).

Pregnancy is experienced by many young adults. It is a time of transition and lifestyle adjustments. Women experience changes in self-concept during pregnancy and may need reassurance that this is normal.

Significance for Nursing

Young adulthood is usually the healthiest time in a person's life. Consequently, concern for health is low, and wellness is taken for granted. Preventive measures fall into two categories:

- Developing health-promoting behaviors (e.g., lifestyle modification)
- Avoiding accident, injury, and violence

By teaching and counseling, the nurse plays an important role in each of these areas of health promotion. Other

CRITICAL THINKING

Sexually Active Adolescents

How would you provide care to sexually active adolescents if you think their behavior is immoral or "wrong"? Is it ethical for you to try to change their values so they become congruent with yours? Should you change your values to be congruent with those of the client?

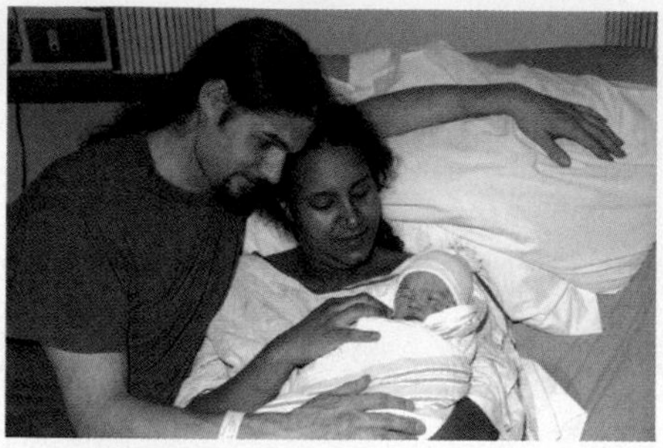

FIGURE 10-10 **Young adulthood is a time for new responsibilities and commitments, including the beginning of a new family.**

developmentally appropriate topics for the nurse to address are vocational counseling and relationship establishment.

Enhancing Wellness Decision making by young adults affects their health status. Young adults often take excessive risks, making them at greater risk for accidents, suicide, or homicide (Edelman & Mandle, 2010). Reckless driving, driving while intoxicated, and unprotected sex are examples that demonstrate a lack of fear by many young adults. Sexually transmitted infections often result in reproductive dysfunction. Nurses should teach women how to perform a breast self-examination (BSE) monthly, and men must learn how to perform a testicular self-examination (TSE). The nurse should confirm currency of tetanus/diphtheria (Td) immunization.

Safety Concerns A health risk to many young adults is sunbathing. Exposure to the radiation resulting from direct sunlight or the lighting used in tanning salons is directly linked to skin cancer. According to the American Cancer Society (2008), more than 1 million new cases of squamous and basal cell skin cancer are diagnosed every year. Nurses can teach and model safe behaviors related to sunbathing.

MIDDLE ADULTHOOD STAGE

Middle adulthood (development from the ages of 40 to 65 years) is characterized by productivity and responsibility. Many physiological changes occur during middle adulthood. Table 10-11 lists the major changes experienced by the middle-aged person. Most activity revolves around family and work with success measured by family life and career accomplishments.

The major developmental task of middle adulthood concerns the conflict of generativity (a sense that one is making a contribution to society) versus stagnation (a sense of nonmeaning in one's life). An individual who successfully resolves this developmental conflict is usually accepting of age-related changes.

TABLE 10-10 Young Adulthood: Growth and Development

DIMENSION	CHARACTERISTICS	NURSING CONSIDERATIONS
Physiological	*Physiological changes:* Physical growth stabilizes. Physical functioning is at an optimum and therefore less likely to be concerned with own health. Maturation of body systems is complete. *Cardiovascular changes:* Men are more likely to have an increased cholesterol level than are women. *Gastrointestinal changes:* After age 30, digestive juices decrease. *Musculoskeletal changes:* At approximately age 25, skeletal growth is complete. *Reproductive changes:* *Women:* Ages 20–30 are optimal years physically for reproduction. *Men:* Beginning at approximately age 24, male hormones slowly decrease (does not affect reproductive ability).	Teach importance of health-promoting behaviors. Encourage a healthy lifestyle.
Psychosocial	*Erikson:* intimacy vs. isolation stage Engages in productive work. Develops intimate relationships.	Emphasize need for social support as the person assumes new roles. Provide sex education information, including information on prevention of STIs.
Cognitive	*Piaget:* formal operations stage Problem-solving abilities are realistic. Manifests less egocentricism. Many engage in formal education.	

TABLE 10-10 Young Adulthood: Growth and Development (Continued)

DIMENSION	CHARACTERISTICS	NURSING CONSIDERATIONS
Moral	*Kohlberg:* postconventional stage Right and wrong are defined in terms of personal beliefs and principles.	Respect the person's value system and beliefs.
Spiritual	*Fowler:* individuative-reflective faith stage Assumes responsibility for own beliefs.	Encourage use of spiritual support system.

Data from *Health Promotion throughout the Lifespan* (7th ed.), by C. L. Edelman and C. L. Mandle, 2010, St. Louis, MO: Mosby Elsevier. Copyright 2010 by Mosby Elsevier.

TABLE 10-11 Middle Adulthood: Growth and Development

DIMENSION	CHARACTERISTICS	NURSING CONSIDERATIONS
Physiological	*Cardiovascular changes:* Decreased capacity for physical activity. Blood vessels lose elasticity. Hypertension (high blood pressure), coronary artery disease, and cerebral vascular accidents ("strokes") may appear.	Encourage to remain physically active. Teach lifestyle modifications related to cardiovascular health: • Quit smoking. • Avoid secondary tobacco smoke. • Practice good nutrition (low fat, low cholesterol). • Engage in physical activity.
	Neurological changes: Impaired sensation of heat and cold.	Explain age-related changes. Teach safety precautions regarding: • Exposure to sunlight • Sensitivity to heat stroke, and frostbite
	Gastrointestinal changes: Slower gastrointestinal motility results in constipation.	Teach to: • Increase high-fiber food intake; drink more fluid • Maintain physical activity
	Genitourinary changes: Nephron units diminish in number and size; blood supply to kidneys diminishes.	Teach signs indicating dehydration. Educate to maintain adequate fluid intake.
	Integumentary changes: Wrinkles develop. Hair may thin and turn gray.	Assess for body image alterations. Employ nonjudgmental listening.
	Musculoskeletal changes: Bone mass and density decreases. Slight loss of height (1–4 inches) may occur.	Educate about: • Need for increased calcium intake • Decreasing caffeine and alcohol consumption • Effects of sedentary lifestyle on osteoporosis
	Generalized decrease in muscle tone; appearance becomes "flabby," and agility lessens, leading to an increased risk of injury.	Instruct about need for proper posture (especially when sitting), exercise, and adequate fluid intake. Educate about need for physical activity.
	Endocrine changes: Reduced production of enzymes and increased hydrochloric acid, leading to acid indigestion and belching.	Instruct client to: • Eat foods that are not spicy or fried. • Avoid eating within 2 hours of bedtime.
	Reproductive changes: *Women:* Estrogen and progesterone production cease at menopause. Secondary sex characteristics regress (decreased breast size, loss of pubic hair). Vaginal secretions decrease.	Teach age-related sexual/reproductive changes.

(Continues)

Table 10-11 Middle Adulthood: Growth and Development (Continued)

DIMENSION	CHARACTERISTICS	NURSING CONSIDERATIONS
Physiological (Continued)	*Men:* Testosterone level decreases as does the amount of viable sperm. Sexual energy declines, and it takes longer to achieve an erection, but it is sustained longer. Adapting to chronic diseases and sexual problems may diminish self-esteem.	Encourage responsible sexual behavior. Teach prevention of sexually transmitted infections.
Psychosocial	*Erikson:* generativity vs. stagnation stage Those who have achieved generativity feel good about themselves and comfortable with their lives. Become involved in altruistic acts (volunteer work). Family roles may change (become caregiver to aging parents, become grandparent).	Provide support as aging occurs. Encourage involvement in community activities. Explain the need to care for self while caring for others.
Cognitive	*Piaget:* Uses all stages, depending on the task. Able to reflect on the past and anticipate the future. Reaction time diminishes. Learning ability remains for motivated person.	Encourage clients who return to school or participate in other intellectually stimulating activities.
Moral	*Kohlberg:* postconventional stage	Be nonjudgmental when discussing values.
Spiritual	*Fowler:* conjunctive faith stage The middle-aged adult is able to appreciate others' belief systems. Middle-aged adults are less dogmatic about own beliefs. Religion is often a source of comfort.	Encourage use of spiritual support. Refer to clergy if desired by client.

Data from *Health Promotion throughout the Lifespan* (7th ed.), by C. L. Edelman and C. L. Mandle, 2010, St. Louis, MO: Mosby Elsevier. Copyright 2010 by Mosby Elsevier; *Health Assessment: A Nursing Approach* (3rd ed.), by J. Fuller and J. Schaller-Ayers, 2000, Philadelphia: Lippincott Williams & Wilkins.

Evaluation of one's life may lead to a midlife crisis, especially if the individual feels that little has been accomplished or self-expectations have not been met.

Significance for Nursing

Middle-aged adults constitute almost half the U.S. population (Edelman & Mandle, 2010). The baby-boom generation has entered this stage, and more nurses will be required to care for them.

Assist middle-aged clients in improving their health by identifying risk factors and providing early intervention. The major risk factors are primarily behavioral and environmental for adults in the middle years, so they can be changed. In assisting the middle-aged client to change unhealthy behaviors, the nurse can work on either a one-on-one or group basis.

CLIENT TEACHING

Self-Care for Middle Adulthood

Self-care topics for the middle-aged adult include:

- Nutrition, exercise, and weight control
- Managing stress
- Recommendations for health screening (cholesterol, prostate exam, mammogram, Pap test)
- Changes related to aging

Enhancing Wellness Encourage middle-aged adults to assume more responsibility for their own health by receiving influenza and pneumococcal immunizations as recommended by their physicians. Confirm currency of tetanus/diphtheria (Td) immunization.

Safety Concerns Middle adulthood is the time when lifelong unhealthy practices, such as smoking, being sedentary, and overuse of alcohol, begin to exhibit their adverse effects. Reversing these practices can greatly improve one's health status. Occupational health hazards are another significant problem.

Most middle-aged individuals have more leisure time for jogging, tennis, golf, or boating, resulting in an increased risk of injuries (Figure 10-11).

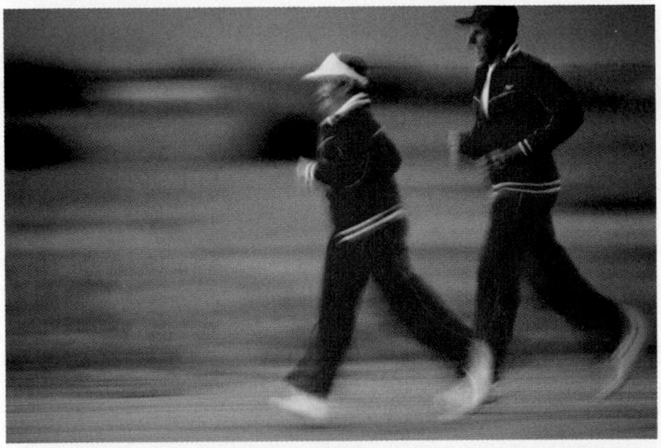

COURTESY OF GETTY IMAGES/PHOTODISC

FIGURE 10-11 Healthy activities such as jogging enhance wellness in the middle-aged adult.

OLDER ADULTHOOD STAGE

Older adulthood is development occurring from age 65 until death. Table 10-12 provides an overview of growth and development in the older adult. Table 10-13 lists common disorders of the older adult.

The CDC (2008) estimates that by 2030, the number of American older adults will more than double to 71 million people. This will be roughly 20% of the U.S. population. The CDC (2008b) states, "An enhanced focus on promoting and preserving the health of older adults is essential if we are to effectively address the health and economic challenges of the aging society" (p. 1). The demands associated with long-term care will pose one of the greatest challenges for both personal/family resources and public resources (CDC, 2003).

Older adults have several psychosocial tasks to accomplish, including:

- Accepting own life as it is (refer to Concept Map 10-1)
- Finding meaningful activities

TABLE 10-12 Older Adulthood: Growth and Development

DIMENSION	CHARACTERISTICS	NURSING CONSIDERATIONS
Physiological	*Respiratory changes:* Respiratory muscles become less flexible resulting in decreased vital capacity of the lungs. Effectiveness of cough mechanism lessons. Alveoli thicken and decrease in size and number. Less effective gas exchange. Structural changes in the chest skeleton such as kyphosis can decrease diaphragmatic expansion.	Educate about the importance of obtaining a pneumovaccine and influenza vaccine. Assess lung sounds, effectiveness of cough mechanism, pulse oximetry, and need for oxygen therapy. Monitor for any signs of respiratory distress.
	Cardiovascular changes: Cardiac output declines. Heart rate slows. Blood flow to all organs decreases. Arterial elasticity decreases causing increased peripheral resistance and a slight increase in systolic and diastolic blood pressure.	Arrange for and encourage regular blood pressure checks. Monitor for signs of fluid retention, and arterial and venous insufficiency. Assess apical and peripheral pulses. Educate the client about limiting dietary intake of fat, cholesterol, sodium, and alcohol. Recommend a smoking cessation program.
	Neurovascular changes: Neurons in brain decrease in number. Decreased production of neurotransmitters. Cerebral blood flow and oxygen utilization decrease.	Monitor general health status. Assess client for cognitive changes. Assess for risk factors for stroke.
	Sensory changes: *Vision:* Lacrimal glands secrete less fluid causing dryness and itching. The lens becomes less pliable causing presbyopia and yellows resulting in distorted color perception. Accommodation of pupil size decreases. Vitreous humor changes cause blurred vision.	Encourage regular examination by an ophthalmologist. Ensure clients have their glasses on when needed.
	Hearing: Cerumen (earwax) production increases. The number of neurons in the cochlea decrease and the blood supply lessons causing the cochlea and the ossicles to degenerate.	Encourage regular hearing testing by an audiologist. Assess for ear pain, drainage, and impacted cerumen. Ensure clients have their hearing aids in when needed.

(Continues)

Table 10-12 Older Adulthood: Growth and Development (Continued)

DIMENSION	CHARACTERISTICS	NURSING CONSIDERATIONS
Physiological (Continued)	*Gastrointestinal changes:* Periodontal disease rate increases and tooth enamel thins. Effectiveness of gag reflex lessons. Esophageal peristalsis slows and hiatal hernia may occur. Gastric emptying slows and peristalsis decreases. Liver size and enzymes decrease, slowing drug metabolism.	Inspect the mouth regularly for signs of dental disorders. Assess nutritional status and gag reflex. Educate the client to avoid the overuse of laxatives. Discuss the importance of dietary fiber and exercise for regular bowel elimination.
	Urinary changes: Glomerular filtration rate decreases resulting in decreased renal clearance of drugs. Bladder capacity decreases. Sodium conserving ability diminishes. Bladder and perineal muscles weaken. Prostate may enlarge.	Monitor fluid intake and output. Complete an assessment for bladder management and implement an appropriate bladder management program as needed. Teach and encourage client to empty the bladder every 3 to 4 hours. Offer absorbent incontinent pads or briefs.
	Integumentary changes: Skin becomes thinner and less elastic. Wrinkles develop. Melanocytes diminish ability to produce even pigmentation, resulting in "age spots." Eccrine, apocrine, and sebaceous glands decrease in size, numbers, and function resulting in dry itchy skin. Body temperature regulation diminishes. Capillary blood flow decreases. Melanin production decreases causing gray-white hair. Facial hair growth occurs on upper lip and chin.	Ensure adequate intake of protein and fluids to promote good skin integrity. Assess client for risk of pressure ulcer formation.
	Musculoskeletal changes: Bone demineralization occurs. Joints undergo degenerative changes. Muscle mass and elasticity diminish.	Assess dietary intake of calcium, protein and vitamin D. Teach, encourage, and assist clients to establish exercise programs appropriate to their capabilities. Teach the client and caregivers about measures to reduce the risk of falling and sustaining fractures.
	Endocrine changes: Alterations occur in the production and reception of hormones. Thyroid changes lower the basal metabolic rate. Blood glucose levels may increase related to the slowing of insulin release by the beta cells of the pancreas.	Monitor for signs and symptoms of hypo-/hyperthyroidism. Assess for signs and symptoms of hypo-/hyperglycemia.
	Reproductive changes: *Women:* Estrogen production decreases with the onset of menopause (the cessation of menses). Uterus, ovaries, and cervix decrease in size. Vaginal lining thins and vaginal secretions decrease. Breast tissue diminishes.	Teach and encourage monthly breast self-exams. Encourage annual gynecological examinations with primary care provider.
	Men: Testosterone production decreases. Sperm count and viscosity of seminal fluid decreases. Prostate gland may enlarge. Impotency may occur.	Teach and encourage monthly testicular self-exams, and yearly digital rectal examinations of the prostate gland by a primary care provider.

TABLE 10-12 Older Adulthood: Growth and Development (Continued)

DIMENSION	CHARACTERISTICS	NURSING CONSIDERATIONS
Psychosocial	*Erikson:* integrity vs. despair stage Accepts own life as it is. A sense of worth is gained from helping others.	Seek the older person's advice. Identify and use the older adult's strengths. Advocate reminiscence. Encourage socialization with peers.
Cognitive	*Piaget:* formal operations stage No decline in IQ is associated with aging. Reaction time slows. *Memory:* *Short-term:* Capacity for recall decreases. *Long-term:* Capacity remains unchanged.	Allow time for responses. Watch for medication-induced confusion.
Moral	*Kohlberg:* postconventional stage Makes moral decisions to fit own principles and beliefs.	Support decision making. Respect values even when different from own.
Spiritual	*Fowler:* universalizing stage Generally satisfied with own spiritual beliefs and tends to act on beliefs.	Listen carefully to determine spiritual needs. Acknowledge losses and encourage appropriate grieving.

Data from Women's Health: *Health Promotion throughout the Lifespan* (7th ed.), by C. L. Edelman and C. L. Mandle, 2010, St. Louis, MO: Mosby Elsevier. Copyright 2010 by Mosby Elsevier; *Health Promotion Strategies through the Life Span* (8th ed.), by R. B. Murray and J. P. Zentner, 2008, Upper Saddle River, NJ: Prentice Hall. Copyright 2008 by Prentice Hall.

TABLE 10-13 Common Disorders of the Older Adult

Respiratory	Respiratory tract infection (RTI) Chronic obstructive pulmonary disease (COPD) Pulmonary tuberculosis (TB)
Cardiovascular	Peripheral vascular disease (PVD) Hypertension Chronic congestive heart failure (CHF)
Neurovascular	Dementia Alzheimer's Depression Transient ischemic attack (TIA)
Sensory	Presbyopia Cataract Glaucoma Hearing impairment
Gastrointestinal	Dental disorders Constipation Dehydration Over/undernutrition
Urinary	Incontinence Urinary tract infections
Integumentary	Skin cancer Pressure ulcers Herpes zoster (shingles)
Musculoskeletal	Osteoporosis Degenerative arthritis Fractured hip
Endocrine	Diabetes mellitus type 2 Hypo/Hyperthyroidism
Reproductive	*Women:* Breast cancer Uterine prolapse *Men:* Benign prostatic hypertrophy (BPH) Impotence

Client Scenerio

65-year-old male with Schizophrenia needs to achieve growth and development tasks for age

Assessment

Does client accept own life as it is?
Proud of current job and role in family
Does client express a sense of worth in helping others?
Minimal contact with others except through employment
Does client participate in meaningful activities?
Attends church, holds job, can read and write
Does client express adjustment to health issues?
Physical decline impacting ability to maintain employment and care for self
How does client cope with changes and losses?
No longer feels safe in own home
Has client planned for own death?
Unknown
Has IQ changed?
Unknown, sister assists with some tasks
Has reaction time slowed?
May need to retire related to physical decline
Assess short- and long-term recall
No identified changes noted
Does client express consistent moral principles and beliefs?
Attends church regularly
Does client express satisfaction with spiritual beliefs?
Attends church regularly
Is home environment safe?
Recently injured during mugging, verbalizes does not feel safe, lives in area with increased crime rate

Nursing Diagnosis

At risk for alteration in achieving age-related growth and development task related to declining physical ability.

Outcome

Growth and developmental tasks achieved as evidenced by:

1. Accepts life as is
2. Maintains current level of physical and cognitive health
3. Maintains current moral principle and beliefs
4. Maintains spiritual beliefs

Evaluation

1. Outcomes met
2. Maintains pride in current abilities including job, spiritual beliefs, and ability to read and write
3. Identifies methods to promote personal safety, attends medical appointments, and utilizes social agencies appropriately

Nursing Interventions

1. Explore with client/significant other (sister) physiological, psychosocial, cognitive, moral, and spiritual characteristics for age that may alter client's ability to achieve growth and developmental tasks.
2. Explore with client/significant other alternative solutions to identified actual or potential alterations in normal growth and developmental tasks.

Activities

1. Identification of risk factors

Activities

1. Compare alternative solutions
2. Refer client to health care providers or social agencies to facilitate achievement of growth and developmental tasks

Concept Map 10-1

COMMUNITY/HOME HEALTH CARE

Home Safety for Older Adults

Encourage the elderly client to make the home environment safe by:

- Ensuring adequate lighting
- Removing all throw or loose rugs
- Clearing all walking paths
- Having a handrail on all stairs
- Installing hand-holds in tubs and showers

- Adjusting to age- and health-related changes
- Coping with changes and losses
- Making preparations for death

Significance for Nursing

Nursing care is important in assisting the aging person to develop a sense of well-being (Eliopoulos, 2004). Nurses working with elderly clients must be aware of their own attitudes, feelings, and beliefs about aging and understand how these may affect care provided to these clients.

CRITICAL THINKING

Retirement

What factors affect an older adult's adjustment to retirement?

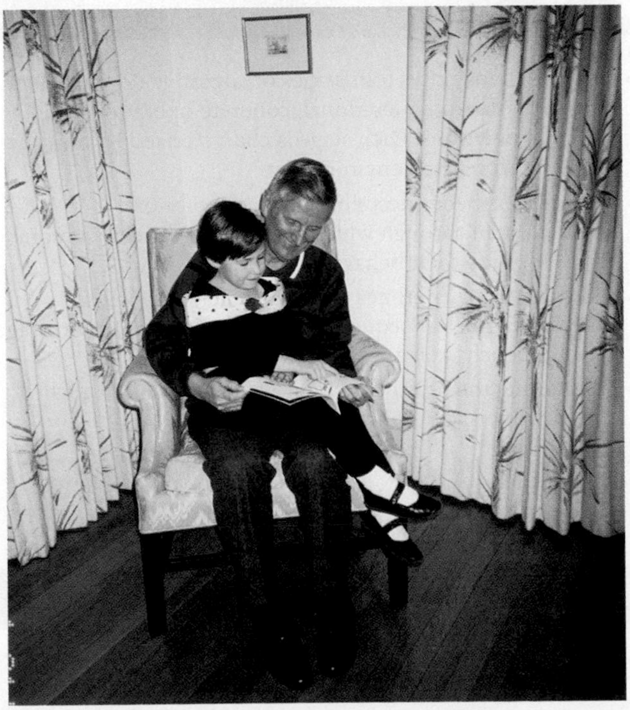

COURTESY OF DELMAR CENGAGE LEARNING

FIGURE 10-12 **Older adults often experience more free time to participate in enjoyable and satisfying activities.**

LIFE SPAN CONSIDERATIONS

Urinary Tract Infections in Older Adults

The older adult frequently does not present with the usual signs and symptoms of a urinary tract infection (UTI). Falling or signs of acute confusion (more than usual) may often be the major clinical manifestations.

Older adults assume new roles such as grandparents. They enjoy spending time with family and friends sharing stories, family history, and wisdom with the younger generation (Figure 10-12).

Assessment of the older adult should include the client's background, family history, work history, achievements, sense of self-worth (refer to Chapter 15 Self-Concept), and hobbies. Encourage clients to talk about their life experiences. Care is more likely to be individualized when the client's unique experiences and assets are recognized.

The issue of caregiving for the older adult has become a national health concern. The 2004 *Caregiving in the U.S.* report (CDC, 2008a) estimated that 44 million men and women provided unpaid care to an older adult family member, friend, or neighbor, resulting in an estimated economic value of $306 billion. Caregivers should be encouraged to respect the client's values, support decision making, encourage the client's socialization with peers, and assist the older adult in accomplishing psychosocial tasks within their developmental stage.

When clients express dissatisfaction and regrets about the past, listen in a nonjudgmental manner. Help older clients put disappointments into perspective by reviewing with them their achievements and accomplishments. Encourage family members to reminisce with the older client. Many nursing interventions for the older adult include introspection and reflection on their lives. Life review (or reminiscence therapy) promotes a positive self-concept in older people.

Enhancing Wellness Health-promotion activities should focus on maintaining functional independence

PROFESSIONALTIP

Polypharmacy

A challenge for many older adults is that side effects from one medication are often treated with another prescription medication. If a client then goes to a different physician, he may prescribe even more medication to address the same or other health concerns. This is called **polypharmacy**, the problem of clients taking numerous prescription and over-the-counter medications for the same or various disease processes, with unknown consequences from the resulting combinations of chemical compounds and cumulative side effects.

and maximizing abilities and strengths. Independent, older adults are generally healthier. Specific topics for discussion with older clients are regular physical activity, use of leisure time, increased socialization, maintaining a positive mental attitude, and adequate nutrition. Encourage the client to obtain influenza and pneumococcal immunizations as recommended and confirm currency of Td immunization.

Safety Concerns Falls pose a major health threat to elderly persons. Teach ways to minimize risk of falling. Confusion with complicated medication regimens causes problems for many elderly. Emerging technology is producing many assistive devices related to safe medication administration.

CRITICAL THINKING

Driving Issues

A 92-year-old female client informs you that her family is planning on moving her into an assisted living apartment. She is alert and oriented and in good physical health. Her family insists that she sell her car before moving. The client adamantly wants to take her car with her, and the assisted living apartment has parking spaces available for residents. Should the client take her car with her to the assisted living apartment? Why or why not? What factors should be taken into consideration when making this decision? How would you handle this situation if the client were your mother?

CASE STUDY

C. W., a 68-year-old female, was admitted to the skilled care facility for rehabilitation following an open reduction internal fixation (ORIF) of the left hip. C. W. had fallen while going down the porch steps in front of her home, suffering a fracture of the left femur. She has no recollection of what caused her to fall. She is widowed and volunteers part time at the local library. While in the hospital, C. W. exhibited signs of disorientation and confusion. Her family reports that she has never had this problem before and has been in good health until the fall. C. W. and her family agree that she will return home after rehabilitation is complete.

1. Write a nursing diagnosis and goal for C. W.
2. List three nursing interventions related to altered mental status.
3. List two outcomes for C. W.
4. Develop a teaching plan for C. W.

SUMMARY

- Growth is the measurable changes in physical size, and development refers to behavioral changes in functional abilities and skills.
- Growth and development of an individual are influenced by heredity, life experiences, health status, and cultural expectations.
- Maturation is the process of becoming fully grown and developed both physically and behaviorally.
- Certain developmental tasks must be achieved during each developmental stage for normal development to occur.
- According to Freud, repressed sexual problems in childhood cause problems later in life.
- Erikson explains that psychosocial development is a series of conflicts occurring during eight stages of life.
- Piaget's theory cites four stages of cognitive development: sensorimotor, preoperational, concrete operations, and formal operations. Each stage is characterized by how the child interprets the environment.
- Kohlberg's theory describes six stages of moral development through which individuals develop a moral code to guide their behavior.
- Fowler's theory outlines six distinct stages of faith development. The sequence remains the same, but the age at which each stage is experienced varies.
- Promoting the health and safety of individuals at each stage of life is an important role for nurses.

REVIEW QUESTIONS

1. The nurse has assessed four children of varying ages. Which one requires further evaluation?
   1. A 5 month old who eats rice cereal.
   2. A 2 year old who is not potty trained.
   3. A 7 year old with a casted broken leg from skateboarding.
   4. A 15 year old who is neglecting personal hygiene.

2. Nursing interventions that enhance neonatal wellness include: (Select all that apply.)
   1. conducting screening tests.
   2. providing a warm environment.
   3. limiting visitation by siblings.
   4. providing a sterile environment.
   5. promoting early parent–neonate interaction.
   6. monitoring nutritional status.
3. The nurse is teaching safety information to the mother of a 22-month-old toddler. Which of the following actions by the mother indicates understanding of the safety needs of a toddler?
   1. Placing a gate at the top of the stairs.
   2. Securing the seat belt properly across the toddler's lap.
   3. Placing all medication on the top shelf of the medication cabinet.
   4. Checking toys for lead-based paint.
4. When a school-aged child experiences changes in height, weight, bone density, and dental structure, this is known as:
   1. accommodation.
   2. critical period.
   3. growth.
   4. assimilation.
5. During this stage of cognitive development, the client's imagination flourishes, thinking begins using representational thought, and events are interpreted in relation to the client's self:
   1. sensorimotor.
   2. preoperational.
   3. formal operational.
   4. concrete operational.
6. During the admission health history, the 22-year-old client informs the nurse that he has been having "safe sex" with his girlfriend for 2 years. This indicates that the client is in which stage of Freud's psychosexual development?
   1. Anal.
   2. Phallic.
   3. Latency.
   4. Genital.
7. A client who graduated from law school and who is beginning her career as a lawyer is in which stage of Erikson's psychosocial development?
   1. Identity vs. role confusion.
   2. Industry vs. inferiority.
   3. Intimacy vs. isolation.
   4. Integrity vs. despair.
8. Respecting authority, believing in rules, seeking approval of others through actions, and maintaining cordial interpersonal relationships occurs in which level of Kohlberg's moral development theory?
   1. Conventional.
   2. Preconventional.
   3. Postconventional.
   4. Preoperational.
9. A 70-year-old client has noticed that his short-term memory recall has decreased, but IQ and long-term memory recall have remained unchanged. Which stage of Piaget's theory is this client in?
   1. Formal operational.
   2. Concrete operational.
   3. Latency operational.
   4. Integrity operational.
10. An 81-year-old client is informed that she has terminal cancer. When her physician leaves the room, she begins to cry and expresses dissatisfaction and regrets about her past to the nurse. Appropriate nursing interventions at this time include all the following except:
   1. listening in a nonjudgmental manner.
   2. contacting hospice to make arrangements for impending death.
   3. providing uninterrupted time for the client to discuss her concerns.
   4. offering to contact the client's religious counselor.

REFERENCES/SUGGESTED READING

American Academy of Child and Adolescent Psychiatry. (2008a). Teenagers with eating disorders. Available: http://www.aacap.org/publications/factsfam/eating.htm

American Academy of Child and Adolescent Psychiatry. (2008b). Teen suicide. Available: http://www.aacap.org/publications/factsfam/suicide.htm

American Academy of Pediatrics. (2007). Adolescent health: critical adolescent health issues—Sexual health. Retrieved November 30, 2008, from http://www.aap.org/sections/adolescenthealth/sexualhealth.cfm

American Academy of Pediatrics. (2008a). Adolescent health. Available: http://www.aap.org/advocacy/washing/chiah/htm

American Academy of Pediatrics (AAP). (2008b). Puberty—Ready or not expect some changes. Available: http://www.aap.org/healthtopics/stages.cfm#adol

American Cancer Society. (2003). *Cancer facts and figures 2003.* Atlanta: Author.

American Cancer Society. (2008). What are the key statistics about squamous and basal cell skin cancer? Retrieved August 30, 2009 from http://www.cancer.org/docroot/CRI/content/CRI_2_4_1X_What_are_the_key_statistics_for_skin_cancer_51.asp?sitearea=

Beare, P. & Myers, J. (1998). *Adult health nursing* (3rd ed.). St. Louis, MO: Mosby.

Bradley-Springer, L. (2001). HIV prevention: What works? *American Journal of Nursing, 101*(6), 45–48.

Centers for Disease Control and Prevention. (2002). AIDS falls from top ten causes of death; teen births, infant mortality, homicides all decline; Updated November 30, 2008. Available: http://www.cdc.gov/od/oc/media/pressrel/r981007.htm

Centers for Disease Control and Prevention. (2003). Public health and aging: Trends in aging—United States and worldwide. *Morbidity and Mortality Weekly Report, 52*(06), 101–106. Retrieved December 14, 2008, from http://www.cdc.gov/mmwr/preview/mmwrhtml/mm5206a2.htm

Centers for Disease Control and Prevention. (2007). Trends in reportable sexually transmitted diseases in the United States, 2006. Retrieved November 30, 2008, from http://www.cdc.gov/std/stats/trends2006.htm

Centers for Disease Control and Prevention. (2008a). Assuring healthy caregivers, a public health approach to translating research into practice: The RE-AIM framework. Retrieved December 14, 2008, from http://www.cdc.gov/aging/caregiving/index.htm

Centers for Disease Control and Prevention. (2008b). The state of aging and health in America 2007 report. Retrieved December 14, 2008, from http://www.cdc.gov/aging/saha.htm

Centers for Disease Control and Prevention. (2008c). Teen pregnancy. Retrieved November 30, 2008, from http://www.cdc.gov/reproductivehealth/AdolescentReproHealth

Connell, R. (2005). Japan messes up with potty training. Retrieved June 21, 2009, from http://www.deeker.com/Articles/japan_messes_up_with_potty_training.html

Edelman, C. & Mandle, C. (2010). *Health promotion throughout the lifespan* (7th ed.). St. Louis, MO: Mosby Elsevier.

Eliopoulos, C. (2004). *Gerontological nursing* (6th ed.). Philadelphia: Lippincott Williams & Wilkins.

Erikson, E. (1968). *Childhood and society.* New York: Norton.

Estes, M. (2010). *Health assessment and physical examination* (4th ed.). Clifton Park, NY: Delmar Cengage Learning.

Firth, P. & Watanabe, S. (1996). *Women's health: Instant nursing assessment.* Clifton Park, NY: Delmar Cengage Learning.

Fowler, J. (1995). *Stages of faith: The psychology of human development and the quest for meaning.* New York: Harper & Row.

Freud, S. (1961). *Civilization and its discontents.* New York: Norton.

Fuller, J. & Schaller-Ayers, J. (2000). *Health assessment: A nursing approach* (3rd ed.). Philadelphia: Lippincott Williams & Wilkins.

Guyton, A. & Hall, J. (2002). *Textbook of medical physiology* (10th ed.). Philadelphia: W. B. Saunders.

Hockenberry, M. & Wilson, D. (2007). *Wong's nursing care of infants and children* (8th ed.). St. Louis, MO: Mosby Elsevier.

Kimbell, S. (2001). Before the fall: Keeping your patient on his feet. *Nursing2001, 31*(8), 44–45.

Kohlberg, L. (1977). *Recent research in moral development.* New York: Holt, Rinehart and Winston.

Levinson, D. (1978). *The seasons of a man's life.* New York: Knopf.

Mayo Clinic. (2008). Children's snacks: 20 tips for healthier snacking. Retrieved December 17, 2008, from http://www.mayoclinic.com/health/childrens-health/HQ00419

Mohr, W. (2009). *Psychiatric-mental health nursing* (7th ed.). Philadelphia: Lippincott Williams & Wilkins.

Murray, R. & Zentner, J. (2008). *Health promotion strategies through the life span* (8th ed.). Upper Saddle River, NJ: Prentice Hall.

Norimatsu, H. (2006). Development of child autonomy in eating and toilet training: One to-three-year-old Japanese and French children. *Early Development and Parenting, 2*(1), 39–50. Retrieved June 22, 2009, from http://www3.interscience.wiley.com/journal/112465782/abstract

Overman, B. (2009). *Older adult concept care map.* Lima, OH.

Piaget, J. (1963). *The origins of intelligence in children.* New York: Norton.

Spangler, A. (2009). Breastfeeding in a bottle-feeding culture. Retrieved June 21, 2009, from http://www.breastfeeding.com/reading_room/bottle_culture.html

World Health Organization. (2008a). The global burden of disease: 2004 update. Retrieved November 30, 2008, from http://www.who.int/child_adolescent_health/media/causes_death_u5_neonates_2004.pdf

World Health Organization. (2008b). Vaccines to prevent pneumonia and improve child survival. Retrieved November 30, 2008, from http://www.who.int/bulletin/volumes/86/5/07-044503/en/index.html

RESOURCES

American Academy of Pediatrics, http://www.aap.org

American Association of Retired Persons, http://www.aarp.org

American Foundation for Suicide Prevention, http://www.afsp.org

American Society on Aging, http://www.asaging.org

Centers for Disease Control and Prevention (CDC), http://www.cdc.gov

Gerontological Society of America, http://www.geron.org

National Institute of Child Health and Human Development, http://www.nichd.nih.gov

Zero to Three: National Center for Infants, Toddlers and Families, http://www.zerotothree.org

CHAPTER 11
Cultural Considerations

MAKING THE CONNECTION

Refer to the following chapters to increase your understanding of cultural considerations and nursing:

Basic Nursing

- ***Holistic Care***
- ***Legal and Ethical Responsibilities***
- ***Communication***
- ***Wellness Concepts***
- ***Spirituality***
- ***Complementary/Alternative Therapies***
- ***Pain Management***

LEARNING OBJECTIVES

Upon completion of this chapter, you should be able to:

- Define key terms.
- Describe the characteristics and components of culture.
- Discuss the impact of cultural beliefs on illness and health.
- Compare and contrast diverse health beliefs of major cultural groups in the United States.
- Describe cultural differences in relation to time and space.
- Identify nutritional preferences held by various cultural groups.
- Identify the general beliefs that account for the differences among religions.
- Describe the way that the nurse's religious beliefs or lack thereof influences nursing care.
- Discuss the nurse's role in meeting the spiritual needs of the client and family.
- Analyze personal values and cultural beliefs.
- Perform a cultural assessment.

KEY TERMS

acculturation
agnostics
atheists
cultural assimilation
cultural diversity
culture
dominant culture
ethnicity
ethnocentrism
minority group
oppression
race
religious support system
spiritual care
spiritual needs
stereotyping
yin and yang

INTRODUCTION

Every aspect of a person's life—including attitudes, values, and beliefs—is influenced by that person's culture. Behavior, including behavior affecting health, is culturally determined. Recognition of cultural differences and their impact on health care becomes even more critical as the population of the United States continues to diversify. Because nurses provide health care to culturally diverse client populations in various settings, knowledge of culturally relevant information is essential for delivery of competent nursing care. This chapter discusses the various concepts related to culture, the influence of culture on health, the relationships between culture and health beliefs, cultural aspects and the nursing process, and illnesses associated with ethnic groups.

CULTURE

Each individual is culturally unique. A person's culture, as influenced by life experiences, education, and creative thought, is the lens through which a person sees everything. The nurse needs a thorough understanding of cultural concepts to provide holistic care.

In society, **culture** refers to an integrated dynamic structure of knowledge, attitudes, behaviors, beliefs, ideas, habits, customs, languages, values, symbols, rituals, and ceremonies that are unique to a particular group of people. This structure provides the group of people with a general design for living.

Individuals often acquire cultural beliefs unconsciously throughout the process of growth and maturation (Giger & Davidhizar, 2004). People are exposed to culture at an early age through the observance of traditions (established customary patterns of thought and behavior). Cultural beliefs, values, customs, and behaviors are transmitted from one generation to another through interaction, daily activities, and celebrations. For instance, the birth of a child is celebrated according to the family's cultural norms and customs, which may include prayers, blessings, special naming ceremonies, religious rites, and so forth. Parents, grandparents, and other elders all teach children cultural norms and expectations through demonstration, discussion, and role modeling (Figure 11-1).

Culture is not static, nor is it uniform among all members within a given cultural group. Culture represents adaptive dynamic processes learned through life experiences. Diversity among and within cultural groups results from individual perspectives and practices. Consider, for example, the way that a family deals with a crisis. A crisis may cause a family that is part of a culture with a strong sense of responsibility to family and blood relatives to become closer; conversely, the same situation may cause a family that is from a culture that values independence and individuality to withdraw and create distance among its members. These reactions are rooted in the family's cultural background and heritage.

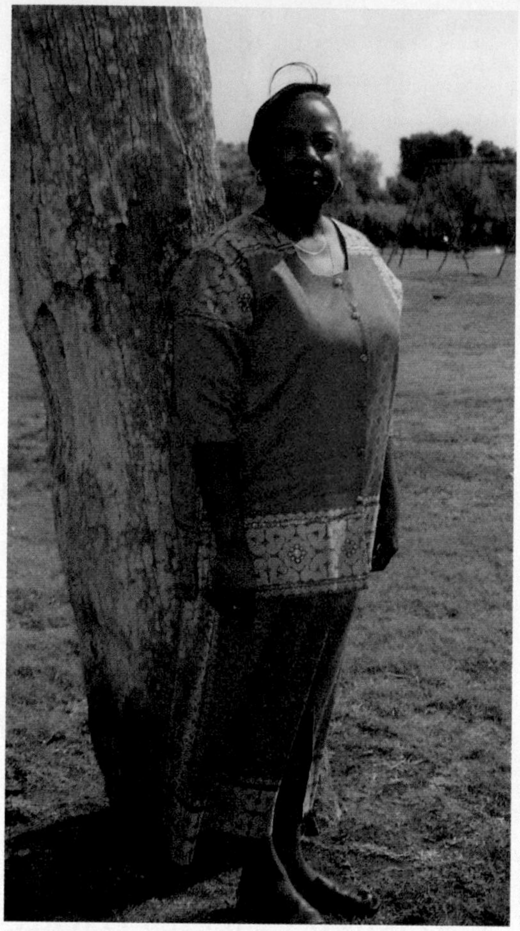

COURTESY OF TIRA BUTLER

FIGURE 11-1 This woman celebrates her African American heritage when wearing this ethnic dress.

CULTURAL CONSIDERATIONS

Sharing Culture

Cultural messages are transmitted in a variety of settings, such as homes, schools, religious organizations, and communities. The various media, such as radio and television, are also powerful transmitters and shapers of culture.

ETHNICITY AND RACE

Ethnicity is a cultural group's perception of itself, or a group identity. Ethnicity is a common social heritage providing a sense of belonging that is passed from one generation to the next. Members of an ethnic group display their sense of identity through common traits and customs. Ethnic identity can be expressed in many ways, including dress; for instance, many African Americans display ethnic pride by choosing clothing that highlights their ethnic origin and shared heritage.

Race is a group of people with biological similarities. Members of a racial group have similar physical characteristics, such as facial features and color of hair, eyes, and skin. Racial and ethnic groups often overlap because the cultural and biological commonalities support one another (Giger & Davidhizar, 2004). The similarities of racial and ethnic group members reinforce a sense of identity and cohesiveness.

Cultural Diversity

Cultural diversity refers to the differences among people resulting from ethnic, racial, and cultural variations. A variety of rich cultural heritages exists within the United States. The sociopolitical climate is enriched by this vast potential of human resources with divergent viewpoints and behaviors. A diverse population provides varied ideas, viewpoints, and problem-solving approaches and an expectation of increased tolerance.

Living and working in such a culturally diverse society has some disadvantages. Problems arise when differences between and within cultural groups are not understood. Apprehension and turmoil often accompany people's expectations of others.

Some cultural groups have historically experienced prejudice or bias in the form of racism (discrimination based on race and biological differences). Individuals may experience sexism (discrimination based on gender) and classism (prejudice based on perceived social class). Society perpetuates these biases consciously or unconsciously. The underlying premise is that one way is superior and that every other way is inferior. **Ethnocentrism**, the assumption of cultural superiority and inability to accept another culture's ways, results in oppression. When the rules, values, and ideals of one group are imposed on another group, it is termed **oppression**. Oppression is based on cultural biases, which stem from beliefs, expectations, and traditions.

Stereotyping is the belief that all people within the same ethnic, racial, or cultural group will act the same way, sharing the same beliefs and attitudes. Stereotyping results in labeling people according to cultural preconceptions, thereby ignoring individual identity.

The group whose values prevail within a given society is the **dominant culture**. The dominant culture of the United States is composed of white, middle-class Protestants of European ancestry. The European values have greatly influenced U.S. culture.

These dominant values may conflict with the values of minority groups. A **minority group** is a group of people constituting less than a numerical majority of the population. Such groups are often labeled and treated differently from others in the society. Minority groups are generally considered to have less power than the dominant group (Giger & Davidhizar, 2004).

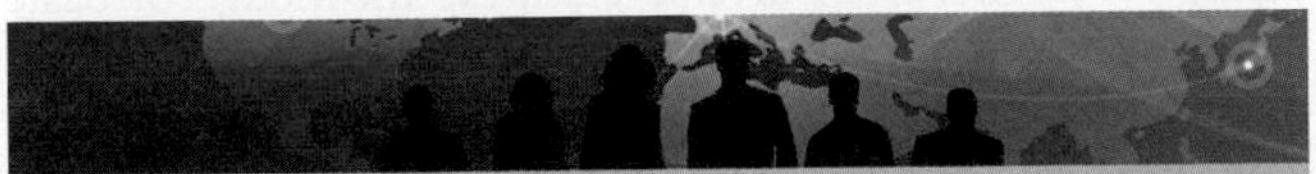

CULTURAL CONSIDERATIONS

Individuality

Remember that each person is first and foremost an individual and second a member of a cultural group. Although similarities may exist within an ethnic or culture group, individual differences are respected.

When people assume the characteristics of the dominant culture, it is called **acculturation** (the process of learning beliefs, norms, and behavioral expectations of a group). **Cultural assimilation** happens when members of a minority group are absorbed by the dominant culture, taking on the characteristics of the dominant culture.

Culture's Components

Stewart identified five components of culture that establish the way people think about life (as cited in Lock, 1992):

- *Perception of self and the individual:* Refers to personal identity, respect for individuals, and value
- *Motivation:* Explains the methods and value of achievement
- *Activity:* Identifies the ways people organize and value work
- *Social relations:* Explains the structure and importance of gender roles, friendships, and class
- *Perception of the world:* Indicates the explanation of religious beliefs and life events

These concepts are particularly helpful to the nurse when planning care for a client from another cultural group. Self-identity, social relationships, work, success, and religion influence the cultural group's definition of health and illness and the response to health events. For example, if a culture values relationships more than work, the culture may sanction an extended period of illness and a lengthy time away from the employment site; however, if a culture measures achievement by output at work, illness may be interpreted negatively. Members of the latter culture may deny illness and delay seeking appropriate health care.

Culture's Characteristics

Leninger (2002) has identified certain characteristics shared by all cultures:

- Culture is "learned behavior." Behavior patterns are picked up as children imitate adults and develop actions and attitudes acceptable in society.
- Culture is a "reflection of shared beliefs." Cultural beliefs are widely known and adopted. The beliefs and values of the group "guide human thought and action."
- Culture defines acceptable behavior. Behavioral patterns are not individually defined but rather are defined, accepted, and practiced by everyone who belongs to the cultural group. Everyone in the cultural group understands acceptable behavior.
- Culture is dynamic. New ideas experienced by each generation may lead to different standards of behavior.
- Culture is an observance of traditions. Traditional observances, ceremonies, and food festivities connect the family and bind group relationships.

CULTURAL INFLUENCES ON HEALTH CARE BELIEFS AND PRACTICES

Culture influences health care decisions and practices and determines the way we react to illness and pain. In cultures where raw foods are not consumed, for instance, the

PROFESSIONALTIP

Cultural Sensitivity

Nurses who are culturally competent provide culturally appropriate care to a diverse population of clients. Cultural diversity presents special challenges for nurses who provide care that is incongruent with personal beliefs and values. Culturally sensitive nurses caring for clients who differ from themselves remember to find out how the client views the event (illness), including the significance (meaning) that the client assigns the event. The culturally diverse nurse honors individual differences.

incidence of shigellosis may be lower than cultures where consumption of raw meat and fish is common. On the other hand, cultural taboos against eating protein during pregnancy have a harmful or destructive effect on fetal development. Cultural values define human responses to illness and determine whether an individual will seek professional care when ill and comply with prescribed treatment.

Beliefs and patterns of behavior affect attitudes about various aspects of health. Beliefs about the definition of health, etiology (cause and origin of disease), health promotion and protection practices, and health practitioners and remedies are all influenced by cultural background. Clients tend to define wellness and illness in the context of their own culture.

Definition of Health

The most widely accepted definition of health, developed by the World Health Organization (WHO), states that health is not only the absence of disease but also complete physical, mental, and social wellness. While this definition of health is broad enough to be global, the physical, mental, and social dimensions are culturally defined. Any deviation from that which is culturally understood to be normal health is considered illness. For example, a biological disease of immediate etiology might not be interpreted as an illness by some cultures; intestinal parasites are so common in some areas in Africa that the presence of ascaris in stools is considered normal. If a cultural group does not perceive certain symptoms or behaviors as illness, members are not likely to seek medical care when these symptoms appear. In this situation, disease conditions may persist untreated, resulting in permanent damage or even death.

Etiology

The noted medical anthropologist Peter Morley presents four views of the origin of disease: supernatural, nonsupernatural, immediate, and ultimate (Morley & Wallis, 1978). The supernatural view of disease traces diseases to metaphysical forces such as witchcraft, sorcery, and voodoo. An individual with this view might attribute illness to evil spirits or to a curse by a powerful spiritual person. The nonsupernatural view holds that diseases have an accepted cause-and-effect relationship, even though that relationship may lack scientific rationale. For example, people of many cultures believe that colic in an infant is caused by breast milk rendered impure when a nursing mother has sexual relations. In such cultures, sexual relations are prohibited for nursing mothers. The immediate view of disease traces diseases to known pathogenic agents, such as chickenpox being caused by *Herpes varicella,* and the ultimate view describes determinates for diseases, such as smoking resulting in lung cancer. Most cultural groups support a multietiologic origin, believing there may be three or four explanations as to why and how diseases occur.

Health Promotion and Protection

Strategies for achieving and maintaining good health vary by cultural group. For example, the dominant U.S. culture has come to endorse a low-fat, high-fiber diet; regular exercise; and appropriate immunizations as means to promote and protect health. Other cultures may place greater value on prayer, meditation, and restored relationships, particularly in those cultures where disease prevention and health maintenance are closely linked to beliefs about disease etiology. For example, disease prevention may require paying homage to ancestral spirits to avoid offending them and seeking their revenge through illness.

Practitioners and Remedies

Variety in health/illness care providers is a natural extension of culturally diverse concepts of etiology and definitions of health and illness. Standard medicine may not be accepted as treatment when a scientific rationale for the etiology of disease is not accepted by a cultural group. Alternative remedies and practitioners are often found in culturally diverse groups. In order to enhance client compliance with treatment regimens, health care providers must make efforts to base therapy and prescribe treatments that respect culturally traditional remedies. Clients who trace disease etiology to a supernatural cause are more likely to seek interventions from spiritual leaders or traditional healers.

The folk medicine system categorizes illnesses as either natural or unnatural (Giger & Davidhizar, 2004). The classification of an illness determines the type of treatment and healer used. Because the folk medicine system (also referred to as alternative medicine) can present challenges to nurses caring for clients from diverse cultures, knowledge of basic beliefs about illness, factors contributing to illness, and home remedies is necessary.

Folk healers are knowledgeable about cultural norms and customs (Edelman & Mandle, 2005). Table 11-1 lists the various healers within the five dominant cultural groups in the United States (European American, African American, Hispanic American, Asian American, and Native American) and the common folk healing practices within these cultures. Nurses must be able to relate care and treatment to the client's cultural context and incorporate informal caregivers, healers, and other members of the client's support system as allies in treatment.

TABLE 11-1 Cultural Groups in Communication, Relationships, Health Values and Beliefs, and Health Practices

CULTURAL GROUP	COMMUNICATIONS STYLES	FAMILY, SOCIAL, AND WORK RELATIONSHIPS	HEALTH VALUES AND BELIEFS	HEALTH CUSTOMS AND PRACTICES
Asian-American				
Chinese	Nonverbal and contextual cues important. Silence after a statement is used by a speaker who wishes the listener to consider the importance of what is said. Self-expression repressed. Value silence. Touching limited. May smile when do not understand. Hesitant to ask questions.	Hierarchical, extended family pattern. Deference to authority figures and elders. Both parents make decisions about children. Value self-reliance and self-restraint. Important to preserve family's honor and save face. Value working hard and giving to society.	Health viewed as gift from parents and ancestors and the result of a balance between the energy forces of *yin* (cold) and *yang* (hot). Illness caused by an imbalance. Blood is the source of life and cannot be regenerated. Lack of blood and chi (innate energy) produces debilitation and long illness. Respect for the body and belief in reincarnation dictates that one must die with the body intact. Believe a good physician can accurately diagnose an illness by simply examining a person using the senses of sight, smell, touch, and listening.	May use medical care system in conjunction with Chinese methods of acupuncture (a *yin* treatment consisting of the insertion of needles to meridians to cure disease or relieve pain) and moxibustion (a *yang* treatment during which heated, pulverized wormwood is applied to appropriate meridians to assist with labor and delivery and other yin disorders). Medicinal herbs, e.g., ginseng, are widely used. Fear painful, intrusive diagnostic tests, especially the drawing of blood. May refuse intrusive surgery or autopsy. May be distrustful of physicians who order and use painful or intrusive diagnostic tests. Accept immunizations as valid means of disease prevention. Heavy use of condiments such as mono-sodium glutamate and soy sauce.
Japanese	Attitude, action, and feeling more important than words. Tend to listen empathically. Touching limited. Direct eye contact considered a lack of respect. Stoic, suppress overt emotion. Value self-control, politeness, and personal restraint.	Close, interdependent, intergenerational relationships. Individual needs subordinate to family's needs. Will endure great hardship to ensure success of next generation. Belonging to right clique or society important to status and success. Obligation to kin and work group. Education highly valued.	Believe illness caused by contact with polluting agents (e.g., blood, skin diseases, corpses), social or family disharmony, or imbalance from poor health habits. Cleanliness highly valued.	Tend to rely on Euro-American medical system for preventive and illness care. Oldest adult child responsible for care of elderly. Care of disabled is a family's responsibility. Take pride in good health of children. Believe in removal of diseased areas. Practice of emotional control may make pain assessment more difficult. When visiting ill, often bring fruit or special Japanese foods.

(Continues)

TABLE 11-1 Cultural Groups in Communication, Relationships, Health Values and Beliefs, and Health Practices (Continued)

CULTURAL GROUP	COMMUNICATIONS STYLES	FAMILY, SOCIAL, AND WORK RELATIONSHIPS	HEALTH VALUES AND BELIEFS	HEALTH CUSTOMS AND PRACTICES
Appalachian	Avoid answering questions related to income, children's school attendance, the affairs of others in the household and of neighbors. May consider direct eye contact impolite or aggressive. Uncomfortable with the impersonal and bureaucratic orientation of the American health system. May evaluate health professional on basis of interpersonal skills rather than on professional competence.	Community interdependence. Stay near home for protection. Keep ties with kin. Guard against strangers and outsiders. Kindness to others valued. Do more for others, less for self.	Disability an inevitable part of life and aging. Severity of illness perceived in terms of degree of dependency it necessitates during the period of illness. Believe cold and lack of personal care cause illness. Frugal; always use home remedies first. The hospital is "the place where people die."	Use folk practices "first and last." Rule for primary prevention: "eat right, take fluids, keep the body strong, stay warm when it's cold." Self-care for minor illnesses. Medical care for serious illnesses. Help from kin as needed for primary care. Help from family members and extended family expected and accepted.

Note: Used by permission from Estes, M., Health Assessment & Physical Examination, 4th edition (2010). Clifton Park, NY: Delmar Cengage Learning. Compiled from information in Transcultural Nursing: Assessment and Intervention *(4th ed.), by J. N. Giger and R. E. Davidhizar, 2004, Baltimore: Mosby*; Transcultural Nursing: Concepts. Theory, Research, and Practice *(3rd ed.), by M. M. Leininger and M. McFarland, 2002, New York: McGraw-Hill Professional*; Pocket Guide to Cultural Assessment *(3rd ed.), by E. M. Geissler, 2003, Baltimore: Mosby-Year Book*; Cultural Diversity in Health and Illness *(6th ed.), by R. Spector, 2003, Norwalk, CT: Appleton & Lange*; Wong's Nursing Care of Infants and Children *(7th ed.), by D. L. Wong, M. J. Hockenberry, D. Wilson, M. L. Winkelstein, and N. E. Kline, 2003, Philadelphia: Mosby*; Transcultural Health Care: A Culturally Competent Approach *(2nd ed.), by L. Purnell and F. Paulanka, 2003, Philadelphia: F. A. Davis.*

Beliefs of Select Cultural Groups

While the population of the United States encompasses innumerable ethnic groups, European Americans, African Americans, Hispanic Americans, Asian Americans, and Native Americans together represent a majority. These groups form the basis for the following brief discussion of specific health beliefs influenced by culture.

European American

In 2000, Americans of European descent represented 71% of the U.S. population (U.S. Census Bureau, 2001). The prevailing value system for many European Americans is based on what is referred to as the white, Anglo-Saxon, Protestant (WASP) ethic (Sue & Sue, 2007). This ethnic group traces its origins to the Caucasian Protestants who came to this country from northern Europe more than 200 years ago. Values that still dominate the Caucasian American middle-class ethic include independence, individuality, wealth, comfort, cleanliness, achievement, punctuality, hard work, aggression, assertiveness, rationality, orientation toward the future, and mastery of one's own fate (Andrews & Boyle, 2008; Edmission, 1997).

Traditionally, most Caucasian Americans have wanted to be recognized as individuals rather than as members of groups. Thus, Caucasian Americans, unlike members of many other cultures, tend to be competitive rather than cooperative with each other. Mainstream American culture also values the nuclear family and its traditions (Luckmann, 2000).

African American

The African American population in 2000 represented 12% of the U.S. population (U.S. Census Bureau, 2001). African American ancestors came to North America from various African countries and the Caribbean as either free immigrants or slaves. The heterogeneous (different) cultural practices among African Americans today may be explained by the diverse countries of origin, disparate educational levels, income, occupations, and religious beliefs.

Traditional African societies may believe that disease is caused by disharmony in relationships. Discord may occur between a client and evil spirits, living relatives, or ancestral spirits. Restoration of harmony may be achieved through prayer, meditation, or other activities, such as wearing a charm, offering a gift, or confessing a wrong, leading to healing.

Disease may be viewed as sent by God or another higher power as a punishment for a serious infraction. Evil forces may be thought to account for illness in other cases. Healing may be found in home remedies and herbs, consultation with a local healer, or prayer.

CULTURAL CONSIDERATIONS

Subculture

Many Caucasian Americans do not belong to the mainstream culture but instead belong to ethnic subcultures that hold strong values of their own (e.g., Irish, Jewish, German, Italian, Norwegian, Appalachian, and Amish subcultures).

Hispanic American

Hispanic Americans also represented 12% of the U.S. population in 2000 (U.S. Census Bureau, 2001). The majority of this group has origins in Mexico, Puerto Rico, and Cuba. Although the Spanish language is common to most Hispanics, cultural patterns vary according to the different countries of origin. The Hispanic American usually belongs to a large extended family system within which females are seen as subservient to males but as having a major role in family cohesiveness (Giger & Davidhizar, 2004).

In Hispanic populations the influence of religion on culture is particularly evident. Most Hispanic Americans have roots in Catholicism blended with traditional Indian beliefs. Illness may be viewed as "an act of God" as punishment for sin, as the result of witchcraft or a curse by an enemy, or as having a natural cause. Diseases may be traced to an imbalance between "hot" and "cold" or "wet" and "dry" forces. Treatment depends on the cause. Western medicine is believed to be appropriate for some diseases, whereas the native healer (curandera) may be called on to intervene for illnesses having supernatural causes. The elders of the community are valued for folk care knowledge, sometimes taking precedence over professional health care advice. Families have an obligation to care for the ill person. Treatment may consist of religious ceremonies, herbal potions, or diets based on hot and cold foods. If the Hispanic client wears an amulet, he believes that the removal of it precedes certain death. The amulet is believed to protect the person from external evils, and the person is reluctant to remove it.

Asian American

Asian Americans, representing 4% of the U.S. population in 2000 (U.S. Census Bureau, 2001), have origins in the Pacific Rim countries: China, Japan, Korea, Vietnam, Laos, the Philippines, and Cambodia. Generalization of a specific Asian culture is not possible; however, certain similarities do exist. Family relations are traced through males. Males as the head of household are the decision makers. Elders are revered and respected. Only physical complaints are acceptable, and maintaining eye contact is considered disrespectful (Estin, 1999).

Asians believe in yin (cold) and yang (hot) as etiology of disease. **Yin and yang** are opposing forces that yield health when in balance. An imbalance in these forces causes illness. Foods are identified as either hot or cold and are used in treatment. For example, if yang is overpowering yin, hot foods are avoided until balance is restored. Illness may be thought to be caused by supernatural powers such as God, ancestral spirits, or evil spirits. In this situation, healing is sought through prayer or treatment by a traditional healer. Many Asian Americans rely on acupuncture, herbal remedies, and cupping and burning. In cupping, the inside and rim of a cup are heated with a candle flame. Then the rim of the cup is applied directly to the client's skin. Blood is drawn to the surface of the skin as the cup cools, causing a bruised appearance. Cupping is used to draw out evil or illness in order to restore yin and yang. The nurse, aware of these cultural practices, views them not as abusive but as an important cultural custom.

Native American

Native Americans represented 1% of the U.S. population in 2000 (U.S. Census Bureau, 2001). These peoples form a very diverse group, descending from more than 200 different tribes across the United States. Although many Native Americans have assumed Euro-American practices with regard to health, some still use traditional practices. Health is believed to result from a harmonious relationship with nature and the universe. Illness is frequently traced to a supernatural origin and discord with the forces of nature. Using witchcraft is believed to cause illness, and treatment may require the exorcism of evil spirits. Disease prevention may be achieved through prayer, charms, and fetishes (objects having power to protect or aid the owner). "Medicine men" are persons believed to have supernatural powers of healing. Health may be restored through herbal drinks, prayers, rituals, and ceremonies.

CULTURAL AND RACIAL INFLUENCES ON CLIENT CARE

Clients' cultural backgrounds and preferences influence the manner whereby they interact with other people and with the world around them. In an unfamiliar situation, such as admission to a health care setting, cultural differences may seem even greater. In these instances of stress, most people hold tightly to that which is familiar in order to protect themselves from the unknown. The nurse can show caring in such a situation by acknowledging the expression of these differences and encouraging the client to retain what is familiar. Providing opportunities for decisions in their care decreases the stress of unfamiliar situations.

The influences of culture and race can be viewed through the phenomena of communication, space and time orientation, social organization, and biological variations.

Communication

Although language is common to all human beings, not everyone shares the same language. This cultural difference can lead to misunderstanding and frustration. The nurse must realize that a client who speaks a different language or with an accent simply has a different means of expressing needs. When communication is restricted because of language differences, alternative methods of communication, such as gestures and flash cards, can be used.

PROFESSIONALTIP

Nonnative Speakers

When interacting with someone who does not understand English well, many people will try to compensate for the lack of understanding by speaking loudly. Speaking slowly, distinctly, and in a normal volume; making eye contact; and avoiding slang and medical jargon are effective measures to ensure communication.

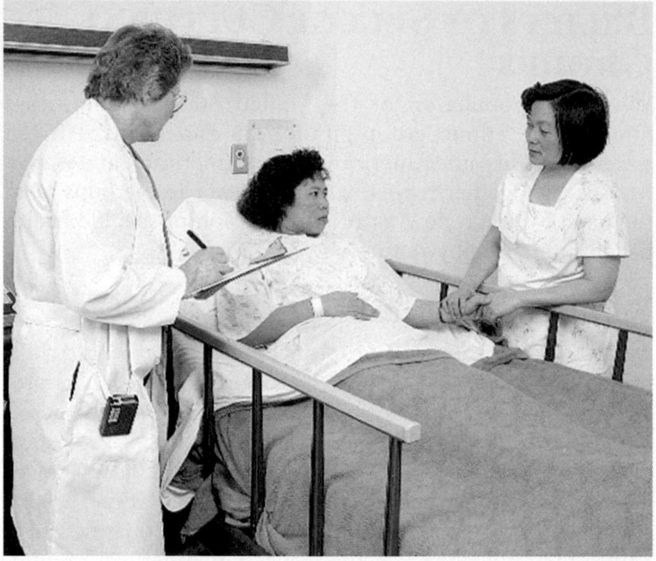

COURTESY OF DELMAR CENGAGE LEARNING

FIGURE 11-2 Family members may serve as interpreters to help clients who do not speak English understand procedures and instructions, and to communicate the client's thoughts and questions to the nurse.

The client's family may be able to assist when there is a block in communication. Family members can interpret procedures and instructions for the client and communicate the client's thoughts and questions to the nurse (Figure 11-2). If no family members are available, the hospital social worker may be able to find an interpreter. Often hospitals will have a pool of staff or people within the community whom they can request to interpret for different clients as needed.

Orientation to Space and Time

Orientation with regard to space and time represents two other culturally influenced variables that may affect a client's attitude toward care. Territoriality, or interpretation of personal space, is a pattern of behavior resulting from an individual's belief that certain spaces and objects belong to that person. The distance that a person prefers to maintain from another is determined by one's culture. In general, people of Arabic, southern European, and African origin frequently sit or stand relatively close to each other (0–18 inches), whereas people of Asian, northern European, and North American origin are more comfortable with a larger personal space (more than 18 inches).

Affection and caring behaviors are not communicated by touch in some cultures. For instance, among Asians, adults seldom touch one another, and the head is believed to be sacred. The nurse should thus not touch an Asian client's head without permission to do so. When working with clients from cultures where personal touch is viewed negatively, the nurse should use the universal sign of caring and acceptance: the smile.

People in U.S. society tend to be future oriented: They plan for the future, establish long-term goals, and, increasingly, are concerned with prevention of future illnesses. In daily life, they are oriented to time of day, constantly referring to clock time for everything from mealtime to time of appointments with health care professionals as well as other obligations. The nurse must also be very attentive to time. Medications are given at scheduled times, and work begins and ends at specified times. Other groups that tend to be future oriented are Japanese, Jews, and Arabs. These groups tend to view time as a commodity for achieving future goals.

Not all cultural groups are future oriented, however. People of some cultures (e.g., Asians) may be oriented to the past. For Asians, this orientation is reflected in the roles that ancestor worship and Confucianism play in the present. Members of other cultural groups, such as Native Americans, tend to be present oriented. Many Native Americans do not own clocks, and they live one day at a time, showing little concern for the future (Giger & Davidhizer, 2004). Mexican Americans and African Americans often value relationships with people in the present more than in the future. African Americans tend to be present oriented in health care behaviors as well. They often express the fatalistic belief that "it's going to happen anyway, so why bother" and fail to seek medical attention until a disabling condition occurs. The African American culture often teaches flexible attention to schedules; whatever is happening currently is most important. Explanations about the necessity of time scheduling (e.g., the need for strict schedules for medication requiring therapeutic blood level maintenance) must be given to the client.

An individual's orientation to time may affect promptness or attendance at health care appointments, compliance with self-medication schedules, and reporting the onset of illness or other health concerns. Clients might not see the necessity for preventive health care measures if they experience no difference in their health today when they follow a special diet or exercise program. The nurse teaches clients when timing is critical in health care situations and practices patience when working with people whose background differs from that of the dominant culture.

Social Organization

Social organization refers to the ways that cultural groups determine rules of acceptable behavior and roles of individual members. Examples of social organization include family structure, gender roles, and religion.

Family Structure

The definition of family has changed dramatically through the years. Until 1920, the norm was the "institutional family," which was organized around economic production and the kinship network. Marriage was not a romantic relationship but a functional one. Family loyalty and tradition were more important than individual romantic interests or goals. Responsibility was the chief value.

From 1920 to 1960, the norm was the "psychological family." Affairs were more private and less tied to the extended family. Family was based on fulfillment of the individual members and personal satisfaction in a nuclear, two-parent arrangement. Satisfaction was the chief value (Figure 11-3).

The social changes of the 1960s caused modifications in the family, including gender equality and personal freedom. The increased divorce rate may have resulted from the sexual revolution and the attitude that the individual deserves more and owes less to the family.

Today, no single family arrangement has a monopoly. Many types of families have emerged and are accepted. Flexibility is the chief value. Family no longer necessarily implies biological relation but rather has come to mean members of

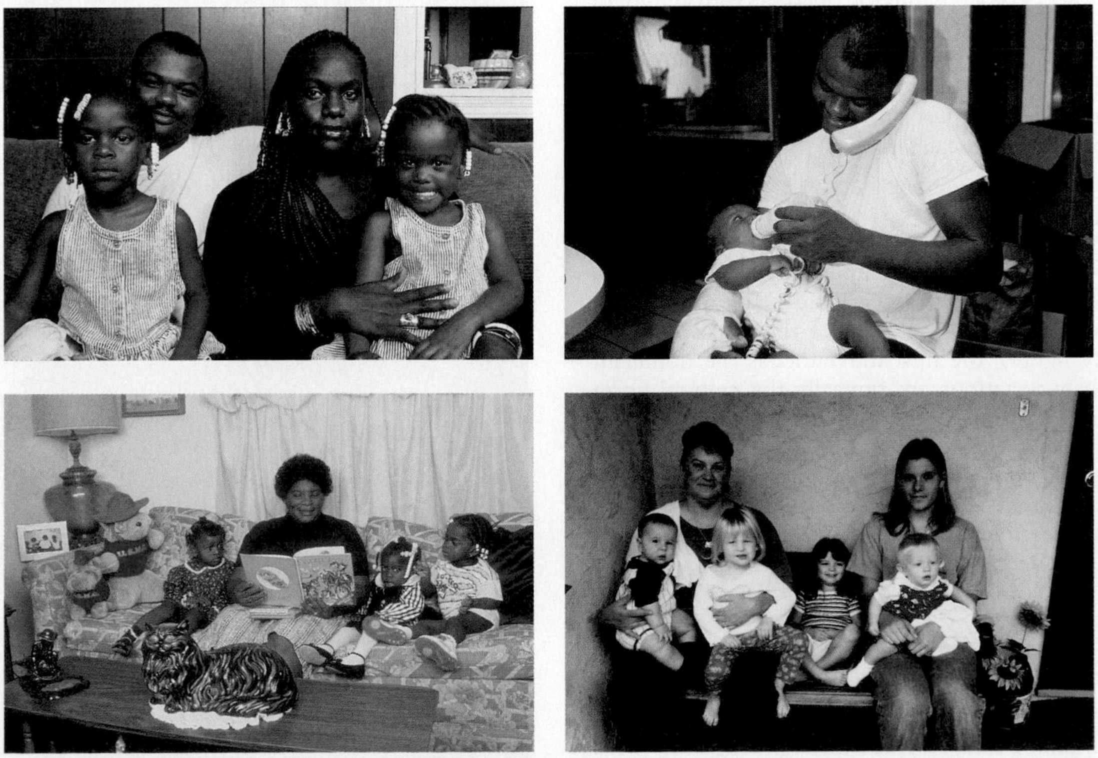

Figure 11-3 Family structures are diverse.

PROFESSIONALTIP

Families

Each individual defines family differently. These definitions are shaped by personal experience and observation of other families. Nurses must remain objective and nonjudgmental when the client's family is different from their idea of family. The client should identify family members so that the nurse knows exactly who the client considers to be family.

a shared household who have similar values and participate in shared goals. Fawcett (1993) cites the following characteristics of family:

- Love and affection
- Caring and compassion
- Sense of belonging and connectedness
- History and linkage to posterity
- Rituals of rejoicing
- Sense of place
- Acceptance of members, including shortcomings
- Honor of elders
- System of earning and spending money
- Competent manner of parenting or caretaking
- Division of chores and labor

Systems theory states that families are considered to be interacting, interdependent individuals related by marriage, birth, or mutual consent. Examples of families with varying lifestyles today are two-parent nuclear (parents with children), attenuated (single parent with children), blended (through remarriage), extended (including grandparents), incipient (married couple with no children), cohabitating (couple having never married), gay or lesbian, divorced, adoptive, multi-adult, and mixed or interracial families.

Gender Roles

Gender roles vary according to cultural context (Figure 11-4). For example, in families organized around a patriarchal structure (with the man being the head of the household and chief authority figure), the husband/father is the dominant member. Such expectations are typically the cultural norm in Latino, Hispanic, and traditional Muslim families. The husband/father is the one who makes decisions regarding health care for all family members. Also, in such cultures, the wife is responsible for child care and household maintenance, whereas the father's role is to protect and support the family members.

Religion

Anthropologists have identified the strength of the influence of religion on culture. In many cases, culture and tradition have been maintained and preserved through religious beliefs. Religion often is the formal organizational structure for social behavior.

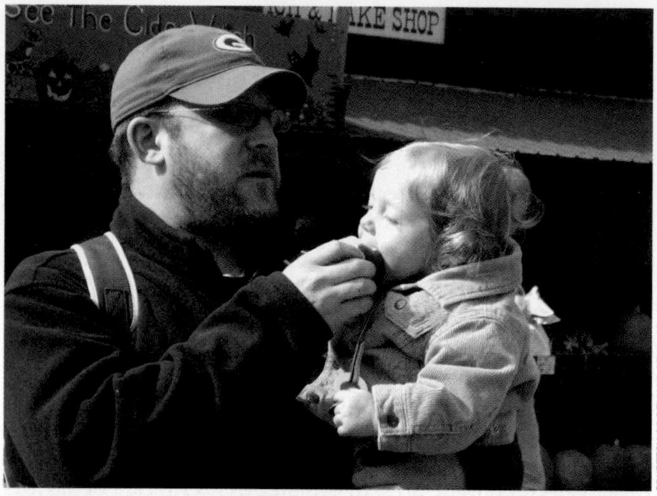

COURTESY OF DELMAR CENGAGE LEARNING

FIGURE 11-4 Fathers assuming more responsibility in caring for children is one example of shifting gender roles.

Religious and spiritual beliefs are important in many individuals' lives. These beliefs can influence attitudes, lifestyle, and feelings about life, pain, and death. Some religions specify practices about diet, birth control, and appropriate medical care. Often, spiritual beliefs assume a greater significance at the time of illness than at other times in a person's life. These

COMMUNITY/HOME HEALTH CARE

Culturally Sensitive Care

To provide culturally sensitive care in the home:

- Remember that the setting for care is controlled not by the health care provider but by the client and family.
- Be aware that the nurse is often viewed as a guest by the client and family. Social communication may be necessary to facilitate rapport.
- Be nonjudgmental about the home (e.g., presence of clutter and disarray).
- Display consideration and respect for the client. For example:
  —Before entering the home, wipe your feet.
  —Before washing your hands, ask permission to use the sink or bathroom.
  —Before moving the client's belongings, ask permission, then replace items when finished.
- Benefit from the home environment by assessing cultural values and norms. Clues to cultural values may include:
  —Possessions and decor on display in the home
  —Family roles and task assignment
  —Interactions among family members
  —Value placed on privacy and possessions

beliefs assist some people in accepting their illnesses and help explain illness for others. Religion can both help people live fuller lives and console or strengthen people during suffering and in preparation for death. Religion, by providing meaning to life and death, can supply the client, the family, and the nurse with a sense of security and strength during a time of need.

Spiritual needs are identified as an individual's desire to find purpose and meaning in life, pain, and death. To provide holistic care, the nurse must be attentive to the spiritual dimension of each client and assist the client in meeting spiritual needs (Figure 11-5).

While spiritual needs are recognized by many nurses, **spiritual care** (recognition of and assistance toward meeting spiritual needs) is often neglected. Spirituality is defined as an individual's search to find purpose and meaning in life. The goal of spiritual nursing care is to empower clients to identify and utilize their spiritual beliefs to cope with a health crisis. Among reasons that nurses give for failing to provide spiritual care are:

- Spirituality is a private matter.
- They are uninformed about the religious beliefs of others.
- They have not identified their own spiritual beliefs.
- Meeting the spiritual needs of the client is a family or clergy responsibility, not a nursing responsibility.

Spiritual nursing care is appropriate when the nurse cares about the client's emotional, physical, and psychosocial health. The nursing diagnosis of *Spiritual Distress* can be apparent in a client who is unable to practice religious or spiritual rituals because of illness or confinement in a health care institution.

The **religious support system** is a group of ministers, priests, nuns, rabbis, shamans, mullahs, or laypersons who are able to meet clients' spiritual needs. The nurse is responsible for working with these individuals and including them in the client care team.

Be aware of the general philosophies of clients' spiritual beliefs and also be aware that some individuals do not believe in a higher being or practice a specific religion. **Agnostics** believe that the existence of God cannot be proved or disproved, whereas **atheists** do not believe in God or any other deity.

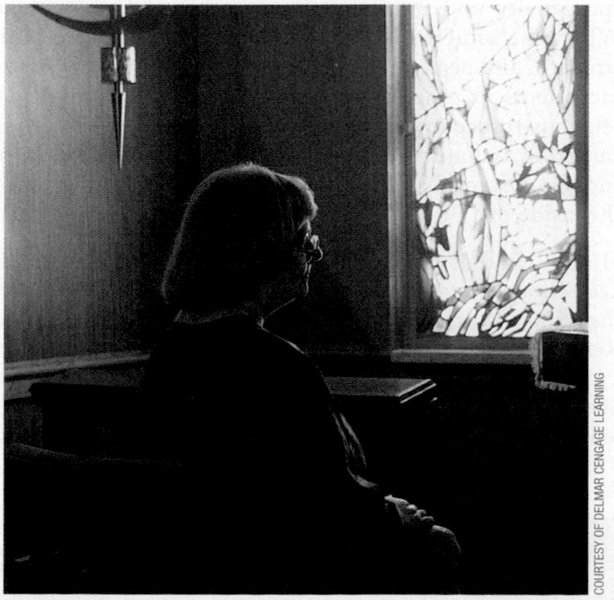

FIGURE 11-5 **Spiritual needs often increase when individuals are sick.**

It is important to identify particular beliefs from various religions that can influence client care activities. Some of these beliefs concern holy day practices, dietary restrictions, birth, death, and organ donation.

Protestant Many separate denominations (more than 1,200) constitute the group known as Protestant. Protestant groups include such denominations as Baptist, Episcopal, Lutheran, Methodist, Presbyterian, and Seventh-Day Adventist. The majority worship on Sunday, and their primary written reference is the Holy Bible.

Baptist Baptists believe that baptism is performed only after the believer reaches an age of understanding and confesses a personal acceptance of Jesus' saving work. Communion is a spiritual act symbolizing the suffering, death, and resurrection of the Lord.

Episcopal Episcopalians have a number of sacraments, including baptism, confession, communion, and anointing of the sick (Holy Unction). Holy Unction is most often given as a healing sacrament. They believe that a dying infant should be baptized, and a nurse may perform the rite. Usually, an Episcopal priest administers these sacraments.

Lutheran Traditionally, Lutherans baptize infants and adults by sprinkling. Any baptized Christian may perform an emergency baptism. The Lutheran churches recognize two sacraments: baptism and Holy Communion. Holy Communion is understood to be the body and the blood of Jesus. It is often administered to the ill or those awaiting surgery. Central to Lutheran doctrine is the belief in "justification by faith." People are redeemed by God solely on the basis of God's grace, which they receive through faith in what God has done for them.

Methodist Methodists practice both infant and adult baptism. For them, religion is a matter of personal belief, and the conscience is used as a guide for living.

Presbyterian Presbyterians also practice baptism and communion, which is a remembering of the death of Jesus Christ for them. Salvation is believed to be a gift from God.

Seventh-Day Adventist Seventh-Day Adventists baptize individuals only after they reach an age of accountability. Some dietary restrictions are followed. Sunset on Friday to sunset on Saturday is observed as their Sabbath. Jobs or worldly pleasures are not pursued during this time.

Roman Catholic Priests perform various rites known as Sacraments (sacred) at various times in the life of the Catholic. Sacraments that might be encountered in the health care setting are baptism, the Eucharist (Communion), confession, and sacrament of the sick. Baptism, administered only once in the life of a Catholic, is believed to be absolutely necessary for salvation. A client preparing for communion is generally asked to abstain from food or drink an hour before the rite. Water and medications are allowed at any time. Confession is a sacrament for forgiveness of sins. It should be respected as a very private matter. The Sacrament of the Sick, in which the client is anointed with holy oil, was formerly given to someone near death and was called the "last rites."

Orthodox Orthodox churches show their love of God through worship liturgies. It is important that followers remain faithful to the teachings of the ancient church. Holy Unction, anointing the body with oil, is used for healing of both bodily and spiritual infirmities. Baptism is important, so in life-threatening situations an unbaptized child should have an emergency baptism.

Jehovah's Witness Receiving any blood or blood products, including plasma, is prohibited. Also, they will not eat anything containing blood. Blood volume expanders that are not derivatives of blood are permissible. To receive blood when a medical condition requiring blood transfusion is life threatening, children have been made wards of the court. They hold a special observance of the Lord's Supper.

Mormon (Church of Jesus Christ of the Latter-Day Saints) Mormons baptize at the age of 8 years. When necessary, baptism of the dead is performed for adults. Mormons wear a special undergarment that symbolizes dedication to God. This may be worn under the hospital gown.

Christian Science Christian Scientists believe that illness will be eliminated through prayer and spiritual understanding. A critically ill Christian Scientist client may wish to have a Christian Science practitioner contacted to provide treatment through prayer. They usually do not use medicine, do not agree to surgical procedures, and do not accept blood transfusions.

Scientology is a study of the interactions of the spirit with itself, others, and life (Church of Scientology International, 2009). The fundamental truths of the scientology religion are that man is an immortal, spiritual being with unlimited capabilities that allow him to solve problems, accomplish goals, gain lasting happiness, and gain higher awareness and abilities (Church of Scientology International, 2009). Man consists of the spirit, called thetan (thought or spirit); mind; and body. The mind is a means of communication between himself and his environment. The body is not the person. The thetan is the most important component making up the spirit or individuality of a person. A main principle of scientology is the ARC Triangle, which guides interpersonal relationships and understanding (Church of Scientology International, 2009). The ARC Triangle consists of affinity, reality, and communication. Affinity is the emotional response of affection or lack of affection. Reality is the real objects in life. Communication is the interchange of ideas. For communication to occur, there must be agreement and affinity. To improve communication, persons find something on which they agree and improve affinity by talk or contact and tangible touch.

An individual applies principles of Scientology through a process called auditing (Church of Scientology International, 2009). During an auditing session, the auditor helps an individual explore and rid oneself of damaging spiritual conditions and thereby improve awareness and ability.

American Indian Religions That all life is sacred and all things are interconnected is the central belief of the various religions. Community importance is emphasized. The individual who is able to communicate with the spirits or the Great Spirit is the spiritual leader. There are no written religious books. Religious traditions are passed on orally and through participation in ceremonies and festivals. Illness may be the result of a sin or a spirit or god who is unhappy.

Judaism Judaism is both an ethnic identity and a religious faith. The religion is based on the five books of Moses called the Torah. Religion and culture are deeply interwoven in the Jewish faith, resulting in ritual, tradition, religious ceremony, and social laws.

There are three groups of Judaism: Orthodox, Conservative, and Reformed. They vary in how strictly they follow the traditions, but all share the fundamental teachings of Judaism. Orthodox Jews strictly observe all traditional practices. The Conservative group observes many of the traditional practices, and the Reformed group loosely interprets the traditions. The spiritual leader of the Jewish congregation is the rabbi and the person to be informed when a client requests it. The Jewish Sabbath, or day of worship, begins at sunset on Friday and ends at sunset on Saturday. Circumcision is performed on the male infant 8 days after birth. It may be done by the pediatrician or by the Mohel, who may also be a rabbi.

Islam Islam is the religion of Muslims. Allah is the supreme deity, and Mohammed, the founder of Islam, is the chief prophet. The Muslim's day of worship lasts from sunset on Thursday to sunset on Friday. Some Muslims pray five times a day (after dawn, at noon, at mid-afternoon, after sunset, and at night). A bed or chair may be positioned facing southeast (in the continental United States) when a client requests that he face Mecca, the holy city of Islam. Muslim clients may wear an article of writing from the Koran on a piece of string around the neck, waist, or arm. This should not be removed or allowed to get wet. Rules of cleanliness involve eating with the right hand and cleansing self with the left hand after defecating or urinating. Hand medications or other materials to the Muslim client with the right hand so as not to offend them.

Some Islamic females wish to be clothed from head to ankle. They may prefer to undress one body part at a time during a physical examination and may refuse to be cared for by male nurses or physicians.

Buddhism Buddhism is a general term indicating a belief in Buddha, "the enlightened one." Nirvana, a state of greater spontaneity and inner freedom, is the goal of existence. When one achieves Nirvana, the mind has supreme purity, strength, and peace. Buddhism does not dictate any specific sacraments or practices. There are no special holy days or religious restrictions for therapy. Buddhists believe in reincarnation but not in healing through faith. The religious support system for the sick is the priest. Figure 11-6 shows the inside of a Buddhist temple.

Hindu Hinduism has no common doctrines or creeds that keep Hindus together. They are free to worship one or more of their 320,000 gods. The Vedas are the Scripture of Hinduism. Reincarnation is central in Hindu thought. Freedom from the cycle of rebirth and death and entrance into what the Hindus, like the Buddhists, call Nirvana is the goal of existence. Hindu temples are dwelling places of deities and where offerings are

CRITICAL THINKING

Religion and Culture

Describe your religious support system.

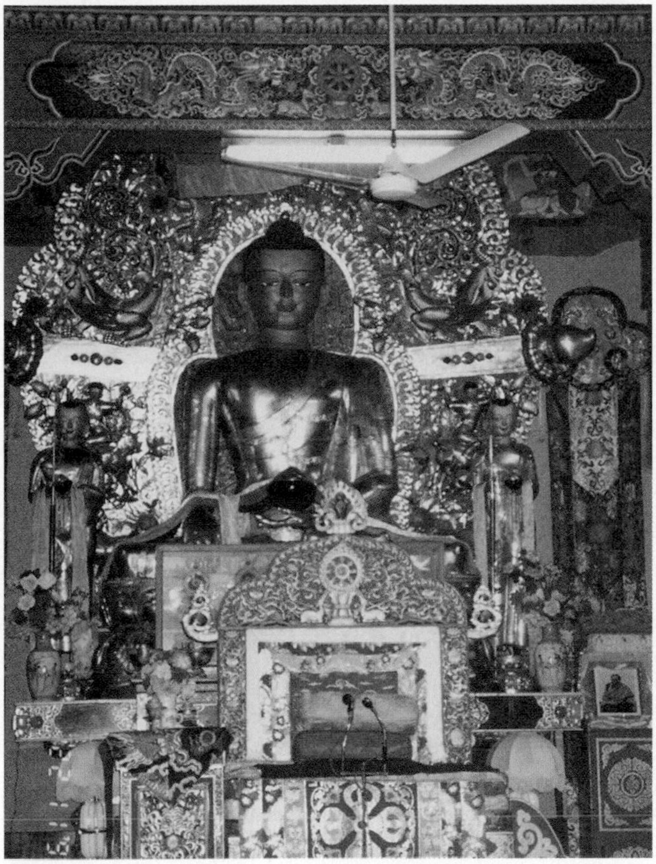

FIGURE 11-6 The inside of a Buddhist temple.

brought. Some Hindus believe that illness is God's way of punishing a person for sins; others believe in faith healing.

BIOLOGICAL VARIATION

Biological variations distinguish one racial or cultural group from another. Easily identified biological variations include skin color, hair texture, eye shape, thickness of lips, and body structure (Degazon, 2000). Less obvious biological variations include enzyme differences and susceptibility to disease (Andrews & Boyle, 2008; Giger & Davidhizar, 2004). Enzyme differences account for varied responses of some groups to dietary and drug therapy (Table 11-2).

According to Kudzma (1999), drug metabolism is genetically determined, and race seems to affect the response. A drug is more efficient in clients who metabolize the drug rapidly. Sometimes it may be metabolized too quickly for the full clinical effect to be achieved. When a drug is metabolized slowly, it is less effective, and the client experiences greater drug toxicity.

CULTURAL ASPECTS AND THE NURSING PROCESS

Each individual comes from a cultural background that, in some way, influences behavior and attitudes about health and illness. Personal attitudes and behaviors determine not only the ways that clients interpret health events and utilize health care but also the ways that nurses interpret health events and

TABLE 11-2 Biological Variations

Cultural Group	Biological Variation
European American	• Liver enzyme differences cause caffeine to be metabolized and excreted faster. • Increased susceptibility for breast cancer, heart disease.
African American	• Isoniazid (drug used to treat tuberculosis) is metabolized rapidly, thereby becoming quickly inactive; occurs in approximately 60% of population. • Increased susceptibility for keloid formation, hypertension, lactose intolerance, sickle cell disease. • Higher doses of antihypertensive drugs (e.g., propranolol) must be administered to produce same effects as in European Americans.
Hispanic American	• Increased susceptibility for diabetes, hypertension, lactose intolerance.
Asian American	• Isoniazid is metabolized rapidly, thereby becoming quickly inactive; occurs in approximately 85% to 90% of population. • Alcohol is rapidly metabolished resulting in excessive facial flushing and other vasomotor symptoms. • Increased susceptibility for hypertension, liver and stomach cancer, lactose intolerance. • Chinese men require half as much propranolol (antihypertensive drug) to produce same effects as in European American men.
Native American	• Isoniazid is metabolized rapidly, thereby becoming quickly inactive; occurs in approximately 60% to 90% of population. • Increased susceptibility for tuberculosis, diabetes, cirrhosis of the liver, heart disease. • Rapid metabolism of alcohol results in excessive facial flushing and other vasomotor symptoms

Data compiled from *Transcultural Concepts in Nursing Care*, by M. Andrews and J. Boyle, 2003, Philadelphia: Lippincott Williams & Wilkins; *Transcultural Nursing: Assessment and Intervention* (4th ed.), by J. Giger and R. Davidhizar, 2004, St. Louis, MO: Mosby-Year Book; Cultural Diversity and Community Health Nursing, by C. Degazon, in *Community Health Nursing* (5th ed.), by M. Stanhope and J. Lancaster (Eds.), 2000, St. Louis, MO: Mosby-Year Book; and *Transcultural Concepts in Nursing Care* (5th ed.), by M. M. Andrews and J. S. Boyle, 2008, Philadelphia, PA: Lippincott Williams & Wilkins.

PROFESSIONAL TIP

Culturally Diverse Coworkers

Many nursing units have a mix of nationalities and cultures. While such a mix has the potential of improving nursing care, in practice it often leads to conflict and poor teamwork. The same cultural differences discussed in relation to clients may also be found among coworkers. Ways to successfully manage diversity in the workplace include:

- Be aware of your own biases and strive to avoid stereotyping others.
- Be aware of the way in which the things you do and say affect others.
- Help others be more sensitive and help correct misconceptions.
- Learn to welcome different opinions and viewpoints.
- Be open to feedback.

Nurses must cultivate a cultural consciousness. There must be a heightened sensitivity and awareness of the uniqueness and diversity of perspective each individual has to offer. Cultural awareness is essential in the process of providing appropriate, effective care (Mullins, 1999). As health care professionals, even if we cannot understand or accept particular cultural practices, it is important to show respect for them. This directly reflects how we value our own beliefs and practices.

their personal views about health and illness before assessing and caring for clients from other cultural groups.

Assessment

Culturally sensitive nursing care begins with an examination of one's own culture and beliefs. It is followed by an assessment of the client's cultural beliefs and background.

Personal Cultural Assessment

Spradley and Allender (2001) suggest five areas to be examined when assessing one's culture and the influence it has on personal beliefs about health care:

- Influences from racial/ethnic background
- Usual verbal and nonverbal communication patterns
- Cultural norms and values
- Religious practices and beliefs
- Health practices and beliefs

They suggest that the nurse identifies information on each issue and then validates this information with another person(s) from the same cultural group.

CRITICAL THINKING

Culture and Health Practices

How has your culture influenced your beliefs about health practices?

If a client put an amulet (religious icon and necklace) around her newborn's neck, how would you approach the client to discuss your concern about the risk of strangulation?

Client Cultural Assessment

After examining one's own culture and the influences it had in developing personal beliefs about health and sickness, then assess the client's cultural background (Figure 11-7). Data about various cultures may be collected from members of the culture to be studied, from others familiar with the culture, or from the local library.

Six categories of information necessary for a comprehensive cultural assessment of the client are suggested by Spradley and Allender (2001):

- *Ethnic or racial background.* Where did the client group originate, and how does that influence the status and identity of group members?
- *Language and communication patterns.* What is the preferred language spoken, and what are the culturally based communication patterns?
- *Cultural values and norms.* What are the beliefs, values, and standards regarding education, roles, leisure, family functions, child rearing, work, aging, death and dying, and rites of passage?
- *Biocultural factors.* Are there genetic or physical traits unique to the ethnic or racial group that predispose group members to certain conditions or illnesses?
- *Religious beliefs and practices.* What are the religious beliefs, and how do they influence roles, life events, health, and illness?
- *Health beliefs and practices.* What are the beliefs and practices regarding treatment, causes, and prevention of illnesses?

Nursing Diagnosis

Any nursing diagnosis may be appropriate for a client of any cultural group. When cultural variables are identified during assessment, the nurse should be as specific as possible when asking questions and determining appropriate nursing diagnoses so that interventions can be individualized with respect to the client's cultural beliefs. For instance, *Decreased Cardiac Output* may be viewed by the nurse or physician as having a medical or physical cause, whereas the client may attribute the origin to an imbalance of yin and yang. Table 11-3 lists select nursing diagnoses that are most likely to have cultural implications.

Planning/Outcome Identification

Cultural variables must be taken into consideration when establishing goals and planning interventions. Care will be

Cultural Assessment Guide

Name: ______________________

Nickname or other names or special meaning attributed to your name: ______________________

Primary language:

When speaking ______________________

When writing ______________________

Date of birth: ______________________

Place of birth: ______________________

Educational level or specialized training: ______________________

To which ethnic group do you belong? ______________________

To what extent do you identify with your cultural group? ______________________

Who is the spokesperson for your family? ______________________

Describe some of the customs or beliefs that you have about the following:

Health ______________________

Life ______________________

Illness ______________________

Death ______________________

How do you learn information best?

☐ Reading

☐ Having someone explain verbally

☐ Having someone demonstrate

Describe some of your family's dietary habits and your personal food preferences. ______________________

Are there any foods forbidden from your diet for religious or cultural reasons? ______________________

Describe your religious affiliation. ______________________

What role do your religious beliefs and practices play in your life during times of good health and poor health? ______________________

Who/what is your primary source of information about your health? ______________________

On whom do you rely for health care services or healing? ______________________

Of what cultural health practices are you aware, and which do you utilize? ______________________

Are there cultural restrictions that your caregiver should know? ______________________

Describe your current living arrangements. ______________________

How do members of your family communicate with each other? ______________________

Describe your strengths. ______________________

Is there anything else that is important about your cultural beliefs that you would like to share? ______________________

(Adapted from Daniels, Grendell, & Wilkins, 2010, *Nursing Fundamentals: Caring and Clinical Decision Making*, Delmar Cengage Learning.)

FIGURE 11-7 Cultural Assessment Guide

TABLE 11-3 Nursing Diagnoses With Cultural Implications

Anxiety
*Disturbed **B**ody Image*
*Ineffective **B**reastfeeding*
*Impaired Verbal **C**ommunication*
*Decisional **C**onflict (specify)*
*Ineffective **C**oping*
*Compromised Family **C**oping*
***F**ear*
*Anticipatory **G**rieving*
*Ineffective **H**ealth Maintenance*
***H**ealth-Seeking Behaviors (specify)*
***N**oncompliance*
*Imbalanced **N**utrition: More Than Body Requirements*
***P**ain*
*Ineffective **R**ole Performance*
*Disturbed **S**leep Pattern*
*Impaired **S**ocial Interaction*
***S**piritual Distress*

CLIENT TEACHING

Culturally Sensitive Teaching Guidelines

Consider the following guidelines for teaching clients from diverse cultures:

- Identify the client's cultural background.
- Evaluate the client's current knowledge by asking the client to state what he knows about the topic.
- Identify the perception of need by asking the client and family what they need and want to learn.
- Observe interactions between the client and family to determine family roles and authority figures. Ask the client which family member they would like included in teaching and care sessions.
- Use language easily understood by the client, avoiding jargon and complex medical terms.
- Clarify your verbal and nonverbal messages with the client.
- Ask the client to repeat the information. Ask the client to do a return demonstration of the material taught.

most effective when the client and family are active participants in planning care and when cultural preferences are respected. Suggested goals to consider when cultural factors are involved include:

PROFESSIONAL TIP

Culturally Appropriate Care

- Respect clients for their beliefs.
- Be sensitive to behaviors and practices different from your own.
- Accommodate differences if they are not detrimental to the client's health. For example, a client might believe that eating onions will resolve his respiratory infection. While eating onions may not be therapeutic, it is also not likely to cause any health problems.
- Listen for cues in the client's conversation that relay a unique ethnic belief about prevention, etiology, transmission, or some other aspect of disease. For example, a client might say, "I knew I would be sick today. I heard an owl last night."
- Use the occasion to teach positive health habits if the client's practices are deleterious to good health. For example, when asked about her diet, a pregnant woman might reply that she never eats meat or eggs while pregnant because she believes that gaining too much weight will increase her risk of a difficult delivery. This situation offers the nurse an opportunity to provide nutritional instruction.

- Client will express health care needs to family and caregiver.
- Client will maintain cultural health practices as appropriate.
- Client and family will understand the effect that health care beliefs have on health status.

IMPLEMENTATION

Cultural aspects are always a factor in a nursing care plan, and effective communication and client education are important nursing responsibilities that can enhance cultural understanding and appreciation. Interventions should be carried out in a manner that will respect, to the degree possible, the preferences and desires of the client. When a client does not speak or understand the native language well, the nurse should arrange to have an interpreter present to explain procedures and tests.

EVALUATION

Evaluation includes feedback from the client and family to determine their reaction to the interventions. Revisions to the plan of care are made with client and family input and alternative sources and resources brought in when needed to enhance communication and exchange of information. Culturally competent nurses perform self-evaluations to identify their attitudes toward caring for clients from diverse cultures.

CASE STUDY

M.G. brings her Catholic, 18-year-old sister, R.G., to the hospital emergency room with a high temperature, chills, vomiting, and complaint of right lower quadrant pain. M.G. brings her three children, ages 3, 2, and 1 year old, with her. M.G. understands and speaks broken English, but R.G. is fluent in Spanish only. The nurse directs M.G. to the waiting room with her children and then takes R.G. to the examination room. R.G. is examined by a male nurse who promptly complains at the nurse's station about how uncooperative R.G. was during the physical examination. R.G. is admitted for inpatient care with a diagnosis of appendicitis requiring emergency surgery. M.G. is left in the waiting room unaware of the difficulty that the nursing staff has had communicating with her sister. R.G. is taken upstairs to her room to prepare her for surgery. M.G. is notified that she can go upstairs for a few minutes but then must leave because her children do not meet the age requirement for visitor privileges. A hospital volunteer was asked to watch the children until M.G. returned. M.G. finds R.G. weeping and nearly hysterical. The nurse informs M.G. that R.G. will not sign the surgical permit form. Tearfully, M.G. tells her sister that the "nurse took my amulet, and she won't let me wear it to surgery." The physician walks in and asks M.G. why she waited so long to bring R.G. in for treatment. He informs her that R.G.'s appendix was close to rupturing and that treatment should have been started 3 days ago when her symptoms began. M.G. informs him that she had taken R.G. to the curandero, who had given her some herbal tea to drink, but when it did not help, she brought R.G. to the hospital.

The following questions will guide your development of a nursing care plan for the case study.

1. Why was communication between M.G., R.G., and the health care professionals a problem?
2. What Hispanic cultural diversities were not addressed by the health care professionals? As a result, what needs of M.G. and R.G. were ignored by the health care professionals?
3. Write three individualized culturally sensitive nursing diagnoses and goals for R.G.
4. Recall the diagnoses and goals identified in question 3 and list pertinent nursing interventions for R.G.
5. List at least three successful client outcomes for R.G.

SAMPLE NURSING CARE PLAN

The Family with Ineffective Coping

M.W., an 82-year-old Asian American housewife, is in the hospital with severe nausea and vomiting related to recurrent breast cancer with bone metastasis treatment. Her appetite is decreasing, although she is able to drink some fluids.

At M.W.'s insistence, her husband of 61 years and their two grown daughters remain at her bedside. She does not bother the nurses for her basic care and insists that the oldest daughter bathe her and walk her to the bathroom. Mr. W. leaves only to go home and shower. Both daughters remain when he goes home.

Mr. W. looks exhausted and appears to have lost weight. The daughters try to relieve their father at night, but he insists on remaining at the bedside.

M.W. has her husband and daughters constantly massaging her back but never voices discomfort. She changes position slowly and grimaces with each movement. M.W. lets her family talk for her. When questioned by the nurse, she denies pain, but she complains of pain to her family. She does not sleep well.

M.W.'s treatment plan is supportive. The hospital staff suggested the idea of hospice care when M.W. stated that she wants to go home.

NURSING DIAGNOSIS 1 *Compromised Family Coping* related to prolonged disease or disability progression that exhausts the supportive capacity of significant people as evidenced by Mr. W.'s looking exhausted

Nursing Outcomes Classification (NOC)	Nursing Interventions Classification (NIC)
Caregiver Emotional Health	*Emotional Support*
Caregiver Stressors	*Family Support*
Family Normalization	*Family Therapy*
Self-Esteem	*Normalization Promotion*

(Continues)

SAMPLE NURSING CARE PLAN (Continued)

PLANNING/OUTCOMES	NURSING INTERVENTIONS	RATIONALE
Family will plan a rotation schedule to meet each one's needs for rest and support while caring for M.W.	Provide empathy and support for the husband and daughters. Provide family with unlimited visitation, adequate space for members who stay overnight, and privacy.	Family is very important in the life of the Asian American. A sense of obligation to intervene and assist is highly valued. Casual help from strangers is avoided.
	Assess family members for signs of fatigue or overexertion.	Self-control and self-sufficiency are highly valued. Asking for help would mean loss of face and dignity.
	Explore with husband and daughters other support persons who would be willing and accepted by M.W. to keep her company.	Prolonged periods of unrelieved vigil will exhaust family members.
	Develop trusting and respectful relationships with M.W. and family members.	Asian Americans tend to be reserved with those whom they view as being in authority.
Client and family will maintain open communication.	Encourage Mr. W. to discuss realistic plans and expectations of daughters, including health care providers as needed.	Asians traditionally value authoritarian styles of leadership, where the father makes unilateral family decisions.
Family will provide care without compromising their own physical and emotional health.	Assess if basic physical and emotional needs of M.W. and family are being met focusing on nonverbal clues.	Silent communication and stoic reactions to pain and other uncertain situations is common. Direct expression of negative feelings is unusual.
	Monitor ability of family members to carry out treatment plan and provide safe care.	Care is provided by family members who are exhausted, which is a safety issue.

EVALUATION

Husband and eldest daughter remain at bedside during daytime hours. Youngest exchanges places with the father and eldest sister at night. M.W. is agreeable. The entire family meets with the primary care nurse to discuss the plan of care. Mr. W. and his daughters continue to provide the physical care for M.W. The daughters express gratefulness that their father is stronger and has taken on the leadership role.

(Continues)

SAMPLE NURSING CARE PLAN (Continued)

NURSING DIAGNOSIS

Impaired Communication related to cultural misunderstandings and lack of communication

NOC: Communication Ability
NIC: Communication Enhancement

CLIENT GOAL

M.W. will communicate personal needs as evidenced by verbally sharing needs with family and nurses by the next day.

NURSING INTERVENTIONS

1. Express that tiredness and loss of weight is noted in family members.
2. State that you notice she is grimacing and moving slowly and offer pain medication.
3. Explain pain physiology and state the benefits of taking pain medication on a routine basis and as needed.
4. State the benefits of accepting medication for nausea and vomiting and offer medication.

SCIENTIFIC RATIONALES

1. When a person does not get the proper rest and nutrition, it may be evidenced by tiredness and loss of weight.
2. Some cultures do not encourage persons to freely express pain.
3. If the pain threshold is not kept under control, it is very difficult to keep the client comfortable and relaxed. Regular assessment and administration of medication keeps the client's pain below a 2 on a 0-10 scale with 0 being no pain and 10 is the most pain one has experienced.
4. If the nausea and vomiting is controlled with medication, the client has more energy for other needed tasks.

EVALUATION

Is the client verbalizing personal needs to family and nursing staff?

Cultural Consideration Care Map 11-1

SUMMARY

- Culture is composed of beliefs about relationships, motivation, activities, perception of the world, and self.
- Culture is learned, shared, integrated, unspoken, and dynamic.
- Beliefs about concepts of health, disease etiology, health promotion and protection, and practitioners and remedies are influenced by culture.
- Unlike opinions, preferences, and attitudes, which can change, cultural characteristics are deeply rooted and are thus difficult to change. Clients reflect their cultural and ethnic heritage every time they interact with the world around them.
- Culture is influenced by religion, which also affects practices and beliefs about health and illness.
- Spiritual and religious beliefs are important in many people's lives. They can influence lifestyle, attitudes, and feelings about illness and death.
- Individuality exists among all peoples; nurses should not make assumptions based on the client's religious and cultural affiliations.
- The focus of nursing care is to help clients maintain their own beliefs when in a health care crisis. Those personal beliefs can be used to strengthen coping patterns.
- It is an important aspect of nursing to understand client differences.
- Response to health and illness varies depending on cultural origin.
- Providing culturally appropriate care begins with an understanding of the nurse's own cultural beliefs.
- Prerequisite to providing appropriate nursing care is performing a cultural assessment.

REVIEW QUESTIONS

1. A mother is observed breastfeeding her 4-year-old son, a client in the hospital. The nurses talk in the nursing station about why a mother would continue to breastfeed a 4-year-old. They state that the American way is better. The nurses are expressing:
   1. stereotyping.
   2. ethnocentrism.
   3. acculturation.
   4. cultural diversity.
2. The nurse knows that the religious group teaching that physical healing comes exclusively through prayers and readings is:
   1. Hindu.
   2. Roman Catholic.
   3. Christian Science.
   4. Seventh-Day Adventist.
3. A blood transfusion would most likely be refused by:
   1. Buddhist.
   2. Orthodox.
   3. American Indian.
   4. Jehovah's Witness.
4. The nursing diagnosis that might be used for a client who is hospitalized and has religious practices that conflict with hospital procedure is:
   1. *Religious Guilt.*
   2. *Guilt and Misery.*
   3. *Spiritual Distress.*
   4. *Spiritual Depression.*
5. If a client says to the nurse, "I need to pray with my group leader to get well," the most appropriate response for the nurse is:
   1. "May I call your group leader for you and ask her to visit you?"
   2. "The medications and treatment will make you well."
   3. "Why do you think your group leader is needed to make you well?"
   4. "When you are released from the hospital, you can go to your group leader and pray."
6. An Egyptian Muslim comes to the emergency room. The examination reveals a diagnosis of pneumonia. The nurse taking care of the client approaches his bed with Tylenol. Holding his hand with her right hand to read his patient ID band, she hands him the Tylenol with her left hand. As the nurse turns to pick up the water glass to hand to the client, she sees him throw the Tylenol away in the bedside wastebasket. How do you explain his behavior?
   1. He does not like taking medication from a female. It is demeaning to him.
   2. He regards the left hand as unclean and refuses to swallow a medication that he feels is contaminated.
   3. He is a fatalist and believes that nothing can be done to reverse the infectious process in his lungs.
   4. He hates European Americans and is unwilling to accept anything that the Caucasian nurse has touched.
7. An Asian American woman is being treated for new-onset diabetes mellitus. The nurse caring for her is attempting to teach her how to inject insulin. The nurse becomes increasingly frustrated because the client will not engage in the lesson. She refuses to look at the nurse's face when she talks to her, and she does not respond quickly to the questions that the nurse asks her. Why will this client not look at the nurse when she is communicating with her?
   1. The client is being defiant.
   2. The client has low self-esteem.
   3. Engaging in eye contact is considered disrespectful.
   4. The client is not ready to learn.
8. A Korean American is being discharged today from the hospital. The nurse is at the bedside giving discharge instructions and also has several prescriptions that the client needs to take home with her. The nurse reviews the instructions and pharmacy orders and extends the papers to the client. She accepts the paperwork initially but then tries to hand them back to the nurse. When you consider cultural perspectives, what could be an explanation for this behavior?
   1. The client does not agree with the doctor's home-going instructions.
   2. The client is trying to communicate to the nurse that she needs to give home-going instructions and prescriptions to the head of the family, her husband.
   3. The client does not work, and she has no money to purchase the prescriptions.
   4. The client thought that the nurse gave her the hospital bill, and she assumed that medical care would be free for her since it was in her home country.
9. A Haitian American is brought to the emergency room with acute stomach pains. She is brought by her supervisor at the grocery store where she works. The examining physician determines that the client has appendicitis and needs surgery immediately. The doctor telephones the client's husband to obtain permission for the surgery. The husband replies that he will come to the hospital as soon as possible. On arrival, the husband refuses to sign the consent form for the operation. He wants his wife discharged immediately so that he can take her home. He promises to bring her back later. The emergency room staff is puzzled. How is this behavior explained?
   1. The couple cannot afford to pay for surgery, but the husband is too embarrassed to say so.

2. The husband does not trust the hospital staff, so he wants to take his wife to their private physician instead.
3. The husband wants to consult the hungan (voodoo priest) to rule out the possibility of spiritual causes for the abdominal pain.
4. The husband wants to give his wife some cold cucumber soup before her surgery.

10. A Chicano (Mexican American) student from Texas volunteers at the gift shop in the hospital. A nurse from the hospital encounters the Mexican student on the street pushing a stroller with a year-old baby. The baby is friendly, smiling and appears well nourished. The student informs the nurse that the baby is her sister. The nurse compliments the student on her solicitous care of her sister "the baby is a beautiful, adorable little girl isn't she?" Without responding, the student immediately turns the carriage away from the nurse, and after a strained moment of silence states, "I must get home to help my mother." How would you explain the student's behavior?

1. The student does not feel that it is respectful to take up the nurse's time, so she feels that she should leave.
2. Seeing the nurse reminds the student that she needs to get ready to volunteer at the gift shop.
3. The student needs to go home to help her mother.
4. The student is afraid that the baby has been given the evil eye, and she wants to tell her mother about it as soon as possible.

REFERENCES/SUGGESTED READINGS

Andrews, M. (2008). Religion, culture, and nursing. In M. M. Andrews & J. S. Boyle (Eds.), *Transcultural concepts in nursing care* (5th ed.). Philadelphia: Lippincott Williams & Wilkins.

Andrews, M., & Boyle, J. (2008). *Transcultural concepts in nursing care* (4th ed.). Philadelphia: Lippincott Williams & Wilkins.

Boyle, J. (2008). Culture, family, and community. In M. M. Andrews & J. S. Boyle (Eds.), *Transcultural concepts in nursing care* (5th ed.). Philadelphia: Lippincott Williams & Wilkins.

Bulechek, G., Butcher, H., McCloskey, J., & Dochterman, J., eds. (2008). *Nursing Interventions Classification (NIC)* (5th ed.). St. Louis, MO: Mosby/Elsevier.

Church of Scientology International. (2009). Introduction to scientology. Retrieved February 12, 2009, from http://www.scientology.org/religion/presentation/pg006.html

Clark, M. (1999). *Community health nursing handbook*. New York: Prentice Hall.

Daniels, R., Grendell, R., & Wilkins, F. (2010). *Nursing fundamentals: Caring and clinical decision making* (2nd ed.). Clifton Park, NY: Delmar Cengage Learning.

Davidhizar, R., Dowd, S., & Giger, J. (1998). Educating the culturally diverse health care student. *Nurse Educator, 23*(2), 38–42.

Degazon, C. (2000). Cultural diversity and community health nursing practice. In M. Stanhope & J. Lancaster (Eds.), *Community and public health nursing* (5th ed.). St. Louis, MO: Mosby.

Doherty, W. (1992). Private lives, public values. *Psychology Today, 25*(3), 27–32.

Doswell, W., & Erlen, J. (1998). Multicultural issues and ethical concerns in the delivery of nursing care interventions. *Nursing Clinics of North America, 33*(2), 353–361.

Edelman, C., & Mandle, C. (2005). *Health promotion throughout the lifespan* (6th ed.). St. Louis, MO: Elsevier/Mosby.

Edmission, K. (1997). Psychosocial dimensions of medical–surgical nursing. In J. M. Black & E. Matassarin-Jacobs (Eds.), *Medical surgical nursing: Clinical management for continuity of care* (5th ed.). Philadelphia: W. B. Saunders.

Estes, M. (2010). *Health assessment and physical examination* (4th ed.). Clifton Park, NY: Delmar Cengage Learning.

Estin, P. (1999). Spotting depression in Asian patients. *RN, 62*(4), 39–40.

Fawcett, C. (1993). *Family psychiatric nursing*. St. Louis, MO: Mosby.

Giger, J., & Davidhizar, R. (2004). *Transcultural nursing: Assessment and intervention* (4th ed.). St. Louis, MO: Mosby-Year Book.

Gonzalez, R. (1999). ANA advocates more diversity in nursing. *American Journal of Nursing, 99*(11), 24.

Gravely, S. (2001). When your patient speaks Spanish—and you don't. *RN, 64*(5), 65–67.

Grossman, D. (1996). Cultural dimensions in home health nursing. *American Journal of Nursing, 96*(7), 33–36.

Kelz, R. (1997). Delmar's English–Spanish pocket dictionary for health professionals. Clifton Park, NY: Delmar Cengage Learning.

Kelz, R. (1999). *Conversational Spanish for health professionals* (3rd ed.). Clifton Park, NY: Delmar Cengage Learning.

Kirkpatrick, M., Brown, S., & Atkins, T. (1998). Using the internet to integrate cultural diversity and global awareness. *Nurse Educator, 23*(2), 15–17.

Kudzma, E. (1999). Culturally competent drug administration. *American Journal of Nursing, 99*(8), 46–51.

Lee, E. (Ed.). (2000). *Working with Asian Americans: A guide for clinicians*. New York: Guilford Press.

Leininger, M., & McFarland, M. (2002).*Transcultural nursing: Concepts, theories, research, and practice* (3rd ed.). New York: McGraw-Hill.

Lock, D. (1992). *Increasing multicultural understanding: A comprehensive model*. Newbury Park, CA: Sage.

Louie, K. (1999). Health promotion interventions for Asian American Pacific Islanders. In L. Zhan (Ed.), *Asian voices* (pp. 3–13). Boston: Jones & Bartlett.

Luckmann, J. (2000). *Transcultural communication in nursing*. Clifton Park, NY: Delmar Cengage Learning.

Malone, B. (1998). Diversity, divisiveness and divinity. *American Nurse, 30*(1), 5.

Marrone, S. (2008). Factors that influence critical care nurses' intentions to provide culturally congruent care to Arab Muslims. *Journal of Transcultural Nursing, 19*(1), 8–15.

Mazanec, P., & Tyler, M. (2003). Cultural considerations in end-of-life care. *American Journal of Nursing, 103*(3), 50–57.

McCaffery, M., & Pasero, C. (1999). Pain control. *American Journal of Nursing, 99*(8), 18.

Miller, J., Leininger, M., Leuning, C., Andrews, M., Ludwig-Beymer, P., & Papadopoulos, I. (2008). Commentary: Transcultural Nursing Society Position Statement on Human Rights. *Journal of Transcultural Nursing, 19*(1), 5–7.

Moorhead, S., Johnson, M., & Maas, M. (2007). *Nursing Outcomes Classification (NOC)* (4th ed.). St. Louis, MO: Mosby.

Morley, P., & Wallis, R. (Eds.). (1978). *Culture and curing: Anthropological perspectives on traditional medical beliefs and practices.* Pittsburgh, PA: University of Pittsburgh Press.

Mullins, M. (1999). Cultural awareness. *OB/GYN Nurse Forum, 7,* 3.

NewsWatch. (2000). Delay in seeking MI treatment is tied to social factors. *RN, 63*(10), 20.

North American Nursing Diagnosis Association International. (2010). *NANDA-I nursing diagnoses: Definitions and classification 2009–2011.* Ames, IA: Wiley-Blackwell.

Competent Care. (2001, September). *Travel Nursing Today* (A supplement to *RN*), 26–32.

Purnell, L., & Paulanka, B. (2008). *Transcultural health care: A culturally competent approach* (3rd ed.). Philadelphia: F. A. Davis.

Rivera-Andino, J., & Lopez, L. (2000). When culture complicates care. RN, 63(7), 47–49.

Shelley, J. (2000). Spiritual care: A guide for caregivers. Downers Grove, IL: Inter Varsity.

Simpson, J., & Carter, K. (2008). Muslim women's experiences with health care providers in a rural area of the United States. *Journal of Transcultural Nursing, 19*(1), 16–23.

Smith, L. (1998). Concept analysis: Cultural competence. *Journal of Cultural Diversity, 5*(1), 4–10.

Spector, R. (2000). *Cultural care: Guides to heritage assessment and health traditions* (2nd ed.). Upper Saddle River, NJ: Prentice Hall.

Spector, R. (2008). *Cultural diversity in health and illness* (5th ed.). Upper Saddle River, NJ: Prentice Hall.

Spradley, B., & Allender, J. (2001). *Community health nursing: Concepts and practice* (5th ed.). Philadelphia: Lippincott Williams & Wilkins.

Stanhope, M., & Knollmueller, R. (2000). *Handbook of community-based and home health nursing practice* (3rd ed.). St. Louis, MO: Mosby.

Stanhope, M., & Lancaster, J. (2003). *Community and public health nursing* (6th ed.). St. Louis, MO: Mosby.

Sue, D., & Sue, D. (2007). *Counseling the culturally diverse: Theory and practice* (5th ed.). New York: Wiley.

U.S. Census Bureau. (2001). Population estimates. Available: http://www.census.gov/population/estimates/nation/intfile3-1.txt

U.S. Department of Commerce, U.S. Census Bureau. (2007). *Statistical abstract of the United States: 2008* (127th ed.). Washington, DC: U.S. Government Printing Office.

RESOURCES

Transcultural Nursing Society, http://www.tcns.org

CHAPTER 12
Stress, Adaptation, and Anxiety

MAKING THE CONNECTION

Refer to the following chapters to increase your understanding of stress, adaptation, and anxiety:

Basic Nursing

- ***Holistic Care***
- ***Communication***
- ***Complementary/Alternative Therapies***
- ***Rest and Sleep***
- ***Infection Control/Asepsis***
- ***Pain Management***

LEARNING OBJECTIVES

Upon completion of this chapter, you should be able to:

- Define key terms.
- Describe how stress, adaptation, and anxiety affect health.
- Identify factors that contribute to the stress response.
- Describe the general adaptation syndrome.
- Detail the effects of stress on the whole individual.
- Explain intrinsic stressors in the change process.
- Describe the role of the nurse as a change agent.
- Discuss nursing interventions that promote positive adaptation to stress.
- Develop an individualized plan for managing stress.

KEY TERMS

adaptation
adaptive energy
adaptive measures
anxiety
burnout
catharsis
change
change agent
cognitive reframing
conditioning
crisis
crisis intervention
defense mechanisms
depersonalization
distress
endorphin
eustress
fight-or-flight response
general adaptation syndrome (GAS)
homeostasis
local adaptation syndrome (LAS)
maladaptive measures
stress
stressor

INTRODUCTION

Stress and anxiety are universal experiences that can be either a catalyst for positive change or a source of discomfort and pain. Nurses help clients cope with the stress of illness, disability, injury, or treatment approaches. Caring for clients experiencing a high level of anxiety can also be stressful for the nurse. Successful stress management is necessary for everyone's well-being. This chapter discusses the major concepts related to stress and anxiety, including strategies for coping with stress.

STRESS

According to Hans Selye (1974), **stress** is a nonspecific response to any demand made on the body. Selye termed such demands **stressors**. Any situation, event, or agent that produces stress is a stressor. A stressor is a stimulus that evokes the need to adapt. Stressors can be internal or external. For example, pain is an internal stressor, whereas loss of a job is an external stressor.

Even pleasant events can be stressful when they evoke the need to adapt. Stressors themselves are neutral, neither good nor bad. It is the individual's *perception* of the stressor that determines whether the effect is positive or negative. Any event can be stressful, depending on how the person views the event.

Responses to Stress

Adaptive energy is the term Selye coined to describe the inner force an individual uses to respond or adapt to stress. All persons have adaptive energy, but the amount of adaptive energy varies. When an individual has used all of his adaptive energy, illness, disease, or even death may result, as he is no longer able to adapt. Reactions to stress are typically categorized as either general (affecting the entire body) or local (affecting only the involved body part).

General Adaptation Syndrome

Stressors cause structural and chemical changes in the body as the body attempts to maintain **homeostasis**, which is the balance or equilibrium among the physiologic, psychological, sociocultural, intellectual, and spiritual needs of the body. Selye called these responses to stressors the **general adaptation syndrome (GAS)**.

Selye divided the GAS into three stages, as illustrated in Figure 12-1. In the first stage, crisis or alarm, the body readies itself to handle the stressors. The physiologic changes may result in symptoms such as cool, pale skin; shivering; and sweating of the palms and soles of the feet. Severe stress may cause dilated pupils, dry mouth, pounding heart, nausea, and diarrhea.

> **PROFESSIONALTIP**
>
> **Anticipatory Stress**
>
> Thoughts can be stressors that trigger the GAS, such as a person worrying about a situation. The body responds as if the person were *actually* experiencing the event, and the individual may feel ill, sweaty, nauseous, or very jittery.

During the second stage, adaptation or resistance, the body attempts to defend against the stressor through the **fight-or-flight response**. The body becomes physiologically ready to defend itself by either fighting or fleeing from the stressor.

The third stage, exhaustion, occurs if adaptive energy is inadequate to deal with prolonged or overwhelming stress.

The physiologic reactions of the body are essentially the same no matter what the source of the stress. For example, an imagined stressor will have the same physiologic response (GAS) as if the stressor had actually been experienced. According to Selye (1976), all stress reactions exhibit similar physiologic reactions.

Local Adaptation Syndrome

Selye also described the **local adaptation syndrome (LAS)**, which is the physiologic response to a stressor (e.g., trauma, illness) on a specific part of the body. For example, if a person cuts a hand, the LAS is initiated, inducing localized inflammation. The classic symptoms of inflammation (redness, swelling, and warmth) occur at the injured site. The LAS is usually a temporary process that resolves when the traumatized area is restored to its preinjury state; however, if the inflammation does not resolve with the LAS, the individual then experiences the GAS as the entire body becomes affected.

Signs and Symptoms of Stress

The signs and symptoms of stress are many and affect every dimension of a person. Common signs and symptoms of stress are outlined in Table 12-1.

Outcomes of Stress

Experiencing stress provides the individual with two possibilities: (a) an opportunity for personal growth or (b) the risk of disorganization and distress. When stressors are handled appropriately, adaptation is attained, and the body returns to normal.

The term **eustress** describes a type of stress resulting in positive outcomes. Consider for example, students who have an examination scheduled the following week. The stress over the impending test motivates them to study early, and they pass the examination. This stress was positive because it motivated them to study (an example of growth) and resulted in positive or desired outcomes.

Stressors evoking an ineffective response cause **distress**. For example, students who have a scheduled examination the next day put studying off until the last minute. They "cram" all night, do not know the material, are not alert, and fail the examination; they experience distress.

ADAPTATION

Adaptation is an ongoing process whereby individuals adjust to stressors and change. The nurse's goal is to identify and support the client's positive adaptive responses. Adaptation is a holistic response that involves all dimensions of an individual. Individuals seek to maintain a steady state in all dimensions of life: physiologic, psychological, cognitive, social, and spiritual. Wellness is an adaptive state; that is, the well person is one who is coping effectively with stressors and thus maintains a high level of wellness. Adaptation may be physiologic, psychological, cognitive, social, or spiritual.

Physiologic adaptation is the way the body responds to stressors affecting the functioning of the body. It may involve the

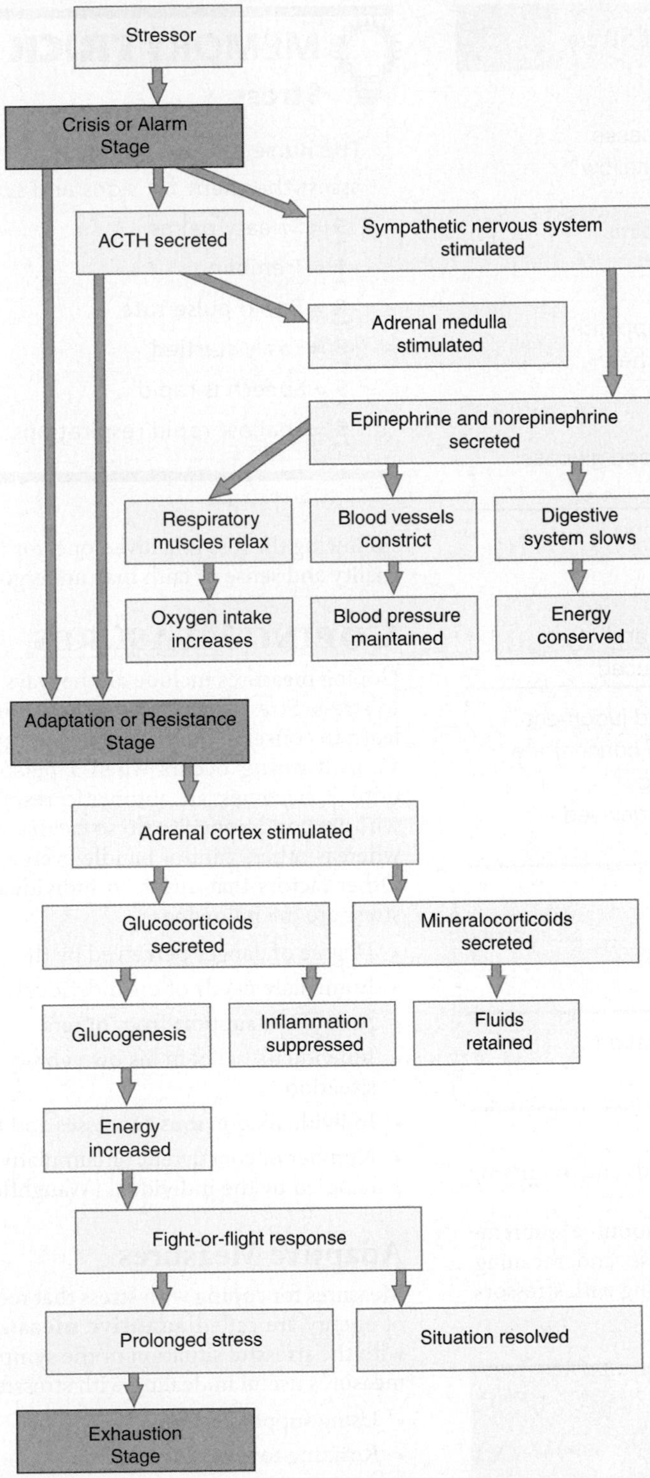

FIGURE 12-1 **Physiological Effects of the General Adaptation Syndrome (GAS)**

entire body (GAS) or only a specific area (LAS). An individual who lives in the mountains (high elevation) produces more red blood cells to carry enough oxygen to meet the body's needs. The chest also enlarges to allow the lungs to expand to accommodate the needed exchange of oxygen and carbon dioxide.

Psychological adaptation involves the use of defense mechanisms and learning to mentally accept new situations. A 55-year-old worker who suddenly finds himself unemployed will need to learn to adapt psychologically to the new situation and decide which steps to take next.

Cognitive adaptation involves education, communication, problem-solving ability, and perception of people and the world. A person gains these methods throughout life. For example, the high school student will have a different perspective of the world and different problem-solving abilities than will this same individual as a college graduate.

Social adaptation involves social relationships with family, friends, and coworkers who may provide support in times of stress (Figure 12-2). A person unable to cope may withdraw socially. An example of social adaptation would be a family

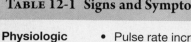

TABLE 12-1 Signs and Symptoms of Stress

Physiologic	• Pulse rate increases • Blood pressure increases • Breathing is rapid, shallow • Blood thickens • Dizziness, sweaty palms • Headache • Pupils dilate • Nausea, change in appetite • Constipation or diarrhea • Increased urination • Twitching, trembling • Increased level of blood glucose and cortisol
Psychological	• Irritability • Feelings easily hurt • Sadness, depression • Feelings of pleasure and accomplishment reduced
Cognitive	• Impaired memory and judgment • Confusion, unable to concentrate • Poor decision making • Altered perceptions, delayed response
Behavioral	• Pacing, rapid speech • Insomnia • Withdrawal • Easily startled
Spiritual	• Alienation, social isolation • Feeling of emptiness

moving to a new town and making new friends and modifying relationships with existing friends.

Spiritual adaptation involves beliefs about a supreme being and a positive sense of life's purpose and meaning. These beliefs are a personal resource for coping with stressors.

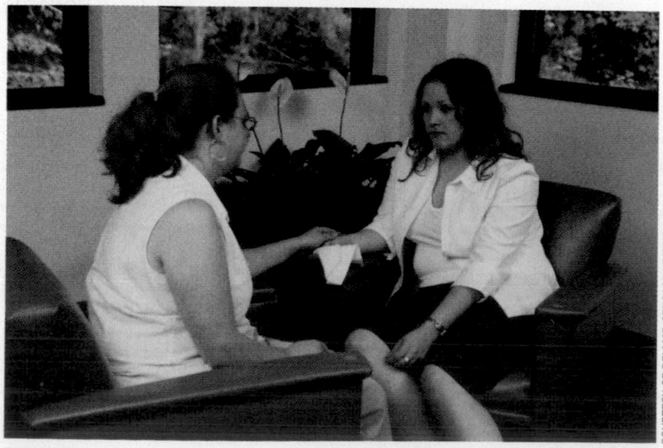

FIGURE 12-2 A coworker providing support is an example of social adaptation.

MEMORYTRICK

Stress

The nurse can use the memory trick **STRESS** to assess the client for signs and symptoms of stress:

S = Sweaty palms
T = Trembling
R = Rapid pulse rate
E = Easily startled
S = Speech is rapid
S = Shallow rapid respirations

Following the loss of a loved one, for instance, a family's spirituality and sense of faith may undergo changes.

COPING MEASURES

Coping measures include all the ways an individual may react to stress. Stress is an automatic response, but individuals can learn to conserve their adaptive energy through conditioning. **Conditioning** occurs when a person is taught a behavior until it becomes an automatic response. Some individuals who are conditioned to do so can handle a great deal of stress, whereas others cannot handle even a small amount of stress. Other factors that affect an individual's ability to cope with stress are the following:

- Degree of danger perceived by the individual
- Immediate needs of the individual
- Amount of support from others
- Individual's belief in his own ability to handle the stressful situation
- Individual's previous successes and failures in coping
- Number of concurrent or cumulative stresses being handled by the individual (Waughfield, 2002)

Adaptive Measures

Measures for coping with stress that require a minimal amount of energy are called **adaptive measures**. They deal directly with the stressful situation or the symptoms thereof. Adaptive measures useful in dealing with stressful situations include:

- Using support people
- Relaxing to relieve tension
- Changing behavior
- Developing more realistic goals
- Solving problems

Defense Mechanisms

Just as the body has physiologic mechanisms (e.g., the immune system, the inflammatory response) to defend against infection and disease, the mind has psychological protective mechanisms. Most **defense mechanisms** are unconscious functions protecting the mind from anxiety. They are used to gain and maintain psychological homeostasis. The individual does not consciously decide to use a defense mechanism; it happens automatically.

LIFE SPAN CONSIDERATIONS

Coping Ability

An individual's ability to cope with stressors depends in part on age and developmental level.

Everyone uses defense mechanisms. Their use does not imply mental illness or psychosocial imbalance. Defense mechanisms are considered maladaptive only when they are the only way an individual responds to a threat or when they limit the individual's ability to function. Table 12-2 describes and gives examples of various defense mechanisms.

Maladaptive Measures

Measures used to avoid conflict and stress are considered **maladaptive measures** because they prevent the individual from making progress toward resolving and accepting stress. They may include somatic disorders (transferring stress to an organ as pain), rituals, excessive use of alcohol or drugs, excessive eating, or withdrawal from reality.

CRISIS

A crisis occurs when stressors surpass the ability to cope. A **crisis** (an acute state of disorganization) occurs when the usual coping mechanisms are no longer adequate. Crisis is characterized by extreme anxiety, disorganized behavior, and inability to function. A crisis is time limited because no one can stay in acute disequilibrium for a long time and experi-

CULTURAL CONSIDERATIONS

Adaptive Measures

Nurses must be sensitive to the fact that culture and ethnicity may influence an individual's choice of coping mechanisms. For instance, moaning and chanting may be an expected response to stress in some cultures; the nurse must be careful to view this behavior not as maladaptive but as a culturally healthy response to a stressor.

TABLE 12-2 Defense Mechanisms

DEFENSE MECHANISM	DESCRIPTION	EXAMPLE
Denial	Refusal to acknowledge the reality of threatening situations despite factual evidence	A person with heart disease continues to eat fatty foods and fried foods despite medical advice to the contrary.
Displacement	Transfer of feelings or reactions from one object to another object, usually one that is "safer"	A husband who is angry with his wife yells at the dog instead of dealing with his anger at his wife.
Projection	Attribution of one's own thoughts, feelings, or impulses to others	An adolescent who does not want to go with the crowd states, "My parents won't let me go."
Rationalization	Intellectual explanation or justification of ideas, feelings, or behavior	A student responds after failing a test that "The test had many trick questions on it; I really know the material."
Reaction formation	Expression of a feeling that is the opposite of one's real feeling	A client brings a gift to a nurse with whom he is really angry.
Regression	A return to a previous developmental level	A child who has not sucked her thumb in 2 years starts to do so again when admitted to the hospital.
Repression	The unconscious blocking from awareness of material that is painful or threatening	Adult's claim, despite evidence, that "I never got angry with my parents; we lived in love and harmony."
Suppression	A conscious or unconscious attempt to keep threatening or unpleasant material out of consciousness	Failure to remember a house fire during childhood.
Sublimation	Channeling of socially unacceptable impulses into socially acceptable activities	A young man who deals with aggression by playing football.

Adapted from *Psychiatric Mental Health Nursing* (4th ed.), by N. Frisch and L. Frisch, 2010. Clifton Park, NY: Delmar Cengage Learning.

PROFESSIONALTIP

Defense Mechanisms

The nurse who is unfamiliar with defense mechanisms may be judgmental about clients who do not respond as the nurse expects. If the nurse tries to break through a client's denial (defense mechanism) too quickly by presenting reality, the client may be overwhelmed by anxiety and will panic.

ence the great discomfort. Given the time-limited nature of crisis, a client in crisis needs immediate intervention for a successful resolution. Crisis intervention is discussed later in this chapter.

Crisis can be a negative experience, but it can also present an opportunity for growth and learning. The outcome depends on each individual's perception and coping abilities. Nurses can guide clients to discover opportunities in the crisis and adapt in positive, healthy ways.

Stressful events do not always result in a crisis. A crisis is *not* a mental illness, even though persons experiencing the acute anxiety and discomfort fear for their sanity. Each crisis is unique to the individual; however, crises have common characteristics (Table 12-3).

ANXIETY

Anxiety is a subjective response that occurs when a person experiences a real or perceived threat to well-being; it is a diverse feeling of dread or apprehension. There is a close relationship between anxiety and stress. Anxiety is the psychological response to a threat, such as the worry that results when oversleeping on a workday. This worry can translate into stress (the person's physiologic response to a stimulus) by rushing, perspiring, and becoming careless. Anxiety can be an activator of stress *and* a response to stress: It is usually activated by stress and may lead to more stress. Anxiety is a major component of mental health disturbances.

TABLE 12-3 Crisis Characteristics

- A loss, actual or perceived, is a part of every crisis.
- A crisis occurs suddenly.
- A crisis has a known precipitating event.
- The situation is seen as overwhelming or life threatening.
- Communication becomes impaired.
- Usual coping skills cannot resolve the situation.
- Intervention is required to reestablish equilibrium.

Data from *Contemporary Psychiatric-Mental Health Nursing*, by H. S. Wilson, C. R. Kneisl, and E. Trigoboff, 2004, Upper Saddle River, NJ: Prentice Hall. Copyright 2004 by Prentice Hall.

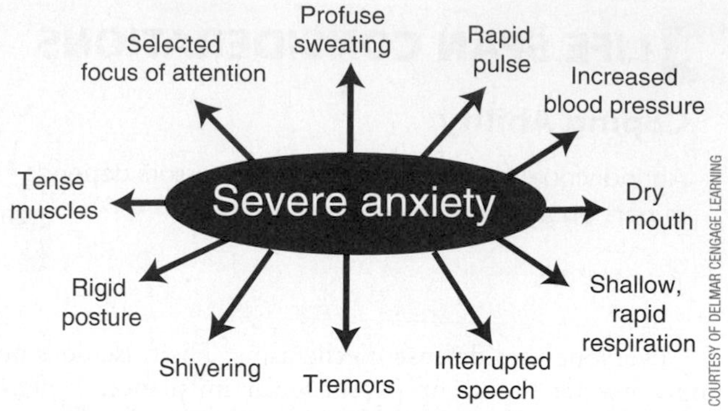

FIGURE 12-3 Physical and Mental Responses to Severe Anxiety

The most common emotional (affective) response to stress is anxiety. Individuals feel anxious when they are threatened, even if the threat is only perceived. Anxiety occurs on a continuum; some degree of anxiety is beneficial as a motivator. A high level of anxiety, however, can overpower a person and diminish the ability to function and think. The person is less able to function as the level of anxiety increases (Figure 12-3). Table 12-4 describes the levels of anxiety.

EFFECTS OF AND ON ILLNESS

Anxiety often increases during illness and recovery. It is often difficult to determine whether illness or stress came first. Illness occurs when adaptive attempts are unsuccessful. Also, an ill person has fewer usable adaptive resources to cope with stressors. Some stressors may not directly cause disease, but stress is a substantial aspect in the onset and progress of many illnesses. Some disorders commonly associated with stress include:

- Arrhythmias
- Asthma
- Back pain
- Decreased libido
- Diabetes
- Eating disorders
- Eczema
- Emphysema
- Fertility problems
- Headache
- Hives
- Hypertension
- Impotence
- Irritable bowel syndrome
- Menstrual disorders
- Periodontal disease
- Psoriasis
- Sleep disturbance
- Ulcers
- Viral activation, herpes, or HIV
- Weight gain or loss

The immune system is impaired during prolonged periods of stress. Steroid production increases as the body fights

COMMUNITY/HOME HEALTH CARE

Reducing Stressors

Remember, as a home health or visiting nurse, you are a guest in the client's home. If changes must be made in the home or the way it is kept, provide suggestions that are directly related to the client or the care of the client. Never criticize the home itself or the way it is kept.

TABLE 12-4 Levels of Anxiety

ANXIETY LEVEL	CHARACTERISTICS OF THE ANXIOUS PERSON	NURSING CONSIDERATIONS
Mild	• Increased degree of alertness • Increased vigilance • Increased motivation • Readiness for action • Slight increase in vital signs	• Best time for client teaching.
Moderate	• Subjective distress (tension) • Decreased perception and attention • Alert only to specific information • Possible tendency to complain or argue • Possible headache, diarrhea, nausea, or vomiting	• Assist client in determining cause and effect between stressor and anxiety.
Severe	• Increased subjective distress • Feeling of impending danger • Selective attention • Distorted communication • Distorted perception • Feelings of fatigue	• Encourage verbalization. • Encourage motor activity (walking, exercise). • Give specific directions.
Panic	• Major perceptual distortion • Immobilization; inability to function • Feelings of terror • Possible harm to self and others	• Provide guidelines and limits. • Maintain client safety (both physical and psychological).

Data from *Interpersonal Relations in Nursing*, by H. E. Peplau, 1952, New York: Putnam; *The Interpersonal Theory of Psychiatry*, by L. S. Sullivan, 1953, New York: Norton.

the perceived or actual threat. Steroids reduce the immune system's ability to function, and the body is less able to protect itself from disease.

All clients in a health care facility have a change in their routine that may cause anxiety and stress. The unfamiliar environment, loss of control over their schedule, and dependence on others for care are issues with which these clients must cope. Each issue is a stressor requiring adaptation by the client to maintain homeostasis. Some clients do not have the adaptive energy to cope with the many changes and cope with their illness. Cues that a person may not be coping well to hospitalization include:

- Increased stress response
- High level of anxiety
- Increased use of coping mechanisms
- Inability to function
- Disorganized behavior

The person having "minor" surgery at an outpatient center, the adolescent being treated by the school nurse, or the employee being treated at an industrial clinic for a work-related injury may also experience client role stressors. Even clients who are treated in their homes may experience stressors from having a health care provider in their personal environment.

The greater the threat (or perceived threat), the higher the level of anxiety. Nurses must be sensitive to stress and many changes caused by illness. This reduces the risk of depersonalizing the client.

Depersonalization is the process of treating an individual as an object instead of a person. It takes away a client's individuality by treating him as a thing. Nursing interventions focus on assisting the client to lessen feelings of loss of control.

CHANGE

Change, a dynamic process whereby an individual's response to a stressor leads to an alteration in behavior, is an inevitable part of life. Whether change is planned or unplanned, it is inevitable and constant. Change can be stressful to individuals and activate the GAS. Characteristics of change are that it:

- May be stressful or distressful
- Can be externally imposed or self-initiated
- Can occur abruptly or have a gradual onset
- Requires energy to effect as well as to resist

CRITICAL THINKING

Stress and Illness

How would you explain the relationship between stress and illness to a client?

PROFESSIONALTIP

Promoting Client Control

- *Communicate clearly.* Avoid using medical jargon.
- *Thoroughly answer questions.* Validate the level of understanding.
- *Teach relaxation techniques,* such as progressive muscle relaxation and guided imagery.
- *Instruct clients how to use* **cognitive reframing** (the individual changes a negative perception of a situation to a less-threatening perception).
- *Provide support and reassurance.* The most therapeutic way to alleviate client anxiety is the nurse's therapeutic use of self (Figure 12-4).

All health care providers should know how to initiate and cope with change. Critical thinking and problem-solving skills are needed to effectively initiate and cope with change.

Types of Change

Change may be unplanned or planned. Unplanned change is unpredictable and may be imposed by others or by uncontrollable events (e.g., losing one's home in a fire). Planned change is a specific effort to modify a situation. A marriage is an example of a planned change. In addition to planned change and unplanned change, there are other types of change.

Developmental changes are physical and emotional alterations occurring at different stages of life. These are usually predictable and occur in a certain order. For instance, a baby will first learn to roll over, then crawl, then walk. The exact age will vary, but the sequence usually does not.

Accidental or reactive changes are adaptive responses to change imposed by others. This may include a change in one's working hours or a child's baseball game being rescheduled.

Covert changes are often subtle and occur without a person's conscious awareness. These might include a gradual shifting of responsibilities as new skills are acquired or developed at work.

Overt changes are obvious and identifiable, and an individual is aware they are occurring. They are usually not under an individual's direct control, such as the restructuring of one's place of employment, but must be adapted to and accepted in order to continue functioning effectively.

Resistance to Change

People tend to resist change because of the energy required to adapt, although energy is also required to resist change, or to maintain the status quo. The ability to tolerate (or even thrive on) change differs in individuals. There are no guarantees that change will lead to a positive outcome. Uncertainty regarding outcome is a major barrier to change.

It is risky to challenge one's own ideas or those of others by initiating change. Questioning is one of the first signs of the need for change. The nurse who wonders "Why?" "What if?" or "Why not?" will likely risk initiating change. Successful risk takers consider the costs and benefits of their ideas and the outcomes relative to available resources.

Because change is inevitable, nurses must learn ways to deal with change. Resistance looks like the individual is rejecting proposed new ideas without critically thinking about the proposal. Nurses must take time to research ideas and make informed decisions as to whether change is worthwhile. Coping with change calls for adaptability, flexibility, and resilience.

Nurse as Change Agent

The nurse often serves as a **change agent** (a person who intentionally creates and implements change). Change agents seek ways to make improvements using critical thinking to develop innovative, creative solutions.

Change should be planned by individuals who are proactive. The proactive individual initiates action rather than waiting for others to solve problems, make decisions, or become rescuers. Reactive persons, on the other hand, respond only to externally imposed change. Proactive nurses are change agents who often affect the entire health care system as well as individual clients.

Change agents work toward a positive outcome. Client education is a powerful tool for initiating change. The client is provided with an opportunity to change when taught a disease process, a treatment modality, or a lifestyle alteration. Learning results in behavioral changes. The change process is similar to the nursing process in that change involves assessment, planning, decision making, implementation, and evaluation.

NURSING PROCESS

Nurses can be instrumental in helping clients both understand their anxiety and learn measures to cope with and control their feelings of stress.

Assessment

The nurse must first ascertain the anxious client's perception of the situation. This is accomplished by directly asking the client and then listening carefully to the client's response (Figure 12-4). Nurses must be aware of their own body language because the nurse's nonverbal behavior can affect the client's anxiety level. Anxiety is a subjective experience and

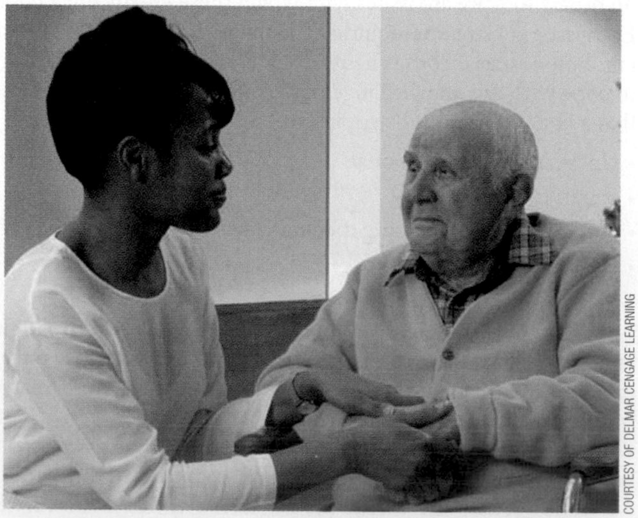

FIGURE 12-4 **Through talking, listening, and touch, the nurse can help relieve the client's feelings of anxiety.**

cannot be directly observed. The nurse must therefore look for signs of anxiety (refer back to Table 12-4).

A thorough assessment of stress and anxiety levels includes asking the client about:

- Types or patterns of stressors
- Usual response to stressful situations
- Cause-and-effect relationships among stressors and thoughts, feelings, and behaviors
- History of successful coping

The client's coping abilities can be assessed in various ways. Open-ended questions can be used to ascertain previously used coping mechanisms. Some sample questions are:

- What is the problem?
- What have you tried before?
- How well did it work?

Appropriate nursing diagnoses and an effective plan of care can be established by identifying the client's coping abilities. Assessment provides the data necessary for identifying nursing diagnoses.

Nursing Diagnosis

Several nursing diagnoses may apply to clients experiencing anxiety; the most common of these are *Anxiety*, *Ineffective **C**oping*, *Ineffective **D**enial*, and ***P**owerlessness*. Additional North American Nursing Diagnosis Association International (NANDA-I, 2010) diagnoses that may also apply include:

- *Impaired **A**djustment*
- *Ineffective **R**ole Performance*
- *Disturbed **T**hought Processes*
- *Defensive **C**oping*
- ***F**ear*
- ***P**ost-Trauma Syndrome*
- *Impaired **S**ocial Interaction*
- ***S**piritual Distress*
- ***H**opelessness*
- ***F**atigue*
- *Disturbed **S**leep Pattern*

Planning/Outcome Identification

Involving clients in planning care is essential because helping clients learn to cope successfully is part of the empowerment process. Planning means exploring with the client self-responsibility issues. A major goal for working with an anxious client is to reduce anxiety so problem solving and learning can occur.

There may be many expected outcomes (goals) appropriate for clients experiencing stress or anxiety. A few basic goals are for the client to:

- Identify situations when stress and anxiety increase.
- Describe ways to decrease the effects of usual stressors.
- Identify positive and negative stressors in the client's life.
- Group stressors into categories: ones that can be eliminated, ones that can be controlled, and ones that cannot be controlled directly by self.
- Demonstrate correct use of select stress-management exercises (e.g., progressive muscle relaxation, guided imagery, thought stopping).

> **SAFETY**
>
> **The Client Experiencing Panic**
>
> Never leave a panic-stricken client alone. The client with panic-level anxiety may harm herself. Stay with this client or have someone else do so.

- Describe the plan for managing stress, including lifestyle modifications.

Implementation

Teaching is part of holistic nursing practice. Stress-management methods can be taught to clients of every age and developmental stage in all health care settings.

A major step in improving self-care is to teach clients how to reduce their own stress level. Education gives clients options. Clients who understand their options can make informed decisions (Figure 12-5). Some of the many interventions that may assist the anxious client follow.

Meet Basic Needs

Stress and basic physiologic needs are closely related. Anything interfering with basic needs being met elicits the stress response, causing anxiety. Clients who are in pain, cold, or hungry have a higher anxiety level than when comfortable. The perception of pain increases with a higher level of anxiety. The nurse actually improves the potential for recovery by reducing client anxiety.

Minimize Environmental Stimuli

An individual's immediate environment can influence stress levels. The nurse should decrease environmental stimuli that may cause anxiety. Environmental stimuli can be reduced by:

- Closing the client's room door
- Turning the television off
- Reducing loudness of the telephone ringer or disconnecting the phone, if feasible

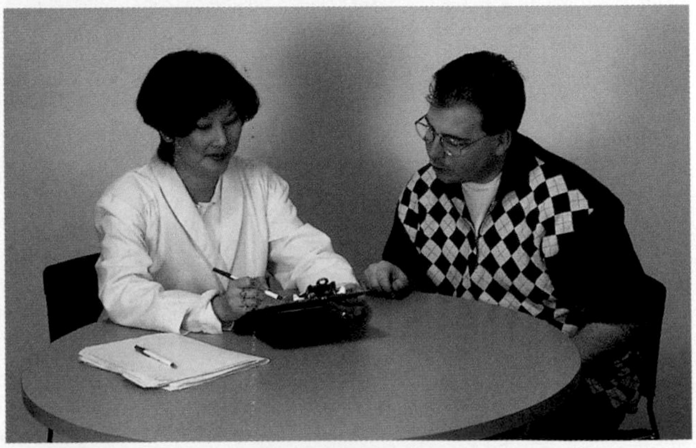

COURTESY OF DELMAR CENGAGE LEARNING

FIGURE 12-5 The nurse discusses the options for care and provides the client with the information needed to plan effective lifestyle changes.

- Dimming the lights or closing the blinds
- Limiting the number of visitors (unless isolation increases the client's anxiety)

Verbalize Feelings

Encouraging clients to express their feelings is especially helpful to reduce stress. Freud (1959) described the process of talking out one's feelings as a **catharsis**. People seem to instinctively know the value of "getting things off their chest." Verbalizing promotes relaxation because (a) a verbalized feeling becomes real and an identified problem can be dealt with, and (b) the activity of talking uses energy and reduces anxiety.

Involve Family/Significant Others

The type of intervention for managing stress is influenced by the client's developmental stage. Children need and rely on their parents or caretakers for security and support. Because families provide essential support for clients, it is important to include the entire family in the care of the client whenever possible (Figure 12-6) to decrease the stress level of everyone involved.

Family members who are anxious may have a negative impact on the client's health status. One way nurses must often help family members relax is to provide information and explanations. Researchers have concluded that both the client and family benefit from family presence during invasive procedures and resuscitation (Meyers et al., 2000).

Several national organizations, such as the American Heart Association, the Society of Critical Care Medicine, the American Association of Critical-Care Nurses, and the Emergency Nurses Association, have developed guidelines and practice statements to advocate family presence during invasive procedures and CPR. Studies have indicated that "family presence doesn't usually interfere with medical interventions when the focus is on a patient's survival" (Briguglio, 2007).

Use Stress-Management Techniques

A variety of stress-management techniques can easily be taught to clients, families, and significant others. Some of the most common approaches for managing stress are discussed next.

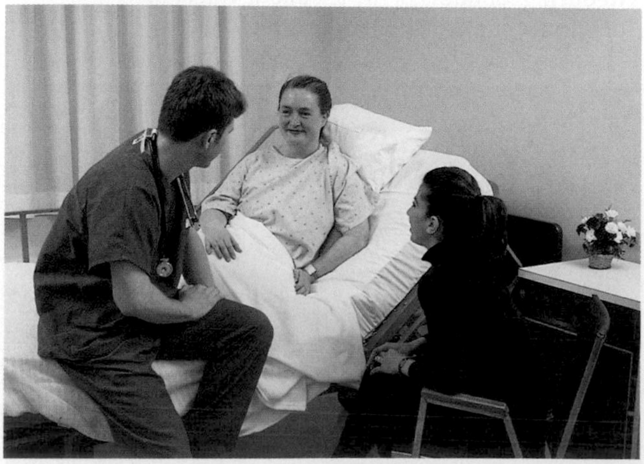

FIGURE 12-6 The nurse encourages interaction between the client and family members and significant others. This involvement helps ease the client's anxiety and keeps the family informed about the client's cares.

Exercise A powerful way to reduce anxiety is physical exercise. The need for incorporating exercise into one's lifestyle should be emphasized in client teaching. To establish an exercise program:

- Explore the different exercise programs available
- Ask a health care provider about the safety of a specific exercise program
- Set realistic goals
- Select a routine allowing warm-up and cool-down periods
- Take up activities that increase heart rate for a period of time

If exercise is to reduce anxiety, it must be done on a regular, ongoing basis. Physiologic benefits of regular exercise are listed in Table 12-5 and include:

- Feelings of well-being are enhanced
- Concentration and memory improve
- Depression is lessened
- Insomnia is lessened
- Dependence on external stimulants or relaxants is reduced
- Self-esteem increases
- Sense of self-control over anxiety is renewed

Relaxation Techniques Several techniques can help individuals relax (Figure 12-7). Complementary and alternative interventions such as progressive muscle relaxation and guided imagery are useful in helping clients learn to relax. Meditation and hypnosis can also be very effective in inducing relaxation and relieving stress.

Cognitive Reframing or Thought Stopping Cognitive reframing is a technique based on Beck's (1976) theory that a person's emotional response to an event is determined by the meaning attached to it. For example, the client is likely to feel anxious if an event is perceived as threatening. The client will be less anxious if the interpretation of the event can be modified. Reframing is used to alter one's perceptions and interpretations by changing one's thoughts.

Crisis Intervention

Some clients will be in an acute crisis state and require **crisis intervention**, a specific technique to help a person regain equilibrium. Crisis intervention views individuals as capable of personal growth and able to influence and control their own lives (Kneisl & Riley, 1996). The five steps of crisis intervention are:

1. Identify the specific problem, including the underlying issues.
2. Identify all possible options.
3. Examine possible outcomes for each option and select an option.
4. Implement the selected option.
5. Evaluate the overall effectiveness of the plan.

Clients sometimes need more assistance than the nurse is able to provide. Prompt consultation with or referral to other health care providers is necessary, such as:

- Psychiatric clinical nurse specialists
- Nurse psychotherapists

TABLE 12-5 Physiological Benefits of Exercise

EFFECT OF EXERCISE	PHYSIOLOGICAL BENEFIT
Promotes metabolism of adrenalin and thyroxine	• Minimizes autonomic arousal and hypervigilance
Reduces musculoskeletal tension	• Decreases feelings of being tense and "uptight"
Improves circulation, resulting in better oxygenation of the brain	• Increases alertness and concentration, and leads to enhanced problem-solving ability
Stimulates **endorphin** (a group of opiate-like substances produced naturally by the brain) production	• Raises the body's pain threshold, and promotes a sense of well-being
Reduces cholesterol level	• Decreases the risk of atherosclerosis
Reduces blood pressure	• Decreases the risk of myocardial infarction (heart attack) and cerebral vascular accident (CVA) (stroke)
Stimulates elimination (through lungs, skin, bowels)	• Reduces toxin buildup in the body

Data from "Nutrition, Exercise, and Movement," by L. Keegan, 2000, in B. Dossey, L. Keegan, and C. Guzzetta (Eds.), *Holistic Nursing: A Handbook for Practice* (3rd ed.), Gaithersburg, MD: Aspen; "Health Promotion and the Individual," by C. Mandle and R. Gruber-Wood, 2002, in C. Edelman and C. Mandle (Eds.), *Health Promotion throughout the Lifespan* (5th ed.), St. Louis, MO: Mosby.

- Psychologists
- Psychiatrists
- Social workers
- Clergy or other counselors

EVALUATION

Evaluation of the client's coping abilities must include client input. The nurse must evaluate client outcomes as well as nursing care. The family can also be a valuable source of information about the effectiveness of the stress-reduction approaches.

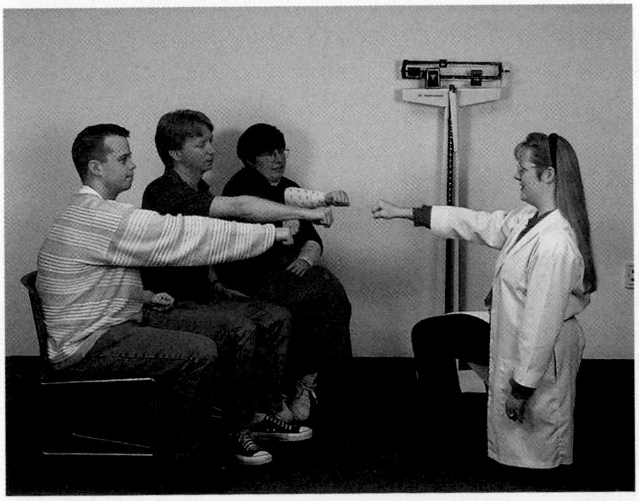

FIGURE 12-7 The nurse demonstrates the technique of progressive muscle relaxation in a client-education program.

STRESS MANAGEMENT FOR THE NURSE

There are many stressors in nursing. It is essential that nurses learn to cope successfully with the stressors (Figure 12-8). Nurses must cope successfully with stress to maintain their own wellness and to model healthy behaviors. Nurses must first be able to manage their own stress before helping clients learn to manage theirs.

High stress levels among nurses often lead to **burnout**, a state of physical and emotional exhaustion occurring when caregivers use up their adaptive energy. In an article by Fink

CLIENT TEACHING

Cognitive Reframing or Thought Stopping

- Listen to self-talk (thoughts).
- Identify negative self-talk.
- Do something physical when a negative thought is detected to stop the train of thought, such as clapping your hands or snapping a rubber band on your wrist.
- Replace the negative thought with one that is both realistic and positive.

Like all other relaxation exercises, thought stopping becomes more effective with repetition.

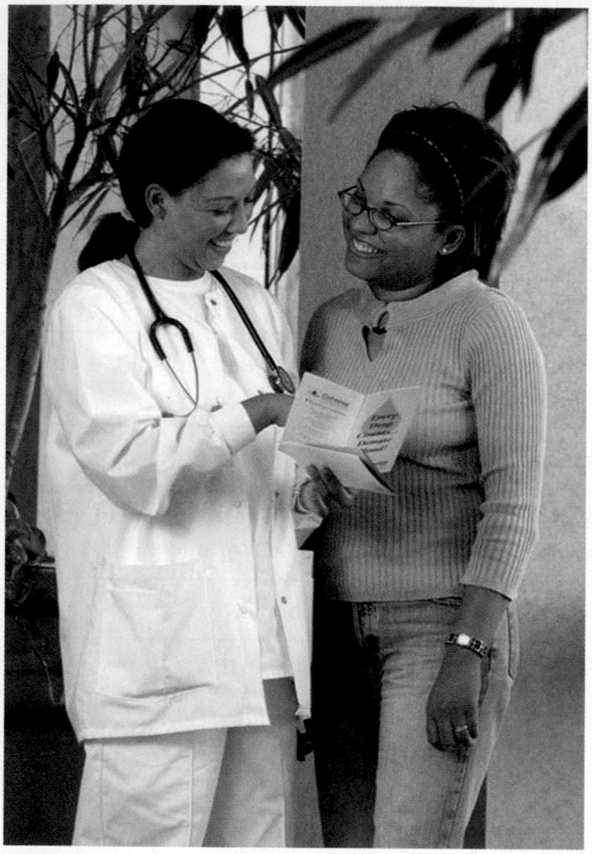

FIGURE 12-8 Sharing a light and humorous moment with a friend is a wonderful way to relieve stress and regain perspective.

CRITICAL THINKING

Burnout

A client is exhibiting panic-level anxiety and should not be left alone. You are experiencing severe burnout because of very long work hours and recent stressful situations. Your stress level is so high that you feel you cannot stay in the room with this client. If you leave the room to find another nurse to stay with him, he may injure himself; if you stay, you risk your own emotional well-being. How do you deal with this situation?

(2005), she discussed a recent study of nurses in five countries in which 30% to 40% stated that they felt burned out. The nurses at highest risk of experiencing burnout were the best and brightest who set high standards for themselves. Nurses experiencing such an overwhelming degree of stress often treat clients in a depersonalizing manner. These nurses also lack feelings of personal accomplishment. Burnout imposes a high price on individual nurses and on the profession as highly qualified professionals leave nursing. The quality of care declines as a result.

Several work-related factors can contribute to burnout:

- Heavy workload (critically ill clients)
- Interpersonal conflict in the work environment
- Mandatory overtime and "floating" to other units
- Little work-related social support

Stress management is the key to burnout prevention and recovery. A stress-management plan begins with self-awareness. It is a continuous process, not the occasional use of a technique or exercise. Nurses often fail to take care of themselves, but it is essential that nurses learn to care for themselves.

TABLE 12-6 Strategies for Managing Professional Stress

STRATEGY	RATIONALE
Develop active support systems at work and away from work.	Non–health care provider friends help maintain a balance in life.
Use time management and decision-making methods.	Viewing personal needs as a priority encourages one to schedule time to meet those needs. Breaking down large tasks into small, realistic ones prevents being overwhelmed.
Focus on accomplishments.	Increases self-esteem.
Know personal limits.	Helps separate the important from the less important.
Avoid harmful substances.	Smoking, overeating, and intake of caffeine, alcohol, or other substances often increase stress and anxiety in the long run.
Nourish the body with healthy diet, exercise, and sleep.	A healthy mind and body is better able to handle stress.
Practice slow, focused breathing.	Muscle tension is alleviated with more oxygen in the blood.
Vary tasks between mental and physical activities.	Conserves energy, reduces fatigue, and maintains a sense of balance.
Maintain a sense of humor.	Helps keep a positive outlook; can be used to reframe a situation.

CRITICAL THINKING

Stressors

Reflect on the past month. List some of the stressors that you have experienced during that time. How did you respond to the stressors? Would you now respond differently in similar situations? If so, what would you change?

There are many strategies to help nurses manage professional and personal stress, as outlined in Table 12-6.

Nurses who cultivate the hardiness factor will likely be resilient to stress. Kobasa (1979) put forth the concept of hardiness in the late 1970s. Hardiness consists of a set of attitudes, beliefs, and behaviors that make individuals more resilient (or hardy) to the negative effects of stress. The three components to stress hardiness are:

- *Commitment:* Become involved in what one is doing
- *Challenge:* Perceive change as an opportunity for growth instead of an obstacle or threat
- *Control:* Believe that one is directing what happens to oneself rather than feeling victimized and helpless

According to studies (Kobasa, 1979; Kobasa, Maddi, & Kahn, 1982), persons having higher degrees of hardiness are healthier than those with low degrees of hardiness. When experiencing multiple stressors, such people develop fewer illnesses.

Many nurses must learn when to stop working and relearn the value of play. Nursing students, spending many hours working and studying, may need to schedule playtime. The student nurse doing so is making a start on managing stress.

SAMPLE NURSING CARE PLAN

The Client Experiencing Severe Anxiety

S.H. is a 38-year-old female in the emergency department of the local hospital. She paces, wrings her hands, and is tearful. She says she has chest pressure, palpitations, and shortness of breath. She is diaphoretic and her hands are trembling. Her blood pressure is 140/90, pulse 110, and respirations 30 and shallow. She says that her husband left her a month ago. She states, "I feel like I'm going crazy! My heart is racing and I can't sit still."

Assessment reveals autonomic hyperactivity (rapid pulse and respirations, elevated blood pressure), verbalized feelings of apprehension, restlessness, and going crazy.

NURSING DIAGNOSIS *Anxiety* related to situational crisis, threat to self-concept, and change in role status as evidenced by statement "I feel like I'm going crazy" and the fact that her husband left her a month ago

Nursing Outcomes Classification (NOC)
Anxiety Control
Coping
Psychosocial Adjustment: Life Change

Nursing Interventions Classification (NIC)
Anxiety Reduction
Coping Enhancement
Simple Relaxation Therapy

PLANNING/OUTCOMES	NURSING INTERVENTIONS	RATIONALE
S.H. will identify effective coping mechanisms.	Establish a trusting relationship.	Reduces anxiety.
	Have S.H. identify and describe physical and emotional feelings.	Is the first step in coping with anxiety.
	Help S.H. relate cause-and-effect relationship between stressors and anxiety.	Enhances S.H.'s sense of power and control over the situation.
	Encourage S.H. to use previously successful coping mechanisms.	Builds confidence in own coping abilities.

(Continues)

SAMPLE NURSING CARE PLAN (Continued)

PLANNING/OUTCOMES	NURSING INTERVENTIONS	RATIONALE
S.H. will report that anxiety has lessened and is manageable.	Using therapeutic communication techniques, encourage S.H. to talk about what has been happening in her life.	Clarifies situation by talking about it.
S.H. will demonstrate relaxation skills.	Teach S.H. relaxation techniques (such as cognitive reframing and imagery).	Counters the physiologic effects of the stress response (lower blood pressure, decreased heart rate, and respirations).

EVALUATION

S.H. looks relaxed. Vital signs are within normal limits. S.H. verbalizes that she feels calmer and no longer afraid that she is "going crazy."

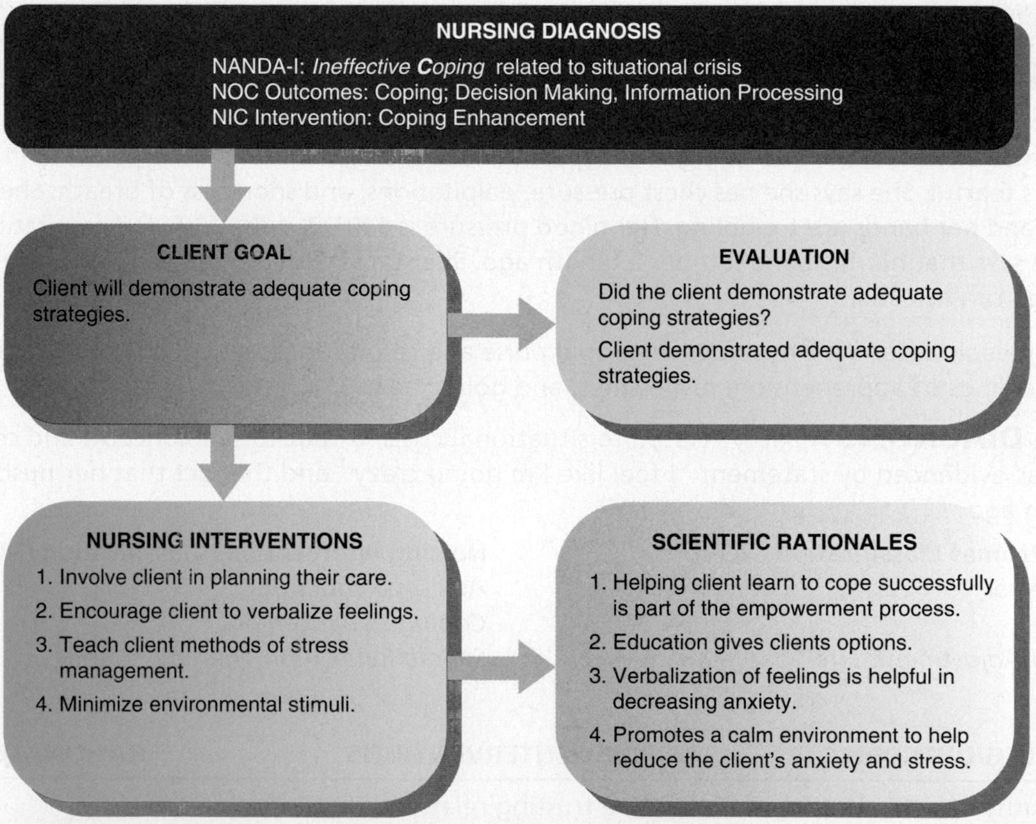

NURSING DIAGNOSIS
NANDA-I: *Ineffective Coping* related to situational crisis
NOC Outcomes: Coping; Decision Making, Information Processing
NIC Intervention: Coping Enhancement
CLIENT GOAL
Client will demonstrate adequate coping strategies.
EVALUATION
Did the client demonstrate adequate coping strategies?
Client demonstrated adequate coping strategies.
NURSING INTERVENTIONS
1. Involve client in planning their care.
2. Encourage client to verbalize feelings.
3. Teach client methods of stress management.
4. Minimize environmental stimuli.
SCIENTIFIC RATIONALES
1. Helping client learn to cope successfully is part of the empowerment process.
2. Education gives clients options.
3. Verbalization of feelings is helpful in decreasing anxiety.
4. Promotes a calm environment to help reduce the client's anxiety and stress.

CONCEPT CARE MAP 12-1 Ineffective Coping

SUMMARY

- Stress is an individual's physiologic response to a demand made on the body.
- Individuals experiencing prolonged periods of stress risk developing stress-related diseases.
- Anxiety, the psychological response to a real or perceived threat to the health and well-being of an individual, activates the stress response.
- An individual seeks equilibrium through adaptation. When adaptation is effective, homeostasis is maintained.
- The general adaptation syndrome (GAS), the physiologic response to stress, consists of three stages: alarm, resistance, and exhaustion. The GAS is the same whether the stressor is actual or imagined, present or potential.

- Major stressors for clients and their families are illness and hospitalization. To alleviate the stress of hospitalization, nursing interventions should reduce the client's feelings of unfamiliarity and loss of control.
- Change can be perceived as stressful because of a fear of failure, a threat to security, or a potential for loss of self-esteem.
- Burnout occurs when the nurse is overwhelmed by stress, resulting in physical, emotional, and behavioral dysfunction, including decreased productivity.
- A stress-management plan for nurses involves maintaining support systems, using time-management and decision-making skills, maintaining a sense of humor, and knowing personal limits.

REVIEW QUESTIONS

1. The client is in an acute crisis state and requires crisis intervention. The nurse recognizes that the client needs more assistance than the nurse is able to provide. Prompt consultation/referral to other health care providers is necessary and would include:
   1. psychologist, psychiatrist, social worker.
   2. family physician, midwife, social worker.
   3. social worker, respiratory therapist, nursing supervisor.
   4. psychologist, nursing supervisor, pharmacist.
2. The general adaptation syndrome (GAS) is the:
   1. behavioral response to stress.
   2. sociocultural response to stress.
   3. psychological response to stress.
   4. physiologic response to stress.
3. The nurse tells her unit supervisor that she is feeling burned out and not sure that she wants to be a nurse anymore. Which of the following work-related factors can contribute to her burnout? (Select all that apply).
   1. Heavy workload.
   2. Mandatory overtime.
   3. Recently divorced.
   4. Little work-related social support.
   5. Child care issues.
   6. Interpersonal conflict in the work environment.
4. The purpose of the first stage of the GAS is to:
   1. alert the individual to danger.
   2. determine the cause of the danger.
   3. mobilize energy needed for adaptation.
   4. prevent the individual from having an unpleasant experience.
5. Which of the following statements is correct when teaching the client about the degree and duration of stress?
   1. A large number of stressors at one time will increase the severity of stress.
   2. The longer a stress lasts, the less severe it becomes for a person.
   3. A large amount of stress will improve performance.
   4. Many persons under severe stress go through life without any psychological effect.
6. While assisting the client with his morning care, the nurse notes that the client is quieter than yesterday and appears to be very anxious. To determine the level of anxiety that the client is experiencing, the nurse should ask which of the following questions?
   1. "You seem worried about something. Would it help to talk about it?"
   2. "Would you like for me to call a family member to come and give you support?"
   3. "Would you like to go down the hall and talk with another client who had the same surgery?"
   4. "How serious do you think your illness is?"
7. A 68-year-old client is in a rehabilitative facility after having had a cerebrovascular accident. The client is noncommunicative, heart rate increases, blood pressure is maintained, and respirations are becoming increased and labored. Which of the stages of the GAS is the client experiencing?
   1. Resistance stage.
   2. Alarm reaction.
   3. Exhaustion stage.
   4. Reflex pain response.
8. A factory worker cuts his arm while trimming a piece of steel, and it bleeds profusely. He quickly applies pressure to his arm and causes a cessation of the bleeding within minutes. Shortly afterward, the factory worker bumps the arm again. The bleeding begins again and will not stop. Which stage of the GAS would the factory worker have experienced if the blood loss continued and he could not obtain assistance?
   1. Stage of alarm reaction.
   2. Stage of resistance.
   3. Stage of exhaustion.
   4. Stage of distress.
9. A client who has been newly diagnosed with a terminal illness and is hospitalized for the first time is exhibiting signs that she is not coping well, which include all of the following except:
   1. increase in stress response.
   2. increased use of coping mechanisms.
   3. inability to function.
   4. increased organizational behavior.
10. Coping mechanisms to avoid dealing directly with stress are called:
    1. adaptive measures.
    2. maladaptive measures.
    3. nonadaptive measures.
    4. progressive measures.

REFERENCES/SUGGESTED READINGS

Aguilera, D. C. (1998). *Crisis intervention: Theory and methodology* (8th ed.). St. Louis, MO: Mosby.

Alfaro-LeFevre, R. (2009). *Critical thinking and clinical judgment* (4th ed.). Philadelphia: W. B. Saunders.

American Institute of Stress. (2002a). America's #1 health problem. Available: http://www.stress.org/problem.htm

American Institute of Stress. (2002b). Job stress. Available: http://www.stress.org/job.htm

American Institute of Stress. (2002c). Stress. Available: http://www.stress.org

Badger, J. M. (1995). Tips for managing stress on the job. *American Journal of Nursing, 95*(9), 31–33.

Beck, A. (1976). *Cognitive therapy and emotional disorders*. New York: International Universities Press.

Briguglio, A. (2007). Should the family stay? *RN, 70*(5), 42–48.

Bulechek, G., Butcher, H., McCloskey, J., & Dochterman, J., eds. (2008). *Nursing Interventions Classification (NIC)* (5th ed.). St. Louis, MO: Mosby/Elsevier.

Cullen, A. (1995). Burnout: Why do we blame the nurse? *American Journal of Nursing, 95*(11), 23–27.

Delaune, S. C., & Ladner, P. K. (2006). *Fundamentals of Nursing Standards & Practice* (3rd ed.)., Clifton Park, NY: Delmar Cengage Learning.

Fink, J. L. W. (2005). Burned out? Here's help. *Nursing, 35*(4), 53.

Freud, S. (1959). Inhibitions, symptoms and anxiety. In J. Strachey (Trans.), *The standard edition of the complete psychological works of Sigmund Freud* (Vol. 20). London: Hogarth.

Frisch, N., & Frisch, L. (2010). *Psychiatric mental health nursing* (4th ed.). Clifton Park, NY: Delmar Cengage Learning.

Keegan, L. (2000). Nutrition, exercise, and movement. In B. M. Dossey, L. Keegan, & C. E. Guzzetta (Eds.), *Holistic nursing: A handbook for practice* (3rd ed.). Gaithersburg, MD: Aspen.

Kneisl, C. R., & Riley, E. (1996). Crisis intervention. In H. S. Wilson & C. R. Kneisl (Eds.), *Psychiatric nursing* (5th ed., pp. 711–731). Menlo Park, CA: Addison-Wesley.

Kobasa, S. C. (1979). Stressful life events, personality and health: An inquiry into hardiness. *Journal of Personality and Social Psychology, 37*(1), 1–11.

Kobasa, S. C., Maddi, S. R., & Kahn, S. (1982). Hardiness and health: A prospective study. *Journal of Personality and Social Psychology, 45*(4), 839–850.

Lyon, B. L. (2000). Situational anger and self-empowerment. *Reflections on Nursing Leadership, 26*(3), 36–37.

Mandle, C. L., & Gruber-Wood, R. (2002). Health promotion and the individual. In C. L. Edelman & C. L. Mandle (Eds.), *Health promotion throughout the lifespan* (5th ed.). St. Louis, MO: Mosby.

Mayo Clinic. (1999). Stress patrol: Stop tension in its tracks. Available: http://www.mayohealth.org/mayo/9912/ htm/stress_patrol.htm

Mayo Clinic. (2000a). Dealing with co-worker conflict. Available: http://www.mayohealth.org/mayo/9704/ htm/stre_1sb.htm

Mayo Clinic. (2000b). Workplace stress: Can you control it? Available: http://www.mayohealth.org/mayo/9704/ htm/stress.htm

Meyers, T. A., Eichhorn, D. J., Guzzetta, C. E., Clark, A. P., Klein, J. D., Taliaferro, E., et al. (2000). Family presence during invasive procedures and resuscitation. *American Journal of Nursing, 100*(2), 32–40.

Moorhead, S., Johnson, M., Maas, M., & Swanson, E. (2007). *Nursing Outcomes Classification (NOC)* (4th ed.). St. Louis, MO: Mosby.

North American Nursing Diagnosis Association International. (2010). *NANDA-I nursing diagnoses: Definitions and classification 2009–2011*. Ames, IA: Wiley-Blackwell.

Page, K. (2002). Panic attack. *Nursing2002, 32*(1), 88.

Peplau, H. (1952). *Interpersonal relations in nursing*. New York: Putnam.

Selye, H. (1974). *Stress without distress*. New York: New American Library.

Selye, H. (1976). *Stress in health and disease* (Rev. ed.). Boston: Butterworths.

Sullivan, H. S. (1953). *The interpersonal theory of psychiatry*. New York: Norton.

Talbott, S. W. (1997). Political analysis: Structure and process. In D. J. Mason, S. W. Talbott, & J. K. Leavitt (Eds.), *Policy and politics for nurses* (2nd ed., pp. 129–148). Philadelphia: W. B. Saunders.

U.S. Preventive Services Task Force. (2002). Screening for depression: Recommendations and rationale. *Annals of Internal Medicine, 136*(10), 760.

Waughfield, C. (2002). *Mental health concepts* (5th ed.). Clifton Park, NY: Delmar Cengage Learning.

Wilson, H. S., & Kneisel, C. R. (1996). *Psychiatric nursing* (5th ed.). Menlo Park, CA: Addison-Wesley.

Wilson, H. S., Kneisel, C. R., & Trigoboff, E. (2004). *Contemporary psychiatric-mental health nursing*. Upper Saddle River, NJ: Prentice Hall.

RESOURCES

American Holistic Nurses Association, http://www.ahna.org

American Institute of Stress, http://www.stress.org

International Stress Management Association UK, http://www.isma.org.uk

CHAPTER 13

End-of-Life Care

MAKING THE CONNECTION

Refer to the following chapters to increase your understanding of loss, grief, and death:

Basic Nursing

- ***Legal and Ethical Responsibilities***
- ***Arenas of Care***
- ***Life Span Development***
- ***Cultural Considerations***
- ***Spirituality***
- ***Complementary/Alternative Therapies***

LEARNING OBJECTIVES

Upon completion of this chapter, you should be able to:

- Define key terms.
- Discuss the various losses that affect individuals at different stages of the life span.
- Identify characteristics of an individual experiencing grief.
- Compare and contrast adaptive grief and pathological grief.
- Discuss the stages of the normal grieving process.
- Describe the holistic needs of the dying person and family.
- Plan care for a dying client.
- Describe nursing responsibilities when a client dies.
- Discuss ways that nurses can cope with their own grief.

KEY TERMS

advance directive
algor mortis
anticipatory grief
autopsy
bereavement
breakthrough pain
Cheyne-Stokes respirations
complicated grief
death rattle
disenfranchised grief
dysfunctional grief
end-of-life care
grief
Health Care Surrogate Law
hospice
life review
liver mortis
loss
maturational loss
mortuary
mourning
palliative care
postmortem care
resuscitation
rigor mortis
shroud
situational loss
traumatic imagery
uncomplicated grief

INTRODUCTION

Individuals are constantly experiencing loss. Episodes of personal crisis, natural disaster, and terrorism result in the experience of loss. The nurse must be aware of the many ways individuals react and adapt to losses.

Individuals are faced with losses throughout the life cycle. Growth and development would not continue to progress without some losses.

Nurses encounter clients every day who are responding to grief associated with losses. An understanding of the major concepts related to loss and grieving is necessary for each nurse. Many people consider loss only in terms of death and dying. Because nurses also care for dying clients, this chapter includes information on meeting the special needs of terminally ill clients and their families.

LOSS

Loss is any situation, either potential, actual, or perceived, wherein a valued object or person is changed or is not accessible to the individual. Everyone experiences losses because change is a major constant in life. Loss can be actual (e.g., a child is lost in the woods) or anticipated (a diabetic client is faced with having a foot amputated). The loss can be tangible or intangible. For example, when a person is not selected for a job, the tangible loss is income, and the intangible loss is self-esteem.

Losses also occur as a person moves from one developmental stage to another. An example of such a **maturational loss** is the toddler who loses the bottle after learning to drink from a glass. A **situational loss** takes place in response to external events generally beyond the individual's control, such as losing a job when the company is bankrupt.

The four major categories of loss are loss of significant other, loss of aspects of self, loss of external objects, and loss of a familiar environment.

LOSS OF SIGNIFICANT OTHER

Losing a loved one is a very significant loss. Such a loss can result from moving to a different area, separation, divorce, or death.

LOSS OF ASPECT OF SELF

Loss of an aspect of self can be physiological or psychological. Physiological loss includes loss of physical function or loss resulting from disfigurement or disappearance of a body part, as is the case with amputation or mastectomy. Loss of a physical aspect of self can result from trauma, illness, or a treatment methodology such as surgery. Psychological aspects of self that may be lost include a sense of humor, ambition, or enjoyment of life. These feelings of loss may result from life events such as losing a job or failing at a task that the individual deems important.

LOSS OF AN EXTERNAL OBJECT

Whenever an object that a person highly values is changed or damaged or disappears, loss occurs. The type and amount of grieving depends on the significance of the lost object to the individual. For instance, an individual who loses a family heirloom in a fire may react not only to the lost financial value of the piece but also to the lost sense of history and heritage that the piece represented.

LOSS OF FAMILIAR ENVIRONMENT

The loss of a familiar environment occurs when a person moves away from familiar surroundings, for instance to another home or a different community, to a new school, or to a new job. A client who is hospitalized or institutionalized may also experience loss when faced with new surroundings. This type of loss evokes anxiety related to fear of the unknown.

GRIEF

Grief is a series of intense psychological and physical responses occurring after a loss. These responses are necessary, normal, natural, and adaptive responses to the loss. Loss moves the individual to the adaptive process of **mourning**, the period during which grief is expressed and integration and resolution of the loss occur. **Bereavement** is the period of grief that follows the death of a loved one (Figure 13-1).

STAGES OF GRIEF

Three stages of grief generally recognized are shock, reality, and recovery.

Shock Stage

The period of shock may last from only days to a month or more. The person may describe feeling "numb." It is an emotional numbness rather than a physical one.

Reality Stage

A painful experience begins when the individual consciously realizes the full meaning of the loss. Anger, guilt, fear, frustration, and/or helplessness may be the expressed reactions.

Recovery Stage

During the last stage, recovery, the loss is integrated into the reality of the individual's life. The person exhibits adaptive

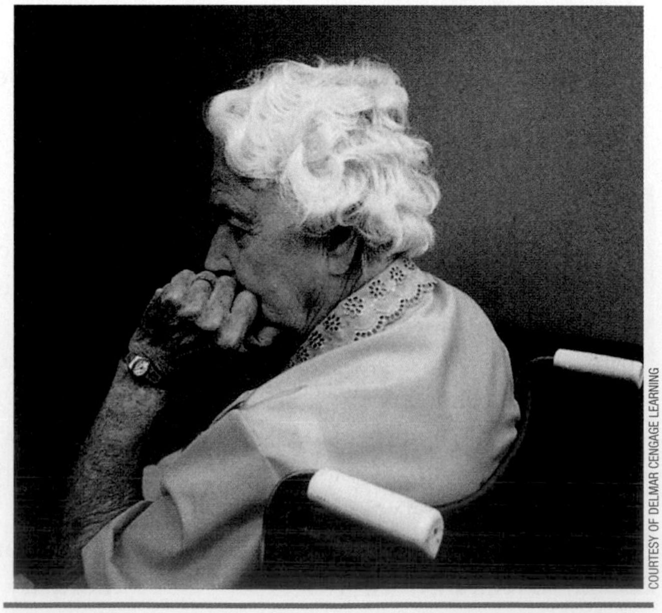

FIGURE 13-1 Older adults may grieve intensely over the loss of a person or situation that has been a part of their lives for many years.

MEMORYTRICK

A memory trick to recall the grief stages is "**SRR**":

S = Shock

R = Reality

R = Recovery

behaviors and begins to live again, doing things that were formerly enjoyed.

Types of Grief

Grief is a normal, universal, response to loss. Grief drains people, both physically and emotionally, and relationships often suffer. Different types of grief include uncomplicated ("normal"), anticipatory, dysfunctional, and disenfranchised grief.

Nurses assist many individuals to understand the normal grieving process. Nurses who understand all types of grief are better prepared to assist others.

Uncomplicated Grief

Uncomplicated grief is what many individuals would refer to as *normal grief*. Engle (1961) proposed the term **uncomplicated grief** to describe the grief reaction normally following a significant loss. Uncomplicated grief has a fairly predictable course that ends with relinquishing the lost object and resuming the duties of life.

The grieving person may feel angry, hopeless, or sad and may express feelings of depression. A person who is grieving may experience loss of appetite, weight loss, insomnia, restlessness, indecisiveness, impulsivity, and inability to concentrate or carry out daily activities.

Anticipatory Grief

Anticipatory grief is the occurrence of grief before an expected loss actually occurs. Anticipatory grief may be experienced by both the person's family and the terminally ill person. This process promotes early grieving, freeing emotional energy for adapting once the loss has occurred. Although anticipatory grieving may be helpful in adjusting to the loss, it also has some potential disadvantages. For example, in the case of the dying client, the family members may distance themselves and not be available for support. Also, if the family members have separated themselves emotionally from the dying client, they may seem cold and distant and, thus, not meet society's expectations of mourning behavior. This response can, in turn, prevent the mourners from receiving their own much-needed support from others (Pritchett & Lucas, 1997b).

PROFESSIONALTIP

Successful Grieving

The person experiencing successful grieving will:

- Consciously recognize that a significant loss has occurred.
- Progress through the stages of grief.
- Use adaptive coping behaviors, such as interacting with others, participating in and completing tasks, and having a positive attitude.

PROFESSIONALTIP

Identifying Dysfunctional Grief

Normal and dysfunctional grief are differentiated in that the person experiencing dysfunctional grief is unable to adapt to life without the deceased person.

Dysfunctional grief can take several forms, specifically chronic grief, delayed grief, exaggerated grief, or masked grief.

Chronic grief is the inability to conclude grieving.

Delayed grief occurs when grief work does not take place at the time of loss.

Exaggerated grief describes the situation when grief is experienced as overwhelming.

Masked grief occurs when grief is covered up by maladaptive behaviors such as apathy, irritability, and unstable moods or a physical symptom such as loss of libido, with the person being unaware of the connection to the loss and grief.

Dysfunctional Grief

Dysfunctional grief is a demonstration of a persistent pattern of intense grief that does not result in reconciliation of feelings. The person experiencing dysfunctional (or pathological) grief does not progress through the stages of grief. The dysfunctionally grieving person cannot reestablish a routine. The professional caregiver must be aware of these behaviors and refer the pathologically grieving person to professional counseling.

Disenfranchised Grief

Disenfranchised grief is described as grief not openly acknowledged, socially sanctioned, or publicly shared. When an individual either is reluctant to recognize the sense of loss and develops guilt feelings or feels pressured by society to "get on with life," grief can become disenfranchised. An example of disenfranchised grief is extreme sadness over the loss of a pet when this mourning might be viewed by others as excessive or inappropriate. A mother's sadness over a miscarriage might also be considered disenfranchised grief because a lengthy period of mourning may not be publicly expected despite the mother's intense feelings of loss and despair.

Factors Affecting Loss and Grief

Variables affecting the intensity and duration of grieving are:

- Developmental stage
- Religious and cultural beliefs

- Relationship with the lost object
- Cause of death

Developmental Stage

Depending on the client's place on the age/development continuum, the grief response to a loss will be experienced differently. For example, a pregnant woman will, to some degree, experience loss after delivery of a first child (loss of freedom, independence, and self-focused life), even when the child is normal and healthy. Certain kinds of loss at key developmental points may have a profound effect on a person's ability to both work through the resulting grief and achieve the tasks of the given developmental stage. For example, an adolescent who has lost a parent may have difficulty forming an intimate relationship with members of the opposite sex.

Childhood Children vary in their reactions to loss and in the ability to comprehend the meaning of death. It is important to understand the way a child's concept of death evolves because the concept varies with developmental level and may affect mastery of developmental tasks (Table 13-1).

Children who are grieving need honest explanations about death using terms they can understand.

Adolescence Physical attractiveness and athletic abilities are valued by most adolescents. Because adolescents seek approval of their peer group, when the adolescent suffers the loss of a body part or function, grief includes fear of being rejected. After a disfiguring accident, grief is usually very intense. Even though they have an intellectual understanding of death, adolescents believe themselves to be invulnerable and, thus, immune to death; they reject the possibility of their own mortality.

Early Adulthood In the young adult, grief is often precipitated by loss of role or status. For example, significant grief may be caused by unemployment or the breakup of a relationship. The concept of death in this age-group reflects primarily spiritual beliefs and cultural values (Figure 13-2).

Middle Adulthood The potential for experiencing loss increases during middle adulthood. The death of parents often occurs during this developmental phase. As an individual ages, it can be especially threatening when peers die, because these deaths force acknowledgment of one's own mortality.

Late Adulthood Most individuals recognize the inevitability of death during late adulthood. It is challenging for elders to experience the death of age-old friends or to find themselves the last one of their peer group left living. Older adults often turn to their children and grandchildren as sources of comfort and companionship. Cultivating friendships in all age-groups helps prevent loneliness and depression.

Table 13-1 Perception of Death by Children and Adolescents

DEVELOPMENTAL STAGE	PERCEPTION	POTENTIAL DEVELOPMENTAL DISRUPTIONS
Infancy, toddlerhood	• Unaware of death • Aware of changes in normal routine • Reacts to family's expressions of grief	• Death of primary caregiver during the first 2 years of life may have significant long-lasting psychosocial implications.
Preschool	• Believes death is a temporary separation • Reacts to the gravity of death as they see parents or others react	• Loss of either parent may have significant psychosocial implications, especially between ages 4 and 6 years (because of magical thinking, wherein children may believe death is their fault). • Problems with development of sexual identity, depending on the gender of the parent lost, the child's identification with that parent, and the child's present state of sexual identity.
School age	• Comprehends that death is inevitable and final • Conjectures about and is inclined to personify death ("the boogie-man")	• Potential nightmares. • Potential death-avoidance behaviors (e.g., hiding under the covers, leaving the lights on, closing closet doors). • Possible intense guilt and a sense of responsibility for the death.
Preadolescence and adolescence	• Acknowledges that death is final • Comprehends that death is inevitable • *Preadolescents:* may worry about dying; *adolescents:* seem to deny that they could die	• Loss of a parent may cause difficulty in forming an intimate relationship with members of the opposite sex.

LIFE SPAN CONSIDERATIONS

Talking with Children about Death

- *Avoid the* use of euphemisms. For example, if a child is told that the deceased person has "gone away," the child may believe that the dead person will return. Also, a child may develop sleep phobia if told that the deceased is "asleep."
- *Do not overexplain.* Keep explanations concise and factual; do not offer lengthy explanations of medical conditions.
- *Use simple, concrete terms.* Young children are not able to conceptualize abstract ideas, such as "grandma is in a better place now."
- *Show them.* Many young children understand something only when they see it. Take them to the funeral service and cemetery.

From *National Directory of Bereavement Support Groups and Services* (3rd ed.), by M. Wong, 1998, New York: ADM Publishing.

Religious and Cultural Beliefs

An individual's grief experience is significantly affected by religious and cultural beliefs. Every culture has rituals for care of the dying and beliefs about the significance of death. Other beliefs regarding an afterlife, redemption of the soul, a supreme being, and reincarnation can assist the individual in grief work.

Relationship with the Lost Person or Object

Generally, the grief experienced is more intense the more intimate the relationship was with the deceased. The risk for dysfunctional grieving is particularly great after the death of a child.

The death of a child is generally thought to be exceptionally painful because it upsets the natural order of things; parents do not expect their children to die before them.

Parents experiencing grief usually have intense responses and reactions (Figure 13-3). Parental grief is unique in that it encompasses both the loss of the perceived potential of that child and the loss of parental hopes for the child. Table 13-2 suggests some characteristics of parents of infants who have died.

The death of a sibling or parent can be a major challenge for children. Adults failing to understand the child's need to mourn may not recognize the child's feelings. Normal reactions of a child when a sibling dies as an infant, and nursing responses to these reactions, are given in Table 13-3.

CRITICAL THINKING

Perceptions of Death

Find a classmate from a different cultural background than yours. How does your classmate's perception of death differ from yours?

Cause of Death

The intensity of the grief response also varies depending whether the cause of death was unexpected, traumatic, or a suicide.

Unexpected Death The bereaved have particular difficulty in achieving closure when the loss occurs as a result of an unexpected death. Survivors are shocked and bereaved after an unanticipated death, such as an aneurysm, heart attack, or stroke. Usually, the bereaved can work through the grieving process without complications.

Traumatic Death Complicated grief is associated with traumatic death such as death by accident, violence, or homicide. Survivors are not necessarily predisposed to complications in mourning but often have more intense emotions than those associated with normal grief.

Following a violent death, the bereaved may undergo **traumatic imagery** (imagining the feelings of horror felt by the victim or reliving the terror of the incident). Traumatic imagery is a common occurrence in cases of traumatic death. Such thoughts, coupled with intense grief, can lead to post-traumatic stress disorder (PTSD) in the survivors. Nurses' awareness of the possibility of PTSD and alertness for the presence of symptoms is important. Symptoms may include:

- Chronic anxiety
- Psychological distress
- Sleep disturbances, such as recurrent, terror-filled nightmares

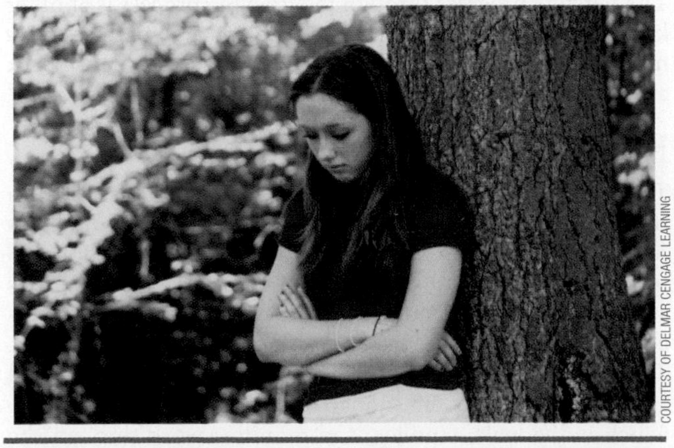

COURTESY OF DELMAR CENGAGE LEARNING

FIGURE 13-2 Young adults usually grieve loss of a role, such as employment or the breakup of a relationship.

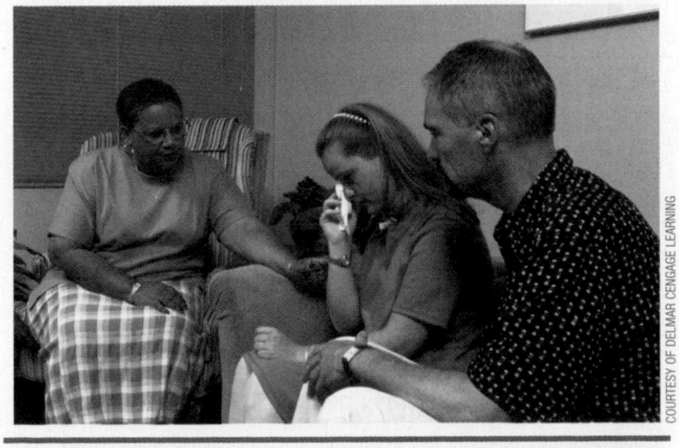

COURTESY OF DELMAR CENGAGE LEARNING

FIGURE 13-3 The couple discusses grief over the loss of a child.

Table 13-2 Characteristics of Parents When a Child Dies

TYPE OF DEATH	PARENTAL CHARACTERISTICS
Spontaneous abortion (miscarriage) and stillbirth	• The mother, especially, may have feelings of intense sadness, guilt, or anger. If the loss occurs in early weeks of pregnancy, the death may be inadequately recognized by others. • The death may be regarded as a personal failure. • Parents may blame themselves or others. • Previous miscarriages may be relived and grieved. • If the condition of the infant was known, anticipatory grief may occur. • Grief may increase if ambivalent about being pregnant. • Despair may be greatest when the parents leave the hospital or birthplace without the baby.
Neonatal death	• Similar reactions as with stillbirth. • The bond between parents and infant intensifies the grief. • Both parents may have intense grief.
Sudden infant death syndrome (SIDS)	• Parents are in a state of shock. • Lack of knowledge and misinformation increases pain. • Because SIDS usually occurs during the first 6 months of life, parental bonding is complete. • May feel guilt. • Grief is acute; parents are not prepared for the loss. • May be engrossed with the details of the death.
Induced Abortion	• Secrecy, guilt, and shame may accompany grief. • May have ambivalent feelings. • May find little support or comfort from others. • Feelings of despair and depression may be present when relief was expected. • If child was not wanted, no guilt may be felt.

From *Healing and the Grief Process*, by S. Roach and B. Nieto, 1997, Clifton Park, NY: Delmar Cengage Learning.

Only when this problem is identified and the survivors are encouraged to express their intense feelings will they be able to move through the normal, adaptive grieving process.

Suicide The loss of a loved one to suicide is frequently compounded by feelings of guilt by the survivors for failing to recognize clues that may have permitted the victim to receive help. The feelings of guilt and self-blame can change into anger at the victim for inflicting such pain. Having a suicide in the family may evoke feelings of shame. Survivors may be prohibited from successfully resolving their grief by the negative stigma of suicide.

Nursing Care of the Grieving Client

Rodebaugh, Schwindt, and Valentine (1999) suggest that grief be thought of as a journey through four broad categories titled reeling, feeling, dealing, and healing. Clients are reeling when experiencing shock or disbelief. Feelings are expressed in various emotions and behaviors. Dealing occurs when they begin to adapt to the loss. Things do not necessarily get better; they just get different. Healing is when the loss becomes part of them, and the acute anguish lessens; it does not mean forgetting. People are changed by grief. Self-esteem is affected, new ways of coping are developed, and a new lifestyle without the deceased is begun. Although it is a painful process, clients must resolve the loss in their own way. As the client moves through the process of mourning, nurses can assist by providing support. The nurse asks the client what he can do to help and listens for needs expressed.

Nurses can assist people to grieve by encouraging them to experience their feelings to the fullest in order to work through them. Providing support and explaining to the bereaved that it will take time to grieve the loss and to gain some closure to the relationship are both important nursing responsibilities.

After the loved one dies, the caregiver feels grief and relief. Caregivers often feel guilty for feeling relieved. Assure them these feelings are very normal, as caregiving is exhausting, leaving one with little emotional and physical reserve. The nurse assists the caregiver to find ways to fill his life with meaningful activities.

Assessment

Determining the personal meaning of the loss is the beginning of a thorough assessment of the grieving client and family. The person's progress through the grieving process is another key assessment area. The stages of grieving are not necessarily mastered sequentially, but instead individuals may move back and forth through the stages of grief.

Nursing Diagnosis

The North American Nursing Diagnosis Association International (NANDA-I) defines *Dysfunctional **G**rieving* as "extended, unsuccessful use of intellectual and emotional responses by which individuals, families, communities attempt to work through the process of modifying self-concept based upon the perception of loss" (NANDA, 2010). The other grieving diagnosis is *Anticipatory **G**rieving*, defined as "intellectual and emotional responses and behaviors by which individuals, families, communities work through the process of modifying self-concept based on the perception of potential loss" (NANDA, 2010).

TABLE 13-3 Reactions of Siblings after Infant Death

NORMAL REACTION	NURSING RESPONSE
• Fear loss of and separation from parents	• Reassure that parents will not leave them
• Guilt, because of feelings of jealousy and anger related to wishing that the infant would go away	• Reassure siblings that they did not influence the cause of death by providing information (at the appropriate level of understanding)
• Fear that parents' intense reactions will hinder parents' ability to take care of them	• Provide assurance that life will go on by continuing routine activities
• Fear of dying soon and concern over own health	• Persuade parents to avoid being overprotective, which will reinforce children's fears

Data adapted from "Supporting Families after Sudden Infant Death," by M. McClain and S. Shaefer, 1996, *Journal of Psychosocial Nursing and Mental Health Services, 34*(4), 30–34.

Planning/Outcome Identification

When planning care for the grieving client, it is important to clarify the expected outcomes. Some expected goals for the person experiencing grief are:

- Accept the loss
- Verbalize feelings of grief
- Share grief with significant others
- Renew activities and relationships

Some of these expected outcomes will take a long time to achieve, and some must be achieved before others are mastered. For example, to accept the loss, the person must begin to share grief with others by verbalizing those feelings. Two of the expected outcomes are discussed below.

Acceptance of the Loss Individuals are able to reach some acceptance and resolution of feelings about the loss only by going through grief work. Often, people try to find some meaning in their situations. This search involves introspection, for which spiritual support may be therapeutic.

Renewal of Activities and Relationships The basis of grief work revolves around accepting the fact that the needs met by key people in life can be met by other people in other ways. Knowing that the deceased cannot be replaced, healing must occur so that new relationships may begin.

Implementation

Basic to therapeutic nursing care is an understanding of the significance of the loss to the client. The nurse must spend time listening to understand the client's perspective. Even if the client does not respond according to the nurse's belief system or expectations, the nurse must demonstrate acceptance. The nurse's nonjudgmental, accepting attitude is essential during the bereaved's expression of all feelings, including anger and despair. The nurse avoids personalizing and using defensive behaviors by communicating an understanding of the client's anger. The expression of grief is not only appropriate but also essential for therapeutic resolution of the loss.

Grieving people need reassurance, support, and counseling. One mechanism of support on a long-term basis is support groups. The nurse must be informed about the availability of such groups within the community in order to make appropriate referrals. Members of support groups have experienced similar losses. Discussions in support groups decrease the feelings of loneliness and social isolation that are so common in the grief experience.

Evaluation

People follow their own time schedule for grief work. Because it takes months or years for grief resolution, nurses usually do not have the opportunity to know when the bereaved family completes its grief work. The nurse does have a unique opportunity to lay the foundation for adaptive grieving by encouraging the family to verbalize their experience and share their feelings with significant others. The foundation for evaluation is the goals mutually established with client and family. It is important for nurses to teach grieving individuals that resolution of the loss is generally a process of lifelong adjustment.

DEATH

Historically, death has been considered as natural as birth, as simply the last stage of life. Significant changes in the perception of death have occurred in the past three decades. In some cases, dying and death are no longer simple matters but are issues involving ethical concerns and, in some cases, legal intervention by the court system.

Each person dies a unique death, just as each person lives a unique life. Death may be sudden and unexpected, caused by accident or heart attack, for example, or death may be prolonged, coming after a distressing long-term illness. For the older person who dies during sleep, death comes quietly. Those who choose to die on their own terms by suicide plan their deaths.

Health care workers must understand the ethical and legal issues surrounding dying and death. Understanding the stages

PROFESSIONALTIP

Adaptive Grieving

How long does the process of adaptive grieving take? The length of time necessary for grief resolution is as individual as the person experiencing it and depends on the intensity of the grief. Grief is considered to be a "long-term process" (Corless, Germino, & Pittman, 2006). Grief work takes time. There are no definite time frames within which grief should occur. Each person grieves in his own way and at his own pace.

CULTURAL CONSIDERATIONS

Cultural Diversity and Death

Cultural Group	Role of Family	Display of Emotion	Care of Dying in Home
African American	Health care providers should communicate with the oldest family member about the dying client.	Expected	Families frequently care for dying elders in the home.
Chinese American	Family may prefer dying client not be told of terminal illness or imminent death or may prefer a family member tell the client.	Express sorrow at parents' funeral; the first son is in mourning for 72 days and cannot wear red clothing or marry during that time.	Some believe bad luck will occur if client dies in the home and others think the client's spirit will get lost if death occurs in the hospital. Family may use amulets or cloths.
Filipino American	Health care providers should communicate with the head of the family and not in the presence of the client.	Expected	Dying client may desire to die in the home.
Hispanic or Latino American	Extended families care for the dying client. Families share information and decision making.	Wailing shows respect for the dead client.	Some believe the spirit will get lost if the client dies in the hospital. Use of amulets, rosary beads, and prayers are common.

Data from "Cultural Considerations in End-of-Life Care" by P. Mazanec and M. Tyler, 2003, *American Journal of Nursing*.

of death and dying and the signs of impending death will help prepare the nurse to render sensitive, effective care, both to the client and family and to the client's body after death. Nurses must also come to terms with their own mortality and feelings about death if they are to provide comfort to dying clients and their families. Health care workers can learn a great deal about life from the dying client.

LEGAL CONSIDERATIONS

The *Patient Self-Determination Act* (PSDA) is part of the Omnibus Budget Reconciliation Act (OBRA) of 1990. This act provides a legal means for individuals to specify the circumstances under which life-sustaining measures should or should not be rendered to them. The individual's choices are identified in advance directives. An **advance directive** is any written instruction recognized under state law, including a durable power of attorney, for health care or living will. The act applies to hospitals, home health agencies, long-term care facilities, hospice programs, and certain health maintenance organizations (HMOs). According to the PSDA, all clients entering the health care system through any of these organizations must be given information and the opportunity to complete advance directives if they have not already done so. In many states, just signing these documents may not be adequate for carrying out client wishes. They may also need to indicate their desires regarding intubation, artificial feeding, blood transfusions, chemotherapy, surgery, and transfer to the hospital (for residents in skilled care facilities).

Although a durable power of attorney for health care and living will are legal documents, they do not prevent **resuscitation** (support measures to restore consciousness and life). The medical record must have a written do-not-resuscitate (DNR) order from a physician if this is in agreement with the client's wishes and with the advance directives. In the absence of such an order, resuscitation will be initiated.

PROFESSIONALTIP

Care of the Dying Client

Dying was once considered to be a normal part of the life cycle. Today, it is often considered to be a medical problem that should be handled by health care providers. Technological advances in medicine have led to depersonalized and mechanical care of those who are dying. Our highly technological world calls for application of high-touch interventions with the dying. In other words, appropriate care of the dying is administered by compassionate nurses who are both technically competent and able to demonstrate caring. Huizdos (2000) learned that death is not the enemy—lack of caring is.

In many states a **Health Care Surrogate Law** is implemented when there is no advance directive. This law varies from state to state but basically provides a legal means for certain individuals to make decisions for the client when the client cannot do so. The spouse is the first person who would act in the interests of the client. Then children in the event there is no spouse.

Ethical Considerations

Death is often fraught with ethical dilemmas that occur almost daily in health care settings. Ethics committees in many health care agencies develop and implement policies to deal with end-of-life issues. These committees are interdisciplinary and may have clergy and attorneys as well as health care providers as members. Ethical decision making is a complex issue. Determining the difference between killing and allowing someone to die by withholding life-sustaining treatment methods is one of the most difficult dilemmas.

The American Nurses Association (ANA) distinguishes mercy killing (euthanasia or assisted suicide) and relieving pain. Euthanasia is viewed as unethical, whereas pain relief is a central value in nursing. The ANA's position is that increasing doses of medication to control pain in terminally ill clients is ethically justified, even at the expense of maintaining life (ANA, 1996, 2008).

Stages of Dying and Death

Elizabeth Kübler-Ross (1997a, 1997d) identified in her classic works five stages of dying that are experienced by clients and their families (Table 13-4). Every client does not move through each stage sequentially. These stages are experienced for varying lengths of time and in varying degrees. The client may express denial and then, a few minutes later, express acceptance of the inevitable and then anger. An important value of Kübler-Ross's work is that it has increased sensitivity to the dying client's needs.

Table 13-4 Kübler-Ross's Stages of Dying and Death

STAGE	EXAMPLE
Denial	*Verbal:* "No, I don't believe that." *Behavioral:* Client diagnosed with leukemia and refuses to consider treatment options.
Anger	*Verbal:* "Why me, why?" *Behavioral:* Client is demanding and demonstrates aggressive behavior.
Bargaining	*Verbal:* Client prays, "Please, just let me live to see my new grandbaby." *Behavioral:* Client makes deals with caregivers or god.
Depression	*Verbal:* "I just want to be alone." *Behavioral:* Client turns away and closes eyes.
Acceptance	*Verbal:* "I am ready. I feel at peace now." *Behavioral:* Client gets legal and financial affairs in order and says goodbye to family and friends.

Data from *On Death and Dying*, by E. Kübler-Ross, 1997a, New York: Macmillan. Copyright 1969 by Macmillan.

Denial

During the first stage of dying, the initial shock can be very overwhelming, making denial a useful tool of coping. It is an essential, protective mechanism that may last for only a few minutes or may manifest for months.

In some clients, denial manifests as "doctor shopping" (not to imply that second opinions are not sometimes necessary) or insisting that there must have been a mix-up or mistake in the diagnostic tests. In other clients, denial manifests as simply avoiding the issue. Their daily routines are the same as though nothing in their lives has changed. Given time, most people will eventually move past the stage of denial.

Clients may choose to be selective in the use of denial. For example, clients try to protect certain family members or friends from the truth by using denial. Clients may also use denial from time to time to set aside thoughts of illness and death in order to focus on living.

Anger

Anger often follows the initial stage of denial. The client's security is threatened by the unknown, with the normal daily routines becoming disrupted. This stage is typically very difficult for family and caregivers because they often feel useless in terms of helping their loved one through the situation. Since the client has no control over the situation, anger is the response. The anger may be directed at self, God, others, the environment, and the health care system. In the client's eyes, whatever is done is not the right thing. Family members may be greeted with silence or with outbursts of anger. Their response, in turn, may be anger, guilt, or despair.

Bargaining

The client attempts to postpone or reverse the inevitable by bargaining. The client's bargaining represents an attempt to

LIFE SPAN CONSIDERATIONS

Reactions to Impending Death

- Persons of all ages generally experience the same feelings and emotions as they progress through a terminal illness.
- Persons of any age who have endured a long illness may view death as a release from their suffering.
- Persons of any age may find it difficult to reach acceptance if they have unfinished business.
- Many people receive satisfaction from **life review** (a form of reminiscence wherein a client attempts to come to terms with conflict or to gain meaning from life and die peacefully).
- Elderly clients may welcome death, especially if they have outlived everyone who was near and dear to them.

MEMORYTRICK

A memory trick for the stages of dying and death is "**DA-B-DA**":

D = Denial

A = Anger

B = Bargaining

D = Depression

A = Acceptance

postpone death and usually has self-imposed limitations. For example, a client may ask to live long enough to see the first grandchild in exchange for giving money to a charity. Most clients bargain in silence or in confidence with their spiritual leader. It is not uncommon for a client to live long enough for some special event (a wedding or birth), then die shortly afterward.

Depression

Depression resulting from the realization that death can no longer be delayed is different from dysfunctional depression because it helps the client detach from life and makes it easier to accept death. Depression in this sense is a therapeutic experience for the dying person. Clients sometimes feel abandoned, as persons who were once friends begin to visit less and less, sometimes severing ties with the client even before death; this may compound the client's feelings of depression and hopelessness.

Acceptance

Every dying client may not reach the final stage, acceptance. Peace and contentment comes with acceptance. The client often expresses feeling that all that could be done has been done. It is important to reinforce the client's feelings and sense of personal worth. Many clients will make an effort to get all of their personal and financial affairs in order.

Sleep is required to fill a physical and emotional need, not to avoid reality. The client may limit visitors to those people with whom he feels comfortable and safe. The most significant forms of communication at this time are touch and moments of silence.

END-OF-LIFE CARE

End-of-life care is nursing care of the terminally ill that focuses on meeting the physical and psychosocial needs of the client and his family. Attention is directed to the control of symptoms, identification of client needs, the promotion of interaction between the client and significant others, and the facilitation of a peaceful death. The nurse focuses on improving the quality of life for the dying client during the final stage of life and ensures a dignified and peaceful death. As a member of the interdisciplinary team responsible for providing end-of-life care, the nurse plays a critical role in identifying client needs and in supporting family members through the end-of-life experience (Hull, 2008).

The decision to abandon aggressive treatment should not be regarded as a sign of "immediate death." Palliative and hospice care evolved over the years to bridge the gap between cure-focused treatments to end-of-life care. Both approaches serve as coordinated, multidisciplinary efforts developed purposefully to address the needs of the client and family facing a terminal illness (Hull, 2008).

Palliative Care

Terminally ill clients are often given **palliative care**, or care that relieves symptoms, such as pain, but does not alter the course of disease. Palliative care is an approach that focuses on the seriously ill client and family and is most often provided in the home, hospital setting, or long-term facilities (Hull, 2008).

In palliative care, the goal is to ensure the highest possible quality of life for the client and family (Hull, 2008). A primary aim is to help the client feel comfortable, safe, and secure. The nurse can do much to increase the client's feelings of safety by being available when needed. Holding the client's hand and listening are therapeutic measures.

Care delivered by an interdisciplinary team emphasizes the management of psychological, social, and spiritual problems experienced by clients and families during end of life. The nurse addresses pain control and the management of other physical problems (Hull, 2008). The client needs to know that he has the nurse's support as an advocate for his care and well-being.

Hospice Care

Hospice is care for the terminally ill founded on the concept of allowing individuals to die with dignity surrounded

CULTURAL CONSIDERATIONS

Rituals Following Death

- Judaism practices burial of the dead within 24 hours. A 7-day period of mourning, called Shiva, begins the day of the funeral.
- In the Islamic faith, men wash the body of a man and women wash the body of a woman after death.
- Buddhists believe that after death, the body should not be disturbed by movement, talking, or crying.
- Hindus pour holy water into the mouth of the dying person. The eldest son arranges for the funeral and cremation within 24 hours of death. Embalming is forbidden.
- Jehovah's Witnesses believe that the soul dies with the body, but 144,000 will be resurrected at the end-time and will be born again as spiritual sons of God.
- Native Americans believe that the spirit lives on after death. Ancestor worship is practiced.

by those who love them. Clients enter hospice care either at home or in a hospice center when aggressive medical treatment is no longer an option or when the client refuses further medical care. Hospice care is based on the belief that meaningful life can be achieved during terminal illness and that care of the dying is best supported in the home setting or hospice center, free from technological interventions to prolong physiologic dying (Hull, 2008).

Hospice is a coordinated program of interdisciplinary services provided by professional caregivers and volunteers. Hospice care does not hasten life, nor does it prolong death through artificial means. Instead, it assists the client and family in understanding the death process and how best to enjoy life until the end (Hull, 2008).

Differentiating Palliative Care and Hospice Care

Although used interchangeably, the terms *palliative care* and *hospice care* are different in several ways. For example, palliative care can start much earlier in the disease process than hospice care, which is usually offered in the last 6 months of life. Table 13-5 explains the two approaches in end-of-life care (Hull, 2008).

NURSING CARE OF THE DYING CLIENT

Despite health care advances, care of the terminally ill client remains a challenging and rewarding reality for many nurses. The death process is typically a very emotional time for clients and their families; compassionate and sensitive nursing care that respects clients' wishes and that meets their physical needs can help bring peace and dignity to this natural process.

PROFESSIONALTIP

Information Gathered in Assessment of the Dying Client

- Client and family goals and expectations
- Client's awareness that illness is terminal
- Client's stage of dying
- Identification of support systems
- History of positive coping skills
- Client perception of unfinished business to be completed

Adapted from "Death and Dying," by K. Pritchett and P. Lucas, 1997a. In *Psychiatric–Mental Health Nursing: Adaptation and Growth* [4th ed., pp. 206–207], by B. S. Johnson [Ed.], Philadelphia: Lippincott Williams & Wilkins.

Assessment

A thorough assessment of the client's holistic needs is the basis for nursing interventions. Assessment of the dying client includes an ongoing collection of data regarding the strengths and limitations of the dying person and the family.

Nursing Diagnoses

The nurse's assessment of the dying client may lead to several diagnoses. One NANDA-I-approved nursing diagnosis that is applicable for many dying clients is ***Powerlessness***, that is, "the perception that one's own action will not significantly affect an outcome; a perceived lack of control over a current situation or

TABLE 13-5 Approaches in End-of-Life Care

DIMENSIONS	PALLIATIVE CARE	HOSPICE CARE
Recipient of care	Anyone with a serious illness regardless of life expectancy	Life expectancy of 6 months or less
Services provided	Symptom management Physical therapy Client and family counseling Spiritual care	Symptom management Provision of medications, medical supplies, and equipment Coverage for short-term inpatient care Grief support Volunteer services
Care settings	Home care Ambulatory/outpatient Acute care Long-term care	Inpatient care Home care
Third-party coverage	Some treatments and medications may be covered by Medicare, Medicaid, and private insurers	Medicare Hospice Benefit Medicaid Hospice Benefit Some private insurers

Data from *Palliative and End of Life Care*, by E. Hull, 2008. Manuscript submitted for publication.

PROFESSIONAL TIP

Planning Care for the Dying Client

- Schedule time to spend with the client.
- Identify areas of special concern to the client and make referrals when appropriate (e.g., social worker consult for information on equipment rental).
- Promote and protect individual self-esteem and self-worth.
- Balance the client's needs for assistance and independence.
- Meet the physiological needs of the client and family.
- Respect the client's confidentiality.
- Provide factual information to the client and family and answer all questions.
- Offer to contact clergy or other spiritual leader.

Adapted from "Death and Dying," by K. Pritchett and P. Lucas, 1997a. In *Psychiatric–Mental Health Nursing: Adaptation and Growth* (4th ed., p. 208), by B. S. Johnson (Ed.), Philadelphia: Lippincott Williams & Wilkins.

immediate happening" (NANDA-I, 2010). Another response that is often experienced by the dying is described by the diagnosis ***Hopelessness***, "a subjective state in which an individual sees limited or no alternatives or personal choices available and is unable to mobilize energy on own behalf" (NANDA-I, 2010). The client may also exhibit *Death Anxiety*, "apprehension, worry, or fear related to death or dying" (NANDA-I, 2010).

Planning/Outcome Identification

The major goals of nursing care are the physical, emotional, and mental comfort of the client. The goals of nursing care for the dying client are the same as those goals developed for all clients who are unable to meet their own needs. The dying client should be treated as a unique individual worthy of respect instead of a diagnosis to be cured. Many dying clients do not fear death but are anxious about a painful death or dying alone.

Promoting optimal quality of life includes treating the client and family with respect and providing a safe environment for expressing their feelings. Planning should focus on meeting the client's and family's holistic needs, as specified in the Dying Person's Bill of Rights (Figure 13-4). It is as relevant today as when it was written in 1975. When planning care, the nurse should make every effort to be sensitive to the rights of the dying client.

Implementation

The first priority is to communicate caring to the client and family. Powell (1999) found that the presence of a comforting nurse made a tremendous difference to the client. LaDuke (2001) suggests holding a client's or family member's hand and saying "I will not leave you." This assurance of the nurse's presence is a powerful way to show caring.

The nurse should approach the client in denial with understanding and the knowledge that moving between the stages of dying is enhanced by a trusting nurse–client relationship.

The Dying Person's Bill of Rights

- I have the right to be treated as a living human being until I die.
- I have the right to maintain a sense of hopefulness, however changing its focus may be.
- I have the right to be cared for by those who can maintain a sense of hopefulness, however challenging this might be.
- I have the right to express my feelings and emotions about my approaching death in my own way.
- I have the right to participate in decisions concerning my care.
- I have the right to expect continuing medical and nursing attention even though "cure" goals must be changed to "comfort" goals.
- I have the right not to die alone.
- I have the right to be free from pain.
- I have the right to have my questions answered honestly.
- I have the right not to be deceived.
- I have the right to have help from and for my family in accepting death.
- I have the right to die in peace and dignity.
- I have the right to retain my individuality and not be judged for my decisions, which may be contrary to beliefs of others.
- I have the right to discuss and enlarge my religious and/or spiritual experiences, whatever these may mean to others.
- I have the right to expect that the sanctity of the human body will be respected after death.
- I have the right to be cared for by caring, sensitive, knowledgeable people who will attempt to understand my needs and will be able to gain some satisfaction in helping me face my death.

FIGURE 13-4 The Dying Person's Bill of Rights (*From The Dying Person's Bill of Rights, by A. Barbus, 1975, American Journal of Nursing, 75[1].*)

Establishing rapport facilitates the client's verbalization of feelings (Figure 13-5). A safe environment established by the nurse allows the client to express those feelings being experienced. Nurses must understand that clients are not angry with them but, rather with the situation they are experiencing.

Physiological Needs Physiological needs are essential for existence, according to Maslow's hierarchy of needs. Therefore, they must be met before all other needs. Areas that are often problematic for the terminally ill client are respirations; fluids and nutrition; mouth, eyes, and nose; mobility; skin care; and elimination.

Respirations Oxygen is frequently ordered for the client experiencing labored breathing. Suctioning may be needed to remove secretions that the client is unable to swallow.

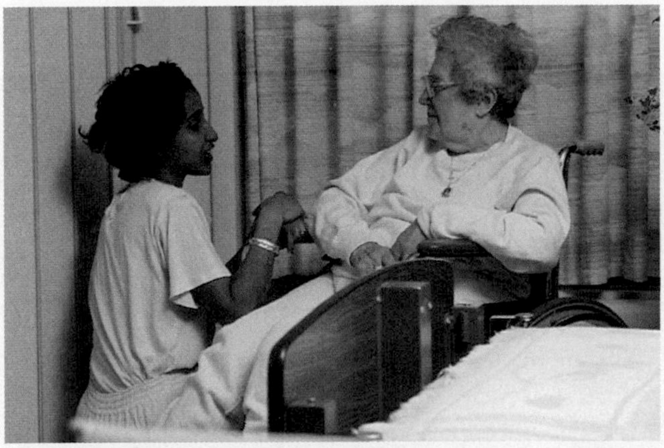

COURTESY OF DELMAR CENGAGE LEARNING

FIGURE 13-5 Establishing a caring and trusting relationship helps the client come to terms with a terminal illness.

Fluids and Nutrition Dying clients are rarely hungry and gradually stop eating and drinking. Refusal of food and fluids is a natural part of the dying process. A study of clients dying of cancer found the clients did not feel hunger or thirst (Robert Wood Johnson Foundation, 2004). In fact, hospice workers found that clients who are not given artificial nutrition and hydration are more comfortable than those who receive it (Robert Wood Johnson Foundation, 2004). When artificial nutrition and hydration are withheld, symptoms of nausea, vomiting, abdominal pain, loss of bladder control, and shortness of breath decrease. Artificial nutrition often increases the client's agitation and risk of aspiration pneumonia. When clients are nearing death and artificial nutrition and hydration are stopped, the client dies within 3 to 14 days. Health care personnel noticed that the dying process was peaceful and that the clients did not experience pain or distress (Robert Wood Johnson Foundation, 2004).

The client's wishes must always take precedence in every situation. Family members must be given truthful and accurate information when a comatose client has not previously made his wishes known. The American Dietetic Association, the American Medical Association, and the ANA agree that it is ethically, legally, and professionally acceptable to discontinue nutritional support if that is the terminally ill client's request.

Mouth, Eyes, and Nose The administration of oxygen and mouth breathing increase the need for meticulous oral care. Saliva substitutes and moisturizers can be used to alleviate discomfort. Regular use of toothpaste and a toothbrush may be adequate. The tongue should be gently brushed. Offer ice chips and sips of favorite beverages frequently. Apply petroleum jelly to the lips to prevent dryness. To maintain the client's comfort, give oral care every 2 to 3 hours.

If the client's eyes remain open, apply an ophthalmic lubricating gel to the conjunctiva every 3 to 4 hours or artificial tears or physiologic saline solution every 15 to 30 minutes. A cotton ball is used to gently wipe the eye from inner to outer canthus (one wipe per cotton ball) to remove any discharge.

The nares may become dry and crusted. Oxygen given by cannula can further irritate the nares. A thin layer of water-soluble jelly applied to the nares alleviates discomfort. The elastic strap of the oxygen cannula is not applied too tightly, lest it cause discomfort. If oxygen tubing is placed behind the ears, the area is assessed for irritation.

Mobility Mobility decreases as the client's condition deteriorates. The client requires more assistance as he becomes less able to move about in bed or get out of bed. Physical dependence increases the risk of complications related to immobility, such as atrophy and pressure ulcers. These complications, which increase both cost of care and client discomfort, can be prevented by attentive nursing care.

Reposition the client at least every 2 hours. Remember that the client may have other disorders that contribute to discomfort related to mobility, such as arthritis or lung disease. Maintain body alignment with the use of pillows and other supportive equipment and use positioning techniques to facilitate ease of breathing. Perform passive range-of-motion exercises at least twice a day to prevent stiffness and aching of the joints. The client may wish to be in a reclining type of chair several times a day. Use a wheelchair to increase the client's environmental space and give the client more mobility, control, and independence.

Skin Care Prevention of pressure ulcers is a priority. They are painful, can cause secondary complications, and are costly to treat. Two preventive measures are passive range-of-motion exercises every 1 to 2 hours and regular repositioning every hour to hour and a half. Turning the client with the use of a draw sheet decreases pain and prevents skin shearing. The use of air mattresses or air beds reduces pressure to all body surfaces. In addition, keeping the skin clean and moisturized will promote healthy tissue. Inspect the skin once or twice daily, with special attention paid to pressure points and areas where skin surfaces rub together. Gentle massages with soothing lotion are comforting and decrease skin breakdown by improving circulation. Areas of nonblanching erythema or actual skin breakdown should not be massaged. Apply hydrocolloid dressings to bony prominences to protect them from pressure and skin breakdown. Bed baths are adequate if the client cannot get into the tub or sit in a shower chair.

Elimination Side effects of pain medications and a lack of physical activity may cause constipation. For clients with adequate oral intake, foods with high-fiber content and fluids can be effective preventive measures. Constipation can also be alleviated by administering suppositories, if necessary, and maintaining a scheduled time for bowel elimination. A commode with padded arms can be more comfortable than a toilet.

The client may become incontinent of bowel and bladder. After each incontinent episode, clean the skin with peri-washes, and apply a moisture barrier. Urine and fecal material on the skin will quickly lead to excoriation and skin breakdown.

Indwelling catheters are not a first choice for bladder management; however, for some clients, the discomfort of

PROFESSIONALTIP

Adjuvant Therapy

Adjuvant therapy may be effective. Nonsteroidal anti-inflammatory agents are beneficial for bone metastases, tricyclic antidepressants and antiseizure medications for neurogenic pain, antidepressants for terminally ill clients, and steroids for headaches related to cerebral edema. Nonpharmacological techniques can be used along with medication. Relaxation techniques, guided imagery, massages, and repositioning may enhance the action of the medications.

using a bedpan, getting out of bed to use the toilet or commode, or the need for frequent cleaning may cause agonizing pain. The benefits of a urinary catheter greatly outweigh the risks in such circumstances.

Comfort The primary activities for promoting physical comfort include pain relief, keeping the client dry and clean, and providing a safe, nonthreatening environment. The nurse who has a caring, respectful attitude increases the client's psychological comfort. Fear of a painful death is almost universal. Pain is a subjective, personal experience, and the client is the best judge of the severity of the pain. Many, but not all, dying clients experience pain. The ANA states in its position statement on pain relief for the terminally ill that promotion of comfort is the major goal of nursing care (ANA, 1996, 2008). Comfort is to be maximized by managing pain and other causes of discomfort.

The client must know that caregivers accept and believe complaints of pain and that they will intervene to alleviate or prevent the pain. Ask the client to rate the pain on a scale from 0 to 10, with 0 being no pain and 10 being severe pain. Pain is defined as what the client states it is, and the nurse administers pain medication according to the client's statement of need.

To maintain therapeutic blood level, medication must be given around the clock and not "as needed." A nonnarcotic analgesic may be effective in early stages for mild, intermittent pain. As the pain increases, the client may need to start on morphine, titrated at increments until adequate pain relief is achieved without severe side effects. Finding the lowest dose and the longest interval that will relieve pain is called titrating the dose. The dosage that should be used is the one that controls the pain to the satisfaction of the client and that causes minimal side effects. The dose is individual and continually assessed to remain therapeutic in controlling pain.

The World Health Organization (WHO) has a three-step ladder that guides pain administration and titration. Clients with mild pain are given acetaminophen (Tylenol) or nonsteroidal anti-inflammatory drugs (NSAIDs); for moderate pain, a weak opioid or combination agents, such as oxycodone/hydrocodone and acetaminophen or tramadol (Ultram); and for severe pain, strong longer-acting opioids, such as morphine, hydromorphone hydrochloride (Dilaudid), fentanyl (Duragesic), or oxycodone (OxyContin) (Webster & Dove, 2007). Figure 13-6 shows some long- and short-acting opioids. Treatment starts at the level of the client's pain and does not have to start at the first step.

Guidelines for administering pain medication in palliative care are:

- Assess the client's pain and note how it affects quality of life
- Give sustained-release medications around the clock
- Treat breakthrough pain with immediate-release medications
- Monitor pain status frequently
- Treat adverse effects as needed
- Know drug–drug and drug–disease interactions
- Reassess pain on a regular basis (Panke, 2002)

When the client cannot verbalize his pain, note the nonverbal behavior. Nonverbal clues of pain are decreased activity or restlessness, furrowed brow, grimacing, crying, moaning, withdrawal from others, guarded or stiffened posture, irritability, elevated blood pressure, and increased pulse. If the furrowed brow comes and goes, it may indicate mental activity of dreams and hallucinations. Assess other nonverbals to obtain the total pain picture.

Opioids

Long Acting	[redacted]
fentanyl transdermal system (Duragesic)	[redacted]
methadone hydrochloride (Metadol)	[redacted]
buprenorphine hydrochloride (Buprenex)	[redacted]
Morphine sulfate	[redacted]
oxycodone hydrochloride (Roxicodone)	[redacted]
oxymorphone hydrochloride (Numorphan)	[redacted]

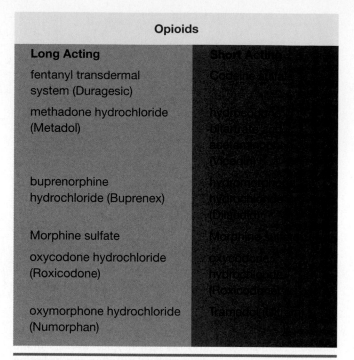

FIGURE 13-6 **Long-Acting and Short-Acting Opioids** ***(Adapted from Optimizing Opioid Treatment for Breakthrough Pain, by L. Webster and M. Dove, 2007, Retrieved October 14, 2007, from http://www.medscape.com.)***

Monitor the client's responses with regard to pain rating and respiratory rate. For example, 30 mg of morphine sulfate given orally may provide pain relief, but if the respiratory rate drops from 12 to 6 per minute, adjust or change the medication. If the same dose given to another client provides minimal relief and the client is alert and displays no change in respirations, the next dose is increased (Webster & Dove, 2007).

Pain medication is given by the least invasive route of administration, preferably oral or buccal mucosa, then IV or subcutaneous, with intramuscular rarely used. The rectal route is also used when medication cannot be given orally (Panke, 2002). If the dying client has diminished liver or renal function, continuous administration of morphine causes an accumulation of active metabolites leading to terminal delirium. Fentanyl is the drug of choice at this point because it has no active metabolites to accumulate and cause toxicity (Webster & Dove, 2007).

Monitor the client for **breakthrough pain**, or sudden, acute, temporary pain that is usually precipitated by a treatment, a procedure, or unusual activity of the client. A supplemental dose of medication is then required. If the precipitating factor is known (e.g., dressing changes), give medication 30 to 60 minutes before the procedure. Table 13-6 describes care given to a client during end-of-life care.

Physical Environment The client's comfort can be significantly increased by a soothing physical environment. Soft lighting may enhance vision. Complying with the client's request for a nightlight is also helpful in creating a pleasant and nonthreatening environment. If possible, the client should be offered the opportunity to have the bed or a chair near a window to increase the range of the environment. Since body temperature falls as circulation becomes more sluggish, a lightweight comforter will increase warmth without adding much weight. Help eliminate environmental odors by ensuring adequate ventilation, daily cleaning of the room, removal of leftover food, and frequent linen changes.

TABLE 13-6 Nursing Management during End-of-Life Care

PHYSIOLOGIC RESPONSE	CONTRIBUTING FACTORS	NURSING INTERVENTIONS
Pain	Terminal illness Fear and anxiety	Assess for pain frequently and thoroughly Administer pain medications in a timely manner and around the clock Address break through pain in a timely manner Do not delay or deny pain medication for the terminally ill client Evaluate effectiveness of pain medication frequently
Dyspnea	Fear and anxiety Primary lung tumors Lung metastases Pleural effusion Restrictive lung disease	Assist with relaxation techniques Administer prescribed medications to relieve dyspnea (anxiolytic, bronchodilators, corticosteroids, diuretics, opioids) Administer prescribed oxygen therapy Teach client and family energy conservation techniques For home or hospice care, offer electric bed, lift chair, and bedside commode
Anorexia	Fear and anxiety Treatment Complications of disease process	Feed the client when hungry Assess for nausea and vomiting Offer culturally appropriate foods Provide frequent mouth care, especially following vomiting episodes
Weakness fatigue	Terminal illness Treatment Change in metabolic demands	Assess loss of tolerance for activities Provide frequent rest periods Time nursing interventions to conserve energy
Constipation	Medications Immobility Dehydration	Encourage foods high in fiber Increase fluid intake as tolerated Encourage activity
Nausea and vomiting	Complications of disease process Medications	Encourage the client to avoid eating if nauseated Suggest small meals of cool nonodorous foods Encourage the client to eat slowly
Delirium	Use of opioids and steroids	Reorient to time, place, and person frequently Ensure frequent nursing rounds Provide a quiet, well-lit room Administer sedatives and benzodiazepines

Data from *Palliative and End of Life Care,* by E. Hull, 2008, Manuscript submitted for publication.

Noise can be distracting and anxiety provoking, so the nurse and visitors should comply with the client's wishes with regard to the use of radio and television. The telephone can be removed from the room if the client finds the ringing disturbing.

Psychosocial Needs Death presents a threat to one's psychological integrity as well as to one's physical existence. The dying person is often tethered to tubes and electronic gadgetry in an intensive care unit. The client is held captive in a tangle of technology and is kept at a distance from the supportive presence and touch of family and friends.

Technology cannot replace concern, touch, compassion, or human companionship. By their presence, nurses and family can humanize the dying person's environment. Invite and encourage families to participate in the client's care if they desire to do so and the client is willing.

For many clients, maintaining a well-groomed appearance is important. When the client can no longer make requests or give directions for care, caregivers should presume that the

COMMUNITY/HOME HEALTH CARE

Equipment to Increase Client Comfort

The following equipment can be rented and may qualify for payment by Medicare or private insurance:

- An electric hospital bed with overhead trapeze allows the client some control of the environment.
- A commode promotes the client's independence in elimination.
- A lifting device eases getting the dependent client out of bed.
- Handheld shower and chair for the bathtub or shower are helpful.
- Devices such as cushions for chairs and special mattresses for the bed provide comfort.
- An overbed table for eating and other activities is useful.
- Comfortable chairs close to the bed facilitate visits of friends and family.

client would prefer to maintain the same grooming habits as were previously preferred. Shaving the male client's beard or cleaning and trimming the client's fingernails and toenails, for instance, will help the client maintain a well-groomed appearance and will also promote client dignity. Combing and brushing the hair not only improves appearance but is also a comforting and relaxing activity for many clients.

Dressing and undressing may become a cumbersome, frustrating, and fatiguing activity. The client who spends time up and about may choose attractive pajamas, housecoats, dusters, or exercise suits. Advise individuals who may be purchasing clothing for the client to select items that are loose fitting, have few fasteners, and are washable.

Spiritual Needs Dying persons may experience confusion, anger at their god, crises of faith, or other types of spiritual distress. Nurses have the opportunity to play a major role in promoting the dying client's spiritual comfort.

Yet a survey on end-of-life care by Ferrell, Virani, Grant, Coyne, and Uman (2000) showed that fewer than 35% of nurses described grief/bereavement support and the attention to spiritual needs as effective; however, 66% of nurses said that care of the dying was better than 5 years prior.

Dying clients are most vulnerable. The moral health and integrity of the broader community can be measured in part by the way we respond to their needs.

Dying is a personal and often a lonely process. Table 13-7 provides information on the views of various religions with regard to withdrawal of life support, death, and organ donation. Listen as a client expresses values and beliefs related to death. Therapeutic nursing interventions that address the spiritual needs of the dying client include:

- Using touch
- Playing music
- Praying with the client
- Communicating empathy
- Contacting clergy if requested by the client
- Reading religious literature aloud at the client's request

Support for the Family The presence of the nurse is extremely important. It shows support and caring not only for the client but for the family as well. Family members may have increased guilt because of feelings of helplessness. The nurse encourages family members to speak to, touch, read to, sing to, pray with, or just sit with the client. This can give family members a sense of purpose, ease feelings of helplessness, and provide more pleasant memories in the future.

Each family group has its unwritten rules, its leaders and followers, and its methods for coping with crises. The family's equilibrium is threatened by the impending death. If family members have limited coping skills and inadequate support systems, they need assistance and guidance from the caregivers. Nurses must remember that the rules and coping mechanisms used by the family may not always coincide with the values and beliefs of the staff and that the client's and family's wishes must be respected to the extent possible.

The relationship with the family does not always end with the client's death. Staff members may attend visitations, funerals, or memorial services. If a hospice was involved, the family may participate in a bereavement support program. If the client was a resident in a long-term care facility, family members may return to visit other residents with whom they became acquainted.

Learning Needs The nurse's role is to provide the client and family members with support and information. For example, they may not realize that the dying person should conserve energy. Family activities are best scheduled early in the morning or following a period of rest by the client. The nurse may need to point out to the family this type of commonsense approach, as simple interventions such as these can be overlooked during this highly charged emotional time.

Client and family learning needs may relate to:

- Information about physical condition and treatment regimen
- Anticipating a medical crisis
- Inexperience with the personal threat of death
- Unfamiliarity with what to do in case of an emergency outside the hospital

CLIENT TEACHING

Guidelines for Teaching a Family Caregiver

- Use adult-education principles.
- Frequently reinforce material.
- Provide information about the nature and extent of the disease process.
- Explain the purpose of palliative care yet maintain a sense of realistic hope.
- Reassure client and family by informing them of available community resources; tell them that they are not alone.
- Discuss steps for caregiver to follow if an emergency arises at home by providing written instructions, including persons to be contacted and important telephone numbers.

TABLE 13-7 Religions and Death and Dying Issues

RELIGION	LIFE SUPPORT WITHDRAWAL IN TERMINAL ILLNESS	DEATH	ORGAN DONATION
Judaism	Allowed under the right circumstances (when life support is serving only to impede a natural death).	• Suicide is forbidden. • Burial should occur within 24 hours. • Cremation is forbidden. • Autopsy is permitted if it will save future lives.	• Permitted because the procedure saves life. • Rejected by Orthodox Jews.
Islam	Permitted if only serving to prolong death or if client's condition is medically hopeless.	• Suicide is forbidden. • Relatives and friends are present. • Autopsy is permitted to solve a crime or provide further medical knowledge.	• Permitted.
Catholicism/ Orthodoxy	Controversial; permitted if client's condition is hopeless.	• Prayers are offered at time of death. • Burial and cremation are permitted. • Autopsy is permitted.	• Permitted.
Protestantism	Permitted if client's condition is hopeless.	• Prayers are offered at time of death. • Burial and cremation are permitted. • Autopsy is permitted.	• Permitted, although may be rejected by some Baptists or Pentecostals.
Jehovah's Witness	Permitted if serving only to prolong death or if quality of life is nonexistent.	• Suicide is not approved. • Autopsy is permitted if legally necessary.	• Individual choice.
Buddhism	Acceptable for those on threshold of death.	• Suicide is criticized. • Cremation is common.	• Controversial.
Hinduism	Supported to allow a natural death.	• Prefer to die at home. • Embalming is forbidden. • Autopsy is discouraged. • Suicide is forbidden.	• Discouraged because of disturbing the body after death.
Mormons	A client or family decision.	• Cremation is discouraged. • Autopsy is a family decision.	• A family decision.
Native Americans	Life support is viewed as unnatural and, therefore, unnecessary.	• Complex beliefs about death and treatment of the body; some are forbidden to touch a dead body. • Ancestral worship. • Often believe the spirit of the person continues to live.	• Discouraged because of death and burial practices.
Christian Science	Most have advance directives to avoid medical treatment; however, no illness is seen as hopeless.	• Practitioner should always be notified at death. • Autopsy is permitted. • Cremation is usual practice.	• Do not donate or receive organs because the spiritual cause of organ failure is not treated with an organ transplant.
Unitarian	Support withdrawal of life support when quality of life is poor and suffering is great.	• Suicide is a tragedy. • Autopsy is permitted as needed.	• Permitted.

Data from *Health Assessment and Physical Examination* (4th ed.), by M. Estes, 2010, Clifton Park, NY: Delmar Cengage Learning. Copyright 2010 by Delmar Cengage Learning.

CRITICAL THINKING

Caring for a Dying Client

Think about caring for a dying client. How can you prepare to care for a dying client?

Impending Death

There is no way to predict how long a client may be in the terminal stages of illness. A client may have signs of impending death and then rally to live several more days. Clients often live until a family member arrives for a last good-bye. The client who has had a long illness and is ready to die may need "permission" to die from a loved one, who says, "It's okay, you can go now." Some clients may not wish to die when anyone is present and will wait to take the last breath until alone in the room.

It is never easy for the family, even when death is expected. The family should be simply and thoroughly informed about what will happen before and after the client's death, including:

- Physical changes that occur just before and following death
- Death pronouncement
- Postmortem care
- Body removal

Impending death is signaled by a series of irrevocable events (Hull, 2008):

- The lungs become unable to provide adequate gas diffusion.
- The heart and blood vessels become unable to maintain adequate tissue perfusion.
- The brain ceases to regulate vital centers.

Cheyne-Stokes respirations (breathing characterized by periods of apnea alternating with periods of dyspnea) most often herald pulmonary system failure. Secretions accumulate in the larynx and trachea, causing noisy respirations, often called the **death rattle**.

COMMUNITY/HOME HEALTH CARE

When the Client Dies at Home (Preparing for an Expected Death)

Have the family prepare:

- A list of names and telephone numbers they wish to notify of the death including the name and telephone number of the funeral director.

Instruct the family:

- Whom to call (physician or hospice nurse or funeral director).
- Whom *not* to call (ambulance and emergency services).
- To record the time of death, last medications given, the condition of the client during the last few hours, and the last time the client was seen by the nurse.

The heart fails in its pumping function, resulting in poor perfusion, ischemia, and cell death. The skin becomes cool and, possibly, very pale, cyanotic, jaundiced, or mottled. The pulse becomes rapid, irregular, weak, and thready. Death is several hours away if a peripheral pulse is strong and easily palpated. Cold, cyanotic extremities and irregular respirations indicate that death is imminent.

Inadequate cerebral perfusion hinders the brain's ability to integrate vital functions. The client may be confused and lethargic and may respond only to direct visual, auditory, or tactile stimulation. Pupils no longer react to light and become fixed. The client may "talk" to dead loved ones. A frown or tight facial muscles may indicate pain or discomfort. A client in a coma will move only in response to deep pain. Analgesics should not be withdrawn from a conscious client in a coma.

The care of the client does not cease during this final stage of life. The nursing actions previously described should be continued. Tell the client in brief, simple terms what is happening as care is rendered. The family should be allowed and encouraged to continue their participation if that is their wish. Caution family members that the dying client can hear even in the absence of verbal response, so all comments and conversation should continue to be respectful.

There may be other indications that death is near. The client may report seeing someone who has died or angels or hearing someone or beautiful music (Pitorak, 2003). These experiences should be accepted as a natural step in the process of dying. When the final breath is taken, the heart stops beating. Within a few minutes, cerebral death (the point at which brain cells die) occurs, and brain activity ceases.

Physical signs of death are:

- Absence of a heartbeat
- Cessation of respirations
- Mottling of skin or skin that is cool to the touch
- Eyelids remain slightly open
- Jaws relaxed and mouth slightly open
- No response to name, touch, or environmental sounds
- Eyes fixed on a certain spot
- No eye blinking in response to touch or air movement over the eyes
- Release of bowel and bladder contents (Hull, 2008)

Care after Death

Meeting the needs of the grieving family and caring for the deceased body are nursing responsibilities. Treat the body of the deceased with respect by maintaining privacy and preventing damage to the body. **Postmortem care** is given immediately after death but before the body is moved to the mortuary (see Professional Tip: Postmortem Care).

After death, several physiological changes occur. Body temperature decreases, resulting in a lack of skin elasticity (**algor mortis**). In order to avoid skin breakdown, the nurse must therefore use caution when removing tape from the body. **Liver mortis**, a bluish-purple discoloration of the skin, is a by-product of red blood cell destruction. It usually begins within 20 minutes of death (Harvey, 2001). This discoloration occurs in dependent areas of the body; the nurse should therefore elevate the head of the bed 30 degrees to prevent discoloration of the head and neck. If the body is moved on a stretcher, keep the head elevated on two pillows. **Rigor mortis**, the natural stiffening of muscles after death, begins about 4 hours after death. The funeral director

PROFESSIONALTIP

Postmortem Care

- Treat the body with dignity and respect.
- Bathe and put a clean gown on the body—and place an incontinent pad under the client's hips.
- Remove dressings and tubes, unless these must remain in place for an autopsy.
- Place the body in alignment with the head elevated.
- Place dentures in a denture cup and send with the body.
- Comb the client's hair.

will have the best results if embalming is completed before rigor mortis sets in (Harvey, 2001). Position the body in a natural position.

When preparing the body for family viewing, endeavor to make the body look natural and comfortable. This means preparing and positioning the body as previously described. According to Harvey (2001), if the client wore dentures, they should not be put in the deceased person's mouth. Jaw muscles relax after death, so dentures often fall out and are lost or broken. Put them in a hospital denture cup without water and send them with the body to the funeral director. After the family has viewed the body, place identification tags on the body's toe and wrist. Sometimes the body is placed is a plastic or fabric **shroud** (a covering for the body after death) and tagged. Next, transport the body to the morgue according to the agency's policy, where it is kept until it is transported to a **mortuary** (funeral home). In some institutions, the body is kept in the room until the funeral director arrives. The nurse is also responsible for returning the deceased's possessions, such as jewelry, eyeglasses, clothing, and all other personal items, to the family.

Information for Funeral Director

Harvey (2001) explains information that is important to the funeral director when preparing the body. The cause of death influences which procedures are used. For example, a client with liver or renal failure has a high level of ammonia in the body. A special solution will have to be used because the ammonia neutralizes the formaldehyde generally used. If the client had tuberculosis (TB) or any other communicable disease, special procedures will be followed to prevent spreading the disease. If the client weighed more than 300 pounds (136 kg), the funeral director will need extra staff for transferring the body.

Legal Aspects

The physician is legally responsible for determining the cause of death and signing the death certificate in most states. In certain situations, the RN may be responsible for certifying the death. Some institutions require two nurses to certify death. Nurses must know their legal responsibilities as defined by their respective state boards of nursing.

Autopsy

An **autopsy** is the examination of the body after death by a pathologist to determine the cause of death. It is mandated in situations where an unusual death has occurred. For example, a violent death or an unexpected death is a circumstance necessitating an autopsy. For an autopsy to be performed in other situations, families must give consent. The funeral director must know whether an autopsy is to be performed.

Organ Donation

Organ donation for transplantation requires sensitivity and compassion from the health care team. Health care facilities must have a policy regarding the referral of a potential organ donor to appropriate organ procurement agencies. The Centers for Medicare and Medicaid Services requires hospitals to notify a local organ-procurement organization (OPO) of a client in imminent death or who has died so that the person who initially approaches the family is an OPO representative or "designated requestor" (Truog, 2008). When an organ(s) is donated, the OPO representative coordinates the entire process, including finding organ recipients (OrganDonor.Gov, 2008).

The organs and tissues that can be transplanted are:

- Liver
- Lungs
- Heart
- Kidneys
- Pancreas
- Skin
- Bones (middle ear bones and long bones)
- Corneas

The average waiting time is 230 days for a heart, 1,068 days for a lung, 796 days for a liver, 1,121 days for a kidney, and 501 days for a pancreas. Transplantation must occur within 4 to 6 hours for heart and lungs, 12 to 24 hours for liver and pancreas, and 48 to 72 hours for kidneys (OrganDonor.Gov, 2008).

Care of the Family

The nurse provides invaluable support to the family of the deceased at the time of death. It is extremely important to inform the family of the circumstances surrounding the death. The nurse offers information about viewing the body and contacts support people (e.g., other relatives, clergy). The nurse may even help the family with decisions regarding transportation, a funeral home, and removal of the deceased's belongings. Sensitive and compassionate interpersonal skills are essential when providing information and support to families. Providing coffee, tissues, and light snacks are small gestures that convey sensitivity to the family and friends and are appreciated.

Nurse's Self-Care

Working with dying clients can evoke both a personal and a professional threat in the nurse. Grief is a common experience for nurses because many nurses are confronted with death and loss daily. Smith-Stoner and Frost (1998) describe a part of the psyche called the shadow self, where stresses are stored. Unresolved sadness is called shadow grief. Everyone has a shadow self and may have some shadow grief. Nurses often have a great deal of shadow grief, which, if not released, may

PROFESSIONALTIP

Care for Yourself during Grief

- Do what nurses do well: care. Help the family and your feelings of helplessness will diminish.
- Plan time for your own grieving.
- Allow for crying to help ease the pain.
- Learn when to ask your coworkers for help.
- Express your feelings of grief to someone you can trust.
- Find support within your facility from counselors, support groups, and clergy.
- Use rituals to say good-bye to the deceased client and bring closure.

From "Please Cry with Me: Six Ways to Grieve," by C. D. Reese, 1996, *Nursing96, 26*(8), 56.

cause illness and burnout. Frequent exposure to death can interfere with the nurse's effectiveness because of subsequent anxiety and denial.

Nurses are at particular risk for experiencing negative effects from caring for the dying, whether working in a hospital, a hospice, a long-term care facility, or the home. They may not wish to confront their grief and will often use some of the common defense mechanisms against grieving, such as being strong, keeping busy, and suffering in silence. Nurses must talk about the intense emotions associated with caregiving instead of pretending that they do not experience grief. According to Smith-Stoner and Frost (1998), shadow grief may be staring to overwhelm a person if that person experiences the following:

- A loss of energy, spark, joy, and meaning in life
- Detachment from surroundings
- A feeling of being powerless to make a difference
- Increased smoking or drinking
- Unusual forgetfulness
- Constant criticism directed toward others
- Consistent inability to get work done
- Uncontrolled outbursts of anger
- Perception of clients and their families as objects
- Surrender of hobbies or interests

To effectively cope with their own grief, nurses need education, support, and assistance when coping with the death of clients. The focus of staff education should be on ways to seek support, decreasing staff anxiety when working with grieving clients and families, and ways to provide support to coworkers. Smith-Stoner and Frost (1998) suggest the following ways to cope:

- Take time to cry with and for clients
- Get physical: run, walk, bike, play tennis
- Ask colleagues to help with tasks; do not try to be "Supernurse"
- Connect to a place of worship; pray
- Look for joy in work—laughter is a great healer
- Create a caring circle of friends
- Listen to music

The nurse's own fears and doubts about death may surface and cause anxiety about feelings of mortality. Caring for the dying client and the client's family is emotionally draining, so nurses must remember to care for themselves.

SAMPLE NURSING CARE PLAN

The Client with a Terminal Illness/Cancer of the Lung

V.P., an 84-year-old widow, was diagnosed with cancer of the right lung 6 months ago. After a right lower lobectomy, she was discharged to a local skilled-care facility and planned to go home after completing her radiation therapy. After completing the treatments, V.P.'s condition began deteriorating. She did not want to go home, so discharge plans were discontinued. Now she is frequently short of breath, has dyspnea, requires pain medication, and needs some assistance with activities of daily living because of fatigue. She frequently grimaces and says, "I hurt." Her nutritional intake is very little because of swallowing difficulties. V.P. gets up only to use the commode. Her two adult children and four grandchildren live nearby and visit often. They want to assist their mother to get her affairs in order, but she resists their efforts. The family is trying to make V.P.'s remaining time as serene and comfortable as possible, but V.P. often defies their attempts.

NURSING DIAGNOSIS 1 *Chronic **P**ain* related to disease progression as evidenced by verbal statements, body language, and the need for pain medication

Nursing Outcomes Classification (NOC)
Pain: Disruptive Effects
Pain: Psychological Response
Pain Control

Nursing Interventions Classification (NIC)
Pain Management
Analgesic Administration
Coping Enhancement

(Continues)

SAMPLE NURSING CARE PLAN (Continued)

PLANNING/OUTCOMES	NURSING INTERVENTIONS	RATIONALE
V.P. will verbalize relief from pain.	Give analgesics as ordered.	Administering regular doses of analgesics is more effective than waiting until the pain begins.
	Have client rate pain on a scale of 0 to 10, with 0 being no pain and 10 being severe pain, to assess the need for morphine. Give morphine as ordered, titrated at increments until adequate pain relief is achieved.	The client should be given analgesics when pain is experienced. Morphine is the drug of choice for severe pain associated with cancer.
	Monitor for signs of breakthrough pain. If the precipitating factor is known, give medication 30 to 60 minutes before the event. Medicate as soon as possible for unpredictable breakthrough pain.	Breakthrough pain is often precipitated by activity or stress and supplemental medication is required.
	Assure V.P. that the nurses will help her manage the pain and keep it under control. Reposition frequently and give back massages for comfort. Assist with relaxation techniques if client agreeable.	Needs reassurance that everything possible will be done to manage the pain. Promotes psychological comfort.
	Monitor bowel elimination.	Pain medication often causes constipation.

EVALUATION
V.P.'s body language and verbal statements indicate freedom from pain

NURSING DIAGNOSIS 2 *Ineffective Coping* related to terminal illness as evidenced by inability to communicate effectively with family members and to accept their help

Nursing Outcomes Classification (NOC)
Coping
Self-Esteem
Social Interaction Skills

Nursing Interventions Classification (NIC)
Coping Enhancement
Counseling
Emotional Support

PLANNING/OUTCOMES	NURSING INTERVENTIONS	RATIONALE
V.P. will express her feelings openly.	Consult V.P. on all aspects of care. Give complete information. Provide opportunities to express feelings. Acknowledge V.P.'s feelings and let her know that crying and grieving are beneficial.	Allows V.P. to express her feelings and validates those feelings as being normal and expected.

(Continues)

SAMPLE NURSING CARE PLAN (Continued)

PLANNING/OUTCOMES	NURSING INTERVENTIONS	RATIONALE
	Listen for clues indicating unfinished business that needs to be completed. Encourage the process of life review.	Life review is a process of reflection and pondering of one's past and accepting one's life as being meaningful and valuable.
V.P. will maintain a satisfying relationship with her family.	Encourage family visits. Provide privacy.	Families need privacy in order to feel free to express their emotions.

EVALUATION

V.P. still resists family's assistance.

NURSING DIAGNOSIS 3

*Ineffective **B**reathing Pattern* related to diminished lung function as evidenced by dyspnea and shortness of breath

NOC: *Respiratory Monitoring, Anxiety Reduction*
NIC: *Vital Signs Status, Anxiety Control*

CLIENT GOAL

V.P. will be free from moderate or severe dyspnea.

NURSING INTERVENTIONS

1. Teaching breathing exercises and effective coughing techniques.
2. Allow adequate time for physical activities. Postpone activity if dyspnea is present. Provide as much assistance as needed.
3. Administer low-flow oxygen if blood gases indicate need.
4. Encourage client to drink 8 to 10 glasses of fluid each day.
5. Humidify the air with a cold-water vaporizer.
6. Assess respiratory system frequently.

SCIENTIFIC RATIONALES

1. Enhances gas exchange in the alveoli.
2. Physical exertion increases dyspnea.
3. Effective only if indicated by blood gases.
4. Liquefies respiratory secretions and promotes hydration.
5. Enhances breathing.
6. Identifies complications at early stages.

EVALUATION

Is V.P. free from moderate and severe dyspnea?

CONCEPT CARE MAP 13-1

SUMMARY

- Loss is when someone (or something) of value is no longer available. It is a universal response.
- Grief is a psychological response to loss evidenced by deep sorrow and mental anguish.
- The difference between pathological and normal grief is the inability of the individual to adapt to life without the loved one.
- Kübler-Ross identified five psychological stages of the dying process: denial, anger, bargaining, depression, and acceptance.
- Complicated grief is associated with traumatic death such as suicide, accident, or homicide.
- Each person dies a unique death.
- Hospice care is an alternative to hospitalization when aggressive medical treatment is no longer an option.
- After death, the nurse's focus is on supporting the family and caring for the deceased body.
- Nurses must care for themselves in order to provide compassionate, quality care to the dying person and family.

REVIEW QUESTIONS

1. S.R., age 11 years, was left with a distant relative 2 weeks ago. Her parents have not returned or called. S.R. is experiencing a/an:
1. physical loss.
2. situational loss.
3. maturational loss.
4. anticipational loss.

2. A defining characteristic of the NANDA-I nursing diagnosis *Anticipatory **Grieving*** is:
1. prolonged denial or depression.
2. unsuccessful adaptation to loss.
3. social isolation or withdrawal from others.
4. an expression of distress at potential loss.

3. The purpose of the Patient Self-Determination Act is to:
1. serve as an order for "do not resuscitate."
2. designate a guardian for an incompetent client.
3. provide a means, instead of a will, to designate what is to be done with a person's property, money, and personal possessions.
4. provide a legal means for individuals to state those circumstances under which life-sustaining treatment should or should not be provided to them.

4. One of the major goals of hospice care is:
1. freedom from pain and other symptoms.
2. free care for all dying clients and their families.
3. to cure the client using very aggressive medical treatment.
4. to transfer all dying clients to the hospital when death is imminent.

5. A client is in the last stages of dying. The nurse assesses for the signs of impending death that include:
1. flushed warm skin.
2. very slow regular pulse rate.
3. inability to hear.
4. Cheyne-Stokes respirations.

6. Nursing care of a grieving client includes: (Select all that apply.)
1. telling the grieving client that he will feel better soon.
2. assuring the grieving client that feeling relief after a long illness is normal.
3. exploring ways to fill his life with meaningful activities.
4. encouraging him to feel his feelings to the fullest so that he can work through the feelings.
5. leaving him alone so that he can work through the feelings on his own.
6. explaining that each person works through grief in his own way and in his own timing.

7. A dying client tells God that he will become a pastor if he is healed. The nurse knows that the client is experiencing what stage of death and dying?
1. Denial
2. Anger
3. Bargaining
4. Depression

8. A client is in hospice care. To meet the physiological comfort needs of the client, the nurse: (Select all that apply.)
1. accepts and believes the client's expressions of pain.
2. cleans the skin and applies a moisture barrier after urination.
3. reads scripture passages as requested by the client.
4. provides soft lighting in the room.
5. applies petroleum jelly to the lips.
6. listens as the client shares his fears.

9. A terminally ill client is agitated and keeps stating, "I want to talk to my children, all of my children!" The nurse's best response is:
1. "I know you are upset. Let me reposition you and make you more comfortable."
2. "You seem agitated. Tell me the reason you want to speak with your children."
3. "I know you want to talk with your family. Tell me how I can help you speak to your children."
4. "It is late at night, and your children are in bed. Try to go to sleep."

10. A terminally ill client enters the hospital and the daughter presents the client's advanced directive papers and states she is the durable power of attorney. The client has not signed a do-not-resuscitate (DNR) form. The daughter leaves the hospital and the client codes. The nursing staff:
    1. starts resuscitation because there is no DNR order from a physician.
    2. does not start resuscitation because the client is terminal.
    3. does not start resuscitation but places a call to the daughter for her decision regarding resuscitation desires.
    4. starts resuscitation but then stops when no DNR order is found.

REFERENCES/SUGGESTED READINGS

American Nurses Association. (1996). Promotion of comfort and relief of pain in dying patients. In *Compendium of ANA position statements.* Washington, DC: Author.

American Nurses Association. (2008). Communique: The newsletter of the Center for Ethics and Human Rights 5(2). Retrieved October 10, 2008, from http://198.65.150.241/readroom/cmqfw97.htm

Andreas, L. (1998). Controlling pain: Keeping a dying patient comfortable. Nursing98, 28(1), 70.

Backer, B., Hannon, N., & Russell, N. (1994). *Death and dying: Understanding and care* (2nd ed.). Clifton Park, NY: Thomson Delmar Learning.

Barbus, A. (1975). The dying person's bill of rights. *American Journal of Nursing, 75*(1), 99.

Boon, T. (1998). Don't forget the hospice option. *RN, 61*(2), 30–33.

Boss, P. (2000). *Ambiguous loss: Learning to live with unresolved grief.* Cambridge, MA: Harvard University Press.

Bowlby, J. (1982). *Attachment and loss: Vol. 2. Separation anxiety and anger.* New York: Basic Books.

Bral, E. (1998). Caring for adults with chronic cancer pain. *American Journal of Nursing, 98*(4), 27–32.

Bulechek, G., Butcher, H., McCloskey, J., & Dochterman, J., eds. (2008). *Nursing Interventions Classification (NIC)* (5th ed.). St. Louis, MO: Mosby/Elsevier.

Caring Connections. (2008). Supporting a grieving caregiver. Retrieved from http://www.caringinfo.org/GrievingALoss/GriefSupport/SupportingAGrieving Caregiver.htm

Castillo, L., & Phoummarath, M. (2009). Culturally competent school counseling with Asian American adolescents. Retrieved April 14, 2009, from http://www.jsc.montana.edu/articles/v4n20.pdf

Cerrudo, J. (1998). Letting go of Abuelo. *American Journal of Nursing, 98*(8), 53.

Corless, I., Germino, B., & Pittman, M. (Eds.). (2006). *Dying, death, and bereavement: A challenge for living* (2nd ed.). New York: Springer Publishing.

Corr, C., Nabe, C., & Corr, D. (2000). *Death and dying, life and living* (3rd ed.). Belmont, CA: Wadsworth.

Dineen, K. (2002). Gift of presence. *Nursing2002, 32*(7), 76.

Durham, E., & Weiss, L. (1997). How patients die. *American Journal of Nursing, 97*(12), 41–46.

Edelman, C., & Mandle, C. (2002). *Health promotion throughout the lifespan* (5th ed.). St. Louis, MO: Mosby.

Egan, K., and Arnold, R. (2003). Grief and bereavement care. *American Journal of Nursing, 103*(9), 42–52.

Emanuel, L., Ferris, F., vonGunten, C., & Roenn, J. (2007). The last hours of living: Practical advice for clinicians. Retrieved April 22, 2008, from http://www.medscape.com/viewprogram/5808_pnt

Engle, G. L. (1961). Is grief a disease? *Psychosomatic Medicine, 23,* 18–22.

Estes, M. (2010). *Health assessment and physical examination* (4th ed.). Clifton Park, NY: Delmar Cengage Learning.

Ferrell, B. (1998a). End-of-life care. *Nursing98, 28*(9), 58.

Ferrell, B. (1998b). How can we improve care at the end of life? *Nursing Management, 29*(9), 41–43.

Ferrell, B., & Coyle, N. (2005). *Textbook of palliative nursing* (2nd ed.). New York: Oxford University Press.

Ferrell, B., Virani, R., Grant, M., Coyne, P., & Uman, G. (2000). End-of-life care: Nurses speak out. *Nursing2000, 30*(7), 54–57.

Forbes, V. (1998). The dying game. *American Journal of Nursing, 98*(9), 50.

Frisch, N., & Frisch, L. (2005). *Psychiatric mental health nursing* (3rd ed.). Clifton Park, NY: Delmar Cengage Learning.

Furman, J. (2000). Taking a holistic approach to the dying time. *Nursing2000, 30*(6), 46–49.

Furman, J. (2001). Living with dying: How to help family caregivers. *Nursing2001, 31*(4), 36–41.

Furman, J. (2002). What you should know about chronic grief. *Nursing2002, 32*(2), 56–57.

Harvey, J. (2001). Debunking myths about postmortem care. *Nursing2001, 31*(7), 44–45.

Haynor, P. (1998). Meeting the challenge of advance directives. *American Journal of Nursing, 98*(3), 27–32.

Hellwig, K. (2000). A family lesson in dying. *RN, 63*(12), 32–33.

Hooks, F., & Daly, B. (2000). Hastening death: Is a natural death always best? *American Journal of Nursing, 100*(5), 56–63.

Huizdos, D. (2000). The tie that binds: Hanging on by a shoelace. *American Journal of Nursing, 100*(7), 25.

Hull, E. (2008). *Palliative and end of life care.* Manuscript submitted for publication.

Kübler-Ross, E. (1989). *To live until we say good-bye.* Upper Saddle River, NJ: Prentice Hall Trade.

Kübler-Ross, E. (1995). *Death is of vital importance: On life, death, and life after death.* Barrytown, NY: Station Hill.

Kübler-Ross, E. (1997a). *On death and dying.* New York: Macmillan.

Kübler-Ross, E. (1997b). *Death, the final stage of growth.* Old Tappan, NJ: Simon & Schuster.

Kübler-Ross, E. (1997c). *Meaning of our suffering.* Barrytown, NY: Barrytown, Ltd.

Kübler-Ross, E. (1997d). *Questions and answers on death and dying.* New York: Macmillan.

Kübler-Ross, E., & Kessler, D. (2001). *Life lessons: Two experts on death and dying teach us about the mysteries of life and living.* Carmichael, CA: Touchstone Books.

Kübler-Ross, E., & Kessler, D. (2007). *On grief and grieving: Finding the meaning of grief through the five stages of loss.* New York: Scribner.

Kubler-Ross, E., & Myss, C. (2008). *On life after death.* Berkeley, CA: Celestial Arts.

Kubler-Ross, E., & Warshaw, M. (1992). *To live until we say good-bye.* New York: Simon & Schuster.

LaDuke, S. (2001). Terminal dyspnea and palliative care. *American Journal of Nursing,* 101(11), 26–31.

Lindemann, E. (1944). Symptomatology and management of acute grief. *American Journal of Psychiatry, 101,* 141–148.

Lynn, J., Schuster, J., & Kabcenell, A. (2000). *Improving care for the end of life: A sourcebook for health care managers and clinicians.* New York: Oxford University Press.

Mazanec, P., & Tyler M. (2003). Cultural considerations in end-of-life care. *American Journal of Nursing, 103*(3), 50–58.

McCaffery, M., & Pasero, C. (1999). *Pain: Clinical manual for nursing practice* (2nd ed.). St. Louis, MO: Mosby.

McClain, M., & Shaefer, S. (1996). Supporting families after sudden infant death. *Journal of Psychosocial Nursing and Mental Health Services, 34*(4), 30–34.

McGowan, D. (1998). The right to say goodbye. *RN, 61*(5), 84.

Moorhead, S., Johnson, M., Swanson, E., & Maas, M. (2007). *Nursing Outcomes Classification (NOC)* (4th ed.). St. Louis, MO: Mosby.

North American Nursing Diagnosis Association International. (2010). *NANDA-I nursing diagnoses: Definitions and classification 2009–2011.* Ames, IA: Wiley-Blackwell.

OrganDonor.Gov. (2008). The matching process—Waiting list. Retrieved October 16, 2008, from http://www.organdonor.gov/transplantation/matching_process.htm

Paice, J. (2002). Managing psychological conditions in palliative care. *American Journal of Nursing, 102*(11), 36–42.

Panke, J. (2002). Difficulties in managing pain at the end of life. *American Journal of Nursing, 102*(7), 26–34.

Pitorak, E. (2003). Care at the time of death: How nurses can make the last hours of life a richer, more comfortable experience. *American Journal of Nursing, 103*(7), 42–51.

Popernack, M. (2000). Are we overlooking a hidden source of organs? *Nursing2000, 30*(1), 44–47.

Powell, C. (1999). Near death: A nurse reflects. *RN, 62*(4), 43–44.

Pritchett, K., & Lucas, P. (1997a). Death and dying. In B. S. Johnson (Ed.), *Psychiatric–mental health nursing: Adaptation and growth* (4th ed., pp. 206–207). Philadelphia: Lippincott Williams & Wilkins.

Pritchett, K., & Lucas, P. (1997b). Grief and loss. In B. S. Johnson (Ed.), *Psychiatric–mental health nursing: Adaptation and growth* (4th ed., pp. 199–218). Philadelphia: Lippincott Williams & Wilkins.

Puopolo, A. (1999). Gaining confidence to talk about end-of-life care. *Nursing99, 29*(7), 49–51.

Reese, C. D. (1996). Please cry with me: Six ways to grieve. *Nursing96, 26*(8), 56.

Robert Wood Johnson Foundation. (2004). When patients cannot eat or drink. Retrieved October 8, 2008 from http://www.rwjf.org/common/templates/printallfriendly.jsp?id+2093&referer+http%3A//

Rodebaugh, L., Schwindt, R., & Valentine, F. (1999). How to handle grief with wisdom, *Nursing99, 29*(10), 52–53.

Scanlon, C. (2003). Ethical concerns in end-of-life care. *AJN, 103*(1), 48–55.

Simmons, S. (1999). Multicultural interview—Grief in the Chinese culture. Grief in a family context—HPER F460F560. Retrieved April 14, 2009, from http://www.indiana.edu/~famlygrf/culture/simmons.html

Slade, J., & Lovasik, D. (2002). Understanding brain death criteria. *Nursing2002, 32*(12), 68–69.

Smalkin, P. (2001). Facing a mother's death. *Nursing2001, 31*(7), 51.

Smith-Stoner, M., & Frost, A. (1998). Coping with grief and loss: Bringing your shadow self into the light. *Nursing98, 28*(2), 49–50.

Smith-Stoner, M., & Frost, A. (1999). How to build your "hope skills." *Nursing99, 29*(9), 49–51

Spicer, T. (2003). Coping with grief when a patient dies. *Nursing2003, 33*(3), 32hn6.

Taylor, M. (1995). Benefits of dehydration in terminally ill clients. *Geriatric Nursing, 16*(6), 271–272.

Thompson, G. (2002). Taking the measure of a father's grief. *Nursing2002, 32*(3), 46–47.

Truog, R. (2008). Consent for organ donation—Balancing conflicting ethical obligations. *New England Journal of Medicine, 358*(12), 1209–1211.

Tutka, M. A. (2001). Near-death experiences: Seeing the light. *Nursing2001, 31*(5), 62–64.

Ufema, J. (1995a). How to help dying clients feel "safe." *Nursing95, 25*(9), 59.

Ufema, J. (1995b). Insights on death and dying. *Nursing95, 25*(11,12), 19, 22–23.

Ufema, J. (1999). Reflections on death and dying. *Nursing99, 29*(6), 56–59.

Ufema, J. (2000a). Death and dying: Bedside vigils. *Nursing2000, 30*(7), 26.

Ufema, J. (2000b). Death and dying: Seeking closure. *Nursing2000, 30*(8), 28.

Ufema, J. (2000c). Death and dying: Setting goals, withholding nutrition, will to die. *Nursing2000, 30*(9), 66–67.

Ufema, J. (2002). Insights on death and dying. *Nursing2002, 32*(10), 28–30.

Vanderbeek, J. (2000). Till death do us part: A firsthand account of family presence. *American Journal of Nursing, 100*(2), 44.

Virani, R., & Sofer, D. (2003). Improving the quality of end-of-life care. *American Journal of Nursing, 103*(5), 52–60.

Webster, L., & Dove, M. (2007). Optimizing opioid treatment for breakthrough pain. Retrieved October 14, 2007, from http://www/medscape.com/viewprogram/7869_pnt

Wong, M. (1996). *The 1996 national directory of bereavement support groups and services.* Forest Hills, NY: ADM.

Wong, M. (2001). *Understanding your grieving heart after a loved one's death.* Forest Hills, NY: ADM.

Zerwekh, J. (2003). End-of-life hydration—Benefit or burden? *Nursing2003, 33*(2), 32hn1–32hn3.

RESOURCES

American Nurses Association Center for Ethics and Human Rights, http://www.nursingworld.org

Americans for Better Care of the Dying, http://www.abcd-caring.org

Association for Death Education and Counseling, http://www.adec.org

Compassion in Dying Federation, http://www.compassionindying.org

Hospice Foundation of America, http://www.hospicefoundation.org

Last Acts, http://www.lastacts.org

National Hospice and Palliative Care Organization, http://www.nhpco.org

Partnership for Caring: America's Voices for the Dying, http://www.partnershipforcaring.org

TransWeb, The Northern Brewery, http://www.transweb.org

United Network for Organ Sharing, http://www.unos.org

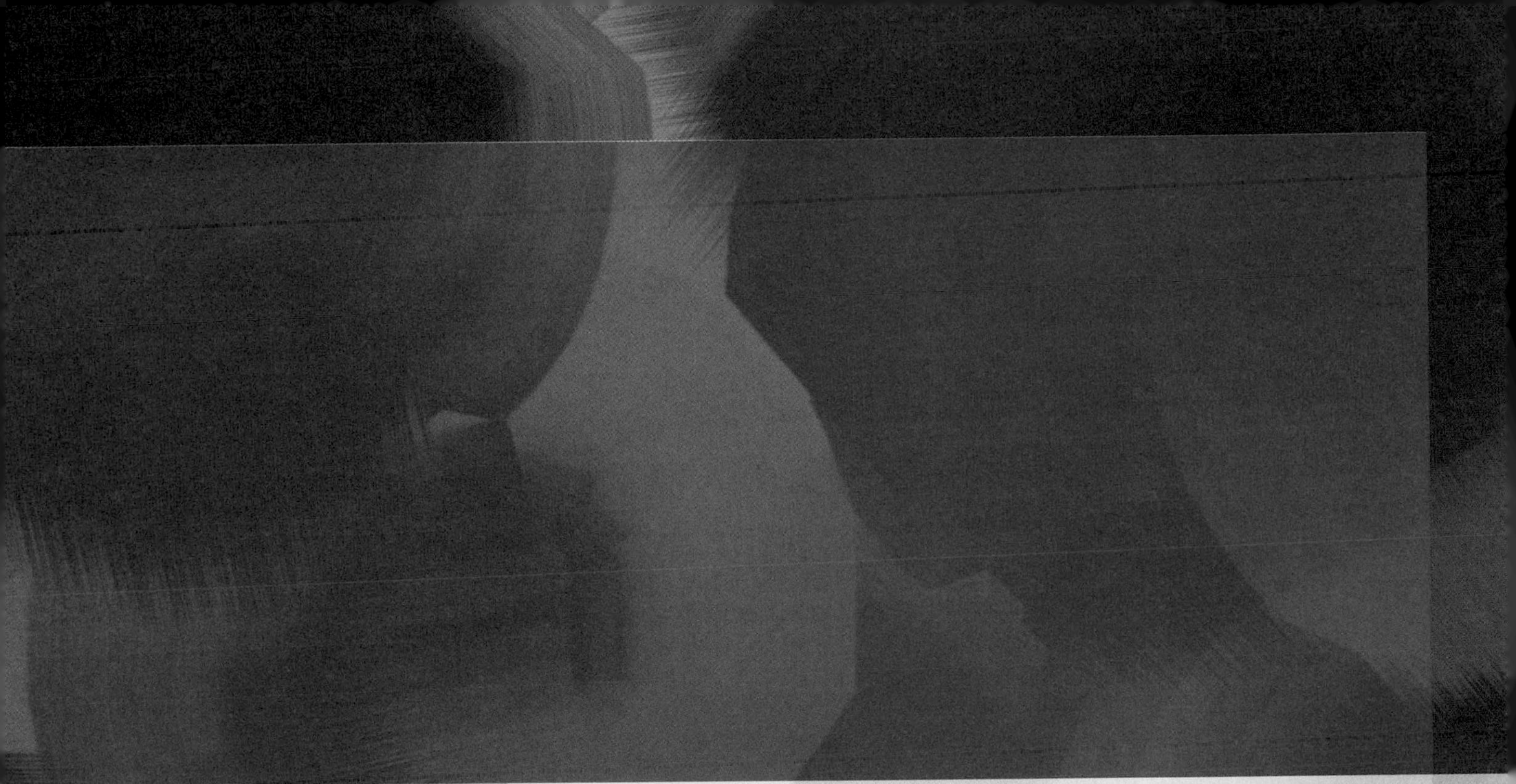

UNIT 5 Health Promotion

CHAPTER 14
Wellness Concepts

MAKING THE CONNECTION

Refer to the following chapters to increase your understanding of wellness concepts:

Basic Nursing

- ***Cultural Considerations***
- ***End-of-Life Care***

LEARNING OBJECTIVES

Upon completion of this chapter, you should be able to:

- Define key terms.
- Explain the importance of *Healthy People 2010*.
- Discuss the scope of prevention.
- Describe the benefits of using a genogram.
- Teach and follow the guidelines for healthy living.
- Make a teaching plan to promote and maintain wellness.

KEY TERMS

genogram
health
prevention
primary prevention
secondary prevention
tertiary prevention
wellness

INTRODUCTION

Individual adults have the responsibility for maintaining their own health, and parents are also responsible for maintaining their children's health and teaching them a healthy lifestyle. Health maintenance includes prevention of disease and early detection and treatment of disease, requiring constant effort focusing on all aspects of a person's life.

In 1896, Dr. Wood Hutchinson wrote in the *Journal of the American Medical Association* that "our system's philosophy might be condensed in the motto 'millions for health care and not a penny for prevention.'" More than 100 years have passed, and still less than 3 cents of each health dollar is spent on prevention and education.

The United States is 31st among nations in life expectancy yet is the world leader in medical science and education (CNN, 2008a). In 2008, the United States reportedly spent more than $2,500 per person per year for health care (CNN, 2008b). In 2005, the average spent on prescription drugs was $1,141 per person (CNN, 2008b). In 1960, the United States ranked 12th in infant mortality, and in 2004, the ranking dropped to 29th (*Harris*, 2008). Yet the United States spends more for health care than any other country. One of the major reasons for these statistics is that many doctors need to move preventive medicine from the sidelines to the forefront of their practice (CNN, 2008b; Cohen, Davis, & Mikkelsen, 2000). The focus is treating the disease rather than preventing the disease.

There is no profit in prevention. Insurance pays for diagnosis and treatment of illnesses, not health maintenance, but often will not pay for preventive testing and treatment. Paying for clinical care makes illness the priority, not wellness.

HEALTH

The generally accepted definition of **health** from the World Health Organization (WHO) defines health as a state of complete physical, mental, and social well-being, not merely the absence of disease or infirmity.

Another concept of health focuses on motivation. The individual is motivated by joy and self-fulfillment and believes that health is the realization of potential, and illness is an obstacle in that realization.

Those who have an adaptive view of health are motivated by altering the risks in self or the environment through diet and exercise or by reducing exposure to environmental hazards. When the individual is unable to cope with the stresses and risks of daily life, illness results.

Some individuals are motivated by being able to meet responsibilities at home, at work, at play, and in the community: Their health focus is role performance. Health is considered achieved when the individual fulfills the responsibilities and obligations to family, job, and community.

Other individuals are motivated by the absence of disease: Theirs is a clinical health focus. As long as no disease is present, the individual considers himself healthy. A person's definition of health influences personal health decisions and life choices.

WELLNESS

Wellness is defined as a state of optimal health wherein an individual maximizes human potential, moves toward integration of human functioning, has greater self-awareness and self-satisfaction, and takes responsibility for health. Floyd, Mimms, and Yelding-Howard (1995), Hoeger, Turner, and Hafen (2001), and Seiger, Kanipe, Vanderpool, and Barnes (2000) describe the behaviors exhibited by individuals in a state of wellness. These researchers outline seven areas of wellness: emotional, mental, intellectual, vocational, social, spiritual, and physical wellness. Various areas of wellness overlap and none is mutually exclusive.

Emotional Wellness

Emotions bridge the gap between body and mind. The individual who is emotionally well understands his own feelings and knows when to express them appropriately. This person accepts limitations, copes with stress in healthy ways, has the ability to adjust to change, is optimistic and happy, enjoys life, and shows respect and affection to others.

Mental Wellness

The person who is mentally well is alert, curious, clear thinking, open-minded, creative, logical, and accepting of others. This person also has a good memory, common sense, and a desire for continual learning.

Intellectual Wellness

Intellectual wellness is revealed by an ability to think, process information, and solve problems. The intellectually well person questions and evaluates information and situations; is creative, flexible, and open to new ideas; and learns from life experiences.

Vocational Wellness

The individual who is satisfied in school and/or job and who works in harmony with others enjoys vocational wellness (Figure 14-1).

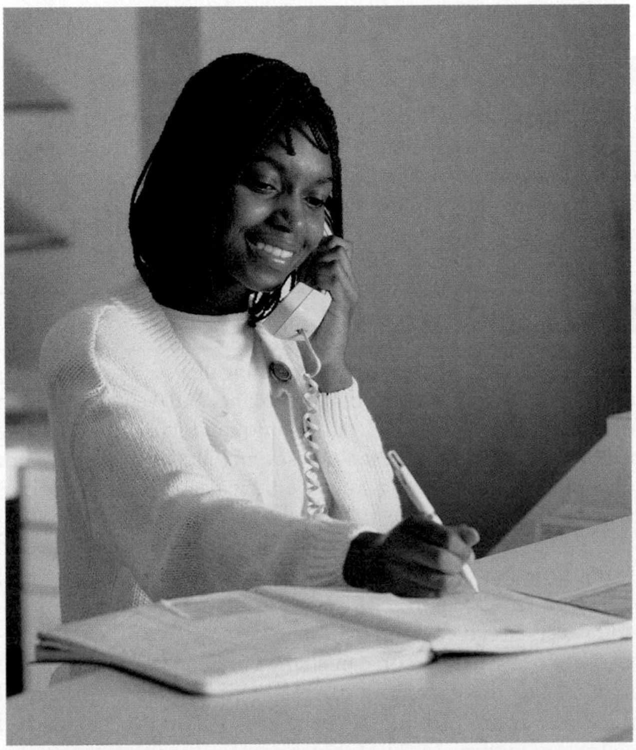

Figure 14-1 Vocational wellness means being content and satisfied with your occupation.

CLIENT TEACHING

Suppressed Anger in Women

Research has shown that women who suppress anger and who have hostile attitudes may be at greater risk for developing cardiovascular disease and physical problems (Meyers, 2008). Nurses can help such women minimize this risk by encouraging them to learn to express negative feelings constructively, to talk calmly about their feelings, to find other women who may share some of the same concerns and stressors, and to engage in regular exercise routines to relieve stress and tension. Encourage the person to change her perception of the situation to lessen the impact on her thoughts and feelings. Learning and using assertive communication allows the person to express her feelings and increase control of the situation. Maintaining positive relationships provides upbeat input into one's life.

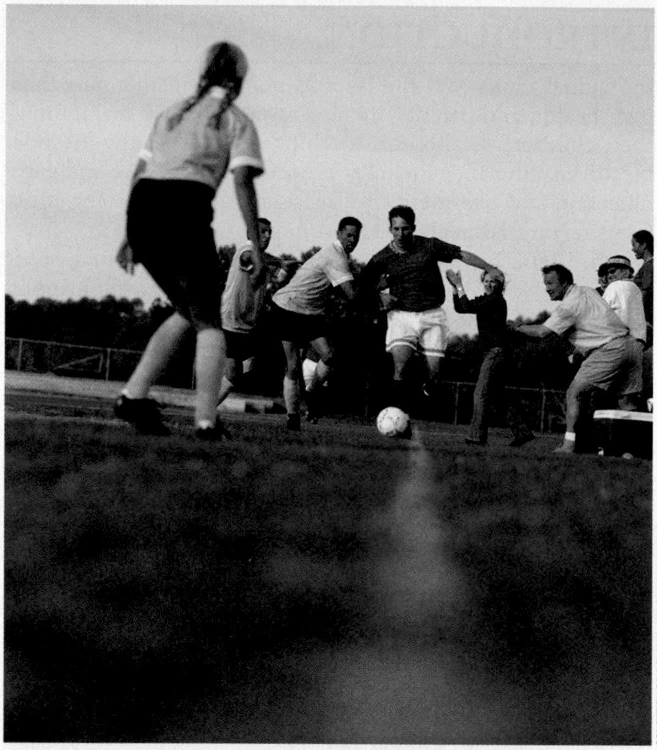

FIGURE 14-2 **A person maintains physical wellness by exercising, eating a well-balanced diet, having a regular physical exam, and avoiding at risk behaviors.**

SOCIAL WELLNESS

The person who shows affection, fairness, concern, and respect for others; communicates effectively; has satisfying relationships; and interacts well with others enjoys social wellness. This person has a network of friends and family, is a member of various organizations, and enjoys working together. Other behaviors exhibited are confidence, loyalty, honesty, and tolerance.

SPIRITUAL WELLNESS

Spiritual wellness gives direction, meaning, and purpose to life through values, morals, and ethics. The spiritually healthy person has optimism, faith, and high self-esteem.

PHYSICAL WELLNESS

Physical wellness is seen in individuals who exercise regularly, eat a well-balanced diet, and have regular physical examinations. They avoid risky sexual behavior, try to limit exposure to environmental contaminants, and restrict the intake of alcohol, tobacco, caffeine, and drugs (Figure 14-2).

HEALTH PROMOTION

Health promotion is more than preventing illness: It means assisting individuals to better health, functioning, and well-being and to maximize their potential. Health promotion focuses on choosing healthy behaviors rather than on escaping illness. The goal is for individuals to control and improve their health. Health promotion is appropriate for the individual and the entire population.

The concept of self-responsibility is important to health promotion. No one else can make a person live a healthy life; self-responsibility is the only way to make changes. An individual can be given information relating to health and wellness, but only that person can change unhealthy or destructive habits. With the exception of small children, each individual must take responsibility for behaviors leading to health and wellness (Figure 14-3). Objectives for healthy living are outlined in the *Healthy People 2000* and *Healthy People 2010* documents issued by the federal government.

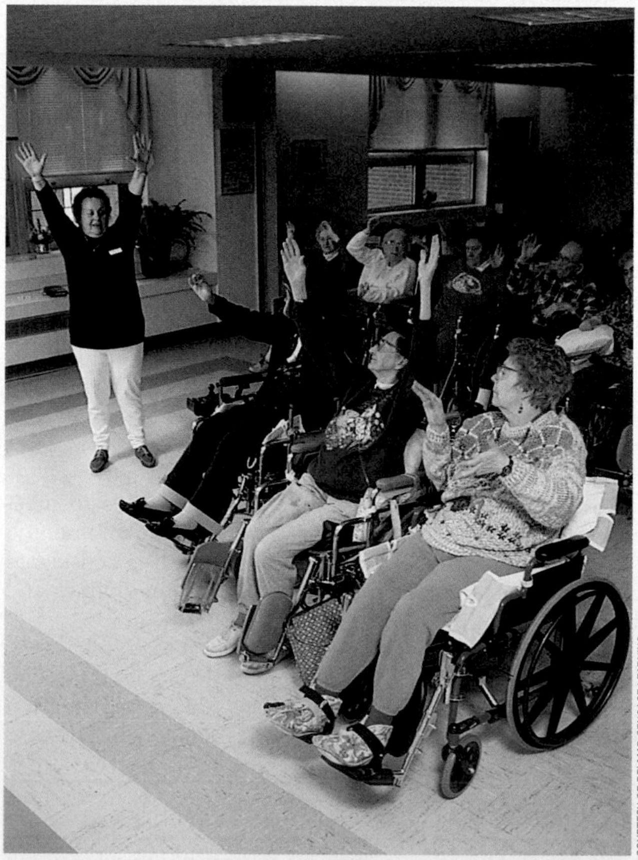

FIGURE 14-3 **Individuals must learn to achieve physical wellness in a manner that accommodates their lifestyles and physical abilities.**

CULTURAL CONSIDERATIONS

Spiritual Well-Being

According to a study by Hall (2006), weekly attendance at religious services add 2 to 3 additional years of life. Stibich (2007) suggests increased social contacts, prayer, and spiritual reflection as possible reasons for longevity. This underscores the importance of religion and spiritual wellness to an individual's overall state of health.

HEALTHY PEOPLE 2000

In 1980 and again in 1990, the U.S. Department of Health and Human Services (DHHS) released a list of objectives for disease prevention and health promotion in 22 priority areas (DHHS, 1990). More than 10,000 individuals representing 300 national organizations met in 1990 to develop the health objectives for the year 2000. More than 300 health objectives were drafted for the nation to achieve by the year 2000. These objectives were published in a document titled *Healthy People 2000: National Health Promotion and Disease Prevention Objectives*, which addresses three important issues:

- *Personal responsibility:* Each individual must be health conscious and must practice informed, responsible, health behaviors (Figure 14-4).
- *Health benefits for all people:* Everyone must have health benefits for the nation to be healthy.
- *Health promotion and disease prevention:* Health care must change from a treatment focus to a prevention focus to increase the quality of life and to cut costs.

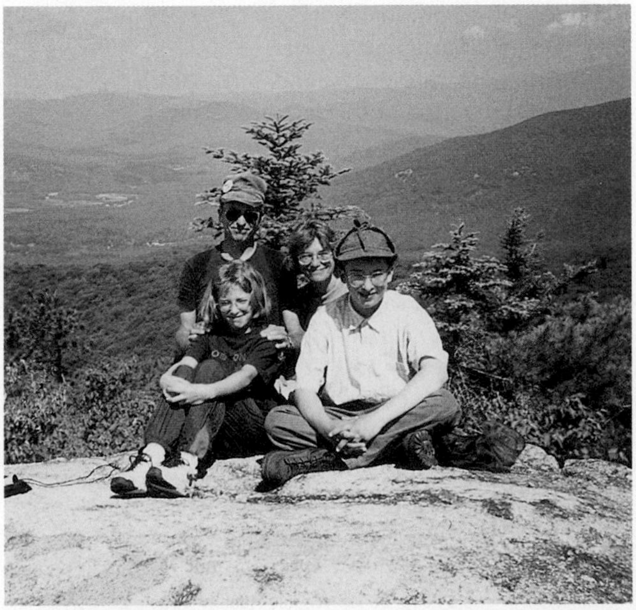
COURTESY OF DELMAR CENGAGE LEARNING

FIGURE 14-4 Families can engage in activities together to achieve wellness.

LIFE SPAN CONSIDERATIONS

Older Adults and Exercise

Health promotion activities in the older client have been shown to contribute to improving the quality if not the quantity of life (Resnick, 2001). Maintaining some type of physical activity benefits the musculoskeletal, cardiac, and respiratory systems for the older adult (Carethers, 1992). Other benefits include decreased bone loss, improved glucose tolerance, improved lipid profile, decreased body fat, and increased self-esteem and cognitive status (Carethers, 1992).

The Agency for Healthcare Research and Quality (AHRQ) suggests that older people can benefit the most from regular physical exercise because they are more at risk of the health problems that exercise prevents (Marshall & Altpeter, 2005). Physical activity improves muscle strength, flexibility, gait, and balance. These positive effects decrease the risk of falls for the older client. More than one-third of adults over the age of 65 fall each year in the United States, and falls are the leading cause of injury and injury-related deaths in the older population (Centers for Disease Control and Prevention, 2006).

The extent of exercise prescribed for the elderly client is dependent on the client's health status. The client with several risk factors for cardiovascular disease or with diagnosed cardiac disease will need to be evaluated by a physician before initiating an exercise program (Resnick, 2001). The level of fitness necessary to produce health benefits in the elderly can be attained through low-intensity activities, including walking, cycling, and swimming (Carethers, 1992). Elderly with functional disabilities can also receive benefits from physical activity, such as range-of-motion exercises, wheelchair push-ups, and isotonic exercises (Carethers, 1992). These activities will prevent joint contractures and muscle atrophy.

There are many exercise programs and gyms that offer programs geared to the exercise needs of the older client. These programs usually combine weight training with aerobic exercise. Encouraging older clients to participate in an exercise program will provide them with a variety of physical and psychosocial benefits and may contribute to an increased quality of life (Smith, in press).

The overall goals included:

- Increasing the span of healthy life for Americans
- Reducing health disparities among Americans
- Achieving access to preventive services for all Americans

PROFESSIONALTIP

Predictors of Healthy Aging

The most consistent predictors of healthy aging are low serum glucose, normal blood pressure, avoidance of smoking, and maintenance of target weight for height (Reed, 1998). To prevent disease in later years, young adults and even adolescents must keep these four factors in check. It is never too late to modify these four factors to improve health.

HEALTHY PEOPLE 2010

Healthy People 2010 is a document developed by the federal government to serve as a "road map" for improving the health of American citizens for the first decade of the 21st century. It is the third such document developed by the DHHS. The underlying premise of *Healthy People 2010* is that the health of the individual is almost inseparable from the health of the larger community (Hunt, 2008). Health care providers in all settings are using this document to guide them in developing programs of care. The DHHS is currently creating *Healthy People 2020,* a document that will address the major health issues of the next decade. They expect to have the framework of the document completed by early 2009 and to have the objectives completed by January 2010. Updates on the progress of the document and ways to provide input to the document can be accessed through the *Healthy People 2010* Web site at http://www.healthypeople.gov.

Overview and General Goals

Healthy People 2010 has two broad goals that it hopes to achieve: to increase the quality and years of healthy life and to eliminate health disparities. The 467-page document was developed with input from a national consortium of health care professionals, citizens, and private and public government agencies (Hunt, 2008). It contains demographic, statistical, and disease-related information that describes current health trends in the country. It is divided into four areas: (a) promoting healthy behaviors, (b) promoting healthy and safe communities, (c) improving systems for personal and public health, and (d) preventing and reducing diseases and disorders (Potter & Perry, 2009).

Healthy People 2010 identifies 10 leading health indicators (LHIs) that are major health issues for the nation. These LHIs include physical activity, overweight and obesity, tobacco use, substance abuse, responsible sexual behavior, mental health, injury and violence, environmental quality, immunization, and access to health care. The document states that improving health behaviors in these areas will move the nation toward an increased level of wellness and achievement of the document's broad goals.

Focus Areas and Specific Goals

Healthy People 2010 identifies 28 focus areas that the country should target to improve its health status. Box 14-1 lists these focus areas. Each focus area has specific goals related to that topic area. For example, two goals related to the focus area of diabetes include:

Goal 5-1: Increase the proportion of persons with diabetes who receive formal diabetes education.

Goal 5-5: Reduce the diabetes death rate.

Most focus areas have at least 15 stated goals, and most goals are statistically measurable. Current statistical information related to each goal is included in the document so that change toward achievement of the goal can be measured (Smith, 2008).

ILLNESS PREVENTION

Prevention (obstructing, thwarting, or hindering a disease or illness) incorporates both new and old ideas. The dietary laws, taboos, and traditions of various ethnic, cultural, and religious groups were begun for a reason. There is no reason not to practice the old ways if scientific research has not proven them incorrect or harmful. New methods of illness prevention emerge as technology expands and health awareness increases.

Preventive health should be practiced in all stages of life, beginning before conception with healthy parents and

Box 14-1 *HEALTHY PEOPLE 2010* FOCUS AREAS

1. Access to quality health services
2. Arthritis, osteoporosis, and chronic back conditions
3. Cancer
4. Chronic kidney disease
5. Diabetes
6. Disability and secondary conditions
7. Education and community-based programs
8. Environmental health
9. Family planning
10. Food safety
11. Health communication
12. Heart disease and stroke
13. Human immunodeficiency virus (HIV)
14. Immunization and infectious disease
15. Injury and violence prevention
16. Maternal, infant, and child health
17. Medical product safety
18. Mental health
19. Nutrition and obesity
20. Occupational safety and health
21. Oral health
22. Physical activity and fitness
23. Public health infrastructure
24. Respiratory diseases
25. Sexually transmitted diseases
26. Substance abuse
27. Tobacco use
28. Vision and hearing

From Healthy People 2010 (2005). What Is Healthy People 2010? Retrieved April 21, 2009, from http://www.healthypeople.gov/About/hpfact.htm

continuing through prenatal care and the life span. Interventions for disease prevention range from lifestyle changes that cost little or nothing to high-tech procedures that are very expensive.

Major changes are needed in health care delivery, funding, and insurance coverage before the full impact of illness prevention can be discovered. The health care system must insist on more research relating to prevention and must then apply the results of the research to insurance practices. Prevention practices must be supported and funded by the health care system in order for a change from illness treatment to illness prevention to occur. Enhanced health, longer life expectancy, and a population that functions better, feels better, and looks better will be the rewards of such a shift.

Types of Prevention

There are three types of prevention: primary, secondary, and tertiary. Primary prevention has not historically been supported by our health care system, whereas secondary and tertiary prevention have been and still are the main focus. They are also the most expensive.

Primary Prevention

Primary prevention includes all practices designed to keep health problems from developing. Primary prevention includes following recommended childhood immunization schedules, eating calcium-rich foods to prevent osteoporosis, and not smoking to prevent lung cancer. Every individual and health care provider should focus on primary prevention. It is usually the least expensive intervention and provides the greatest benefits.

Secondary Prevention

Secondary prevention includes activities related to early identification and treatment of disease processes. At this level of prevention, when taking the client's history, the nurse would focus on identification of family history, risk factors, and signs and symptoms of possible disease in the client. The client would also be screened for a variety of conditions as appropriate for age and evidence of risk. For example, all adults are screened for hypertension on every physician visit, and school-age children are screened for hearing and vision problems. The American Cancer Society has determined the age and frequency that certain cancer screenings should occur in adults. It is recommended that women over the age of 40 have a baseline mammography and then have a clinical breast examination and mammography yearly thereafter. If it was determined that the client has a strong family history of breast cancer, these screening recommendations may be increased to detect a problem at an earlier age. Secondary preventive activities often result in early detection of disease and the ability to obtain a quick and effective resolution of the illness (Smith, in press).

Tertiary Prevention

Tertiary prevention focuses on maximizing recovery after an illness or injury and preventing long-term complications. Rehabilitative and educational activities are common at this level of prevention. The client who has experienced a stroke usually undergoes intensive physical rehabilitation to promote independence with activities of daily living. They may learn how to utilize adaptive equipment, such as a quad cane or splint to improve mobility. They may also benefit from a stroke support group to help cope with the psychosocial issues they are facing as a result of their current illness (Smith, in press).

Prevention Health Care Team

The individual assisted by nurses, the nurse practitioner, and the primary physician make up the prevention health care team.

Individual

The center of the prevention health care team is the individual. The individual must combine the knowledge of preventive health care with behavioral changes necessary to live a healthier life.

Individuals should decide those things that they want and expect from health care. Clients must be honest with self, the nurses, and physician; be assertive and ask questions of the physicians and nurses; and be active, informed health care consumers. Ultimately, responsibility for health care rests with the individual.

Nurses

Nurses, especially nurse practitioners, often do the initial health screening in clinics and physicians' offices. This provides a great opportunity to inquire about the preventive health habits and

CLIENTTEACHING

Health Promotion Teaching

- Infancy: Teach parents about healthy lifestyle during prenatal period, infant feeding, basic infant care, and infant safety.
- Childhood: Teach parents about immunizations, nutrition, growth and development, building self-esteem in children, and childhood safety.
- Adolescence: Teach parents and adolescents about sexual health; avoidance of drug, alcohol, and tobacco use; motor vehicle safety and other adolescent safety issues; support of mental health; and prevention of suicide.
- Adulthood: Teach adults about nutrition, physical activity, stress management, sexual health, avoidance of tobacco and substance abuse, recommended cancer screenings, and risk factor reduction for heart disease, stroke, and cancer.
- Older Adults: Teach older adults about changing nutritional requirements, exercise, stress management, safety issues related to mobility and sensory changes, promotion of independence and self-esteem, and prevention of suicide.

From Nettina, S. (2001) *The Lippincott Manual of Nursing Practice*. Philadelphia: Lippincott.

lifestyle of the client. Nurses can use their excellent listening skills to give clients time to discuss health care habits and ask questions. Nurses are also great teachers of preventive health habits and health promotion activities.

Primary Physicians

Primary physicians usually are family practitioners, internists, or pediatricians. These are the family doctors seen on a regular basis. They have the opportunity and obligation to discuss and inquire about preventive health habits. They refer clients to specialists for specific problems when necessary. When the problem is resolved, the client returns to the primary physician for further care.

FACTORS AFFECTING HEALTH

The many factors affecting health can be categorized into four broad topics:

- Genetics and human biology
- Environmental influences
- Personal behavior
- Health care

Genetics and Human Biology

Inherited traits and the way the human body functions have an impact on an individual's state of health and wellness. An individual's genetic makeup may include inherited disorders, such as sickle-cell anemia, or chromosomal anomalies, such as Down syndrome. Both of these may ultimately affect the individual's quality of life and level of health.

Human biology affects health because normal body functioning prevents some illnesses and makes us more susceptible to others.

Environmental Influences

Environmental factors that may influence health are numerous, can be natural or man-made, and vary depending on geographic location and living conditions. Exposure to or ingestion of certain natural biological irritants can cause disease, such as results from exposure to poison ivy, and even death, such as results from ingestion of poisonous mushrooms. Exposure to chemicals such as asbestos in older buildings, lead paint in older houses, and mercury in polluted water sources also are health hazards. Radiation from the sun and some types of machinery can be harmful; extreme, prolonged exposure to solar radiation can even result in death. Natural disasters, such as hurricanes, floods, volcanic eruptions, droughts, heat waves, blizzards, and other extreme weather conditions, pose health risks, as do man-made environmental crises, including wars, bombings, pollution, and overpopulation.

Personal Behavior

Personal behavior is the area with the most factors affecting health and wellness, and they are controlled entirely by the individual. It is the individual's decision to use or not to use these factors to promote health and wellness. Factors typically deemed to be under the individual's control include diet, exercise, personal care, sexual relationships, level of stress, tobacco and drug use, alcohol use, and safety.

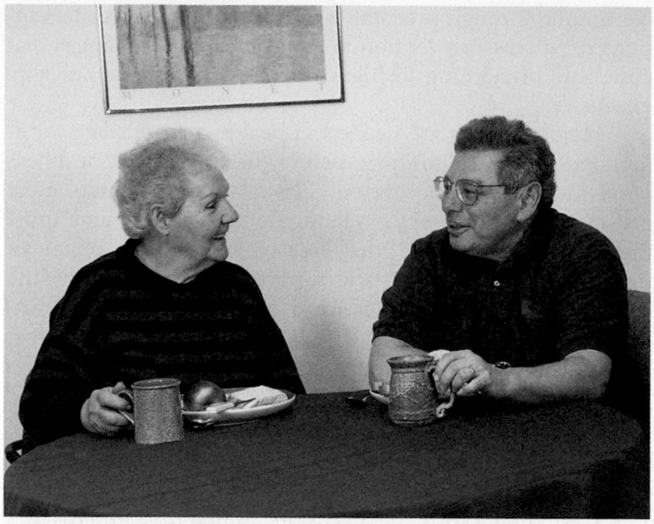

FIGURE 14-5 Sharing meals together is a wonderful means of meeting both physical and interpersonal needs.

Diet

Healthy eating habits and a proper diet greatly enhance an individual's overall state of health and well-being. Eating both fulfills the basic biological needs of sustenance, nutrition, and hydration and allows individuals to meet social and interpersonal needs (Figure 14-5). All of these factors contribute to overall wellness.

Exercise

Integrating physical activity into daily life is one of the best ways of promoting health. Exercise improves muscle strength, circulation, and emotional well-being; increases endurance; lowers blood pressure; and reduces the chances of heart attack, osteoporosis, and stroke. The individual who exercises regularly feels better and looks healthier.

Health clubs are used by many people in an effort to meet their need for exercise. Health clubs are a wonderful place for regular exercise but also can be a source of disease. For example, perspiration on exercise machines is a prime source of impetigo. Clients should be made aware of such dangers so that they can practice safety precautions, such as wearing thigh-length shorts and always keeping a towel between the body and the exercise equipment.

Personal Care

The skin works with the immune system to defend the body against harmful allergens, bacteria, fungi, and viruses by protecting the body from outside elements. Regular skin, hair, and nail care will enhance wellness and foster self-esteem. Personal care also includes such wellness habits as proper posture, proper body mechanics, adequate sleep, and dental hygiene.

Sexual Relationships

Establishing intimacy and a sexual relationship with another person is a natural step in growth and development. To maintain health and wellness, the individual will use values, ethics, and morals to guide the development of the relationship. A healthy sexual relationship is based on mutual satisfaction of the parties, a consensual approach to pleasurable activities, and mutual respect for preferences and personal choices.

CULTURAL CONSIDERATIONS

Parents' Beliefs about Feeding Children

Many parents:

- Believe that milk alone will not satisfy their babies' hunger, so they begin feeding cereal and other solid foods earlier than recommended.
- Use food to console children.
- Believe that a plump child is a healthier child.
- View a heavy infant or toddler as evidence of parental competence (Baughcum, 1998).

Nurses can work with these clients by respecting their cultural beliefs while enforcing the notion that a healthy child is a child who is satisfied following a meal and who shows a healthy, normal physical and emotional growth pattern. These factors, not plumpness, are indicators of wellness.

One role of the nurse is to educate the client on ways to prevent sexually transmitted infections.

Level of Stress

Not all stress is harmful. Limited stress raises one's energy level and makes one more alert. The way one responds to or copes with stressors dictates whether the situation is healthy or harmful. For instance, one individual may enjoy the challenge of balancing work and family, while another may feel torn by these seemingly conflicting demands and will experience undue stress. Stress results not from an individual's life situation but from that individual's reaction to and perception of the life situation.

Tobacco and Drug Use

Refraining from tobacco use is a strong step toward health promotion and maintenance. Even when a longtime smoker gives up the habit, the health risks begin to decrease at once, although it will take 10 to 15 years to eliminate all the effects of smoking from the lungs. The person who smokes exhales secondhand smoke, which presents a health risk to those who do not smoke. According to the Office of the Surgeon General (2007), exposure to secondhand smoke at home or work increased one's risk of developing heart disease by 25% to 30% and lung cancer by 20% to 30%.

Abuse of both illegal and prescription drugs is a serious medical and social problem in our society. Drugs prescribed by a physician are abused if they are not taken as directed or if they are taken by anyone other than the client for whom they were prescribed. If not taken as directed, many prescribed drugs can be addictive. Health can be maintained when clients understand the effects, indications, side effects, and interactions of the prescription medications they are taking.

Alcohol Use

The decision to consume alcohol is a personal choice that can influence an individual's state of health. The amount of alcohol consumed will affect sobriety, decision-making ability, and, in many instances, safety. The use of alcohol can play a prominent role in drownings, suicides, traffic fatalities, adult fire deaths, and falling fatalities.

CLIENTTEACHING

Dietary Guidelines for Americans

- Consume a sufficient amount of fruits and vegetables while staying within energy needs. Two cups of fruit and 2½ cups of vegetables per day are recommended for persons consuming a 2,000-calorie intake.
- Choose a variety of fruits and vegetables each day. In particular, select from all five vegetable subgroups (dark green, orange, legumes, starchy vegetables, and other vegetables) several times a week.
- Consume three or more ounce equivalents of whole-grain products per day, with the rest of the recommended grains coming from enriched or whole-grain products. In general, at least half the grains should come from whole grains.
- Consume 3 cups per day of fat-free or low-fat milk or equivalent milk products.
- Include lean meats, poultry, fish, beans, eggs and nuts in your diet.
- Limit saturated fats, trans fats, cholesterol, sodium and added sugars.

From Office of Disease Prevention and Health Promotion. (2006). *Dietary Guidelines for Americans 2005.* Retrieved December 2, 2006, from http://www.odphp.osophs.dhhs.gov

Safety

Personal choices concerning safety affect many areas of an individual's life and can be viewed collectively more as a lifestyle

CLIENTTEACHING

Preventing Food-Borne Diseases

Share the following tips with clients to educate them in ways to prevent food-borne diseases:

- Allow cooked foods to sit at room temperature for no more than 2 hours.
- Date leftovers, refrigerate, and eat within 2 to 3 days.
- Wash dirty dishes in hot (120°F) water, as dirty dishes are an ideal place for bacteria to multiply.
- Keep dishcloths and sponges clean and allow to dry between uses.
- Use a bleach solution to clean cutting boards and countertops.
- Wash all fruits and vegetables in a diluted bleach solution (a bleach to water ratio of 1:100).

PROFESSIONAL TIP

Moderate Exercise Reduces Stroke Risk

- Individuals who burn 1,000 to 1,999 calories per week by exercising moderately have a 24% lower risk of suffering a stroke than do those who burn less.
- Individuals who burn 2,000 to 2,999 calories per week by exercising moderately have a 46% lower risk.
- Burning over 2,999 calories a week through moderate exercise lowered the risk of having a stroke by only 20%.
- Moderate exercise includes activities such as brisk walking, dancing, and cycling (Krarup et al., 2008; Lee & Paffenbarger, 1998).

choice than individually as separate acts to promote safety. For example, individuals who embrace safety as a fundamental element of health and well-being will ensure safety in their homes by having smoke detectors, fire extinguishers, carbon monoxide detectors, practiced escape plans, locked medicine cabinets, and gates blocking dangerous stairways. These individuals will also most likely buckle their car seat belts, secure their children in child car seats, and obey speed limits when driving. All these elements of safety support a healthy lifestyle.

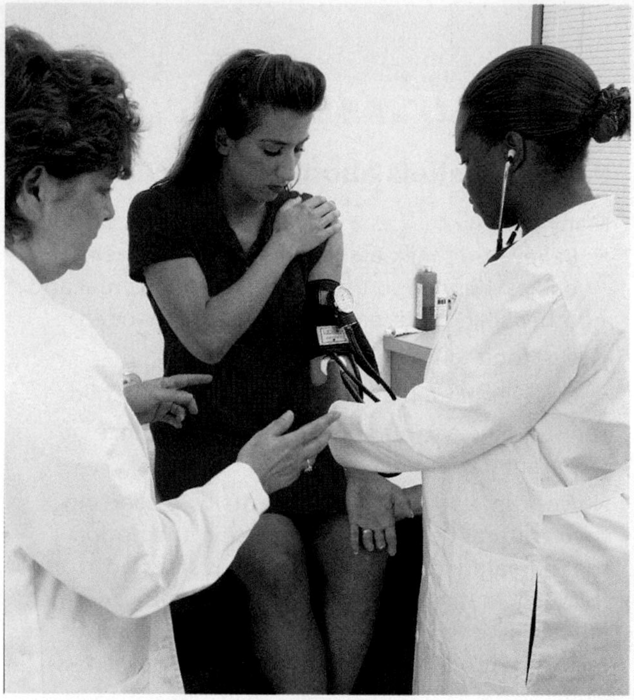

FIGURE 14-6 **Routine physical examinations are essential to maintaining health and preventing disease.**

HEALTH CARE

Most people use the health care system to treat their illness or condition. However, health promotion and disease prevention are a more effective use of the health care system. Routine physical examinations with minimal testing are beneficial for preventing disease and maintaining health (Figure 14-6). Healthy adults should consider health care services based on family health history, personal habits, or personal health history. The presence of symptoms will alter the time frame for suggested health care services.

Physical Exam

The physical examination begins with a review of family health history, personal health history, personal habits (sexual practices, tobacco, alcohol, and drug use), and concerns or questions the client may have. The client should write down questions and concerns before visiting the physician so that none will be forgotten. Between the ages of 20 and 39 years, individuals should have a complete physical exam every 1 to 3 years; those 40 to 49 years of age, every 1 to 2 years; and those older than 50 years of age, every year.

Immunizations

Adults who did not have the recommended immunizations as children should discuss this with their primary physicians. The physician may recommend having the immunizations as an adult based on the client's risk factors.

Every adult should have a tetanus booster every 10 years for life. Health care workers and college students; those with high risk of exposure; those with chronic heart, pulmonary, or kidney disease; those with diabetes; and those 65 years of age and older should have an influenza immunization every year and a pneumococcal pneumonia immunization every 6 years.

Tests

The following tests should be done with every physical exam: complete blood count, blood sugar, cholesterol, urinalysis, stool for blood, and, for women, a Papanicolau (Pap) smear. An electrocardiogram (EKG or ECG) should be done at ages 20 and 40 and every 5 years thereafter (yearly if the client is at high risk). Women should have a breast exam with every physical exam and a baseline mammogram (Figure 14-7) at age 40 and yearly thereafter. Men should have a testicular exam and a rectal exam to check the prostate with every physical exam after age 40. A breast self-exam should be done by every woman after each menstrual period. A testicular self-exam should be done monthly by every male.

PROFESSIONAL TIP

Mammograms

The Centers for Disease Control and Prevention (2005) reports that in 2002, 68.4% of women, age 40 and older, at less than $15,000 annual income, had a mammogram, as did 75.3% with annual incomes of $15,000 to $34,999 and 82.5% with annual incomes of $50,000 or more. Women with less than a high school education, never being married, and with no health insurance had fewer mammograms than those who were college graduates, married, and had health insurance.

PROFESSIONALTIP

Hepatitis B Vaccine

Health care personnel who may be exposed to blood and body fluids are at risk for contracting the hepatitis B virus. Health care employers are required by law to offer the hepatitis B vaccination without cost to employees who are in direct care positions. Employees have the option of having or refusing this immunization. The vaccine is not contraindicated during pregnancy, and there are no apparent adverse effects to developing fetuses; however, the vaccine may cause shock in individuals who are allergic to baker's yeast.

Dental Exam

Throughout life, a dental exam, prophylaxis, and needed treatment should be performed every 6 to 12 months.

Eye Exam

An eye exam, including tonometry for glaucoma, should be performed every 2 to 3 years from ages 40 to 49 years and every 1 to 2 years after the age of 50.

MAKING A GENOGRAM

A **genogram** is a way to visualize family members, their birth and death dates or ages, and specific health problems. At least four generations should be included: the individual, the parents, the grandparents, and the children. Then it is easy to follow health problems through the generations. Health problems that may be encountered can be identified and steps taken to prevent them. Figure 14-8 shows a sample genogram.

GUIDELINES FOR HEALTHY LIVING

Because of their education and training, nurses are in a unique position to practice healthy living habits themselves and to promote such habits in their clients. Table 14-1 identifies the top 9 causes of death and the controllable factors that most contribute to these types of deaths. While it is important to remember that certain health variables such as gender and race cannot be controlled or changed, others, such as diet and tobacco use, result from individual choice. These lifestyle choices are based on individual preference, and nurses can help clients make the

CRITICAL THINKING

Wellness

How can you assist clients to assess their state of wellness?

What preventive health care should be received by a person 20 years old, 42 years old, and 65 years old?

How does the nurse's state of wellness affect client care?

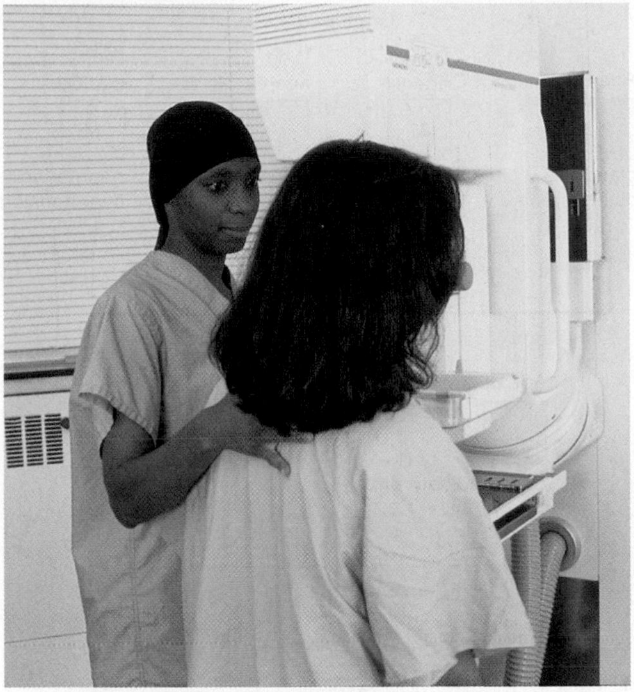

FIGURE 14-7 Mammograms are a key element to wellness promotion for all women older than 40 years of age.

CLIENTTEACHING

Crucial Health Practices

Simon (1992) states that all the medical progress in the United States from 1900 to 1990 increased the life span of an average adult by 4 years but that simple lifestyle changes increased the life span of an average adult by 11 years. His 10 crucial health practices are still applicable today:

- Use no tobacco or drugs.
- Consume no more than 2 ounces of alcohol per day.
- Eat a diet low in fat, cholesterol, and salt but high in fiber, fruits, vegetables, and fish.
- Exercise regularly—1 hour each week is helpful, 3 is ideal.
- Stay lean.
- Drive cars with air bags and wear seat belts; drive prudently, and never drink before driving.
- Avoid excessive stress.
- Minimize exposure to radiation, ultraviolet rays, chemical pollutants, and other environmental hazards.
- Protect self from sexually transmitted diseases.
- Obtain regular medical care including immunizations and screening tests.

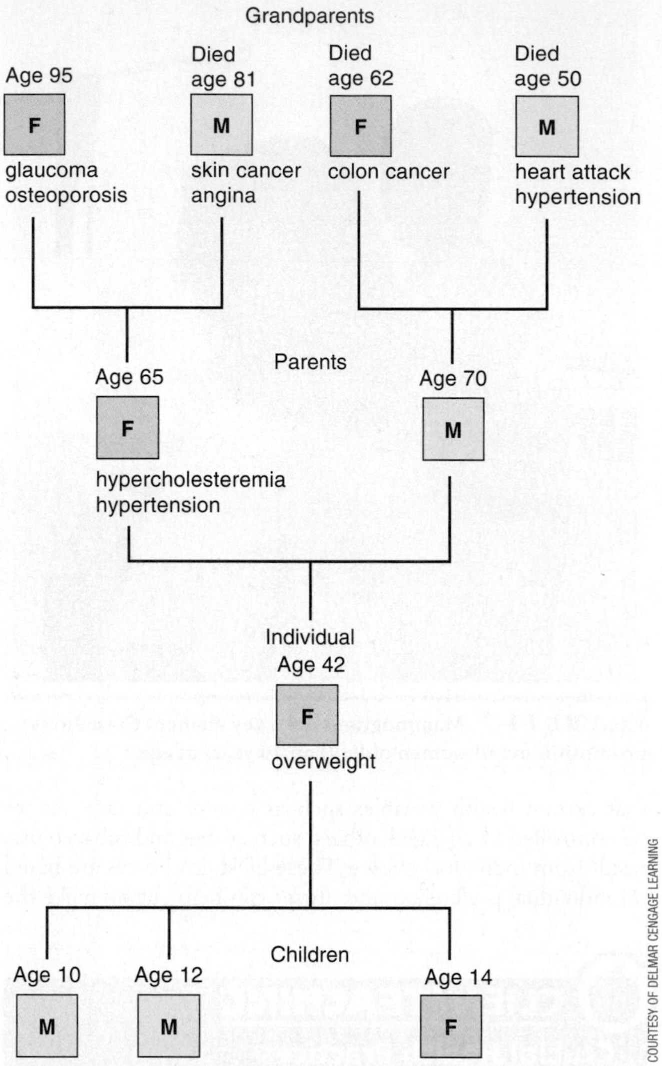

FIGURE 14-8 **Sample Genogram**

best choices to promote wellness and optimal functioning. Following is a list of select guidelines, for nurses and their clients, to promote healthy living and wellness in daily life.

Heart Disease:

- Eat a diet low in fat and cholesterol and high in fiber.
- Exercise regularly, 30 minutes three to five times a week (walking, swimming, cycling).
- Quit smoking or do not start to smoke.
- Reduce stress; use relaxation or meditation.
- Do not use caffeine or alcohol excessively.
- Maintain appropriate height-to-weight ratio.
- Maintain normal blood pressure.
- Have a physical exam regularly.

Osteoporosis:

- Throughout life, eat a balanced diet and calcium-rich foods (milk and milk products).
- Get plenty of exercise.
- Discuss with the primary care physician the need for a calcium supplement and estrogen replacement therapy (females).
- Do not smoke.

Cancer:

- Do not smoke.
- Avoid unnecessary exposure to radiation.
- Protect skin from ultraviolet rays; use sunscreen.
- Avoid exposure to harmful chemicals.
- Minimize exposure to pesticides, herbicides, and poisons.
- Limit alcohol intake.
- Eat a well-balanced diet with adequate fiber.
- Exercise regularly.
- Practice safe sex.
- Have cancer screening tests—mammogram, Pap smear, rectal exam—fecal occult blood test with each physical exam.

Low-Back Pain:

- Exercise regularly.
- Practice good posture and proper body mechanics.

Colds and Flu:

- Wash hands frequently.
- Use paper tissues and dispose of properly.
- Have flu shots yearly.
- Eat a balanced diet.
- Drink plenty of fluids.

Breast Cancer:

- Eat a diet low in fat.
- Exercise regularly.
- Limit alcohol and caffeine intake.
- Perform monthly breast self-examinations.
- Have mammograms as recommended by the American Cancer Society.

Sexually Transmitted Infections:

- Practice monogamous sex between noninfected individuals.
- Use latex condoms.

Tuberculosis (especially for health care workers):

- Take a Mantoux test.
- Receive isoniazid preventive therapy; any newly exposed and infected individual should take a full course of therapy.

Urinary Tract Infections:

- Drink plenty of water.
- Empty bladder frequently, especially before and after sexual intercourse.
- Wear cotton-crotch underwear.
- Wipe from front to back.
- Drink cranberry juice.
- Avoid bubble bath, douches, and colored or scented toilet paper.

Sickle-Cell Anemia and Thalassemia:

- Request genetic screening and counseling if a high-risk group.

Cataracts:

- Wear a brimmed hat and sunglasses.
- Eat a well-balanced diet.
- Do not smoke.

Glaucoma:

- Have tonometry performed.
- Have an optic nerve exam.

TABLE 14-1 Controllable Risk Factors for Top 9 Causes of Death

CAUSE OF DEATH	CONTROLLABLE RISK FACTORS
Heart disease	Tobacco use, high blood pressure, high cholesterol, lack of exercise, excessive stress, diabetes, obesity
Cancer	Tobacco use, radiation, alcohol abuse, improper diet, environmental exposure
Stroke	Tobacco use, high blood pressure, high cholesterol, lack of exercise
Chronic lung disease	Tobacco use, environmental exposures
Accidents	Alcohol abuse, drug abuse, tobacco use, failure to use seat belts, fatigue, stress, recklessness
Diabetes	Obesity, improper diet, lack of exercise, excessive stress
Alzheimer's disease	Prevent head injuries by wearing seat belts, helmets, and decreasing fall risks; control heart disease risk factors as there is a link between heart damage and vascular disease and Alzheimer's; stay socially involved; exercise mind and body; avoid tobacco and excess alcohol use; maintain healthy weight
Pneumonia and influenza	Chronic lung disease, environmental exposures, tobacco use, alcohol abuse, lack of immunizations
Kidney disease	Blood pressure and blood sugar control as a diabetic; maintain blood pressure within normal limits; avoid urinary system blockages; limit use of nonsteroidal anti-inflammatory drugs (NSAIDs) and acetaminophen (Tylenol); avoid heroin and cocaine use; promptly treat *Streptococcus* infections

From Risk factors. By Alzheimer's Association, 2008. Retrieved April 21, 2009, from http://www.alz.org/alzheimers_disease_causes_risk_factors.asp; National vital statistics report, vol. 15, no. 5. By National Center for Health Statistics, 2001. Retrieved April 21, 2009, from http://www.cdc.gov/nchs/data/nvsr/nvsr51/nvsr51_05.pdf; National vital statistics report, vol. 57, no. 14. By National Center for Health Statistics, 2001. Retrieved April 21, 2009, from http://www.cdc.gov/nchs/products/nvsr.htm#vol57

Sunburn:

- Always wear suncreen (with a minimum SPF of 15) when out in the sun.

Dental Caries and Periodontal Disease:

- Floss daily and brush after each meal.
- Use toothpaste with fluoride.
- Have a professional cleaning twice a year.
- Have a dental exam yearly.

Home Safety:

- Lock cupboards containing medicines and cleaning materials.
- Keep smoke alarms and fire extinguishers working.
- Use a carbon monoxide alarm in the presence of gas appliances and heaters.
- Plan escape routes in case of fire and have fire drills.
- Safety-proof home against falls.
- Know water safety rules.

Work Safety:

- Follow safety regulations at work.
- Report unsafe practices or equipment.

Travel Safety:

- Wear seat belts.
- Do not drive and drink.
- Drive defensively and safely.
- Use infant and child seats and restraints.
- Wear a helmet when riding a motorcycle or bicycle.
- Never swim alone.

Weight:

- Follow the Dietary Guidelines for Americans for a balanced diet.
- Exercise daily for 30 minutes.
- If overweight, eat the least number of servings recommended and use raw fruits or vegetables as snacks between meals.
- If underweight, eat the largest number of servings recommended and eat a nutritious snack between meals.

Stress:

- Identify sources of stress.
- Establish realistic expectations and goals.
- Try to be flexible.
- Express feelings and thoughts.
- Do not use alcohol or drugs for relaxation.
- Exercise regularly.
- Practice muscle relaxation and deep breathing.
- Get enough sleep.
- Have a sense of humor—laugh.
- Obtain professional help when needed.

After reading this chapter and especially the "Guidelines for Healthy Living," list three behaviors you could change to improve your health. What actions could you take to improve these behaviors? Write three specific measurable goals to achieve improved health. At the end of the semester, evaluate your achievement.

CASE STUDY

At a geriatric clinic in a low-income inner-city neighborhood, the nurse is providing care to an 80-year-old African American woman. She is diagnosed with hypertension, adult-onset diabetes, and congestive heart failure. She is obese with a BMI of 31 and is consistently noncompliant with her 1,800-calorie, carbohydrate-controlled diet. On this visit, her primary concerns are increased pedal edema and elevated blood sugar levels. Her vital signs are T-98.6 P-112 R-28 BP-163/96.

1. List some questions you would ask the client to assess how her lifestyle behaviors are affecting her health status.
2. List some primary, secondary, and tertiary preventive interventions the nurse would recommend for this client.

SUMMARY

- Wellness encompasses prevention, early detection, and treatment of health problems.
- The best way to maintain health is to follow the Dietary Guidelines for Americans, reduce stress, exercise regularly, prevent accidents, and receive routine health exams.
- Lifestyle changes can significantly reduce the leading causes of death.
- Physical, emotional, mental, social, and spiritual aspects all play key roles in the ability to resist disease and maintain health and wellness.

REVIEW QUESTIONS

1. Health maintenance and disease prevention are the responsibility of the:
   1. nurse.
   2. physician.
   3. individual.
   4. nurse practitioner.
2. Primary prevention:
   1. is the nurse's job.
   2. is curing a disease in 5 days.
   3. occurs before a disease begins.
   4. includes all diseases or conditions.
3. Health can be improved by:
   1. not smoking.
   2. drinking alcohol.
   3. eating more pasta.
   4. sleeping 4 to 5 hours each night.
4. The nurse is aware that a genogram is used for:
   1. identifying a family tree.
   2. identifying potential health problems.
   3. preventing most diseases and illnesses.
   4. acknowledging the genes a person inherits.
5. Clients should be made aware that colds and flu can best be prevented by:
   1. smoking.
   2. staying warm and dry.
   3. washing hands frequently.
   4. having a flu shot every three years.
6. A nurse working in a primary care clinic in an inner-city hospital is providing health promotion teaching to a 56-year-old woman. The patient has been diagnosed with hypertension for 10 years and is currently taking antihypertensive medications. She is overweight and noncompliant with dietary teaching. Which of the following statements indicate that the nurse is providing teaching at the secondary level of prevention?
   1. "Losing 20 pounds will bring you to your ideal weight."
   2. "You should have blood work drawn to screen for elevated cholesterol levels."
   3. "If you don't make some lifestyle changes, you may have a heart attack or stroke."
   4. "Exercise will decrease your risk of heart disease."
7. The overall goal of *Healthy People 2010* is:
   1. identifying health disparities.
   2. predicting the health status of the country in 2010.
   3. identifying unhealthy lifestyle practices.
   4. increasing quality and years of healthy life.
8. As B.D. is riding his bike around the community, he speaks to several neighbors and stops to help an elderly woman carry a large box into her home. He is a member of the Lions Club and has good interactive relationships at work. B.D. is exhibiting:
   1. emotional wellness.
   2. mental wellness.
   3. physical wellness.
   4. social wellness.
9. A client fell on the ice and suffered a strained muscle and pulled tendons. To prevent an imbalanced gait and further damage to the musculoskeletal system, the client went to physical therapy three times a week for 6 weeks to mend and strengthen the injured muscle and tendons. The client is practicing:
   1. primary prevention.
   2. secondary prevention.
   3. tertiary prevention.
   4. control of risk factor.

10. What statements describe *Health People 2010*? (Select all that apply.)
1. The basis of *Healthy People 2010* is healthy individuals make a healthy larger community and finally a nation.
2. *Healthy People 2010* is a grassroots organization that mandates healthy behavior of all in the community.
3. *Healthy People 2010* identified leading health indicators that are major health issues in the United States.
4. *Healthy People 2010* singles out groups with poor health and pays them to try activities to improve their health.
5. *Healthy People 2010* is a nationalized health care plan that goes into effect in 2010.
6. *Healthy People 2010* attempts to eliminate health inequalities within the nation.

REFERENCES/SUGGESTED READINGS

Alzheimer's Association. (2008). Risk factors. Retrieved April 21, 2009, from http://www.alz.org/alzheimers_disease_causes_risk_factors.asp

Baughcum, A. (1998). Mom's beliefs may cause child obesity. *Archives of Pediatric and Adolescent Medicine, 152,* 1010–1014.

Browder, S. (1998). Attention, women over 50. Available: http://www.seniornews.com/new-choices/article593.html

Carethers, M. (1992). Health promotion in the elderly. *American Family Physician, 45*(5), 2253–2260.

Centers for Disease Control and Prevention. (2005). Breast cancer screening and socioeconomic status—35 metropolitan areas, 2000 and 2002. *Morbidity and Mortality Weekly Report, 54*(39), 981–985. Retrieved on October 22, 2008, from http://www.cdc.gov/mmwr/preview/mmwrhtml/mm5439a2.htm

Centers for Disease Control and Prevention. (2006). Falls among older adults: An overview. Retrieved December 19, 2006, from http://www.cdc.gov/ncipc/factsheets/adultfalls.htm

Cerrato, P. (1999). A radical approach to heart disease. *RN, 62*(4), 65–66.

Chopra, D., & Simon, D. (2001). *Grow younger, live longer.* New York: Harmony Books.

CNN. (2008a). U.S. life expectancy still trails 30 countries. Retrieved October 21, 2008, from http://cnn.site.printthis.clickability.com/pt/cpt?action=cpt&title=U.S.+life+expectancy+st

CNN. (2008b). WHO slams global health care, calls for universal coverage. Retrieved October 21, 2008, from http://cnn.site.printthis.clickability.com/pt/cpt?action=cpt&title=WHO+slams+global+he

Cohen, L., Davis, R., & Mikkelsen, L. (2000, March/April). Comprehensive prevention: Improving health outcomes through practice. *Minority Health Today.* Retrieved October 20, 2008, from http://preventioninstitute.org/minorityhealth.html

Edlin, G., Golanty, E., & McCormack-Brown, K. (1999). *Essentials for health and wellness.* Boston: Jones & Bartlett.

Floyd, P., Mimms, S., & Yelding-Howard, C. (1995). *Personal health: A multicultural approach.* Englewood, CO: Morton.

Hall, D. (2006). Religious attendance: More cost-effective than Lipitor? *Journal of the American Board of Family Medicine, 19,* 103–109.

Harris, G. (2008, October 16). Infant deaths drop in U.S., but rate is still high. *New York Times.* Retrieved October 20, 2008, from http://www.nytimes.com/2008/10/16/health/16infnat.html?_r=1&em=&oref+slogin&pag

Healthy People 2010. (2005). What is Healthy People 2010? Retrieved April 21, 2009, from http://www.healthypeopel.gov/About/hpfact.htm

Hoeger, W., & Hoeger, S. (2000). *Lifetime physical fitness and wellness* (5th ed.). Belmont, CA: Wadsworth.

Hoeger, W., Turner, L., & Hafen, B. (2001). *Wellness: Guidelines for a healthy lifestyle* (3rd ed.). Belmont, CA: Wadsworth.

Hoffman, E. (1996). *Our health, our lives.* New York: Pocket Books.

Hunt, R. (2008). *Introduction to Community-Based Nursing* (4th ed.). Philadelphia: Lippincott Williams & Wilkins.

Krarup, L. et al. (2008). Prestroke physical activity is associated with severity and long-term outcome from first ever stroke. *Neurology, 71*(17), 1313–1318.

Lee, I., & Paffenbarger, R. (1998). Exercise can cut stroke risk 50%. *Stroke, 29,* 2049–2054.

Lifeoptions. (2009). Risk factors for CKD. Retrieved April 21, 2009, from http://www.lifeoptions.org/kidneyinfo/ckdinfo.php?page=3

Lyon, B. (2000). Conquering stress. *Reflections on Nursing Leadership, 26*(1), 22–23, 43.

Malaty, H. (1998). Twin study: *H. pylori* tied to hygiene. *American Journal of Epidemiology, 148,* 793–797.

Marshall, V., & Altpeter, M. (2005) Cultivating social work leadership in health promotion and aging: Strategies for active aging interventions. *Health and Social Work, 30*(2), 135–145.

Matthews, K. (1998). Suppressed anger hard on women's hearts. *Psychosomatic Medicine, 60,* 633–638.

Maville, J., & Huerta, C. (2002). *Health promotion in nursing.* Clifton Park, NY: Delmar Cengage Learning.

McEwen, M. (2002) *Community-based nursing: An introduction* (2nd ed.). Philadelphia: W. B. Saunders.

Meyers, S. (2008). Anger and health—An update. Retrieved October 21, 2008, from http://www.extension.umn.edu/distribution/familydevelopment/components/7269ai.html

National Center for Health Statistics. (2001a). National vital statistics report, vol. 51, no. 5. Retrieved April 21, 2009, from http://www.cdc.gov/nchs/data/nvsr/nvsr51/nvsr51_05.pdf

National Center for Health Statistics. (2001b). National vital statistics report, vol. 57, no. 14. Retrieved April 21, 2009, from http://www.cdc.gov/nchs/products/nvsr.htm#vol57

Nettina, S. (2001) *The Lippincott manual of nursing practice.* Philadelphia: Lippincott.

Office of Disease Prevention and Health Promotion. (2006). Dietary guidelines for Americans 2005. Retrieved December 2, 2006, from http://www.odphp.osophs.dhhs.gov

Office of the Surgeon General. (2007). The health consequences of involuntary exposure to tobacco smoke: A report of the surgeon general, U.S. Department of Health and Human Services—6 major conclusions of the surgeon general report. Retrieved October 22, 2008, from http://www.surgeongeneral.gov/library/secondhandsmoke/factsheets/factsheet6.html

Oman, D., & Reed, D. (1998). Religious elderly tend to live longer. *American Journal of Public Health, 88,* 1469–1475.

Payne, W., & Hahn, D. (2000). *Understanding your health* (6th ed.). New York: McGraw-Hill.

Poliafico, F. (1999). Abstinence is not the only answer. *RN, 62*(1), 58–60.

Potter, P., & Perry, A. (2009). *Fundamentals of nursing* (7th ed.). St Louis, MO: Mosby.

Reed, D. (1998). Four factors predict "healthy aging." *American Journal of Public Health, 88*, 1463–1469.

Reichler, G., & Burke, N. (1999). *Active wellness: A personalized 10 step program for a healthy body, mind and spirit.* Richmond, VA: Time Life.

Resnick, B. (2001). Geriatric health promotion. *Topics in Advanced Practice Nursing eJournal.* Retrieved October 20, 2008, from http://www.medscape.com/viewarticle/408406

Seiger, L., Kanipe, D., Vanderpool, K., & Barnes, D. (2000). *Fitness and wellness strategies* (2nd ed.). New York: McGraw-Hill.

Simmerman, J. M., & Mauzy, C. (2001). Finally! Babies can get this vaccine. *RN, 64*(7), 28–32.

Simon, H. (1992). *Staying well.* Boston: Houghton Mifflin.

Smith, C., & Maurer, F. (1999). *Community health nursing: Theory and practice* (2nd ed.) Philadelphia: W. B. Saunders.

Smith, R. (in press). *Promoting health and wellness.*

Stibich, M. (2007). Religion might add years to your life. Retrieved October 21, 2008 from http://longevity.about.com/od/longevityboosters/a/religion_life.htm?p=1

U.S. Department of Agriculture, U.S. Department of Health and Human Services. (2000). *Home and Garden Bulletin No. 232* (5th ed.).

U.S. Department of Health and Human Services. (1990). *Healthy People 2000: National health promotion and disease prevention objectives* (DHHS Publication No. [PHS] 91-50212). Washington, DC: Author.

U.S. Department of Health and Human Services, Public Health Service. (1998). Healthy People 2000: National health promotion and disease prevention objectives and first draft Healthy People 2010: National health promotion and disease prevention objectives. Available: http://web.health.gov/healthypeople

U.S. Department of Health and Human Services, Public Health Service. (2000a). Healthy People 2010: National health promotion and disease prevention objectives. Available: http://web.health.gov/healthypeople

U.S. Department of Health and Human Services, Public Health Service. (2000b). *1998–1999 progress review.* Available: http://odphp.osophs.dhhs.gov/pubs/hp2000

Wash your hands (to help prevent colds). (1996, January). *Consumer Reports on Health, 2*(1).

Weil, A. (1998). *Natural health, natural medicine* (2nd ed.). Boston: Houghton Mifflin.

Weil, A. (2001). *Eating well for optimum health: The essential guide to bringing health and pleasure back to eating.* Camperdown, New South Wales, Australia: Quill.

Weil, A., & Daley, R. (2002). *The healthy kitchen: Recipes for a better body, life and spirit.* Westminster, MD: Knopf.

RESOURCES

Aerobics and Fitness Association of America, http://www.afaa.com

American Dietetic Association, http://www.eatright.org

American Health Care Association, http://www.ahcancal.org

American Heart Association, http://www.ahs.org

American Holistic Nurses' Association, http://www.ahna.org

Center for Science in the Public Interest, http://www.cspinet.org

Centers for Disease Control and Prevention, http://www.cdc.gov

Environmental Protection Agency, http://www.epa.gov

Food and Drug Administration, http://www.fda.gov

Food and Nutrition Information Center, http://www.nal.usda.gov

Healthy People 2010, http://www.cdc.gov/nchs/hphome.htm

Medic Alert Foundation International, http://www.medicalert.org

National Highway Traffic Safety Administration, http://www.nhtsa.dot.gov

National Institute for Occupational Safety and Health, http://www.cdc.gov/niosh

National Institute on Aging, http://www.nih.nia.gov

National Institutes of Health, http://www.nih.gov

National Safety Council, http://www.nsc.org

National Wellness Institute, http://www.nationalwellness.org

National Women's Health Network, http://www.nwhn.org

U. S. Consumer Product Safety Commission, http://www.cpsc.gov

U.S. Department of Agriculture, http://www.usda.gov

U.S. Department of Health and Human Services, http://www.hhs.gov

World Health Organization, http://www.who.int

CHAPTER 15
Self-Concept

MAKING THE CONNECTION

Refer to the following chapters to increase your understanding of self-concept:

Basic Nursing

- ***Communication***
- ***Life Span Development***
- ***Stress, Adaptation, and Anxiety***
- ***End-of-Life Care***
- ***Spirituality***
- ***Complementary/Alternative Therapies***

LEARNING OBJECTIVES

Upon completion of this chapter, you should be able to:

- Define key terms.
- Discuss the development of self-concept throughout the life span.
- Describe four major components of self-concept.
- Identify factors affecting self-concept.
- Delineate nursing interventions that promote self-concept.

KEY TERMS

body image
empowerment
ideal self
identity
public self
real self
role
role performance
self-awareness
self-concept
self-esteem

SELF-CONCEPT

Self-concept is the way people think about themselves. It is unique, dynamic, and always evolving. This mental image of oneself influences a person's identity, self-esteem, body image, and role in society. As a global understanding of oneself, self-concept shapes and defines who we are, the decisions we make, and the relationships we form (Figure 15-1). Self-concept is perhaps the basis for all motivated behavior (Franken, 1994).

COMPONENTS OF SELF-CONCEPT

Self-concept is an individual's perception of self, including self-esteem, body image, and ideal self. A person's self-concept is often defined by self-description such as "I am a mother, a nurse, and a volunteer." Client self-descriptive statements such as these help the nurse gain insight into the client's perception of self. The nurse should be observant for self-descriptive statements when assessing the client's self-concept. A healthy self-concept is necessary for overall physical and mental wellness.

Three basic components of self-concept are the ideal self, the public self, and the real self (Figure 15-2). The **ideal self** is the person the client would like to be, such as a good, moral, and well-respected person. Sometimes, this ideal view of how a client would like to be conflicts with the **real self** (how the client really thinks about oneself, such as "I try to be good and do what's right, but I'm not well respected"). This conflict can motivate a client to make changes toward becoming the ideal self. However, the view of the ideal self needs to be realistic and obtainable, or the client may experience anxiety or be at risk for alterations in self-concept. **Public self** is what the client thinks others think of him and influences the ideal and real self. Positive self-concept and good mental health results when all three components are compatible.

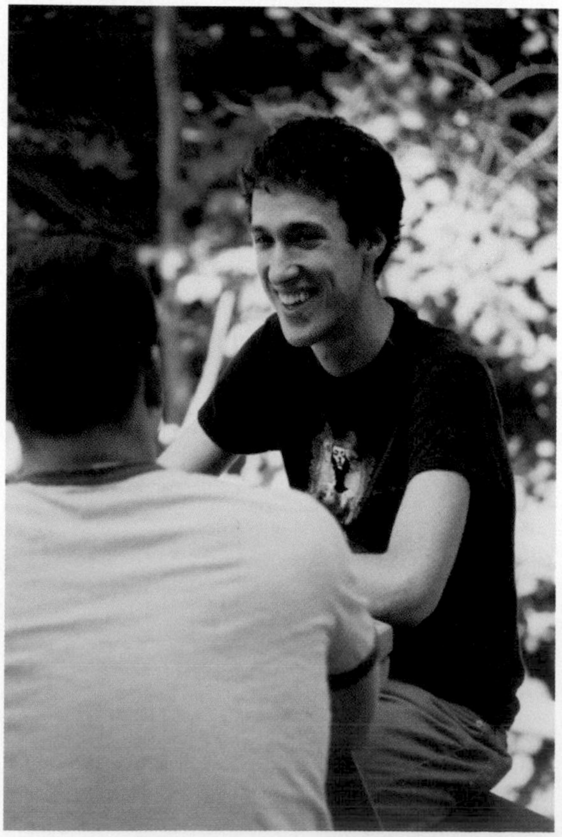
COURTESY OF DELMAR CENGAGE LEARNING

FIGURE 15-1 A positive self-concept enhances healthy relationships.

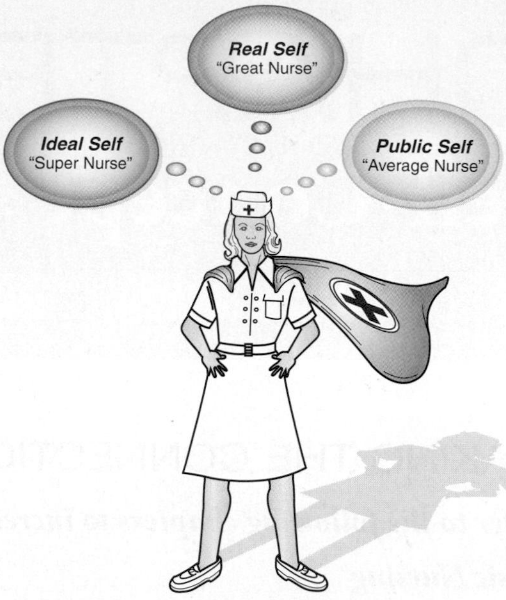

COURTESY OF DELMAR CENGAGE LEARNING

FIGURE 15-2 Example of how a nurse may view her ideal self, real self, and public self.

A positive self-concept is an important part of a client's happiness and success. Individuals with a positive self-concept have self-confidence and set goals they can achieve. Achieving their goals reinforces their positive self-concept. A client with a positive self-concept is more likely to change unhealthy habits (such as sedentary lifestyle and smoking) to promote health than a client with a negative self-concept.

A person's self-concept is composed of evolving subjective conscious and unconscious self-assessments. Physical attributes, occupation, knowledge, and abilities of the person will change throughout the life span, contributing to changes in one's self-concept. Memory Trick 15-1 lists nursing interventions to promote positive self-concept.

PROFESSIONALTIP

Characteristics of a Positive Self-Concept

Characteristics of a client with a positive self-concept include:

- Self-confidence
- Ability to accept criticism and not become defensive
- Setting obtainable goals
- Willingness to take risks and try new experiences

MEMORY TRICK

I LIKE ME

The memory trick "**I LIKE ME**" lists nursing interventions to promote a positive self-concept in clients:

- **I** = Identify client's strengths.
- **L** = Listen to the client's self-description.
- **I** = Involve the client in decision making.
- **K** = Keep goals realistic.
- **E** = Encourage client to think positively.
- **M** = Maintain an environment conducive to client self-expression.
- **E** = Explain to the client how to use positive self-talk instead of negative self-talk.

CLIENT TEACHING

Positive Self-Talk

Positive self-talk can be used to change negative inner messages to positive ones.

1. Send yourself positive thoughts.
2. Say the positive thoughts out loud.
3. Remind yourself of your positive attributes and accomplishments.
4. Recall memories of success.
5. Tell yourself out loud something new that you learned or something good that you did today.

PROFESSIONAL TIP

Emotional Intelligence

Emotional intelligence (EI) refers to the ability to perceive, understand, control/manage, and evaluate emotions. A number of quizzes and testing instruments have been developed to measure EI. To take a fun and quick quiz to learn more about your emotional intelligence, go to http://psychology.about.com and search for Emotional Intelligence Test.

IDENTITY

Identity is an individual's conscious description of who he is. A client's identity is assessed by asking the person to describe oneself. This description of oneself provides the nurse with insight into whether the client is comfortable with one's identity. A client who uses positive self-descriptions will exhibit a healthy self-identity.

An individual's identity is developed over time, constantly evolving, and influenced by self-awareness. **Self-awareness** involves consciously knowing how the self thinks, feels, believes, and behaves at any specific time (Figure 15-3). According to Burkhardt and Nathaniel (2008), we can enhance self-awareness by developing the ability to step back and look at any situation while being aware of ourselves and how we are reacting to the situation. A client needs to be able to identify one's personal and emotional feelings of a situation without judging oneself.

BODY IMAGE

An individual's perception of physical self, including appearance, function, and ability, is known as one's **body image**. Normal growth and developmental changes may influence and alter body image, such as the physical and hormonal changes that occur during puberty and adolescence. The onset of puberty involves the emergence of secondary sex characteristics in the female and male client. While these are normal expected physical changes that occur during the adolescent stage, these changes will impact an adolescent's body image, thus affecting self-concept.

In later adulthood, physical and hormonal changes present as thinning and graying of hair, wrinkling and loss of skin elasticity, weight gain, decrease in hearing and vision, and decrease in mobility. While some adults accept these changes as the normal process of aging, others may find themselves resisting or feeling negatively about them. These changes will naturally cause the adult to reevaluate the image they have of their body and how they feel about it. A person's body image will continue to change throughout the growth and developmental life span stages.

Health-related factors that may affect body image include stroke, spinal cord injury, amputation, mastectomy, burns, surgical and/or procedural scarring, and loss of a body part or function. Other common physical changes that affect body image involve the development of acne and weight gain and/or loss. According to the Centers for Disease Control and Prevention (CDC, 2007), approximately 66% of American adults are overweight or obese. These physical issues may add stress and anxiety on the client, lowering their self-esteem and self-confidence.

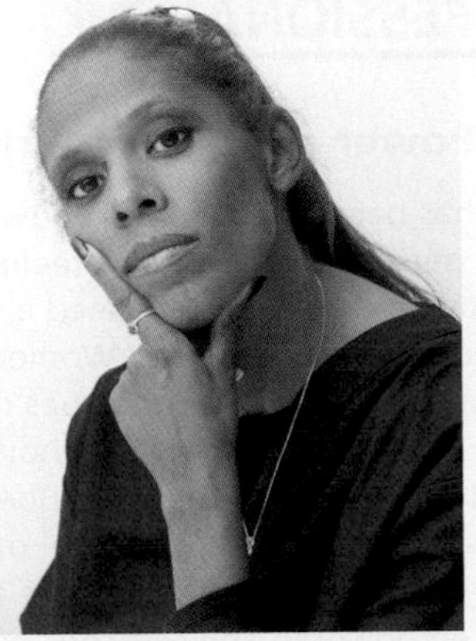

COURTESY OF DELMAR CENGAGE LEARNING

FIGURE 15-3 Self-awareness involves reflecting on feelings, thoughts, and reactions to situations.

CRITICAL THINKING

Body Image versus Self-Esteem

What are the differences between body image and self-esteem? How do they affect each other?

SELF-ESTEEM

Self-esteem is a personal opinion of oneself and is shaped by individuals' relationships with others, experiences, and accomplishments in life. A healthy self-esteem is necessary for mental well-being and a positive self-concept. This is achieved by setting attainable goals and successfully accomplishing the goals, resulting in an increase in self-confidence, assertiveness, and feeling valued. Since self-esteem impacts all aspects of life, it is important to establish a healthy, realistic view of oneself (Mayo Clinic, 2009).

Individuals with low self-esteem put little value on themselves and their accomplishments. They feel that they are not good enough and that they are worth less than others and often feel ashamed of themselves. They engage in negative self-talk, frequently apologize, and seek constant reassurance. Often this type of person is a perfectionist who struggles with failure.

One method of improving an individual's low self-esteem is for the nurse to empower the client. Burkhardt and Nathaniel (2008) define **empowerment** as "a helping process and partnership, enacted in the context of love and respect for self and others, through which individuals and groups are enabled to change situations, and are given skills, resources, opportunities, and authority to do so" (p. 542). Chamberlin (2008) recognized that empowerment has elements in common with concepts of self-esteem and self-efficacy. As a client becomes more empowered, one will feel more confident in one's ability to manage one's life, resulting in improved self-esteem and self-image. Box 15-1 lists the elements of empowerment that nurses may teach clients to use to increase their self-esteem.

Research and assessment has been conducted on self-esteem for several decades. The Rosenberg Self-Esteem Scale was originally developed to assess self-esteem among adolescents (Rosenberg, 1965). This self-report consists of statements related to feelings of self-worth or self-acceptance to measure global self-esteem. The scale has been validated to be used with male and female adolescents, adults, and elderly populations and remains in use today.

PROFESSIONALTIP

Healing Power of Journal Writing

Journaling has been found to be a powerful way to bridge a person's thoughts and feelings. Merrill Devito at Stanford University formed a support group of women titled "Hungry Women Writing" to assist women struggling with issues of food, confidence, and self-image to learn how to use journal writing to explore their attitudes toward their bodies (Hanson, 2004). The goal of each participant is to overcome his negative thoughts and to feel empowered and self-confident about himself and his body image.

CRITICAL THINKING

Feelings of Empowerment

1. Consider a situation in which you felt empowered. List and describe factors that contributed to your feelings of empowerment.
2. Reflect on a situation in which you felt disempowered. What would have helped you feel more empowered?

ROLE

We experience many roles in our lifetime. As we pass from birth to death, we will become a child, teenager, friend, worker, and perhaps spouse or parent. Many of our roles are defined by our success, education, relationships, and career. An individual's **role** is defined as an ascribed or assumed expected behavior in a social position or group. Specific behaviors that a person exhibits within each role make up **role performance.**

Illness, injury, and aging can lead to alterations in a person's role. Additional alterations may include pregnancy, loss of a job, retirement, or death of a significant other. How the individual views these changes or losses will determine the impact on one's self-concept. Individuals who view these alterations negatively are at risk for ineffective role performance and a decreased self-concept.

DEVELOPMENT OF SELF-CONCEPT

Various psychosocial theories have been developed to explain the development of self-concept. A discussion of Erikson's

BOX 15-1 ELEMENTS OF EMPOWERMENT

A client's self-esteem will increase when using the following elements:

- Having decision-making power
- Having access to information and resources
- Having a range of options from which to make choices
- Using assertiveness skills
- Feeling that oneself can make a difference
- Feeling part of a group, not alone
- Effecting change in one's life and one's community
- Learning skills that the individual defines as important
- Self-initiated growth and change
- Increasing one's positive self-image

From A Working Definition of Empowerment. By J. Chamberlin, 2008. Retrieved February 1, 2009, from http://www.power2u.org/articles/empower/working_def.html

CLIENTTEACHING

Activities That Increase Self-Esteem

The following are activities that the nurse can teach the client to engage in to increase one's self-esteem:

- Taking good care of self
- Taking time to do enjoyable activities
- Journaling
- Getting something done that has been put off
- Spending time with people that make you feel good about yourself
- Learning something new
- Forgiving yourself
- Doing something nice for someone else
- Positive self-talk
- Giving yourself rewards

theory of psychosocial development related to self-concept follows.

Erikson's Theory

Erikson's (1963) psychosocial theory states that an individual's development proceeds throughout life. Each of his eight developmental stages includes psychosocial tasks that need to be mastered (see Chapter 10, "Life Span Development").

Newborn and Infant

At birth, the newborn does not differentiate itself from the parents. As the parents begin to care for the newborn, their feelings and attitudes toward the newborn will begin to develop the baby's self-concept. The parents will experience a change in their own self-concept. Parental roles are being established, body images are formed in the mother before and after giving birth, and emotional changes will affect the parents' self-concept.

The nurse will need to teach the family about the infant's emotional needs in developing a trusting relationship to promote the infant's feelings of security and trust in the parents. A sense of security and trust is especially important for the infant if it becomes ill and is hospitalized. Parents need to be encouraged to spend as much time as possible with the infant and provide routine care and developmental interventions for the infant to facilitate the continued healthy development of self-concept.

Toddler and Preschooler

The toddler needs a supportive environment for body image and self-esteem to develop positively. The parents should provide the toddler with an environment to practice his newly learned skills. The toddler needs to be encouraged to try his skills again (such as learning to walk or potty training) if not successful at first. Praising the toddler for mastery of learning his new skill is important in developing a positive self-concept.

Preschoolers begin to exhibit a sense of sexual curiosity. As they hear the names and functions of their body parts, they may ask a lot of questions. How the parents answer a preschooler's questions may have an impact on his self-concept and body image. As preschoolers develop their self-concept, they will often imitate parents and siblings.

School Age and Adolescence

The school experience has a major impact on a child's development of self-concept, identity, body image, self-esteem, and role. Parents, teachers, and peers have a direct influence on the child's developing feelings, views, and sense of self. Children compare their physical appearance, academic and athletic abilities, and social status to those of their peers and seek approval and acceptance from this group. Bullying by verbal, emotional, or technological methods (e-mail, chatting, blogging, texting, or twittering) is common in this age group and negatively affects a child's developing self-concept. The school-age child places importance on receiving acceptance and approval by one's peer group to feel included and positive about oneself.

Adolescence marks numerous physical and hormonal changes, including in the female the onset of menses, pubic and axillary hair growth, breast development, and an increase in height, and in the male a slow, progressive deepening of the voice; pubic, axillary, and chest hair growth; enlargement of the testicles and penis; and thinning and reddening of the scrotum. The development of acne and body odor will also occur at this age. These changes influence the adolescent's view of one's body and oneself. Adolescents look to their peers, parents, role models, and the media to view what is expected of them (Figure 15-4).

Many adolescents are experiencing issues with the image of their body weight, shape, size, hair, acne, or height. Negative

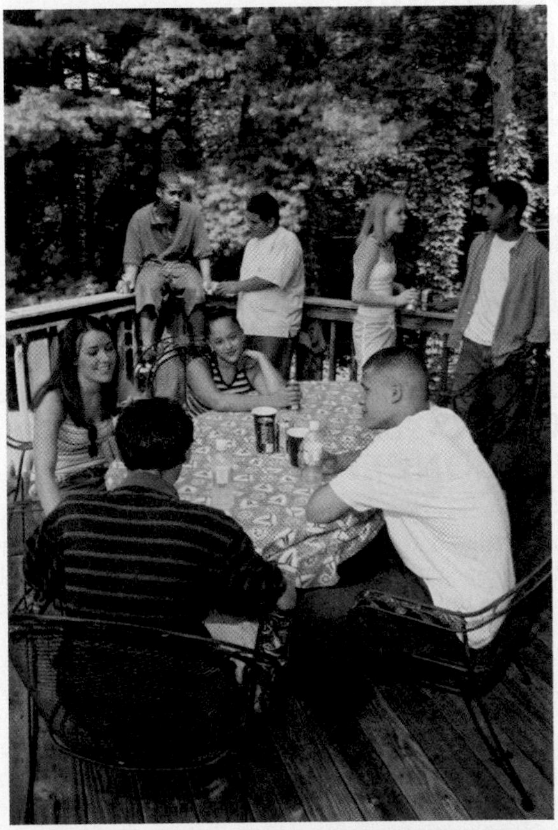

COURTESY OF DELMAR CENGAGE LEARNING

FIGURE 15-4 Peer relationships are important during adolescence.

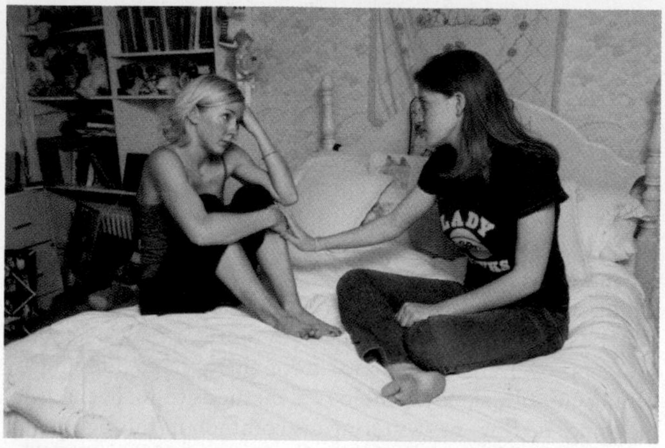

COURTESY OF DELMAR CENGAGE LEARNING

FIGURE 15-5 Support from friends promotes a healthy self-concept during adolescence.

comments and reactions from their peers can cause them to participate in substance abuse, inappropriate sexual behavior, and eating disorders as an attempt to fit in. Adolescents struggling with how to deal with anxiety and depression due to these expectations may use self-injury (self-mutilation) as a method of coping or even attempt suicide.

The development of a healthy self-concept for the adolescent often lies in parental involvement and support. As the adolescent becomes more independent, the parents may need to adapt and change their parenting style. While adolescents may begin to attain more independence, they still require the love, support, and involvement of their family and friends (Figure 15-5).

ADULTHOOD

The natural process of aging will lead to significant changes in a person's self-concept. Over the course of a lifetime, an adult will experience changes in one's roles, body, and identity. Young adults strive to develop relationships, careers, and often a family. Older adults attempt to define themselves by their accomplishments. Major life events in adulthood will continuously shape a person's self-concept, such as obtaining a college degree, getting a job, marriage, divorce, losing a job, retirement, and the death of a significant other. How the individual views and copes with these changes will determine the influence and impact they have on the person's self-concept.

FACTORS AFFECTING SELF-CONCEPT

Self-concept can be affected by an individual's life experiences, heredity and culture, stress and coping, health status, and developmental stage. The nurse needs to evaluate each of these factors and the influence each has on the client's achievement of a healthy self-concept (Figure 15-6).

LIFE EXPERIENCES

Life experiences, including success and failure, will develop and influence a person's self-concept. Experiences in which the individual has accomplished a goal and achieved success will positively reinforce the development of a healthy self-concept. Difficult experiences and/or failures can negatively impact a person's self-concept unless they have established coping strategies to deal effectively with these challenges to their self-concept. Coping strategies are learned as a person encounters and deals with various situations in life.

SAFETY

A mental health professional needs to be consulted immediately when self-injury, suicide, or eating disorders are suspected or committed.

Self-injury: Self-injury involves intentional self-inflicted tissue damage, such as cutting, burning, skin picking, or pulling one's hair out. This disorder occurs in either sex and in any religion or race and is not limited by education, age, or social status. Statistics are difficult to obtain because of the secretive nature of this disorder (Cleveland Clinic, 2005). Search online at http://www.clevelandclinic.org for more information.

Suicide: Suicide is the third-leading cause of death in clients aged 10 to 24. Boys, Native Americans/Alaskan Natives, and Hispanic youth have the highest rates of suicide. Approximately 32,000 suicides (one every 16 minutes) are committed in the United States each year (CDC, 2008b). Search online at http://www.cdc.gov for more information.

Eating disorders: Anorexia nervosa, bulimia, and binge eating are the three most common eating disorders. Anorexia nervosa and bulimia can lead to life-threatening conditions, resulting in permanent damage to major organs of the body. Statistics are difficult to obtain because of the secretive nature of these disorders (CDC, 2009). Search online at http://www.cdc.gov for more information.

HEREDITY AND CULTURE

Individuals typically grow up learning and integrating their family's heredity and culture into their life. Beginning at birth, heredity and culture shape and influence a person's self-concept. Individuals who have integrated their heredity and culture into their life tend to have a healthier self-identity and self-concept (Figure 15-7).

STRESS AND COPING

Everyone experiences stress at some level each day. Common stressors include financial, work-related, relationship, and health issues. Individuals react and deal with stress in different ways depending on their past experiences and success and failure with dealing with stress. Individuals who learn and use effective coping strategies to deal with stress will most likely develop a positive self-concept. People who become overwhelmed with stress may feel hopeless and powerless, leading to a feeling of low self-confidence and self-esteem (Figure 15-8). The nurse may need to teach the client effective coping strategies and techniques for handling stress.

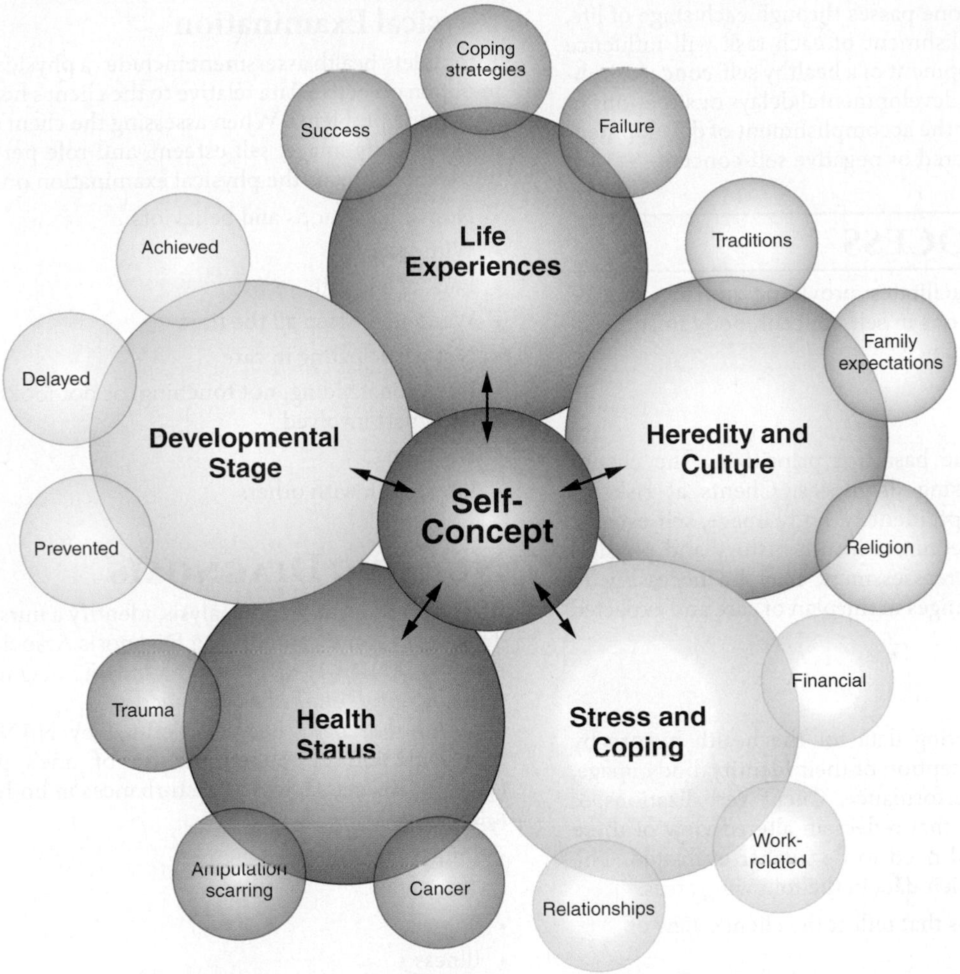

COURTESY OF DELMAR CENGAGE LEARNING

FIGURE 15-6 Concept Map Depicting Factors That Affect Self-Concept

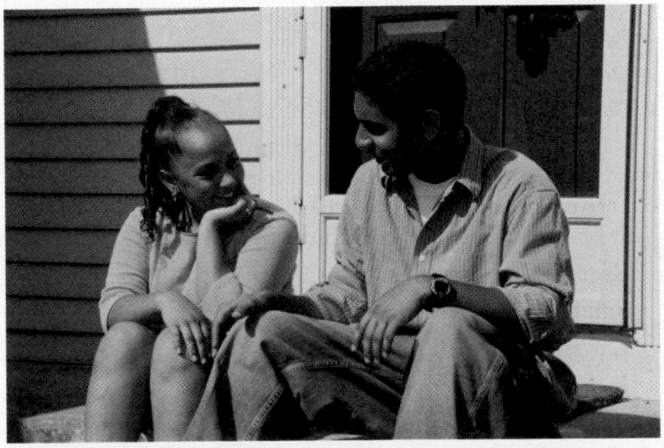

COURTESY OF DELMAR CENGAGE LEARNING

FIGURE 15-7 Self-concept is influenced by an individual's heredity and culture.

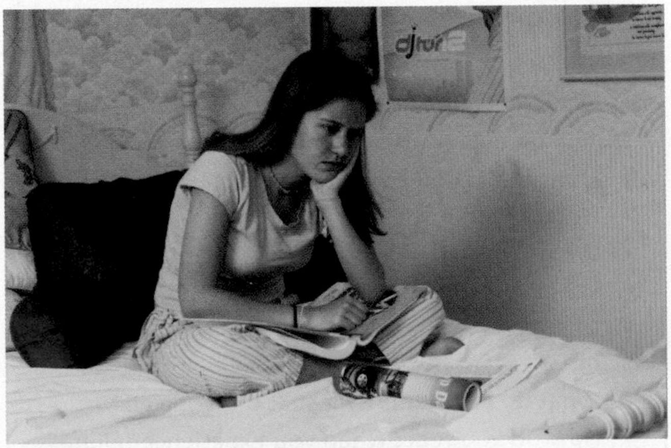

COURTESY OF DELMAR CENGAGE LEARNING

FIGURE 15-8 Ineffective coping and stress may lead to feelings of low self-confidence and self-esteem.

HEALTH STATUS

People tend to take their good health for granted. When they become ill, their altered health status can change their self-identity and self-concept. Alterations in body image can result from such health issues as amputation, cancer, mastectomy, trauma, or scarring. The nurse needs to monitor for changes in the client's self-concept due to alterations in their health status.

DEVELOPMENTAL STAGE

Growth and development begins at birth and continues into adulthood. Typically a person will achieve specific developmental tasks as one passes through each stage of life. The successful accomplishment of each task will influence and reinforce the development of a healthy self-concept. Individuals who experience developmental delays or situations in life that prevent or delay the accomplishment of developmental tasks can have an altered or negative self-concept.

NURSING PROCESS

The nursing process facilitates providing nursing care to clients at risk for alterations in self-concept, body image, self-esteem, and role performance.

ASSESSMENT

Assessment data are the basis for prioritizing the client's problems and the nursing diagnoses. Clients at risk for alterations in self-concept, identity, body image, self-esteem, and role performance require a health history and physical examination. Frequent reassessment may be necessary to facilitate appropriate changes in the plan of care and expected outcomes.

Health History

The nurse begins gathering data for the health history by assessing the client's perception of their identity, body image, self-esteem, and role performance. Client verbalizations of feelings and perceptions that reflect an altered view of these areas of self-concept will need to be further evaluated. The nursing history should elicit data in the following areas:

- Feelings or perceptions that reflect the client's view of oneself
- Client report of any changes in body image, self-esteem, or role
- Feelings of powerlessness and/or hopelessness related to any of these changes

BOX 15-2 QUESTIONS TO USE IN OBTAINING A HEALTH HISTORY

Obtaining a Client History of Self-Concept

- How would you describe yourself?
- How do others describe you?
- What has been your greatest accomplishment?
- How does this make you feel?
- When you receive praise, do you feel worthy of it?
- What do you admire most about yourself?
- How do you react when you experience failure?
- How do you cope with failure?
- Have you experienced past or recent changes in body image, self-esteem, or role performance?
- Have you experienced feelings of powerlessness or hopelessness?
- Who do you consider your support group?
- What do you do to make yourself laugh or feel good about yourself?

Physical Examination

A complete health assessment includes a physical examination to obtain objective data relative to the client's health status and presenting problems. When assessing the client's self-concept, identity, body image, self-esteem, and role performance, the nurse should focus the physical examination on:

- Nonverbal actions and behaviors
- Withdrawal
- Lack of appetite
- Wanting to sleep all the time
- Not participating in care
- Intentional hiding, not touching, or not looking at the body part involved
- Isolation
- Interaction with others

NURSING DIAGNOSIS

After data collection and analysis, identify a nursing diagnosis. The North American Nursing Diagnosis Association International (NANDA-I) identifies the nursing diagnosis related to self-concept: *Disturbed **B**ody Image.*

*Disturbed **B**ody Image* is defined by NANDA-I (2010) as "Confusion in mental picture of one's physical self" (p. 197). Related factors to disturbances in body image are as follows:

- Injury
- Trauma
- Surgery
- Illness
- Illness treatment
- Perceptual
- Cognitive
- Spiritual
- Cultural
- Psychosocial
- Developmental changes
- Biophysical

Clients who are at risk for disturbances in body image may have other associated physiological and psychological concerns. The common nursing diagnoses that often accompany *Disturbed **B**ody Image* include:

*Readiness for Enhanced **S**elf-Concept*
*Situational Low **S**elf-Esteem*
*Chronic Low **S**elf-Esteem*
*Ineffective **R**ole Performance*
*Social **I**solation*
***P**owerlessness*
***H**opelessness*
*Disturbed Personal **I**dentity*
*Risk for Compromised Human **D**ignity*
*Risk for **L**oneliness*
*Readiness for Enhanced **P**ower*

The list identifies related diagnoses for alterations in self-esteem and role performance that must be considered when planning care for a client at risk for alterations in self-concept.

PLANNING/OUTCOME IDENTIFICATION

Holistic nursing care requires collaborating with each client to identify goals for each nursing diagnosis. Planning and outcome identification for the client focuses on promoting a healthy self-concept or facilitating change in an altered self-concept. These individualized goals should reflect the client's abilities and limitations.

Nursing interventions are selected and prioritized to support the client's achievement of expected outcomes based on the goals. For example, if the client states that she considers herself overweight, unattractive, and undesirable to others, this leads to a nursing diagnosis of *Disturbed Body Image*, and the goals might include expressing positive feelings about herself and integrating a realistic body image.

IMPLEMENTATION

Several interventions can promote a positive healthy self-concept in clients; they are as follows:

- Encourage client to list past and current accomplishments
- Ask client to describe how they and others would describe them
- Assess the client's report of changes in their self-concept, body image, self-esteem, or role performance
- Encourage verbalization of the positive and negative feelings and perceptions of the changes that have occurred to their self-concept, body image, self-esteem, or role
- Acknowledge normalcy of changes in the emotional response and grieving stages to changes
- Assist client in incorporating the necessary changes into their daily life
- Assist the client in identifying methods of coping that have been useful in the past
- Assist client in contacting appropriate support groups and/or counseling as needed

EVALUATION

Evaluation of the effectiveness of nursing care is based on the achievement of goals and expected outcomes. The plan of care must be updated on a regular basis with additional interventions used as needed.

SAMPLE NURSING CARE PLAN

The Client with Alterations in Self-Concept

T.H., a 38-year-old male, had surgery for placement of a cardiac pacemaker. Two days postoperatively, T.H. refused to participate in his care and appeared quiet and withdrawn. When the nurse asked T.H. if he would like to talk about it, he replied, "I don't want to look at it or touch it. I will never be able to take my shirt off in the summer again. Why did the scar have to be so big?"

NURSING DIAGNOSIS *Disturbed Body Image* related to scarring from surgical pacemaker placement

Nursing Outcomes Classification (NOC)
Body Image
Self-Esteem

Nursing Interventions Classification (NIC)
Body Image Enhancement
Grief Work Facilitation
Coping Enhancement

PLANNING/OUTCOMES	NURSING INTERVENTIONS	RATIONALE
T.H. will be able to look at, touch, and talk about the surgical scar on his chest where the cardiac pacemaker was inserted.	Encourage T.H. to verbalize his feelings and perceptions regarding the scar on his chest.	Verbalizing feelings and perceptions may help T.H. express and identify his concerns.
	Assist T.H. to identify effective coping strategies.	Identifying coping strategies may assist T.H. to deal effectively with his body image issues.
	Acknowledge T.H.'s emotional response to the changes in the appearance of his chest.	Acknowledging a client's emotional response promotes trust and is validating their feelings and thoughts.
	Provide empathy and support to T.H.	Providing empathy and support are necessary to facilitate a positive nurse–client helping relationship.

EVALUATION

T.H. states that he does not like the scar on his chest, but he can live with it. He has participated in his activities of daily living and washed and dried his chest during morning hygiene care.

SUMMARY

- A positive self-concept is important in achieving happiness, success, and a healthy self-identity.
- The four main components of self-concept are identity, body image, self-esteem, and role performance.
- A variety of activities are available for the nurse to teach the client to promote a positive self-concept.
- Body image continuously changes throughout an individual's growth and developmental life stages.
- Self-esteem is shaped by relationships with others, experiences, and accomplishments in life.
- A variety of factors affecting self-concept include life experiences, heredity and culture, values and beliefs, stress and coping, health status, and developmental stage.

REVIEW QUESTIONS

1. A 16-year-old female client tells the nurse, "I am fat, ugly, and stupid." This statement best reflects the client's:
   1. ideal self.
   2. real self.
   3. public self.
   4. other self.
2. The nurse knows that a positive self-concept is an important part of a client's happiness and success. Individuals with a positive self-concept exhibit all of the following except:
   1. difficulty accepting criticism.
   2. setting goals they can achieve.
   3. changing unhealthy habits.
   4. self-confidence.
3. A 78-year-old male client presents with thinning and graying of hair, wrinkling and loss of skin elasticity, weight gain, decrease in hearing and vision, and a decrease in mobility. These data are describing which component of self-concept?
   1. Self-esteem.
   2. Body image.
   3. Role performance.
   4. Identity.
4. The nurse knows that activities to promote and enhance a client's self-esteem include: (Select all that apply.)
   1. empowering the client.
   2. encouraging negative self-talk.
   3. providing support and counseling as needed.
   4. using passive skills.
   5. including the client in decision making.
   6. proving information and resources as needed.
5. A 43-year-old male client tells the nurse, "In the last year, my wife has divorced me, my father passed away from cancer, and now last week I lost my job because of downsizing in the company. I really don't know who I am anymore." This statement best reflects a change in the client's:
   1. role.
   2. body image.
   3. self-esteem.
   4. self-awareness.
6. A 12-year-old female client experiencing the onset of menses, pubic and axillary hair growth, breast development, and an increase in height would be identified as being in which of Erikson's stages of development?
   1. Trust versus mistrust.
   2. Autonomy versus shame.
   3. Identity versus role confusion.
   4. Integrity versus despair.
7. A 65-year-old retired schoolteacher states that she is enjoying retirement by traveling and playing more with the grandchildren. According to Erikson's theory, she would be in the stage of:
   1. trust versus mistrust.
   2. autonomy versus shame.
   3. identity versus role confusion.
   4. integrity versus despair.
8. While the nurse is completing a physical exam on a 15-year-old male client, he notices unusual straight razorlike cuts on his forearm. On questioning, the client informs the nurse that he has been cutting himself for the past 6 months because of "unbearable stress" in his life. Which of the following nursing diagnoses is appropriate for the client?
   1. Hopelessness.
   2. Powerlessness.
   3. Disturbed personal identity.
   4. All of the above.
9. A 52-year-old female client has recently been diagnosed with breast cancer. The factor most likely to affect the client's self-concept is:
   1. her health status.
   2. her developmental stage.
   3. her culture.
   4. her ethnicity.
10. The nurse is obtaining a health history on self-concept for a 45-year-old male client who has recently lost his job. Which of the following questions is the most appropriate to ask the client when gathering data regarding self-concept?
    1. "When did you lose your job?"
    2. "Why did the company terminate your work position?"
    3. "How would you describe yourself?"
    4. "How many years did you work there?"

REFERENCES/SUGGESTED READINGS

Bulechek, G., Butcher, H., McCloskey, J., & Dochterman, J. (2008). *Nursing Interventions Classification (NIC)* (5th ed.). St. Louis, MO: Mosby/Elsevier.

Burkhardt, M., & Nathaniel, A. (2008). *Ethics and issues*. Clifton Park, NY: Delmar Cengage Learning.

Cappeliez, P. (2008). An explanation of the reminiscence bump in dreams of older adults in terms of life goals and identity. *Self and Identity, 7*(1), 25–33.

Centers for Disease Control and Prevention. (2005). Self-injury. Retrieved February 7, 2009, from http://www.clevelandclinic.org/disorders/self-injury/hic_self-injury.aspx

Centers for Disease Control and Prevention. (2007). Fastfacts a to z: Overweight. Retrieved February 1, 2009, from http://www.cdc.gov/nchs/fastats/overwt.htm

Centers for Disease Control and Prevention. (2008a). NCHS data on adolescent health. Retrieved February 7, 2009, from http://www.cdc.gov/nchs/data/infosheets/infosheet_adoleshealth.htm

Centers for Disease Control and Prevention. (2008b). Suicide prevention: youth suicide. Retrieved February 7, 2009, from http://www.cdc.gov/ncipc/dvp/suicide/youthsuicide.htm

Centers for Disease Control and Prevention. (2009). College health and safety. Retrieved February 7, 2009, from http://www.cdc.gov/family/college

Chamberlin, J. (2008). A working definition of empowerment. Retrieved February 1, 2009, from http://www.power2u.org/articles/empower/working_def.html

Classen, S., Velozo, C., & Mann, W. (2007). The Rosenberg self-esteem scale as a measure of self-esteem for the noninstitutionalized elderly. *Clinical Gerontologist, 31*(1), 77–93.

Daniels, R., Grendell, R., & Wilkins, F. (2010). *Nursing fundamentals: Caring and clinical decision making* (2nd ed.). Clifton Park, NY: Delmar Cengage Learning.

Delaune, S., & Ladner, P. (2006). *Fundamentals of nursing: Standards and practice* (3rd ed.). Clifton Park, NY: Delmar Cengage Learning.

Erikson, E. (1963). *Childhood and society* (2nd ed.). New York: W. W. Norton

Franken, R. (1994). *Human motivation* (3rd ed.). Pacific Grove, CA: Brooks/Cole.

Hanson, K. (2004). Battling the burden of body image: The healing power of journal writing. Retrieved February 2, 2009, from http://daily.stanford.edu/article/2004/11/17/battlingTheBurdenOfBodyImageTheHealingPowerOfJournalWriting

Hermann, A., & Lucas, G. (2008). Individual differences in perceived esteem across cultures. *Self and Identity, 7*(2), 151–167.

Koch, E., & Shepperd, J. (2008). Testing competence and acceptance explanations of self-esteem. *Self and Identity, 7*(1), 54–74.

Maslow, A. (1987). *Motivation and personality* (3rd ed.). New York: Harper & Row.

Mayo Clinic. (2009). Self-esteem check: Too low, too high or just right? Retrieved February 1, 2009, from http://www.mayoclinic.com/health/seelf-esteem/MH00128

Moorhead, S., Johnson, M., Maas, M., & Swanson, E. (2007). *Nursing Outcomes Classification (NOC)* (4th ed.). St. Louis, MO: Mosby.

National Institutes of Health. (2007). NIH news in health: Stressed out? Stress affects both body and mind. Retrieved February 1, 2009, from http://newsinhealth.nih.gov/2007/January/docs/01features_01.htm

North American Nursing Diagnosis Association International. (2010). *NANDA-I nursing diagnoses: Definitions and classification 2009–2011*. Ames, IA: Wiley-Blackwell.

Rosenberg, M. (1965). *Society and the adolescent self-image*. Princeton, NJ: Princeton University Press.

Wilburn, V., & Smith, D. (2005). Stress, self-esteem, and suicidal ideation in late adolescence. *Adolescence, 40*(157), 33.

RESOURCES

National Alliance on Mental Illness (NAMI), http://www.nami.org

National Empowerment Center, http://www.power2u.org

National Institute of Mental Health, http://www.nimh.nih.gov

National Mental Health Consumers' Self-Help Clearinghouse, http://www.mhselfhelp.org

SAMHSA's National Mental Health Information Center, http://mentalhealth.samhsa.gov

CHAPTER 16
Spirituality

MAKING THE CONNECTION

Refer to the following chapters to increase your understanding of the health care delivery system:

Basic Nursing

- ***Cultural Considerations***
- ***Complementary/Alternative Therapies***

LEARNING OBJECTIVES

Upon completion of this chapter, you should be able to:

- Define key terms.
- Discuss spiritual health concepts.
- List the defining characteristics of spiritual distress.
- Assess the spiritual needs of clients utilizing spiritual assessment models.
- Contribute to a plan of care for a client experiencing spiritual distress.
- Evaluate client outcomes for attainment of spiritual health.

KEY TERMS

faith
hope
meditation
prayer
religion
spiritual distress
spirituality
transcendence
values

INTRODUCTION

Spirituality has come to the forefront of nursing as an important aspect of client care. A growing body of evidence suggests a connection between spirituality and health (Hay, 2002; Park, 2007). **Spirituality** is the core of a person's being, a higher experience or **transcendence** (a state of being or existence above and beyond the limits of material experience) of oneself. The medical advances can make nursing seem more science and technology based (Cavendish et al., 2004). But over the past few years, an increasing number of nurses are advocating care involving the whole person. Assessing and meeting a client's spiritual needs has long been an inherent part of nursing. Incorporating a client's spiritual and religious values in the planning and delivering of care encompasses the art of nursing: caring and being there for the client.

The ever-increasing diverse and mobile society exposes nurses to different values, beliefs, and health care practices. Nurses can find themselves faced with clients who may speak different languages, eat different foods, and believe in healing practices far removed from Western medicine. This diversity may also result in a range of values and beliefs that are vastly different from what nurses believe. Nurses need to find ways to provide nursing care that respects a client's values and offers health care options that will enhance the client's wellness, provide care and comfort during times of illness, and protect and respect the client's choices.

Caring for clients whose values and beliefs are considerably different may pose a dilemma for the nurse if there is conflict with what the nurse believes. Even if there is little conflict, it may be difficult for the nurse to understand or support choices that seem different. In order to provide care that is respectful of beliefs and values, it may be helpful for the nurse to take her personal beliefs and values into consideration. Having a clear understanding of personal principles and convictions will enable the nurse to put the client's beliefs into perspective. Providing spiritual care requires the nurse to have a comfort level with this type of care and also requires conscientious thought and personal reflection.

SPIRITUALITY

For many years, scholars have been attempting to define spirituality. It is difficult to put into words something that cannot be seen, touched, or heard. According to Wilt and Smucker (2001), "The spiritual dimension is one beyond and yet somehow within, the physical and material world" (p. 4). People may have spiritual experiences or feel spiritual, and the experience or feeling is different for every person. Although the word "spirit" may be used in everyday conversation, many nurses find it difficult to describe how spirituality is an integral part of their client's being. Spirituality is often represented in pictures and paintings as a light in the sky (see Figure 16-1).

CRITICAL THINKING

Disclosure

When would it be an appropriate situation for the nurse to disclose her personal values and beliefs to a client?

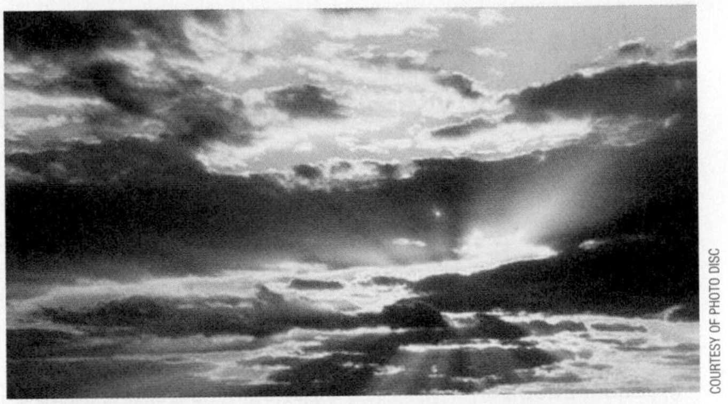

FIGURE 16-1 **An abstract concept like spirituality is sometimes depicted as the sky, indicating a higher power.**

Over the past 30 years, many nursing authors have defined spirituality. Most agree that spirituality applies to all persons. However, more complex definitions of spirituality have been developed. Table 16-1 lists some of the definitions of spirituality taken from the nursing literature. While there are some differences within the definitions, there is general agreement within the nursing profession regarding spirituality.

For practicing nurses, however, it is important to remember that spirituality is at the core of a person's being and includes the feelings and thoughts that bring purpose and meaning to that person's life. If a nurse can come to understand the client's purpose and meaning, nursing care can support the needs specific for that person. Providing individualized care that is in harmony with the client's spirituality may result in a health care experience that is positive for both the client and the nurse.

SPIRITUAL HEALTH CONCEPTS

A variety of spiritual health concepts are used in describing an individual's spirituality. Nurses need an understanding of these various concepts to better understand their client's personal views of spiritual health.

Faith

The concept of **faith** is closely linked to beliefs. Faith is a confident belief in the truth, value, or trustworthiness of a person, idea, or thing. Faith allows people to hold beliefs that cannot be observed (Mauk & Schmidt, 2004). A client may have faith that God will heal the injury or have faith that the physician will make a correct diagnosis. Faith is frequently referred to in terms of religion such as "faith in God." For the nurse, it is important to note that there are beliefs linking spirituality to health.

LIFE SPAN CONSIDERATIONS

Spirituality in Older Adults

Several research studies have shown that older people believe having a relationship with God supports their psychological well-being (Barton, Grudzen, & Zielske, 2003; Mackenzie, Rajagopal, Meilbohn, & Lavizzo-Mourney, 2000).

TABLE 16-1 Definitions of Spirituality

LITERATURE SOURCE	DEFINITION
(Macrae, 1995)	In her manuscript "Suggestions for Thought," Nightingale attempted to integrate science and mysticism. She wrote that the universe is the incarnation of a divine intelligence that regulates all things through law. For Nightingale, the laws of science are the "Thoughts of God."
(Burkhardt & Jacobson, 2000)	Spirituality is known and experienced relationships. (p. 95)
(Friesen, 2000)	Spirituality is described as one's quest for vision, meaning, insight, or inspiration. It is the way one sees the world, lives in the world, and derives meaning from the world. Each person's spiritual journey is a highly personalized experience that is different from another's. (p. 13)
(Dossey & Guzzetta, 2000)	Spirituality is a unifying force of a person; the essence of being that permeates all of life and is manifested in one's being, knowing, and doing; the interconnectedness with self, others, nature and God/life. (p. 7)
(Wilt & Smucker, 2001)	Spirituality is the recognition or experience of a dimension of life that is invisible and both within us yet beyond our material world, providing a sense of connectedness and interrelatedness with the universe.
(Carson & Koenig, 2004)	Spirituality is relational even in its focus on meaning and purpose. When people ask questions such as "Why me?," "Why now?," or "What does it mean?," they are attempting to define the relationship of their lives to ultimate truth and reality. (p. 74)
(Galek, Flannelly, Vane, & Galek, 2005)	The Eight Gates of Zen provide a comprehensive model of spirituality including meditation, study with a teacher, academic study, liturgy, right action, art practice, body practice, and work practice. All Zen paths are interrelated: together they provide a more balanced spiritual life. (p. 64)

Prayer

Prayer is defined as a human being's communication with spiritual and divine entities (Gill, 1987). Since prayer is intended for divine beings, humans have very different conceptions of what prayer is and how it should be enacted. Figure 16-2 demonstrates a prayer enactment by showing a spiritual counselor praying with an older adult. However, prayer can occur within and outside a religious context. Thus, a person not affiliated with **religion** (a system of organized beliefs, rituals, and practices with which a person identifies and wishes to be associated) can still engage in prayer (Taylor, 2002). Nurses may be asked to pray with a client, yet prayer can also benefit the nurse in promoting spiritual health.

When questioned about how they cope with the difficulties of illness, many clients report that prayer and faith is what gets them through (Taylor, 2002). Hence, it may also benefit nurses to encourage their own spiritual health. Whether prayer is done in private or communally with a body of believers, the purpose for the nurse is to find the connectedness and meaning for spiritual health.

CRITICAL THINKING

Faith

How can a client's faith help or hinder her recovery from an illness episode?

Meditation

To some, meditation may seem similar to prayer. The main distinguishing feature is that prayer is directed toward a divine entity, whereas **meditation** is an activity that brings the mind and spirit in focus on the present (Mauk & Schmidt, 2004). Meditation also provokes a sense of peace, relaxation, and self-awareness (see Figure 16-3). Meditation has been practiced for thousands of years in many different forms. Taylor (2002) has some introductory suggestions for an individual who is new to meditation (see Box 16-1). It is important to remember that the purpose of using meditation is to help the nurse develop a connectedness to the universe and to experience peacefulness and relaxation.

Values

Values are principles, standards, or qualities considered worthwhile or desirable. Individuals may not always be aware of their values, yet each person has a core set of personal values. Values can encompass a wide range of situations with common values involving such matters as the belief in hard work and punctuality. At the other end of the spectrum are psychological values, such as self-reliance, concern for others, and harmony of purpose (Posner, 2006). The way a person behaves or spends time or money can be indicative of the

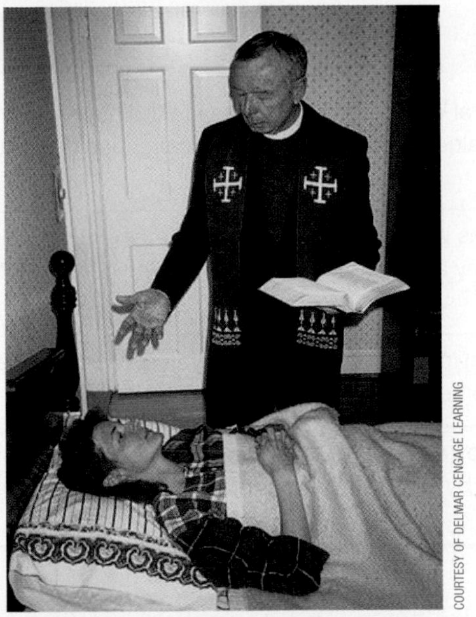

FIGURE 16-2 Today, spiritual counselors freely pray with their clients as part of providing spiritual care.

values he holds. Thus, someone who claims to value the environment can be expected to endorse recycling programs.

Values are formed over a person's lifetime and at first are learned from parents. Over the years, these can change as a child is exposed to friends, school, the media, and the community. Simon, Howe, and Kirschenbaum (1978) identified four ways parents and adults may transmit values to their children (see Table 16-2).

When a person needs to make an important decision, personal values help determine what choice the person will make. Awareness of the client's values will help the nurse

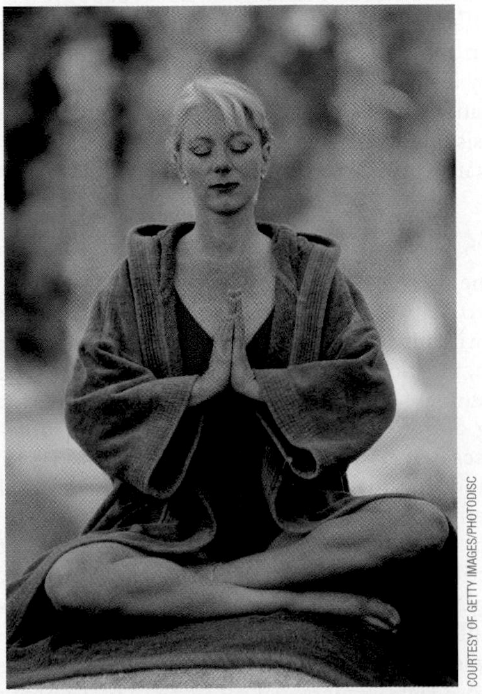

FIGURE 16-3 Developing Self-Awareness in Quiet Meditation

Box 16-1 Introductory Suggestions for Meditation

- Select a short phrase to repeat during the meditation. Some people select a prayer or verse that is meaningful.
- Assume a comfortable position.
- Close the eyes.
- Relax the muscles.
- Maintain a passive attitude.
- Develop an awareness of breathing and concentrate on a slow and rhythmic pattern.

provide care that will be supportive of the client's decisions. Moreover, the nurse's awareness of her own values will add a stronger dimension of understanding regarding the client's choices. A nurse who has gone through the process of becoming aware of her values, like embracing diversity, will be able to better understand her client's reluctance to be cared for by a nurse whose ethnicity is different from the client's.

The Joint Commission Spiritual Care Criteria

The Joint Commission, a major accrediting agency for hospitals, includes spiritual care criteria in their accreditation criteria. Specifically, the Joint Commission recommends that "healthcare organizations 1) acknowledge patient's rights to spiritual care and 2) provide for these needs through pastoral care and a diversity of services that may be offered by certified, ordained, or lay individuals" (La Pierre, 2003, p. 219). Nursing organizations have also crafted statements reflecting the need to incorporate spiritual care in everyday practice. The International Council of Nurses (2006), a federation of national nurse's organizations, include spiritual care in their code of ethics stating that, "in providing care, the nurse promotes an environment in which the human rights, values, customs and spiritual beliefs of the individual, family and community are respected." Furthermore, the American Association of Colleges of Nursing (1995) advocates teaching students how to conduct spiritual care assessments, nursing diagnoses, interventions, and outcomes. For these reasons, developing spiritual awareness can be a key step toward providing care that encompasses the client's need for the search for meaning during times of illness.

American Nurses Association Code of Ethics

The American Nurses Association (ANA, 2005) *Code of Ethics* clearly states the ethical responsibility for providing spiritual care. Specifically, the code states, "An individual's lifestyle, value system and religious beliefs should be considered in planning health care with and for each patient. Such consideration does not suggest that the nurse necessarily agrees with or condones certain individual choices, but that the nurse respects the patient as a person" (ANA, 2005, Provision 1:1.2). Furthermore, the code also addresses spirituality by stating,

TABLE 16-2 Four Ways Parents Transmit Values to Children

Moralizing	From an early age, some parents teach their own moral values to their children in the hopes of preparing them to lead productive lives. Moralizing instills the values without giving the recipient an opportunity to compare different values.
Laissez-faire	This attitude allows the child to explore different values without parental or adult intervention. Children, however, may become confused and conflicted as they attempt to make sense of the different values they encounter.
Modeling	Children learn values from those who exhibit the behavior associated with the value. Modeling can lead to both socially acceptable and socially unacceptable behavior.
Values clarification	Helps young people develop their own value system by answering questions that may be confusing. Values clarification assists by providing a mechanism by which adolescents can make decisions when faced with conflicting values.

"The measures nurses take to care for the patient enable the patient to live with as much physical, emotional, social and spiritual well-being as possible" (Provision 1:1.3). Thus, nurses are ethically bound to provide care for the spiritual well-being of the client. It is then up to the nurse to ensure that spiritual assessment and interventions are provided for the client's well-being. Under no circumstances should nurses engage in the promotion of personal religious beliefs. Any act that resembles proselytizing is an unethical practice and should be avoided at all times.

As stated previously, the ANA's (2005) *Code of Ethics* explicitly deals with the provision of spiritual care. The code also provides nurses with a guide for managing diversity of beliefs and values. "The nurse strives to provide patients with opportunities to participate in planning care, assures that patients find the plans acceptable and supports the implementation of the plan" (Provision 2:2.1). Furthermore, the code states, "Nurses must examine the conflicts arising between their own personal and professional values, the values and interests of others who are also responsible for patient care and health care decisions, as well as those of patients. Nurses strive to resolve such conflicts in ways that ensure patient safety, guard the patient's best interests and preserve the professional integrity of the nurse" (Provision 2:2.2). Key in this section is the reference to protecting the patient's interests while preserving one's own professional integrity.

An example of how the *Code of Ethics* can help a nurse is illustrated with the birth process. A Hmong family may participate in spiritual practices designed to protect their children from evil spirits. One of these consists of tying strings on a child's wrist to bind the child's soul to the body. Over time, these strings may become soiled (Fadiman, 1997). The nurse believes this practice is not appropriate and wants to cut them off, believing circulation could be impaired. This then results in a conflict between the family and the nurse. A review of the *Code of Ethics* reveals that the nurse's responsibility is to examine the conflict and then to resolve it with the client. An assessment of the family's beliefs related to the behavior is of utmost importance to resolve this conflict. When the nurse begins to understand the rationale behind the religious practice, the differences between the nurse and the client can be managed in a way that respects the client.

SPIRITUAL DISTRESS

Many clients experience spiritual distress when faced with a health care crisis. This spiritual distress causes various responses in many areas of the client's life, including physical, mental, psychosocial, and spiritual.

DEFINITION

Spiritual distress is defined as "disruption in the life principle that pervades a person's entire being and that integrates and transcends one's biologic and psychosocial nature" (Cox et al., 2002, p. 683) A similar definition of spiritual distress suggests an "impaired ability to experience and integrate meaning and purpose in life through a person's connectedness with self, others, art, music, literature, nature, or a power greater than oneself" (Wilkinson, 2005, p. 507). While somewhat different, these two definitions share the notion that a client in this situation may have a troubled, fragmented, or possibly disintegrating spirit (Wilt & Smucker, 2001). Given the relationship between health and spirituality, expedient diagnosis and intervention for a client experiencing spiritual distress may possibly enhance recovery and promote wellness.

DESCRIPTION

Over the past 30 years, nurses have been developing ways in which to help clients with their spiritual needs. Recognizing that spirituality is personal and not necessarily grounded in religion, the North American Nursing Diagnosis Association International (NANDA-I) first developed spirituality-related nursing diagnoses in 1979 (Mauk & Schmidt, 2004). These diagnoses were labeled "spiritual concerns," "spiritual distress," and "spiritual despair." Over the years, these labels have been refined, and today, "spiritual distress" is the accepted label for addressing the needs of the client. Another way of describing this diagnosis is distress of the human spirit, essentially conveying the idea that there are factors causing disequilibrium for the client. The factors can be the response to disease, family altercations, self-doubt, or reasons a client might lose sight of personal meaning. Nurses now routinely assess the client's spirit, and spiritual care needs are addressed as part of holistic nursing care.

Defining Characteristics

A client experiencing spiritual distress will most likely exhibit signs and symptoms indicating distress. Just as a client with impaired gas exchange may exhibit signs of cyanosis or confusion and symptoms of dyspnea, the client experiencing spiritual distress will show evidence of the distress. Box 16-2 summarizes the defining characteristics of spiritual distress.

The defining characteristics related to spiritual distress stem from both subjective and objective data. Thus, clients may verbally express concerns such as conflicting feelings about previously held religious beliefs. Furthermore, the nurse may be the one to whom the client turns, as she may feel uncomfortable talking to a family member about these conflicts. Other signs of spiritual distress may be evident as behavior that will require additional assessment as to the cause.

When dealing with clients who may be experiencing spiritual distress, the nurse needs to use all manner of assessment skills since the signs and symptoms may be subtle. A client may initiate the discussion by asking the nurse, "Why is this happening to me? Why must I suffer so much?" An opening statement such as this is like an invitation for the nurse to further explore the client's illness experience from a spiritual perspective. Other cues, however, are not as straightforward and may require the nurse to be attuned to subtle innuendos. For example, a client experiencing spiritual distress may complain only of sleeplessness and not feeling rested. A nurse who suggests the client take a sleeping aid may be missing an opportunity to assist the client through a difficult period.

Box 16-2 Spiritual Distress: Defining Characteristics

- Expresses lack of acceptance
- Expresses lack of courage
- Expresses lack of hope
- Expresses lack of love
- Expresses lack of meaning in life
- Expresses lack of purpose in life
- Expresses lack of serenity (e.g., peace)
- Guilt
- Poor coping
- Displacement of anger toward religious representative
- Expresses anger toward God

From *Nursing Diagnoses: Definitions and Classification 2009–2011*, by North American Nursing Diagnosis Association International, 2010, Ames IA: Wiley-Blackwell.

NURSING PROCESS

The nursing process is used in the same way as for other client problems. One of the major differences is in the data collection methods and tools used. Conducting a spiritual care assessment requires sensitivity and compassion.

ASSESSMENT

To assess the person's spirit requires a consideration of both subjective and objective data. While the objectivedata may seem unrelated, subtle objective signs may be evident and would cue the nurse that additional assessment may be necessary. For example, a client who has been communicative and outgoing in the past may show episodes of silence and disinterest. The spiritually aware nurse, seeing the change in behavior, can explore the client's feelings using a spiritual assessment tool. At times it may be difficult for the nurse not to feel intrusive. However, nurses have a moral responsibility to address and manage all aspects of client care.

Spiritual Assessment Models

Various authors and researchers have developed models that can assist the nurse to assess spirituality. A comprehensive spiritual assessment tool provides a valuable mechanism to address these sometimes sensitive issues. Novice nurses are encouraged to use these tools until they find a way that works well for them in actual practice. There are many spiritual care models available, with many originating from the fields of psychology and pastoral care. Assessment guides developed from these models can be a valuable tool to help the nurse gather relevant spirituality data. Limiting spiritual care assessments questions to religious preference restricts the focus of spirituality. Therefore, making use of a spiritual care model will allow the nurse to conduct a comprehensive spiritual assessment leading to identification and management of client needs (Taylor, 2002). The following models provide useful tools for nurses conducting spiritual assessments.

CASE STUDY: FAMILY EXPERIENCING SPIRITUAL DISTRESS

M.B., a 73-year-old widow, has been admitted to the intensive care unit with the diagnosis of a massive cerebrovascular accident. She is experiencing both dysphagia and dysphasia. Over the past 3 days, her condition has deteriorated, and the family has decided to stop all heroic measures. M.B. has four daughters, and at least two have been at her bedside around the clock. At 9:00 A.M., the cardiac monitor shows a bradycardia with subsequent asystole. All four daughters are present, tearfully saying good-bye to their mother. A nurse enters the room, places her hand on one daughter's shoulder, and begins to sing the hymn "Amazing Grace." The daughter angrily shrugs off the nurse's hand and tells her to leave the room.

The following questions will guide your development of contributions to the nursing care plan for the case study:

1. After making these observations, what nursing diagnosis and goals might the nurse identify for M.B.'s family?
2. List the nursing interventions to be performed in caring for M.B.'s family.

Stoll (1979) developed one of the first nursing spiritual care models for nursing. This model is predicated on the notion that not all clients have clearly identified and articulated religious beliefs, and some may find the discussion threatening. The model has four distinct dimensions and suggests guiding questions to elicit the information. Spiritual issues can be burdened with emotions, so conducting the assessment at the latter part of the nursing interview may be more comfortable for both the client and the nurse (Stoll, 1979).

Another spiritual assessment model uses the acronym FICA to guide assessment questions (Puchalski & Romer, 2000). This basic model allows the health care practitioner to incorporate the spiritual assessment questions in the initial client interview. Additionally, the model provides an avenue for the client to be in control of the way in which her spiritual issues are addressed. The FICA model is straightforward to use and provides a method to document the results simply and straightforward. Moreover, the acronym is easy to remember and gives the nurse the ability to conduct a spiritual assessment when a sudden opportunity arises (Mauk & Schmidt, 2004).

Another spiritual assessment tool incorporates the dimensions of meaning and purpose, inner strengths, and interconnections (Dossey, 1998). Although not a specific model, the dimensions of this tool provide ways to elicit client information regarding spirituality. Relying heavily on the concept of holistic nursing, the tool focuses on determining how a person makes sense of meaning in her life. While there is some focus on divinity, this tool may be especially useful for clients who are not affiliated with a formal religion. Furthermore, using these questions, the nurse can easily perform a spiritual self-assessment (see Table 16-3).

MEMORY**TRICK**

FICA represents the following:

F = Faith or beliefs
What is your faith? Do you consider yourself religious? What gives meaning to your life?

I = Importance and influence
Is it important in your life? What influence does it have on how you take care of yourself? Have your beliefs influenced your behavior during this illness? What role do your beliefs play in regaining your health?

C = Community
Are you part of a spiritual or religious community? Is this a support to you and how? Are there people who support you or are really important to you?

A = Address
How would you like me to address these issues in your nursing care?

A model developed for use by physicians is also useful for nursing. Created by Maugans (1996), the model utilizes the acronym SPIRIT. The acronym makes this model easy to remember and may afford the nurse the opportunity to implement this when the opportunity presents itself. Using this model, the nurse can ask questions appropriate to the client's developmental level and specific situation (Maugans, 1996;

TABLE 16-3 Spiritual Assessment Tool

The following reflective questions may assist you in assessing, evaluating, and increasing spirituality in yourself and others.

Meaning and Purpose These questions assess a person's ability to seek meaning and fulfillment in life, manifest hope, and accept ambiguity and uncertainty.	• What gives your life meaning? • Do you have a sense of purpose in life? • Does your illness interfere with your life goals? • Why do you want to get well? • How hopeful are you about obtaining a better degree of health? • Do you feel that you have a responsibility in maintaining your health? • Will you be able to make changes in your life to maintain your health? • Are you motivated to get well? • What is the most important or powerful thing in your life?
Inner Strengths These questions assess a person's ability to manifest joy and recognize strengths, choices, goals, and faith.	• What brings you joy and peace in your life? • What can you do to feel alive and full of spirit? • What traits do you like about yourself? • What are your personal strengths? • What choices are available to you to enhance your healing? • What life goals have you set for yourself? • Do you think that stress in any way caused your illness? • How aware were you of your body before you became sick? • What do you believe in? • Is faith important in your life? • How has your illness influenced your faith? • Does faith play a role in recognizing your health?

(Continues)

TABLE 16-3 Spiritual Assessment Tool (Continued)

Interconnections These questions assess a person's positive self-concept, self-esteem, and sense of self; sense of belonging in the world with others; capacity to pursue personal interests; and ability to demonstrate love of self and self-forgiveness.	• How do you feel about yourself right now? • How do you feel when you have a true sense of yourself? • Do you pursue things of personal interest? • What do you do to show love for yourself? • Can you forgive yourself? • What do you do to heal your spirit?
These questions assess a person's ability to connect in life-giving ways with family, friends, and social groups and to engage in the forgiveness of others.	• Who are the significant people in your life? • Do you have friends or family in town who are available to help you? • Who are the people to who you are the closest? • Do you belong to any groups? • Can you ask people for help when you need it? • Can you share your feelings with others? • What are some of the most loving things that others have done for you? • What are the loving things that you do for other people? • Are you able to forgive others?
These questions assess a person's capacity for finding meaning in worship or religious activities and a connectedness with a divinity.	• Is worship important to you? • What do you consider the most significant act of worship in your life? • Do you participate in any religious activities • Do you believe in God or a higher power? • Do you think that prayer is powerful? • Have you ever tried to empty your mind of all thoughts to see what the experience might be? • Do you use relaxation or imagery skills? • Do you meditate? • Do you pray? • What is your prayer? • How are your prayers answered? • Do you have a sense of belonging in this world?
These questions assess a person's ability to experience a sense of connectedness with life and nature, an awareness of the effects of the environment on life and well-being, and a capacity or concern for the health of the environment.	• Do you ever feel a connection with the world or universe? • How does your environment have an impact on your state of well-being? • What are your environmental stressors at work and at home? • What strategies reduce your environmental stressors? • Do you have any concerns for the state of your immediate environment? • Are you involved with environmental issues such as recycling environmental resources at home, work, or in your community? • Are you concerned about the survival of the planet?

From Holistic Modalities and Healing Moments, by B. Dossey, 2008, *American Journal of Nursing, 98*(6), 44–47.

Mauk & Schmidt, 2004). Although this model is focused primarily on religious affiliation, it can provide a starting point for a spiritual assessment. Once this information has been gathered, the nurse can conduct a more in-depth assessment addressing life meaning, connectedness, and client strength.

Cultural Differences When conducting assessments, the nurse should include the cultural uniqueness of the client. Culture, religion, and spirituality are closely related in that these concepts frequently are intertwined in a client's life. Thus, religion, health, spirituality, and healing are highly interdependent and require compassionate attention when caring for clients from different cultures. Sensitivity in matters concerning religion and healing is necessary in order to protect the client's autonomy. Moreover, it is important for nurses to recognize that addressing religious issues during times of

> **MEMORY TRICK**
>
> Spiritual assessment using the **SPIRIT** model:
>
> **S** = Spiritual belief system
>
> **P** = Personal spirituality
>
> **I** = Integration and involvement in a spiritual community
>
> **R** = Ritualized practices and restrictions
>
> **I** = Implications for medical (nursing) care
>
> **T** = Terminal events planning (advance directives)

health crisis may not be beneficial for the client. Instead, it may be more appropriate to engage the help of the client's spiritual leader (Mauk & Schmidt, 2004).

Determining spiritual needs from clients from other cultures is not much different from the basic spiritual assessment. Special attention to the client's environment may provide information that religion is part of the person's spiritual makeup. Religious items, get-well cards, or special clothing can alert the nurse to focus the assessment. Client behavior and verbalization also may indicate the presence of religion or spirituality in the client's life. Special attention may need to be given to health situations, such as death and bereavement, which include spiritual and religious components (Andrews & Boyle 2003; Spector, 2004).

Nursing Diagnoses

Once the assessment has been completed, the nurse analyzes the subjective and objective data to determine if a spiritual problem exists. Based on the assessment, the nurse selects either ***Spiritual** well-being, **Spiritual** Distress, or Risk for **Spiritual** Distress.*

For clients who are spiritually healthy, there are actions the nurse can take to increase spiritual well-being. The appropriate nursing diagnosis is ***Spiritual** well-being, readiness for enhanced,* and is defined as "the ability to experience and integrate meaning and purpose in life through a person's connectedness with self, others, art, music, literature, nature, or a power greater than oneself" (Wilkinson, 2005, p. 513).

Wilkinson (2005) divides the defining characteristics of this nursing diagnosis into four categories: connections to self; connections with art, music, literature, and nature; connections with others; and connections with power greater than self. The descriptions under each category may be helpful for the nurse in determining if the client is ready for enhanced spiritual well-being (see Concept Map 16-1).

At times it may be difficult to differentiate between the diagnoses. It may help to remember that spiritual distress is an actual problem occurring at the time of the assessment. Clients with spiritual distress exhibit characteristics that can cue the nurse. A review of the defining characteristics can help the nurse sort through the assessment data to make the clinical judgment.

Clients who are at risk for spiritual distress may not state or indicate that they have a disruption of the spirit. These clients are experiencing situations where spiritual distress may occur. Thus nurses must be aware of their client's circumstances and behavior and note when spiritual distress may occur. The diagnosis of risk for spiritual distress will allow the nurse to intervene and assist the client to avert actual spiritual distress. Table 16-4 illustrates the differences between *Spiritual Distress* and ***Risk** for Spiritual Distress.*

Clients can respond to illness experiences in a variety of ways. The psychosocial responses may be difficult to categorize and treat. The following are diagnoses related to spiritual distress:

- *Ineffective individual coping*
- *Anxiety*
- *Chronic sorrow*
- *Decisional conflict*
- *Powerlessness*

Individuals sometimes have difficulty coping with the effects of illness. If this is the case, a more appropriate diagnosis would be *Ineffective Individual **Coping*** (Cox et al., 2002; Wilkinson, 2005). A diagnosis that may be more appropriate to the client's situation is anxiety, especially if the situation is related to death and dying. *Chronic **Sorrow** and Decisional **Conflict*** are two more diagnoses that may be used with clients who are having difficult illness experiences (Wilkinson, 2005). Another diagnosis that may be used is ***Powerlessness.*** Client's may feel powerless during illness but express this in terms of disruption of the spirit.

Planning/Outcome Identification

Contributing to the plan of care requires careful thought and design. Matters of the spirit are personal, and the nurse needs to ensure that goals and interventions are acceptable to the client. As such, some of the suggested goals and interventions are intended to place the nurse in the role of a supporter.

If the nurse has conducted an empathetic assessment and used sound clinical judgment in determining the nursing diagnosis, the client will most likely be in agreement with the plan of care. The goal should be client focused and realistic. Since clients may be believe that all people have a spirit, some expressing this through formal religion and others through connectedness with the universe, a wide variety of possible outcomes exist. Table 16-5 depicts some outcomes that would be appropriate to manage spiritual distress.

As can be seen, the goals or outcomes for managing spiritual distress are not necessarily measurable or time limited. That is because spirituality is dynamic, and change may take months or even years. Wilkinson (2005) suggests short-term or immediate goals that are appropriate for the hospitalized client (see Box 16-3).

For clients experiencing spiritual distress, these goals can seem more realistic and easier to attain. Once the client feels comfortable with these smaller steps, she may be ready to address spirituality on a more long-term basis.

Implementation

The second step for contributing to a plan of care is designing the interventions. There is a vast difference between interventions for a biological problem and interventions for a spiritual problem. For spiritual care, the nurse uses a different type of intervention. This is due to the very unique nature of spirituality. If a client has no **hope** (to look forward to with confidence or expectation), the nurse cannot give a client hope. Instead, the nurse can support the hoping abilities of the client.

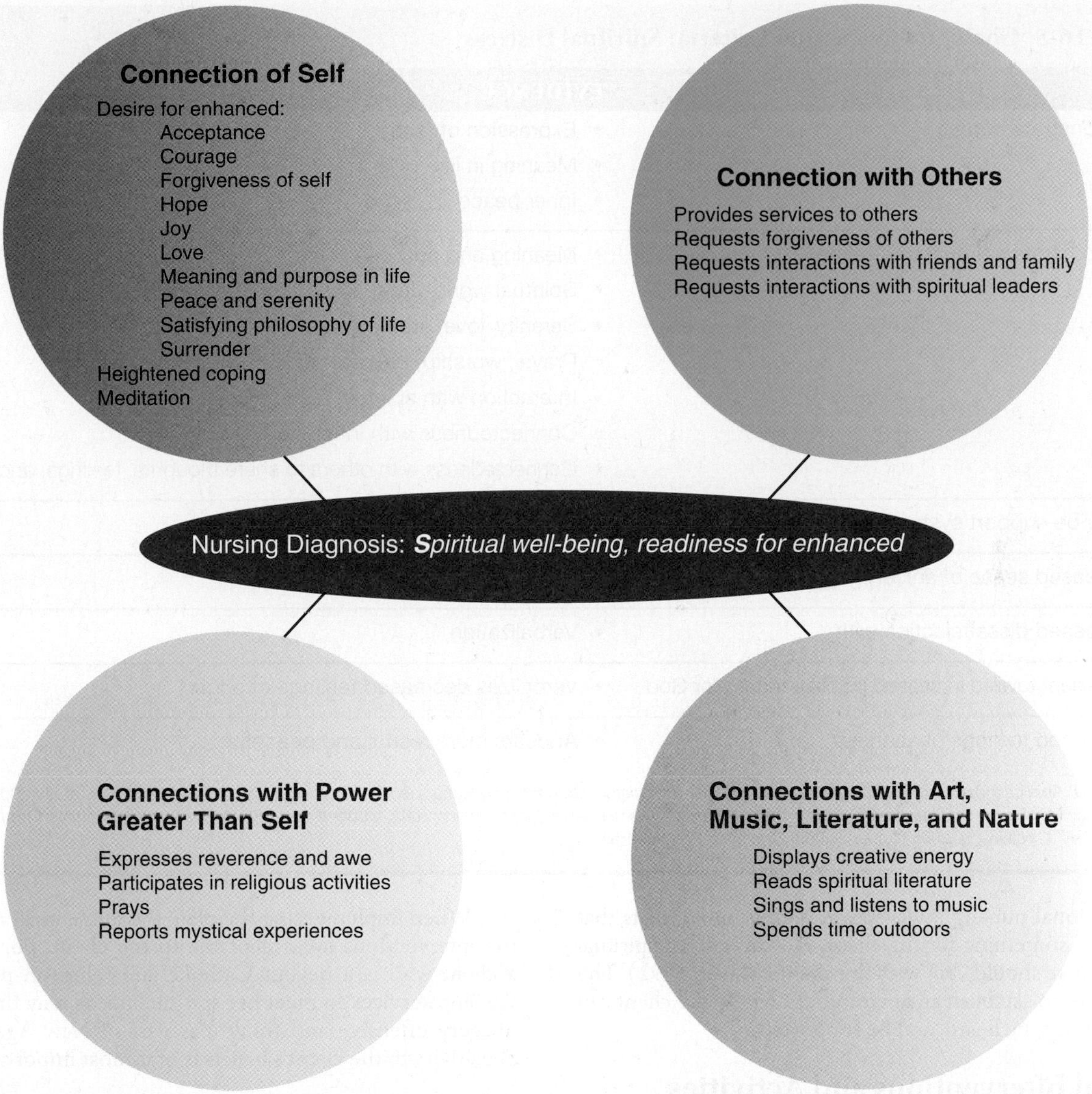

Concept Map 16-1

Table 16-4 Differences Between Spiritual Distress and Risk for Spiritual Distress

SPIRITUAL DISTRESS	RISK FOR SPIRITUAL DISTRESS
T.M., a 33-year-old married woman, is recovering from a total abdominal hysterectomy. She has a 12-year-old son. She is crying and says to the nurse, "I signed the form saying I know I won't be able to have more children. Everyone tells me how to recover from surgery. But no one has talked to me about what I feel like. I wanted more children, and now that's impossible. I feel like part of what I am as a woman is missing."	P.B. had a total prostatectomy 5 years ago. Two years ago, he underwent radiation treatment for a rise in prostate-specific antigen (PSA). After 18 months of a stable PSA, he has just been told that the latest PSA level has risen to 2.6. He tells the nurse, "I just don't understand it; I have done everything right. I had routine PSA screenings, my surgery was done in a timely manner, I underwent radiation, and I eat right and exercise. What else could I have done? I am so frustrated. The next treatment will be so much worse. What else do I have to do to keep this cancer from coming back?"
Diagnosis statement: ***S****piritual Distress* related to questioning about the meaning of her role in life.	*Diagnosis statement:* ***S****piritual Distress,* risk for, related to recurring elevated PSA levels and future uncertainty.

TABLE 16-5 Goals and Evaluation Criteria: Spiritual Distress

GOAL	EVIDENCE
• Demonstrate hope	• Expression of faith • Meaning in life • Inner peace
• Demonstrate spiritual well-being	• Meaning and purpose in life • Spiritual world view • Serenity, love, and forgiveness • Prayer, worship, or meditation • Interaction with spiritual leaders • Connectedness with inner self • Connectedness with others to share thoughts, feelings, and beliefs
• Describe support systems	• Access during times of spiritual crisis
• Decreased sense of anxiety regarding . . .	• Verbalization
• Decreased dissatisfaction with . . .	• Verbalization
• Movement toward increased positive regard for God	• Verbalizes decreased feelings of anger
• Decreased feelings of sadness	• Appears more restful and peaceful

From *Clinical Applications of Nursing Diagnosis: Adult, Child, Psychiatric, Gerontic, and Home Health Considerations* (4th ed.), by H. Cox et al., 2002, Philadelphia: F. A. Davis; *Spiritual Care, Nursing Theory, Research, and Practice,* by E. Taylor, 2002, Upper Saddle River, NJ: Prentice Hall; *Nursing Diagnosis Handbook,* by J. Wilkinson, 2005, Upper Saddle River, NJ: Prentice Hall.

The traditional nursing intervention definition suggests that nurses "do" something for the client. However, with spiritual care, the nurse should "be" with the client (Mayer, 1992). The nurse strives to establish an environment where the client can share concerns, be heard, and be supported.

General Interventions and Activities

Some of the interventions useful for managing spiritual care are those designed to "boost the spirit" (Taylor, 2002). These interventions are used with other nursing diagnoses, such as ***P**owerless, Chronic **S**orrow, and **A**nxiety*. General interventions should be used by nurses as part of standardized nursing care since these are the hallmark of caring (see Box 16-4).

Box 16-3 Appropriate Goals for the Hospitalized Client

These goals or outcomes suggest that the client will do the following:

- Acknowledge that illness is a challenge to belief system
- Acknowledge that treatment conflicts with belief system
- Demonstrate coping techniques to deal with spiritual distress
- Express acceptance of limited religious or cultural ties
- Discuss spiritual practices or concerns

When implementing the plan, the nurse must make sure the interventions are acceptable to the client. For example, a client who is a devout Catholic and relies on prayer and worship services to meet her spiritual needs may find guided imagery offensive and think it is part of New Age religion. Sensitivity to the client's beliefs is of utmost importance.

Role of Prayer

Some nurses may question whether they should pray with a client. Prayer is a very personal and private act and should be approached with respect. If a client requests that the nurse pray, it is important to determine what the client's prayer habits are. A Muslim client may not appreciate a Christian nurse's prayer to Jesus. Some religious traditions support ritualized prayer, while others incorporate a conversational style. A nurse can offer to pray with a client, but permission should be obtained first.

Seeking out peers with more experience can be beneficial for the novice nurse. For example, a novice nurse was caring for an elderly client who asked her to pray with him. The novice nurse asked, "What religion are you?" The client responded by saying he was Catholic. The novice nurse had no idea what kind of prayer Catholics used, so she solicited the help of a

PROFESSIONALTIP

Today, spiritual care is a recognized nursing activity. One key point for nurses to remember is that every person experiences spirituality in a unique way.

Box 16-4 General Interventions

General interventions used by nurses include the following:

- Active listening
- Caring touch
- Guided imagery
- Use of humor
- Meditation
- Client involvement in care and decision making
- Calm environment

fellow nurse who was a practicing Catholic. Both nurses came to the client's bedside, and while the Catholic nurse prayed, the other held the client's hand and listened. Even though the novice nurse had little experience, she was able to use her caring concern to provide spiritual care to the client.

Being Present

A new nurse may find attending to spiritual needs daunting. One intervention that requires no special training is being present. Presence can be defined as a giving of one's self in the present moment. It also includes listening with full awareness of the privilege of being there for a person—to be available with all the self in a way that is meaningful to another person (Pettigrew, 1990). Presence is an active intervention and suggests more than a physical presence. The nurse who makes eye contact while listening instead of writing notes on the clipboard is exhibiting presence. The client is the one who can most accurately identify nurses who are present.

PROFESSIONALTIP

The history of nursing demonstrates strong support for spiritual care as an integral part of nursing care. The past 20 years have shown a renewed interest in spiritual care. This renewed interest is based on the results from nursing research that demonstrates the positive outcomes when nurses engage in spiritual care (Taylor, 2002).

PROFESSIONALTIP

Most hospitals have a spiritual care or similar department frequently staffed by someone who has had formal or informal spiritual training. The hospital chaplain may be the most immediate resource available to the nurse. Before any professionals are notified, it is important for the nurse to ask the client if he or she wishes a visit from a clergy of their choice.

Evaluation

At times, it may be difficult to evaluate the outcomes of spiritual distress. Evaluating the outcome for airway clearance is objective: either the airway is clear or it is not. However, Mauk and Schmidt (2004) point out that a person cannot truly observe the spirit. It is therefore imperative that the nurse first involve the client when writing the outcome statements. This will allow the client to state whether the goal was met.

Family Involvement

Up to now, the recommended resources for spiritual care have been personnel trained in spiritual care. Clergy, spiritual leaders, and parish nurses can provide valuable assistance for the client in spiritual distress. However, the family can also be included as spiritual care resources. The family may understand the client's situation and the client's religious and spiritual preferences and share the rituals and celebrations of faith. Family can pray with the client, be present, and provide love and empathy. The nurse's role can be to encourage family participation. The nurse can also be the one who can arrange the client's activities to include private time for prayer and reflection. Keeping the client at the center of concern, the nurse can help the family continue to provide the support they wish to give.

SAMPLE NURSING CARE PLAN

The Client with Spiritual Distress

R.G. is a 53-year-old man diagnosed with colon cancer. He was admitted with severe rectal bleeding, and tests showed that surgery needed to be done soon. R.G. has been married to his wife for 12 years. They have one daughter. This is R.G.'s first marriage but his wife's second. She has two sons from a previous marriage who no longer live at home. Both R.G. and his wife are practicing Catholics. His wife's first marriage was conducted by a priest in the Catholic Church. When that marriage broke up, she chose not to ask for annulment, believing it was in the best interest of her children. Six years later, she met and married R.G. However, because she was a divorced woman, they were not allowed to marry in the Church.

(Continues)

SAMPLE NURSING CARE PLAN (Continued)

Over the past 12 years, they have attended Sunday mass and taken communion. According to Catholic Church doctrine, couples like R.G. and his wife may not receive communion. The couple has decided that since the church is large, they could just quietly do so anyway. Now R.G. is facing a serious surgery, and he wants the priest to bring him communion. The church they attend is very strict and follows the rules and regulations prescribed by the Church in Rome. Although they will send a priest to visit, the senior priest will not allow R.G. to take communion. R.G. is devastated and tells his primary nurse that he just doesn't understand. He believes in the Catholic Church with all his heart yet believes he has done nothing wrong marrying his wife. After all, it is his first marriage. "How can they deny me access to God?" he asks.

NURSING DIAGNOSIS *Spiritual Distress* related to separation from religious practices

Nursing Outcomes Classification (NOC)
Hope
Spiritual
Emotional Support

Nursing Interventions Classification (NIC)
Spiritual Support
Well-Being Coping Enhancement

PLANNING/OUTCOMES	NURSING INTERVENTION	RATIONALE
R.G. and his family will demonstrate spiritual well-being as evidenced by prayer.	Conduct a focused assessment regarding R.G.'s faith, prayer life, relationship to spiritual leaders, and receptiveness to a visit from the hospital chaplain.	Obtaining assessment data that are pertinent to R.G. specific to his religion or spiritual beliefs and practices will improve the nurse's understanding of the client's needs.
R.G. and his family will discuss spiritual concerns with a spiritual leader.	Conduct an indirect assessment of R.G.'s spiritual status by observing R.G.'s concept of God through books, exploring R.G.'s meaning in life, determining R.G.'s source of hope and strength, asking "Who is most important to you?" and observing for signs of prayer and meditation.	Obtaining indirect assessment data will improve the nurse's understanding of the client's needs.
	Request spiritual consultation.	During a time of crisis, R.G. may not have the inner strength to call for spiritual consultation without assistance.
R.G. and his family will verbalize connectedness to God.	Involve his wife in spiritual care conferences.	This facilitates communication between R.G. and his wife, may reduce the feeling of isolation, and may facilitate a resolution of the spiritual distress that he is feeling.
	Encourage his wife to pray and be with R.G.	This faciliates communication and interaction between R.G. and his wife and may facilitate a resolution of the spiritual distress.
	Be open to R.G.'s expressions of anger and disappointment.	Allowing R.G. to express his emotions creates a supportive climate and demonstrates caring.
	Assure R.G. you will be available for support.	Being present and allowing the opportunity to express emotions creates a supportive climate and sends a message of caring.

(Continues)

SAMPLE NURSING CARE PLAN (Continued)

EVALUATION

Evidence of R.G.'s progress toward relieving spiritual distress is his verbalization of a closer relationship with God. He might also indicate that he would like to visit with a spiritual leader, such as the hospital chaplain. A continued close relationship with his wife indicates that he does not blame her.

SUMMARY

- Spirituality is the core of a person's being, the dimension of life that is invisible, and brings meaning to one's life.
- Research studies have shown that spirituality is closely related to health.
- Values and beliefs are closely connected to spirituality: the search for meaning and making sense of life.
- Beliefs and spirituality may have strong ties to religion.
- Religion is not necessary for spirituality.
- Nurses should be sensitive to clients experiencing spiritual distress.
- Several spiritual care models exist that can help nurses conduct a spiritual assessment.
- A trusting nurse–client relationship is necessary and provides an environment where the client feels free and safe to share private thoughts and feelings.
- Family involvement can be beneficial for the client experiencing spiritual distress.

REVIEW QUESTIONS

1. Which of the following statements is correct regarding spirituality?
   1. A growing body of evidence does not suggest a connection between spirituality and health.
   2. Spirituality is the core of a person's being, a higher experience or transcendence of oneself.
   3. Assessing and meeting a client's spiritual needs is a new concept in nursing.
   4. The Four Gates of Zen provide a comprehensive model of spirituality.
2. When discussing spirituality with a client, the nurse knows that the definition of values is/are:
   1. principles, standards, or qualities considered worthwhile or desirable.
   2. a confident belief in the truth, value, or trustworthiness of a person, idea, or thing.
   3. human communication with divine and spiritual entities.
   4. an activity that brings the mind and spirit in focus on the present.
3. The nurse is assessing a client for spiritual distress. Defining characteristics indicative of spiritual distress in the client include: (Select all that apply.)
   1. lack of hope.
   2. poor coping.
   3. anger toward God.
   4. displacement of anger toward family.
   5. maintaining feelings of love and courage.
   6. lack of purpose in life.
4. A 33-year-old married female client is recovering from a total abdominal hysterectomy. She states, "I wanted more children and now that's impossible. I feel like part of what I am as a woman is missing." Which of the following nursing diagnoses is the most appropriate for the client?
   1. Anxiety related to ineffective individual coping and lack of spousal support.
   2. Decisional conflict related to powerlessness and inability to make decisions.
   3. Spiritual distress related to questioning about the meaning of her role in life.
   4. Ineffective coping related to anxiety and powerlessness due to a total abdominal hysterectomy.
5. Appropriate assessment questions for the nurse to ask a client include: (Select all that apply.)
   1. Are there any religious practices that are important to you?
   2. Who is an important person to you?
   3. Why do you pray?
   4. What religious books or symbols are helpful to you?
   5. Why are you refusing to speak with the hospital chaplain?
   6. What is your source of hope or strength?
6. The nurse observes a terminally ill client crying as she reads from her Bible. Which of the following interventions is the most appropriate?
   1. Contact the client's family.
   2. Provide quiet uninterrupted time.
   3. Contact the client's clergy.
   4. Provide a distraction.

7. A client has recently been in a serious car accident in which his wife and two children were killed. He tells the nurse that he does not understand why God has done this to him and that he feels like God has abandoned him. Which of the following nursing diagnoses is the most appropriate for this client?
   1. Chronic sorrow.
   2. Readiness for enhanced religiosity.
   3. Readiness for enhanced spiritual well-being.
   4. Spiritual distress.
8. Specific nursing actions to promote spiritual well-being in a client who has recently been diagnosed with a terminal illness include all the following except:
   1. make referrals to clergy when appropriate.
   2. respect the client's beliefs.
   3. listen actively to the client's concerns.
   4. provide sympathy to the client and family.
9. Which of the following need interferences would receive the highest priority when providing care to a client experiencing spiritual distress?
   1. The client has difficulty falling asleep.
   2. The client has disturbed body image.
   3. The client has a decreased appetite.
   4. The client has suicidal thoughts.
10. A recently hospitalized client states, "I believe that God and my doctor will heal my injury and make me all better." This is an example of:
   1. hope.
   2. values.
   3. faith.
   4. wellness.

REFERENCES/SUGGESTED READINGS

American Association of Colleges of Nursing. (1995). A model for differentiated nursing practice. Retrieved September 23, 2006, from http://www.aacn.nche.edu/Publications/pdf/DIFFMOD.PDF.

American Nurses Association. (2005). Code of ethic for nurses with interpretive statements. Retrieved October 25, 2008, from http://www.nursingworld.org/ethics/ecode.htm

Andrews, M. M., & Boyle, J. S. (2003). *Transcultural concepts in nursing care*. Philadelphia: Lippincott Williams & Wilkins.

Barton, J., Grudzen, M., & Zielske, R. (2003). *Vital connections in long-term care: Spiritual resources for staff and residents*. Baltimore: Health Professions Press.

Burkhardt, M., & Jacobson, M. (2000). Spirituality and health. In B. M. Dossey, L. Keegan & C. E. Guzzetta (Eds.), *Holistic Nursing: A handbook for practice* (pp. 91–121). Gaithersburg: Aspen.

Carson, V., & Koenig, H. (2004). *Spiritual caregiving: Healthcare as ministry*. Philadelphia: Templeton Foundation Press.

Cavendish, R., Kraynyak-Luise, B., Russo, D., Mitzeliotis, C., Bauer, M., McPartlan-Bajo, M., et al. (2004). Spiritual perspectives of nurses in the United States relevant for education and practice. *Western Journal of Nursing Research, 26*(2), 196–212.

Cox, H., Hinz, M., Lubno, M., Scott-Tilley, D., Newfield, S., Slater, M., et al. (2002). *Clinical applications of nursing diagnosis: Adult, child, psychiatric, gerontic, and home health considerations* (4th ed.). Philadelphia: F. A. Davis.

Dossey, B. (1998) Holistic modalities and healing moments. *American Journal of Nursing, 98*(6), 44–47.

Dossey, B., & Guzzetta, C. E. (2000). Holistic nursing practice. In B. M. Dossey, L. Keegan & C. E. Guzzetta (Eds.), *Holistic nursing practice: A handbook for practice* (pp. 5–26). Rockville: Aspen.

Fadiman, A. (1997). *The spirit catches you and you fall down*. New York: Farrar, Straus & Giroux.

Friesen, M. (2000). *Spiritual Care for Children Living in Specialized Settings*. Binghamton: Haworth Press.

Galek, K., Flannelly, K., Vane, A., & Galek, R. (2005). Assessing patient's spiritual needs. *Holistic Nursing Practice, 19*(2), 62–69.

Gill, S. (Ed.). (1987). *Prayer*. New York: Macmillan.

Hay, D. (2002). The spirituality of adults in Britain: Recent research. *Scottish Journal of Healthcare Chaplaincy, 5*(1), 4–8.

International Council of Nurses. (2006). The ICN code of ethics for nurses. Retrieved September 23, 2006, from http://www.icn.ch/icncode.pdf

La Pierre, L. (2003). JCAHO safeguards spiritual care. *Holistic Nursing Practice, 17*(4), 219.

Mackenzie, E., Rajagopal, D., Meilbohn, M., & Lavizzo-Mourney, R. (2000). Spiritual support and psychological well-being: Older adults' perceptions of religion and health connection. *Alternative Therapies in Health and Medicine, 6*(6), 37–45.

Macrae, J. (1995). Nightingale's spiritual philosophy and its significance for modern nursing. *Image: The Journal of Nursing Scholarship, 27*(1), 8–10.

Maugans, T. (1996). The SPIRITual history. *Archives of Family Medicine, 5*(1), 11–16.

Mauk, K., & Schmidt, N. (2004). *Spiritual care in nursing practice*. Philadelphia: Lippincott Williams & Wilkins.

Mayer, J. (1992) Wholly responsible for a part, or partly responsible for a whole? The concept of spiritual care in nursing. *Second opinion, 17*(3), 26–55.

Park, C. (2007). Religiousness/spirituality and health: A meaning systems perspective. *Journal of Behavioral Medicine, 30*, 319–328.

Pettigrew, J. (1990) Intensive nursing care: Four ways of being there. *Critical Care Nursing Clinics of North America, 2*, 503–508.

Posner, R. (2006). The power of personal values. Retrieved July 13, 2006, from http://gurusoftware.com/Gurunet/Personal/Topics/Values.htm

Puchalski, C., & Romer, A. L. (2000). Taking a spiritual history allows clinicians to understand patients more fully. *Journal of Palliative Medicine, 3*(1), 129–137.

Simon, S., Howe, L., & Kirschenbaum, H. (1978). *Values clarification: A handbook of practical strategies for teachers and students*. New York: Hart.

Spector, R. (2004). *Cultural diversity in health and illness*. Upper Saddle River, NJ: Prentice Hall.

Stoll, R. (1979). Guidelines for spiritual assessment. *American Journal of Nursing, 79*(9), 1574–1577.

Taylor, E. (2002). *Spiritual care, nursing theory, research, and practice*. Upper Saddle River, NJ: Prentice Hall.

Wilkinson, J. (2005). *Nursing diagnosis handbook*. Upper Saddle River, NJ: Prentice Hall.

Wilt, D. & Smucker, C. (2001). *Nursing the spirit*. Washington, DC: American Nurses Association.

RESOURCES

American Academy of Family Physicians, http://www.aafp.org

Duke University Center for Spirituality, Theology and Health, http://www.dukespiritualityandhealth.org

Johns Hopkins Medicine, http://www.hopkinsmedicine.org

Mayo Clinic, http://www.mayoclinic.com

MedlinePlus, http://www.medlineplus.gov

National Cancer Institute, http://www.cancer.gov

National Center for Complementary and Alternative Medicine, http://www.nccam.nih.gov

Spirituality & Practice, http://www.spiritualityandpractice.com

University of Minnesota Center for Spirituality and Healing, http://www.csh.umn.edu

WholeHealthMD, http://www.wholehealthmd.com

CHAPTER 17
Complementary/Alternative Therapies

MAKING THE CONNECTION

Refer to the following chapters to increase your understanding of complementary/alternative therapy:

Basic Nursing

- ***Holistic Care***
- ***Cultural Considerations***
- ***Wellness Concepts***
- ***Spirituality***
- ***Rest and Sleep***

LEARNING OBJECTIVES

Upon completion of this chapter, you should be able to:

- Define key terms.
- Describe the influences of history on current complementary/alternative modalities.
- Discuss the connection between mind and body and how this affects a person's health.
- Explain the concept of the nurse as an instrument of healing.
- Identify the various mind-body, body-movement, energy healing, spiritual, nutritional, and other modalities that can be used as complementary therapies in client care.
- Discuss the use of complementary/alternative modalities.

KEY TERMS

acupressure
acupuncture
allopathic
alternative therapies
antioxidant
aromatherapy
biofeedback
bodymind
complementary therapies
curing
energy therapy
free radicals
healing
healing touch
hypnosis
imagery
meditation
neuropeptides
neurotransmitters
phytochemicals
psychoneuroimmuno-endocrinology (PNIE)
shaman
shamanism
therapeutic massage
therapeutic touch
touch

INTRODUCTION

Our Western society generally equates health and healing with medicine, surgery, and other technological interventions. Many other cultures, however, promote healing through faith, ritual, magic, and other nonmedical approaches.

The use of **complementary therapies** (therapies used *in conjunction with* conventional medical therapies) and **alternative therapies** (therapies used *instead of* conventional or mainstream medical modalities) is becoming more prevalent among the general public (National Center for Complementary and Alternative Medicine [NCCAM], 2008a).

This chapter addresses complementary/alternative (C/A) treatment methods that are currently being used in holistic nursing practice. Nurses must think critically before recommending or implementing any of these therapies. Whether simply discussed with clients or performed, nurses should understand the ramifications. The abbreviation C/A will be used in this chapter.

LEGAL ASPECTS

Because more and more states are regulating C/A therapies, nurses must know the laws that govern these therapies in the states in which they work. Some states have outlawed certain therapies or consider them experimental procedures, whereas other states require licensure or certain educational standards before allowing practitioners to perform C/A therapies. Nurses who perform C/A therapies not in accordance with the laws of their respective states could have legal charges filed against them (Lorenzo, 2003).

Employer policy and the nurse's job description must also be checked to confirm that performing C/A therapies is within the nurse's scope of practice at that agency. Employer malpractice insurance policies typically do not cover situations where a client is injured as a result of a C/A therapy. The financial risk of any nurse who engages in C/A therapies will be lowered by having insurance that specifically covers those therapies.

HISTORIC FOUNDATION

People have tried to relieve pain and cure ills throughout history. Early cave drawings depict healers. Primitive healers believed that magic and superstition caused diseases, resulting in the intertwining of religious beliefs and health practices. Practices and remedies based in ancient traditions are being rediscovered and used. A brief look at ancient Greek, Far Eastern, Indian, and shamanistic practices will highlight their influences on modern C/A modalities.

ANCIENT GREECE

In the ancient Greek culture, health was perceived as maintaining balance in all dimensions of life. In Greek mythology, Asclepius was the god of healing. Temples (called Ascleipions) were beautiful places for people (regardless of ability to pay) to worship, rest, and restore themselves. Their system of healing used symbols, myths, and rites administered by specially trained priest-healers. Illnesses were treated by restoring balance to a person's life through baths, massage, music, laughter, art, herbs, and simple surgery (Keegan, 1994). Many of our current therapies, such as massage, art therapy, and herbal therapy, have origins in ancient Greek traditions.

THE FAR EAST

Healing systems of the Far East have traditionally integrated body, mind, and spirit into a system balancing energy between the individual and the universe. The practices of traditional Chinese medicine (TCM) have been used for centuries and are not considered to be an alternative therapy in Asia. It is a lived philosophy of health and well-being. Restoring and maintaining a balance of vital energy is the goal of TCM. Life energy *qi* (pronounced "key") or *chi* (pronounced "chee") are the words used to describe the vital energy that is the focus of the philosophical principles of TCM. Fundamental elements include balancing opposing forces of *yin* and *yang* (e.g., light–dark, cold–hot, and female–male). Assessment and diagnostic techniques of the TCM practitioner are very different from the **allopathic** (traditional medical and surgical treatment) approach of Western medicine. The five senses are used to assess the client by looking, listening, feeling, smelling, and tasting (if needed).

Chinese medicine is used to treat a range of human diseases and illnesses, such as allergies, asthma, headaches, infertility, and cancer. The nurse's role in care of the client who may integrate TCM with allopathic medicine for treatment of disease is to be sure that the client is aware of potential interactions of prescribed medications and treatments with prescribed herbs.

Herbs are an important part of traditional Chinese healing practice. A discussion of the use of herbs in contemporary health practices appears later in this chapter.

Traditional Chinese healing techniques are being studied and used by contemporary Western health care providers. **Acupuncture**, one technique of traditional Chinese medicine, applies needles and heat to various points on the body to alter the energy flow (Figure 17-1). The Mayo Clinic (2007) acknowledged the efficacy of acupuncture in treating pain and nausea after surgery, low back pain, headaches, fibromyalgia, migraines, osteoarthritis, postoperative dental pain, chemotherapy-induced nausea and vomiting, chronic menstrual cramps, and tennis elbow. Acupuncture may not be safe for clients with bleeding disorders or those taking anticoagulants.

INDIA

For more than 5,000 years, the people of India have practiced Ayurvedic medicine emphasizing "certain lifestyle interventions and natural therapies to regain a balance between the

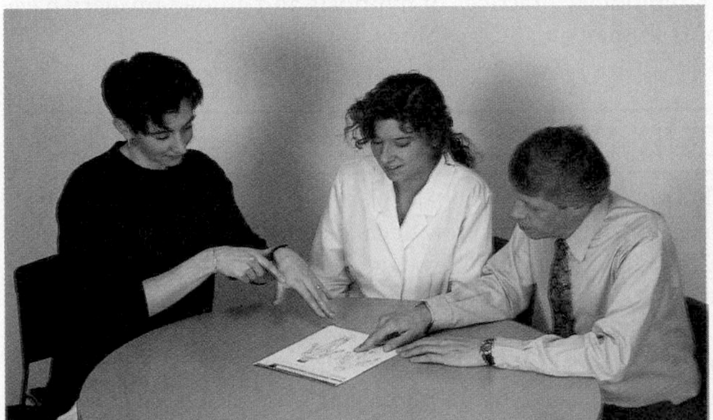

COURTESY OF DELMAR CENGAGE LEARNING

FIGURE 17-1 Acupuncturist, Nurse, and Client

body, mind, and the environment" (Bloomington Hospital, 2008a). The term *ayurveda* ("the science of life") refers to India's traditional medicine, which has an underlying spiritual basis. The life energy (prana) is moved through the body by a "wind," or Vata, which regulates every type of movement.

Vata, Kapha, and Pitta are the three metabolic principles (doshas) that "express particular patterns of energy-unique blends of physical, emotional, and mental characteristics" (Chopra, 2008). Kapha is the energy responsible for body structure. Pitta is the transformative process between Vata and Kapha. Each person is born with a unique balance of the three doshas. The dominant dosha determines temperament, body type, and susceptibility to certain illnesses.

The areas of energy concentration in the body are called chakras. Like the Chinese pathways (or meridians), these areas can become blocked and stagnant, causing illness. Ayurvedic healers try to activate chakra energy for self-healing.

The primary goals in the Ayurvedic system are preventing illness and restoring health by inner searching and spiritual growth. In contemporary practice, Ayurvedic intervention may consist of yoga, herbs, diet, and exercise; methods to cleanse the body, such as steam baths, cathartics, and detoxifying massage; and nasal purging.

Shamanistic Practices

Part of being human is a need to understand and explain life processes (i.e., birth, health, illness, and death). In many cultures, both modern and ancient, ritualized practices have been used to keep peace with the great spirits, to harness their power, to promote power, and to prevent death.

Shamanism refers to the practice of entering an altered state of consciousness with the intent to help others. The **shaman** is a folk healer–priest who uses natural and supernatural forces to help others and who is skilled in many forms of healing, has an extensive knowledge of herbs, and serves as guardian of the spirits. Illness is believed to be the result of spirit loss. Shamans work with the spirits to encourage their full return to the individual. The shaman functions as both priest and healer and has access to the supernatural.

Seeking wisdom about the universe, establishing a relationship with the creator, and avoiding death are all feats accomplished through ritualized processes performed by the shaman. The shaman uses special objects, such as power animals, fetishes, and totems, as well as dances, ritual songs, food, and clothing. Ritual chants, imagery, drumming, and hallucinogenic drugs may be used to create a trancelike state through which the shaman contacts the spirit world. The contemporary practices of hypnosis and guided imagery have roots in shamanistic traditions.

CURRENT TRENDS

The public perception of C/A treatment methods has been changing over the past few decades. In the late 1960s and early 1970s, the "natural," "new age," and "self-help" movements began to attract followers, first among consumers and later among health care practitioners. During that time period, there was a growing trend toward rejection of traditional medicine because of its perceived invasiveness, painfulness, cost, and ineffectiveness. A rekindled interest in Eastern religions, lifestyle, and medicine has fueled the development of contemporary holistic, C/A modalities.

In 1992, the U.S. government established the Office of Alternative Medicine (OAM) at the National Institutes of Health and allocated $2 million to disseminate information about complementary and alternative medicine to practitioners and the public. Congress increased the OAM's budget to $20 million for fiscal year 1998 (NCCAM, 2002).

Then in late 1998, Congress established the National Center for Complementary and Alternative Medicine (NCCAM), which replaced the OAM. Its budget for fiscal year 2002 was $104.6 million (NCCAM, 2008a). The NCCAM has the added responsibility of conducting and supporting basic and applied research and research training on C/A therapies. The NCCAM (2000) reported that as many as 42% of the U.S. population in 1997 used some type of C/A therapy, with a conservative estimate of spending $21.2 billion on these therapies.

In 2008, the NCCAM reported that 36% of American adults are using some form of C/A. When prayer and megavitamin therapy are included, that number rises to 62%. The profession of nursing is evolving from a traditional Western medical model of client care to an integrative model that incorporates healing tools from cultures and customs other than our own (Fontaine, 2005). Current nursing practice is advancing toward a holistic approach to healing the whole person through integration of complementary and alternative practices with conventional medical treatments into client health care for individuals, families, and communities (Dossey, Keegan, & Guzzetta, 2004; Falsafi, 2001).

Mind/Body Research

Traditional medicine is founded on the belief that the body, mind, and spirit are separate entities. A relatively new field of science, called **psychoneuroimmunoendocrinology (PNIE)**, describes the connection of thought with physical reactions. This word envelops the relationship of neural messages from thoughts, emotions, feelings, and attitudes into molecular responses from the immune and endocrine systems (Dossey et al., 2004). The power of thought is the basis of mindfulness-based healing therapies.

All body cells have receptor sites for **neuropeptides**, amino acids produced in the brain and other sites in the body that act as chemical communicators. Neuropeptides are released when **neurotransmitters** (chemical substances produced by the body that facilitate nerve-impulse transmission) signal emotions in the brain. Pert, of the National Institutes of Health, wrote in 1986 that "the more we know about neuropeptides, the harder it is to think in the traditional terms of a mind and a body. It makes more sense to speak of a single integrated entity, a 'body-mind'" (Pert, 1986).

Cells can be directly affected by emotions. This means that people can affect their health by what they feel and think. There are many examples of terminally ill persons hanging on to life until the occurrence of a specific event, such as a child coming to visit or a grandchild's graduation or marriage.

This complex, intermeshed system of psyche and body chemistry is now called the **bodymind**, an inseparable connection and operation of thoughts, feelings, and physiological functions.

Holism and Nursing

The growing acceptance of the concept that body, mind, and spirit are interconnected is the basis for the expansion of the holistic health movement. The physiological, psychological, sociocultural, intellectual, and spiritual aspects of each individual are considered in holism. Holistic nursing has been described by the American Holistic Nurses' Association (AHNA) as embracing "all nursing practice which has healing the whole person as its goal" (Dossey et al., 2004). Nurses who embrace their personal and professional lives within a holistic perspective are aware that their presence, attention, and intention are essential elements of wholeness and healing. Living within the framework of holism, nurses use their knowledge, nursing concepts and theories, expertise, and intuition to discover patterns of health for themselves and their clients that promote health and well-being. As the nurse and client become therapeutic partners, wholeness and healing is achieved for the client, family, group, and community.

Nurses as holistic caregivers may use C/A techniques to promote clients' well-being. The focus of care in these practices is healing as opposed to curing. The word **healing** comes from the Anglo-Saxon word *hael*, meaning "to make whole, to move toward, or to become whole." It is important to understand that healing is not **curing** (ridding one of disease) but is instead a process activating the individual's forces from within. The nurse as a healing facilitator enters into a relationship with the client to assist the client by being a guide. The objective is to assist the client in releasing inner resources for healing.

CRITICAL THINKING

Alternative Methods

A close friend has AIDS and is experiencing a great deal of pain and discouragement. She wants to find alternative methods to ease the pain. She confides to you that she believes there may be a cure available at the holistic health center. How do you best help your friend in this situation?

Nurses have an important role to educate clients about nontraditional interventions throughout the life span (Table 17-1).

COMPLEMENTARY/ ALTERNATIVE THERAPIES

Many C/A therapies are used in holistic nursing practice. These interventions are categorized as mind/body, spiritual, manipulative and body based, energy therapies, biologically based, and other methodologies.

TABLE 17-1 Suggested Complementary Therapies through Life

STAGE OF LIFE	SUGGESTED COMPLEMENTARY THERAPIES	
Infants	• Massage (modified) • Movement (rocking)	• Music
Young Children	• Massage • Music • Play	• Humor • Imagery • Art/drawing
School-Age Children	• Massage • Music • Play • Humor • Animal-assisted therapy	• Imagery • Aromatherapy • Yoga • Tai chi
Adolescents	All therapies discussed in this chapter, as appropriate to the condition	
Adults	All therapies discussed in this chapter, as appropriate to the condition	
Older Adults	• Massage (lighter pressure and other modifications for body's status) • Animal-assisted therapy • Aromatherapy (with precautions) • Any other therapy discussed in this chapter, as appropriate to the condition and with precautions	
Terminally Ill	• Massage • Reflexology • Energy therapies • Music	• Prayer • Any other therapies discussed in this chapter, as appropriate to the condition and with precautions

CASE STUDY

Complementary Therapies

A female client is diagnosed with stage 3 breast cancer. She is considering surgery to remove the tumor and cancer therapy options, yet she would like to know more about complementary therapies (CT) for health recovery and health promotion. Her medical team is not familiar with complementary and alternative therapies.

1. As the nurse on the health care team for this client, what interventions can be provided to promote support for this client during this time?
2. How can the nurse create a more informed health care team when clients ask about CT?

Mind/Body Interventions

Mind/body interventions are methods by which an individual can, independently or with assistance, consciously control some sympathetic nervous system functions (e.g., heart rate, respiratory rate, and blood pressure). When the client is learning the way to perform these techniques, an assistant is involved; later, however, the client can perform them independently. Self-regulatory techniques include meditation, relaxation, imagery, biofeedback, and hypnosis.

Meditation

Meditation, a quieting of the mind by focusing attention on a sound or image or one's own breathing, is an ancient art. The person is no longer aware of worries or preoccupations, and stress is reduced. Health benefits from reduced stress include decreased respiration, heart rate, and oxygen consumption; improved mood; spiritual calm; and heightened awareness.

Nurses can assist clients with meditation by explaining what it is and answering any questions. When the client is in a comfortable position, instruct in a calm voice to concentrate on inhaling and exhaling. If the client's mind wanders, a refocus on breathing is needed. This should be practiced every day for 15 minutes.

PROFESSIONALTIP

Use of Complementary/Alternative (C/A) Therapy

Nurses wanting to use C/A therapies should:

- Ask the client if he or she is currently using C/A and, if so, which therapy, the purpose of using the therapy, and the outcome.
- Educate the client about C/A prior to using it.
- Create a supportive environment of healing conducive to C/A therapy.
- Obtain the necessary training, certification, or licensure.
- Be aware of the potential risks.
- Provide nonjudgmental supportive counsel.

CLIENTTEACHING

Progressive Muscle Relaxation

Explain the purpose and process of progressive muscle relaxation, then have the client:

- Assume a comfortable position in a quiet environment.
- Close eyes and keep them closed until the exercise is completed.
- Breathe in deeply to a count of 4.
- Hold breath for a count of 4.
- Breathe out to a count of 4.
- Continue to breathe slowly and deeply.
- Tense both feet until muscle tension is felt.
- Hold a gentle state of tension in both feet for a count of 5.

Tighten the muscles only until tense, but not painful.

- Slowly release the tension from the feet.
- Recognize the difference between tension and relaxation.
- Repeat the previous three steps.
- Gently tense the muscles of both lower legs.
- Continue the process with all muscle groups in a toe-to-head direction.
- After tensing and releasing all muscle groups, take in a few more deep relaxing breaths and scan your body for any areas that remain tense. Concentrate on tensing and relaxing the muscles in those areas.
- Breathe in deeply to a count of 4.
- Hold breath for a count of 4.
- Breathe out to a count of 4.
- Resume your usual breathing pattern.
- Slowly stretch and open your eyes.

This takes approximately 20 to 30 minutes and is most effective with repetition.

Meditation has proved particularly beneficial for clients in labor.

Relaxation

Progressive muscle relaxation (PMR) is one method for achieving relaxation. It employs the alternate tensing and relaxing of muscles. Clients are instructed to concentrate on a certain body area (the jaw, for instance), tense the muscles for a count of 5, then relax the muscles for a count of 5. This process is repeated for muscle groups over the entire body until the client has achieved a state of overall relaxation. Nurses can use relaxation techniques to reduce pain and stress in clients.

Imagery

Imagery is a technique of using the imagination to visualize a pleasant, soothing image. The client is encouraged to use as

BOX 17-1 GUIDED IMAGERY

- Allow 10 to 20 minutes for this exercise.
- Provide a quiet comfortable environment.
- Set a goal for the session such as "pain relief" or "relaxation."
- Assess the client by asking him [or her] to describe a relaxing setting.
- Allow the client to use sensory details of the setting that include a visual image, the feeling (e.g., temperature, wind, sun), and the scents (e.g., evergreen, ocean breeze, lavender). Add music or be quiet for the auditory sense.
- Once the client is in a comfortable position. soften your voice to say:

  Bring your attention to the rhythm of your breathing. As you breathe in and out, allow an image to develop of a comfortable setting. In this setting you are relaxed and feel a sense of peace. Bring to mind the colors of the setting, the feel of the environment, the details of the setting as they surround you, and any comforting scents or aromas that allow you to feel at peace. Take a moment to enjoy this image.

  When you are ready, allow yourself to image the pain or areas of tension as a round ball of light. Bring your awareness to this light. Then, become aware of your ability to dim this light, slowly turning the light down to release the pain and tension. (Allow 2–3 minutes of quiet.)

  When you are ready, allow yourself to create a memory of this feeling of relaxation and comfort. As you rest, bring your awareness to areas of your body that need healing. Allow this feeling to facilitate healing throughout your body.

Downey, M. (2009). *Understanding Complementary and Alternative Therapies.* Manuscript submitted for publication.

many of the senses as possible to enhance the formation of vivid images. Table 17-2 presents examples of using all five senses in imagery.

Nurses can use guided imagery with clients capable of hearing and understanding the nurse's suggestions. For example, show and explain a chart of the stages of bone healing to a client who has suffered a fracture and ask the client to imagine this sequential activity in his body.

With guided imagery, the nurse can promote a sense of well-being in clients and help them change their perceptions about their disease, treatment, and healing ability (Dossey, 1999a). Research has shown positive effects of imagery when used with guidance from a trained health care practitioner (Dossey et al., 2004). Although imagery and visualization are effective complementary therapies for health and healing, contraindications should be noted for clients with mental disorders who are sensitive to traumatic images.

TABLE 17-2 Using All Five Senses in Imagery

SENSE	IMAGERY
Visual	See the white, fluffy clouds.
Auditory	Hear the waves on the beach.
Kinesthetic	Feel yourself floating in the water.
Gustatory	Taste the tartness of the lemonade.
Olfactory	Smell the hotdogs cooking on the grill.

BIOFEEDBACK

Biofeedback measures physiological responses, which assist individuals to improve their health by using signals from their own bodies. The biological functions commonly measured are muscle tension, skin temperature, heart rate, sweat gland activity, and brain wave activity. Biofeedback works by teaching clients to "recognize how their bodies are functioning and to control patterns of physiological functioning" (Association for Applied Psychophysiology and Biofeedback [AAPB], 2008). Biofeedback is effective for migraine and tension headaches, urinary incontinence, hypertension, chronic pain, sleeping problems, epilepsy, and Raynaud's disease (AAPB, 2008).

Hypnosis

The practice of hypnosis was once overshadowed by mystery and misconception. Today, with the expanding knowledge of the human mind, hypnosis is being used more. Therapeutic **hypnosis** induces an altered state of consciousness or awareness resembling sleep and during which the person is more receptive to suggestion. Hypnosis does not magically cure anything. Nurses desiring to use hypnosis in their practices must be aware of their scope of practice as defined by their respective state boards of nursing.

Spiritual Therapies

A state of health depends on one's relationship not only to the physical and interpersonal environments but also to the spiritual part of self. The idea of a relationship between spirituality and health is not new. "From the earliest time of the shaman we have witnessed the mysterious spiritual element of healing . . . the connection of the healer with the divine" (Keegan, 1994).

Many cultures accept the inseparable link between the state of one's soul (life energy or spirit) and the state of one's health. Scientists (especially psychoneuroimmunologists) are beginning to validate that individuals have inner mechanisms of healing. Many religions have ideologies about health, illness, and healing.

Faith Healing At the heart of spiritual or faith healing is the belief that practitioners must purify themselves and reach a state of unity with God or a higher power before faith healing can occur. This process is usually accomplished through prayer. When preparing for healing, the practitioner adapts a passive and receptive mood to be a channel for divine power. The ill person's belief enhances but is not necessary for healing.

Healing Prayer When praying, people believe they are communicating directly with God or a higher power. Prayer, an integral part of a person's spiritual life, can affect well-being. Florence Nightingale recognized that prayer helps connect individuals to nature and the environment (Nightingale, 1969). Medical research is currently investigating the effects of prayer on physical health.

Shamanism Shamanism was discussed earlier in this chapter.

Manipulative and Body-Based Methods

Body-based methods use techniques of manipulating or moving various body parts to achieve therapeutic outcomes. Movement/exercise, yoga, tai chi, and chiropractic treatment are discussed in the following sections.

Movement/Exercise

The therapeutic intervention and health-promoting activity of movement is associated with athletic exercise, dance, celebration, and healing rituals. The primary goal of exercise is fitness (muscle strength, endurance, flexibility, and cardiovascular and respiratory health). There are many other positive outcomes of exercise, such as sleeping better and having more energy.

Nurses can help clients use movement as therapy through range-of-motion exercises, stretching exercises, and physical therapy. Movement is an effective method through which people of all ages can improve their level of functioning.

Yoga/Yoga Therapy

Yoga (meaning "union" in Sanskrit) integrates mental, physical, and spiritual energies to promote health and wellness. The basic elements of yoga are proper breathing, posture, and movement. The breathing is believed to promote relaxation and enhance the flow of prana (vital energy). Yoga develops proprioception (an awareness of where the body is in space and time) and an awareness of movement, weight distribution, and position (Davis, 2002).

Traditional yoga has always been primarily concerned with healthy individuals and promoting health by maintaining the balance and flow of life forces.

Yoga therapy is an effort to integrate traditional yogic concepts and techniques with Western medical and psychological knowledge (Feuerstein, 1998). The focus of yoga therapy is to holistically treat various psychological or somatic dysfunctions ranging from back problems to emotional distress. Both yoga and yoga therapy are based on the understanding that the human being is an integrated body/mind system that best functions in a state of dynamic balance (Feuerstein, 1998). Yoga is used for a variety of health conditions, including depression, high blood pressure, stress, and asthma. Research suggests that yoga may reduce heart rate and blood pressure, increase lung capacity, positively affect specific brain or blood chemical levels, and improve body composition and muscle relaxation (NCCAM, 2008b). Yoga improves overall strength, flexibility, and fitness.

Tai Chi

The philosophy of looking for harmony with nature and the universe through complementary (yin and yang) balance is the basis for tai chi. When there is perfect harmony, everything functions spontaneously, effortlessly, perfectly, and according to the laws of nature. If one moves to the right, one must also move to the left. Tai chi is a series of slow, graceful, nonaerobic movements with controlled rhythmic breathing (Bloomington Hospital, 2008b).

Those who regularly practice tai chi believe that it enhances agility, stamina, and balance and that it boosts energy and bestows a sense of well-being. The entire tai chi form can take as little as 7 minutes or as long as an hour to practice. Tai chi has been shown to decrease blood pressure; increase muscle tone, stamina, and flexibility; and improve balance, muscle mass, posture, and strength in older people (Bloomington Hospital, 2008b).

> **LIFE SPAN CONSIDERATIONS**
>
> **Tai Chi Chih**
>
> A research trial conducted by the University of California (Irwin, Olmstead, & Motivala, 2008) concluded that tai chi chih can improve sleep quality in older adults ages 59 to 86 years with moderate sleep complaints. Tai chi chih can be considered a useful nonpharmacological approach to improve sleep quality in older adults.

Chiropractic Therapy

Chiropractic therapy is based on the principle that the brain sends vital energy to every organ in the body via the nerves originating in the spinal column. Disease, body disharmony, or malfunction results from vertebral subluxation complex (spinal nerve stress). The body is rebalanced and realigned using chiropractic "spinal adjustment" techniques.

The goal of chiropractic care is to awaken the client's own natural healing ability by correcting any areas of vertebral subluxation complex. Vitality, strength, and health are thus promoted. The Chiropractic Arts Center (2007) reports case histories of clients recovering from heart trouble, hyperactivity, fatigue, digestive problems, and many other conditions.

Stedman (1999) explains that chiropractic practitioners fall into one of two groups: the "straights" and the "mixers." The straights believe in the chiropractic therapy just described. The mixers use spinal adjustments mainly to relieve back pain, neck stiffness, and headaches, conditions that have sometimes been shown to be alleviated by chiropractic therapy. Most mixers are willing to work closely with a client's medical doctor.

Chiropractic services have gained increasing acceptance in the United States. Insurance coverage for chiropractic services is extensive. All state workers' compensation systems and many health maintenance organizations and private health insurance companies provide coverage for chiropractic therapy

> **PROFESSIONALTIP**
>
> **Preparing for Chiropractic Therapy**
>
> Encourage clients considering the use of chiropractic services to first undergo a comprehensive health assessment to rule out any contraindications.

(NCCAM, 2007). The client should check with their insurance company prior to seeking treatment to verify coverage.

Energy Therapies

One category of C/A therapies incorporated into nursing practice in the past 25 years is the **energy therapies**, or the use of the hands to direct or redirect the flow of the body's energy fields and enhance balance within those fields. These therapies are effective for many problems and can restore harmony in all aspects of health. These therapies can be used with persons of all ages and all stages of wellness and illness.

Energy therapies have their roots in traditional Chinese, ancient Eastern, and Native American philosophies. The fundamental concept is that individuals have a life force, energy not confined to physical skin boundaries. Figure 17-2 illustrates the energy field that extends beyond a person's physical body.

An individual's energy field consists of energy layers in constant flux. They can be reduced or otherwise adversely affected by any type of trauma, illness, or distress. The energy system can also be positively affected intentionally by the use of a practitioner's hands. The primary focus is to restore the optimal flow of life energy through the energy fields.

Many energy therapies are being used by nurses today, such as touch, therapeutic massage, therapeutic touch, and healing touch. Other therapies are acupressure and reflexology, both of which involve deep-tissue body work and require advanced training for the practitioners.

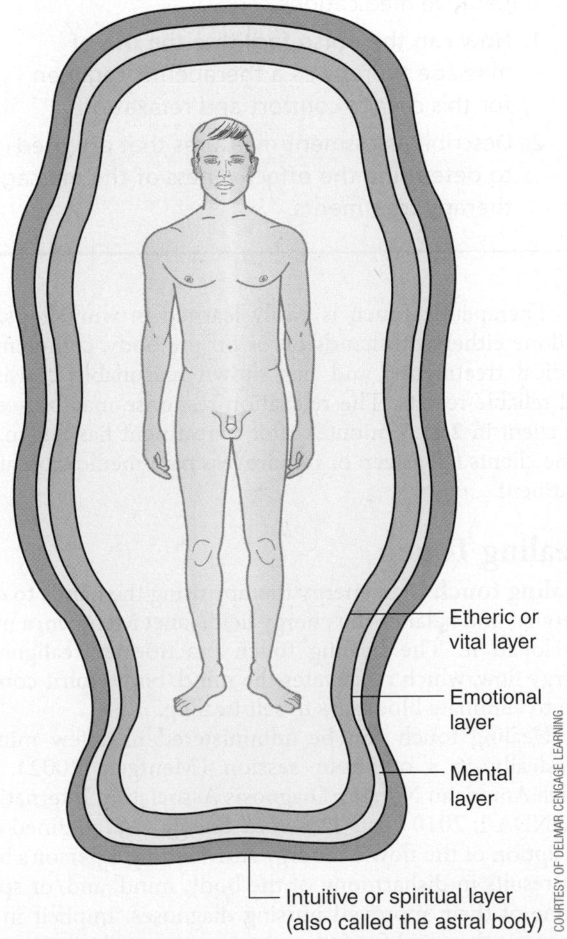

FIGURE 17-2 Layers of the Human Energy Field Extending Beyond the Physical Boundaries

CULTURAL CONSIDERATIONS

Touch

- Ask permission before touching a client.
- Tell the client what is going to happen.
- The meaning of touch and the body areas acceptable to touch vary from culture to culture.

Touch

The most universal C/A therapy is touch. **Touch** is the means of perceiving or experiencing through tactile sensation. Although it was used in all ancient cultures and shamanistic traditions for healing, the advent of scientific medicine and Puritanism led many healers away from the purposeful use of touch. It should be noted that touch carries with it taboos and prescriptions that are culturally dictated. Some cultures are very comfortable with physical touch; others specify that touch may be used only in certain situations and within specified parameters.

The nurse must be sure to convey positive intentions when touching. If in doubt, the nurse should not touch until establishing effective communication with the client. Touch is important in nursing practice, because it:

- is an integral part of assessment.
- promotes bonding between nurse and client (Figure 17-3).
- is an important means of communication, especially when other senses are impaired.
- assists in soothing, calming, and comforting.
- helps keep the client oriented.

Therapeutic Massage

Therapeutic massage is the application of hand pressure and motion to improve the recipient's well-being. It involves rubbing, kneading, and using friction.

Massage therapy is recognized as highly beneficial and is prescribed by many physicians. Many states now have licensing requirements for massage practitioners.

Traditionally, back rubs were given by nurses to provide comfort to hospitalized clients. Massage techniques can be used with all age-groups and are especially beneficial to those

PROFESSIONALTIP

Contraindications for Touch

It is important to know when *not* to touch.

- It may be difficult for persons who have been neglected, abused, or injured to accept touch therapy.
- Touching those who are distrustful or angry may increase negative behaviors.
- Persons with burns or overly sensitive skin may not benefit from touch.

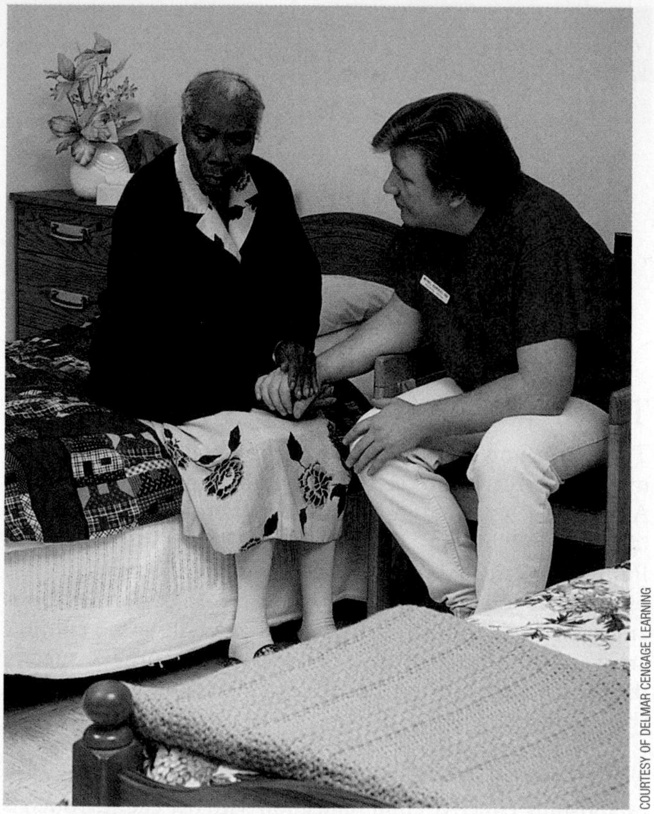

FIGURE 17-3 Touch promotes bonding between nurse and client.

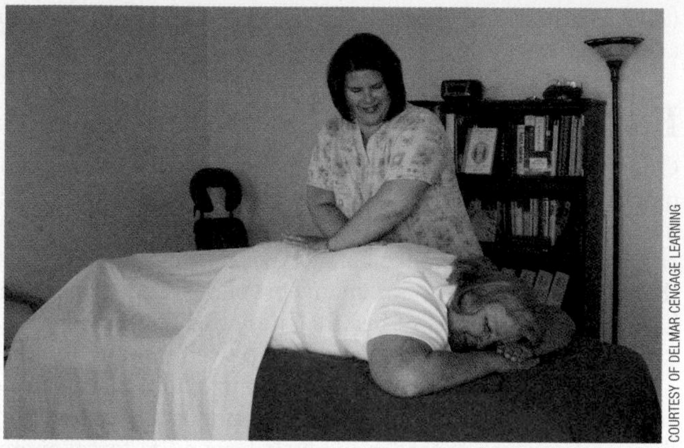

FIGURE 17-4 Therapeutic massage promotes relaxation, health, and well-being for the client.

who cannot move. A back rub or massage results in relaxation, increased circulation of the blood and lymph, and relief from musculoskeletal stiffness, spasm, and pain (Figure 17-4).

Therapeutic Touch

Therapeutic touch, based on the ancient practice of the laying on of hands, consists of finding alterations in a person's energy field and using the hands to direct energy to achieve a balanced state. Therapeutic touch is based on four assumptions:

- A human being is an open energy system.
- Anatomically, a human being is bilaterally symmetrical.
- Illness is an imbalance in an individual's energy field.
- Human beings have natural abilities to transform and transcend their conditions of living (Krieger, 1993).

SAFETY

Precautions for Massage

- Increased circulation may be harmful in people with heart disease, diabetes, hypertension, or kidney disease.
- Never attempt massage in areas of circulatory abnormality, such as aneurysm, varicose veins, phlebitis, thrombus, or necrosis, or in areas of tissue injury, inflammation, open wounds, dermatitis, joint or bone injury, recent surgery, or sciatica.

CASE STUDY

Massage Therapy

A 42-year-old male is admitted to the cardiovascular observation unit prior to his fourth cardiac bypass surgery. He is experiencing a great deal of anxiety in anticipation of his postoperative pain related to this procedure. The client proposes that he be given massage therapy along with the customary preoperative medications.

1. How can the nurse facilitate the use of massage therapy as a therapeutic regimen for this client's comfort and relaxation?
2. Describe assessment measures that are used to determine the effectiveness of the massage therapy treatments.

Therapeutic touch is easily learned in workshops, can be done either with hands on or off the body, complements medical treatments, and has shown reasonably consistent and reliable results. The relaxation response may be seen in the client in 2 to 5 minutes after a treatment has begun, and some clients fall asleep or require less pain medication after a treatment.

Healing Touch

Healing touch is an energy therapy using the hands to clear, energize, and balance the energy field. Janet Mentgen, a nurse, developed it. The healing touch practitioner realigns the energy flow, which reactivates the mind/body/spirit connection to eliminate blockages to self-healing.

Healing touch can be administered in a few minutes or, ideally, in a one-hour session (Mentgen, 2002). The North American Nursing Diagnosis Association International (NANDA-I, 2010) lists *Disturbed Energy Field,* defined as "a disruption of the flow of energy surrounding a person's being that results in disharmony of the body, mind, and/or spirit," as one of their approved nursing diagnoses. Implicit in this therapy is the need for follow-up or sequential treatments as well as discharge planning and referral to assist the client in adequately meeting goals.

CRITICAL THINKING

Reflexology

A client asks the nurse to rub his foot in a particular spot because that is where his reflexologist rubs to relieve his abdominal pain. How should the nurse handle this situation?

Acupressure and Shiatsu

Both acupressure and shiatsu are based on the Chinese meridian theory, which states that the body is divided into meridian channels through which qi, or energy, flows. Cold, damp, fire, bacteria, or viruses may block the flow of qi, causing disease in the body. **Acupressure** is a technique of releasing blocked energy within an individual when specific points (Tsubas) along the meridians are pressed or massaged by the practitioner's fingers, thumbs, and heel of the hands. When the blocked energy is freed, the disease subsides. Shiatsu, a Japanese form of acupressure, also uses the forearm, elbow, knee, and foot to activate the points. Both acupressure and Shiatsu relieve tension and many stress-related ailments. Contraindications include venous stasis, phlebitis, and traumatic and deep-tissue injuries (Sutherland, 2000).

Shiatsu treatment is holistic, with the aim of aiding the whole body to heal rather than focusing on the area where symptoms are most obvious. The aim is for the Shiatsu practitioner to assist the client's body to naturally heal by encouraging the client's energy to move into a more balanced state (Shiatsu Society, 2008).

Reflexology

Reflexology is a noninvasive complementary modality that involves the application of pressure by the use of the practitioner's hands, fingers, and thumb to the client's feet, hands, and ears with specific thumb, finger, and hand techniques. The fundamental concept of reflexology divides the body into 10 equal, longitudinal zones running the length of the body, from the top of the head to the tip of the toes. These 10 zones correspond to the 10 fingers and toes. The foot is viewed as a microcosm of the entire body (Figure 17-5). Reflexology theory states that illness is evident as calcium deposits and acids in the corresponding part of the person's feet. Pressing certain points on the feet brings an autonomic nervous system response or reflex. Reflexology induces an optimal state of relaxation, which is conducive to healing. It promotes health by relieving pressures and accumulation of toxins in the corresponding body part.

Reflexology can be used as a complementary therapy for chronic conditions such as asthma, sinus infections, migraines, irritable bowel syndrome, constipation, and kidney stones.

Biologically Based Therapies

In the past 20 to 30 years, nutritional interventions for prevention and treatment of disease have generated increasing interest among consumers and health care providers. This section addresses the C/A nutritional and herbal approaches.

Phytochemicals

Currently, certain foods are being studied for their medicinal value. **Phytochemicals** are "non-nutritive plant chemicals that have protective or disease preventive properties"

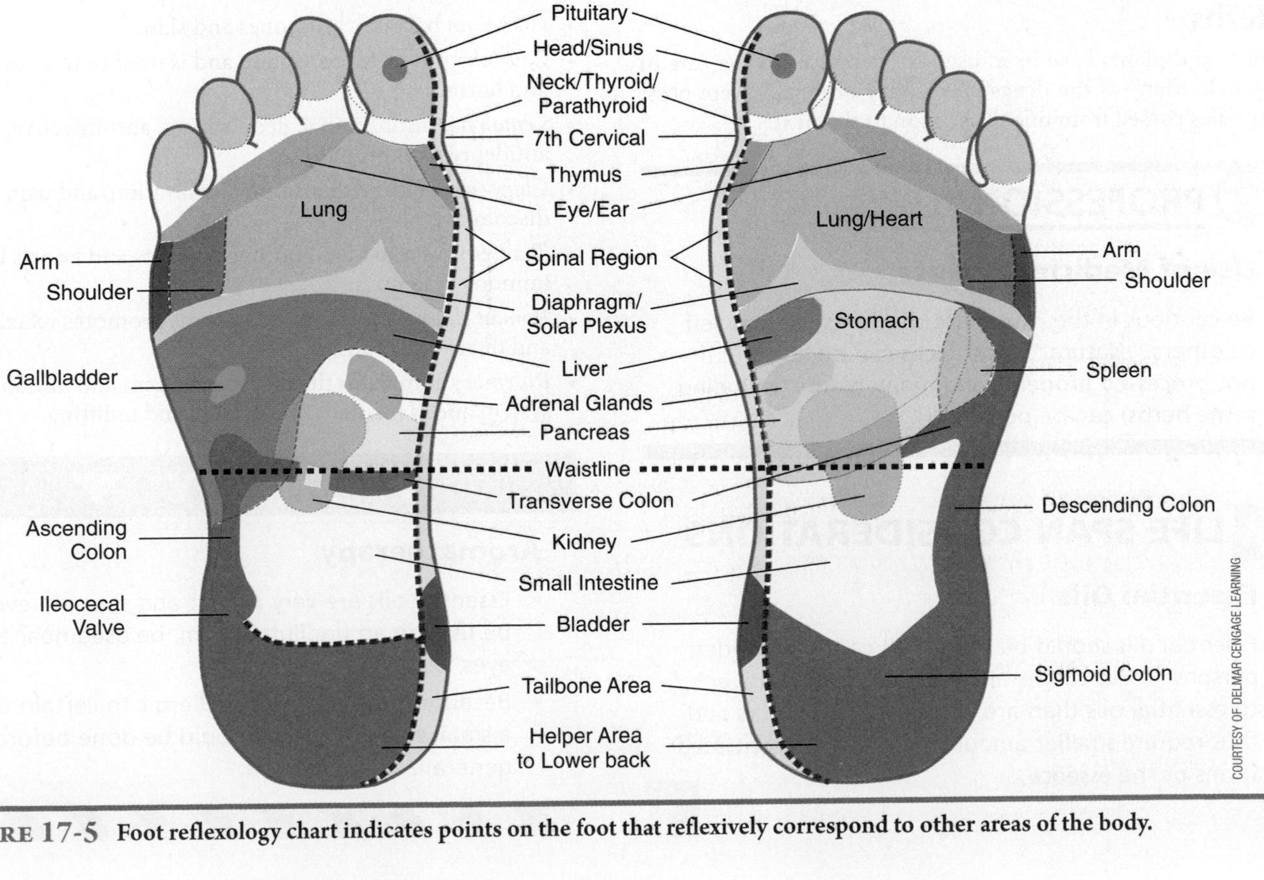

FIGURE 17-5 Foot reflexology chart indicates points on the foot that reflexively correspond to other areas of the body.

(Phytochemicals, 2008). *Phyto* is the Greek word for "plant." Therefore, phytochemicals are plant chemicals. These chemicals have several functions, including storage of nutrients and provision of structure, aroma, flavor, and color. Phytochemicals protect against cancer and prevent heart disease, stroke, and cataracts. Phytochemicals are found in fruits and vegetables.

No single fruit or vegetable contains all phytochemicals. The consumption of a wide variety of fruits and vegetables provides the best supply. The major sources of phytochemicals are onions, garlic, leeks, chives, carrots, sweet potatoes, squash, pumpkin, cantaloupe, mango, papaya, tomatoes, citrus fruits, grapes, strawberries, raspberries, cherries, legumes, soybeans, tofu, and the cruciferous vegetables (broccoli, cauliflower, brussels sprouts, and cabbage). Nurses can use this information to encourage clients to eat more fruits and vegetables.

Antioxidants

Antioxidants are substances that prevent or inhibit oxidation, a chemical process whereby a substance is joined to oxygen. In the body, antioxidants prevent tissue damage related to **free radicals**, which are unstable molecules that alter genetic codes and trigger the development of cancer growth in cells. Vitamins C and E, beta-carotene (which is converted to vitamin A in the body), and selenium are antioxidants. Antioxidants may prevent heart disease, some forms of cancer, and cataracts. Other vitamins, minerals, trace elements, and enzymes are being investigated for their possible therapeutic value. Phytosterols (plant sterols) are structurally similar to cholesterol and act in the intestine to decrease cholesterol absorption. Research has shown that phytosterols effectively reduce low-density-lipoprotein (LDL) cholesterol when given as supplements (Ostlund, 2004). Increasing the intake of phytosterols may reduce coronary heart disease with minimum risk.

Herbs

Herbs and plants have been used for centuries in the care of the sick. Many of the drugs used today originally were plant remedies passed from one generation to the next.

PROFESSIONALTIP

Use of Medicinal Plants

Be cautious in the casual use of plants to treat self or others. "Natural" substances can be harmful if not processed properly, and many plants (including some herbs) can be poisonous.

LIFE SPAN CONSIDERATIONS

Essential Oils

Essential oils should be used with caution in elderly persons. These clients are usually more sensitive to essential oils than are adults and teenagers and thus require smaller amounts and less concentrated forms of the essence.

Although herbs may have medicinal value (Table 17-3), some can cause potentially harmful herb–drug interactions when used with prescribed medications. It is important to ask during assessment specifically about the client's use of herbal and vitamin supplements. Feverfew, ginseng, and garlic prolong the clotting time. Encourage clients to reveal the use of herbs to their primary care provider.

OTHER METHODOLOGIES

Iridology, aromatherapy, humor, animal-assisted therapy, music therapy, and play therapy are also used by holistic practitioners.

Iridology

According to Caradonna (2008), iridology began more than 100 years ago when two physicians began observing eyes and organizing their findings. Iridology is the study of the iris, or colored part, of the eye. It is theorized that the fibers and pigmentation of the iris reflects information about a person's physical and psychological makeup.

Aromatherapy

Aromatherapy is the therapeutic use of concentrated essences or essential oils extracted from plants and flowers. Essential oils diluted in oil for massage or in warm water for inhalation may be stimulating, relaxing, or soothing. According to the National Association for Holistic Aromatherapy (NAHA, 2008b), the top 10 essential oils are the following:

- *Peppermint* is useful in treating headaches, muscle aches, and digestive disorders.
- *Eucalyptus* boosts the immune system, relieves muscle tension, and treats respiratory problems.
- *Ylang-ylang* aids in relaxation and depression.
- *Geranium* balances hormones and skin.
- *Lavender* promotes relaxation and is used to treat wounds and burns.
- *Lemon* has antibacterial, deodorizing, anti-infective, and antidepressant properties.
- *Clary sage* helps with insomnia, relaxation, and pain/discomfort.
- *Tea tree* is said to have antifungal effects and boosts the immune system.
- *Roman chamomile* decreases anxiety, promotes relaxation, and treats infections.
- *Rosemary* stimulates the digestive system and immune system and is mentally stimulating and uplifting.

SAFETY

Aromatherapy

- Essential oils are very potent and should never be used in an undiluted form, be used near the eyes, or be ingested orally.
- Because some people are allergic to certain oils, a small skin-patch test should be done before generalized application.

TABLE 17-3 Common Herbs for Health Promotion

HERB	REPORTED USES	ADMINISTRATION/ AVAILABILITY	CAUTIONS/INTERACTIONS	CLINICAL CONSIDERATIONS AND ASSESSMENTS
Aloe (*Aloe vera*)	Used topically to treat minor burns, sunburn, cuts, abrasions, acne, and stomatitis. Internally used as a stimulant laxative (little evidence base). Possible antidiabetic action related to the thromboxane inhibitor (TXA2) effects.	Capsules, cream, extract, gel, jelly, and juice. Teach client to use aloe internally only under the supervision of a qualified herbalist.	Internal administration of dried aloe juice is contraindicated for pregnancy and lactation and for children under 12 years of age. Avoid with kidney and cardiac disease and bowel obstruction. Aloe may enhance the effects of cardiac medications, diuretics, and steroids. Hypersensitivity (allergy) to garlic, onions, or tulips may indicate sensitivity to aloe.	• Assess clients for cardiac or renal disease/medications, steroids, and diuretics. • Assess for pregnancy and lactation. • Assess fluid and electrolyte balance. • Assess for allergy (see contraindications).
Bilberry (*Vaccinium myrtillus*)	Improvement of night vision, prevention of cataracts, macular degeneration, diabetic retinopathy, myopia, and glaucoma. Treatment of varicose veins, hemorrhoids, and postoperative hemorrhage.	Bilberry can be taken orally in the form of capsules, tinctures, fluid extract, and fresh berries.	Contraindicated for pregnancy, lactation, and children. Interactions: Anticoagulants (heparin, warfarin), antiplatelet agents (aspirin), nonsteroidal anti-inflammatory drugs (NSAIDs), insulin, and oral antidiabetics.	• Assess clients for use of anticoagulants, antidiabetics, and antiplatelets. • Assess and monitor vision changes. • Monitor blood glucose. • Assess for pregnancy and lactation.
Black cohosh (*Cimicifuga racemosa*)	Used as a smooth-muscle relaxant, antispasmodic, diuretic, antidiarrheal, astringent, antitussive, and antiarthritic; more commonly known for hormone balance in perimenopause and for dysmenorrhea. Possible decreased uterine spasms in first trimester of pregnancy and, for children, as an antiasthmatic.	Capsules, extract, powdered extract, and tincture. Standardized products should be used for administration of black cohosh.	Contraindicated for use in pregnancy after first trimester because of uterine stimulation. This herb should not be used during lactation and for children. Interactions: Black cohosh may interfere with antihypertensive and hormone replacement therapies.	• Assess for menopausal and menstrual irregularities: duration of cycle, flow, pain, and hot flashes. • Assess history of client for fibroids and ovarian cysts. • Assess use of other hormonal products such as estrogen, progesterone, and oral contraceptives.

(Continues)

TABLE 17-3 Common Herbs for Health Promotion (Continued)

HERB	REPORTED USES	ADMINISTRATION/ AVAILABILITY	CAUTIONS/INTERACTIONS	CLINICAL CONSIDERATIONS AND ASSESSMENTS
Capsicum (cayenne, chili, or hot peppers) (*Capsicum annum*)	Capsicum (peppers) can be used topically for treatment of arthritis, diabetic neuropathy, herpes zoster, peripheral circulation, psoriasis, and Raynaud's disease. Internal use for promotion of cardiovascular health, arthritic and muscular pain, gastric protection for peptic ulcers, and cold and flu symptoms.	Capsules, tablets, and tincture, topical cream/gel/lotion (0.025%–0.075% concentration) for approximately 2 weeks for pain relief (up to q.i.d.).	Minimal research has been done to support the use of capsicum during pregnancy and lactation or for children. Hypersensitivity (allergic reaction) is a contraindication. Capsicum in any form should not be used on open wounds, on abrasions, and near the eyes. Interactions: For internal application, avoid concurrent use with alpha-adrenergic blockers, clonidine, monoamine oxidase inhibitors (MAOIs), and methyldopa.	• Assess for use of alpha-adrenergic blocking agents, clonidine, MAOIs, and methyldopa. • Assess for improvement of symptoms in topical use such as psoriasis, peripheral vascular effects, diabetic neuropathy, or herpes zoster. • Assess for gastrointestinal conditions such as peptic ulcers and irritable bowel syndrome.
Chamomile (*Matricaria chamomilla*)	Used to treat anxiety and insomnia, as a digestive aid and an anti-inflammatory, and to promote wound healing.	Capsules, cream, fluid extract, lotion, tea, and tinctures.	Contraindicated for pregnancy and lactation. Allergies to sunflowers, ragweed, or asters (echinacea, feverfew, milk thistle) may cause hypersensitivity to chamomile. Asthmatics should avoid chamomile. Interactions: Avoid using alcohol, anticoagulants, and sedatives when taking chamomile because of the enhanced effects of these substances when used with this herb.	• Assess for hypersensitivity (see contraindications). • Assess client's sleeping patterns if taking chamomile. • Assess for use of alcohol, sedatives, and anticoagulants before administering this herb.
Cinnamon (*Cinnamomum*)	Used as an antifungal, analgesic, appetite stimulant, and antidiarrheal. Cinnamon is also reported to treat the common cold, abdominal pain, passive internal bleeding, hypertension, and bronchitis.	Essential oil, fluid extract, powder, and tincture. Dosage for passive bleeding is to use the essential oil in combination with Erigeron oil, diluted in carrier oil.	Contraindicated for pregnancy, lactation, and small children. No known drug interactions.	• Assess for hypersensitivity in the form of wheezing or a rash. Discontinue this herb if these symptoms are present and administer an antihistamine.

Echinacea purpura (*Echinacea angustifolia*)	Primarily used as an immune support for the common cold, influenza, and bacterial infections. Echinacea may be used to promote wound healing, bruises, burns, scratches, and leg ulcers.	Capsules, fluid extract, juice, powder, sublingual tablets, tea, and tincture. For prevention of colds and infections, the root tincture is recommended at ½ teaspoon b.i.d. Do not use this herb longer than 8 weeks.	Contraindicated for pregnancy, lactation, and children under 2 years of age. Caution should be used for persons with autoimmune diseases (HIV/AIDs), lupus erythematosus, multiple sclerosis, tuberculosis, and hypersensitivity. Interaction: Echinacea may decrease the action of econazole vaginal cream.	• Assess for hypersensitivity to this herb and to daisies. • Teach clients not to use this herb longer than 8 weeks.
Feverfew (*Chrysanthemum parthenium*)	Used to treat arthritis, fever, menstrual irregularities, and threatened miscarriages. It may be effective for prevention of migraine headaches.	Capsules, fresh herb, extract, tablets, and tinctures.	Contraindicated for pregnancy, lactation, and children. Avoid if hypersensitive to feverfew. Interactions: None known.	• Assess client for hypersensitivity to feverfew. • Assess for effects of this herb. • Assess for side effects such as mouth ulcers and muscle and joint pain.
Garlic (*Allium sativum*)	Cholesterol-lowering effects for decreasing low-density lipoprotein (LDL) and triglycerides raises high-density lipoproteins (HDL). It may regulate blood sugar and decrease blood pressure and platelet aggregation.	Capsules, extract, fresh garlic bulbs, oil, powder, and syrup.	Do not use with anticoagulants because of prolongation of bleeding. Because of potentiation of insulin and oral antidiabetics when taking garlic, insulin dosages may need to be adjusted. Garlic may stimulate labor and cause colic in infants and is contraindicated for pregnancy and lactation. Persons with hyperthyroidism should avoid consuming garlic because of the side effect of reducing iodine uptake. Garlic increases clotting time and should be avoided for persons undergoing surgery.	• Assess client for hypersensitivity to garlic. • Assess lipid levels if used for lipid lowering or cholesterol reduction. • Assess client's diabetic regimen (insulin or oral antidiabetics). • Assess coagulation studies and CBC. • Assess for use of anticoagulants.

(*Continues*)

Table 17-3 Common Herbs for Health Promotion (Continued)

HERB	REPORTED USES	ADMINISTRATION/ AVAILABILITY	CAUTIONS/INTERACTIONS	CLINICAL CONSIDERATIONS AND ASSESSMENTS
Ginger root (*Zingiber officinale*)	Prevents nausea and vomiting and acts as a digestive aid, peripheral circulatory stimulant, and antioxidant. May treat migraine headaches and induce platelet aggregation.	Capsules, extract, fresh and dried root, powder, tablets, tea, and tincture.	Contraindicated for pregnancy, lactation, and hypersensitivity reactions. Not recommended for persons with cholelithiasis. Interactions: It may potentiate bleeding if used with anticoagulants and antiplatelets.	• Assess client for allergies to ginger. • Assess for use of anticoagulants and antiplatelets. • Assess for effectiveness of ginger for intended use (i.e., nausea).
Ginkgo (*Ginkgo biloba*)	An antioxidant that may improve peripheral vascular circulation. Used to reduce peripheral vascular insufficiency and cerebral dysfunction in Alzheimer's disease. Also used for treatment of arthritis, mild depression, dizziness, headaches, and intermittent claudication.	Capsules, fluid extract, tablets, tea, and tincture.	Ginkgo is contraindicated for pregnancy, lactation, and children. Avoid use in persons with coagulation disorders and hemophilia or with allergies to ginkgo. Interactions: This herb may increase bleeding. Use with anticoagulants, platelet inhibitors, and MAOIs should be avoided.	• Assess clients for allergic reaction to this herb. • Assess for use of anticoagulants, platelet inhibitors, and MAOIs.
Horse chestnut (*Aesculus hippocastanum*)	Decreases capillary permeability. Used to treat venous insufficiency, phlebitis, and varicose veins. Possible effectiveness for edema, hemorrhoids, inflammation, and prostate enlargement.	Standard forms of horse chestnut include extract and tincture.	Contraindicated for pregnancy, lactation, and children. May cause hepatotoxicity and renal dysfunction in high doses. Interactions: Anticoagulants, aspirin, and salicylates.	• Assess client for allergic reaction. • Assess for bleeding tendencies. • Assess lab values for hepatic (AST, ALT, and bilirubin levels) and renal (BUN and creatinine) functioning.
Kava kava (*Piper methystium*)	Sedative and sleep enhancer. Used for anxiety, stress, restlessness, depression, and muscle relaxation. Possible effectiveness as an antiepileptic and antipsychotic.	Beverage, capsules, extract, tablets, and tinctures.	Do not combine with alcohol or central nervous system (CNS) depressants. Persons with Parkinson's disease, allergies, and major depressive disorders should not use this herb. Kava is contraindicated for pregnancy, lactation, and children under 12 years of age. Interactions: Sedatives, CNS depressants, antiparkinsonians.	• Assess clients for allergies. • Assess for use of alcohol, antidepressants, barbiturates, Parkinson's medications, benzodiazepines, sedatives, and CNS depressants.

Milk thistle (*Silybum marianum*)	Used for treatment of liver toxicity due to poisonous mushrooms, cirrhosis of the liver, chronic hepatitis C, and liver transplantation.	Tincture.	Contraindicated for pregnancy, lactation, and children. Avoid use with allergies to herbs and plants from the aster family. Interactions: Drugs that are metabolized via the liver.	• Assess client for allergies to this herb. • Monitor liver lab values (AST, ALT, and bilirubin). • Assess for use of drugs that are metabolized by the liver.
St. John's Wort (*Hypericum perforatum*)	Used to treat mild to moderate depression and anxiety. Used topically as an anti-inflammatory for hemorrhoids, vitiligo, and burns.	Capsules (sublingual), cream, and tincture.	Contraindicated for pregnancy, lactation, and children. Avoid use with allergies to this herb. Interactions: Alcohol, amphetamines, immunosuppressants, antiretroviral agents, MAOIs, selective serotonin reuptake inhibitors (SSRIs), sedatives, and tricyclics.	• Assess for allergies to St. John's Wort. • Assess for use of antidepressants, antiretrovirals, and sedatives.
Saw palmetto (*Sabal serralata*)	Reports of effectiveness for chronic cystitis and to increase breast size, sperm count, and sexual potency are related to saw palmetto use. Most notably, this herb is used for treatment of benign prostatic hypertrophy (BPH).	Berries, capsules, extract, tablets, and tea.	Contraindicated for pregnancy, lactation, and children. Interactions: Anti-inflammatories, hormones, immunostimulants.	• Assess for allergic reaction. • Assess for urinary retention, frequency, urgency, and nocturia. • Assess client's use of anti-inflammatory drugs, hormones, and immunostimulants.

Adapted from *Understanding Complementary and Alternative Therapies*, by M. Downey, 2009, manuscript submitted for publication.

Aromatherapists have used oils to treat specific ailments. Some essential oils have antibacterial properties and are used in a variety of pharmaceutical preparations. These oils should be used intelligently and with caution.

A growing phenomenon in aromatherapy is called Raindrop Therapy (NAHA, 2008a). This type of aromatherapy uses seven single undiluted oils that are dripped onto the spinal area of a client's back. The therapist uses his fingertips to work the oil into the skin. These treatments have become common in homes and spas, and clients have claimed a variety of healing properties from their use. However, there is controversy and warning regarding the use of Raindrop Therapy because of the possibility of serious skin rashes, irritation, and burns from the undiluted oils.

Humor

Therapeutic humor includes any intervention that promotes health and wellness by stimulating a playful discovery, expression, or appreciation of the absurdity or incongruity of life's situations (Association for Applied and Therapeutic Humor, 2008). It is probably the least understood but the easiest to do.

To avoid giving offense, it is important to determine the client's perception of what is humorous. Whether a given situation is considered humorous or offensive will vary greatly from culture to culture and person to person. Good taste and common sense should serve as guides.

Nurses can promote humor in various ways. A humor cart (cart filled with cartoon and joke books, silly noses, and magic tricks) allows clients to select their own humor tools. A "humor room" may be made available where clients can watch comedy videos or play fun games with visitors or other clients.

Humor has many therapeutic outcomes. Norman Cousins, former chairperson of the Task Force in Psychoneuroimmunology at the School of Medicine at UCLA, tells how his recovery from an incurable connective tissue disorder, ankylosing spondylitis, was enhanced by watching films and movies that made him laugh daily (Cousins, 1979). Humor can effectively relieve anxiety, improve respiratory function, promote relaxation, enhance immunological function, and decrease pain by stimulating endorphin production.

Animal-Assisted Therapy

Animals were used in England in 1792 at York Retreat, where psychiatric clients cared for rabbits and poultry (McConnell, 2002). It was 1944 before animals were used in a therapeutic setting in the United States.

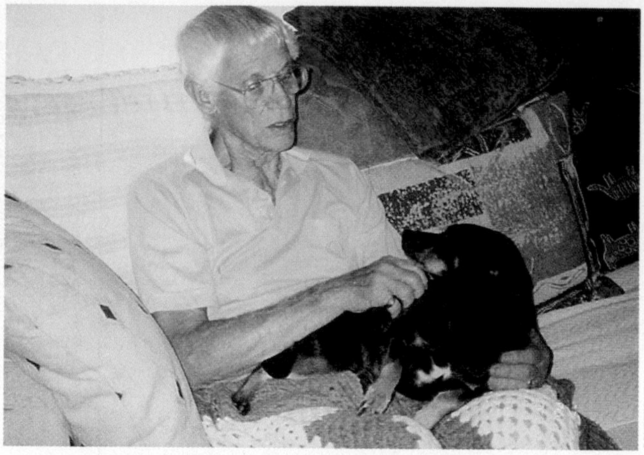

FIGURE 17-6 Pet therapy provides health benefits.

In animal-assisted therapy (AAT), a prepared handler and trained animal work one-on-one with a client toward identified short- and long-term goals.

Currently, AAT is used as a complementary therapy for people in both acute and long-term care settings (Figure 17-6).

Dogs are the animals most often used in AAT. Cats are less predictable, and many people are allergic to cat dander (Miller & Connor, 2000). Animal-assisted therapy has many applications, including overcoming physical limitations, improving mood, lowering blood pressure, and improving socialization skills and self-esteem.

Music Therapy

Therapeutic use of music consists of playing music to elicit positive changes in behavior, emotions, or physiological response. Music encourages clients to actively participate in their health care and recovery and complements other treatment modalities.

Music is good to use with imagery, as it enhances the relaxation response and heightens images. All music influences human behavior by triggering brain processes that affect a client's cognitive, emotional, and physical functions. Music radiates throughout society and culture and is easily accessible (Center for Music Therapy, 2007).

A CD player, iPod, or MP3 player with headphones playing music can be a useful tool for immobilized clients, those

LIFE SPAN CONSIDERATIONS

Creative Therapies

Modalities such as aromatherapy, music therapy, art therapy, humor, and pet therapy are among the group of creative and sense-complementary interventions in health care. These therapies are therapeutic in a variety of clinical situations and especially for children and elderly who may have difficulty verbally expressing their feelings.

CULTURAL CONSIDERATIONS

Music and Culture

- Each culture and each generation within each culture has its own preferred type of music.
- Music that is soothing to one client may be irritating to another.
- Either ask which type of music the client would prefer or allow the client to bring music.

waiting for diagnostic tests, or those waiting for surgery. Some facilities allow clients to choose the type of music played while they undergo procedures such as cardiac catheterization. Pleasurable sound and music can reduce stress, perception of pain, anxiety, and feelings of isolation. Music can be very useful to help adolescents relax.

Play Therapy

Play therapy is especially useful with children. Toys are used to allow children to learn about what will be happening to them and to express their emotions and their current situations. Drawing and artwork also provide a way for children to share their experiences. When language ability is reduced or not yet well developed, play therapy and drawings constitute a method for children to communicate their needs and feelings to care providers.

CRITICAL THINKING

Comfort Therapies

In the hospice setting, it is common for family members to ask about comfort therapies that they may be able to provide for the client.

1. What complementary therapies can a nurse teach family members?
2. What precautions would the nurse include in the teaching of these complementary therapies?
3. What evaluative measures can the nurse teach the family members to determine whether the complementary therapy that is provided is effective for the client?

SUMMARY

- More and more health care consumers are using nontraditional treatment modalities.
- Healing is not curing. It is regaining balance and finding harmony and wholeness as changes take place within the individual.
- No one can heal another, but a nurse can act as a guide and support system for the client.
- Some of the mind/body modalities used by nurses are meditation, relaxation, imagery, biofeedback, and hypnosis.
- Body-movement modalities include movement and exercise and chiropractic therapy.
- Energy therapies can be used with clients of all ages and in various stages of illness and wellness.
- Nutritional/medicinal therapies include the use of antioxidants and herbal therapy.
- Other modalities such as aromatherapy, humor, animal-assisted therapy, music therapy, and play therapy are valuable adjuncts to conventional treatment.

REVIEW QUESTIONS

1. Therapies that are used instead of mainstream medical practice are called:
   1. alternative therapies.
   2. contemporary therapies.
   3. complementary therapies.
   4. nontraditional therapies.
2. When assessing a client's use of complementary and alternative therapies for pain management, the nurse would gain more information from the client when asking which of the following questions in the interview?
   1. Which pain medications have you used in the past?
   2. What therapies are most effective for managing your pain?
   3. Have you discussed acupuncture with your medical physician?
   4. What is your experience with traditional Chinese medicine?
3. A 40-year-old female client is being treated for high blood pressure and diabetes. She tells the nurse that she has read about herbal preparations that may enhance metabolism of insulin in the body. The nurse's response should be:
   1. "There is no evidence that this herbal therapy is effective for diabetes."
   2. "You must consult your physician about this herb."
   3. "The type of diabetes that you have is controlled only with diet, exercise, and insulin injections."
   4. "You should search for studies that investigate the effects of this herb on diabetes management."
4. One of the most universal complementary/alternative modalities is:
   1. touch.
   2. massage.
   3. nutrition.
   4. faith healing.
5. A 17-year-old male is admitted to the emergency department following a skateboarding accident. He sustained a fractured pelvis and possible skull fracture. The physician has requested low doses of pain medication until the client's neurological status is stable. The client is restless and complaining of pain at a 9/10. Which of the following methods of relaxation

can the nurse use to complement the effects of the pain medication and increase the client's comfort?
1. Imagery, gentle massage to nontraumatized areas, and music.
2. Herbs, Ayurvedic medicine, and biofeedback.
3. Chiropractic, craniosacral therapy, and yoga.
4. Hypnosis, prayer, and naturopathy.

6. In contemporary practice, Ayurvedic interventions include: (Select all that apply.)
   1. antibiotics.
   2. herbs.
   3. detoxifying massage.
   4. nasal purging.
   5. chemotherapy.
   6. yoga.

7. The nurse explains the basic elements of yoga to a client who is considering taking a yoga class. Which of the following statements indicates that the client needs further teaching?
   1. "Yoga integrates mental, physical, and spiritual energies to promote my health and wellness."
   2. "The basic elements are proper breathing, posture, and movement."
   3. "Yoga can holistically treat my back problems and emotional distress."
   4. "The nurse will use her hands to redirect my energy flow."

8. A client informs the nurse that he would like to use aromatherapy in treating his headaches. The most appropriate response from the nurse is:
   1. "Lavender is useful in treating headaches, muscle aches, and digestive disorders."
   2. "I encourage you to inform your physician that you are considering using aromatherapy to treat your headaches."
   3. "Aromatherapy has not been scientifically proven to work."
   4. "You will want to try eucalyptus and clary sage, as they work well together to treat headaches."

9. The nurse knows that which of the following complementary and alternative therapies should not be performed on a client who is diagnosed with a deep-vein thrombosis?
   1. Massage.
   2. Music therapy.
   3. Hypnosis.
   4. Aromatherapy.

10. Chamomile tea is contraindicated in which of the following clients?
    1. A client with a stage 3 decubitus ulcer.
    2. A client who has insomnia.
    3. A client who is 7-months pregnant.
    4. A client who has a history of heartburn.

REFERENCES/SUGGESTED READINGS

Achterberg, J. (2002). *Imagery in healing: Shamanism and modern medicine.* Boston: Shambhala.

Achterberg, J., Dossey, B., & Kolkmeier, L. (1994). *Rituals of healing: Using imagery for health and wellness.* New York: Bantam.

Association for Applied Psychophysiology and Biofeedback. (2008). Potential clients. Retrieved August 26, 2008, from http://www.aapb.org

Association for Applied and Therapeutic Humor. (2008). Purpose. Retrieved August 26, 2008, from http://www.aath.org

Astin, J. (1998). Why patients use alternative medicine: Results of a national study. *Journal of the American Medical Association, 279*(19), 1248.

Avis, A. (1999). Aromatherapy in practice. *Nursing Standard, 13*(24), 14–15.

Benson, H. (1975). *The relaxation response.* New York: Morrow.

Bloomington Hospital. (2008a). Ayurveda: What is it? Retrieved August 28, 2008, from http://www.bloomingtonhospital.org

Bloomington Hospital. (2008b). Body movement. Retrieved August 26, 2008, from http://www.bloomingtonhospital.org

Brett, H. (1999). Aromatherapy in the care of older people. *Nursing Times, 95*(33), 56–57.

Brown, H., Cassileth, B., Lewis, J., & Renner, J. (1994, June 15). Alternative medicine—Or quackery? *Patient Care,* 80–98.

Byers, D. (2001). *Better health with foot reflexology* (10th ed.). St. Petersburg, FL: Ingham.

Byrd, C., & Sherrill, J. (1995). The therapeutic effects of intercessory prayer. *Journal of Christian Nursing, 12*(1), 21–23.

Caradonna, B. (2008). Iridology: An introduction. Available: http://www.iridologyassn.org/index.php?page=2887

Carpenter, D. (2008). Basic iridology. Available: http://www.iridologyassn.org/index.php?page=2889

Center for Music Therapy. (2007). Center for Music Therapy philosophy. Retrieved August 29, 2008, from http://www.centerformusictherapy.com

Cerrato, P. (1998). Aromatherapy: Is it for real? *RN, 61*(6), 51–52.

Cerrato, P. (1999a). A radical approach to heart disease. *RN, 62*(4), 65–66.

Cerrato, P. (1999b). Tai chi: A martial art turns therapeutic. *RN, 62*(2), 59–60.

Cerrato, P. (2000). Diet and herbs for BPH? *RN, 63*(2), 63–64.

Cerrato, P. (2002). Complementary therapies update. *RN, 65*(9), 23.

Chiropractic Arts Center. (2007). Frequently asked questions. Available: http://www.chiroarts.com/faqs.html

Chopra, D. (1998). *Ageless body, timeless mind.* New York: Harmony.

Chopra, D. (2008). The wisdom of Ayurveda. Retrieved August 25, 2008, from http://www.chopra.com

Cousins, N. (1979). *Anatomy of an illness.* New York: Norton.

Davis, J. (2002). Yoga finds new twists in the U.S. Available: http://aolsvc.health.webmed.aol.com/content/article/1668.51358?SRC=aolkw&K W=yoga

Dossey, B. (Ed.). (1997). *Core curriculum for holistic nursing.* Gaithersburg, MD: Aspen.

Dossey, B. (1999a). Imagery: Awakening the inner healer. In B. Dossey, L. Keegan, C. Guzzetta, & L. Kolkmeier (Eds.), *Holistic nursing: A handbook for practice* (3rd ed.). Gaithersburg, MD: Aspen.

Dossey, B. (1999b). The psychophysiology of bodymind healing. In B. Dossey, L. Keegan, C. Guzzetta, & L. Kolkmeier (Eds.), *Holistic nursing: A handbook for practice* (3rd ed.). Gaithersburg, MD: Aspen.

Dossey, B., Keegan, L., & Guzzetta, C. (2004). *Holistic nursing: A handbook for practice.* (4th ed.). Boston: Jones & Bartlett.

Dossey, L. (1997). *Healing words: The power of prayer and the practice of medicine.* San Francisco: Harper.

Dossey, L. (1999). *Prayer, healing, and medicine: An evening with Larry Dossey.* Arvada, CO: Lutheran Medical Center Community Foundation, Arvada Center.

Dossey, L. (2003). *Healing beyond the body: Medicine and the infinite reach of the mind.* Boston: Shambhala.

Dossey, L., Polkinghorne, J., & Benson, H. (2002). *Healing through prayer: Health practitioners tell the story.* Toronto: Anglican Book Centre.

Downey, M. (2009). *Understanding Complementary and Alternative Therapies.* Manuscript submitted for publication.

Evans, B. (1999). Complementary therapies and HIV infection. *American Journal of Nursing, 99*(2), 42–45.

Falsafi, N. (2001). The use of holistic concepts in professional practice. *Journal of Holistic Nursing, 19*(4), 390–392.

Feuerstein, G. (1998). Yoga and yoga therapy. Available: http://members.aol.com/yogaresearch/yogatherapy.htm

Floyd, J., & Fernandes, J. (2003). Making a place for CAM in the ICU. *RN, 66*(7), 44–47.

Fonnesbeck, B. (1998). Are you kidding? *Nursing98, 28*(3), 64.

Fontainc, K. (2005). *Complementary and alternative therapies for nursing practice* (2nd ed.). Upper Saddle River, NJ: Prentice Hall.

Frisch, N. (1997). Changing of the guard. *Beginnings, 17*(1), 1, 11.

Frisch, N., & Frisch, L. (2010). *Psychiatric mental health nursing* (4th ed.). Clifton Park, NY: Delmar Cengage Learning.

Gates, R. (1997). Legal issues in alternative medicine. *Alternative Therapies in Clinical Practice, 4*(4), 143.

Geiter, H. (2002). The spiritual side of nursing, *RN, 65*(5), 43–44.

Geller, U. (2002). *Mind medicine: The secret of powerful healing.* Boston: Element Books.

Guinness, A. (1993). *Family guide to natural medicine: How to stay healthy the natural way.* Pleasantville, NY: Reader's Digest.

Hatcher, T. (2001). The proverbial herb. *American Journal of Nursing, 101*(2), 36–43.

Herbert-Ashton, M. (2002, September). Getting a handle on herbals. *Travel Nursing Today* (Supplement to *RN*), September, 16–24.

Hodge, P., & Ullrich, S. (1999). Does your assessment include alternative therapies? *RN, 62*(6), 47–49.

Hover-Kramer, D. (2002). *Healing touch: A resource for health care professionals* (2nd ed.). Clifton Park, NY: Delmar Cengage Learning.

Hutchison, C. (1999). Healing touch: An energetic approach. *American Journal of Nursing, 99*(4), 43–48.

Irmin, M., Olmstead, R., & Motiva, S. (2008). Improving sleep quality in older adults with moderate sleep complaints: A randomized controlled trial of tai chi chih. *Sleep, 31*(7), 1001–1008.

Japsen, B. (1995, August 21). Cost-conscious providers take to holistic medicine. *Modern Healthcare,* 138–142.

Kane, J. (2001). *The healing companion: Simple and effective ways your presence can help people heal.* San Francisco, CA: Harper.

Keegan, L. (1994). *The nurse as healer.* Clifton Park, NY: Delmar Cengage Learning.

Keegan, L. (1998). Alternative and complementary therapies. *Nursing98, 28*(4), 50–53.

Keegan, L. (1999a). Nutrition, exercise, and movement. In B. Dossey, L. Keegan, C. Guzzetta, & L. Kolkmeier (Eds.), *Holistic nursing: A handbook for practice* (3rd ed., pp. 257–285). Gaithersburg, MD: Aspen.

Keegan, L. (1999b). Touch: Connecting with the healing power. In B. Dossey, L. Keegan, C. Guzzetta, & L. Kolkmeier (Eds.), *Holistic nursing: A handbook for practice* (3rd ed.). Gaithersburg, MD: Aspen.

Keegan, L. (2001). *Healing with complementary and alternative therapies.* Clifton Park, NY: Delmar Cengage Learning.

King, M., Pettigrew, A., & Reed, F. (1999). Complementary, alternative, integrative: Have nurses kept pace with their clients? *Medsurg Nursing, 8*(4), 249–56.

Klein, A. (2001). How can you laugh at a time like this? Available: http://aath.org/art_klein.html

Kolkmeier, L. (1999). Relaxation: Opening the door to change. In B. Dossey, L. Keegan, C. Guzzetta, & L. Kolkmeier (Eds.), *Holistic nursing: A handbook for practice* (3rd ed.). Gaithersburg, MD: Aspen.

Krieger, D. (1993). *Accepting your power to heal: The personal practice of therapeutic touch.* Santa Fe, NM: Bear.

Levin, J. (2001). *God, faith and health: Exploring the spirituality-healing connection.* Hoboken, NJ: Wiley.

Lorenzo, P. (2003). Complementary therapies—They're not without risk. *RN, 66*(1), 65–68.

Marwick, C. (1995). Should physicians prescribe prayer for health? Spiritual aspects of well-being considered. *Journal of the American Medical Association, 273*(20), 1561–1562.

Mason, J. (1999). Massage: The nursing touch. In C. Hutchinson, Healing touch: An energetic approach. *American Journal of Nursing, 99*(4), 44.

Maxwell, J. (1997). The gentle power of acupressure. *RN, 60*(4), 53–56.

Mayo Clinic. (2007). Acupuncture: Can it help? Retrieved August 25, 2008, from http://www.mayoclinic.com

McConnell, E. (2002). Myths and facts about animal-assisted therapy. *Nursing2002, 32*(3), 76.

McGhee, P. (1998). Rx: Laughter. *RN, 69*(7), 50–53.

McGhee, P. (1999). *Health, healing, and the amuse system* (3rd ed.). Dubuque, IA: Kendall/Hunt.

Mentgen, J. (2002). The clinical practice of healing touch. In D. Hover-Kramer (Ed.), *Healing touch: A resource for health care professionals* (2nd ed.). Clifton Park, NY: Delmar Cengage Learning.

Miller, J., & Connor, K. (2000). Going to the dogs . . . for help. *Nursing2000, 30*(11), 65–67.

Mills, E. M. (1994). The effect of low-intensity aerobic exercise on muscle strength, flexibility, and balance among sedentary elderly persons. *Nursing Research, 43,* 206–211.

Moyers, B. (1995). *Healing and the mind.* New York: Doubleday.

National Association for Holistic Aromatherapy. (2008a). *Aromatherapy undiluted—Safety and ethics.* Retrieved August 28, 2008, from http://www.naha.org

National Association for Holistic Aromatherapy. (2008b). Top 10 essential oils. Retrieved August 28, 2008, from http://www.naha.org

National Center for Complementary and Alternative Medicine. (2002). Funding: Appropriations history. Available: http://nccam.nih.gov/about/appropriations/index.htm

National Center for Complementary and Alternative Therapy. (2007). Insurance coverage. Retrieved August 26, 2008, from http://www.ncaam.nih.gov

National Center for Complementary and Alternative Medicine. (2008a). The use of complementary and alternative medicine in the United States. Retrieved August 25, 2008, from http://nccam.nih.gov/news/camsurvey_fs1.htm

National Center for Complementary and Alternative Medicine. (2008b). Yoga for health: An introduction. Retrieved August 26, 2008, from http://www.nccam.nih.gov

Nightingale, F. (1969). *Nursing: What it is and what it is not.* New York: Dover.

Nontraditional Choices. (2001a). Discovering yoga. *Nursing2001, 31*(2), 20.

Nontraditional Choices. (2001b). Potentially dangerous herbs. *Nursing2001, 31*(10), 92.
Nontraditional Choices. (2001c). Trying therapeutic massage. *Nursing2001, 31*(6), 26.
Nontraditional Choices. (2001d). When patients ask about . . . reflexology. *Nursing2001, 31*(9), 68.
Nontraditional Choices. (2002a). Learning about acupuncture. *Nursing2002, 32*(1), 28–29.
Nontraditional Choices. (2002b). Learning about tai chi chuan. *Nursing2002, 32*(12), 86.
Nontraditional Choices. (2002c). Practicing meditation. *Nursing2002, 32*(4), 70.
Nontraditional Choices. (2002d). Understanding biofeedback. *Nursing2002, 32*(6), 88–90.
Nontraditional Choices. (2003a). Putting imagery to work for your patient. *Nursing2003, 33*(6), 73.
Nontraditional Choices. (2003b). Understanding echinacea. *Nursing2003, 33*(1), 76.
North American Nursing Diagnosis Association International. (2010). *NANDA-I nursing diagnoses: Definitions and classification 2009–2011.* Ames, IA: Wiley-Blackwell.
Ostlund, R. Jr. (2004). Phytosterols and cholesterol metabolism. *Current Opinion in Lipidology*, 15(1), 37–41.
Payne, M. (2002). Power of touch. *Nursing2002, 32*(6), 102.
Pert, C. (1986). The wisdom of the receptors: Neuropeptides, the emotions, and bodymind. *Advances, 3*, 8–16.
Phytochemicals. (2008). What are phytochemicals? Retrieved August 30, 2008, from http://www.phytochemicals.info
Renner, J., Dillard, J., & Edelberg, D. (1999). Should the FDA regulate alternative medicines? *Hospital Health Network, 73*(10), 24.
Rosing, M. (2001). Warm hands, warm heart. *Nursing2001, 31*(12), 32.
Schroeder-Shecker, T. (1994). Music for the dying. *Journal of Holistic Nursing, 12*(1), 83–99.
Shiatsu Society. (2008). Frequently asked questions. Retrieved August 29, 2008, from http://www.shiatsusociety.org
Smith, M., Kemp, J., Hemphill, L., & Vojir, C. (2002). Outcomes of therapeutic massage for hospitalized cancer patients. *Journal of Nursing Scholarship, 34*(3), 257–262.
Snyder, J. R. (1999). Therapeutic touch in hospice care. In C. Hutchison, Healing touch: An energetic approach. *American Journal of Nursing, 99*(4), 46.
Spencer, J., & Jacobs, J. (Eds.) (1999). *Complementary/alternative medicine: An evidence-based approach.* St. Louis, MO: Mosby.
Stanley-Hermanns, M., & Miller, J. (2002). Animal-assisted therapy. *American Journal of Nursing, 102*(10), 69–76.
Stedman, M. (1999). Alternatives: You'd better shop around. *Health, 13*(1), 60–66.
Sutherland, J. (2000). Getting to the point. *American Journal of Nursing, 100*(9), 40–43.
Trevelyan, J. (1993). Aromatherapy. *Nursing Times, 89*(25), 38–40.
Vacca, V. (1998). Back to high touch. *RN, 69*(7), 88.
Weil, A. (1998). *Natural health, natural medicine: A comprehensive manual for wellness and self-care* (Rev. ed.). New York: Houghton Mifflin.
Weil, A. (2000). *Spontaneous healing: How to discover and enhance your body's natural ability to maintain and heal itself.* New York: Ivy Books.

RESOURCES

Acupressure Institute, http://www.acupressureinstitute.com
American Academy of Medical Acupuncture (AAMA), http://www.medicalacupuncture.org
American Holistic Nurses Association (AHNA), http://www.ahna.org
American Massage Therapy Association (AMTA), http://www.amtamassage.org
Association for Applied Psychophysiology and Biofeedback (AAPB), http://www.aapb.org
Association for Applied and Therapeutic Humor (AATH), http://www.aath.org
Healing Touch International, Inc., http://www.healingtouchinternational.org
International Iridology Practitioners Association, http://www.iridologyassn.org
National Center for Complementary and Alternative Medicine, National Institutes of Health, http://www.nccam.nih.gov
Tai Chi Association, http://www.tai-chi-association.com
Yoga Research and Education Foundation (YREF), http://www.yref.org

CHAPTER 18
Basic Nutrition

MAKING THE CONNECTION

Refer to the following chapters to increase your understanding of nutrition:

Basic Nursing
- ***Life Span Development***
- ***Cultural Considerations***
- ***Diagnostic Tests***

Basic Procedures
- ***Hand Hygiene***
- ***Measuring Intake and Output***

Intermediate Procedures
- ***Feeding and Medicating via Enteral Tube***

LEARNING OBJECTIVES

Upon completion of this chapter, you should be able to:

- Define key terms.
- Describe the role of the nurse in promoting proper nutrition.
- Explain how the body uses nutrients.
- Compare the six types of nutrients for functions, sources, digestion, absorption, storage, and signs of deficiency and excess.
- Describe factors affecting kilocalorie needs.
- Explain the food guide pyramid.
- Explain the purposes of the Dietary Guidelines for Americans and the recommended dietary allowances (RDAs).
- Discuss factors influencing nutrition.
- Explain the dietary needs and nutritional assessments for infancy, childhood, adolescence, older adulthood, pregnancy, and lactation.
- Explain the relationship between health and nutrition.
- Discuss weight management.
- Explain how to determine energy (kcal) needs.
- Describe three ways to promote food safety.
- Describe the standard hospital diets: regular, soft, liquid, mechanical, and pureed.

- Cite the proper procedure for serving a meal tray.
- List important points to follow when feeding a client.

KEY TERMS

absorption
anabolism
anthropometric measurements
atherosclerosis
basal metabolism
body mass index
calorie
catabolism
cholesterol
chyme
complete proteins
deglutition
dehydration
diet therapy
dietary prescription/order
digestion
enriched
enteral nutrition
euglycemia
excretion
extracellular fluid
fat-soluble vitamins
fortified
gluconeogenesis
glycogenesis
glycogenolysis
hyperglycemia
hypoglycemia
incomplete proteins
ingestion
insensible water loss
insulin
interstitial fluid
intracellular fluid
ketosis
kilocalories
kwashiorkor
lipids
marasmus
mastication
metabolic rate
metabolism
monounsaturated fatty acids
nutrition
obesity
oxidation
parenteral nutrition
peristalsis
phospholipids
polyunsaturated fatty acids
satiety
sensible water loss
triglycerides
vitamins
water-soluble vitamins

INTRODUCTION

Nutrition encompasses all of the processes involved in consuming and utilizing food for energy, maintenance, and growth. These processes are ingestion, digestion, absorption, metabolism, and excretion. Much of the discussion throughout this chapter focuses on ingestion because this is the process that the individual can control and with which the nurse can be of assistance to the client. Basic information is presented about proper nutrition and the role of the nurse in assisting clients to meet their nutritional needs. Topics covered include specific nutrients and their functions in the body; phytochemicals; promoting proper nutrition; factors influencing nutrition; nutritional needs during the life cycle; nutrition and health; weight management; food labeling, quality, and safety; food allergies; and nutrition and the nursing process.

PHYSIOLOGY OF NUTRITION

Five processes are involved in the body's use of nutrients: ingestion, digestion, absorption, metabolism, and excretion.

INGESTION

Nutrition begins with **ingestion**, taking food into the digestive tract, generally through the mouth. In special circumstances, ingestion occurs directly into the stomach, through a feeding tube; this situation is discussed later in the chapter.

DIGESTION

Digestion refers to the mechanical and chemical processes that convert nutrients into a physically absorbable state. Mechanical digestion includes **mastication** (chewing), breaking food into fine particles and mixing it with enzymes in saliva, and **deglutition** (swallowing food), the peristaltic waves and mucus secretions that move the food down the esophagus.

PROFESSIONAL TIP

Role of the LP/VN in Meeting Nutritional Needs

There are several aspects to the role of the licensed practical/vocational nurse (LP/VN) in meeting a client's nutritional needs. These are discussed throughout the chapter and are summarized as follows:

- Teach clients ways to meet their nutritional needs.
- Receive and implement physician's orders.
- Help clients understand their diets.
- Assist clients with eating their meals.
- Report and record observations about nutrient intake and the nutritional status of clients.
- Act as a communication link between the client, the physician, and the dietitian.

Chemical digestion is the process whereby enzymes, gastric and intestinal juices, bile, and pancreatic juices change food into the individual nutrients that can be used by the body.

Digestion begins in the stomach (except in the case of some starches, for which digestion begins in the mouth) and is completed in the intestines. **Peristalsis** (rhythmic, coordinated, serial contractions of the smooth muscles of the GI tract) forces **chyme** (an acidic, semifluid paste) through the small and large intestines. Only carbohydrates, proteins, and fats require chemical digestion to make the nutrients available for absorption. Figure 18-1 illustrates the basic elements and functions of the digestive system.

Absorption

Absorption is the process whereby the end products of digestion (i.e., individual nutrients) pass through the epithelial membranes in the small and large intestines and into the blood or lymph systems. The nutrients are absorbed and taken to the parts of the body that need them. Most nutrients are water soluble and can be absorbed directly through the villi (fingerlike projections that line the small intestine) and into the blood. Fats, which are not water soluble, are absorbed first into the lymph system and eventually enter the circulatory system.

Metabolism

The conversion of nutrients into energy by the body is called **metabolism**; this process is the sum total of all the biological and chemical processes in the body as they relate to the use of nutrients in every body cell. Metabolism involves two processes: anabolism and catabolism. **Anabolism** is the constructive process of metabolism, wherein new molecules are synthesized and new tissues are formed, as in growth and repair. This process requires energy. **Catabolism** is the destructive process of metabolism, wherein tissues or substances are broken into their component parts. This process releases energy. During metabolism, energy is also produced by the process of **oxidation**, which is the chemical process of combining nutrients with oxygen. The energy produced by the body is used in a number of ways: electrical energy for brain and nerve activities, chemical energy for metabolism, mechanical energy for muscle contractions, and thermal energy to keep the body warm.

Metabolic rate is the rate of energy utilization in the body; it is expressed in units called calories. One **calorie** is the amount of heat required to raise the temperature of one gram of water by 1° Celsius. Because of the large quantity of energy released during metabolism, the energy is expressed in **kilocalories** (kcal), each of which is equal to 1,000 calories.

Basal metabolism is the amount of energy needed to maintain essential physiologic functions, when a person is at *complete* rest. It is the lowest level of energy expenditure.

The major factor affecting basal metabolism is body composition. Lean muscle tissue has a higher metabolic rate and thus produces more energy than does fatty tissue. Generally, women have a lower metabolism than men because they

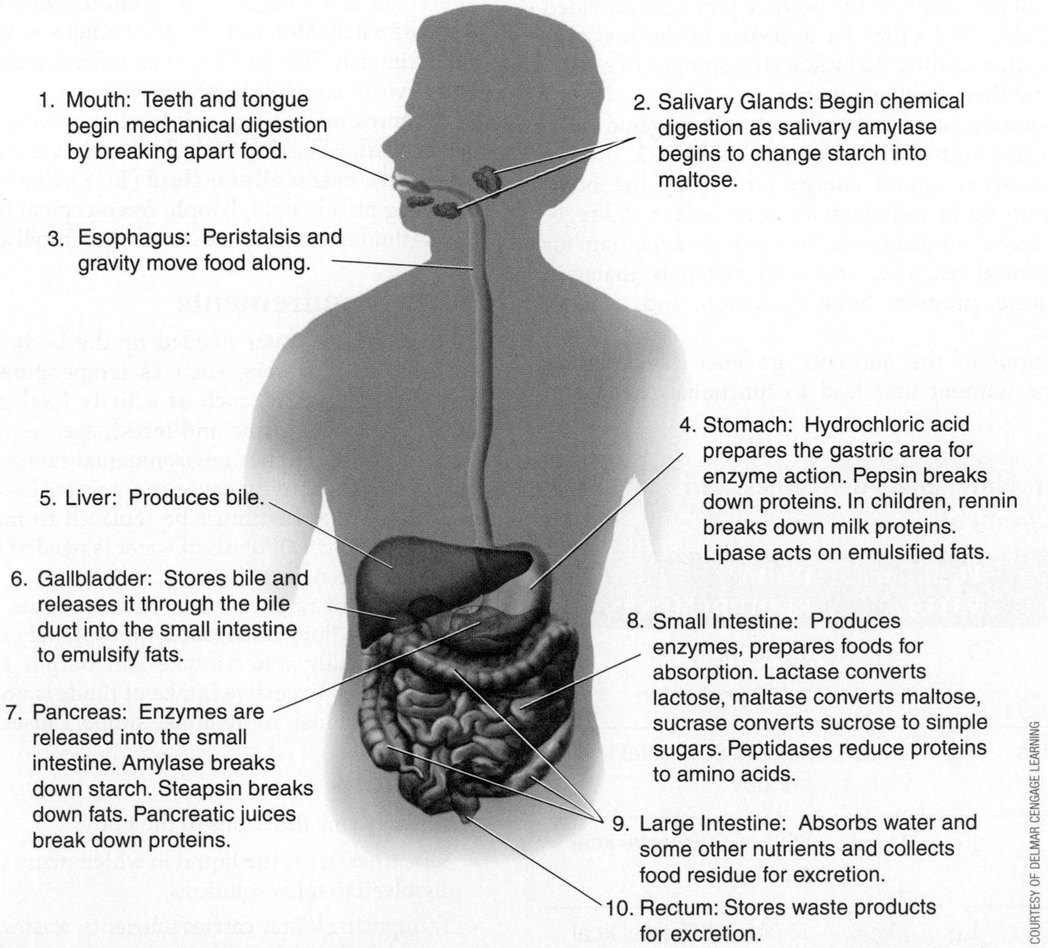

1. Mouth: Teeth and tongue begin mechanical digestion by breaking apart food.
2. Salivary Glands: Begin chemical digestion as salivary amylase begins to change starch into maltose.
3. Esophagus: Peristalsis and gravity move food along.
4. Stomach: Hydrochloric acid prepares the gastric area for enzyme action. Pepsin breaks down proteins. In children, rennin breaks down milk proteins. Lipase acts on emulsified fats.
5. Liver: Produces bile.
6. Gallbladder: Stores bile and releases it through the bile duct into the small intestine to emulsify fats.
7. Pancreas: Enzymes are released into the small intestine. Amylase breaks down starch. Steapsin breaks down fats. Pancreatic juices break down proteins.
8. Small Intestine: Produces enzymes, prepares foods for absorption. Lactase converts lactose, maltase converts maltose, sucrase converts sucrose to simple sugars. Peptidases reduce proteins to amino acids.
9. Large Intestine: Absorbs water and some other nutrients and collects food residue for excretion.
10. Rectum: Stores waste products for excretion.
COURTESY OF DELMAR CENGAGE LEARNING

FIGURE 18-1 Functions of the Digestive System

have a higher percentage of fat tissue; however, metabolism increases during menstruation, pregnancy, and lactation. Age is also an influence because growth periods increase metabolism. Glandular activity, especially of the thyroid gland, affects metabolism. The rate of metabolism is governed primarily by the hormones triiodothyronine (T3) and thyroxine (T4). Hypothyroid activity, a decrease in the secretion of thyroid hormones, causes a lower rate of metabolism, whereas hyperthyroid activity, an increase in the secretion of thyroid hormones, causes a higher rate of metabolism.

Excretion

Excretion is the process of eliminating or removing waste products from the body. Dietary fiber and other indigestible materials, salts, and other products such as bile and water are formed into feces and excreted from the body as solid waste. Other excretory organs that aid the digestive system in the elimination of wastes include the kidneys, bladder, sweat glands, skin, and lungs. Most liquid waste is sent through the kidneys and bladder to be excreted as urine. Some liquid waste is removed through the sweat glands of the skin as perspiration. Gaseous waste is eliminated through the lungs.

NUTRIENTS

The body must have six types of nutrients to function efficiently and effectively. These are water, carbohydrates, fats, proteins, vitamins, and minerals. If a person eats a well-balanced diet, all the nutrients the body requires are provided by the food. Table 18-1 offers an overview of the first four nutrients in relation to their fuel value (the amount of energy they supply) and their daily requirements.

Nutrients are classified as energy nutrients, organic nutrients, and inorganic nutrients, as shown in Table 18-2.

Energy nutrients release energy for use by the body. Organic nutrients build and maintain body tissues and regulate body processes. Inorganic nutrients provide a medium for the body's chemical reactions, transport materials, maintain body temperature, promote bone formation, and conduct nerve impulses.

The functions of the nutrients are interrelated. Intake changes in one nutrient may lead to functional changes in another. Some examples of interrelated functions include that (a) iron is better absorbed when vitamin C is present and that (b) calcium absorption depends on the presence of vitamin D.

Table 18-1 Nutrients, Fuel Values, and Daily Requirements

NUTRIENT	FUEL VALUE	DAILY REQUIREMENTS
Water	0	1,000 mL/ 1,000 kcal eaten
Carbohydrates	1 g = 4 kcal	50% to 60% total kcal per day
Fats	1 g = 9 kcal	25% to 30% total kcal per day
Protein	1 g = 4 kcal	15% to 20% total kcal per day

COURTESY OF DELMAR CENGAGE LEARNING

Table 18-2 Classification of Nutrients

CLASSES	NUTRIENTS
Energy nutrients	Carbohydrates Fats (Lipids) Proteins
Organic nutrients	Carbohydrates Fats (Lipids) Proteins Vitamins
Inorganic nutrients	Water Minerals

COURTESY OF DELMAR CENGAGE LEARNING

Water

Water is the most important nutrient. It is more vital to life than is food. Virtually all body functions require water. An individual may live for weeks without food but for only approximately 10 days without water.

Water is the major constituent in every cell of the body. Approximately 55% to 65% of an adult's weight is water, and approximately 70% to 75% of an infant's weight is water. The body's water content decreases with age.

Approximately two-thirds of the water in the body is **intracellular fluid** (ICF), fluid within the cells. The other one-third is **extracellular fluid** (ECF), fluid outside the cells, including plasma fluid, lymph, cerebrospinal fluid, **interstitial fluid** (fluid in tissue spaces around each cell), and GI fluids.

Daily Requirements

The amount of water needed by the body varies based on environmental factors, such as temperature and humidity, and physical factors, such as activity level, metabolic need, functional losses (urine and feces), age, respiratory rate, and state of health. Higher environmental temperatures and vigorous physical activity cause more water loss as perspiration increases. Water lost must be replaced to maintain metabolism. Generally, 1,000 mL of water is needed to process every 1,000 kcal eaten.

A state of relative water balance exists when the body has adequate fluid distributed appropriately as ICF and ECF. A person's daily water intake and output should be equal (Figure 18-2). Excessive intake of fluids is not a problem in a healthy individual; more intake simply causes more output.

Functions

Water has many functions in the body:

- *Solvent:* Water is the liquid in which many substances are dissolved to form solutions.
- *Transporter:* Water carries nutrients, wastes, and other materials throughout the body and to and from each cell via blood, tissue fluids, and body secretions.

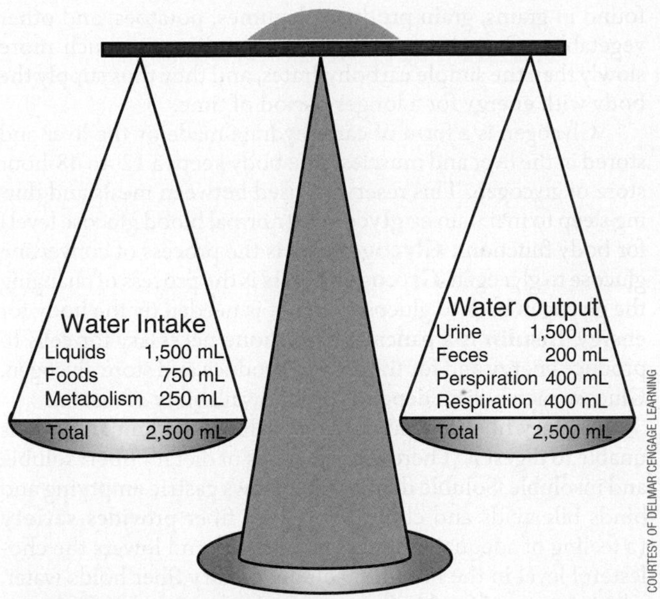

FIGURE 18-2 Body Water Balance (Approximate Figures for a Sedentary Adult)

- *Regulator of body temperature:* Water is excreted as perspiration when the temperature goes up. Evaporation of perspiration cools the body.
- *Lubricant:* Water is a component of fluid within the joints, called synovial fluid, which provides smooth movement of the many joints in the body.
- *Component of all cells:* Water gives structure and form to the body.
- *Hydrolysis:* Water breaks apart substances, especially in metabolism.

Classification and Sources

There are three sources of water for the body:

- Liquids consumed, including water, coffee, juice, tea, milk, and soft drinks
- Foods consumed, especially vegetables and fruits
- Metabolism, which produces water when oxidization occurs

Digestion, Absorption, and Storage

Water is not digested but, rather, is absorbed and used by the body as we drink it. It is not stored by the body and is excreted daily. Water losses are classified as **sensible**, the person is aware of the loss, or **insensible**, the person is not generally aware of the loss. There are four ways the body normally loses water:

- *Urine:* accounts for the greatest amount of water lost from the body (sensible loss)
- *Feces:* contains a small amount of water (insensible loss, except in cases of diarrhea)
- *Perspiration:* varies with temperature, but some fluid is always lost (insensible or sensible loss)
- *Respiration:* releases moisture with every breath (insensible loss)

> **LIFE SPAN CONSIDERATIONS**
>
> **Dehydration**
>
> Infants, small children, and elderly persons are more susceptible to dehydration. For them, dehydration occurs more rapidly and is more severe.

Signs of Deficiency and Excess

Abnormal water losses from the body include profuse sweating, vomiting, diarrhea, hemorrhage, wound drainage (burns), fever, and edema. With edema, the water is still in the body but is not usable.

A deficiency of water is called **dehydration**. Prolonged dehydration results in death. Some conditions cause an excessive accumulation of fluid in the body. This condition is called *positive water balance.* It occurs when more water is taken in than is used and excreted, and edema results. Hypothyroidism, congestive heart failure, hypoproteinemia (low amounts of protein), some infections and cancers, and some renal conditions can cause water retention because sodium is not being excreted normally.

CARBOHYDRATES

Carbohydrates are made of the elements carbon, hydrogen, and oxygen. In nutrition, the first letters of these three elements are used as the abbreviation: CHO.

Carbohydrates constitute the chief source of energy for all body functions. They are also the major food source for all people because they are the least expensive and the most abundant foods.

> **PROFESSIONALTIP**
>
> **Signs and Symptoms of Dehydration**
>
> - Health history reveals inadequate intake of fluids.
> - Urine output is decreased.
> - Urine specific gravity is greater than 1.035.
> - Weight loss (% body weight) is 3% to 5% for mild, 6% to 9% for moderate, and 10% to 15% for severe dehydration.
> - Eyes appear sunken; tongue displays increased furrows and fissures.
> - Oral mucous membranes are dry.
> - Skin turgor is decreased.
> - Venous filling and emptying times are delayed (longer than 3 to 5 seconds).
> - In infants, fontanels are sunken.
> - Changes in neurological status may occur with moderate to severe dehydration.
>
> (From *Health Assessment and Physical Examination* [4th ed.], by M. E. Z. Estes, 2010, Clifton Park, NY: Delmar Cengage Learning.)

Daily Requirements

It is recommended that carbohydrates make up 50% to 60% of an individual's kcal intake per day. For example, if an individual's total energy requirement is 2,000 kcal, 50% of this number is 1,000; this number is then divided by 4 (the number of kcal in each gram of carbohydrate; Table 18-1), for an estimated carbohydrate requirement of 250 g/day. It is estimated that current U.S. diets contain only 45% of their kcal from carbohydrates (Roth, 2006).

Functions

Carbohydrates constitute the primary source of energy for the body. The body must maintain a constant supply of energy; therefore, it stores approximately one-half a day's supply of carbohydrates in the liver and muscles for use as needed. A sufficient supply of carbohydrates spares proteins from being used for energy, thus allowing proteins to perform their primary function of building and repairing body tissues. Carbohydrates are needed to oxidize fats completely and for synthesis of fatty acids and amino acids. The central nervous system and erythrocytes rely solely on carbohydrates for energy.

Classification and Sources

Carbohydrates are classified as either simple or complex. Simple carbohydrates are single sugars (monosaccharides) such as glucose, fructose, and galactose found in fruits, honey, and corn syrup. Monosaccharides require no digestion, are quickly absorbed, and are either used for energy or stored as glycogen.

Double sugars (disaccharides), such as sucrose, maltose, and lactose, are two single sugars joined together. They are found in milk, sweeteners, sugar, and molasses. Before they can be absorbed by the body, disaccharides must be separated into monosaccharides through digestion.

Complex carbohydrates (polysaccharides) are composed of many single sugars joined together. Those important in nutrition are starch, glycogen, and dietary fiber (cellulose). The most significant of these in the diet is starch, which is found in grains, grain products, legumes, potatoes, and other vegetables. Complex carbohydrates are digested much more slowly than the simple carbohydrates, and they thus supply the body with energy for a longer period of time.

Glycogen is a form of carbohydrate made by the liver and stored in the liver and muscles. The body keeps a 12- to 48-hour store of glycogen. This reserve is used between meals and during sleep to maintain **euglycemia** (normal blood glucose level) for body functions. **Glycogenesis** is the process of converting glucose to glycogen. **Glycogenolysis** is the process of changing the glycogen back to glucose when it is needed by the body for energy. **Insulin** is a pancreatic hormone necessary for cells to produce energy and for the liver to produce and store glycogen. Glucose metabolism depends on the availability of insulin.

Dietary fiber has no nutritive value: The human body is unable to digest it. There are two types of dietary fiber: soluble and insoluble. Soluble dietary fiber slows gastric emptying and binds bile acids and cholesterol. This fiber provides **satiety** (a feeling of adequate fullness from food) and lowers the cholesterol level in the blood. Insoluble dietary fiber holds water, which increases fecal bulk and stimulates peristalsis for better elimination. Good sources of both kinds of dietary fiber are whole grains, whole-grain products, legumes, and fruits and vegetables with their skins.

PROFESSIONAL TIP

Insulin Levels and the Client Who Is Diabetic

When the secretion of insulin is impaired or absent, the glucose level in the blood becomes excessively high. This condition is called **hyperglycemia** and is usually a symptom of diabetes mellitus. If control by diet is ineffective, insulin injections or an oral hypoglycemic must be used to control blood sugar. When insulin is given, the client's intake of carbohydrates must be carefully controlled to balance the prescribed dosage of insulin. **Hypoglycemia** occurs when blood glucose levels are unusually low. A mild form of hypoglycemia may occur if one waits too long between meals or if the pancreas secretes too much insulin. Symptoms include fatigue, shaking, sweating, and headache.

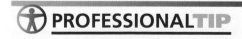

Digestion, Absorption, and Storage

Digestion of cooked starches begins in the mouth, when the salivary enzyme ptyalin mixes with the starch in food during chewing. Little digestion takes place in the stomach. Carbohydrate digestion is completed in the small intestine by pancreatic and intestinal enzymes present there. Carbohydrates leave no waste for the kidneys to eliminate.

Glucose and other monosaccharides, the final products of carbohydrate digestion, are absorbed into the blood through the capillaries in the villi of the intestinal mucosa. Fructose and other monosaccharides are converted to glucose in the liver.

Glucose not needed for immediate energy is converted to glycogen by the liver and stored there and in the muscles. Any remaining glucose is then converted to fatty acids and stored as adipose tissue (fat). The body has no way to rid itself of excess carbohydrates; they are either used or stored.

Signs of Deficiency and Excess

A mild deficiency of carbohydrates can result in weight loss and fatigue. A diet seriously deficient in carbohydrates causes

PROFESSIONAL TIP

Lactose Intolerance

Many adults are unable to digest lactose and suffer from bloating, abdominal cramps, and diarrhea after drinking milk or consuming milk-based food products such as processed cheese. This reaction is called lactose intolerance. It is caused by insufficient lactase, the enzyme required for digestion of lactose. Special low-lactose milk products can be used instead of regular milk. Lactase-containing products are also available.

extra fat to be metabolized to meet the body's energy needs. Without carbohydrates, fat is incompletely oxidized, producing ketones, an acid by-product, which accumulates in the blood and urine causing **ketosis**. Ketosis can result from uncontrolled insulin-dependent diabetes mellitus, starvation, or diets extremely low in carbohydrates. It can lead to coma and even death.

Excess carbohydrate consumption is one of the most common causes of obesity. Although some of the surplus carbohydrate is changed to glycogen, the major part of any surplus becomes adipose tissue. Too many carbohydrates may cause tooth decay, irritate the lining of the stomach, or cause flatulence.

FATS

Fats constitute the most concentrated source of energy in the diet, providing 9 kcal per gram of fat. People in developed countries tend to eat diets relatively high in fat. Although fat is an essential nutrient, too much fat is a hazard to good health. *Lipids* is the descriptive word for fats of all kinds. **Lipids** are organic compounds that are insoluble in water but soluble in organic solvents, such as ether and alcohol, and include true fats and fatlike compounds such as lipoids and sterols. Fats provide slightly more than twice the calorie content of carbohydrates. Like carbohydrates, fats are composed of carbon, hydrogen, and oxygen, but they have a substantially lower proportion of oxygen.

Daily Requirements

It is recommended that fats make up no more than 25% to 30% of an individual's caloric intake per day. For example, assuming that one's total energy requirement is 2,000 kcal/day, one-quarter (25%) of this would be 500 kcal. Dividing 500 kcal by 9 (the number of kcal in each gram of fat; Table 18-1) yields an estimated fat requirement of 55.5 g/day.

Functions

Fat has many functions in the body. It:

- Provides a concentrated source of energy (more than twice the kcal of carbohydrates)
- Assists in the absorption of fat-soluble vitamins
- Is a major component of cell membranes and myelin sheaths
- Improves the flavor of food and delays the stomach's emptying time, providing a feeling of satiety
- Protects and helps hold organs in place
- Insulates the body, thus assisting in temperature maintenance

CLIENTTEACHING

Fats

The average American fat intake has decreased to 33% of the total daily caloric intake. The total fat intake should be less than 30% of an individual's daily caloric intake with no more than 10% of total kcal as saturated fats, 10% polyunsaturated fats, and 10% monounsaturated fats. For example, if an individual consumes 2,000 calories a day, she should eat no more than 65 grams of fat, or about 600 calories of fat (University of Iowa Health Care, 2006).

Classification and Sources

Fat is formed by one molecule of glycerol being joined to one, two, or three fatty-acid molecules. The most important lipids are:

- **Triglycerides** (true fats), composed of one glycerol molecule attached to three fatty-acid molecules. Most dietary fat and body fat are triglycerides.
- **Phospholipids** (lipoids), composed of glycerol, fatty acids, and phosphorus. They are structural components of cells, for example, myelin (insulating covering of many nerves) and lecithin (a part of cell membranes).
- **Cholesterol** (a sterol), not essential in the diet because the liver manufactures approximately 1,000 mg every day. Cholesterol is found in all cell membranes, in brain and nerve tissue, and in blood, and it is excreted in bile. Cholesterol is required to produce several hormones, including estrogen, testosterone, adrenalin, and cortisone. The intake of dietary cholesterol from animal food products may affect the serum (blood) cholesterol level.

Fats can also be classified by source, visibility, and saturation. The source of fats can be either animal or plant (vegetable). Examples of animal fat are lard, butter, milk, cream, egg yolks, and the fat in meat, poultry, and fish. Examples of plant fat are oils (corn, safflower, olive, cottonseed, peanut, palm, and coconut), nuts, and avocado.

Fats are either visible or invisible. Visible fats are easy to identify, such as butter, oils, margarine, lard, shortening, bacon, salt pork, and the fat around beef. Examples of invisible fats are those in egg yolks, whole milk and whole-milk

CLIENTTEACHING

Blood Cholesterol

- Blood cholesterol level should not exceed 200 mg of cholesterol/dL of blood.
- To decrease the blood cholesterol level, the client should follow a diet low in saturated fat.
- Weight loss and exercise also help lower blood cholesterol level.
- A diet high in saturated fat increases the blood cholesterol by 15% to 25%.

LIFE SPAN CONSIDERATIONS

Children and Cholesterol

If children are not fed high-cholesterol foods on a regular basis, their chance of overusing these foods as adults lessens, as does their risk of heart attack and stroke.

products, cheeses, nuts, seeds, olives, avocados, many desserts, and baked goods.

The saturation of a fat refers to its chemical composition. When fatty acids, the main building blocks of fats, contain all the hydrogen ions possible in the molecule, they are said to be saturated. Saturated fats tend to be solid at room temperature. Generally, animal fats are saturated. Plant fats that are saturated are coconut, palm kernel, and palm oils. Unsaturated fats are missing a hydrogen ion at one or more places in the molecule. They tend to be soft or liquid at room temperature. Plant fats are generally unsaturated, with the exceptions already mentioned. Unsaturated fats are subdivided into monounsaturated and polyunsaturated fats. **Monounsaturated fatty acids** are those that form glycerol esters with one double or triple bond; foods in this category are nuts, fowl, and olive oil. **Polyunsaturated fatty acids** form glycerol esters that have many carbons unbonded to hydrogen atoms. Foods such as fish, corn, sunflower seeds, soybeans, cottonseeds, and safflower oil contain polyunsaturated fat.

There are three essential fatty acids (linoleic, linolenic, and arachidonic) necessary for growth, cholesterol metabolism, and heart action. They are found primarily in vegetable oils, egg yolks, and poultry.

Digestion, Absorption, and Storage

No chemical breakdown of fats occurs in the mouth, and very little fat digestion takes place in the stomach. When fat reaches the small intestine, digestion begins. The digestive agents for fat are bile, from the gallbladder, and enzymes, from the pancreas and the small intestine. The final products of fat digestion are fatty acids and glycerol. Approximately 95% of dietary fat is absorbed in the small intestine.

Fats not immediately needed by the body are stored as adipose tissue. Approximately 5 g of fat are excreted daily in the feces.

Signs of Deficiency and Excess

Deficiency symptoms occur when fats provide less than 10% of the total daily kcal requirement. Gross deficiency may result in eczema (inflamed and scaly skin condition), retarded growth, and weight loss.

Excess fat in the diet can lead to overweight and heart disease. In addition, studies point to an association between high-fat diets and cancers of the colon, breast, uterus, and prostate.

An elevated level of cholesterol in the blood is thought to be a contributing factor in heart disease, because hypercholesterolemia (high serum cholesterol) is common in clients with atherosclerosis. **Atherosclerosis** is a cardiovascular disease wherein plaque (fatty deposits containing cholesterol and other substances) forms on the inside of artery walls, reducing the space for blood flow.

> **LIFE SPAN CONSIDERATIONS**
>
> **Proteins**
>
> By the age of 4 years, body protein content reaches the adult level of approximately 18% of body weight.

PROTEIN

Proteins are made of the elements carbon, hydrogen, oxygen, and nitrogen. In nutrition, the first letters of these four elements are used as the abbreviation: CHON.

Protein is the only nutrient that can build, repair, and maintain body tissues. An adequate supply of proteins in the daily diet is essential. All tissues and fluids in the body, with the exception of bile and urine, contain some protein. The basic building materials of protein are amino acids.

Daily Requirements

Daily protein requirement is determined by size, age, gender, and physical and emotional condition. A large person has more body cells to maintain than does a small person. A growing child, a pregnant woman, or a woman who is breastfeeding needs more protein for each pound of body weight than does the average adult. When digestion is inefficient, fewer amino acids are absorbed by the body; consequently, the protein requirement is higher. This is sometimes thought to be the case with elderly clients. Extra proteins are usually required after surgery or severe burns or during infections to replace lost tissue and manufacture antibodies. In addition, emotional trauma can cause the body to excrete more nitrogen than it normally does, thus increasing the need for protein-rich foods.

The National Research Council of the National Academy of Sciences considers the average adult's daily requirement to be 0.8 g of protein for each kilogram of body weight. Daily protein requirement is determined by multiplying body weight in kilograms (weight in pounds divided by 2.2) by 0.8. For instance:

$$\begin{aligned} 130 \text{ lb. woman} \div 2.2 \text{ lb/kg} &= 59.1 \text{ kg} \times 0.8 \text{ g/kg} \\ &= 47.3 \text{ g protein/day} \end{aligned}$$

Functions

The primary function of protein in the diet is to provide the amino acids necessary for the synthesis of body proteins, which are used to build, repair, and maintain the body tissues. Protein composes most of the muscles, skin, hair, nails, brain, nerves, and internal organs.

Another function of protein is to assist in regulating fluid balance. Proteins are a vital part of enzymes, hormones, and blood plasma. Many body processes are regulated by enzymes and hormones. Plasma proteins help control water balance between the circulatory system and surrounding tissues. Protein is also used to build antibodies, which help defend the body against disease and foreign substances.

In the event of insufficient stores of carbohydrate and fat (the body's primary and secondary sources of energy), protein, in the form of amino acids, can be converted into glucose and used for energy. This process is called **gluconeogenesis**; however, when protein is used for energy, it is not available for its primary function. Using protein for energy also results in waste products that are difficult for the kidneys to excrete.

Classification and Sources

Protein is classified by source and completeness. Animal sources include meat, fish, poultry, eggs, milk, and dairy products. Plant sources are grains, legumes, nuts, and seeds. The completeness of a protein refers to its quality. Of the 22 amino acids, nine are called essential amino acids (i.e., they must be present in the diet because the body cannot synthesize them). **Complete proteins** contain all nine essential amino acids. All animal proteins, with the exception of gelatin, are complete proteins; the only complete plant protein is soybeans.

Plant proteins (with the exception of soybeans) are **incomplete proteins** (i.e., one or more of the essential amino acids are missing). Because all plant proteins do not lack the same essential amino acids, they can be combined in various ways to provide all the essential amino acids. When two plant protein foods are combined to provide the essential amino acids, they are said to be complementary. Some of the common complementary plant proteins are rice and beans (legumes), corn and beans, wheat bread and beans, toast and pea soup, and rice and lentils. Complementary proteins are a very important part of planning a healthy vegetarian diet.

Digestion, Absorption, and Storage

Chemical digestion of protein begins in the stomach, when hydrochloric acid activates the enzyme pepsin; however, most of the digestion takes place in the small intestine with the action of pancreatic and intestinal enzymes. The end product of protein digestion is amino acids. The body can then combine the amino acids to build, repair, and maintain body tissues.

The amino acids are absorbed into the blood by the capillaries in the villi of the intestinal mucosa. Amino acids not used to build proteins are converted to glucose, glycogen, or fat and are stored.

Signs of Deficiency and Excess

When people are unable to obtain an adequate supply of protein for an extended period, muscle wasting occurs, and arms and legs become very thin. At the same time, albumin (protein in blood plasma) deficiency causes edema, resulting in an extremely swollen appearance. The edema decreases when sufficient protein is eaten. Clients with edema become lethargic and depressed. These signs are seen in grossly neglected children or in the elderly poor or incapacitated. Children who lack sufficient protein do not grow to their potential size. Infants born to mothers eating insufficient protein during pregnancy can have permanently impaired mental capacities (Roth, 2006).

Two deficiency diseases that affect children are caused by a grossly inadequate supply of protein, energy, or both. **Marasmus**, a condition resulting from severe malnutrition, afflicts very young children who lack both energy and protein foods as well as vitamins and minerals. The infant with marasmus appears emaciated but does not have edema; hair is dull and dry, and the skin is thin and wrinkled. **Kwashiorkor** results when there is a sudden or recent lack of protein-containing food (such as during a famine). This disease results in edema, painful skin lesions, and changes in the pigmentation of skin and hair (Roth, 2006).

It is easy for people living in the developed parts of the world to ingest more protein than the body requires. This should be avoided because the saturated fats and cholesterol common to complete protein foods may contribute to heart disease and provide more kcal than needed. Some studies indicate a connection between long-term high-protein diets and colon cancer and high calcium excretion, which depletes the bones of calcium and may contribute to osteoporosis. People who eat excessive amounts of protein-rich foods may ignore essential fruits and vegetables, and excess protein intake may put more demands on the kidneys than they can handle (Roth, 2006).

PROFESSIONALTIP

Daily Allowance of Protein

The National Research Council recommends that protein intake represent no more than 15% to 20% of one's daily kcal intake and not exceed double the amount given in the table of Recommended Dietary Allowances.

PROFESSIONALTIP

Vegetarians and Protein

It is essential that clients following vegetarian diets carefully calculate the types and amount of protein in their diets to prevent protein deficiency.

VITAMINS

Vitamins are organic compounds essential to life and health. They regulate body processes and are needed in very small amounts. They have no fuel value but are required for the metabolism of fats, carbohydrates, and proteins.

Daily Requirements

The Food and Nutrition Board of the National Academy of Sciences—National Research Council prepared a list of recommended dietary allowances for the 11 vitamins for which it considers current scientific research to be adequate for determining daily recommendations. Vitamin allowances are given by weight in milligrams (mg) or micrograms (mcg).

Vitamins taken in addition to the diet are called vitamin supplements. Lifestyle choices may affect the need for vitamin supplementation (Table 18-3).

Functions

The functions of vitamins are unique to each individual vitamin. Tables 18-4 and 18-5 list the functions of each type of vitamin.

TABLE 18-3 Supplements for Lifestyle Choices

LIFESTYLE CHOICE	SUGGESTED SUPPLEMENT
Restricted diets	B_{12} (cobalamin)
Extensive exercise program	Riboflavin
Oral contraceptives	Pyridoine, niacin, vitamin C
Smoking	Vitamin C
Alcohol	Thiamine, folate
Caffeine	B vitamins, vitamin C

TABLE 18-4 Fat-Soluble Vitamins

VITAMIN	FUNCTION	SOURCES	DEFICIENCY	TOXIC EFFECTS
A	• Aids in night vision • Promotes growth of bones and teeth • Maintains skin and mucous membranes	• Fish oils • Carrots • Sweet potatoes • Broccoli • Cantaloupe • Green leafy vegetables	• Night blindness • Dry, scaly skin • Diarrhea • Respiratory infections	• From supplementation: anorexia, diarrhea, hair loss, bone pain, liver damage
D	• Stimulates absorption of calcium and phosphorus for good bone mineralization	• Yeast • Fish liver oils • Fortified milk and cereals	• Rickets • Malformed teeth • Bone deformities	• Hypercalcemia • Kidney stones • Cardiovascular damage
E	• Acts as an antioxidant • Maintains cell membrane integrity • Protects red blood cells (RBCs) from hemolysis	• Vegetable oils • Leafy vegetables • Wheat germ	• Increased RBC hemolysis • Rare, except in cases of fat malabsorption	• Depression • Fatigue • Diarrhea • Cramps • Headaches
K	• Responsible for synthesis of prothrombin, needed for normal blood clotting	• Dark-green leafy vegetables • Made by intestinal bacteria	• Rare, except in newborns • Delayed blood clotting	• No toxic effects

COURTESY OF DELMAR CENGAGE LEARNING

TABLE 18-5 Water-Soluble Vitamins

VITAMIN	FUNCTION	SOURCES	DEFICIENCY	TOXIC EFFECTS
C (asorbic acid)	• Builds and maintains strong tissues • Promotes wound healing • Aids in resisting infection • Enhances iron absorption	• Citrus fruits • Green and red peppers • Tomatoes • Melons • Cabbage • Broccoli • Strawberries	• Scurvy • Easy bruising • Delayed wound healing • Swollen, inflamed gums • Secondary infections	• Megadoses: excessive iron absorption • Nausea • Diarrhea
B_1 (thiamine)	• Promotes CHO metabolism • Ensures normal nervous system functioning	• Enriched grains and cereals • Pork • Legumes	• Beriberi • Mental confusion • Anorexia • Fatigue • Muscle weakness	• None known
B_2 (riboflavin)	• Promotes CHO, protein, and fat metabolism • Promotes deoxyribonucleic acid (DNA) synthesis • Aids in protein synthesis	• Milk and milk products • Meat, poultry, fish • Enriched grains and cereals	• Oral lesions • Dermatitis • Cheilosis • Red, swollen tongue • Reddening of cornea	• None known

(Continues)

TABLE 18-5 Water-Soluble Vitamins (Continued)

VITAMIN	FUNCTION	SOURCES	DEFICIENCY	TOXIC EFFECTS
Niacin (nicotinic acid)	• Aids in oxidation • Promotes CHO, protein, and fat metabolism • Aids tissue protein building	• Meat, poultry, fish • Legumes • Enriched grains • Peanuts	• Pellegra • Anorexia • Apathy • Weakness • Dermatitis • Diarrhea • Dementia	• Large doses: flushing, itching, hypotension, tachycardia
B_6 (pyridoxine)	• Is necessary for amino acid metabolism • Promotes blood formation • Maintains nervous tissue	• Chicken, fish, pork • Eggs • Whole grains	• Depression • Dermatitis • Abnormal brain wave patterns • Convulsions • Anemia	• Clumsiness • Nerve degeneration
B_{12} (cobalamin)	• Promotes normal function of all cells, especially those of the nervous system • Promotes blood formation • Promotes CHO, protein, and fat metabolism • Aids in synthesis of ribonucleic acid (RNA) and DNA • Is necessary for folate metabolism	• Fresh shrimp, oysters, meats, milk, eggs, and cheese	• Pernicious anemia • Anorexia • Indigestion • Paresthesia of hands and feet • Poor coordination • Depression	• None known
Folate (folic acid)	• Is necessary for synthesis of RNA and DNA • Promotes amino acid metabolism, RBC and white blood cell (WBC) formation • Prevents neural tube defects	• Green leafy vegetables • Milk • Eggs • Yeast	• Glossitis • Diarrhea • Macrocytic anemia	• None known
Pantothenic acid	• Promotes CHO, protein, and fat metabolism	• Animal tissues • Whole-grain cereals • Legumes • Milk	• Not observed in humans	• None known
Biotin	• Promotes CHO and fat metabolism • Is necessary for glycogen formation	• Egg yolk • Yeast • Milk • Soy flours • Cereals • Legumes • Made by intestinal bacteria	• Only induced with long-term total parenteral nutrition (TPN)	• None known

LIFE SPAN CONSIDERATIONS

Vitamins

Vitamin needs vary with the life cycle. Vitamin supplements are generally needed for pregnant or lactating women and for infants, and elders.

Classification and Sources

Vitamins are commonly grouped according to solubility. Vitamins A, D, E, and K are fat soluble, and vitamin C and the B-complex vitamins are water soluble.

Fat-Soluble Vitamins The **fat-soluble vitamins** (A, D, E, and K) require the presence of fats for their absorption from the GI tract into the lymphatic system and for cellular metabolism. They must attach to protein carriers to be transported through the blood. The body's stored reserve makes daily intake unnecessary. In fact, the reserve can result in toxic levels if large supplemental doses are taken, especially in the case of vitamin A. Deficiencies can occur in conditions that interfere with fat absorption.

Water-Soluble Vitamins The **water-soluble vitamins** (C and the B-complex vitamins) require daily ingestion in normal quantities because they are not stored in the body. They are absorbed by the capillaries in the intestinal villi directly into the circulatory system. Deficiency symptoms develop quickly in response to inadequate intake. Foods should be cooked in the least amount of water possible, because the water-soluble vitamins are released into the cooking water: when the water is discarded, the vitamins are lost.

MEMORY TRICK

Fat-Soluble Vitamins

To remember the fat soluble vitamins A, D, E, and K, memorize "Fat **ADEK**," as in "fat addict."

CLIENT TEACHING

Natural or Synthetic Vitamins

Some people believe that natural vitamins are superior in quality to synthetic vitamins. According to the U.S. Food and Drug Administration (FDA), however, the body cannot distinguish between a vitamin of plant or animal origin and one manufactured in a laboratory. The two types of the same vitamin are chemically identical.

CRITICAL THINKING

Vitamin Supplements

What recommendations should be made to a client regarding vitamin supplements?

Digestion, Absorption, and Storage

Vitamins do not require digestion. Fat-soluble vitamins are absorbed into the lymphatic system, whereas water-soluble vitamins are absorbed directly into the circulatory system. Excess amounts of fat-soluble vitamins cannot be excreted but are stored in the liver and adipose tissue. Water-soluble vitamins are excreted through urine, when excess amounts are taken into the body.

Signs of Deficiency or Excess

Vitamin deficiencies can occur and result in disease. Those persons inclined to vitamin deficiencies because they do not eat balanced diets include alcoholics, the poor, incapacitated elders, clients with serious diseases that affect appetite, mentally retarded persons, and young children who receive inadequate care. Deficiencies of fat-soluble vitamins occur in clients with chronic malabsorption diseases such as cystic fibrosis, celiac disease, and Crohn's disease.

Vitamins consumed in excess amounts can be toxic to the body (Tables 18-4 and 18-5).

MINERALS

Minerals are inorganic elements that help regulate body processes and/or serve as structural components of the body. Like vitamins, they have no fuel value.

Chemical analysis shows that the human body is made up of specific chemical elements. Four of these elements—oxygen, carbon, hydrogen, and nitrogen—make up 96% of body weight. All the remaining elements are minerals, making up 4% of body weight. Nevertheless, these minerals are essential for good health.

Daily Requirements

Major minerals are required in amounts greater than 100 mg/day. Trace minerals are those required in amounts less than 100 mg/day. See list of major and trace minerals in Table 18-6.

Functions

The functions of minerals are unique to each individual mineral. Table 18-7 outlines the functions, sources, deficiencies, and toxic effects of each mineral.

Classification and Sources

Minerals are generally classified as major minerals and trace elements. Minerals are found in water and in natural (unprocessed) foods, together with proteins, carbohydrates, fats, and vitamins. Minerals in the soil are absorbed by growing plants. Humans obtain minerals by eating plants grown in mineral-rich soil or by eating animals that have eaten such plants.

Table 18-6 Major Minerals and Trace Elements

MAJOR MINERALS	TRACE ELEMENTS	
	Essential	**Questionable**
Calcium (Ca)	Iron (Fe)	Arsenic (As)
Phosphorus (P)	Iodine (I)	Boron (B)
Sodium (Na)	Zinc (Zn)	Cadmium (Cd)
Potassium (K)	Selenium (Se)	Nickel (Ni)
Magnesium (Mg)	Copper (Cu)	Silicon (Si)
Chlorine (Cl)	Manganese (Mn)	Tin (Sn)
Sulfur (S)	Fluorine (Fl)	Vanadium (V)
	Chromium (Cr)	
	Molybdenum (Mo)	
	Cobalt (Co)	

Highly processed or refined foods such as sugar and white flour contain almost no minerals. Iron, together with the vitamins thiamin, riboflavin, niacin, and folate, is commonly added back to some flour and cereals, which are then labeled enriched.

Most minerals in food occur as salts, which are soluble in water. Therefore, the minerals leave the food and remain in the cooking water when foods are cooked in water. Foods should be cooked in as little water as possible or, preferably,

LIFE SPAN CONSIDERATIONS

Mineral Supplements

- During adolescence, calcium may be needed if the diet is insufficient.
- Pregnant and lactating women require added calcium, phosphorus, and iron.

Table 18-7 Minerals

MINERAL	FUNCTION	SOURCES	DEFICIENCY	TOXIC EFFECTS
Calcium (Ca)	• Aids in bone and teeth formation • Promotes muscle contraction and relaxation • Aids blood clotting • Aids in nerve transmission • Promotes normal heart rhythm • Needs vitamin D for Absorption	• Milk • Cheese • Sardines • Salmon • Green, leafy vegetables • Whole grains	• Rickets • Osteoporosis • Tetany • Poor tooth formation	• Kidney stones • Deposits in joints and soft tissue • May inhibit iron and zinc absorption
Phosphorus (P)	• Aids in bone and teeth formation • Involved in energy metabolism • Regulates acid–base balance • Ensures structure of cell membranes • Is part of nucleic acids	• Fish, beef, pork, poultry • Cheese • Legumes • Milk • Carbonated beverages	• Rickets • Osteoporosis • Poor tooth formation • Disturbed acid base balance	• Low serum calcium • Kidney stones
Sodium (Na)	• Helps regulate fluid balance and acid–base balance • Regulates cell membrane irritability • Regulates nerve Transmission	• Table salt • Milk • Meat • Processed foods • Carrots • Celery	• Hyponatremia • Nausea • Headache • Mental confusion • Hypotension • Anxiety • Muscle spasms	• Hypernatremia • Hypertension • Cardiovascular disturbance • Edema

(Continues)

Table 18-7 Minerals (Continued)

MINERAL	FUNCTION	SOURCES	DEFICIENCY	TOXIC EFFECTS
Potassium (K)	• Maintains fluid balance • Maintains acid–base balance • Regulates muscle activity • Aids in protein synthesis • Aids in CHO metabolism	• Fruits, especially oranges, bananas, and prunes • Red meats • Vegetables • Milk and milk products • Coffee	• Hypokalemia • Fluid and electrolyte imbalances • Tissue breakdown • Cardiac weakness • Muscle cramps	• Hyperkalemia • Muscle weakness • Severe dehydration • Mental confusion • Hypotension • Cardiac arrest
Magnesium (Mg)	• Is necessary for muscle–nerve action • Regulates CHO, CHON, and fat metabolism • Activates enzymes • Aids in bone formation	• Green, leafy vegetables • Whole grains • Legumes	• Hypomagnesemia • Tremors • Spasms • Convulsions	• Hypermagnesemia • Central nervous system (CNS) depression • Coma • Hypotension
Chlorine (Cl)	• Helps regulate fluid balance and acid–base balance • Aids digestion as part of hydrochloric acid in stomach	• Table salt • Milk • Meat • Processed foods	• Rare	• Rare
Sulfur (S)	• Serves as component of amino acids • Aids vitamin, enzyme, and hormonal activity • Is part of skin, hair, nails, and soft tissue	• Cheese • Eggs • Poultry • Fish	• None specific	• None specific
Iron (Fe)	• Aids in formation of hemoglobin • Aids in antibody formation	• Meat • Whole grains • Egg yolk • Legumes • Prunes • Raisins • Apricots	• Iron deficiency • Anemia	• Hemochromatosis • GI cramping • Vomiting • Nausea • Shock • Convulsions • Coma
Iodine (I)	• Is a component of thyroid hormones	• Iodized salt • Seafood (salt water) • Milk	• Cretinism • Goiter	• Hyperthyroidism • Fatal in large amounts
Zinc (Zn)	• Is a component of DNA and RNA • Aids in physical and sexual development • Helps ensure normal taste and smell • Aids in wound healing	• Meats, oysters • Eggs • Milk • Whole grains	• Poor wound healing • Decreased taste and smell • Growth retardation	• Muscle incoordination • Vomiting • Diarrhea • Renal failure

(*Continues*)

TABLE 18-7 Minerals (Continued)

MINERAL	FUNCTION	SOURCES	DEFICIENCY	TOXIC EFFECTS
Selenium (Se)	• Acts as an antioxidant • Works with vitamin E	• Seafoods • Meats	• Muscle weakness • Cardiomyopathy	• Selenosis • Nausea • Peripheral neuropathy • Fatigue
Copper (Cu)	• Aids in bone and blood formation • Promotes iron absorption • Is part of myelin sheath	• Seafood • Nuts • Legumes	• Iron-deficiency anemia • Hypocholesterol-emia	• None known
Manganese (Mn)	• Aids bone growth • Aids reproduction • Acts as enzyme activator	• Whole-grain cereals • Legumes • Tea	• Unknown	• Unlikely
Fluorine (Fl)	• Protects against dental caries • Contributes to bone formation and integrity	• Fluoridated water • Tea • Seafood	• Dental caries	• Mottled stains on teeth
Chromium (Cr)	• Associated with glucose metabolism	• Whole grains • Brewers yeast	• Insulin resistance • Impaired glucose tolerance	• Dietary: unlikely
Molybdenum (Mo)	• Helps ensure normal body metabolism	• Milk • Legumes • Whole grains	• Decreased production of uric acid	• Interferes with copper metabolism
Cobalt (Co)	• Is a component of vitamin B_{12} • Aids in RBC formation	• Meat, as B_{12}	• Associated with vitamin B_{12} deficiency	• Unknown

steamed, and any cooking liquid should be saved to be used in soups, gravies, and white sauces. Using this liquid improves the flavor as well as the nutrient content of foods to which it is added.

Supplemental minerals may be required during growth periods and in some clinical situations. Individuals with iron-deficiency anemia require extra iron. Persons taking potassium-losing diuretics need a potassium supplement.

Digestion, Absorption, and Storage

Minerals are absorbed in their ionic forms (i.e., carrying a positive or negative electrical charge). The amount of a mineral absorbed by the body is influenced by three factors:

- *Type of food:* Minerals in foods that come from animals are more readily absorbed than those in foods that come from plants.
- *Need of body:* If there is a deficiency of a mineral in the body, more will be absorbed.
- *Health of absorbing tissue:* If absorbing tissue (intestine) is affected by disease, less will be absorbed.

Signs of Deficiency and Excess

Because it is known that minerals are essential to good health, some people think "more is better." More can be hazardous to one's health when it comes to minerals. In a healthy individual eating a balanced diet, there will be some normal mineral loss through perspiration and saliva, and amounts in excess of body needs will be excreted in urine and feces. When concentrated forms of minerals are taken regularly over a period of time, however, they become more than the body can handle, and toxicity develops. An excessive amount of one mineral sometimes causes a deficiency of another mineral. Excessive amounts of minerals can cause hair loss and changes in the blood, hormones, bones, muscles, blood vessels, and nearly all tissues. Concentrated forms of minerals should be used only on the advice of a physician. Refer to Table 18-7 for specific signs of deficiency and toxicity of each mineral.

PROFESSIONALTIP

Vitamins, Minerals, and Herbs

Since July 1994, the federal Food and Drug Administration has placed limitations on marketing claims for vitamins, minerals, and herbs. The rules are aimed at deterring false or unproven health claims and require that companies selling these products make only claims that are substantiated by broad scientific consensus. Labeling requirements of dietary supplements began in July 1995.

PROMOTING PROPER NUTRITION

Through the years, various ways to promote proper nutrition have been devised. The best known are the four food groups, the food guide pyramid, the *Dietary Guidelines for Americans*, the recommended daily allowances, and the dietary reference intakes.

Four Food Groups (Historical)

For many years, the four food groups assisted people in eating a well-balanced diet. Eating foods from the four groups—milk, meat, fruit/vegetable and bread/cereal—provided most nutrients required in a daily diet. The minimum number of servings yielded approximately 1,200 kcal. Additional servings were to be added depending on the individual's age and activity level.

Food Guide Pyramid

In 2005, the U.S. Department of Agriculture (USDA) created the new MyPyramid and recommended the food pyramid in Figure 18-3 for a person with regular dietary needs. Each bandwidth represents a guide to the proportion of food from that group. The stepping person in the pyramid represents the importance of balancing the diet with activity. The steps in the pyramid represent the activity of an individual and recommend that the amount consumed, balance the physical activity of the person. The new pyramid has six categories of food groups represented by the six colored bands (Mathew, 2008).

Each food group of the food guide pyramid provides some but not all of the nutrients needed each day. Foods in one group cannot replace foods in another group. No one group is more important than another: all are needed.

The Orange Band: Grains or Carbohydrates

The orange band represents grains or carbohydrates and includes whole-grain bread, cereal, crackers, rice, and pasta. The nutrients contributed by this group are complex carbohydrates, incomplete protein, the B vitamins, and iron, if the product is whole grain or **enriched** (nutrients that are removed during processing are added back) with iron. Six to 11 servings a day should come from this group. Examples of serving sizes from this group are one slice of bread, one tortilla, 1 ounce (1 cup) dry cereal, and ½ cup cooked cereal, rice, or pasta.

The Green Band: Vegetables

The nutritional contributions of vegetables are carbohydrates, vitamins, minerals, water, and very small amounts of proteins and fats. Dietary fiber, important for elimination, is found in the skin of many foods in this group. Three to five servings a day from the vegetable group are suggested. Among the vegetables eaten daily, one should be a dark-green (collards

WHAT COUNTS AS A SERVING?

Bread, Cereal, Rice, and Pasta Group (Grains Group)—whole grain and refined
- 1 slice of bread
- About 1 cup of ready-to-eat cereal
- 1/2 cup of cooked cereal, rice, or pasta

Vegetable Group
- 1 cup of raw leafy vegetables
- 1/2 cup of other vegetables—cooked or raw
- 3/4 cup of vegetable juice

Fruit Group
- 1 medium apple, banana, orange, pear
- 1/2 cup of chopped, cooked, or canned fruit
- 3/4 cup of fruit juice

Milk, Yogurt, and Cheese Group (Milk Group)*
- 1 cup of milk** or yogurt**
- 1 1/2 ounces of natural cheese** (such as Cheddar)
- 2 ounces of processed cheese** (such as American)

Meat, Poultry, Fish, Dry Beans, Eggs, and Nuts Group (Meat and Beans Group)
- 2–3 ounces of cooked lean meat, poultry, or fish
- 1/2 cup of cooked dry beans# or 1/2 cup of tofu counts as 1 ounce of lean meat
- 2 1/2-ounce soyburger or 1 egg counts as 1 ounce of lean meat
- 2 tablespoons of peanut butter or 1/3 cup of nuts counts as 1 ounce of meat

NOTE: Many of the serving sizes given above are smaller than those on the Nutrition Facts Label. For example, 1 serving of cooked cereal, rice, or pasta is 1 cup for the label but only 1/2 cup for the Pyramid.

* This includes lactose-free and lactose-reduced milk products. One cup of soy-based beverage with added calcium is an option for those who prefer a non-dairy source of calcium.

** Choose fat-free or reduced-fat dairy products most often.

Dry beans, peas, and lentils can be counted as servings in either the meat and beans group or the vegetable group. As a vegetable, 1/2 cup of cooked, dry beans counts as 1 serving. As a meat substitute, 1 cup of cooked, dry beans counts as 1 serving (2 ounces of meat).

FIGURE 18-3 Daily appropriate intake of nutrition and exercise makes one healthy. MyPyramid (*Courtesy of United States Department of Agriculture [USDA, 2008] and United States Department of Health and Human Services [HHS]. Nutrition and your health: Dietary guidelines for American, 2000. Food Guide Pyramid, A Guide to Daily Food Choices [Home and Garden Bulletin No. 232]. Washington, DC: U.S. Department of Agriculture and U.S. Department of Health and Human Services*).

and spinach) or orange vegetable (sweet potato or carrot) to provide vitamin A. Sample serving sizes from the vegetable group include 1 cup of raw leafy vegetables, ½ cup of cooked or chopped raw vegetables, or ¾ cup of vegetable juice.

The Red Band: Fruits

The red band represents fruits and includes fresh, frozen, canned, or dry fruits limiting the amount of fruit juices. The nutritional contributions of fruits are carbohydrates, vitamins, minerals, and fiber. Each person should have two or four servings of fruit every day. Citrus fruits, melons, and berries should be eaten regularly, as they are high in vitamin C. Examples of serving sizes from the fruit group are one medium-sized apple, pear, banana, or orange; ½ cup of cooked, chopped, or canned fruit; or ¾ cup of fruit juice.

The Yellow Band: Oils

The yellow band represents oils. Consume most of the daily calories from plant foods (grains, fruits, and vegetables). The recommended fat sources are fish, nuts, and vegetable oils, limiting butter, margarine, shortening, and lard.

The Blue Band: Milk, Yogurt, and Other Milk Products

The blue band represents calcium-rich food, such as low-fat or fat-free milk and dairy products. The nutritional contributions of the milk group are calcium, protein, riboflavin, fat, carbohydrates, phosphorus, sodium, vitamin B_{12}, and vitamin A. If skim milk or skim milk products are used, there is no fat and significantly fewer kcal. All commercial milk products are **fortified** (a nutrient not naturally occurring in a food is added to the food) with vitamin D. Vitamin D, not naturally found in milk, is added because the calcium provided by milk is better absorbed when vitamin D is present.

Two to three servings a day are suggested from the milk group. Eight ounces of milk is considered one serving. Other milk products and their serving sizes to provide the equivalent nutrients of 8 ounces of milk are 1½ ounces of cheese, 1 cup of yogurt, 1½ cups of cottage cheese, and 1½ cups of ice cream. The kcal content of these foods varies, with ice cream containing more kcal than the other foods in the milk group.

The Purple Band: Meat and Beans

The purple band represents meat and beans, which include lean meats or poultry, fish, beans, peas, nuts, or seeds. The meat and beans group contributes complete protein, fats, iron, most other minerals, and the B vitamins. Cheese and bacon are not considered part of this group: cheese has too little iron and bacon has too much fat.

The suggested number of servings from the meat group is two to three each day. A serving size is 2 to 3 ounces of meat, fish, or poultry. Other foods that can be substituted for one serving of meat are two eggs, 4 tablespoons of peanut butter, or 1 cup cooked beans or peas (legumes). Legumes such as dried peas, beans, or lentils can be used instead of meat because of their high protein content. Peanuts as well as many other nuts are high in protein, but they are also high in fats and should be used sparingly.

Number of Servings

The number of servings for an individual depends on the number of calories the individual needs. The number of calories needed by a person depends on age, gender, size, and activity. Almost everyone should have the minimum number of servings for each group. The serving recommendations for three general calorie levels are listed in Table 18-8.

The Vegetarian Diet

There are several vegetarian diets. The common factor among them is that they do not include red meat. When carefully planned, these diets can be nutritious. They can even contribute to a reduction in obesity, high blood pressure, heart disease, some cancers, and, possibly, diabetes (Roth, 2006). They must be carefully planned so they include all the needed nutrients.

Lacto-ovo vegetarians use dairy products and eggs but no meat, poultry, or fish. Lacto vegetarians use dairy products but no meat, poultry, or eggs. Vegans avoid all animal foods.

TABLE 18-8 How Many Servings Do You Need Each Day?

FOOD GROUP	CHILDREN AGES 2 TO 6 YEARS, WOMEN, SOME OLDER ADULTS (ABOUT 1,600 CALORIES)	OLDER CHILDREN, TEEN GIRLS, ACTIVE WOMEN, MOST MEN (ABOUT 2,200 CALORIES)	TEEN BOYS, ACTIVE MEN (ABOUT 2,800 CALORIES)
Bread, Cereal, Rice, and Pasta Group (Grains Group)—especially whole grain	6	9	11
Vegetable Group	3	4	5
Fruit Group	2	3	4
Milk, Yogurt, and Cheese Group (Milk Group)—preferably fat free or low fat	2 or 3*	2 or 3*	2 or 3*

(Continues)

Table 18-8 How Many Servings Do You Need Each Day? (Continued)

FOOD GROUP	CHILDREN AGES 2 TO 6 YEARS, WOMEN, SOME OLDER ADULTS (ABOUT 1,600 CALORIES)	OLDER CHILDREN, TEEN GIRLS, ACTIVE WOMEN, MOST MEN (ABOUT 2,200 CALORIES)	TEEN BOYS, ACTIVE MEN (ABOUT 2,800 CALORIES)
Meat, Poultry, Fish, Dry Beans, Eggs, and Nuts Group (Meat and Beans Group)—preferably lean or low fat	2, for a total of 5 ounces	2, for a total of 6 ounces	3, for a total of 7 ounces

* The number of servings depends on your age. Older children and teenagers (ages 9 to 18 years) and adults over the age of 50 need 3 servings daily. Others need 2 servings daily. During pregnancy and lactation, the recommended number of milk group servings is the same as for nonpregnant women.

Adapted from U.S. Department of Agriculture, Center for Nutrition Policy and Promotion, The Food Guide Pyramid, Home and Garden Bulletin Number 252, 1996. United States Department of Agriculture (USDA) and United States Department of Health and Human Services (HHS). Nutrition and your health: Dietary guidelines for Americans (Home and Garden Bulletin No. 232, 2000).

They use soybeans, chickpeas, meat analogues, and tofu. It is important that their meals be carefully planned to include appropriate combinations of the essential amino acids. For example, beans served with corn or rice, or peanuts eaten with wheat, are complementary proteins. Vegans can show deficiencies of calcium; vitamins A, D, and B_{12}; and, of course, proteins.

Dietary Guidelines

The *Dietary Guidelines* developed by the U.S. Department of Agriculture and the U.S. Department of Health and Human Services were last revised in 1990. They are now stated in positive terms (i.e., "eat . . ."; "consume . . .") instead of negative terms ("avoid . . ."). These guidelines attempt to prevent overnutrition by incorporating some of the concepts of the food guide pyramid (Table 18-9).

Recommended Dietary Allowances

Recommended dietary allowances (RDAs) of essential nutrients are the recommended intake levels judged adequate to meet the known nutrient needs of practically all healthy people. Recommendations are grouped according to infants, children, males, females, and pregnant/ lactating women, and are subdivided within those groups according to age. The RDAs are compiled by the Food and Nutrition Board of the National Academy of Sciences and are periodically revised.

Dietary Reference Intakes

The dietary reference intakes (DRIs) are nutrient-based reference values for use in planning and assessing diets. They are intended to replace the old RDAs. The DRIs focus on decreasing the risk of chronic disease through nutrition, rather than on protecting against deficiency diseases, as do the RDAs.

The DRIs encompass four categories:

- *Estimated average requirement* (EAR) is the amount that meets the estimated nutrient need of 50% of the individuals in a specific group.
- *Recommended dietary allowance* (RDA) is the amount that meets the nutrient need of almost all (97% to 98%) healthy individuals in a specific age and gender group. It is the EAR plus an increase, based on scientific evidence, to account for variation within the specific group. The RDA should be used to achieve adequate nutrient intake aimed at decreasing the risk of chronic disease.
- *Adequate intake* (AI) is set when there is insufficient scientific evidence to estimate an average requirement. It is derived through experimental or observational data that show a mean intake that appears to sustain a desired indicator of health, such as calcium retention in bone.
- *Tolerable upper intake level* (UL) is the maximum intake by an individual that is unlikely to pose risks of adverse health effects in almost all healthy individuals in a specified group. It is not intended to be a recommended level of intake. There is no established benefit for individuals to consume nutrients at levels above the RDA or AI.

FACTORS INFLUENCING NUTRITION

Many factors influence nutrition. Some of the major factors are culture, religion, socioeconomics, fads, and superstitions.

Culture

A person's culture encompasses a total way of life including values, attitudes, and practices. Food practices are a substantial part of a culture. These food habits are based on availability of foods, preparation techniques, methods of serving, and the personal meaning of food (Figure 18-4). American cuisine (cooking style) is a marvelous composite of countless national, regional, cultural, and religious food customs. Consequently, categorizing a client's food habits can be difficult. People who are ill commonly have little interest in food, and sometimes foods that were familiar to them during their childhood and youth are more tempting than other types. The following section briefly discusses some food patterns typical of various cultures, regions, and countries. Of course, there can be and usually are enormous variations within any one classification.

Native American

It is thought that approximately one-half of the edible plants commonly eaten in the United States today originated with the Native Americans. Examples are corn, potatoes, squash, cranberries, pumpkin, peppers, beans, wild rice, and cocoa beans. In addition, wild fruits, game, and fish were used. Foods were

TABLE 18-9 Dietary Guidelines for Americans

	DIETARY GUIDELINES	EXPLANATION
Aim *for Fitness*	• Aim for a healthy weight. • Be physically active each day.	Following these two guidelines will help keep you and your family healthy and fit. Healthy eating and regular physical activity enable people of all ages to work productively, enjoy life, and feel their best. They also help children grow, develop, and do well in school.
BUILD *a Healthy Base*	• Use the food guide pyramid to make your food choices. • Choose a variety of grains daily, especially whole grains. • Choose a variety of fruits and vegetables daily. • Keep food safe to eat.	Following these four guidelines builds a base for healthy eating. Let the food guide pyramid guide you so that you get the nutrients your body needs each day. Make grains, fruits, and vegetables the foundation of your meals. This forms a base for good nutrition and good health and may reduce your risk of certain chronic diseases. Be flexible and adventurous, try new choices from these three groups in place of some less nutritious foods or in place of higher calorie foods that you usually eat. Whatever you eat, always take steps to keep your food safe to eat.
CHOOSE *Sensibly*	• Choose a diet that is low in saturated fat and cholesterol and moderate in total fat. • Choose beverages and foods to moderate your intake of sugars. • Choose and prepare foods with less salt. • If you drink alcoholic beverages, do so in moderation.	These four guidelines help you make sensible choices that promote health and reduce the risk of certain chronic diseases. You can enjoy all foods as part of a healthy diet as long as you do not overdo it on fat (especially saturated fat), sugars, salt, and alcohol. Read labels to identify foods that are higher in saturated fats, sugars, and salt (sodium).

From U.S. Department of Agriculture (USDA) and U.S. Department of Health and Human Services (HHS), 2000. *Nutrition and your Health: Dietary Guidelines for Americans* (Home and Garden Bulletin No. 232, 5th ed). Washington, DC: USDA.

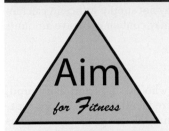

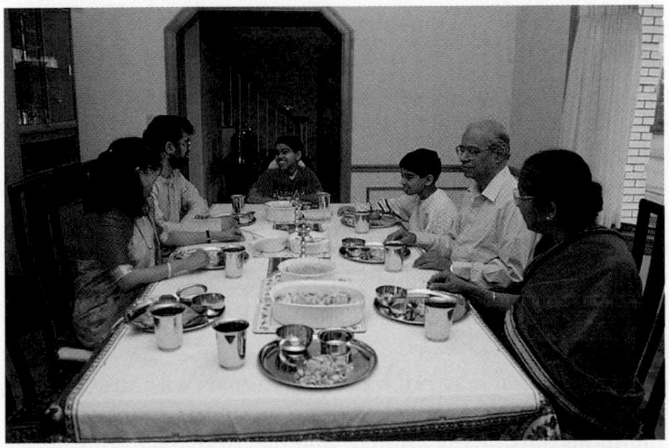

COURTESY OF DELMAR CENGAGE LEARNING

FIGURE 18-4 Family and cultural values often affect diet.

commonly prepared as soups and stews or were dried. The original Native American diets were probably more nutritionally adequate than current diets. Native American diets today may be deficient in calcium, vitamins A and C, and riboflavin (Roth, 2006).

U.S. Southern

Hot breads such as corn bread and baking powder biscuits are common in the U.S. South because the wheat grown in this area does not make good-quality yeast breads. Grits and rice are also popular carbohydrate foods. Favorite vegetables include sweet potatoes, squash, green beans, and lima beans. Watermelon, oranges, and peaches are popular fruits. Fried fish is served often, as are barbecued and stewed meats and poultry. These diets have a great deal of carbohydrate and fat and limited amounts of protein in some cases. Iron, calcium, and vitamins A and C may be deficient (Roth, 2006).

Mexican

Mexican food is a combination of Spanish and Native American foods. Beans, rice, chili peppers, tomatoes, and corn meal are favorites. Meat is often cooked with a vegetable, as in chili con carne. Cornmeal or flour is used to make tortillas, which are served as bread. The combination of beans and corn makes a complete protein. Corn tortillas filled with cheese (called enchiladas) provide some calcium, but the use of milk should be encouraged. Additional green and yellow vegetables and vitamin C–rich foods would also make these diets more well-balanced.

Puerto Rican

Rice is the basic carbohydrate food in Puerto Rican diets. Vegetables commonly used include beans, plantains, tomatoes, and peppers. Bananas, pineapple, mangoes, and papayas are popular fruits. Favorite meats are chicken, beef, and pork. Additional milk would make a more balanced diet (Roth, 2006).

Italian

Pastas with various tomato or fish sauces and cheese are popular Italian foods. Fish and highly seasoned foods are common southern Italian cuisine; whereas meat and root vegetables are common northern cuisine. The eggs, cheese, tomatoes, green vegetables, and fruits in Italian diets provide excellent sources of many nutrients. Added fat-free milk and low-fat meat would make the diet more complete (Roth, 2006).

Northern and Western European

Northern and Western European diets are similar to those of the U.S. Midwest, but with a greater use of dark breads, potatoes, and fish, and fewer green-vegetable salads. Beef and pork are popular, as are various cooked vegetables, breads, cakes, and dairy products. The addition of fresh vegetables and fruits would add vitamins, minerals, and fiber to these diets.

Central European

Citizens of Central Europe obtain the greatest portion of their calories from potatoes and grain, especially rye and buckwheat (Roth, 2006). Pork is a popular meat. Cabbage cooked in many ways is a popular vegetable, as are carrots, onions, and turnips. Eggs and dairy products are used abundantly. Limiting the number of eggs consumed and using fat-free or low-fat dairy products would reduce the fat content in this diet. Adding fresh vegetables and fruits would increase vitamins, minerals, and fiber.

Middle Eastern

Grains, wheat, and rice provide energy in Middle Eastern diets. Chickpeas in the form of hummus are popular. Lamb and yogurt are commonly used, as are cabbage, grape leaves, eggplant, tomatoes, dates, olives, and figs. Black, very sweet coffee is a popular beverage. There may be insufficient protein and calcium in this diet, depending on the amounts of meat and calcium-rich foods eaten. Fresh fruits and vegetables should be added to the diet to increase vitamins, minerals, and fiber.

Chinese

The Chinese diet is varied. Rice is the primary energy food and is used in place of bread. Vegetables are lightly cooked, and the cooking water is saved for future use. Soybeans are used in many ways, and eggs and pork are commonly served. Soy sauce is extensively used, but it is very salty and could present a problem for clients needing low-salt diets. Tea is a common beverage, but milk is not. This diet is typically low in fat (Roth, 2006).

Japanese

Japanese diets include rice, soybean paste and curd, vegetables, fruits, and fish. Food is frequently served tempura style, which means fried. Soy sauce (shoyu) and tea are commonly used. Current Japanese diets have been greatly influenced by Western culture. Japanese diets may be deficient in calcium, given the near-total lack of milk in the diet (Roth, 2006). Although fish is eaten with bones, this may not supply sufficient calcium to meet needs. Japanese diets may contain excessive amounts of salt.

Indian

Many Indians are vegetarians who use eggs and dairy products. Rice, peas, and beans are frequently served. Spices, especially curry, are popular. Indian meals are generally served as one course with many dishes.

Thai, Vietnamese, Laotian, and Cambodian

Rice, curries, vegetables, and fruit are popular in Thailand, Vietnam, Laos, and Cambodia. Meats and fish are used in small amounts. The wok (a deep, round fry pan) is used for sautéing many foods. A salty sauce made from fermented fish is commonly used. Thai, Vietnamese, Laotian, and Cambodian diets may be deficient in protein and calcium (Roth, 2006).

Religion

Religious beliefs often influence nutrition by placing restrictions on the foods eaten and their preparation. A few examples follow.

Jewish

Interpretations of the Jewish dietary laws vary. Persons who adhere to the Orthodox view consider tradition important and always observe the dietary laws. Foods prepared according to these laws are called kosher. Conservative Jews are inclined to observe the rules only at home. Reform Jews consider their dietary laws to be essentially ceremonial and thus minimize their significance. Essentially the laws require the following (Roth, 2006):

- Slaughtering must be done by a qualified person and in a prescribed manner.
- Meat and meat products may not be prepared with milk or milk products.
- The dishes used in the preparation and serving of meat products must be kept separate from those used for dairy foods.
- Dairy products and meat may not be eaten together. Six hours must elapse after eating meat before eating dairy products, and at least 30 minutes to 1 hour must elapse after eating dairy products before eating meat.
- The mouth must be rinsed after eating fish and before eating meat.
- The following may not be eaten: animals without cloven (split) hooves or animals that do not chew their cud, hindquarters of any animal, shellfish or fish without scales or fins, birds of prey, creeping things and insects, and leavened (containing ingredients that cause it to rise) bread during Passover.

There are prescribed fast days: Passover Week, Yom Kippur, and Feast of Purim. Chicken and fresh smoked and salted fish are popular, as are noodles, eggs, and flour dishes. These diets can be deficient in fresh vegetables and milk.

Roman Catholic

Although the dietary restrictions of the Roman Catholic religion have been liberalized, meat is not allowed on Ash Wednesday and Fridays during Lent.

Eastern Orthodox

The Eastern Orthodox religion includes Christians from the Middle East, Russia, and Greece. Although interpretations of the dietary laws vary, meat, poultry, fish, and dairy products are restricted on Wednesdays and Fridays and during Lent and Advent.

Seventh-Day Adventists

In general, Seventh-Day Adventists are lacto-ovo vegetarians, meaning that they use milk products and eggs, but no meat, fish, or poultry. Nuts, legumes, meat analogues (substitutes), and tofu (made from soybeans) may be used. Coffee, tea, and alcohol are considered to be harmful.

Mormon (Latter-Day Saints)

The only dietary restriction observed by the Mormons is the prohibition of coffee, tea, and alcoholic beverages.

Islamic

Adherents of Islam are called Muslims. Dietary laws prohibit the use of pork and alcohol, and other meats must be slaughtered according to specific laws. During the month of Ramadan, Muslims do not eat or drink during daylight hours.

Hindu

To the Hindus, all life is sacred, and animals contain the souls of ancestors. Consequently, most Hindus are vegetarians and do not use eggs in food preparation because eggs represent life.

Socioeconomics

The amount of money available to purchase food certainly influences nutrition. More money, however, does not always mean better nutrition. Persons with less money often plan their meals and buy food more carefully than do those with higher incomes. Expensive food does not mean better nutrition. Many times, persons with no monetary worries eat what they want, when they want, without paying attention to nutritional value, thereby shortchanging themselves nutritionally.

Fads

Food fads are beliefs that persist for a period of time about certain foods and that generally have no scientific basis. Often, these fads are translated into diets that can be harmful if basic nutrients are missing or are in excess. One of the most popular diets some years ago was the grapefruit and egg diet. One of the more recent fads was the liquid-protein diet. This diet overloaded the body with protein, yet other nutrients were lacking. The excessive amount of protein damaged the kidneys of many people. Indeed, some people died from this fad diet (American Heart Association, 1999).

High-protein, low-carbohydrate diets, such as the Atkins diet, have been around for over a century. An individual can lose weight very quickly on the diet, but it is not the diet of choice in the long run, as individuals usually prefer to revert to more varied and desirable choices. Once carbohydrates are reintroduced into the diet, weight gain returns. High-protein diets are not recommended for clients with liver or kidney conditions and may leave the person with depleted glycogen stores. The long-term issues encountered with this diet are uncertain at this point (Brown, 2005).

Superstitions

Superstitions are irrational beliefs about a food that are generally passed down from generation to generation. The nurse should be aware of the beliefs and the facts that contradict them so as to be knowledgeable and respectful. Examples of such superstitions are:

- *Superstition:* Toast is less fattening than bread.
- *Fact:* Only moisture is removed during toasting.
- *Superstition:* "Cravings" during pregnancy should be satisfied, or the infant will be marked or deformed.
- *Fact:* Foods eaten or not eaten by the mother do not directly affect the infant; only the nutrients or lack thereof affect the unborn child.

NUTRITIONAL NEEDS DURING THE LIFE CYCLE

As a person grows and develops from birth to old age, nutritional needs change. These changes generally are based on growth needs, energy needs, and utilization of nutrients. A nutritional assessment should be conducted to ascertain the nutritional needs of the individual.

Infancy

Food and its presentation are extremely important during the baby's first year. Physical and mental development depend on the food itself, and psychosocial development is affected by the time and manner whereby the food is offered.

Although babies have been fed according to prescribed time schedules in the past, it is preferable to feed infants on demand. Feeding on demand prevents the frustrations that hunger can bring and helps the child develop trust in people. The newborn may require more frequent feedings, but, normally, the demand schedule averages approximately every 4 hours by the time the baby is 2 or 3 months old (Roth, 2006).

Nutritional Requirements

The first year of life is a period of the most rapid growth in one's life. A baby doubles its birth weight by 6 months of age and triples it within the first year. This explains why the infant's energy, vitamin, mineral, and protein requirements are higher per unit of body weight than are those of older children or adults.

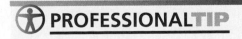

PROFESSIONALTIP

Nutritional Needs of Infants

It is important to remember that growth rates vary from child to child. Nutritional needs depend largely on a child's growth rate.

During the first year, the normal child needs approximately 100 kcal per kilogram of body weight each day. This is approximately two to three times the adult requirement. Infants who have suffered from low birth weight, malnutrition, or illness require more than the normal number of kcal per kilogram of body weight.

The nutritional status of infants is reflected in many of the same characteristics as those of adults.

The American Academy of Pediatrics recommends breast milk for the first 12 months of life, although parents must decide on the method of feeding based on their lifestyle, values, and personal feelings (Gartner et al., 2005).

Breast Milk Breastfeeding is nature's way of providing a good diet for the baby. It is, in fact, used as the guide by whom nutritional requirements of infants are measured.

Mother's milk provides the infant with temporary immunity to many infectious diseases. It is sterile, easy to digest, and usually does not cause GI disturbances or allergic reactions. Breastfed infants grow more rapidly during the first few months of life than do formula-fed babies, and they typically have fewer infections (especially ear infections). Because breast milk contains less protein and minerals than infant formula, it reduces the load on the infant's kidneys. Breastfeeding also promotes oral motor development in infants because sucking requires more and different muscles than does bottle-feeding (Roth, 2006).

One can be quite confident the infant is getting sufficient nutrients and kcal from breastfeeding if (a) there are six or more wet diapers per day, (b) there is normal growth, (c) there are one or two mustard-colored bowel movements per day, and (d) the breast becomes soft during nursing.

CLIENTTEACHING
Breastfeeding

If the mother works and cannot be available for every feeding, breast milk can be expressed earlier, refrigerated or frozen, and used at the appropriate time, or a bottle of formula can be substituted. Never warm the breast milk in a microwave oven because the antibodies will be destroyed. Instead, warm a cup of water and place the bag of breast milk in the water to heat it.

CLIENTTEACHING
Cow's Milk

Infants younger than 1 year of age should not be given regular cow's milk. Its protein is more difficult and slower to digest than that of human milk and can cause GI blood loss. The kidneys are challenged by its high protein and mineral content, and dehydration and even damage to the CNS can result. In addition, the fat is less bioavailable, meaning it is not absorbed as efficiently as that in human milk (Roth, 2006).

Formula If the baby is bottle-fed, the pediatrician provides information on commercial formulas and feeding instructions. Formulas are usually based on cow's milk because it is abundant and easily modified to resemble human milk in nutrient and kcal values.

When an infant is extremely sensitive or allergic to infant formulas, a synthetic formula made from soybeans may be given. Formulas with predigested proteins are used for infants unable to tolerate all other types of formulas (Roth, 2006).

Formulas are available in ready-to-feed, concentrated, or powdered forms. Sterile water must be mixed with the concentrated and powdered forms. The most convenient type is also the most expensive.

If the type purchased requires the addition of water, it is essential that the amount of water added be correctly measured. Too little water will create too heavy a protein and mineral load for the infant's kidneys; too much water will dilute the nutrient and kcal value such that the infant will not thrive.

Solid Foods Introducing solid foods before the age of 4 to 6 months is not recommended. The child's GI tract and kidneys are not sufficiently developed to handle solid food before that age. Furthermore, it is thought that the early introduction of solid foods may increase the likelihood of overfeeding and the possibility of food allergies developing, particularly in children whose parents suffer from food allergies.

An infant's readiness for solid foods will be demonstrated by (a) the physical ability to pull food into the mouth rather than always pushing the tongue and food out of the mouth, (b) a willingness to participate in the process, (c) the ability to sit up with support, (d) having head and neck control, and (e) the need for additional nutrients. An infant drinking more than 32 ounces of formula or nursing 8 to 10 times in 24 hours should be started on solid food.

CLIENTTEACHING
Honey

Honey should never be given to an infant under 12 months because it could be contaminated with *Clostridium botulinum* bacteria.

CLIENTTEACHING
Nursing Bottle Syndrome

Infants should not be put to bed with a bottle. Saliva, which normally cleanses the teeth, diminishes as the infant falls asleep. The milk then bathes the upper front teeth, causing tooth decay. Also, the bottle can cause the upper jaw to protrude and the lower to recede. The result is known as the baby bottle mouth, or nursing bottle syndrome. It is preferable to feed the infant the bedtime bottle, cleanse the teeth and gums with some water from another bottle or cup, and then put the infant to bed.

Solid foods must be introduced gradually and individually. One food is introduced and then no other new food for 4 or 5 days. If there is no allergic reaction, another food can be introduced, a waiting period allowed, then another, and so on. The typical order of introduction begins with cereal, usually iron-fortified rice, then oat, wheat, and mixed cereals. Cooked and pureed vegetables follow, then cooked and pureed fruits, egg yolk, and, finally, finely ground meats. Avoid giving infants egg whites before 1 year of age. Between 6 and 12 months, toast, zwieback, teething biscuits, and Cheerios can be added.

When the infant learns to drink from a cup, juice can be introduced. Juice should never be given from a bottle because babies will fill up on it and not get enough calories from other sources. Pasteurized apple juice is usually given first. Only 100% juice products are recommended because they are nutrient dense (Roth, 2006).

By the age of 1 year, most babies are eating foods from all the food guide pyramid's groups and may have most any food that is easily chewed and digested; however, until the age of 2, precautions must be taken to avoid offering foods that might cause the child to choke. Examples include hotdogs, nuts, whole peas, grapes, popcorn, small candies, and small pieces of tough meat or raw vegetables. Cautiously introduce nuts, as these cause severe allergic responses in some people. Foods should be selected according to the advice of the pediatrician.

CHILDHOOD

Although specific nutritional requirements change as children grow, nutrition always affects physical, mental, and emotional growth and development. Studies indicate that the mental ability and size of an individual are directly influenced by nutrition during the early years.

Eating habits develop during childhood. Once developed, poor eating habits are difficult to change. They can exacerbate emotional and physical problems such as irritability, depression, anxiety, fatigue, and illness. Good eating habits formed in early childhood will generally last a lifetime (Figure 18-5).

Parents should be aware that children's appetites vary. The rate of growth is not constant. As the child ages, the rate of growth actually slows. The approximate weight gain of a child during the second year of life is only 5 pounds. Children between the ages of 1 and 3 years learn to feed themselves.

As children continue to grow and develop, their likes and dislikes may change. New foods should be introduced gradually, in small amounts, and as attractively as possible.

Children should be offered nutrient-dense foods because the amount eaten will be small. Fats should not be limited before the age of 2 years, but meals and snacks should not be fat laden either. Whole milk is recommended until the age of 2, but low fat or fat free should be served from 2 years on. The guideline for fat intake after the age of 2 is the same as that for adults. Children should not salt their food at the table or have foods prepared with a lot of salt (Roth, 2006).

Children are especially sensitive to and reject hot (temperature) foods, but they like crisp textures, mild flavors, and familiar foods. They are wary of foods covered by sauce or gravy. Parents should set realistic goals and expectations as to the amount of food a child needs. A good rule of thumb for preschool children is one tablespoon of new food for each year of age. Table 18-10 details serving sizes according to age.

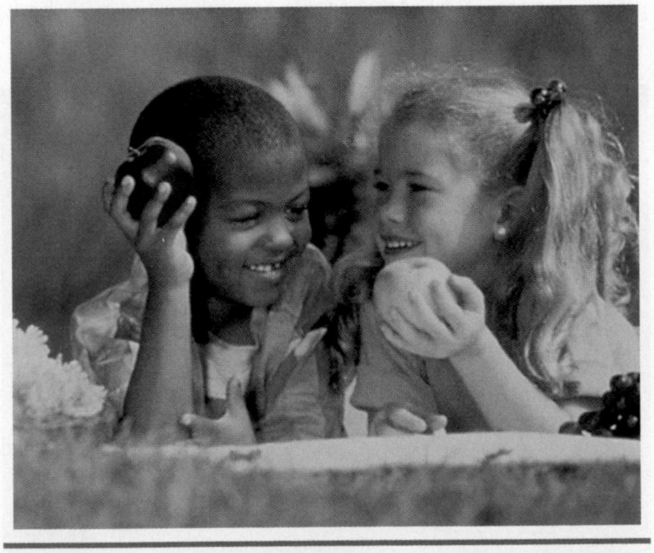

FIGURE 18-5 **Good health radiates from these two children.** *(Photo by Keith Weller, ARS.USDA.)*

CLIENTTEACHING
Introducing New Foods

Allowing the child to assist in purchasing and preparing a new food is often a good way of arousing interest in the food and a desire to eat it.

PROFESSIONALTIP
Snacks

A child needs a snack every 3 to 4 hours for continued energy. Children often prefer finger foods for snacks. Snacks should be nutrient dense and as nutritious as food served at mealtimes. Cheese, saltines, fruit, milk, and unsweetened cereals make good snacks.

CLIENTTEACHING
Preventing Choking

Instruct parents to:

- Avoid the use of foods that may cause choking in infants and small children (up to 3 years old), such as corn, nuts, raw peas and carrots, celery, small candies, hotdogs, popcorn, and any other small, hard food.
- Offer peanut butter only on bread or a saltine.
- Stress the importance of sitting upright while eating.
- Prohibit running with food or objects in the mouth.

TABLE 18-10 Food Plan for Preschool and School-Age Children Based on the Food Guide Pyramid

		APPROXIMATE SERVING SIZE*			
FOOD GROUP	NUMBER OF SERVINGS	AGES 1–2	AGES 3–4	AGES 5–6	AGES 7–12
Milk, yogurt, and cheese	3	½ to ¾ cup or 1 oz	¾ cup or 1½ oz	1 cup or 2 oz	1 cup or 2 oz
Meat, poultry, fish, dry beans, eggs, and nuts	2 or more	1 oz or 1 to 2 Tbsp	1½ oz or 3 to 4 Tbsp	1½ oz or ½ cup	2 oz or ½ cup
Vegetables	3 or more	1 to 2 Tbsp	3 to 4 Tbsp	½ cup	½ cup
Fruits	2 or more	1 to 2 Tbsp or ½ cup juice	3 to 4 Tbsp or ½ cup juice	½ cup or ½ cup juice	½ cup or ½ cup juice
Bread, cereal, rice, and pasta	6 or more	½ slice or ½ cup	1 slice or ½ cup	1 slice or ¾ cup	1 slice or ¾ cup

*Use as a starting point. Increase serving size as energy yields dictate, but maintain variety in the diet by making sure all food groups are still appropriately represented.

Adapted from Food and Nutrition Services, U.S. Department of Agriculture: *Meal Plan Requirements and Offer versus Serve Manual*, FNS-265, 1990.

Calorie needs depend on rate of growth, activity level, body size, metabolism, and health.

Nutritional Requirements

The rate of growth diminishes from the age of 1 year until about age 10; thus, the kcal requirement per pound of body weight also diminishes during this period. For example, at 6 months, a girl needs approximately 54 kcal per pound of body weight, but by age 10, she will require only 35 kcal per pound of body weight.

Nutrient needs, however, do not diminish. From the age of 6 months to 10 years, nutrient needs actually increase because of the increased body size. Therefore, it is especially important that young children are given nutritious foods they will eat.

In general, the young child will need 2 to 3 cups of milk each day, or the equivalent in terms of calcium; however, excessive use of milk should be avoided because it can crowd out other iron-rich foods and possibly cause iron deficiency. The number of servings of the other food groups is the same as for adults, but the sizes will be smaller. The use of sweets should be minimized because children generally prefer them to nutrient-rich foods. Sweetened fruit juices should especially be avoided. Children also need water and fiber in their diets. They need to drink 1 mL of water for each kcal. If 1,200 kcal is eaten, five 8-ounce glasses of water are needed. Fiber needs are calculated according to age. After age 3 years a child's fiber needs are "age + 5g" and no more than "age + 10g." A child eating more fiber than that might be too full to eat enough other foods providing the kcal needed for growth and development. Fiber should be added slowly, if not already in the diet, with fluids also increased. Childhood is a good time to develop the lifelong good habit of getting enough dietary fiber to prevent constipation and diseases such as colon cancer and diverticulitis (Roth, 2006).

ADOLESCENCE

Adolescence is a period of rapid growth that causes major physiologic changes. The growth rate may be as much as 3 inches per year for girls and 4 inches for boys; nutrition plays a role in overall healthy adolescent development. Bones grow and gain density, muscle and fat tissue develop, and blood volume increases (Roth, 2006).

Adolescents typically have enormous appetites. When good eating habits have been established during childhood and there is nutritious food available, the teenager's food habits should present no serious problem. Peer pressure is great at this time, and good eating habits may be forgotten. Many adolescents skip breakfast and/or lunch and then eat at fast-food places (Figure 18-6). Adolescents are concerned with body

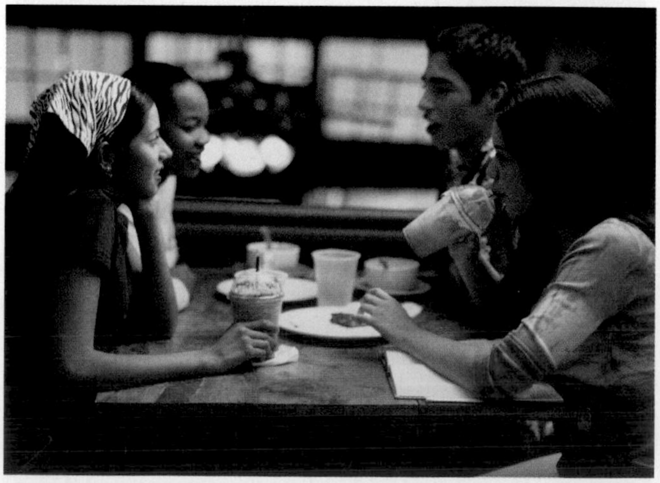

COURTESY OF GETTY IMAGES/PHOTODISC

FIGURE 18-6 Adolescents are vulnerable to peer pressure.

image and often compare their bodies to those of peers and popular media figures. They may restrict food intake, leading to inadequate nutrient intake.

Nutritional Requirements

Because of adolescents' rapid growth, kcal requirements naturally increase. Boys' kcal requirements tend to be greater than girls' because boys are generally bigger, tend to be more physically active, and have more lean muscle mass than do girls (Roth, 2006).

Except for vitamin D, nutrient needs increase dramatically at the onset of adolescence. Because of menstruation, girls have a greater need for iron than do boys. The RDAs for vitamin D, vitamin C, vitamin B_{12}, calcium, phosphorus, and iodine are the same for both sexes. The RDAs for the remaining nutrients are higher for boys than they are for girls (Roth, 2006).

Young and Middle Adulthood

The period of young adulthood ranges from approximately 18 years to 40 years of age. They appear to have boundless energy for both social and professional activities and are usually interested in exercise for its own sake, often participating in athletic events.

The middle adulthood period ranges from approximately 40 years to 65 years of age. This is a time when the physical activities of young adulthood typically begin to decrease, resulting in lowered kcal requirement for most individuals. During these years, people seldom have young children to supervise, and the strenuous physical labor of some occupations may be delegated to younger people. Middle-age people may tire more easily than they did when they were younger. They may not get as much exercise as they did in earlier years. Because appetite and food intake may not decrease, there is a common tendency toward weight gain during this period (Roth, 2006).

Nutritional Requirements

Physical growth is usually complete by the age of 25 years. Consequently, except during pregnancy and lactation, the essential nutrients are needed only to maintain and repair body tissue and to produce energy. During these years, the nutrient requirements of healthy adults change very little.

Despite men's generally larger size, only 11 of the given RDAs are greater for men than for women. Six of the RDAs are the same for both sexes. The iron requirement for women throughout the childbearing years remains higher than that for men. Extra iron is needed to replace blood loss during menstruation and to help build both the infant's and the extra maternal blood needed during pregnancy. After menopause, this requirement for women matches that of men (Roth, 2006).

The kcal requirement begins to diminish after the age of 25 years, as basal metabolism is reduced by approximately 2% to 3% per decade. This is a small amount each year, but, after 25 years, a person will gain weight if the total kcal value of the food eaten is not reduced accordingly. An individual's actual need, of course, will be determined primarily by activity and amount of lean muscle mass. Those who are more active will require more kcal than those with a high proportion of fat tissue.

A normal healthy adult should eat a variety of foods as shown on the food guide pyramid. This, along with following the *Dietary Guidelines for Americans*, should provide a healthy diet for the adult.

PROFESSIONALTIP

Preventing Eating Disorders

- Encourage healthy dietary habits and adequate exercise.
- Emphasize a healthy lifestyle over physical appearance and weight loss.
- Encourage increased self-esteem and stress a positive self-worth.
- Avoid pressuring children to achieve perfection or perform beyond their abilities.
- Recognize signs and symptoms of eating disorders, and seek professional help when suspected.

(From *Health Assessment and Physical Examination* [4th ed.], by M. E. Z. Estes, 2010, Clifton Park, NY: Delmar Cengage Learning.)

Older Adulthood

Physical changes of aging affect nutrition in several ways. The body's functions slow with age, and its ability to replace worn cells likewise diminishes. Metabolic rate slows; bones become less dense; lean muscle mass lessens; eyes do not focus on nearby objects as they once did, and some grow cloudy from cataracts; poor dentition is common; the heart and kidneys become less efficient; and hearing, taste, and smell are less acute.

Digestion is affected because the secretion of hydrochloric acid and enzymes diminishes. This, in turn, decreases the intrinsic factor synthesis, which may lead to a vitamin B_{12} deficiency. The tone of the intestines is reduced, possibly resulting in constipation or, in some cases, diarrhea (Roth, 2006).

Healthy eating habits throughout life, an exercise program suited to one's age, and enjoyable social activities can prevent or delay physical deterioration and depression during the senior years. They give purpose to the day, joy to the heart, and zest to the appetite. Nutrition and lifestyle should be carefully reviewed in any elderly client suspected of having depression.

Food–drug interactions must be monitored closely in the elderly client. Frequently, specific foods will prevent, decrease, or enhance the absorption of a particular drug.

Drug–drug interactions as well as food–drug interactions can contribute to decreased nutritional status. These interactions could affect both appetite and the absorption of nutrients from the food eaten. Careful monitoring is recommended.

Nutritional Requirements

In general, most elderly persons decrease their activity; thus their kcal needs also decrease.

The kcal requirement decreases approximately 2% to 3% per decade because both metabolism and activity slow. If kcal intake is not reduced, weight will increase. Additional weight increases the work of the heart and puts increased stress on the skeletal system. An exercise plan appropriate to one's age and health can be helpful in burning excess kcal and in toning and strengthening the muscles.

PROFESSIONALTIP

Food–Drug Interactions

Dairy products should not be consumed within 2 hours of taking the antibiotic tetracycline or the drug will not be absorbed. A person taking a blood clot–reducing drug such as warfarin sodium (Coumadin) must consume vitamin K–rich food in moderation, as this vitamin counteracts blood thinners. Even vitamin supplements can cause interactions. The antioxidant vitamins are not to be taken with blood clot–reducing medications, because they also have a tendency to thin the blood (Roth, 2006).

CLIENTTEACHING

Special Dietary Considerations for the Elderly

- Give special attention to water needs, regardless of physical activity, because the thirst mechanism is less responsive than in younger people.
- Decrease the kcal requirements in relation to activity: 10% for ages 51 to 75 and 20% to 25% for ages 75 and older. Bedridden and immobilized persons need a further reduction in kcal. Limit the quantities of empty-kcal foods (e.g., sugars, sweets, fats, oils, and alcohol).
- Maintain protein requirements, with 12% to 14% of kcal intake being derived from protein food (meat, eggs, poultry, milk, and cheese).
- Ensure adequate consumption of unsaturated fats, to provide a source of energy, provide the essential fatty acids, utilize the fat-soluble vitamins, and serve as a lubricating agent.
- Select carbohydrates as follows: limit concentrated sweets; use moderate amounts of simple sugars (candy, sugar, jams, jellies, preserves, and syrups); select most sources from complex carbohydrates (fruits, vegetables, cereals, and breads).
- Ensure adequate amounts of vitamin D, calcium, and phosphorus to maintain bone integrity (fortified milk is a good source).
- Consume high-fiber foods (dried fruits, whole-grain cereals, nuts, fresh fruit, and vegetables) to increase satiety and maintain intestinal motility and thereby prevent constipation.
- Maintain a safe, adequate intake of sodium, avoiding canned foods and salted or cured meats high in sodium content for those with cardiac problems and hypertension.
- Include foods from the food guide pyramid in the amounts that meet the RDAs for ages 51 and older.

Protein needs remain the same or may increase during illness. A well-balanced diet of a variety of foods should supply adequate amounts of vitamins and minerals. An increase in water and dietary fiber is often needed to maintain proper elimination.

Pregnancy and Lactation

Good nutrition during the 38 to 40 weeks of a normal pregnancy is essential for both mother and child. In addition to her normal nutritional requirements, the pregnant woman must provide nutrients and kcals for the fetus, the amniotic fluid, the placenta, and the increased blood volume and breast, uterine, and fat tissue.

The pregnant woman who follows a nutritionally adequate diet is more apt to feel better, retain her health, and bear a healthy infant than one who chooses her foods thoughtlessly (Roth, 2006).

Studies have shown a relationship between the mother's diet and the health of the baby at birth. It is also thought that the woman who consumes a nutritious diet before pregnancy is more apt to bear a healthy infant than one who does not. Malnutrition of the mother is believed to cause growth and mental retardation in the fetus. Infants with low birth weight (less than 5.5 pounds) have a higher mortality (death) rate than those of normal birth weight.

Nutritional Requirements

Despite the saying, the pregnant woman is not "eating for two." No increase in kcal is required during the first 12 weeks of pregnancy. After that time, an extra 300 kcal/day is recommended. This increase can almost be accomplished by drinking two *extra* 8-ounce glasses of 2% milk each day, which supplies 240 kcal. Those two extra glasses of milk also supply the extra calcium, protein, and vitamin D required during pregnancy. The other nutrients that should be increased during pregnancy are folic acid and iron. Folic acid is necessary to prevent neural tube deformities in the fetus. Folic acid has been approved as a supplement for pregnant women. Good sources of folic acid are beef, legumes, wheat germ, and eggs. Good sources of iron are red meat, dried fruit, egg yolk, and whole-grain products.

To ensure that the nutritional requirements of pregnancy are met, vitamin supplements may be prescribed in addition to an iron supplement; however, it is not advisable for the mother to take any unprescribed nutrient supplement, as an excess of vitamins or minerals can be toxic to mother and infant. Excessive vitamin A, for example, can cause birth defects (Roth, 2006).

The mother's kcal requirement increases during lactation. The kcal requirement depends on the amount of milk produced. Approximately 85 kcal are required to produce 100 mL (3⅓ oz) of milk. During the first 6 months, average daily milk production is 750 mL (25 oz), and for this, the mother requires approximately 640 extra kcal a day. During the second 6 months, when the baby begins to eat food in addition to breast milk, average daily milk production slows to 600 mL (20 oz), and the kcal requirement reduces to approximately 510 extra kcal a day.

NUTRITION AND HEALTH

An individual who embraces good nutrition is more likely to have good health than is someone who does not follow good nutritional practices. Of course, all situations of disease or ill health cannot be prevented by good nutrition.

The nutrients in the food we eat may be thought of as the building materials, fuel, and regulators necessary to keep the body functioning. When the body is supplied with nutrients in the proper amounts, it is most likely to function efficiently and effectively. The body is very adaptable and keeps functioning, although less effectively, even when not supplied with the proper amounts of nutrients. In this situation, however, the body is more susceptible to some diseases.

Primary Nutritional Disease

A primary nutritional disease occurs when nutrition is the cause of the disease. Usually, there is an inadequate intake of one or more nutrients. Some examples of such diseases are scurvy, from inadequate intake of vitamin C; rickets, from insufficient intake of vitamin D; and anemia, from a deficiency of iron in the diet.

Excesses of nutrients can also cause illness. These, however, occur when nutrient supplements are taken in excess, rather than from food intake. For instance, excess vitamin D may cause nausea, diarrhea, weight loss, and calcification of the renal tubules, blood vessels, and bronchi. Excess niacin may cause flushing, itching, and hypotension.

Secondary Nutritional Disease

Most nutritional diseases are secondary diseases; that is, they are a complication of another disease or condition. The original disease or condition interferes with digestion or absorption, or there is an increased need for one or more nutrients. For instance, in pregnancy, the body's need for iron increases. Not receiving the increased amount may cause anemia in the mother. In malabsorption disorders, the body is unable to absorb sufficient amounts of certain nutrients. The amount ingested may be adequate, but the body is unable to use it. Rapid excretion from the body, as in diarrhea, does not allow the nutrients to be absorbed and utilized. Uncontrolled diarrhea can lead to dehydration along with electrolyte and acid–base imbalance.

WEIGHT MANAGEMENT

Maintaining weight at a desired level can be very difficult for some people. Weight management is based on the relationship between the intake and use of kcal. When these two elements are balanced, weight is maintained at a steady level. A range of 10% over or under the desired weight is considered appropriate.

Determining Caloric Needs

The number of kcal needed to achieve or maintain a desired weight is based on two factors: basal energy needs and total energy requirements.

Basal Energy Needs

Basal energy need refers to the number of kcal required to keep an individual alive when at rest. There are two ways to determine basal energy (kcal) needs. One is based on the person's desired weight (Table 18-11), the other on the person's actual weight.

Calculation using desired weight is as follows:

Basal energy needs = desired weight × 10

Table 18-11 Determining Desired Weight

BUILD	WOMEN	MEN
Medium	100 lb for 5 ft of height, plus 5 lb for each additional inch	106 lb for 5 ft of height, plus 6 lb for each additional inch
Small	Subtract 10%	Subtract 10%
Large	Add 10%	Add 10%

Examples

Female: 5 ft 5 in tall
5 ft = 100 lb
5 in = 25 lb
125 lb desired weight
125 × 10 = 1,250
Basal energy needs = 1,250 kcal

Male: 5 ft 9 in tall
5 ft = 106 lb
9 in = 54 lb
160 lb desired weight
160 × 10 = 1,600
Basal energy needs = 1,600 kcal

Calculation using actual weight is as follows:

Female weight in kg × 0.9 × 24 = basal kcal
Male weight in kg × 1 × 24 = basal kcal
(Weight in lb ÷ 2.2 = weight in kg)

Examples

Female weighs 130 lb
130 ÷ 2.2 = 59.1 kg
59.1 kg × 0.9 × 24 = 1,276.6
Basal energy needs = 1,276.6 kcal

Male weighs 170 lb
170 ÷ 2.2 = 77.3 kg
77.3 kg × 1 × 24 = 1,855.2
Basal energy needs = 1,855.2 kcal

Total Energy Requirements

People do not live their lives at rest. They are active! Kilocalories must be added to the basal metabolic requirement in order to meet the needs of activity. All activity is not equal in kcal needed, however. A person's overall activity level can be divided into sedentary (light, such as watching television), moderate (such as playing tennis), or strenuous (such as running a marathon). The following formulas can be used to determine the number of kcal to add given the activity level:

Sedentary: basal kcal × 1.3 = total kcal
Moderate: basal kcal × 1.5 = total kcal
Strenuous: basal kcal × 2.0 = total kcal

Example: The 125-lb woman in the preceding example who is planning on running a marathon would need the following:

1,250 (basal kcal) × 2 = 2,500 kcal

Factors in addition to activity that have an effect on the total kcal need are state of health and climate. A person who is ill needs more kcal to repair tissue. A cold climate requires a person to take in more kcal to provide more thermal energy to maintain body temperature.

OVERWEIGHT

A person is considered to be overweight when 11% to 19% above the desired weight. **Obesity** is considered present in a person who is 20% or more above the desired weight. Overweight conditions can become serious health hazards by placing increased strain on the heart, lungs, muscles, bones, and joints. Overweight and obese people are more susceptible to diabetes and hypertension and tend to have a shorter life span.

According to the Centers for Disease Control and Prevention (CDC, 2006), obesity is a major problem in the United States, with an increase of overweight and obesity in children and adults throughout the world. In the United States, children between the ages of 2 and 19 years are 17.1% overweight. Among adults, 32.2% are overweight with almost 5% extremely obese.

Causes

There is no single cause of obesity. Genetic, physiologic, biochemical, and psychological factors may all contribute to overweight conditions. Most often, the cause of being overweight or obese is an energy imbalance. That is, more kcal are being taken in than are being used. When this occurs, the body stores the excess kcal as adipose tissue. Hypothyroidism is a possible but rare cause of obesity. In this condition, basal metabolism is low, thereby reducing the number of kcal needed for energy. Unless corrected, this condition can result in excess weight (Roth, 2006).

Treatment

Treatment for an overweight person involves two parts: revised eating habits and exercise. Revised eating habits include reducing daily kcal intake at mealtime, limiting between-meal snacks to fresh fruits or vegetables, and restricting or eliminating empty calories.

One pound of body weight equals 3,500 kcal. Therefore, to lose 1 pound per week, a person must reduce kcal intake by 500 kcal each day. Weight loss should be limited to 1 to 2 pounds per week, unless the client is under strict medical supervision. Diets should be planned according to the minimum servings of the food guide pyramid and should not be reduced to below 1,200 kcal/day in order for the dieter to receive adequate nutrients to sustain health.

Attention should also be given to food preparation. Frying adds many kcal from fat to a food item. Broiling, grilling, baking, roasting, boiling, and poaching are healthy ways to prepare foods. Vegetables should be eaten raw or steamed; the addition of butter, margarine, or sauces should be avoided. Eating habits may be adapted to decrease the amount eaten and yet provide satisfaction: place food on a smaller plate, cut food into smaller bites, chew each bite at least 12 times, and place the fork on the plate between bites.

Exercise, particularly aerobic exercise, is an excellent adjunct to any weight-loss program. Aerobic exercise uses energy from the body's fat reserves, as it increases the amount of oxygen the body takes in. Examples of aerobic exercise are dancing, jogging, bicycling, skiing, rowing, and power walking. Such exercise helps tone the muscles, burns kcal, increases the basal metabolism so that food is burned faster, and is fun for the participant. Any exercise program must begin slowly and increase over time so that no physical damage occurs.

CRITICAL THINKING

Weight Loss

What should the nurse know about nutrition in order to help an obese client lose weight?

Exercise alone can only rarely replace the need to be mindful of diet, however. The dieter should be made aware of the number of kcal burned by specific exercises to avoid overeating after the workout.

UNDERWEIGHT

Persons are considered to be underweight when their weight is 10% to 15% below the desired weight. An underweight person is more likely to have nutritional deficiencies because of the decreased intake of food. For women, this can cause complications during pregnancy. Being underweight may lower a person's resistance to infection. Being severely underweight may even cause death.

Causes

There are several possible causes of being underweight, such as an inadequate intake of food, excessive exercise, poor absorption of nutrients, or severe infection. Occasionally, hyperthyroidism may be the cause. After the adequacy of food intake and the appropriate activity level are ascertained, specific diagnostic tests must be done to determine whether poor absorption, infection, or hyperthyroidism are present.

Treatment

Dietary treatment for an inadequate intake of food is to gradually increase the amount of food eaten. Also, higher-kcal foods can be eaten. Between-meal snacks and a bedtime snack can help increase the intake of food.

If the individual is to gain 1 pound per week, 3,500 kcal in addition to the individual's basic normal weekly kcal requirement are prescribed. This means an extra 500 kcal must be taken in each day. If a weight gain of 2 pounds per week is required, an additional 7,000 kcal each week, or an additional 1,000 kcal per day, are necessary. This diet cannot be immediately accepted at full kcal value. Time will be needed to gradually increase the daily kcal value by increasing intake of foods rich in carbohydrates, some fats, and protein. Vitamins and minerals are supplied in adequate amounts. If there are deficiencies of some vitamins and minerals, supplements are prescribed (Roth, 2006).

FOOD LABELING

In 1990, Congress passed the Nutrition, Labeling and Education Act (NLEA). This was the first legislation on labeling since the 1970s. Before this newest legislation, labeling was required only if a nutrient was added or a nutritional claim was made about the product. Now labeling is required on virtually all retail food products, including bulk foods, fresh produce, and seafood. The nutrition information for fresh produce and seafood is to be displayed or made available at the point of purchase through counter cards, booklets, loose-leaf binders, signs, or tags.

The labels must follow the approved uniform format and use standard serving sizes and household measurements.

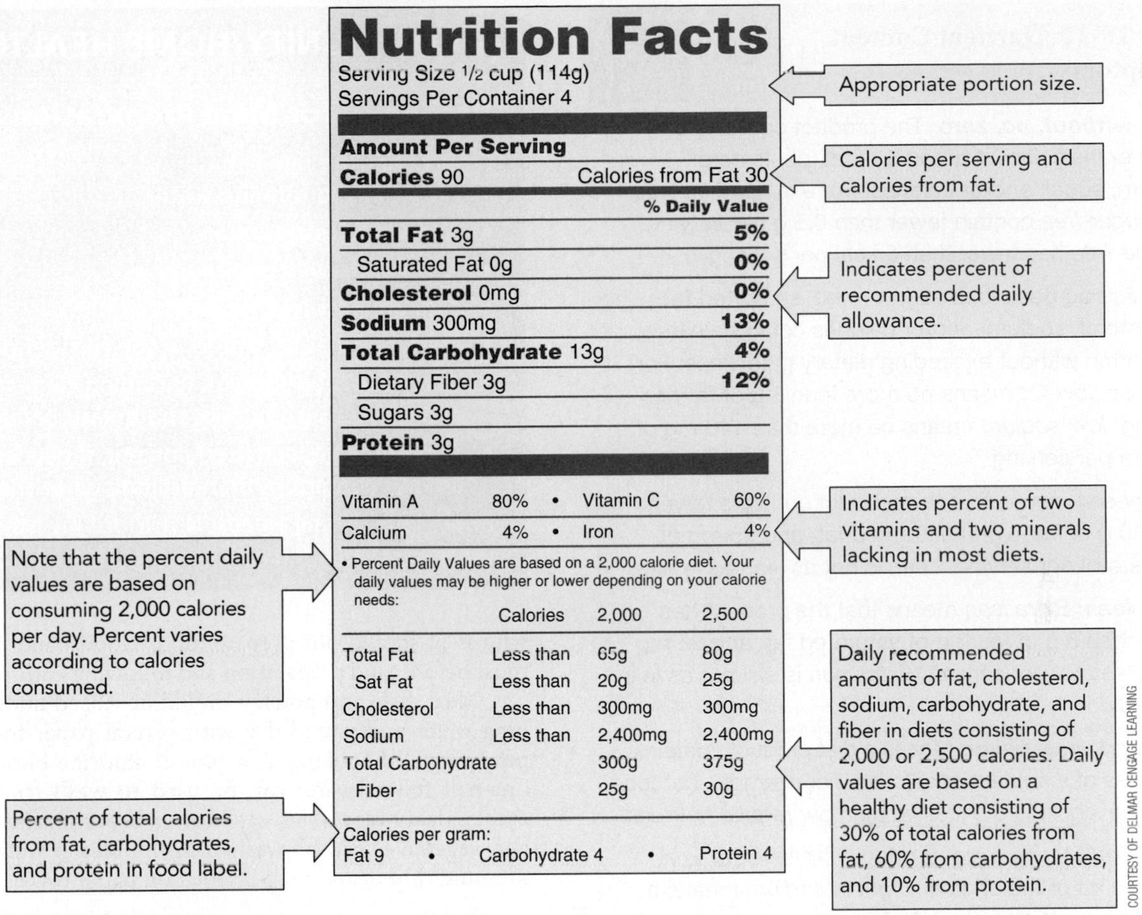
Nutrition Facts
Serving Size 1/2 cup (114g)
Servings Per Container 4
Amount Per Serving
Calories 90 Calories from Fat 30
% Daily Value
Total Fat 3g 5%
Saturated Fat 0g 0%
Cholesterol 0mg 0%
Sodium 300mg 13%
Total Carbohydrate 13g 4%
Dietary Fiber 3g 12%
Sugars 3g
Protein 3g
Vitamin A 80% • Vitamin C 60%
Calcium 4% • Iron 4%
• Percent Daily Values are based on a 2,000 calorie diet. Your daily values may be higher or lower depending on your calorie needs:
Calories 2,000 2,500
Total Fat Less than 65g 80g
Sat Fat Less than 20g 25g
Cholesterol Less than 300mg 300mg
Sodium Less than 2,400mg 2,400mg
Total Carbohydrate 300g 375g
Fiber 25g 30g
Calories per gram:
Fat 9 • Carbohydrate 4 • Protein 4
Appropriate portion size.
Calories per serving and calories from fat.
Indicates percent of recommended daily allowance.
Indicates percent of two vitamins and two minerals lacking in most diets.
Daily recommended amounts of fat, cholesterol, sodium, carbohydrate, and fiber in diets consisting of 2,000 or 2,500 calories. Daily values are based on a healthy diet consisting of 30% of total calories from fat, 60% from carbohydrates, and 10% from protein.
Note that the percent daily values are based on consuming 2,000 calories per day. Percent varies according to calories consumed.
Percent of total calories from fat, carbohydrates, and protein in food label.
COURTESY OF DELMAR CENGAGE LEARNING

FIGURE 18-7 **Sample Food Label**

Information on the label includes calories per serving; calories from fat; total fat, saturated fat, and cholesterol; total sodium; total carbohydrate, dietary fiber, and sugar; amount of protein; and percentages of vitamins A and C, calcium, and iron. A sample food label is shown in Figure 18-7.

Words used to describe nutrient content, such as low, light, lean, or reduced, now have specific, consistent definitions (Table 18-12).

The standardized label and word definitions make it easier for the consumer not only to know the amount of specific nutrients in a food or food product, but also to easily compare foods and food products.

FOOD QUALITY AND SAFETY

When planning an adequate diet, the quality and safety of the food is considered in addition to the types of foods and serving sizes. To ensure the quality (nutrient content) and safety of food, proper storage, preparation, sanitation, and cooking are necessary; such measures prevent or reduce the risk of food-borne illnesses.

> **CRITICAL THINKING**
>
> **Evaluating Food Labels**
>
> Evaluate the health value of the food described in Figure 18-7. For example, calculate the serving size, read the total fat content, and decide if the food is a good value or lesser value to eat.

Quality of Food

Foods usually begin to lose nutrients when they are harvested, so they are best purchased when fresh in appearance and of bright color. Dates should be checked on all processed foods such as dairy products, lunch and other processed meats, crackers, and breads; all foods should be used before their expiration dates. All produce should be cooked until tender and thoroughly done, in the smallest amount of water possible to prevent loss of vitamins. Cooking meats via stewing increases mineral loss, so cooking methods that retain the most nutrients should be used instead; these include stir-frying, steaming, microwaving, or pressure cooking.

Safety of Food

There are three aspects to food safety: proper storage, proper sanitation, and proper cooking.

Proper Storage

Foods must be properly stored before and after purchase. Packages and jars should be tightly sealed, and cans should not leak or bulge. Any foods that look or smell unusual or show signs of mold or deterioration should be discarded. Hot foods should be kept hot—above 140°F—and cold foods should be kept below 40°F. Foods allowed to stand at temperatures

TABLE 18-12 Nutrient Content Descriptors

- ***Free, without, no, zero:*** The product contains only a tiny or insignificant amount of fat, cholesterol, sodium, sugar, and/or calories. For example, *fat-free* and *sugar-free* contain fewer than 0.5 g per serving. *Calorie-free* has fewer than 5 kcal per serving.
- ***Low:*** A food described as *low* in fat, saturated fat, cholesterol, sodium, and/or calories could be eaten fairly often without exceeding dietary guidelines. For instance, *low-fat* means no more than 3 g of fat per serving; *low-sodium* means no more than 140 mg of sodium per serving.
- ***Lean:*** *Lean* means that the product contains fewer than 10 g of fat, 4 g of saturated fat, and 95 mg of cholesterol per serving. *Lean* is not as lean as is *low.*
- ***Extra lean:*** *Extra lean* means that the product has fewer than 5 g of fat, 2 g of saturated fat, and 95 mg of cholesterol per serving. *Extra lean* is still not as lean as is *low.*
- ***Reduced, less, fewer:*** Means a diet product contains 25% less of a nutrient or calories. For example, hotdogs might be labeled *25% less fat than our regular hotdogs.*
- ***Light/lite:*** Means a diet product with ⅓ fewer kcal or ½ the fat of the original. *Light in sodium* means a product with ½ the usual sodium.
- ***More:*** A food in which one serving has at least 10% more of the daily value of a vitamin, mineral, or fiber than usual.
- ***Good source of:*** One serving contains 10% to 19% of the daily value for a particular nutrient.
- ***High:*** One serving contains 20% or more of the daily value for a particular nutrient.
- ***Trans fat free:*** Indicates that the product has less than 0.5 grams of trans fat and less than 0.5 grams of saturated fat.
- ***Healthy:*** *Healthy* means that the serving does not have more than 60 milligrams of cholesterol, 3 grams of fat, 1 gram of saturated fat, 360 milligrams or less of sodium, and more than 10% of the daily value of vitamin A, vitamin C, iron, calcium, protein, or fiber.

between 40°F and 140°F provide an ideal breeding ground for pathogens. Leftovers must be refrigerated promptly and not allowed to cool before refrigerating.

Proper Sanitation

Proper sanitation means that all cooking utensils, pots, pans, and cutting boards, as well as the cook's hands, have been washed with soap and hot water before preparation begins. To prevent contamination of one food by another, cutting boards, utensils, and the cook's hands should be washed well with soap and hot water between preparation of different foods. A person who is ill should not prepare food. Good hand hygiene is a must before food preparation and following bathroom use.

Meat, fish, and poultry should be rinsed under cold running water and patted dry with several paper towels before preparing and cooking. A capful of chlorine bleach in a sink one-half full of water can be used to wash fruits and vegetables: leafy vegetables, cauliflower, broccoli, and other fruits and vegetables can be washed in the bleach water for a few minutes, rinsed, and then drained on paper towels.

COMMUNITY/HOME HEALTH CARE

Resources for Meal Preparation

Ensure that the family has:

- Hot and cold running water
- A working refrigerator
- A working oven and range
- A clean, pest-free kitchen
- Fresh perishables stored in the refrigerator
- Adequate food supplies (including canned goods and staples, such as milk and bread), safely stored
- Appropriate adaptive equipment, if needed, such as low countertops that facilitate wheelchair access

Data from "Home Health Nutrition" by M. Costello, 1996, *MedSurg Nursing 5*(4), 229–238.

Proper Cooking

Meats, fish, shellfish, and eggs should be cooked well done to ensure that harmful microorganisms are destroyed (Figure 18-8).

FOOD-BORNE ILLNESSES

When proper storage, sanitation, or cooking are not maintained, food-borne illnesses often occur. These illnesses range in severity from fairly mild (such as staphylococcal food poisoning) to potentially fatal (such as botulism and *E. coli*). The important thing to remember is that food-borne illness is highly preventable with proper handling, preparation, and storage of food.

Nutrition involves the appropriate kinds and amounts of a variety of available foods so that a properly functioning body can digest and use the nutrients in the foods. If the foods are unsafe, they cannot adequately nourish the body.

NURSING PROCESS

Collection of subjective and objective data regarding the client's nutrition serves as the basis for determining the type of nutritional care the client requires.

ASSESSMENT

Proper assessment allows the health care team to determine the degree to which the client's nutritional needs are met. Assessment must be performed logically and should include a nutritional history, physical examination, and the results of laboratory tests.

Age and pregnancy determine some specific items to be included in the nutritional assessment.

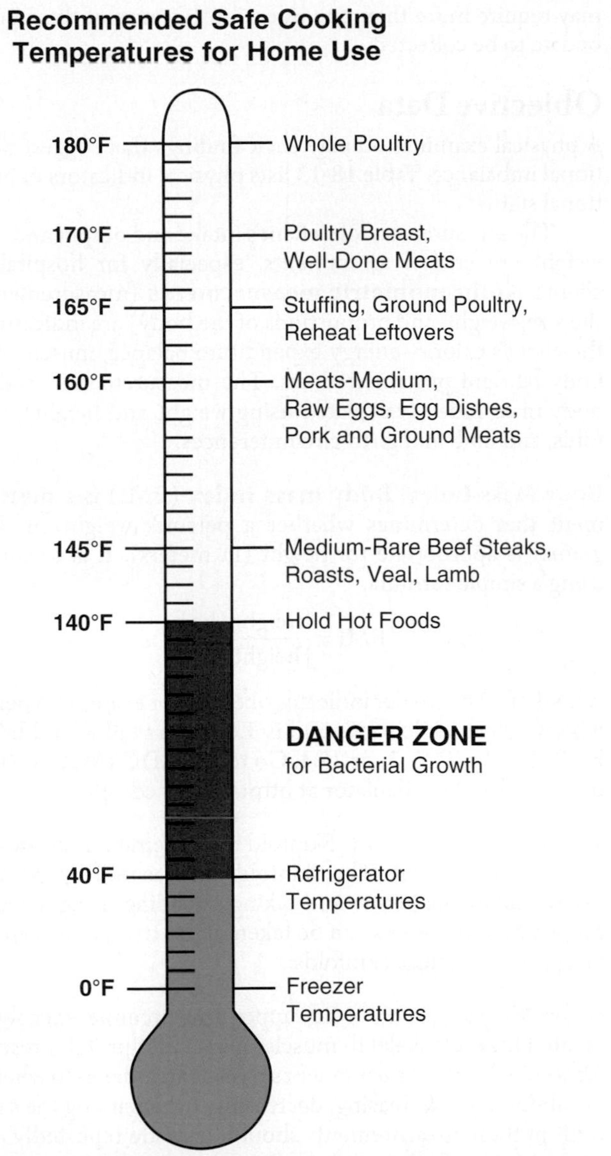

FIGURE 18-8 Bacterium can increase from one to 2,097,152 bacteria within one hour at temperatures between 40 and 140° F. Cook foods at temperatures as indicated on the thermometer. *(From United States Department of Agriculture [USDA] and United States Department of Health and Human Services [HHS], 2000. Nutrition and your health: Dietary guidelines for Americans [Home and Garden Bulletin, No. 232, 5th ed.]. Washington, DC: U.S. DA and HHS.)*

Nutritional assessment for an infant should include:

- Height and weight
- Sleeping habits
- Type of feeding (breast- or bottle-fed)
- If breastfeeding, the mother's nutritional status and use of alcohol, tobacco, caffeine, and drugs; infant's feeding schedule (how often fed and for how long)
- If formula feeding, type, frequency, and method of preparation and storage; feeding schedule; amount taken at each feeding
- Use of vitamin/mineral supplements
- If on solid foods, age at introduction, and any reactions or allergies
- Family attitudes about eating, food, and weight

The basic nutritional assessment for everyone over 1 year old should include:

- Nutritional status
- Height and weight
- Meal and snack pattern (food record or 24-hour recall)
- Adequacy of intake based on the food guide pyramid
- Food allergies
- Physical activity
- Cultural, ethnic, and family influences
- Use of vitamin/mineral supplements

In addition to the basic nutritional assessment, during childhood dental health is also assessed.

In addition to the basic nutritional assessment, the following is assessed for the adolescent client:

- Use of alcohol, tobacco, caffeine, and drugs
- Use of fad diets
- Family attitude toward thinness and the adolescent's weight

In addition to the basic nutritional assessment, the following is assessed for the adult client:

- Use of alcohol, tobacco, caffeine, and drugs
- Use of fad diets
- Prescribed restricted diet

In addition to the basic nutritional assessment, the following is assessed for elderly clients:

- Undesirable change in weight
- Dentition and swallowing
- Appetite
- Vision
- Hand–eye coordination
- Adequacy of daily intake of food
- Ability to self-feed
- Prescribed restricted diet
- Use of alcohol, tobacco, caffeine, and drugs

In addition to the basic nutritional assessment, the following is assessed for the pregnant client:

- Weight and rate of weight gain
- Diet changes in response to pregnancy
- Cravings for foods or nonfoods (pica)
- Intake of supplemental vitamins/minerals
- Feeding plans (breast or formula)
- Use of alcohol, caffeine, tobacco, or drugs

Subjective Data

Subjective data are obtained through a nutritional history by asking clients questions. Several methods are used in collecting these subjective data: 24-hour recall, food-frequency questionnaire, food record, and diet history. Although the history data may indicate adequate nutrition, clients must be reassessed periodically to prevent nutritional problems.

24-Hour Recall The 24-hour recall requires client identification of everything consumed in the previous 24 hours. It is performed easily and quickly by asking pertinent questions; however, clients may be unable to accurately recall their intake or anything atypical in the diet. Family members can often assist with these data, if necessary.

PROFESSIONALTIP

Nutritional History

Food preferences are an expression of an individual's likes and dislikes. They may be related to the texture of food, how it is prepared, or what was served to the individual during childhood; however, preferences can also be an expression of the person's economic, ecological, ethical, or religious beliefs.

Peer pressure often dictates what teenagers eat. Stress, depression, and alcohol abuse alter the appetite. Medications can alter food absorption and excretion and affect the taste of food. Gastrointestinal disorders can cause anorexia, nausea, vomiting, diarrhea, constipation, discomfort, and pain, all of which may alter eating habits and food preferences.

Food-Frequency Questionnaire The food-frequency method gathers data relative to the number of times per day, week, or month that the client eats particular foods. The nurse can tailor the questions to particular nutrients, such as cholesterol and saturated fat. This method validates the accuracy of the 24-hour recall and provides a more complete picture of foods consumed.

Food Record The food record provides quantitative information regarding all foods consumed, with portions weighed and measured for three consecutive days. This method requires full client or family member cooperation.

Diet History The diet history elicits detailed information regarding the client's nutritional status, general health pattern, socioeconomic status, and cultural factors. This method incorporates information similar to that collected by the 24-hour recall and food-frequency questionnaire. The history may require more than one interview because of the amount of data to be collected.

Objective Data

A physical examination may elicit findings that suggest nutritional imbalance. Table 18-13 lists physical indicators of nutritional status.

The measurement of a client's intake and output and daily weight are critical assessments, especially for hospitalized clients. **Anthropometric measurements** (measurement of the size, weight, and proportions of the body) are indicative of the client's calorie–energy expenditure balance, muscle mass, body fat, and protein reserves. The measurements used are body mass index (calculated using weight and height), skinfolds, and limb and girth circumferences.

Body Mass Index **Body mass index** (BMI) is a measurement that determines whether a person's weight (in kilograms) is appropriate for height (in meters). It is calculated using a simple formula:

$$\text{BMI} = \frac{\text{weight (kg)}}{[\text{height (m)}]^2}$$

A BMI of 27 or greater indicates obesity. For example, a person who weighs 65 kilograms and is 1.6 meters tall would have a BMI of 65 kg/(1.6)2, or 25.4. Go to the CDC's Web site for a body mass index calculator at http://www.cdc.gov.

Skinfold Measurement Skinfold measurement indicates the amount of body fat. The skinfold is measured by grasping the subcutaneous tissue and taking a reading using a special caliper. Measurements can be taken of the tricep, subscapular, bicep, and suprailiac skinfolds.

Other Measurements Mid–upper-arm circumference serves as an index of skeletal muscle mass and protein reserve. Abdominal-girth measurement serves as an index as to whether the abdomen is increasing, decreasing, or remaining the same. Both of these measurements should be made repeatedly over a span of time, for best assessment.

TABLE 18-13 Physical Indicators of Nutritional Status

BODY AREA	GOOD NUTRITION	INADEQUATE NUTRITION
General	Alert, responsive, sleeps well, energetic, seldom ill	Apathetic, easily fatigued, looks tired, often ill
Weight	Appropriate for age, height, body build	Overweight, underweight
Skeleton	Good posture, no malformations	Poor posture
Skin	Good color, no rashes or swelling, smooth, moist, good turgor	Rough, dry, pale, poor turgor
Muscles	Firm, good tone	Flaccid, poor tone
Nails	Pink, firm	Pale, brittle
Eyes	Clear, bright, moist	Dull, pale, dry
Hair	Shiny, smooth	Dull, dry, brittle
Elimination	Regular, soft	Diarrhea or constipation

PROFESSIONALTIP

Creatinine Excretion

Record the client's height and gender on the laboratory request for a creatinine excretion test because the normal values are standardized on the basis of these variables.

Laboratory Tests Several laboratory tests provide information about a client's nutritional status. These include the protein indices of serum albumin, prealbumin, and serum transferrin; hemoglobin; total lymphocyte count; blood urea nitrogen (BUN); and urine creatinine. The serum albumin blood test is used to measure prolonged protein depletion that occurs in chronic malnutrition, liver disease, and nephrosis. The prealbumin test indicates protein depletion in acute conditions such as trauma and inflammation. Serum transferrin also measures the protein level as indicated by iron stores. Hemoglobin is a measurement of the oxygen- and iron-carrying capacity of the blood. Total lymphocyte count may reflect protein-calorie malnutrition, which inhibits lymphocyte synthesis. Blood urea nitrogen is a nitrogen balance study that indicates the degree to which protein is being depleted or replaced, and urine creatinine excretion indicates the amount of creatinine eliminated by the kidneys.

NURSING DIAGNOSIS

Nursing diagnoses (NANDA-I, 2010) related specifically to nutrition include:

*Imbalanced **N**utrition: Less Than Body Requirements*
*Imbalanced **N**utrition: More Than Body Requirements*
*Risk for Imbalanced **N**utrition: More Than Body Requirements*

Other possible nursing diagnoses related to nutritional problems include the following:

*Disturbed **B**ody Image*
*Ineffective **B**reastfeeding*
*Impaired **D**entition*
*Deficient **K**nowledge* (specify)
*Impaired **O**ral Mucous Membrane*
*Acute **P**ain, Chronic **P**ain*
*Feeding **S**elf-Care Deficit*
*Chronic Low **S**elf-Esteem*
*Risk for Impaired **S**kin Integrity*

PLANNING/OUTCOME IDENTIFICATION

A plan should be formulated by the nurse and client to achieve mutually agreed-upon goals. The plan is individualized to meet the client's specific needs. These needs may include achieving desired weight, correcting nutritional deficiencies, maintaining a special diet, preventing nutritional disorders secondary to a particular therapy, or improving nutrition to promote health and prevent disease.

Goals for clients with nutritional alterations might be as follows:

Client will maintain intake and output balance.
Client will comply with diet therapy, avoiding high-sodium foods.
Client will gain 2 pounds in 4 weeks.

IMPLEMENTATION

The nurse and client actually carry out the plan through specific actions. Interventions to accomplish the goals may include diet therapy, assistance with meals, weight and intake monitoring, and nutritional support.

Diet Therapy

Diet therapy is the treatment of a disease or disorder with a special diet. A **dietary prescription/order** is an order written by the physician for food, including liquids. This is similar to a medication prescription written for medications a client receives. A client must not be given anything to eat or drink without an order. The dietary prescription is written for one or more of the following purposes:

- Provide the client with nutrients needed for maintenance or growth
- Prepare a client for diagnostic tests
- Treat the client with a disease or condition

When the dietary prescription has been received, the dietary department is notified so that the proper food is sent to the client.

Many times a client needs some help in understanding changes in the diet and the reasons the changes are necessary. A basic knowledge of nutrition and diet therapy contributes to the nurse's ability to competently answer the client's questions about nutrition and diet. It is important, however, for the nurse to recognize when to refer questions to the dietitian.

The dietary prescription may be for nothing by mouth, a standard diet, or a special diet.

Nothing by Mouth Nothing by mouth (nil per os, NPO) status is a type of diet modification as well as a fluid restriction. This is often prescribed before surgery and certain diagnostic procedures, to rest the GI tract, or when the client's nutritional problem has not been identified.

Standard Diets Each health care agency has standard or house diets. The standard diets include general (sometimes called regular), soft, clear liquid, full liquid, mechanical soft, and pureed.

General or Regular Diet The general or regular diet is planned according to the food guide pyramid. There are no restrictions of any kind. It is an adequate diet providing approximately 2,000 kcal a day.

Soft Diet A soft diet provides foods that are easy to chew and swallow, thus promoting mechanical digestion of foods. Foods avoided on this diet include nuts, seeds (tomatoes and berries with seeds), raw fruits and vegetables, fried foods, and whole grains. The food guide pyramid is the basis for this diet, although fewer kcal, usually approximately 1,800, are provided.

Clear-Liquid Diet The clear-liquid diet, also called the surgical liquid diet, is ordered as preparation for diagnostic tests or as the first meal or two after surgery. It consists mostly of water and carbohydrates, providing approximately 500 kcal/day. This is a very nutritionally inadequate diet but does relieve thirst, aids in hydration, and mildly stimulates peristalsis.

Liquids included are water; clear, fat-free broth; tea; coffee; clear and strained fruit juices; jello; popsicles; and carbonated drinks such as lemon-lime soda.

Full-Liquid Diet A full-liquid diet provides approximately 800 to 1,000 kcal per day. It includes all foods that are liquid at room temperature. In addition to the liquids on a clear-liquid diet, milk; milk drinks; cream soups; strained, cooked cereals; ice cream; puddings; all fruit and vegetable juices; and custard are included.

Mechanical Soft or Edentulous Diet A mechanical soft or edentulous diet consists of food fixed especially for a person who has no teeth or has difficulty chewing. The food is either ground or chopped into very small pieces and cooked very soft, to ease the work of chewing.

Pureed Diet A pureed diet uses foods that have been blended to a smooth consistency. It is prescribed for clients who have difficulty swallowing.

Special Diets A special diet restores or maintains a client's nutritional status. These diets are variations of the general diet; however, they still must provide all the nutrients of the general diets. Special diets may provide specific amounts of nutrients or may increase or restrict certain foods. Low-residue, high-fiber, liberal bland, fat-controlled, and sodium-restricted are types of special diets.

Low-Residue Diet The low-residue diet of 5 to 10 g of fiber a day reduces the normal work of the intestines by reducing food residue. Some low-residue diets limit tough or coarse meats, milk, and milk products. The low-residue diet is prescribed to decrease GI mucosal irritation in clients with diverticulitis, ulcerative colitis, and Crohn's disease. Foods to be avoided include raw fruits (except bananas), vegetables, seeds, plant fiber, and whole grains. Dairy products are limited to two servings per day.

High-Fiber Diet A high-fiber diet contains 25 to 35 g or more of dietary fiber. A high-fiber diet is an integral part of the treatment regimen for diverticulosis because it increases the forward motion of the indigestible wastes through the colon. This diet prevents constipation, hemorrhoids, and colon cancer, along with helping to treat diabetes mellitus and atherosclerosis.

The recommended foods for this diet include coarse and whole-grain breads and cereals, bran, all fruits, vegetables (especially raw), and legumes. This nutritionally adequate diet must be introduced gradually to prevent the formation of gas and the discomfort that accompanies it. Eight 8-oz glasses of water also must be consumed along with the increased fiber.

Liberal Bland Diet A liberal bland diet eliminates chemical and mechanical food irritants such as fried foods, alcohol, and caffeine. This diet is prescribed for clients with gastritis and ulcers because it reduces GI irritation.

PROFESSIONALTIP

Opening a Food Tray

Remove the tray cover before moving the over-bed table in front of the client. The concentration of odors when the lid is first removed can be nauseating to the client.

Fat-Controlled Diet The fat-controlled diet reduces the total fat ingested by replacing saturated fats with monounsaturated and polyunsaturated fats and restricting cholesterol. This diet is prescribed for clients with atherosclerosis, heart disease, and obesity. Saturated-fat foods to be avoided include animal fats, gravies, sauces, chocolate, and whole-milk products.

Sodium-Restricted Diet Sodium-restricted diets tailor the level of sodium to mild (2 to 3 g), moderate (1,000 mg), strict (500 mg), or severe (250 mg). This diet is prescribed for clients with fluid volume excess, hypertension, heart failure, myocardial infarction, or renal failure.

Assistance with Meals

Assisting with meals consists of preparing the client, preparing the environment, serving the tray, and assisting with eating.

Preparing the Client Before taking a meal tray into a client's room, the nurse must ensure that the client is ready to eat: face and hands are washed, oral hygiene completed, and, if necessary, the bladder emptied. The nurse should help the client into a comfortable eating position; this must be individualized to each client, as not everyone is allowed or able to sit up to eat a meal.

Preparing the Environment The nurse should make every effort to see that the physical environment is as conducive to a pleasant mealtime atmosphere as possible. This may necessitate cleaning and clearing the over-bed table so that the tray can be placed on it, tidying the room to remove offensive sights and smells, and brightening the room.

Serving the Tray The nurse checks that the tray contains the diet ordered, that everything on the tray is appropriate for the diet, and that nothing has spilled. For example, if a low-sodium diet tray has a salt packet, the packet is removed. The nurse checks the client's ID band against the name on the tray; it is very important that the correct meal is served to each client. The nurse prepares the food by opening cartons or cutting food, if necessary.

Assisting with Eating The client who needs assistance in eating is served last. This way, the nurse will have ample time and not have to hurry the client through the meal (Figure 18-9).

PROFESSIONALTIP

Feeding a Client

- Position yourself at the same level as the client (stand if the bed is high, sit if the bed is low).
- Allow time for prayer, if the client wishes.
- Protect the client's clothing with a napkin.
- Allow time for chewing (do not hurry the client).
- Give bite-size portions.
- Warn about hot foods (do not blow on food to cool).
- Use a separate straw for each liquid.
- Allow the client to choose the order in which the food is eaten.
- Offer pleasant conversation.

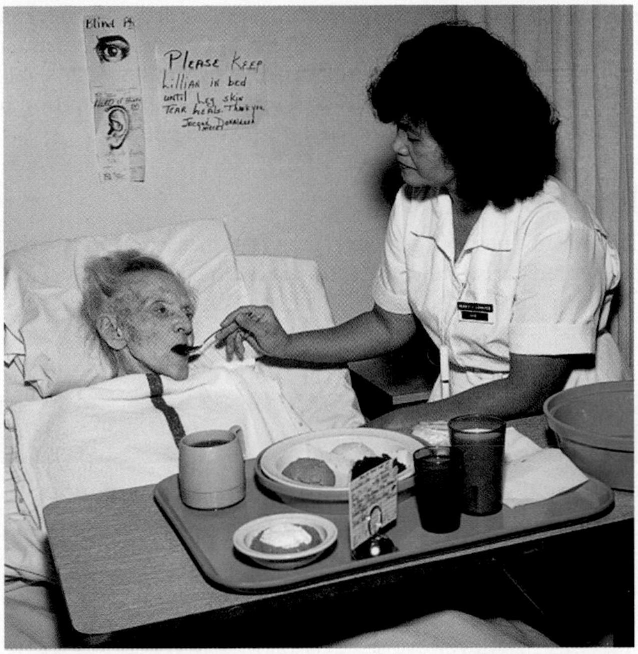

COURTESY OF DELMAR CENGAGE LEARNING

FIGURE 18-9 **Older adults may have health problems that affect their ability to self-feed.**

Weight and Intake Monitoring

Measuring weight daily or weekly and measuring the amount of food and fluid intake monitors therapy effectiveness.

Recording and Reporting

After the client has finished eating, the tray is promptly removed. The amount of food eaten is recorded, usually as the percentage of the meal eaten. When a client with diabetes does not eat all the food on the tray, both the charge nurse and the dietitian must be notified so that a supplemental feeding is sent later. If the client is on intake and output (I&O), the amount of fluids consumed during the meal is recorded. Any problems or difficulty in eating as well as likes and dislikes are reported and documented on the client's medical record.

Nutritional Support

There are two ways nutritional support for adult clients are delivered: enteral nutrition and parenteral nutrition. **Enteral nutrition** includes both the ingestion of food orally and the delivery of nutrients through a GI tube, but is generally used to mean the latter. **Parenteral nutrition** refers to nutrients bypassing the GI system and entering the blood directly.

PROFESSIONALTIP

The Visually Impaired Client and Eating

Clients with impaired vision need an explanation of what is on the plate. For example, using the face of a clock, describe where each food is located. The plate should have a raised edge so the food can be scooped to the outside of the plate. Serving liquids in either a glass or a cup with a lid and straw is helpful to prevent spills.

Enteral Nutrition When clients cannot or will not take food by mouth, but their GI tracts are working, they are given tube feedings (TF). Sometimes, this may be necessary because of unconsciousness, surgery, stroke, severe malnutrition, or extensive burns. Tube feedings maintain the structural and functional integrity of the GI tract, enhance the utilization of nutrients, and are a safe, economical way to provide nutrients.

Usually, for periods that do not exceed 6 weeks, tube feeding is administered through a nasogastric (NG) tube inserted through the nose and into the stomach or small intestine. When the tube cannot be placed in the nose or when tube feedings are required for more than 6 weeks, an opening called an ostomy is surgically created into the esophagus (esophagostomy), the stomach (gastrostomy), or the intestine (jejunostomy) (Figure 18-10). The physician selects the route and type of feeding tube. The tubes used for these feedings are soft, flexible, and as small as they can be and still allow the feeding to pass through. Numerous commercial formulas are available, with varying types and amounts of nutrients.

There are three methods for administering tube feedings: intermittent, bolus, and continuous. Usually, tube feedings are administered by the continuous infusion method, preferably with a pump. This means the feeding is continuous over a 18- to 24-hour period. Sometimes, the formula is given at half

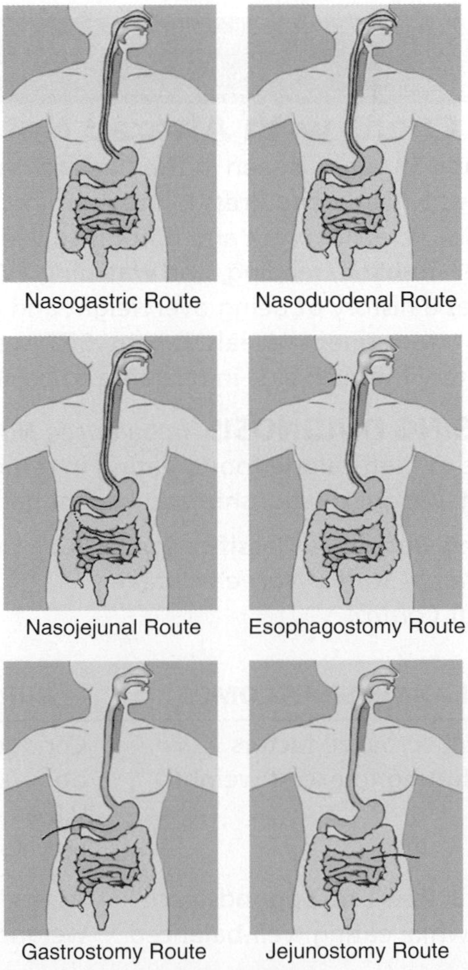

COURTESY OF DELMAR CENGAGE LEARNING

FIGURE 18-10 **Enteral Feeding Routes**

strength at a rate of 30 to 50 mL per hour. This rate may be increased by approximately 25 mL every 4 hours until tolerance has been established. As soon as the client tolerates the half-strength formula, a full-strength formula is initiated at the appropriate rate. When clients are ready to return to oral feedings, the transfer must be done gradually.

Parenteral Nutrition Parenteral nutrition is the infusion of a solution of nutrients directly into a vein to meet the client's daily requirements. It is used if the GI tract is not functional or if normal feeding is not adequate for the client's needs. Formerly called hyperalimentation, it is now generally referred to as total parenteral nutrition (TPN). The solution used in this intravenous infusion contains dextrose, amino acids, fats, essential fatty acids, vitamins, and minerals. Administration of TPN is generally a function of the registered nurse.

EVALUATION

The effectiveness of the plan is evaluated in relation to attaining the desired goals. The nurse assesses whether the goals were met. The plan is continued or modified based on the evaluation.

CASE STUDY

L.J. is an 18-year-old female brought in by her parents with a history of steady weight loss, failing in school, poor interest with social groups, and increasingly staying home and spending time alone. L.J. is 5 feet 3 inches tall and weighs 80 pounds. L.J. lost more than 10 pounds in the past several months.

1. Calculate L.J.'s BMI.
2. Identify risk factors for an eating disorder in L.J.
3. Write a nursing diagnosis for L.J.
4. What are other nursing diagnoses for clients with malnutrition?
5. Write a nursing goal for L.J.
6. List nursing interventions with rationales for L.J.

SAMPLE NURSING CARE PLAN

The Client with Altered Nutrition

V.B., age 58 years, is seen in the clinic for her yearly physical examination. She says, "I hardly have the energy to get up and dress in the morning. Cleaning the house and doing the laundry make me exhausted." She does not work and is not involved in community activities. Her daily routine involves cooking for her husband, reading, and watching TV for 6 to 8 hours. She loves to bake fresh breads and pastry. She has a history of being overweight and does not exercise. She says, "I eat because I have nothing else to do." Assessment reveals: height, 5′3″; weight, 166 pounds; weight gain, 14 pounds in the past year; sedentary lifestyle; eats in response to having nothing to do

NURSING DIAGNOSIS *Imbalanced Nutrition: More Than Body Requirements*, related to excess intake of high-calorie foods, eating in response to boredom, and sedentary lifestyle as evidenced by height–weight relationship and weight gain

Nursing Outcomes Classification (NOC)
Nutritional Status: Nutrient Intake
Weight Control

Nursing Interventions Classification (NIC)
Nutrition Management
Weight Reduction Assistance

PLANNING/OUTCOMES	NURSING INTERVENTIONS	RATIONALE
V.B. will verbalize factors contributing to excess weight.	Conduct a dietary history, using open-ended questions to assist V.B. in exploring factors that may contribute to excess eating.	Encourages client trust and honesty.
V.B. will lose 1 to 2 pounds each week while eating well-balanced meals.	Assess V.B.'s motivation to lose weight.	Will influence success.

(Continues)

SAMPLE NURSING CARE PLAN (Continued)

	Suggest methods to adapt eating habits to decrease amount of intake (smaller servings, taking small bites and chewing each bite 12 times, placing the fork on the plate between bites, drinking water with meals, eating only at mealtime, chewing sugar-free gum when watching TV).	Helps the client eat to satisfy hunger, not boredom.
	Ask V.B. to maintain a daily dietary intake log: time, food, and amount.	Helps the client recognize her eating patterns and note healthy and unhealthy behaviors.
	Provide and review the food guide pyramid and *Dietary Guidelines*; plan with V.B. a diet for 1 week, taking into consideration food preferences.	Ensures that the client has information necessary to plan healthy meals within recommended guidelines.
V.B. will engage in 20 to 30 minutes of exercise three times a week.	Review with V.B. age-appropriate exercises; emphasize the need for walking.	Increases self-esteem, burns calories, increases energy level, and decreases boredom.
V.B. will explore outside interests to decrease boredom and increase feelings of self-worth.	Review with V.B. community interests outside the home, unrelated to cooking and eating.	Helps the client focus on activities not involving food, thereby decreasing boredom and increasing self-esteem.

EVALUATION

V.B. verbalized boredom as the main reason for eating. V.B. is drinking water with meals, chewing her food slowly, and chewing gum while watching TV. She has lost 1.5 pounds in 1 week. V.B. now walks 30 minutes 4 days a week. V.B. will begin volunteering 2 hours three times a week at the church's child care center.

SUMMARY

- The LP/VN plays an important role in promoting proper nutrition.
- The six types of nutrients are water, carbohydrates, fats, protein, vitamins, and minerals.
- Water is the most vital nutrient.
- There must always be a balance between water intake and output to maintain health.
- Nutrients build, repair, and maintain body tissue; provide energy; and regulate body processes.
- The food guide pyramid identifies the five food groups for a well-balanced diet along with a range of servings to meet varying kcal needs.
- Nutritional needs vary as an individual moves through the life cycle.
- Nutrition is influenced by culture, religion, socioeconomics, fads, superstitions, age, and health.
- The kcal needs of an individual are based on basal energy needs plus activity.
- Weight management is based on the relationship between the intake and the use of kcal.
- Food safety is based on proper storage, proper sanitation, and proper cooking.
- Food-borne illnesses can be fairly mild or fatal.

REVIEW QUESTIONS

1. The role of the LP/VN in meeting the nutritional needs of the client includes:
   1. writing the diet order.
   2. preparing food for clients.
   3. preparing a complete diet plan.
   4. answering questions about nutrition.
2. Which of the following would most likely be on a clear liquid diet?
   1. Milkshake.
   2. Tomato soup.
   3. Orange juice.
   4. Cranberry juice.
3. Which of the following is the best source of dietary fiber?
   1. Popcorn.
   2. Chicken.
   3. Tomato juice.
   4. Macaroni and cheese.
4. Cholesterol:
   1. is made in the body.
   2. has no function in the body.
   3. is not important in any disease.
   4. should not be included in the diet.
5. Why should the nurse advise a client to take an iron supplement with orange juice?
   1. To prevent heartburn.
   2. To prevent constipation.
   3. To improve absorption of the iron.
   4. To improve digestion of the orange juice.
6. R.E. is a 45-year-old woman whose weight has been steadily rising over the past 12 years since the birth of her two children. She currently suffers from arthritis in both knees. Her BMI based on her height and weight is 35, placing her in class II obesity. R.E. is concerned about her weight and arthritis. R.E. eats a balanced diet and walks regularly. She enjoys eating out one or two nights a week. She would most likely benefit from:
   1. skipping a meal a day.
   2. eliminating eating out.
   3. exercising every day.
   4. decreasing the amount of food consumed during meals.
7. A positive outcome of management of a client with malnutrition is demonstrated when the client:
   1. states that "I am feeling better."
   2. eats an increased amount of food.
   3. has a steady increase in weight.
   4. expresses a concern over weight gain.
8. An excessively overweight client expressing a desire to lose weight must be advised initially to:
   1. follow a weight-loss diet and increase activity level.
   2. start a treatment combination of exercise, drugs, and weight-loss diet.
   3. consider a referral for surgical intervention.
   4. participate in vigorous exercise.
9. A client with severe malnutrition is admitted to an acute care unit exhibiting many clinical manifestations of malnutrition. While planning a meal for this client, the nurse understands that:
   1. the patient must be given total parenteral nutrition.
   2. the patient must be on a high-calorie, high-protein diet.
   3. allowed to plan own meal and provided privacy to eat.
   4. the nurse and nutritionist must plan the diet for the patient.
10. D.G., a 76-year-old with Parkinson's disease, has difficulty swallowing and handling utensils because of tremors. When preparing to feed D.G., the nurse: (Select all that apply.)
    1. offers a urinal to D.G. and leaves it on the bedside rail after use.
    2. pushes items to one end of the over-bed table with the meal tray.
    3. assists with washing face and hands and oral hygiene prior to eating.
    4. checks that the tray has the diet ordered.
    5. cuts the meat since he is on a pureed diet.
    6. checks his ID band against the name on the tray.

REFERENCES/SUGGESTED READINGS

American Heart Association. (1999). Non-AHA-approved diets. Retrieved October 18, 1999 from http://www.deliciousdecisions.org/ff/tsd_nondiets_fad.html

American Heart Association. (2002). Delicious decisions. Available: http://www.deliciousdecisions.org

Brown, J. (2005). *Nutrition now* (4th ed.). Belmont, CA: Thomson Wadsworth.

Bulechek, G., Butcher, H., McCloskey, J., & Dochterman, J., eds. (2008). *Nursing Interventions Classification (NIC)* (5th ed.). St. Louis, MO: Mosby/Elsevier.

Centers for Disease Control and Prevention. (1997). Update: Prevalence of overweight among children, adolescents, and adults—United States, 1988–1994. *Morbidity and Mortality Weekly Report, 46*(9), 199.

Centers for Disease Control and Prevention. (2002). Body mass index Web calculator. Available: http://www.cdc.gov/nccdphp/dnpa/bmi/calc-bmi.htm

Centers for Disease Control and Prevention. (2006). Obesity still a major problem. Retrieved December 6, 2008, from http://www.cd.gov/nchs/pressroom/06facts/obesity03-04.htm

Cerrato, P. (1999). When food is the culprit. *RN, 62*(6), 52–56.

Cobb, M. (1997). Improving your patient's nutritional status. *Nursing97, 27*(6), 32hhr, 32hh6.

Collins, J. (2002). Helping an older patient eat well to stay well. *Nursing2002, 32*(11), 32hn6–32hn8.

Costello, M. (1996). Home health nutrition. *MedSurg Nursing, 5*(4), 229–238.

Craig, W. (1997). Phytochemicals: Guardians of our health. *Journal of the American Dietetic Association, 97*(10, Suppl. 2), S199–S204.

Dudek, S. (2000). Malnutrition in hospitals: Who's assessing what patients eat? *American Journal of Nursing, 100*(4), 36–42.

Dudek, S. (2006). *Nutrition essentials for nursing practice* (5th ed.). Philadelphia: Lippincott Williams & Wilkins.

Estes, M. (2010). *Health assessment and physical examination* (4th ed.). Clifton Park, NY: Delmar Cengage Learning.

Gartner, L., Eidelman, A., Morton, J., Lawrence, R., Naylor, A., O'Hare, D., et al. (2005) Breastfeeding and the use of human milk. *Pediatrics, 115*(2), 496–506.

Gartner, L., & Greer, F. (2003). Prevention of rickets and vitamin D deficiency: New guidelines for vitamin D intake. *Pediatrics, 111* (4, Pt. 1), 908.

Goldrick, B. (2003). Foodborne diseases. *American Journal of Nursing, 103*(3), 105–106.

Institute of Medicine & Food and Nutrition Board. (1997). *Dietary reference intakes for calcium, phosphorus, magnesium, vitamin D, and fluoride.* Washington, DC: National Academies Press. Available: http://www.nap.edu/books/0309063507/html/index.html

Institute of Medicine & Food and Nutrition Board. (2000a). *Dietary reference intakes for thiamin, riboflavin, niacin, vitamin B6, folate, vitamin B12, pantothenic acid, biotin, and choline.* Washington, DC: National Academies Press. Available: http://www.nap.edu/books/0309065542/html/index.html

Institute of Medicine & Food and Nutrition Board. (2000b). *Dietary reference intakes for vitamin C, vitamin E, selenium, and carotinoids.* Washington, DC: National Academies Press. Available: http://www.nap.edu/books/0309069351/html

Institute of Medicine & Food and Nutrition Board. (2002). *Dietary reference intakes for vitamin A, vitamin K, arsenic, boron, chromium, copper, iodine, iron, manganese, molybdenum, nickel, silicon, vanadium, and zinc.* Washington, DC: National Academies Press. Available: http://www.nap.edu/books/0309072694/html

Kohn-Keeth, C. (2000). How to keep feeding tubes flowing freely. *Nursing2000, 30*(3), 58–59.

Kurtzwell, P. (1998). Staking a claim to good health. Available: http://www.fda.gov/fdca/features/1998/698_labl.html

Loan, T., Magnuson, B., & Williams, S. (1998). Debunking six myths about enteral feeding. *Nursing98, 28*(8), 43–48.

Mathew, L. (2008). *Caring for clients with lower gastrointestinal disorders.* Manuscript submitted for publication.

McConnell, E. (1998). Administering parenteral nutrition. *Nursing98, 28*(7), 18.

McConnell, E. (2001). Administering total parenteral nutrition. *Nursing2001, 31*(11), 17.

McConnell, E. (2002). Measuring fluid intake and output. *Nursing2002, 32*(7), 17.

Metheny, N., & Titler, M. (2001). Assessing placement of feeding tubes. *American Journal of Nursing, 101*(5), 36–45.

Moorhead, S., Johnson, M., Maas, M., & Swanson, E. (2007). *Nursing Outcomes Classification (NOC)* (4th ed.). St. Louis, MO: Elsevier, Health Sciences Division.

North American Nursing Diagnosis Association International. (2010). *NANDA-I nursing diagnoses: Definitions and classification 2009-2011.* Ames, IA: Wiley-Blackwell.

National Academy of Sciences. (1989). *Recommended dietary allowances: 10th edition.* Washington, DC: National Academies Press. Available: http://bob.nap.edu.books/0309046335/html

Nix, S. (2008).*Williams' basic nutrition and diet therapy* (13th ed.). St. Louis, MO: Mosby.

Obarzanek, E., Kimm, S., Barton, B.,Horn, L., Kwiterovich, P., Simons-Morton, D. (2001). Long-term safety and efficacy of a cholesterol-lowering diet in children with elevated low-density lipoprotein cholesterol: Seven-year results of the Dietary Intervention Study in Children (DISC). *Pediatrics, 107*(2), 256.

Roth, R. (2006). *Nutrition and diet therapy (8th ed.).* Clifton Park, NY: Delmar Cengage Learning.

Sheff, B. (2002). Salmonella. *Nursing2002, 32*(7), 81.

Simons, S. (1997). *Vegetables and fruits: Natural "phyters" against disease.* College Station, TX: Texas Agriculture Extension Service.

Stanfield, P., & Hui, Y. (2003). *Nutrition and diet therapy* (4th ed.). Sudbury, MA: Jones and Bartlett.

U.S. Department of Agriculture. (1996). *The food guide pyramid* (Home and Garden Bulletin, No. 252). Washington, DC: U.S. Department of Agriculture, Center for Nutrition Policy and Promotion. Available: http://www.usda.gov/cnpp/pyrabklt.pdf

U.S. Department of Agriculture. (2008). *Inside the pyramid.* Retrieved December 5, 2008, from http://www.mypyramid.gov/pyramid/index.html

U.S. Department of Agriculture & U.S. Department of Health and Human Services. (2000). *Nutrition and your health: Dietary guidelines for Americans* (Home and Garden Bulletin No. 232) (5th ed.). Washington, DC: U.S. Department of Agriculture and U.S. Department of Health and Human Services. Retrieved December 4, 2008, from http://www.cnpp.usda.gov/Publications/DietaryGuidelines/2000/2000DGProfessionalBooklet.pdf

U.S. Food and Drug Administration. (1999). The food label. Available: http://www.fda.gov/opacom/backgrounders/foolaabel/newlabel.html

University of Iowa Health Care. (2006). Fat makes you fat. Iowa City: University of Iowa Hospitals and Clinics. Retrieved December 5, 2008, from http://www.uihealthcare.com/topics/weightcontrol/weig5290.html

Washington, H. (1998). The vitamin revolution. *Health, 12*(6), 104–110.

Wilkes, G. (2000). Nutrition: The forgotten ingredient in cancer care. *American Journal of Nursing, 100*(4), 46–51.

Williams, S. (2001). *Basic nutrition and diet therapy* (11th ed.). St. Louis, MO: Mosby.

RESOURCES

American Dietetic Association, http://www.eatright.org

Food and Nutrition Board, http://www.iom.edu

Food and Nutrition Information Center, http://www.nal.usda.gov

Nestlé Nutrition, http://www.nestle-nutrition.com

U.S. Department of Agriculture, MyPyramid.gov, http://mypyramid.gov

CHAPTER 19
Rest and Sleep

MAKING THE CONNECTION

Refer to the following chapters to increase your understanding of rest and sleep:

Basic Nursing

- ***Communication***
- ***Client Teaching***
- ***Nursing Process/Documentation/Informatics***
- ***Stress, Adaptation, and Anxiety***
- ***Complementary/Alternative Therapies***
- ***Pain Management***

LEARNING OBJECTIVES

Upon completion of this chapter, you should be able to:

- Define key terms.
- Describe the phases and stages of sleep.
- Identify factors that affect normal sleep.
- Discuss age-related sleep variations.
- State the outcomes of sleep deprivation.
- Delineate nursing interventions that promote rest and sleep.

KEY TERMS

biological clock
bruxism
cataplexy
chronobiology
circadian rhythm
hypersomnia
insomnia
narcolepsy
parasomnia
REM movement disorder
rest
restless leg syndrome (RLS)
sleep
sleep apnea
sleep cycle
sleep deprivation
sleep hygiene
somnambulism

INTRODUCTION

The quality of rest and sleep can have a significant impact on a person's health, including physical well-being, mental status, and coping effectiveness. This chapter discusses the importance of rest and sleep and nursing care to assist clients to maintain optimal health when disturbances in rest and sleep occur.

REST AND SLEEP

Rest and sleep are basic to health well-being. Age, developmental level, health status, activity level, and cultural norms influence the need for rest and sleep. **Rest** is a state of mental and physical relaxation and calmness. Rest can take place when lying down, reading a book, or taking a quiet walk. The nurse should try to ascertain which activities and places the client finds restful (Figure 19-1).

Sleep is a state of altered consciousness during which a person has minimal physical activity, changes in level of consciousness, and a slowing of physiologic processes. Sleep is cyclical, usually lasting for several hours. Disruptions in the usual sleep routine can be distressing to clients and often prevent further sleep. Sleep is a restorative function needed for physiologic and psychological healing. It is important that health care providers, clients, and their significant others understand the normal sleep–wake cycle and how sleep affects healing and mood.

PHYSIOLOGY OF SLEEP

Centers in the brain control the cycles of wakefulness and sleep, which are influenced by environmental factors and routines. An individual's biological clock helps determine the specific cycles of wakefulness and sleep.

Phases and Stages of Sleep

The stages of sleep are identified by electroencephalograph (EEG) patterns, eye movements, and muscle activity. Sleep phases are classified as non–rapid eye movement (NREM) and rapid eye movement (REM) sleep (see Box 19-1).

NREM Sleep The first phase of sleep is called non– rapid eye movement, or NREM, sleep and consists of four stages. *Stage 1 sleep* is a light sleep, in which muscles relax and brain waves are rapid and irregular. In adults with normal sleep patterns, stage 1 sleep usually lasts 10 minutes or so. During this stage, it is easy to awaken a sleeper.

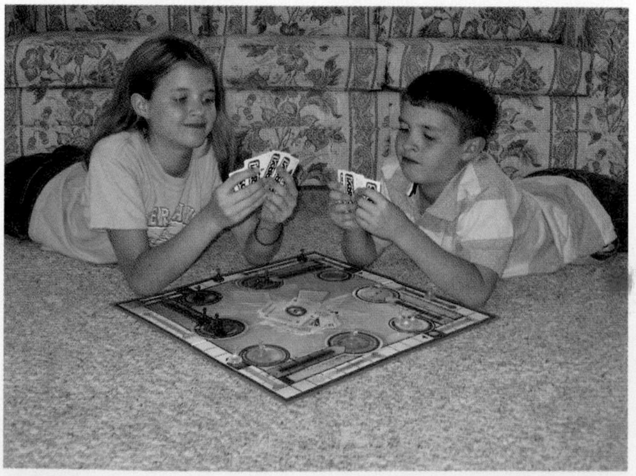

FIGURE 19-1 Playing a quiet board game can be a relaxing activity for children.

BOX 19-1 STAGES OF SLEEP

NREM Stage 1
- The lightest stage of sleep.
- Client is easily aroused by light or noise.

NREM Stage 2
- This stage is deeper than stage 1.
- Client is still easily aroused.
- Blood pressure and respirations decrease.

NREM Stage 3
- Beginning of deep sleep.
- Muscles relax.
- Blood pressure and respirations continue to decrease.

NREM Stage 4
- The deepest and most restful stage of sleep.
- Physical and mental restoration occurs during this stage.
- Sleepwalking and enuresis may occur.

REM
- Vivid, full-color dreaming (dreaming may occur in all other stages but not as vivid).
- REM stage occurs at the end of each NREM cycle.
- Eyes dart rapidly under closed eyelids.

Stage 2 sleep is still fairly light sleep. Brain waves become larger with bursts of electrical activity. Half of normal adult sleep may be spent in stage 2. After 20 minutes or so in stage 2 sleep, a deep sleep is entered.

Stage 3 and *stage 4* sleep are usually discussed together because they are difficult to identify and separate. Stage 3 is a medium-deep sleep, and stage 4 is the deepest sleep. Each stage lasts 15 to 30 minutes. During these stages large, slow waves are seen on the EEG. Vital signs are significantly lower than when awake. It is difficult to awaken a person in this stage of sleep.

Stages 3 and 4 sleep are thought to have restorative value, needed for physical recovery. Human growth hormone is secreted mainly at night, especially during stages 3 and 4 sleep, near the beginning of a sleep period. Growth hormone is necessary for growth and also for normal tissue repair in individuals of all ages. About 75% of sleep is NREM sleep.

REM Sleep After the first 60 to 90 minutes of NREM sleep in adults, the individual enters rapid eye movement, or REM, sleep. The brain waves are almost the same as when awake. This is a highly active time with rapid eye movements, heart rate, respiratory rate, and blood pressure similar to when awake; large muscle tone is decreased, and the person is "virtually paralyzed" (American Academy of Sleep Medicine, 2005; Harvard Medical School, 2007); and muscles are flaccid, making the body paralyzed. This is the time when dreams occur. Dreams are ways for individuals to consolidate memories, solve problems, adapt behaviors, and clarify thoughts and emotions. About 25% of sleep is REM sleep, with REM-sleep periods becoming longer as the night goes on.

Sleep Cycle

The **sleep cycle** is the sequence of sleep beginning with the four stages of NREM sleep, a return to stage 3 and then stage 2 (the first phase), followed by the first REM sleep (Figure 19-2). The duration of a sleep cycle is usually 60 to 90 minutes, and the sleeper will generally go through four to six sleep cycles during a sleep period of 7 to 8 hours.

The length of the NREM and REM periods of sleep change as the sleep period progresses, and dreams during REM sleep may become more vivid and intense. Whenever the sleep cycle is broken, a new sleep cycle starts, beginning again at NREM sleep stage 1.

Biological Clock

The **biological clock** is an internal mechanism in a living organism capable of measuring time. It controls the daily variations in hundreds of physiologic processes, including body temperature, respiratory rate, alertness, performance, and the level of several hormones. According to Coleman (1986), the major characteristics of biological clocks are:

- They are internal physiologic systems that measure the passage of time.
- They have their own daily cycle length, which is close to, but not exactly, 24 hours.
- When exposed to normal environmental cues, such as the day–night cycle, they adapt to a 24-hour day.
- When free of environmental cues, such as the day–night cycle, the organism's internal cycle length determines its behavior.

When external time cues such as day–night, mealtimes, and sleep–wake are inconsistent, a desynchronization of the circadian biological rhythms occurs. This internal desynchronization disrupts the timing of physiologic and behavioral activity, which, in turn, causes disrupted sleep patterns, chronic fatigue, and decreased performance and coping abilities. An example of desynchronization is shift workers who try to sleep in the daytime when activities around them and their own biological clock tell them to be awake.

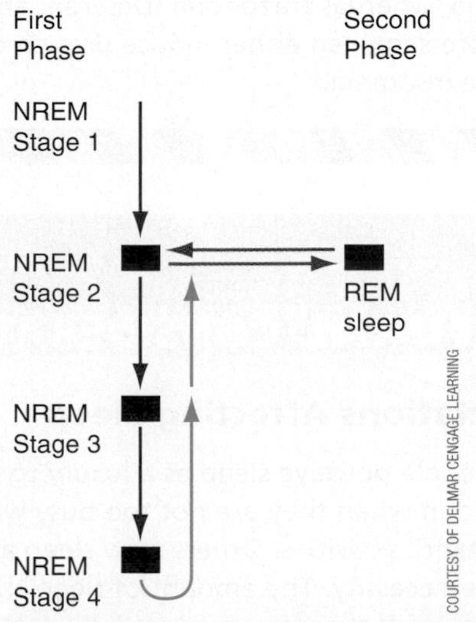

FIGURE 19-2 The two phases and four stages of the sleep cycle.

PROFESSIONAL TIP

Biorhythms

Chronobiology is a relatively new branch of science that studies the rhythms controlled by our biological clocks, or biorhythms. The **circadian rhythms**, those that cycle on a daily basis, such as the sleep–wake cycle, are the most widely studied. Other biological rhythms include:

- **Ultradian:** those lasting much shorter than a day, such as the milliseconds it takes for a neuron to fire
- **Infradian:** those lasting a month or more, such as the monthly menstrual cycle
- **Circannual:** those requiring approximately 1 year to complete, such as seasonal affective disorder, which causes depression in susceptible people during the short days of winter

Factors Affecting Rest and Sleep

Several factors can influence the quality and quantity of both rest and sleep. Often, sleep problems result from a combination of many factors.

Physical Factors

Comfort is a very subjective experience. The nurse must make sure the client's physical and psychological needs are met. When basic needs are not met, the person encounters discomfort, which leads to physiologic tension and anxiety and, possibly, disturbed rest and sleep. For example, a client

PROFESSIONAL TIP

Assessing the Effect of Pain on Sleep

Questioning clients about the effect pain has on their sleep habits will help clarify the intensity of the pain and its effect on the clients' patterns of daily living. The nurse should ask the client whether the pain:

- Prevents the client from falling asleep
- Makes finding a comfortable sleeping position difficult
- Wakes the client from a sound sleep
- Keeps the client from falling back asleep once awakened
- Leaves the client feeling tired and unrefreshed after a sleeping session (White & Duncan, 2002)

experiencing hunger or pain may become restless and irritable and will focus on getting these needs met instead of getting restful sleep.

Some physical problems can interfere with the ability to fall asleep or stay asleep. Conditions that cause discomfort or pain, such as arthritis, make it difficult to sleep well, as can breathing disorders such as sleep apnea and asthma. Hormonal changes that cause premenstrual syndrome (PMS) or menopause with its hot flashes can disrupt sleep. Even pregnancy, especially during the last few weeks, may make sleeping difficult.

Psychological Factors

An active mind and restless body interfere with the ability to sleep. Many individuals have intrusive thoughts or muscle tension, which interferes with rest and sleep. Anxiety related to family demands, work pressures, and other stressors does not necessarily cease when an individual tries to go to sleep and often results in difficulty falling or staying asleep. Usually, sleep problems disappear when the stressful situation is resolved.

Environment

Temperature, lighting, ventilation, odors, and noise level can interrupt sleep when different from the person's usual sleep environment. The comfort and size of the bed, firmness of the pillow, and habits (snoring or movements) of a sleep partner may all interfere with sleep.

Sleep is especially disrupted when a person is hospitalized. Some factors associated with hospitalization that lead to sleep impairment include:

- Physical or emotional pain
- Unfamiliar surroundings
- Change in routine
- Fear of the unknown
- Timing of assessments, procedures, and treatments
- Intrusive lighting or equipment
- Noise level (especially unfamiliar noises)
- Lack of privacy

Lifestyle Stressors

A fast-paced life with many stressors may result in a person being unable to relax easily or fall asleep quickly. Relaxation precedes healthy sleep. Vigorously exercising within an hour of going to bed or performing mentally intense activities just before or after getting into bed often work against getting a good night's sleep.

A work schedule that does not fit with an individual's biological clock (e.g., working at times other than the day shift) may interfere with sleep. More than 15 million Americans are shift workers (National Sleep Foundation [NSF], 2008c). Individuals who frequently change work shifts or travel across several times zones face a real challenge in trying to stabilize their biological rhythms and rest comfortably.

Diet

Foods high in caffeine, such as coffee, colas, and chocolate, are stimulants and often delay sleep. Consuming a large, spicy, or heavy meal just before bedtime may cause indigestion, which often interferes with sleep. Going to bed when hungry can also delay sleep because the individual will be focused on food and hunger pangs instead of on sleep.

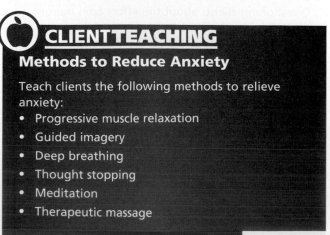

CLIENT TEACHING

Methods to Reduce Anxiety

Teach clients the following methods to relieve anxiety:

- Progressive muscle relaxation
- Guided imagery
- Deep breathing
- Thought stopping
- Meditation
- Therapeutic massage

CRITICAL THINKING

Client Assessment

During morning report, the night nurse tells the day nurse that the client "slept through the night." However, during the morning assessment, the client tells the nurse that she didn't sleep well and is very tired. What are some possible explanations for the discrepancy between what the night nurse and the client told the day nurse?

SAFETY

Medications and Sleep

Some medications used to treat high blood pressure, asthma, or depression may cause sleeping difficulties. For instance, captopril (Capoten) and theophylline (Theomar), used to treat high blood pressure and asthma, respectively, may cause insomnia, whereas trazodone (Desyrel), an antidepressant, can either induce drowsiness or cause insomnia.

CULTURAL CONSIDERATIONS

Expectations Affecting Sleep

Some people perceive sleep as a luxury to be indulged in when they are not too busy with "important" activities. Others view sleep as an absolute necessity. The amount of sleep that a person considers necessary is partially determined by the attitudes of family and culture.

CRITICAL THINKING

Age-Related Sleep Variations

What age-related sleep variations should be considered when assessing the sleep habits of neonates, infants, toddlers, school-age children, adolescents, and elders?

Medications and Other Substances

Many medications, both prescription and over-the-counter, list fatigue, restlessness, sleepiness, agitation, or insomnia as side effects. A small amount of alcohol may help some people fall asleep; however, alcohol may interrupt sleep later in the night. Nicotine, a stimulant, also delays sleep.

Age/Aging

Some sleep variations are based on age.

The neonate (birth–1 month) sleeps 16 to 20 hours per day in 3- to 4-hour intervals. The newborn usually sleeps very soundly and with little activity occurring during sleep ("sleeping like a baby"). There is often no difference in day and night sleep patterns.

As the infant gets older, the amount of sleep needed decreases. When infants begin to sleep through the night, they will usually have two or three naps during the day.

Toddlers typically sleep 10 to 12 hours at night with one or two daytime naps (Figure 19-3). Bedtime rituals such as a bath, brushing teeth, and reading books help establish expectations and provide nighttime security.

During preschool years, daytime napping decreases or ceases, and vivid dreams and nightmares may occur at night. These often awaken the child several times during the night.

School-age children need 10 to 12 hours of sleep daily but may resist bedtime as they struggle for independence. They may develop a fear of the dark and need reassurance and a system to cope with this fear.

Adolescents need 8 to 10 hours of sleep per day. Irregular sleeping habits often become the norm as their high activity level often interferes with regular sleep patterns.

The young adult requires about 8 hours of sleep per day. Sleep may be interrupted by their young children or by work responsibilities. Lifestyle stressors cause difficulties in falling or staying asleep.

Most middle-age adults sleep 6 to 8 hours each day. Daily stressors may result in insomnia and the use of sleep-inducing medications.

Most older adults sleep less at one time than do those who are younger, although overall sleep needs remain constant at 7 to 9 hours (National Institute on Aging, 2007). They may go to sleep earlier, wake up more often, get less deep sleep, and rise earlier (NSF, 2003). Often, a daytime nap is taken. The quality of sleep may diminish because of frequent waking and physical discomfort. The percentage of REM sleep remains fairly constant.

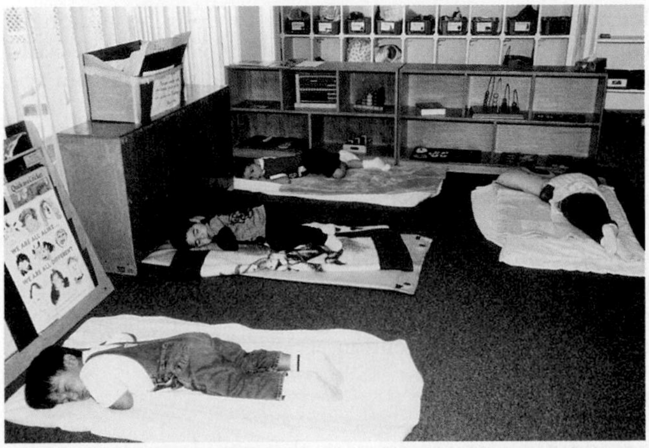

COURTESY OF DELMAR CENGAGE LEARNING

FIGURE 19-3 **Young children require naps and rest periods throughout the day.**

CRITICAL THINKING

Caffeine

Which foods and beverages have the most and least caffeine? Check out the National Sleep Foundation's (NSF) Caffeine Calculator on its Web site at www.sleepfoundation.org.

LIFE SPAN CONSIDERATIONS

Sleep and Aging

- Sleep needs do not decline with age but stay fairly constant at 7 to 9 hours per day.
- Middle-aged and elderly clients are more likely to experience sleep apnea, restless leg syndrome, and periodic limb movement disorder (NIA, 2007).

Sleep Pattern Alterations

Sleep disturbances are varied and are quite common. Sleep pattern alterations are either primary sleep disorders (those where the fundamental problem is the sleep alteration) or secondary sleep disorders (those where a medical or clinical cause results in or contributes to the sleep alteration). The most common sleep alterations include insomnia, hypersomnia, narcolepsy, sleep apnea/snoring, sleep deprivation, parasomnias, restless leg syndrome, and periodic limb movement disorder.

Insomnia

Insomnia refers to difficulty falling asleep or staying asleep (American Academy of Sleep Medicine [AASM], 2008). According to NSF (2008a), approximately 30 million American adults are affected by chronic insomnia each year. Insomnia is not a disease, but it may be a manifestation of many illnesses. Causes may include stress, depression, medical problems, caffeine, alcohol, pain, poor sleep habits, or changes in sleep patterns related to travel or shift work. The person experiencing insomnia often gets caught up in a vicious cycle of not being able to sleep, trying harder to fall asleep, and experiencing increasing anxiety about not sleeping, which, in turn, increases the inability to fall asleep.

Symptoms of insomnia include difficulty falling asleep, waking frequently during the night, waking very early and not being able to go back to sleep, feeling unrested in the morning and/or tired during the day, and becoming anxious and restless as bedtime arrives. Many who have insomnia actually sleep significantly more than they think they do.

Often, insomnia may occur only for a night or two. If it continues or is viewed as very disturbing or disruptive by the individual, a health care provider should be consulted for relief. Treatment is best focused on modifying the factors or behaviors causing it.

Hypersomnia

Hypersomnia is characterized by excessive sleep, especially in the daytime. Persons with hypersomnia often feel they do not sleep enough at night, so they sleep late into the morning and nap several times during the day. Causes of hypersomnia can be physical (such as a disease or medication) or psychological (such as a self-imposed short sleep time); treatment must address the underlying cause.

Narcolepsy

Narcolepsy is a sudden, irresistible urge to fall asleep during the daytime. Approximately 1 in 2,000 people have narcolepsy (National Institute of Neurological Disorders and Stroke, 2008). These "sleep attacks" can occur during a conversation or while driving, and last from a few seconds to more than 30 minutes. The hallmark symptom of narcolepsy is **cataplexy**, a sudden loss of muscle tone without loss of consciousness, which may cause the person to fall (Stansberry, 2001).

Individuals with narcolepsy often sleep adequately at night. There is no cure, but symptoms may be controlled by taking scheduled daytime naps, waking at the same time each morning, and avoiding caffeine, food, and alcohol after 8:00 P.M. (Stansberry, 2001).

Sleep Apnea/Snoring

Apnea is a Greek word meaning "without breath." **Sleep apnea** is a period, during sleep, of not breathing following a period of loud snoring. People with untreated sleep apnea may stop breathing hundreds of times for up to 60 seconds or more. Sleep apnea affects 18 million people in the United States (NSF, 2008a) and is most common in obese, middle-aged men (NSF, 2002).

> **PROFESSIONAL TIP**
>
> **Sleep Apnea**
>
> There are a number of factors that increase the risk for sleep apnea. These risk factors include having a small upper airway (or large tongue, tonsils, or uvula); being overweight; having a recessed chin, a small jaw, or a large overbite; having a large neck size (17 inches or greater in a man or 16 inches or greater in a woman); smoking and alcohol use; being age 40 or older; and ethnicity (African Americans, Pacific Islanders, and Hispanics) (NSF, 2005).

> **PROFESSIONAL TIP**
>
> **Sleep Deprivation**
>
> Sleep deprivation can be deadly, and the price tag is staggering. According to the National Sleep Foundation (NSF, 2001), the costs of drowsy drivers are estimated to be $12.5 billion per year. Drowsy drivers are blamed for 100,000 police-reported crashes and kill more than 1,500 Americans each year.
>
> The person who is deprived of restful sleep is less alert, less attentive, less able to perform even simple tasks, and more irritable and has poorer concentration and judgment and mood problems that make relationships with family, friends, and coworkers difficult. No matter the cause of sleep deprivation, inadequate sleep reduces the quality of life and is harmful to health.

There are three types of apnea: obstructive, caused by relaxation of muscles in the back of the throat that block the airway; central, caused by a failure of the brain to signal the muscles to breathe; and mixed, a combination of the two (American Sleep Apnea Association, 2008).

The unaware sleeper stops breathing repeatedly during sleep and as frequently as 100 times per hour, often for a minute or longer. Usually, those with sleep apnea have no idea that they are not breathing or that they are continually waking up (AASM, 2008).

Sleep apnea results in REM-sleep deprivation, manifesting as excessive daytime sleepiness. Sleep apnea can cause hypertension and an increased risk of heart attack or stroke. A nasal continuous positive airway pressure (CPAP) device, which maintains airflow with a small compressor, may give relief. Dental appliances that reposition the tongue may also help. With some individuals, surgical intervention is required to correct the cause of the apnea.

Sleep Deprivation

Sleep deprivation is a term used to describe prolonged inadequate quality and quantity of sleep, either of the REM or of the NREM type. Sleep deprivation can result from age, prolonged hospitalization, drug and substance use, illness, and frequent changes in lifestyle patterns. Sleep and dreaming have a restorative value necessary for mental and emotional recovery, and they appear to enhance the ability to cope with emotional problems. Therefore, sleep deprivation can cause symptoms ranging from irritability, hypersensitivity, and confusion to apathy, sleepiness, and diminished reflexes. Treating or minimizing the factors that cause the sleep deprivation is the most effective intervention.

Parasomnia

Parasomnia refers to disorders that intrude on sleep in very active ways. **Somnambulism** (sleepwalking), sleep talking, night terrors, REM movement disorder, bed-wetting, and

bruxism (teeth grinding) are the most common parasomnias; the first four are discussed in more detail in the following. Treatment for parasomnias varies, and the client and family should be helped to understand the disorder and its potential safety problems.

Somnambulism Sleepwalking, done mostly by children, is typically not remembered by the individual the next morning. The sleepwalker usually moves around furniture very safely. Doors and windows must be kept locked at night to protect the sleepwalker from harm. Sleepwalkers are difficult to rouse during an episode and if awakened are often confused and without any specific recall of events that led to their behavior. Sleepwalking tends to run in families and usually stops at puberty.

Sleep Talking Sleep talking can occur at any age. It may be a word or two or a long speech, sometimes understandable and sometimes gibberish. The person has no memory of talking, but the sleep partner may have been awakened.

Sleep Terrors Sleep terrors are more common in children and seldom continue into adulthood. The child suddenly appears to awaken, thrashes about, sweats, and may even cry. This can last anywhere from 1 minute to approximately 15 minutes. The child remembers nothing in the morning. Reassurance by the parents during the episode is the only treatment; the child will eventually outgrow the behavior.

REM Movement Disorder **REM movement disorder** results when the normal paralysis of REM sleep is absent or incomplete and the sleeper acts out the dream. It is most common among older men. Violent behavior and injuries may result. The person can remember the dream in the morning. Medication usually is effective in controlling the physical movements.

Restless Leg Syndrome

Restless leg syndrome (RLS) is the uncomfortable sensations of tingling or crawling in the muscles and twitching, burning, prickling, or deep aching in the foot, calf, or upper leg when at rest. The sensations return in seconds or minutes. The legs frequently jump involuntarily if they are not moved. Symptoms worsen at night. If sleep does come, the leg movements awaken the person frequently.

Although the cause is unknown, some cases of RLS have been linked to iron deficiency, dialysis treatment, peripheral neuropathy, pregnancy, excessive caffeine intake, alcohol dependence, and smoking. The disorder is more common among women who have passed middle age. Avoiding or reducing smoking, caffeine, and alcohol intake may help. Symptoms may be relieved by opiates, benzodiazepines, or L-dopa.

Periodic Limb Movements in Sleep

Periodic limb movements in sleep (PLMS) is a condition of repetitive leg movements every 20 to 40 seconds throughout the night. It is typically not uncomfortable for the affected person but may be distressing to the sleep partner. Multiple sleep interruptions occur, leading to daytime sleepiness and nighttime insomnia.

The disorder is quite common in persons older than age 65 years. Approximately 35% of elders have at least a mild form of PLMS, which occurs only during sleep and is not as uncomfortable as RLS (NSF, 2008a).

Nocturnal Sleep-Related Eating Disorder

Nocturnal sleep-related eating disorder (NSRED) is rapid and chaotic eating when partially or fully awake with variable recall of the episode. An estimated 4 million people have this disorder, with two-thirds being women (Montgomery, Haynes, & Garner, 2002). This combination sleep and eating disorder may be misdiagnosed as anorexia, bulimia, or depression.

Clients gain weight with only moderate daytime eating, are not hungry in the morning, and are chronically tired. They typically eat food high in calories and fat at night, often foods they do not eat in the daytime. A spouse, partner, or family member may be able to shed light on the situation.

NURSING PROCESS

All standardized nursing history tools include questions related to a client's rest and sleep patterns. Care of the client who is diagnosed with a sleep disorder is collaborative, with the nurse participating in an interdisciplinary team providing treatment. Concept Map 19-1 identifies key components of the nursing process for clients with a *Disturbed* **S***leep Pattern.*

ASSESSMENT

The nursing assessment includes a history of sleep and rest patterns; **sleep hygiene**, or the client's personal habits in preparing for sleep; and a physical exam. Sleep survey tools such as the Pittsburgh Sleep Quality Index can be administered by the nurse to assess for sleep disturbances or deficits (Smyth, 2008). The client with a sleep disturbance should be thoroughly assessed to determine the types of disturbance, sleep alterations, and impact of sleep problems. Usually, the client is a reliable source for this information,

> **PROFESSIONAL TIP**
>
> **Sleep History**
>
> To help detect a sleep disorder, ask the client:
> - What time do you usually go to bed?
> - How long does it take to fall asleep?
> - What wakes you up in the morning?
> - What time do you wake up in the morning?
> - Do you take a nap during the day? When? How long?
> - How much food do you eat in the evening?
> - Do you drink caffeinated beverages? How much? In the evening?
> - Do you drink alcohol? How much? In the evening?
> - Do you take medications or herbal supplements to help you sleep?

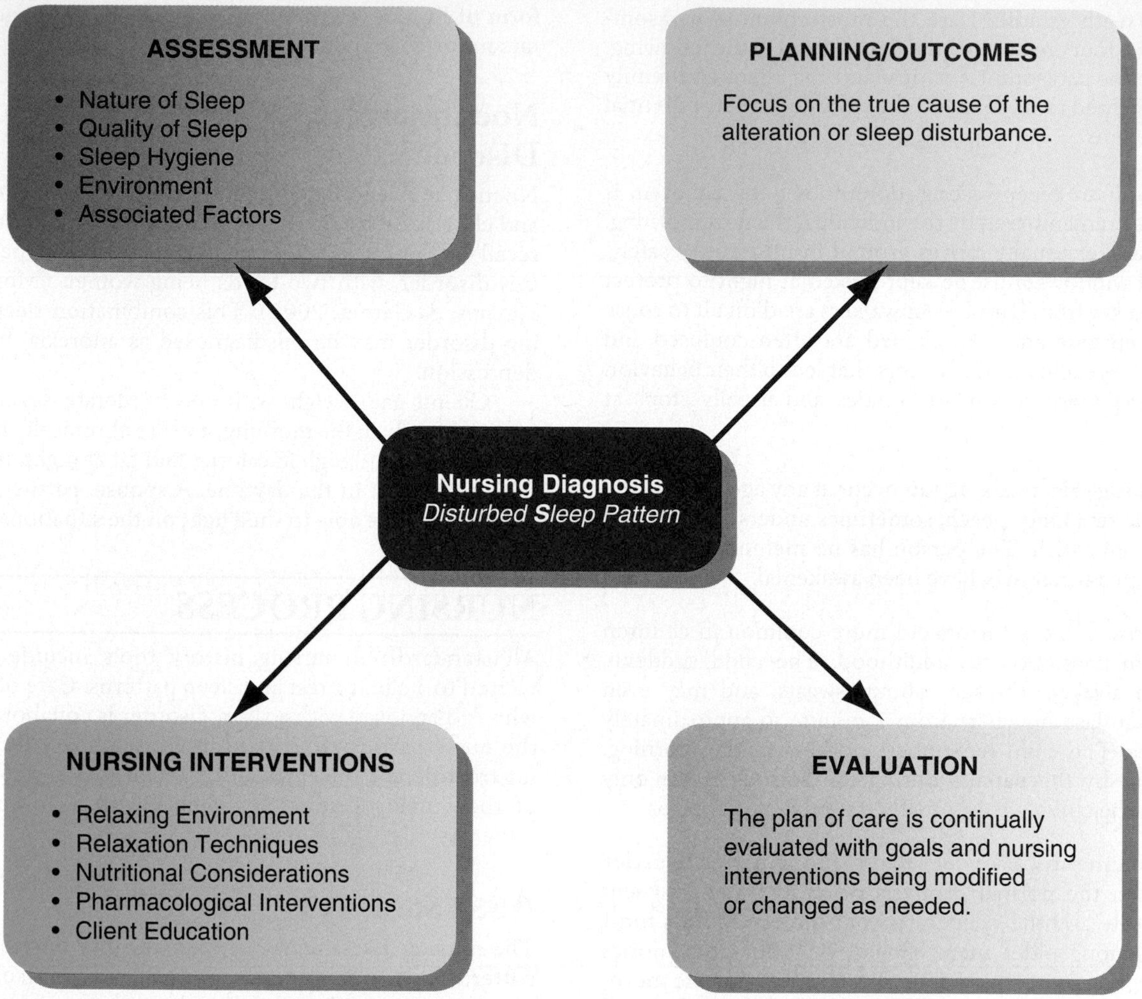

Concept Map 19-1 Nursing Process for Clients with a *Disturbed Sleep Pattern*

but a spouse or partner sharing sleeping arrangements may add valuable information to the client's report. Questions regarding the client's usual sleep patterns should focus on the following:

- Nature of sleep (restful, uninterrupted)
- Quality of sleep (feeling on waking)
- Sleep environment (description of room, temperature, noise level)
- Associated factors (bedtime routines, use of sleep medications or any other sleep inducers)
- Opinion of sleep (adequate, inadequate, problematic)

To discover information about altered sleep patterns, ask questions about:

- Type of problem (inability to fall asleep, difficulty remaining asleep, inability to fall asleep after awakening, restless sleep, daytime sleepiness)
- Quality of the problem (number of hours of sleep versus number of hours spent trying to sleep, duration and frequency of naps, number of awakenings per sleep period)
- Environmental factors (lighting, bed, noise level, surrounding stimulation, sleep partner)
- Other factors (relation to meals eaten, activity before retiring, life stressors, work stressors, anxiety level, pain, recent illness or surgery)
- Alleviating factors (mild diet, warm drink before retiring, reading, listening to quiet music, taking a hot bath)
- Effect of problem (fatigue, irritability, confusion)

A daily journal of their sleep patterns may be helpful for clients whose sleep problems are not well defined. Other factors, such as age, medical diagnosis, occupation, allergies, and psychiatric disorders, must also be considered when assessing sleep problems.

Nursing Diagnosis

After information about the sleep impairment has been collected, the data must be analyzed to formulate appropriate nursing diagnoses. Alterations in sleep can manifest as verbal complaints on the part of the client, physical signs such as yawning or dark circles under the eyes, or alterations in mood, such as apathy or irritability. The primary diagnosis for individuals experiencing sleep problems is *Disturbed **S**leep Pattern*. Another diagnosis related to rest and sleep is ***S**leep Deprivation*

PROFESSIONALTIP

Communicating with the Client Who Is Sleep-Impaired

- Thoroughly explain procedures before implementation.
- Encourage the client and significant others to verbalize feelings and ask questions.
- Answer questions honestly and completely.
- Identify and support coping mechanisms of the client and family.
- Spend adequate time with the client to facilitate communication.
- Assess and incorporate the client's preferences as much as possible into the plan of care.

(North American Nursing Diagnosis Association International, 2009).

If the client has problems in addition to a sleep disturbance, think about the possibility that the sleep disturbance is the cause (not the effect) of another problem. For example, a client may be experiencing *Activity Intolerance* related to lack of sleep as evidenced by verbal complaint, extreme fatigue, disorientation, confusion, and lack of energy.

Planning/Outcome Identification

Client input should be incorporated into the plan and goals. The plan of care and the goals must focus on the true cause of the alteration or sleep disturbance. For example, if the client is experiencing *Disturbed Sleep Pattern* because of bed-wetting, the bed-wetting should be the focus of intervention.

Many sleep disturbances require long periods of time (weeks or months as opposed to days) to correct. Sleep is by nature habitual and part of the person's lifestyle patterns. When planning care, the nurse should time procedures and treatments so they do not disturb sleep time.

Implementation

Several interventions can promote rest and sleep in clients; these are discussed next.

Trusting Nurse–Client Relationship

The client's ability to rest and sleep can be enhanced by the quality of the nurse–client relationship. Knowing that the nurse is trustworthy and genuinely cares about the client allows the client to relax and feel secure. Anxiety can be minimized by the nurse's use of therapeutic communication skills. The therapeutic use of self helps allay client anxiety.

Relaxing Environment

A place to sleep should be inviting. The immediate surroundings should be arranged to promote sleep for the sleep-impaired client. The nurse should ascertain what environment the client finds relaxing, then try to provide this environment in the inpatient setting or help the client establish this type of environment in the home setting.

CLIENTTEACHING

Managing Sleep Disturbance

To facilitate rest and sleep, the client should be encouraged to:

- Select regular times for going to bed and awakening and try to observe them.
- Drink a warm cup of milk before bed.
- Eat a light healthy snack at bedtime.
- Take a warm bath before going to bed.
- Avoid stimulating activities, such as strenuous exercise or demanding intellectual activity, during the hour before bedtime and use the time instead to wind down with relaxing activities such as taking a warm bath, reading a book, or sitting by the fire.
- Use bedtime rituals on a consistent basis.
- Void before going to bed.
- Use the bed only for sleeping.
- Avoid caffeine, spicy foods, and heavy meals in the several hours before bedtime.

PROFESSIONALTIP

Noise Control in Health Facilities

- Keep the door to the client's room closed.
- Reduce the volume of paging and telephone systems, especially at night.
- Ensure that unused equipment in the client's room is turned off.
- Turn off or lower the volume on radios and televisions.
- Workers should keep noises to a minimum, especially at night.
- Hold discussions and conferences away from the client's room.

Relaxation Techniques

The client's mood before sleep is very important. Believing that one can and will sleep affects both sleep quality and quantity. The calm, relaxed client is likely to fall asleep quickly and stay asleep all night. Relaxation techniques are useful sleep aids (Figure 19-4). Progressive muscle relaxation may be helpful for the person who has tense muscles. A warm bath may be relaxing.

Nutritional Considerations

Some foods enhance sleep. Tryptophan, an amino acid in milk, promotes sleep by stimulating the brain's production of serotonin. Scientific data support the old wives' tale that drinking warm milk promotes sleep. Other ways to promote sleep are to avoid caffeine after noon, avoid large or heavy meals close to bedtime, and refrain from eating foods that cause gastrointestinal distress.

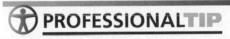

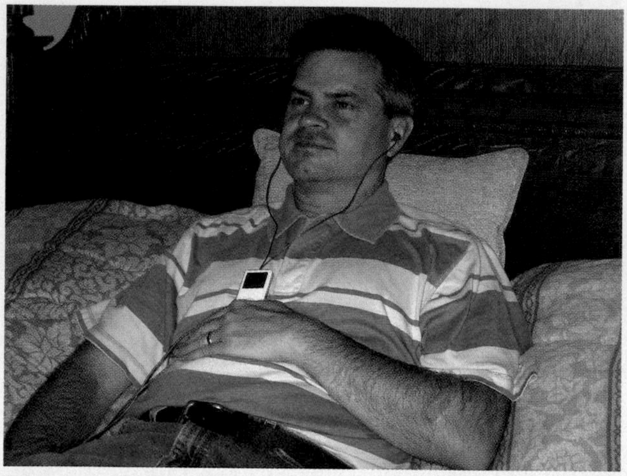

FIGURE 19-4 Listening to favorite music can be very relaxing before going to bed.

Pharmacologic Interventions

If pain is a reason for sleep disturbance, interventions should first focus on pain management. Some nonpharmacologic relaxation and imagery interventions may be effective.

Pharmacologic agents such as tricyclic antidepressants, antihistamines, and short-acting hypnotics may be helpful for clients with sleep disturbances (McCaffery & Pasero, 1999). The tricyclic antidepressant amitriptyline (Elavil) improves the client's ability to fall asleep and stay asleep by causing sedation when given 1 to 3 hours before bedtime; doses are significantly less than those given for depression.

If given at bedtime, antihistamines such as hydroxyzine (Vistaril, Atarax) and diphenhydramine (Benadryl) have mild sedative effects that can promote sleep.

The last group are the short-acting hypnotics. These are not recommended for long-term or routine use, as they may cause insomnia; however, for short-term treatment they may be effective. When used, a hypnotic with a short half-life is recommended.

Client Education

Educating the client about sleep-promoting activities is a good investment of the nurse's time. The nurse can use the memory trick "**REST**" to teach the client interventions that promote rest and sleep. By providing clients with ways of promoting good sleep habits, the nurse helps them gain a sense of control over their sleep disturbances and boosts their confidence so that they can successfully meet their sleep and rest needs.

PROFESSIONALTIP

Variables to Consider in Evaluation

When evaluating the care of the client experiencing a sleep disorder, consider the following questions:

- Were the client's basic needs met?
- Did client education include the family or significant others?
- Was an environment conducive to rest maintained?
- Were therapeutic activities balanced with the client's need for rest and sleep?
- Were the client's bedtime rituals followed as closely as possible?
- Were anxiety-reduction techniques used appropriately?

MEMORYTRICK

"**REST**" stands for:

R = Read a relaxing book

E = Enjoy listening to soothing music

S = Sip a warm glass of milk

T = Take a warm bath

EVALUATION

The plan of care must be updated on a regular basis with additional interventions used as needed.

SAMPLE NURSING CARE PLAN

The Client with Trouble Sleeping

Six-year-old C.R. is brought to your clinic by his father, who states that C.R. has trouble sleeping at night. In the evenings after a dinner of hotdogs, corn or baked beans, and chocolate milk, C.R. reads some books, then watches his favorite superhero video. Afterward, he runs and plays, mimics the actions he sees in the video, and refuses to take a bath or cooperate when getting ready for bed. After being put to bed at 9:00 P.M., he is up several times for any number of reasons and often is not asleep until midnight. When his father wakes him at 7:00 A.M. for school, C.R. is disagreeable, tired, and difficult to get moving.

NURSING DIAGNOSIS *Disturbed **S**leep Pattern* (less than age-normal total sleep time) related to environmental factors (excessive stimulation) and parental lack of knowledge of sleep-promoting behaviors as evidenced by parental complaint, ineffective bedtime rituals, and insufficient hours of sleep for developmental age

SAMPLE NURSING CARE PLAN (Continued)

Nursing Outcomes Classification (NOC)
Rest
Sleep

Nursing Interventions Classification (NIC)
Sleep Enhancement
Energy Management

PLANNING/OUTCOMES	NURSING INTERVENTIONS	RATIONALE
C.R. and his family will determine those sleeping behaviors they would like to achieve.	Explain that the normal sleep requirement for a child of C.R.'s age is 10 to 12 hours each day.	Helps family understand C.R.'s sleep requirements.
C.R. and his family will develop bedtime rituals to help C.R. wind down from the day.	Teach the family about the effect that certain foods can have on digestion and sleep habits and identify with them those foods that are good choices for dinner.	Informs family about potential adverse effects of certain foods and allows them to plan meals more appropriately.
	Discuss those bedtime activities that can be detrimental to sleep induction.	Assists the family in modifying pre-bedtime behaviors.
	Suggest appropriate bedtime rituals such as taking a bath, brushing the teeth, reading a book, or listening to calming music.	Helps the body and mind prepare for bedtime.
C.R. and his family will identify behaviors that are helpful before bedtime.	Explain that overstimulation close to bedtime, such as watching superhero movies and engaging in rowdy play, prevents the body and mind from slowing down and preparing for sleep.	Helps the family in choosing more appropriate bedtime activities.
	Emphasize the importance of establishing a calming bedtime routine that is followed every night, especially for the school-age child.	Helps C.R. know what is expected of him by practicing appropriate bedtime routines.
	Describe an appropriate sleep environment for C.R., such as a calm room kept at a comfortable temperature and lit only by a night-light.	Such an environment promotes sleep and does not interfere with falling back asleep once awake.

EVALUATION

C.R. and his family have decided they would like C.R. to cooperate in getting ready for bed and to be asleep in 30 minutes. Together they have established a bedtime ritual that begins with playing quietly, followed by taking a warm bath, reading two books, brushing teeth, and then going to bed. The behaviors identified as helpful include no watching of stimulating videos after 7:00 P.M. and engaging in quiet play such as reading, arts and crafts, or writing. Some modification to C.R.'s diet is planned for the next few weeks.

SUMMARY

- Sleep has two phases: non–rapid eye movement (NREM) and rapid eye movement (REM).
- The biological clock controls the daily variations of many physiologic processes.
- Nonpharmacologic interventions should be used in promoting rest and sleep.
- The amount of sleep required differs according to developmental stage.
- Pharmacologic agents can be therapeutic for clients experiencing sleep pattern disturbances. However, the medications should not be the only interventions used.

REVIEW QUESTIONS

1. The nurse is teaching the client interventions to promote sleep. Which of the following interventions are appropriate for the nurse to teach a client? (Select all that apply.)
   1. Drink a warm cup of milk before bed.
   2. Eat a light healthy snack at bedtime.
   3. Exercise within 2 hours of going to bed to relax muscles.
   4. Take a brief nap during the day.
   5. Take a warm bath at bedtime.
   6. Void before going to bed.
2. Which of the following questions is the least appropriate to ask a client when gathering subjective data regarding sleep disturbances?
   1. Why are you having difficulty sleeping?
   2. What are your bedtime rituals?
   3. Can you describe your pain to me?
   4. Do you have frequent dreams or nightmares?
3. What stage of sleep is occurring when a client falls asleep and experiences a decrease in large muscle tone and becomes virtually paralyzed?
   1. REM
   2. NREM stage 2
   3. NREM stage 3
   4. NREM stage 4
4. A client informs the nurse that he is having difficulty falling asleep at night and does not understand why. The nurse asks the client to share which activities he uses to promote relaxation and sleep. Which of the following statements made by the client indicates that he needs further teaching?
   1. "I go for a walk after dinner to relax and unwind from the day."
   2. "I sit on a park bench in the evening and watch the sunset."
   3. "I drink a cup of hot tea and read my favorite relaxing book."
   4. "I always try to go to bed at the same time every night."
5. A client's wife informs the nurse that her husband will sometimes stop breathing for up to 30 seconds in his sleep and then begins snoring so loudly that she cannot sleep. This is an example of:
   1. hypersomnia.
   2. bruxism.
   3. cataplexy.
   4. apnea.
6. A client informs the nurse that she has not been able to sleep for 3 days. Which of the following objective assessment findings supports the client's statement?
   1. The client states that she needs a prescription for sleeping medication.
   2. The client informs the nurse that she is exhausted.
   3. The client yawns frequently and has red puffy eyes.
   4. The client appears calm and coordinated with clear speech.
7. To facilitate rest and sleep, the client should be encouraged to:
   1. practice relaxation techniques.
   2. watch television while lying in bed.
   3. eat a big meal to prevent hunger in the night.
   4. perform a daily exercise workout.
8. Which of the following factors affect the quality and quantity of rest and sleep? (Select all that apply.)
   1. Work schedule.
   2. Age.
   3. Room ventilation.
   4. Nicotine.
   5. Muscle tension.
   6. Hormonal changes.
9. Individuals have several rhythms controlled by their biological clocks. The circadian rhythm cycle occurs:
   1. daily.
   2. every year.
   3. every month or so.
   4. several times a day.
10. A new sleep cycle for a client who is awakened during stage 4 NREM sleep will begin in:
    1. REM sleep.
    2. stage 1 sleep.
    3. stage 2 sleep.
    4. stage 3 sleep.

REFERENCES/SUGGESTED READINGS

American Academy of Sleep Medicine. (2005). *Sleep as we grow older* [Brochure]. Westchester, IL: Author.

American Academy of Sleep Medicine. (2008). Insomnia. Available: http://www.aasmnet.org

American Sleep Apnea Association. (2008). Information about sleep apnea. Available: http://www. sleepapnea.org/geninfo.html

Bulechek, G., Butcher, H., McCloskey, J., & Dochterman, J., eds. (2008). *Nursing Interventions Classification (NIC)* (5th ed.). St. Louis, MO: Mosby/Elsevier.

Coleman, R. (1986). *Wide awake at 3:00 a.m.: By choice or by chance?* New York: Freeman.

Coren, S. (1997). *Sleep thieves: An eye-opening exploration into the science and mysteries of sleep*. New York: Free Press.

Harvard Women's Health Watch (2007). Repaying your sleep debt. Harvard Medical School, *14*(11).

Hogstel, M. (2001). *Gerontology: Nursing care of the older adult* (4th ed.). Clifton Park, NY: Delmar Cengage Learning.

McCaffery, M., & Pasero, C. (1999). *Pain: Clinical manual* (2nd ed.). St. Louis, MO: Mosby.

Merritt, S. (2000). Putting sleep disorders to rest. *RN, 63*(7), 26–30.

Montgomery, L., Haynes, L., & Garner, L. (2002). An unusual sleep disorder. *RN, 65*(4), 41–43.

Moorhead, S., Johnson, M., Maas, M., & Swanson, E. (2007). *Nursing Outcomes Classification (NOC)* (4rd ed.). St. Louis, MO: Mosby.

National Institute on Aging. (2007). Sleep and aging. Retrieved August 23, 2008, from http://www.nia.nih.gov/HealthInformation/Publications/sleep.htm

National Institute of Neurological Disorders and Stroke. (2008). Narcolepsy fact sheet. Retrieved August 23, 2008, from http://www.ninds.nih.gov/disorders/narcolepsy/detail_narcolepsy.htm

National Sleep Foundation. (2001). Sleep facts and stats. Retrieved August 23, 2008, from http://www.sleepfoundation.org/site/c.huIXKjM0IxF/b.2419253/k.7989/Sleep_Facts_and_Stats.htm

National Sleep Foundation. (2002). Sleep apnea—An unknown epidemic? Retrieved August 23, 2008, from http://www.sleepfoundation.org/site/apps/nlnet/content3.aspx?c=huIXKjM0IxF&b=2464479&content_id=%7BA9D2F632-83A5-405D-98E2-63F389C095BF%7D&notoc=1

National Sleep Foundation. (2003). Health and aging: The experts speak. Retrieved August 23, 2008, from http://www.sleepfoundation.org/site/c.huIXKjM0IxF/b.2419293/k.23CA/Health_and_Aging_The_Experts_Speak.htm

National Sleep Foundation. (2005). Sleep apnea basics. Retrieved August 23, 2008, from http://www.sleepfoundation.org/site/c.huIXKjM0IxF/b.2464479/apps/nl/content3.asp?content_id=%7B3E9E479E-4C8E-4C35-9564-363A6918C391%7D&notoc=1

National Sleep Foundation. (2008a). Facts about PLMS. Retrieved August 23, 2008, from http://www.sleepfoundation.org/site/apps/nlnet/content3.aspx?c=huIXKjM0IxF&b=2464461&content_id=%7BB0211B38-4864-49EA-A322-E511477EFE71%7D&notoc=1

National Sleep Foundation. (2008b). Sleeping smart. Retrieved August 23, 2008, from http://www.sleepfoundation.org/site/c.huIXKjM0IxF/b.4389513/k.9A3E/Sleeping_Smart.htm

National Sleep Foundation. (2008c). Strategies for shift workers. Retrieved August 17, 2008, from http://www.sleepfoundation.org/site/c.huIXKjM0IxF/b.2421189/k.DF93/Strategies_for_Shift_Workers.htm

North American Nursing Diagnosis Association International. (2010). *NANDA-I nursing diagnoses: Definitions and classification 2009-2011.* Ames, IA: Wiley-Blackwell.

Penland, K. (2009). Caring for clients with sleep disorders. Manuscript submitted for publication.

Smyth, C. (2008). Evaluating sleep quality in older adults. *American Journal of Nursing, 108*(5), 42–45.

Sorrell, J. (1999). Taking steps to calm restless legs syndrome. *Nursing99, 29*(9), 60–61.

Stansberry, T. (2001). Narcolepsy: Unveiling a mystery. *American Journal of Nursing, 101*(8), 50–53.

Tate, J., & Tasota, F. (2002). More than a snore: Recognizing the danger of sleep apnea. *Nursing2002, 32*(8), 46–49.

White, L., & Duncan, G. (2002). *Medical-surgical nursing: An integrated approach* (2nd ed.). Clifton Park, NY: Delmar Cengage Learning.

RESOURCES

American Sleep Apnea Association, http://www.sleepapnea.org

American Academy of Sleep Medicine, http://www.aasmnet.org

Narcolepsy Network, http://www.narcolepsynetwork.org

National Sleep Foundation, http://www.sleepfoundation.org

Restless Legs Syndrome Foundation, Inc., http://www.rls.org

CHAPTER 20

Safety/Hygiene

MAKING THE CONNECTION

Refer to the following chapters to increase your understanding of safety/hygiene:

Basic Nursing

- ***Holistic Care***
- ***Legal and Ethical Responsibilities***
- ***Communication***
- ***Nursing Process/Documentation/ Informatics***
- ***Cultural Considerations***
- ***Stress, Adaptation, and Anxiety***
- ***Wellness Concepts***
- ***Self-Concept***
- ***Complementary/Alternative Therapies***
- ***Infection Control/Asepsis***
- ***Standard Precautions and Isolation***
- ***Assessment***
- ***Diagnostic Tests***

Basic Procedures

- ***Hand Hygiene***
- ***Bed Making: Unoccupied Bed***
- ***Bed Making: Occupied Bed***
- ***Bathing a Client in Bed***
- ***Perineal Care***
- ***Oral Care***
- ***Eye Care***
- ***Giving a Back Rub***
- ***Shaving a Client***
- ***Application of Restraints***

Intermediate Procedures

- ***Assisting with Crutches, Cane, or Walker***

LEARNING OBJECTIVES

Upon completion of this chapter, you should be able to:

- Define key terms.
- Describe the kinds of accidents that can occur in health care settings.
- Describe the importance of and procedure for correctly identifying clients.
- Identify safety factors to be considered before using equipment.
- Recount safety measures related to the use of protective restraints.
- Detail safety measures related to preventing fire when oxygen is in use.
- Discuss the factors influencing a client's personal hygiene practices.
- Explain how assessment maintains a safe environment.
- Describe the modifications that can be used to resolve environmental hazards in institutional and home settings.

KEY TERMS

body image
chemical restraints
dental caries
gingivitis
halitosis
hygiene
perineal care
physical restraints
poison
pyorrhea
restraints
self-care deficit
sensory overload
stomatitis

INTRODUCTION

Safety is basic to the care of all clients. Nurses are responsible for providing professional, quality nursing care to the client in a safe environment. This involves both safety precautions and hygiene assistance. The nurse's role in these areas is described in this chapter.

SAFETY

Safety is the number-one priority when providing client care. The first step is to raise nurses' awareness regarding risk factors because prevention is the key to safety. Nurses must be aware of those factors that have the potential to endanger a client's safety. Constant attention to these factors enables the nurse to maintain a safe environment for the client.

A safety committee is required in all health care facilities, with the purpose of maintaining an overall safe facility for clients, employees, and visitors. The committee is composed of representatives from all departments of the facility. Responsibilities range from analyzing environmental safety in the facility to researching illness rates.

Safety is associated with health promotion and illness prevention. A safe environment reduces the risk of accidents and subsequent alterations in health and lifestyle; it also helps contain the cost of health care services (Figure 20-1). Many factors in the environment can threaten safety.

FACTORS AFFECTING SAFETY

Client safety and health are influenced by several factors, including age, lifestyle/occupation, mobility, sensory and perceptual alterations, and emotional state.

AGE

Injury risk varies with chronological age and developmental stage. Education about preventive measures can prevent injury among clients of various ages.

The potential for injury increases as infants mature. Most accidents occur as infants, toddlers, and preschoolers explore the environment. These can be prevented with careful adult supervision.

The risk for injury increases when school-age children explore the environment outside the home. During this stage, preventive measures should focus on stranger awareness; traffic safety rules; bicycle, skating, and swimming safety; protective equipment; and avoidance of substance abuse.

While good physical health is usually enjoyed by adolescents and young adults, their lifestyle may put them at risk for injury. Because this age-group spends much time away from home, educational efforts of parents, schools, and community health care providers must focus on environmental safety. High-risk factors for injury and death are automobile accidents, substance abuse, violence, unwanted pregnancies, and sexually transmitted diseases.

The injury risk for adults is usually related to lifestyle, behaviors, and work practices. Preventive measures for adults emphasize exercise, nutrition, and occupational safety. High-risk factors for this age-group include anxiety, fatigue, caregiver role strain, sleep pattern disturbances, and altered health maintenance.

The older adult is prone to falls, especially in the bathroom, bedroom, and kitchen because of poor vision and mobility; loss of muscle strength and flexibility; changes in the inner ear that upset the sense of balance; effects of medications; and chronic diseases such as osteoarthritis, Parkinson's disease, and Alzheimer's disease. Preventive measures for older adults include good lighting, using hand rails, changing

PROFESSIONAL TIP

Workplace Safety

EMPLOYEE RIGHT-TO-KNOW LAWS

Under the authority of the Occupational Safety and Health Administration (OSHA) of the Department of Labor and Industry, several states have passed employee right-to-know laws, which state that employees are legally entitled to information regarding hazardous substances or harmful agents in the workplace. Such substances include skin and eye irritants, flammables, poisons, carcinogens, pathogens, and harmful rays (radiation).

REGULATIONS RELATING TO HAZARDOUS MATERIALS

OSHA also outlines and enforces regulations that all health care facilities must follow with regard to employees' exposure to and handling of potentially infectious materials.

MATERIAL SAFETY DATA SHEET

As part of conforming to OSHA regulations, all facilities must have a material safety data sheet (MSDS) for each hazardous substance. The MSDS describes the substance in question, including the associated dangers. Protective equipment, safe handling techniques, and first-aid information are also given. The MSDSs for toxic materials must be kept on site for no fewer than 30 years. All employees must know how to use the MSDS.

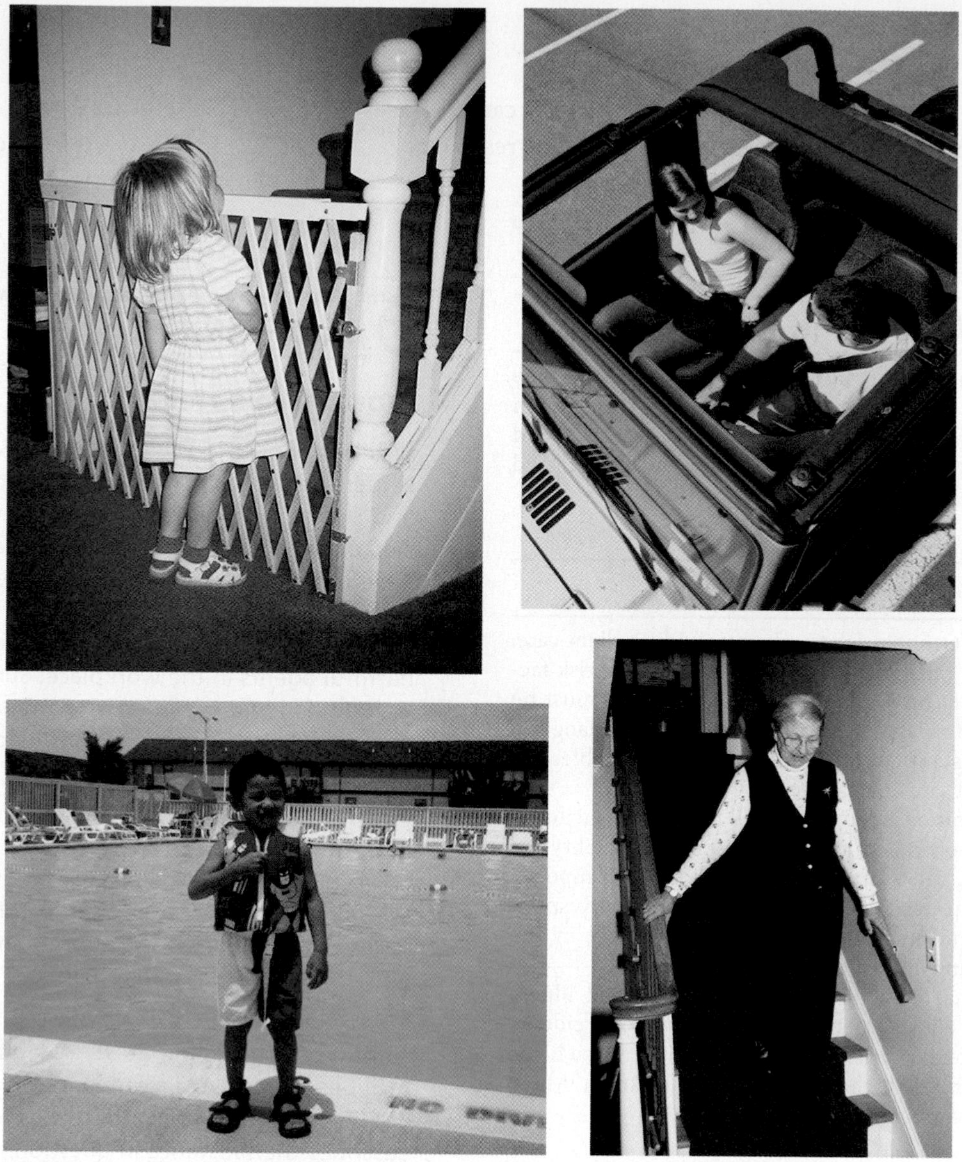

PHOTOS COURTESY OF DELMAR CENGAGE LEARNING

FIGURE 20-1 **Use of stair gates, life vests, seat belts, and hand rails minimizes safety risks.**

position slowly, skidproof mats in bathtub or shower, and removing throw rugs and loose carpets.

According to the Centers for Disease Control and Prevention (CDC, 2002a), one in three adults older than age 65 falls each year. The CDC (2008) states that in 2005, 15,800 people 65 and older died from injuries related to unintentional falls, and about 1.8 million people 65 and older were treated in emergency departments for nonfatal injuries from falls. More than 433,000 of these patients were hospitalized.

Lifestyle/Occupation

Lifestyle practices, reflecting an individual's personal choices about activities or habits to pursue, can increase a person's risk for injury and potential for disease. For instance, individuals who operate machinery; experience excessive stress, anxiety, and fatigue; use alcohol and drugs (prescription and nonprescription); and live in high-crime neighborhoods are at increased risk for injury and alterations to health. Risk-taking behaviors, such as participating in daredevil activities, driving vehicles at high speeds, and not wearing seat belts, are factors that pose a threat to an individual's safety and well-being. Unlike other factors such as age, however, lifestyle/occupation practices are modifiable.

The National Institute for Occupational Safety and Health (2002) reports that an average of 9,000 U.S. workers sustain disabling injuries each day, costing $145 billion each year. Compare this cost to $33 billion for AIDS and $170.7 billion for cancer.

Sensory/Perceptual Changes

Sensory functions are essential for environmental safety. Clients having visual, hearing, smell, taste, communication, or touch impairments have an increased risk for injury because they may not be able to perceive a potential danger.

Mobility

A client with impaired mobility has an increased risk for injury, especially from falls. Impaired mobility may result from poor balance or coordination, muscle weakness, or paralysis. Immobility may lead to physiologic and emotional complications such as pressure ulcers and depression.

PROFESSIONALTIP

Accidents in the Health Care Setting

In the health care setting, accidents are categorized by their causative agent: client behaviors, therapeutic procedures, or equipment:

- **Client behavior accidents** result from the client's behavior or actions. Examples include poisonings, burns, and self-inflicted cuts and bruises.
- **Therapeutic procedure accidents** result from the delivery of medical or nursing interventions. Examples include medication errors, client falls during transfers, contamination of sterile instruments or wounds, and improper performance of nursing activities.
- **Equipment accidents** result from the malfunction or improper use of medical equipment such as electrocution and fire. National and institutional policies establish safety standards with regard to equipment. For example, a facility may attempt to minimize the risk of equipment accidents by requiring the biomedical engineering department to check equipment before use.

All accidents and incident reports must be fully documented according to institutional protocol.

EMOTIONAL STATE

Emotional states such as depression and anger affect the perception of environmental hazards and the degree of risk associated with certain behaviors. These emotional states alter a person's thinking patterns and reaction time. During periods of emotional stress, usual safety precautions may be forgotten.

HYGIENE

Hygiene is the study of health and ways of preserving health. Hygiene provides comfort and relaxation, improves self-image, and promotes cleanliness and healthy skin. Client hygiene is part of client safety in that proper hygiene protects the client against disease. The body's first line of defense, the skin and mucous membranes, is kept healthy by proper hygiene. Nurses are responsible for ensuring that client hygiene needs are met. The care provided depends on the client's needs, ability, and practices.

FACTORS INFLUENCING HYGIENE PRACTICES

Hygiene practices are unique to each client. Nurses provide individualized care based on needs and these practices. Hygiene practices are influenced by body image, personal preferences, social and cultural practices, knowledge, and socioeconomic status.

CULTURAL CONSIDERATIONS

Hygiene

- Some cultures do not permit women to submerge their bodies in water during menstruation because of a fear that the woman may drown.
- In North America, people typically bathe daily and use deodorant products.
- In Europe, many people do not bathe daily, nor do they use deodorant products. They do not consider the smell of human perspiration offensive.

Body Image

Body image is the individual's perception of physical self, including appearance, function, and ability. Body image is linked to the person's attitude, mood, emotions, and values. Body image directly affects the practice of personal hygiene, which may change if the client's body image is altered because of surgical procedures or illness. At these times, the nurse should assist the client to maintain the client's preillness level of hygiene and personal preferences.

Personal Preferences

Personal preferences include the timing of bathing, products used for bathing, and how bathing is performed. For example, some men shave before bathing, whereas others shave after bathing; some people bathe in the morning, whereas others bathe at bedtime to encourage relaxation and sleep. The client should be permitted to practice usual routines and to use preferred hygiene products unless the client's health is adversely affected. Individualized nursing care incorporates the client's personal hygiene preferences.

Social and Cultural Practices

Social and cultural practices and beliefs come from family, religious, and personal values developed during maturation. Clients learn hygiene practices in early childhood. Later, hygiene practices are influenced by socialization outside the family. For example, teenagers often follow the trends in personal hygiene accepted by their peers.

Clients from various cultural backgrounds have differing hygiene practices. A nonjudgmental attitude must be maintained when assessing or providing hygiene care to clients from different social or cultural backgrounds.

Knowledge

The client's understanding of the hygiene and health relationship is influenced by knowledge. For clients to practice basic hygiene, however, they must have more than knowledge; they must be motivated and believe that they are capable of self-care.

An illness or surgical procedure frequently results in a knowledge deficit about the correct hygiene procedure or type of hygiene that can be used. Providing the necessary education about hygiene during an illness is the nurse's responsibility. The nurse may have to perform all hygiene care for a client during an illness until the client is able to do so again.

Socioeconomic Status

A client's hygiene practices may also be influenced by socioeconomic status. Limited economic resources may affect the frequency, extent, and type of hygiene practiced. Some clients may not be able to afford soap, shampoo, toothpaste, and deodorants. The nurse can advocate for the client by contacting social services for referrals to community agencies providing assistance to needy persons.

NURSING PROCESS

The nursing process facilitates providing nursing care to clients at risk for injury or a self-care deficit.

ASSESSMENT

Assessment data are the basis for prioritizing the client's problems and the nursing diagnoses. Clients at risk for injury require frequent reassessment, so appropriate changes can be made in the plan of care and expected outcomes.

The health history and physical examination data correlated with laboratory data identify those clients at risk for problems relating to safety or hygiene. Appropriate risk appraisals may be incorporated into the nursing health history interview.

Subjective Data

The nursing health history interview provides the client's subjective account of specific health data. It is important for the nurse to gather complete, pertinent, and relevant information at this point.

PROFESSIONALTIP

Key Interview Questions about Safety and Hygiene

- What do you do to stay healthy?
- How do you usually spend the day (e.g., home or work)?
- What health care concerns do you have?
- Do you need assistance with bathing and dressing?
- How often do you visit the dentist and eye doctor?
- How often do you use dental floss?
- Do you wash your hands before preparing food?
- Do you keep meats and dairy products refrigerated until ready to use?
- Is there a smoke detector and fire extinguisher in your home?
- Are emergency phone numbers readily available?

Health History Key elements of relevant data regarding the client at risk for injury and infection are obtained in the health history. A health history questionnaire may be used, but depending on the client's status, the nurse may have to perform an interview to obtain these data. When the client cannot provide the subjective data, the nurse must specify, either on the questionnaire or in the nursing progress notes, who provided the information.

During the nursing health history interview, the client's general health perception and management status should be assessed to ascertain how the client manages self-care. This information will provide data regarding the client's routine self-care and health-promotion needs.

Objective Data

Objective data are gathered through the physical examination and the diagnostic and laboratory findings.

Physical Examination When assessing the client specifically for the level of risk for injury and hygiene deficits, the nurse should focus on the following areas and signs:

- Level of consciousness: The Glasgow Coma Scale (GCS) is an objective measurement tool (Neurological System chapter).
- Range of motion: Immobilization of an extremity and/or limited mobility are risk factors for developing skin breakdown, joint contractures, and muscle atrophy.
- Secretions or exudate of the skin or mucous membranes.
- Condition of the skin: Skin condition provides data about a client's nutritional and hydration status, skin integrity, hygiene practices, and overall physical abilities.

Risk Appraisals Specifically developed risk assessment tools appraise the client for potential risks. The client's self-care abilities are appraised during the health history. An analysis of relevant risk factors identifies actual or possible risks. For instance, the risk of impaired skin integrity increases when a person is placed on bed rest. A skin integrity risk appraisal (Table 20-1) should be completed to assist with planning care.

Client in an Inpatient Setting Inpatient clients should be assessed for skin and fall risk factors. The client's risk of falling is identified after gathering specific assessment data, as shown in Table 20-2. Each of these indicators carries a specific weight to determine the client's risk. Special safety measures are implemented as required.

The client should be assessed for safety risks every shift or according to institutional policy. Nurses ensure a safe environment by leaving the bed in low position, side rails up, nurse call light and personal belongings within easy reach, and assistive devices (e.g., a walker) nearby, as shown in Figure 20-2.

Client in the Home Injuries in the home result primarily from falls, poisonings, fires, suffocation, and malfunctioning household equipment (Stanhope & Knollmueller, 2000). Home health nurses may use a safety risk appraisal to determine the client's level of safety knowledge.

The safety risk data assessed in the home direct the nurse's planning for the client's and caregiver's education. Assessment, teaching, and outcome evaluation of the safety hazards can take several home visits.

Diagnostic and Laboratory Data Appraising the client's risk for injury also involves evaluating laboratory findings related to an abnormal blood profile (e.g., anemia, infection). Malnourished clients are at risk for injury.

TABLE 20-1 Skin Breakdown Potential Checklist

_____	(1)	Fair: Major underlying disease, controlled
_____	(2)	Poor: Uncontrolled underlying disease
Mental Status		
_____	(1)	Lethargic: Listless
_____	(2)	Confused: Inappropriate communication
_____	(4)	Comatose: Unresponsive
Mobility/Activity		
_____	(2)	Minor Deficit: Some limitation in movement Needs assistance with ADLs
_____	(4)	Major Deficit: Movement requires assistance
_____	(6)	Immobile: No voluntary movement
Incontinence		
_____	(1)	Mild: Stress incontinence, 1 BM per day
_____	(4)	Frequent: No bladder control, BMs >2–4 per day
_____	(6)	Total: No bladder control, frequent/continuous BM
Nutrition		
_____	(2)	Fair: Intake < body requirements, eats 75% or less
_____	(3)	Poor: Eats 50% or less, started on TPN or tube feeding
_____	(4)	Compromised: No intake, dehydrated
Skin Integrity		
_____	(2)	Fair: Single stage I or II
_____	(4)	Poor: More than one break in skin integrity
_____		TOTAL SCORE OF 8 OR ABOVE, ENTER SKIN INTEGRITY POTENTIAL ON PCP PROBLEM LIST, INITIATE PREVENTATIVE ADLs

Excerpt from Patient Admission Data Base, *Courtesy of CHRISTUS Spohn Health System, Corpus Christi, TX.*

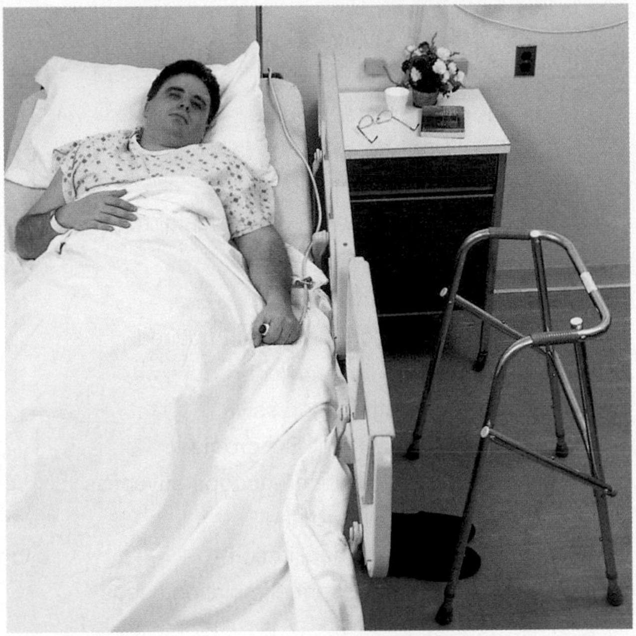

COURTESY OF DELMAR CENGAGE LEARNING

FIGURE 20-2 This client's safety risk has been assessed and responded to through the measures shown here.

NURSING DIAGNOSIS

Following data collection and analysis, the nurse formulates a nursing diagnosis. The main nursing diagnoses that relate to safety and hygiene deficits are *Risk for **I**njury* and the ***S**elf-Care Deficit* diagnoses.

Risk for Injury

The primary nursing diagnosis *Risk for **I**njury* exists when the client is "at risk of injury as a result of environmental conditions interacting with the individual's adaptive and defensive resources" (North American Nursing Diagnosis Association International [NANDA-I], 2010). Although this diagnostic label has no defining characteristics set forth by NANDA, it is categorized as having either internal or external risk factors. An internal biochemical risk factor for a client with impaired vision would be stated as *Risk for **I**njury* related to the risk factor of sensory dysfunction (visual). In contrast, medications on a nightstand in a home with a toddler present should be identified by a home health nurse as creating an external chemical risk factor for the toddler; the nursing diagnosis would be stated as *Risk for **I**njury* related to the risk factor of medications in the environment.

Examples of the other risk nursing diagnoses that may be a risk factor for *Risk for **I**njury* are:

*Risk for **A**spiration:* **risk for entry of gastrointestinal secretions, oropharyngeal secretions, or solids or fluids into the tracheobronchial passages**

*Risk for **D**isuse Syndrome:* **at risk for deterioration of body systems as the result of prescribed or unavoidable musculoskeletal inactivity**

*Risk for **F**alls:* **increased susceptibility to falling that may cause physical harm**

*Risk for Latex **A**llergy Response:* **at risk for allergic response to natural latex rubber products**

*Risk for **P**oisoning:* **at accentuated risk of accidental exposure to, or ingestion of, drugs or dangerous products in doses sufficient to cause poisoning**

*Risk for **S**uffocation:* **accentuated risk of accidental suffocation (inadequate air available for inhalation)**

*Risk for **S**uicide:* **at risk for self-inflicted, life threatening injury**

*Risk for **T**rauma:* **accentuated risk of accidental tissue injury (e.g., wound, burn, fracture)**

These eight nursing diagnoses allow specific nursing interventions to be related to the diagnosed problem. For example, the specific nursing diagnosis for the toddler encountering medications on a nightstand in the home would be *Risk for **P**oisoning,* related to the risk factor of medications accessible to children. The level of risk would be higher if the medications were in open containers or if the closed containers did not have childproof caps. This diagnosis points to specific nursing interventions directed toward the need for client teaching.

TABLE 21-2 Safety Assessment

❑ (5) Age greater than 60	Medications
❑ (5) History of previous falls	❑ (5) Diuretics
❑ (3) From nursing home	❑ (5) Laxatives/G.I. preps
❑ (3) Has had sitter/companion at home	❑ (3) Antihypertensives
	❑ (3) Antiseizures
Status: Mental/Physical	❑ (5) Sedative/hypnotics
❑ (5) Confused/judgement Impaired	❑ (3) Analgesics
❑ (5) Sensory impairment	❑ (3) Antipsychotics/antidepressants
❑ (5) Combative/aggressive	
❑ (5) "Sundowners" Syndrome	
❑ (5) Noncompliance/uncooperativeness	
❑ (5) Paralysis/amputee	❑ LEVEL 1 (0–17)
❑ (5) Weakness/debilitation	❑ LEVEL 2 (18–24)
❑ (5) Urgent/frequent elimination needs	❑ LEVEL 3 (25 or greater)
____ TOTAL	
❑ Safety precautions implemented	❑ Patient/family instructed
❑ Restraints per protocol	❑ Color coded band on

Excerpt from Patient Admission Data Base (*Courtesy of CHRISTUS Spohn Health System, Corpus Christi, TX.*)

Self-Care Deficits

A **self-care deficit** exists when an individual is not able to perform one or more activities of daily living (ADLs). Three self-care deficits related to hygiene practices are identified by NANDA-I (2010). These nursing diagnoses, definitions, defining characteristics, and related factors are presented in Table 20-3.

Other Nursing Diagnoses

The client at risk for injury or having a self-care deficit may have other associated physiologic or psychological problems. The following nursing diagnoses may also be appropriate:

Imbalanced ***N****utrition:* less than body requirements
Imbalanced ***N****utrition:* more than body requirements
Ineffective ***P****rotection*
Impaired ***T****issue Integrity*
Impaired ***S****kin Integrity*
S*ocial Isolation*
Risk for ***L****oneliness*
Ineffective ***C****oping*
Impaired Bed ***M****obility*
Impaired Physical ***M****obility*
Impaired Wheelchair ***M****obility*
H*opelessness*
P*owerlessness*
Deficient ***K****nowledge (specify)*
Acute ***P****ain*
A*nxiety*
F*ear*

Planning/Outcome Identification

The primary nursing goal is to provide safe care by identifying actual or potential risks and implementating safety measures. The nurse reviews assessment data with the client and records what the client indicates are needs for change and health teaching. These findings, when incorporated into the plan of care, reflect the individualized needs of each client. Identified outcomes provide direction for nursing care implemented to reduce the risk of injury.

Another important part of the care plan is client/caregiver education related to identifying potential risks and health-promotion practices. The nursing care plan should include educating the client about preventive actions and changes for an unsafe environment.

Implementation

Implementation involves continual assessment of client health risks and prioritization of nursing interventions aimed at risk reduction, such as:

- Promoting adequate rest and exercise
- Teaching client about health risks
- Administering prescribed medications
- Providing balanced nutritional intake

Implementation of safety measures may require an alteration in the physical environment, as identified by agency fall prevention protocol.

Identify Client

In order to provide safe care, it is essential that nurses correctly match clients with the activity, medication, diet, or treatment

TABLE 20-3 Self-Care Deficits Related to Hygiene Practices

NURSING DIAGNOSIS AND DEFINITION	DEFINING CHARACTERISTICS	RELATED FACTORS
Bathing/Hygiene ***S****elf-Care Deficit:* Impaired ability to perform or complete bathing/ hygiene activities for oneself	Inability to get bath supplies, wash body or body parts, obtain or get to water source, regulate the temperature or flow of bath water, get in and out of bathroom, dry body	Decreased or lack of motivation; weakness and tiredness; severe anxiety; inability to perceive body part or spatial relationship; perceptual or cognitive impairment; pain; neuromuscular impairment; musculoskeletal impairment; environmental barriers
Dressing/Grooming ***S****elf-Care Deficit:* Impaired ability to perform or complete dressing and grooming activities for oneself	Inability to choose clothing, use assistive devices, use zippers, remove clothes, put on socks, put clothing on upper body, maintain appearance at a satisfactory level, put clothing on lower body, pick up clothing; put on shoes, impaired ability to put on or take off necessary items of clothing, obtain or replace articles of clothing, fasten clothing	Decreased or lack of motivation; pain; severe anxiety; perceptual or cognitive impairment; neuromuscular impairment; musculoskeletal impairment; discomfort; environmental barriers; weakness or tiredness
Toileting ***S****elf-Care Deficit:* Impaired ability to perform or complete own toileting activities	Inability to manipulate clothing, carry out proper toilet hygiene, sit on or rise from toilet or commode, get to toilet or commode, flush toilet or commode	Environmental barriers; weakness or tiredness; decreased or lack of motivation; severe anxiety; impaired mobility status; impaired transfer ability; musculoskeletal impairment; neuromuscular impairment; pain; perceptual or cognitive impairment

From *Nursing Diagnoses: Definitions and Classification 2009–2011*, by North American Nursing Diagnosis Association, 2009, Indianapolis, IN: Wiley-Blackwell.

ordered for them. The client's well-being is placed in jeopardy by administering unordered care.

The identification (ID) band or bracelet is the primary means of correctly identifying a client. It lists the client's name, room number, bed number, hospital number, and doctor and may include other information such as age, sex, and religion.

This band is placed on the client's wrist on admission to the hospital. Each time care is given, the band must be checked against the assignment sheet, order sheet, diet card, and medication and treatment sheet or card (Figure 20-3). The client's identity should always be further verified by one other method, such as stating the client's name, asking the client to state his name, or obtaining a positive identification from another person. None of these methods is safe when used alone but, when used with the ID band, can help the nurse verify identity.

If a client is discovered without an ID band, care should be withheld until positive identification is made. A new ID band should be placed on the client's wrist as soon as identity is verified.

Most nursing home residents also wear ID bands. Some, however, do not, and other methods of identification, such as photographs, are used. Nurses working in such long-term care facilities must learn to safely use the identification system. Whatever the system, client identification is essential before rendering any care.

Increase Safety Awareness

In all settings, nurses must show an awareness of safety hazards and teach clients accordingly. Clients must be made aware of safety precautions such as specific information about the use of heating devices, oxygen, intravenous equipment, and automatic bed controls.

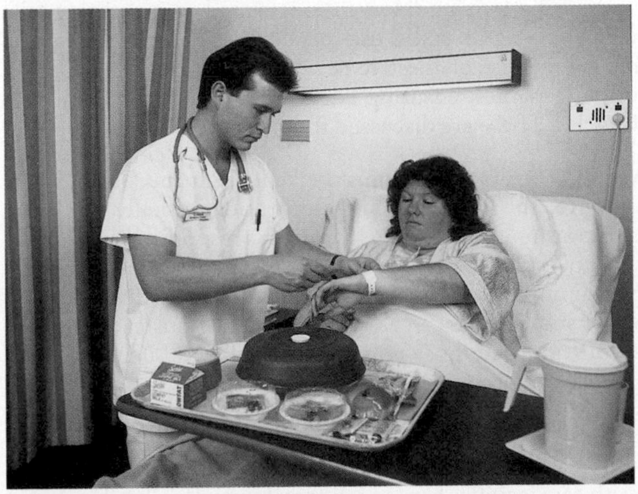

FIGURE 20-3 **Checking the client's ID band ensures that the correct person receives care.**

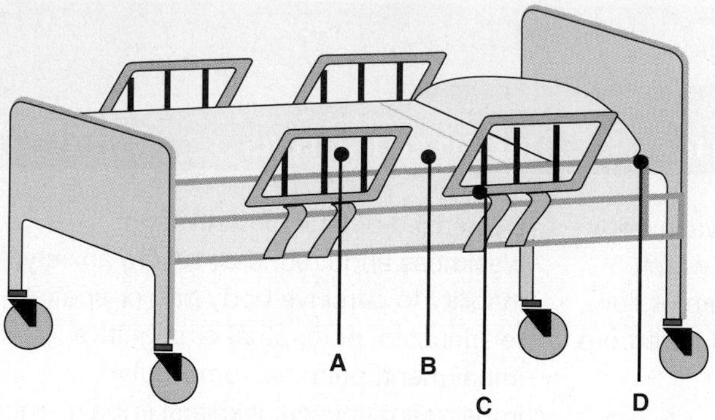

FIGURE 20-4 Entrapment Hazards Associated with Hospital Bed Side Rails; *A*, Between the Bars of the Side Rail; *B*, Between two Side Rails; *C*, Between the Side Rail and Mattress; *D*, Between the Headboard or Footboard, Side Rail, and Mattress (*Source: Food and Drug Administration, Safety Alert, August 1996.*)

A 2008 Food and Drug Administration (FDA) safety alert discussed entrapment hazards related to side rails on hospital beds. The FDA received 772 reports of head and body entrapment incidents resulting in 460 deaths, 136 injuries, and 176 entrapments without injury (FDA, 2008). These incidents occurred in private homes, hospitals, and long-term care facilities. Entrapment hazards associated with hospital bed side rails are illustrated in Figure 20-4.

Prevent Falls

Most falls occur when clients are weak, uncoordinated, fatigued, confused, paralyzed, or disoriented. The data obtained from the safety risk appraisal identifies those clients requiring special measures to prevent falls. The risk for falls can be reduced by:

- Properly supervising clients
- Orienting clients to the environment and the call system
- Providing ambulatory aids (e.g., a wheelchair or walker)
- Keeping personal items and call light in easy reach
- Keeping beds in lowest position and side rails up
- Using rubber mats in shower and tub
- Having adequate lighting

Specific nursing interventions aimed at preventing falls include wiping up spills, use of side rails, applying restraints, encouraging use of assistive devices for walking, using proper body mechanics, ensuring adequate lighting, and removing obstacles. These are discussed following.

Wipe Up Spills Floors must be kept clean and free of spills. Although the housekeeping department usually does the actual washing of floors, it is the nurse's responsibility to either wipe up a spill when it occurs or mark the area as a safety hazard and notify the appropriate person for immediate cleanup. Wet or sticky floors can easily cause a weak, unsteady client to slip or trip. Even those unimpaired by illness, such as visitors and hospital personnel, are at risk.

Use Side Rails Side rails have been used to prevent falls from hospital beds for more than 50 years. Since the 1970s, health care facilities have had side rails on virtually all beds and written policies for the routine use of side rails with all clients. Side rails may be full length, half length, or one-third length.

Clients use side rails to help turn from side to side in bed or to sit up on the edge of the bed and as a support when standing (Figure 20-5). Some clients feel more secure in a strange bed and environment with the side rails up.

Injuries and deaths have occurred with side rail use when clients try to get out of bed by climbing over the rails or when the client becomes entrapped in the rail or between the rail, mattress, and bed frame (Figure 20-4). Many cognitively impaired or older clients feel that they are "in jail" or being "treated like a child" and resist the use of side rails.

The Centers for Medicare and Medicaid Services (CMS) have identified that if the client cannot easily remove or release a side rail, it is considered a restraint and must meet the requirements for restraints (discussed in the next section) (CMS, 2008).

Talerico and Capezuti (2001) suggest safe alternatives to side rail use, including low-height beds, motion sensors, hip pads, floor mats alongside the bed, full-length body pillows, adequate nighttime pain control, individualized nighttime toileting rounds, bed alarms, treating depression and sleep disorders, and individualized sleep regimens. Choosing the appropriate alternative to restrictive side rails (restraint) requires a thorough client assessment. *Clients at risk for falls must always be closely monitored.*

Use Restraints **Restraints** are devices used to limit the physical activity of a client or to immobilize a client or extremity. Restraints are used to protect the client from falls, protect a body part, keep the client from interfering with therapies (e.g., pulling out tubes, disconnecting intravenous setups, or removing wound coverings), and reduce the risk of injury to self and others. Restraints should *never* be used as a substitute for close observation and supervision by nursing personnel.

Before using restraints, find the cause of the problem and then intervene appropriately. Alternatives to restraints may include assessing for pain or other discomfort, using diversional activities, reducing stimuli, coordinating care to minimize sleep interruptions, adjusting room temperature, providing extra pillows and blankets, lowering bed to lowest level, placing call bell within client's reach, having a clock with large numbers and a calendar with large print at the bedside, reintroducing yourself each time you enter the room, providing bathroom breaks every 2 hours, and keeping fluids available and within reach (unless contraindicated) (Napierkowski, 2002; Sweeney-Calciano, Solimene, & Forrester, 2003).

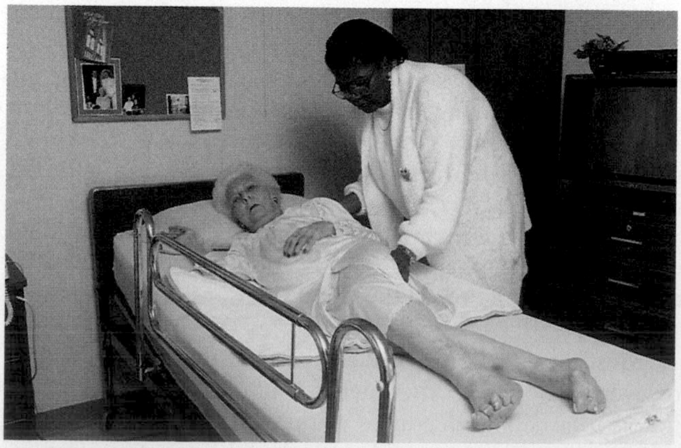

FIGURE 20-5 The use of side rails can contribute to a safe and secure environment.

PROFESSIONALTIP

Key Elements of Restraint Documentation

- Reason for using a restraint
- Type of restraint
- Explanation given to client and family
- Date and time of and client's response to application
- Length of time restraint used
- Frequency of monitoring and client's response
- Safety (release from the restraint along with periodic, routine exercise and assessment for circulation and skin integrity)
- Assessment for continued need of restraint
- Outcome of restraint use

Restraint use is very controversial because of client injuries related to these devices. The Omnibus Budget Reconciliation Act (OBRA) of 1987 defines clients' rights and choices and gives the following as acceptable reasons for using physical restraints:

- Restraints are part of the medical treatment.
- All other interventions have been tried first.
- Other disciplines have been consulted for assistance with the problem.
- Supporting documentation has been provided.

The Joint Commission has also updated its guidelines on physical restraints. Citing studies, the Joint Commission stated that the use of restraints may violate clients' rights and cause "physical and psychological harm, loss of dignity . . . and even death" (Joint Commission, 2001).

Since 1999, the CMS has had regulations regarding the use of restraints. A physician or other licensed independent practitioner (LIP) must conduct a face-to face assessment of the client before writing a restraint order. Each order has a maximum limit of 4 hours for adults, 2 hours for children ages 9 to 17, and 1 hour for clients younger than age 9. They can be written for a shorter time frame. Nurses must continually assess, monitor, and reevaluate the client so that the restraint can be removed at the earliest possible time. The physician or LIP may be telephoned for an order renewal based on the nurse's most recent assessment. The physician or LIP must perform another face-to-face assessment every 24 hours if the restraint is still used (CMS, 2008).

Once restrained, clients are rendered less able to care for their own basic needs; thus, the nurse's responsibility in meeting these needs increases. Facility policy regarding use of restraints, care of the client in restraints, and method of documentation must be followed precisely.

Restraints can be physical or chemical. **Physical restraints** reduce the client's movement through the application of a device (Figure 20-6). **Chemical restraints** are medications used to control the client's behavior. Anxiolytics and sedatives are commonly used chemical restraints.

The nursing plan of care should include safety measures to reduce the potential for injury from restraints. Additional safety measures to observe when using restraint devices are as follows:

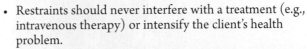

SAFETY

Restraints

- Placing a jacket or belt restraint too tightly on the diaphragm will inhibit lung expansion.
- To avoid accidental injury in the event that the side rail is released, the restraint strap should be secured to the bed frame, not to the side rail.

- Restraints should never interfere with a treatment (e.g., intravenous therapy) or intensify the client's health problem.
- At least once every 2 hours, the nurse must assess the color, temperature, sensation, motion, and capillary refill in the area distal to the restraint and perform range-of-motion exercises.
- The client and significant others should be provided psychological support, as needed.

Use Assistive Devices for Walking Devices used to assist walking include canes, crutches, walkers, and wheelchairs.

Canes Canes are curved walking devices that provide support to the weak side of the body. Three common types of canes are the single stick, the tripod (three footed), and the quad (four footed). All types should have a sturdy grip and rubber tips. The tips should be checked frequently for signs of wear.

Canes should be held on the strong side of the body (Figure 20-7). The affected side and the cane should move simultaneously while the weight is supported on the strong side. The strong side is moved while the weight is supported on the cane and the weaker side.

Crutches Crutches are wooden or metal staffs used either temporarily or permanently to increase mobility. There are two types of crutches: the axillary crutch and the Lofstrand, or forearm, crutch. The axillary crutch, the type most commonly used, fits under the axilla, with the weight being placed on the handgrips. The Lofstrand crutch has a handgrip and a metal cuff that fits around the arm. This type of crutch is more convenient but not as stable as the axillary crutch.

CRITICAL THINKING

Restraints

An 83-year-old widow fractured her hip when she fell in the bathtub. She had hip replacement surgery yesterday. Tonight she is very confused and is trying to dislodge the bandage and stitches. She is now being restrained for her protection. What other nursing activities could have been implemented before use of restraints? Do you think restraints will affect her mental status? If so, in what way(s)? What are some other effects she may experience as a result of being restrained?

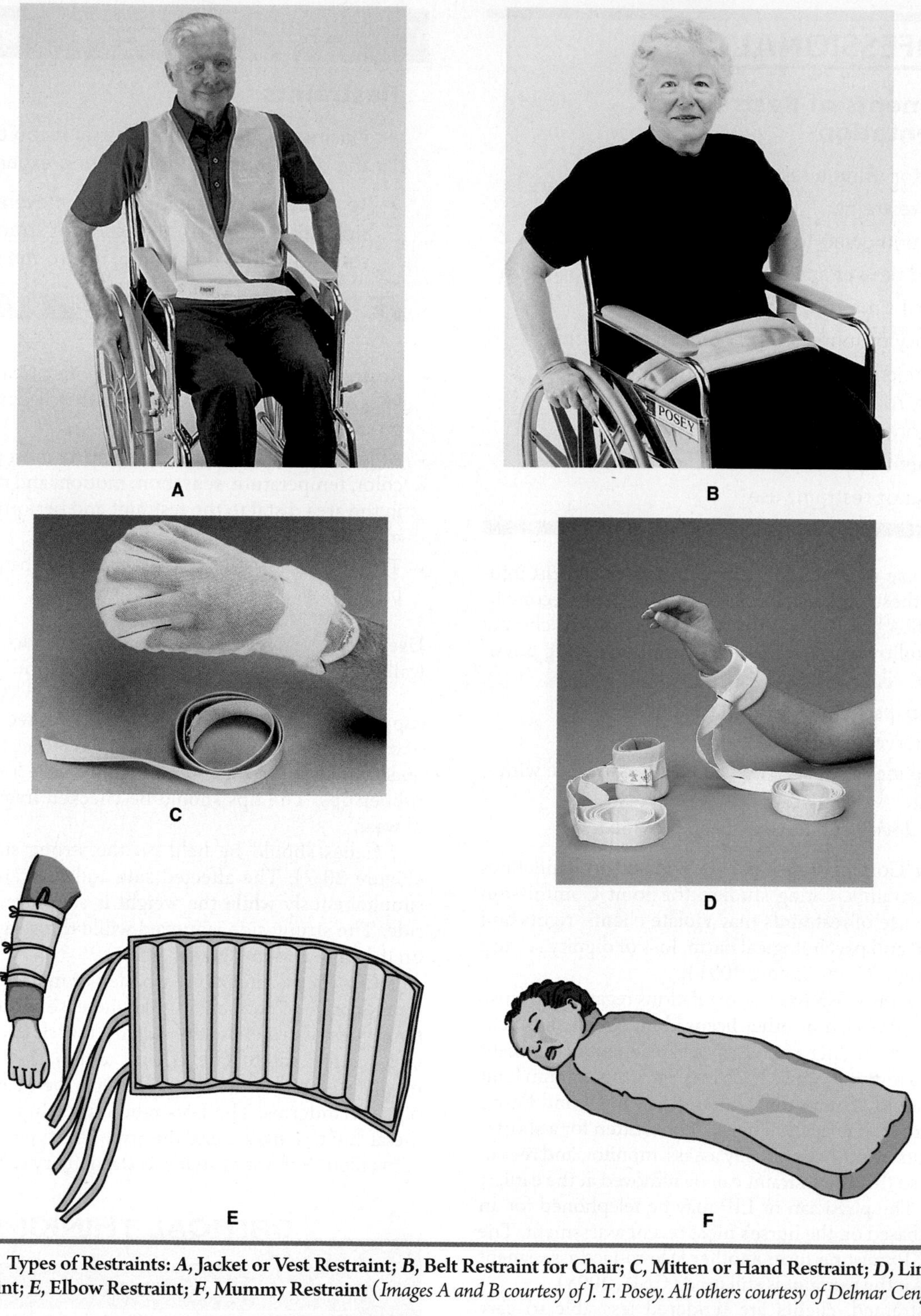

FIGURE 20-6 **Types of Restraints: *A,* Jacket or Vest Restraint; *B,* Belt Restraint for Chair; *C,* Mitten or Hand Restraint; *D,* Limb or Extremity Restraint; *E,* Elbow Restraint; *F,* Mummy Restraint** (*Images A and B courtesy of J. T. Posey. All others courtesy of Delmar Cengage Learning.*)

To prevent slipping, crutches have rubber tips, which must be kept dry. The tips should also be inspected regularly. If tips become loose or worn, they must be replaced immediately. The structure of the crutch must also be inspected regularly. The person's weight will not be properly dispersed if there are cracks or bends in the crutch.

Walkers A walker is a waist-high metal tubular device with a handgrip and four legs. Some walkers have wheels on the front two legs, whereas other walkers have rubber tips on all four legs. Walkers give a sense of security and extra support, as well as independence, to clients. The client first moves the walker forward and then takes a step while balancing weight on the walker.

Wheelchairs A wheelchair is a means of ambulation for clients who are unable to support their weight while standing. The nurse should instruct the client in the safe use of a wheelchair by reminding the client to keep the wheelchair locked when not moving and to lift the footrests out of the way when getting in or out of the wheelchair. The wheelchair should be pushed slowly from behind and should be backed into doorways and into and out of elevators.

Use Proper Body Mechanics The human body is able to move in many different ways, some more efficient than others. The most effective, safest way of lifting and moving things is

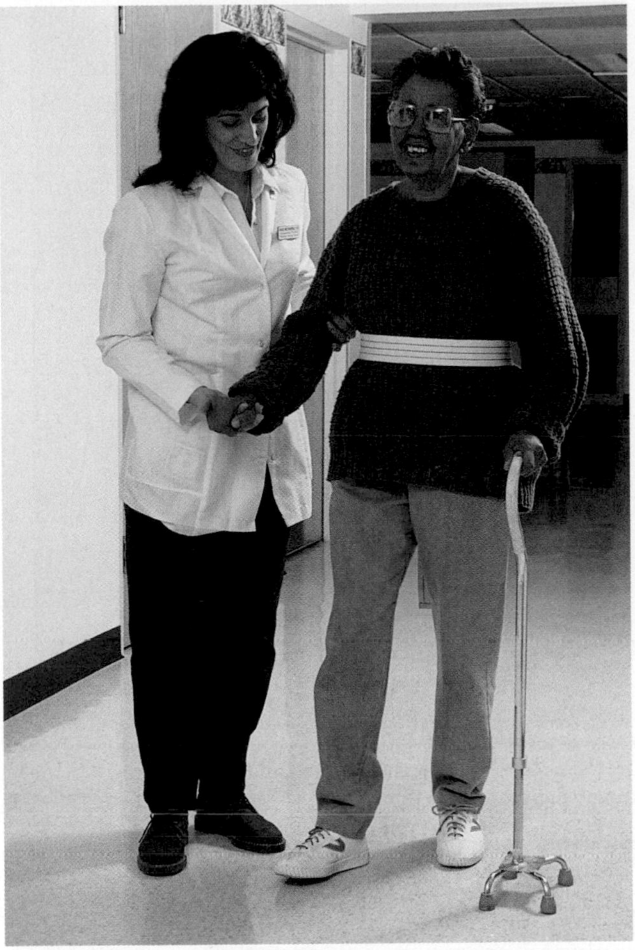

FIGURE 20-7 **A nurse ensures the safety of a client using the quad cane.**

by using the principles of body mechanics, including center of gravity, base of support, and body alignment.

Center of Gravity The center of gravity is located in the center of the body, in the pelvic area. Body weight is approximately equal above and below this area. All movement should pivot around this central point. This keeps the weight over the base of support, making it easier to stay balanced. Keeping the back straight and bending at the knees and hips helps maintain the center of gravity in the pelvic area. If the center of gravity shifts, the body tends to fall.

Base of Support Feet are the base of support. The feet should be kept wide apart when lifting heavy items because it is easier to stay balanced with a wide base of support. Furthermore, one foot should be kept a little forward of the other to give stability from front to back. Keeping the knees slightly bent allows for quick movement and for jolts to the body to be absorbed. When turning, the feet rather than the body should be moved, in order to prevent injury to the back.

Body Alignment Proper body alignment requires that the various parts of the body be kept in proper anatomic relationship to each other.

Ensure Adequate Lighting Adequate lighting helps people see environmental hazards. Rooms should have adequate light so the client can safely perform ADLs and health care providers can perform procedures.

Remove Obstacles Obstacles in heavily traveled areas represent a risk to the client's safety. Older adults and persons unfamiliar with the environment have the greatest risk of injury from obstacles.

SAFETY

Body Mechanics

- Stoop to lift objects from the floor: bend at the hips and the knees, keeping the back straight and base of support wide. The large muscles of the legs can then be used to straighten the body and lift the object.
- Avoid bending from the waist because doing so strains the lower back muscles.
- To prevent undue stress and strain on the back when caring for clients, adjust the height of the bed to one of comfort and ease.
- Carry objects close to the midline of the body.
- Avoid stretching to reach objects.

Reduce Bathroom Hazards

Bathrooms pose a threat to the client because of the presence of water. Accidents common to the bathroom are falls, scalds,

COMMUNITY/HOME HEALTH CARE

Preventing Fires and Burns

- Turn handles of pots and pans toward the center of the stove to prevent children from pulling them down and burning themselves.
- Keep matches in a metal can and in a place where children cannot reach them.
- Be aware of loose, flowing clothing when cooking, especially over an open flame.
- Avoid using candles for light or heat and never leave a burning candle unattended.
- Install smoke alarms near bedrooms and check batteries twice a year.
- Do not place portable heaters near curtains, which can easily catch on fire.
- Allow only certified electricians to work on wiring in the home.
- Do not place electrical cords under carpeting.
- Do not use multiple-plug outlets.
- Do not stick anything into appliances that are plugged in (e.g., a fork in the toaster).
- Teach family members routes of escape from the house, pick a place to meet outside to verify that everyone is safe, and conduct practice fire drills.
- Teach *stop, drop, and roll* to extinguish fire on clothing.

or burns. Accidents can be reduced by using grab bars near the tub, shower, and toilet; nonslip mats in the tub and shower; and a secured bathroom rug near the tub or shower; always check the temperature of the water before entering the tub or shower. Medications should be stored in a locked cabinet, out of reach of children and disoriented or confused adults.

Prevent Fire

Fire is a potential danger in institutional and home environments. Fire requires the interaction of three elements: sufficient *heat* to ignite the fire, combustible material (*fuel*), and *oxygen* to support the fire.

Immobilized or incapacitated clients are at great risk during a fire. Common causes of fire are smoking in bed, discarding cigarette butts in trash cans, and faulty electrical equipment. Because smoking is a health hazard, most health care facilities are now smoke free.

Goals regarding fire are twofold: fire prevention and client protection during a fire. Interventions to prevent or reduce the risk of fire are:

- Make sure fire exits are clearly marked.
- Identify the locations and demonstrate the operation of fire extinguishers.
- Practice fire evacuation procedures.
- Post emergency phone numbers near all telephones.
- Keep open spaces and hallways clear of obstacles.
- Check electrical cords for exposed or damaged wires.
- Teach clients about fire hazards.

When there is a fire, follow institutional policy and procedures for fire containment and evacuation (Figure 20-8). During a fire, nursing interventions are focused on protecting the client from injury and containing the fire. When a fire occurs, nurses should ensure client safety, immediately report the exact location and type of fire, and evacuate if necessary. Nurses should know the locations and operation of fire extinguishers (Figure 20-9). The four types of fire extinguishers are water, carbon dioxide, dry chemical, and Halon. Each type of fire extinguisher is used for a specific class of fire, as outlined in Table 20-4.

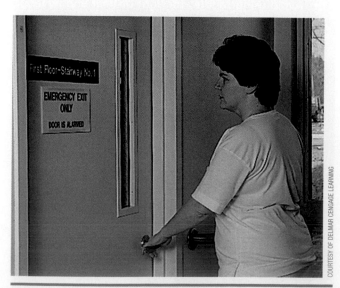

FIGURE 20-8 All personnel should be familiar with the evacuation plan and emergency exits.

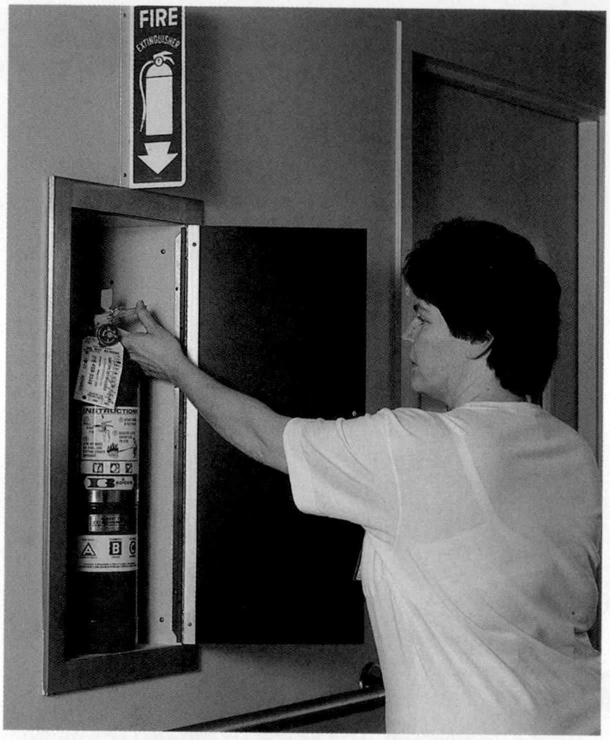

FIGURE 20-9 Know the location and use of fire extinguishers.

MEMORY**TRICK**
RACE

If you discover a fire or see flame or smoke, follow the **RACE** procedures:

R = Rescue individuals directly threatened by the fire
A = Activate alarm and call 911 or have someone call 911
C = Confine the fire by closing doors
E = Evacuate/Extinguish the fire

MEMORY**TRICK**
PASS

By using the memory trick "**PASS**," a nurse will know how to correctly use a fire extinguisher when needed (U.S. Department of Energy, 2001):

P = Pull the pin at the top of the fire extinguisher
A = Aim the nozzle of the fire extinguisher at the base of the fire while standing approximately 8 feet away
S = Squeeze the handle to discharge the fire extinguisher
S = Sweep the nozzle back and forth aiming at the base of the fire

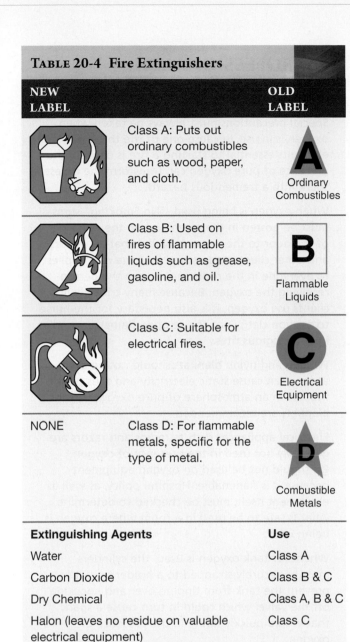

TABLE 20-4 Fire Extinguishers

NEW LABEL		OLD LABEL
	Class A: Puts out ordinary combustibles such as wood, paper, and cloth.	A Ordinary Combustibles
	Class B: Used on fires of flammable liquids such as grease, gasoline, and oil.	B Flammable Liquids
	Class C: Suitable for electrical fires.	C Electrical Equipment
NONE	Class D: For flammable metals, specific for the type of metal.	D Combustible Metals

Extinguishing Agents	Use
Water	Class A
Carbon Dioxide	Class B & C
Dry Chemical	Class A, B & C
Halon (leaves no residue on valuable electrical equipment)	Class C

Data from *HFD: All You Ever Wanted to Know about Fire Extinguishers*, 2001, U.S. Department of Energy, available: http://www.hanford.gov/fire/safety/extingrs.htm, and *Types of Fire Extinguishers*, 2007, Occupational Safety and Health Administration, available: http://www.osha.gov/SLTC/etools/evacuation/portable_about.html#Types.

Ensure Equipment Safety

Checking all equipment and supplies carefully before use and refusing to use any damaged goods or equipment can prevent many accidents. A good rule to follow is *never use any piece of equipment that is damaged in any way or not working properly.* If a wheel comes off an over-bed table, do not attempt to prop the table up but remove it from the room and send it to the appropriate area for repair. The same holds true for smaller supplies given to or used on clients. The safety of clients must always come first.

Glass and Plastic Glass and plastic equipment and supplies should be inspected for cracks and chips before use. The nurse should also check that there are no rough edges that may injure clients.

Disposable Sterile Supplies When using disposable sterile supplies, the nurse should first always check that the package is intact. Any break in or wetness of the wrapper renders it unsterile. Expiration dates should also be verified before use.

Electrical Equipment The hospital environment has a variety of electrical equipment such as bed controls and intravenous and patient-controlled analgesia (PCA) pumps. Each piece of electrical equipment should have a three-pronged, grounded electrical plug. A grounded plug transmits any stray electrical current from equipment to ground. To protect the client from electrical injury, the nurse should read the warning labels on all equipment, check for frayed electrical cords, use only grounded electrical equipment, avoid overloading circuits, and report any shocks received from equipment to the biomedical department (Figure 20-10).

Personal electrical appliances that the client is allowed to keep at the bedside, such as shavers, hair dryers, or curling irons, should be safety checked by the biomedical department before being used.

If a client receives an electrical shock, the electricity should be turned off before touching the client. Then the client's pulse should be checked; if no pulse, CPR should be initiated. The nurse should assess vital signs, mental status, and skin integrity for burns on the client with a pulse. The physician should be notified of the event, and an incident report filled out.

Reduce Exposure to Radiation

Injury from radiation can occur to clients during diagnostic testing and therapeutic interventions if overexposure or exposure to untargeted tissues occurs. Dislodged radiation implants can result in exposure to untargeted tissues. Time, distance, and shielding are the basis of radiation exposure and protection. Protection from radiation therapy involves the following:

- Minimize the time spent in contact with the radiation source (implant or client).
- Maximize the distance from the radiation source (implant or client).
- Use appropriate radiation shields.
- Monitor radiation exposure with a film badge.
- Label all potentially radioactive material.
- Never touch dislodged implants or the body fluids of a client receiving radiation therapy.

The client's risk for injury can be reduced by following all instructions and precautions. The nurse's risk for injury can be

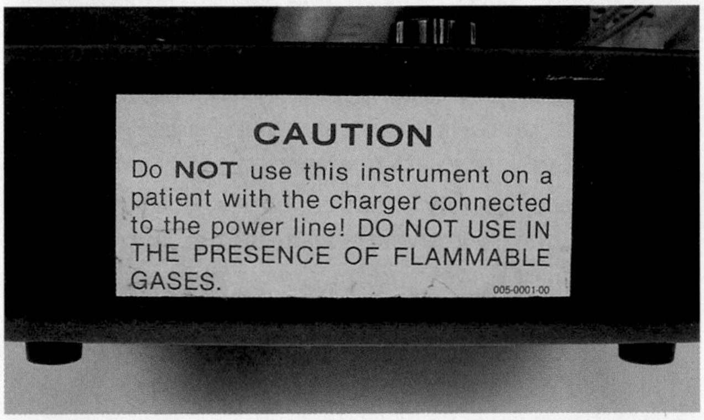

COURTESY OF DELMAR CENGAGE LEARNING

FIGURE 20-10 Heed warning labels on electrical equipment.

SAFETY

Locked Cabinets

Locked cabinets should be used to store all poisonous substances away from children or mentally confused persons.

reduced by observing all radioactive labels, wearing gloves when handling radioactive body discharges, wearing a lead apron, washing hands, disposing of radioactive substances in special containers, reducing the length of client contact, and wearing a badge that measures the amount of radiation exposure.

Prevent Poisoning

A **poison** is any substance that, when taken into the body, interferes with normal physiologic functioning. Poisons may be inhaled, injected, ingested, or absorbed into the body. Many substances can be poisonous if taken in sufficient quantity.

Dangerous chemicals may be found in any workplace, but some are specific to the health care industry, such as radioactive isotopes, laboratory dyes, antiseptics, irrigating solutions, disinfectants, and therapeutic drugs. The nurse must ensure that potentially dangerous materials are never left unattended in clients' rooms. Alcohol and other antiseptics or medications used for dressing changes or other procedures must be removed from the client's room after use.

On admission, clients are asked whether they have brought any medications to the facility. If so, these medications must be either removed to a safe place or sent home with the client's family. Family members sometimes bring in remedies that the client used at home. The nurse should be observant for potentially harmful substances in client rooms.

When poisoning is suspected, the poison control center should be notified. The number can generally be found on the inside cover or first few pages of the telephone book. The person reporting the poisoning should know the amount and type of poison inhaled, ingested, or injected and the client's age and symptoms. Anyone ingesting poison should be turned on the side to prevent aspiration while awaiting further treatment (Stanhope & Knollmueller, 2000).

SAFETY

Medication and Cleaning Carts

- Medication carts and cleaning and supply carts should never be left unattended.
- Confused, visually impaired, or very young clients may help themselves to something harmful or something they may use in a harmful way.
- Medication cupboards and carts must be kept locked when not in use.

PROFESSIONALTIP

Oxygen Use

Special precautions must always be taken when oxygen is in use. Because one of the three elements essential to starting a fire is oxygen, the presence of pure oxygen can transform the tiniest spark into a tremendous hazard.

When oxygen is being used, "No Smoking" signs must be posted in the room and on the outside of the door to the room. It is vital that all visitors and other clients understand that the rule applies to everyone in the room, not just to the person receiving the oxygen. Because many critically ill clients use oxygen, it is also necessary for the nurse to caution clergy not to use open flames or candles in any religious rites.

Woolen and nylon blankets should not be used, as they can cause static electricity and thus pose a fire risk in an atmosphere of pure oxygen. Cotton blankets are recommended.

Electrical appliances such as radios and razors are generally not used in the presence of oxygen. Oil should not be used on oxygen equipment because it is flammable. Hospital policy, as well as equipment itself, must be checked to determine what is safe to be used in a room where oxygen is being used.

Whenever tank oxygen is used, the cylinders must be securely strapped to a holder or cart to prevent the tank from tipping over and knocking off the valve, which could in turn cause a spark that would quickly ignite in the presence of oxygen.

Prevent Choking

To prevent choking on food, special techniques are used when feeding clients in at-risk categories. Nothing should ever be given by mouth to an unconscious client because the epiglottis does not function, and choking and suffocation are likely. Likewise, to prevent aspiration of vomitus, food and drink are usually withheld before the induction of general anesthesia. After some tests, such as a bronchoscopy, food and drink are withheld until the gag reflex returns.

LIFE SPAN CONSIDERATIONS

Vitamins and Minerals

Adult iron preparations are especially poisonous to young children and should be stored in a locked cabinet out of the reach of children.

COMMUNITY/HOME HEALTH CARE

Proper Storage and Use of Medications

Teach clients about:

- Childproofing cupboards where medications are stored.
- The proper use and dosages of medications.
- The use of special medication containers that are divided into days and times (to help prevent the client from duplicating a medication dose).

CLIENT TEACHING

Prevent Accidental Poisonings

- Store medications in child-resistant containers.
- Do not take medications in front of children.
- Never call medicine "candy."
- Place toxic substances in a locked cabinet.
- Keep labels on containers.
- Never put poisonous substances in food or beverage containers.
- Place poison stickers on toxic substances.
- Display poison control center phone numbers near telephones.

Prevent Suffocation

Smothering can be prevented by proper nursing observation of at-risk clients such as infants, those who are impaired with regard to ADLs, and paralyzed or unconscious clients. Such clients should be repositioned frequently and checked for a patent (open) airway. Soft pillows, mattresses, and comforters, in which they might bury their faces, should not be used. In the presence of oral secretions, the client's head should be turned to the side to prevent choking. Monitors that beep if breathing ceases should be used for at-risk clients.

Prevent Drowning

Infants, young children, and weak or confused clients are most at risk for drowning. These clients should never be left alone in the bathtub. If the nurse must leave for any reason, either the client must be removed from the tub or another member of the health care team must stay with the client until the nurse returns or the bath is completed.

Clients should be instructed in the use of call systems installed in tub and shower rooms. Clients should also be instructed to first pull the plug in the tub and then call the nurse should they feel weak or faint.

Reduce Noise Pollution

Noise pollution, an uncomfortable noise level, often occurs in health care facilities from visitor traffic, personnel, and medical equipment. It can result in sensory overload and a disorganized environment. **Sensory overload** is an increased rate and intensity of auditory and visual stimuli. Sensory overload can alter a client's recovery by increasing or causing anxiety, paranoia, hallucinations, and depression.

SAFETY

Noise Pollution

- Maintain a quiet environment.
- Control traffic.
- Provide earplugs.

Provide for Client's Bathing Needs

An essential component of nursing care is bathing clients. The nurse is responsible for ensuring that the hygiene needs of the client are met whether the nurse performs the bath or delegates the activity to another health care provider. The purpose of the bath and the client's self-care abilities determine the type of bath provided. The two general types of baths are cleansing and therapeutic.

Cleansing Baths Cleansing baths are routine client care for personal hygiene. The five types of cleansing baths are shower, tub bath, self-help bath, complete bed bath, and partial bath.

Shower Most ambulatory clients are capable of taking a shower. Clients with physical limitations can use a waterproof chair in the shower. The nurse may provide some assistance with the shower.

Tub Bath Some clients may prefer and enjoy a tub bath. Tub baths can also be therapeutic. Clients with physical limitations should be assisted when entering and exiting the tub.

Self-Help Bath A self-help bed bath provides hygiene care to clients confined to bed. The nurse prepares the bath equipment and assists in washing difficult-to-reach body areas such as the back, legs, feet, and perineal area.

Complete Bed Bath A complete bed bath is provided for dependent clients who are confined to bed. The nurse washes the client's entire body.

SAFETY

Tub Bath

Water temperature must be checked in the bathtub before allowing the client to enter.

PROFESSIONAL TIP

Bathing

- Baths are an excellent time to assess the skin.
- Bathing provides time to meet the client's psychosocial needs through assessment and counseling and to educate the client on basic and special hygiene needs.

Partial Bath In a partial bath, only those body areas that would cause discomfort or odor are cleansed. These areas are the face, hands, axillae, and perineal area. The client or nurse may perform a partial bath, depending on the client's self-care abilities. Partial baths may be performed with the client in bed or standing at the sink.

Therapeutic Baths A physician's order is required for therapeutic baths, stating the type of bath, body surface to be treated, temperature of the water, and type of medicated solutions to be used. A therapeutic bath is usually taken in a tub and lasts approximately 20 to 30 minutes. They are classified as hot, warm, tepid, or cool; soak or sitz; and oatmeal (Aveeno), cornstarch, or sodium bicarbonate.

Hot- or warm-water tub baths reduce muscle spasms, soreness, and tension but can cause skin burns. Cool or tepid baths relieve tension and lower body temperature. To prevent chilling and rapid temperature fluctuations during a tepid or cool bath, the nurse must not leave the client in the tub too long.

A soak is usually limited to a body part but can involve the entire body. Water, with or without a medicated solution, is applied to reduce irritation, pain, or swelling or to soften or remove dead tissue.

Sitz baths reduce inflammation and cleanse the perineal and anal areas. Sitz baths are usually used for hemorrhoids or anal fissures and after perineal or rectal surgery. Skin irritations can be soothed with oatmeal (Aveeno), cornstarch, or sodium bicarbonate baths.

Provide Clean Bed Linens

Clean linens are placed on the bed to promote comfort after a bath. Clients able to be out of bed can sit in a chair while the nurse makes the bed.

If the client cannot be out of bed, the nurse will make an occupied bed. If the client cannot be turned or is in traction, assistance will be needed. Care must be taken to avoid disturbing any traction weights.

Provide Perineal Care

Perineal care is the cleansing of the external genitalia, the perineum, and surrounding area. Perineal care may be called *peri-care*. Perineal care prevents or eliminates infection and odor, promotes healing, removes secretions, and provides comfort. Perineal care can be provided as part of the bath or separately.

Offer Back Rubs

Back rubs and massages stimulate the client's circulation, relieve muscle tension, and relax muscles and give the nurse an opportunity to assess the skin. Cream and lotion facilitate the rubbing and skin lubrication during a back rub or massage.

The client lies either on the side or prone. The nurse uses friction and pressure when rubbing the hands on the client's skin. Friction creates heat, which dilates the peripheral blood vessels and increases the blood supply to the skin. Pressure stimulates the muscle fibers, which relaxes the muscles. The nurse must check for contraindications before giving a back rub or massage. Be cautious when massaging limbs, especially the lower limbs. A thrombus (blood clot) might be dislodged, resulting in an embolus (circulating blood clot). Bony prominences should be massaged lightly to prevent damage to underlying tissue.

Provide Foot and Toenail Care

Proper foot and toenail care are necessary for standing and ambulation. Often, foot and toenail care are ignored until problems arise. Foot and toenail problems may result from poorly fitted shoes, inadequate foot and toenail hygiene, incorrect nail trimming, and exposure to harsh chemicals. These problems may cause a loss of skin integrity and potential for infection.

Pain or tenderness is usually the first sign of foot and toenail problems. These symptoms may result in limping, causing strain to certain muscle groups. Clients with diabetes mellitus have changes in circulation predisposing them to foot problems requiring special foot and toenail care.

Foot and toenail care prevents infection and soft tissue trauma from ingrown or jagged nails and eliminates odor. Hygiene care of feet and toenails includes regular cleansing, rinsing, and drying the feet and toenails; trimming the toenails; cleaning under the toenails; and wearing properly fitted shoes.

Soaking facilitates cleansing dirty or thickened toenails. Use an orangewood stick to clean under the toenails because a metal instrument roughens the nail and causes harboring of dirt. The nail clipper is the safest instrument to trim the toenails; however, some people think that cutting the nails makes them brittle. The client who chooses not to cut the nails should file them straight across with an emery board. The

CRITICAL THINKING

Perineal Care

What is the best way to approach providing perineal care to someone of the opposite sex or of your similar age?

PROFESSIONALTIP

Perineal Care

Perineal care may be embarrassing for both the client and the nurse, especially if the client is of the opposite sex. In this situation, the nurse may provide the client with warm water, a moistened washcloth, soap, a dry towel, and privacy. The nurse is responsible for providing perineal care in a professional and private manner if the client is unable to do so.

PROFESSIONALTIP

Foot and Toenail Care

- Soak feet in warm water and wash with soap.
- Clean under the nails with an orangewood stick.
- Cut or file the nails straight across.
- Trim the cuticles when needed.
- Dry feet and between toes.
- Apply lotion or cream.

areas between the toes should be carefully dried. An emollient, such as cold cream, helps keep toenails and cuticles soft.

Callused areas should never be cut. Lotion applied to the feet maintains moisture and softens callused areas. Soaking also facilitates callus removal. If the client's feet are excessively moist (sweat), water-absorbent powder can be applied between the toes.

Everyone should wear clean, properly fitted shoes. Shoes should not be too tight but should be snug enough to provide support to the feet and have arch supports. Shoes should be half an inch longer than the longest toe.

Provide Oral Care

The oral cavity takes in food, chews it, secretes mucus to moisten and lubricate the food, and secretes a digestive enzyme. Common problems occurring in the oral cavity include:

- Bad breath (**halitosis**)
- Cavities (**dental caries**)
- Inflammation of the gums (**gingivitis**)
- Inflammation of the oral mucosa (**stomatitis**)
- Periodontal disease (**pyorrhea**)
- Plaque

Poor oral hygiene and loss of teeth affects a person's social interaction, body image, and nutritional intake. Daily oral care is vital to maintain the integrity of the mucous membranes, gums, teeth, and lips. Preventive measures can preserve the oral cavity and teeth. Preventive oral care consists of flossing, brushing, and rinsing with fluoride.

Fluoride Research has determined that fluoride can prevent dental caries so communities add fluoride to their water supplies. Fluoride is common in toothpastes and mouthwashes, but persons with very dry or irritated mucous membranes should not use commercial mouthwashes because the alcohol content further dries the mucous membranes.

Infants can be given fluoride drops as early as 2 weeks of age to prevent dental caries. Nurses should inform clients that excessive fluoride can darken the color of tooth enamel. Fluoride should be administered with a dropper directed toward the back of the throat to prevent discoloration of the tooth enamel.

Flossing Flossing should be done daily before brushing the teeth. Flossing prevents the formation of plaque and removes plaque and food debris between the teeth. Regular flossing can prevent dental caries and periodontal disease.

Brushing Brushing promotes blood circulation in the gums and removes plaque and food debris. Tooth brushing should follow flossing. Brush teeth after each meal using a dentifrice (toothpaste) containing fluoride. Brush the tongue to remove bacteria and prevent halitosis. Dentures are brushed the same way as teeth. The oral cavity of a client who wears dentures must also be cleansed. Dentures should be kept moist by putting back in the mouth or immersing in water after cleansing.

CULTURAL CONSIDERATIONS

Influences on Hygiene

- All self-care and hygiene practices are influenced by the client's cultural values and background.
- Ask clients about preferences before performing care and show sensitivity about those practices that may differ from your own.

PROFESSIONALTIP

Oral Care for the Unconscious Client

Special care should be taken when doing oral care for the unconscious client to prevent both client aspiration and injury to the nurse (from the client biting because of the gag reflex).

- Never use your fingers to hold a client's mouth open; use a bite block or padded tongue blade.
- Assess for gag reflex.
- Turn the client's head to one side with a basin under the mouth.
- Use only a small amount of liquid and oral suctioning to facilitate removal of secretions.
- Brush the teeth and tongue in the usual manner. Exercise caution to prevent aspiration.

Provide Hair Care

Hair affects a person's appearance and body image. Hair maintains body temperature and is a receptor for the sense of touch. Hair texture, growth, and distribution provide information on a person's general health status. Common hair problems include hair loss, dandruff, tangled or matted hair, and infestations such as lice. Daily hair care can reduce hair problems and promote hair growth; prevent hair loss, infections, or infestations; promote circulation to the scalp; evenly distribute oils along hair shafts; and maintain the client's physical appearance. Hair care consists of brushing and combing, shampooing, shaving, and mustache and beard care.

Brushing and Combing Hair should be brushed or combed daily in the client's preferred manner. A clean brush or comb should be used to brush from the scalp toward the hair ends. Be gentle when brushing or combing sensitive scalps.

Some clients may have tangled or matted hair. Prevent pain when combing tangled or matted hair by holding the tangled hair near the scalp while combing. The hair can be loosely braided to prevent tangling or matting if the client permits. Tight braids may cause pain and hair loss. Written informed consent must be received before cutting a client's hair.

Shampooing Hair should be shampooed according to the client's usual routine. Shampooing removes soil from the hair, stimulates scalp circulation, and facilitates brushing and combing. Depending on the client's abilities and preferences, hair can be shampooed in the tub, in the shower, at the sink, or in the bed.

Hair can be shampooed with water or with shampoos not requiring water. Use the fingertip pads to gently massage the scalp. Thoroughly rinse and dry with an absorbent towel, comb and style as the client desires.

SAFETY

Shaving

- Review the client's medical record and the facility's policy regarding the use of razors for shaving.
- Clients prone to bleeding should use only electrical razors for shaving.
- The nurse should wear gloves unless using an electric razor.

Shaving Shaving is the removal of hair from the skin surface. Men often shave to remove facial hair, and women may shave to remove leg and/or axillary hair. Operative procedures may also require shaving an area of the body.

Shaving may be performed before, during, or after the bath. The area should be washed with soap and warm water to soften the hair before shaving. Apply shaving cream or mild soap to the area to ease hair removal. Pull the skin taut, hold the razor at a 45-degree angle, and move the razor over the skin in firm, short strokes in the direction of hair growth. Care should be taken to avoid cutting the skin. Wash, rinse, and pat the skin dry following shaving.

Mustache and Beard Care Mustaches and beards need daily care to keep the hair clean, trimmed, and combed. They can be washed with soap or shampoo but often require only gentle wiping with a moist washcloth. A mustache or beard should never be shaved off by the nurse without written informed consent from the client.

Provide Eye, Ear, and Nose Care

Eye, ear, and nose care should be included in routine hygiene care.

Eye Care Eyes are continually cleansed by tears and the movement of the eyelids over the eyes. Eyelids should be washed daily with a warm washcloth and from the inner to the outer canthus.

Eyelashes prevent foreign material from entering the eyes and conjunctival sacs. Eyelashes and eyebrows should be washed with the face.

Although some artificial eyes (prosthetics) are permanently implanted, others may require daily removal and cleaning: The eye is removed from the eye socket and washed.

Comatose clients lack a blink reflex and need special eye care. Lubricants or eyedrops should be frequently instilled to prevent corneal abrasions.

INFECTION CONTROL

Eye Care

In order to prevent the transfer of pathogens, a new, clean corner of the washcloth should be used for each eye and with each stroke.

PROFESSIONAL TIP

Eye Care for the Comatose Client

- At least every 4 hours, use a warm washcloth to cleanse eyelids, eyelashes, and eyebrows. Clean from the inner to the outer canthus.
- Liquid tear solutions should be instilled to prevent corneal drying and ulcerations if eyes remain open and the blink reflex is absent.
- If eye patches or shields are used, they should be removed at least every 4 hours to assess the eyes and provide eye care.

Clients who can insert, remove, and manage the care of their contact lenses require little assistance from the nurse. The client who also has corrective eyeglasses may wish to wear eyeglasses during hospitalization. There are hard and soft types of contact lenses. Each type requires different cleansing and care. The lenses should be removed during emergency situations and placed in the appropriate solution.

Ear Care Foreign material or wax in the external ear canal can affect hearing. Cleansing the ears involves cleansing the external ear canal and auricles. No objects should be inserted into the ear canal. Excess wax or foreign material may be removed with a warm washcloth while pulling the ear up and back in the adult client. The ear is pulled down and back in children under the age of 3. Irrigation of the ear may be necessary to remove dried wax; this will require a physician's order.

Hearing aids amplify sound. Hearing aids should be cleansed regularly to ensure proper functioning.

If the hearing aid is not functioning properly, the nurse should check the on–off switch and volume control, the battery (and replace as necessary), the plastic tubing for cracks and loose connections, and the telephone switch, which should be in the off position unless the client is using the phone. Hearing aids should be handled carefully because bumping or dropping them can damage their delicate mechanisms. The hearing aid should be stored in a container when not in use because dust and dirt can damage the mechanism.

Nose Care The nose is the organ of smell, which humidifies inhaled air, facilitates breathing, and prevents entrance of foreign material into the respiratory tract. Excessive or dried secretions may impair nasal function. If the client cannot blow the nose, insert a cotton-tip applicator moistened with water or saline into the nostrils but not beyond the cotton tip. A suction bulb can remove excessive nasal secretions in infants. The client with a nasogastric tube should receive meticulous skin care to the nose area to prevent skin breakdown.

EVALUATION

Evaluation looks for achievement of goals and expected outcomes.

The client should be not only kept free of injury during hospitalization but also helped to develop an awareness of the factors increasing the risk for injury. In the home, modifications to ensure a safe environment serve as evidence for the home health nurse that learning has taken place.

The therapeutic value of hygiene is greatest when the client participates and is free from infection and changes in skin integrity. Evaluation identifies the client's level of functioning in self-care activities. At the time of discharge, appropriate referrals can be made to home health care agencies to assist the client in safety and hygiene practices.

CASE STUDY

K.H., an 80-year-old male, was involved in a motor vehicle accident (MVA) 1 month prior to being admitted to a rehabilitation facility. The MVA resulted in chest contusions from the seat belt and injury to the lungs, which resulted in general muscle weakness and a medical diagnosis of pneumonia. Before coming to the rehabilitation facility, K.H. lived independently at home and plans on returning home on discharge. When assessed by the nurse, he was alert; oriented to person, place, and time; wheelchair dependent; and ambulating 60 feet once a day with assistance from physical therapy. K.H.'s hand grasp, pedal push/pull, and muscle strength are grade 3. K.H. stated, "I feel so weak. I need to strengthen my muscles if I want to be able to go home."

1. What would be an appropriate nursing diagnosis for this client?
2. What goal/outcome would be appropriate for K.H.?
3. List four nursing interventions and provide rationale for each intervention.
4. When evaluating the plan of care, what data support that the goal/outcome criteria was met?

SAMPLE NURSING CARE PLAN

The Client at Risk for Injury

M.S., age 75 years, presents with coronary heart disease (CHD) on being admitted to the hospital. He has a family history of CHD. He smokes two packs of cigarettes per day, has diabetes mellitus, and is obese. He has gained 7 pounds in the past month and exhibits diminished visual acuity, decreased bladder tone, weakness, and syncope. His blood cholesterol is 320 mg/dL, and his high-density lipoprotein (HDL) level is 28 mg/dL. On the Glasgow Coma Scale (GCS), he received a score of 12 (15 is fully oriented; 7 is comatose). His blood pressure is 186/116.

NURSING DIAGNOSIS 1 *Risk for Injury* related to failure to adapt to sensory dysfunctions as evidenced by diminished visual acuity and a GCS score of 12

Nursing Outcomes Classification (NOC)
Risk Control: Cardiovascular Health
Neurological Status

Nursing Interventions Classification (NIC)
Surveillance
Surveillance: Safety

PLANNING/OUTCOMES	NURSING INTERVENTIONS	RATIONALE
M.S. will be protected from injury during hospitalization.	Initiate fall-prevention protocol.	Identifies and reduces the risk for injury.
	Place M.S. in a room as close as possible to the nurses' station.	Facilitates faster response time to the client's needs.
	Place fall-alert signs on M.S.'s door and head of bed.	Alerts other health care workers to the client's risk status.
	Turn the bed alarm on.	Helps monitor client status and facilitates prompt response if the client tries to get out of bed unassisted.
	Monitor M.S. and the environment every 2 hours and whenever a caregiver passes by his room.	Provides information on status, progress, and needs of the client; encourages team approach to client care.

(Continues)

SAMPLE NURSING CARE PLAN (Continued)

PLANNING/OUTCOMES	NURSING INTERVENTIONS	RATIONALE
	Reassess M.S.'s status every 4 hours.	Identifies changes and, thus, the need to modify the plan of care.
	Instruct all caregivers to respond promptly to the call light.	Ensures rapid response to the client's needs.
	Teach M.S. to use the call light; reinforce teaching each time before leaving him alone.	Ensures that the client has the means and knowledge to call for assistance if necessary.

EVALUATION

The fall prevention protocol was implemented. When discharged on the third day of hospitalization, M.S. was free of injury.

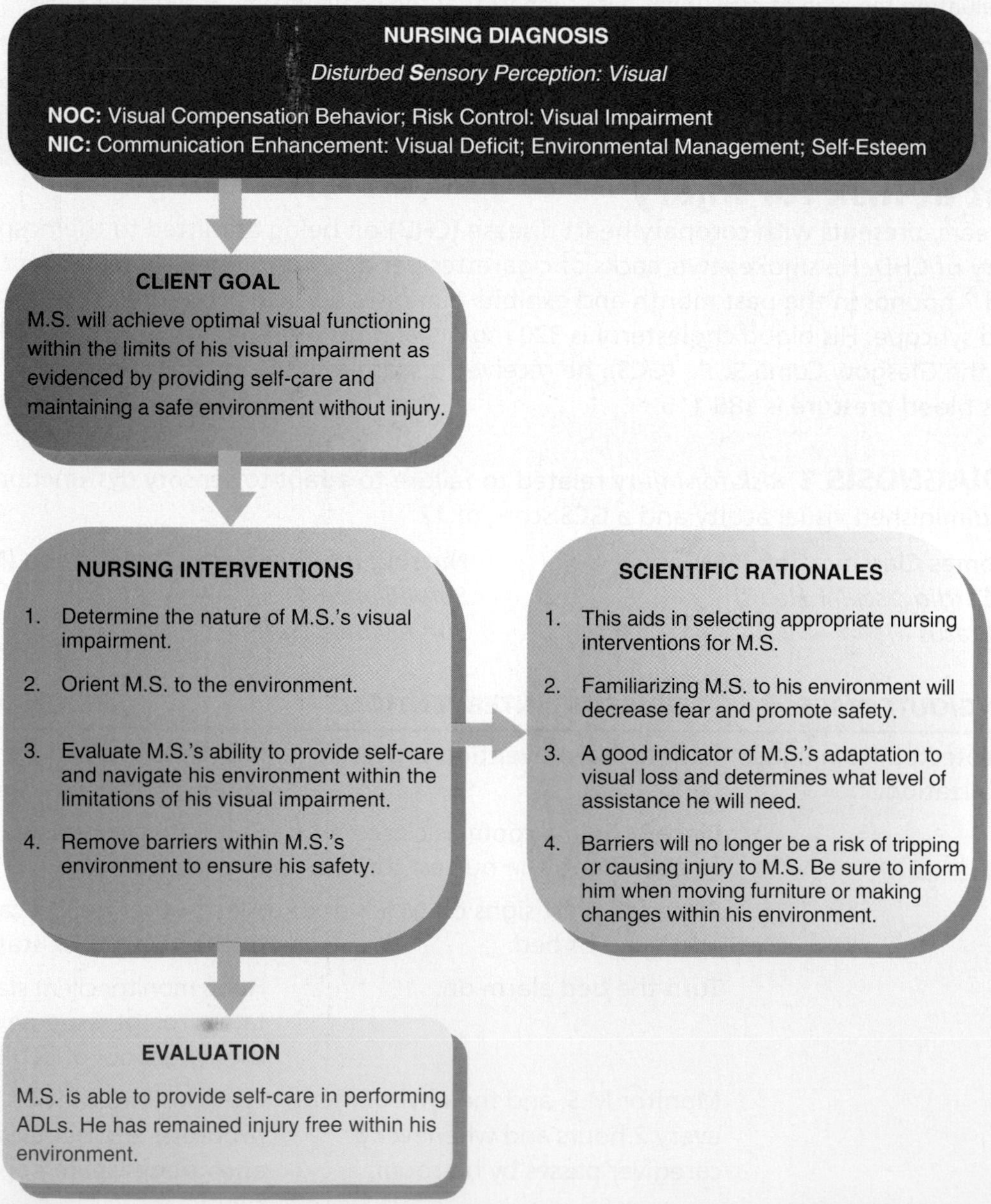

NURSING DIAGNOSIS
Disturbed Sensory Perception: Visual
NOC: Visual Compensation Behavior; Risk Control: Visual Impairment
NIC: Communication Enhancement: Visual Deficit; Environmental Management; Self-Esteem
CLIENT GOAL
M.S. will achieve optimal visual functioning within the limits of his visual impairment as evidenced by providing self-care and maintaining a safe environment without injury.
NURSING INTERVENTIONS
1. Determine the nature of M.S.'s visual impairment.
2. Orient M.S. to the environment.
3. Evaluate M.S.'s ability to provide self-care and navigate his environment within the limitations of his visual impairment.
4. Remove barriers within M.S.'s environment to ensure his safety.
SCIENTIFIC RATIONALES
1. This aids in selecting appropriate nursing interventions for M.S.
2. Familiarizing M.S. to his environment will decrease fear and promote safety.
3. A good indicator of M.S.'s adaptation to visual loss and determines what level of assistance he will need.
4. Barriers will no longer be a risk of tripping or causing injury to M.S. Be sure to inform him when moving furniture or making changes within his environment.
EVALUATION
M.S. is able to provide self-care in performing ADLs. He has remained injury free within his environment.

CONCEPT CARE MAP 20-1

SUMMARY

- Maintaining a safe environment for clients must be the highest priority for nurses.
- The best way to ensure safety is to recognize hazards and eliminate them. Prevention is the best safety measure.
- Clients having a high risk factor for injury must be provided extra protection measures.
- Factors influencing client safety are age, lifestyle, sensory and perceptual alterations, mobility, and emotional state.
- Accidents occurring in health care settings are related to client behavior, therapeutic procedures, and equipment.
- A safety risk appraisal is part of an assessment of a safe environment.
- Nurses can help clients maintain a safe environment by eliminating hazards related to falls, lighting, obstacles, the bathroom, fire, electricity, radiation, poisoning, and noise pollution.
- Safety precautions should be explained thoroughly to clients and/or families.
- Hygiene practices are influenced by personal preference, social and cultural practices, body image, socioeconomic status, and knowledge.
- Basic hygiene practices include bathing, skin care, perineal care, back rubs, foot and nail care, oral care, hair care, and eye, ear, and nose care.

REVIEW QUESTIONS

1. A 60-year-old diabetic client had his left leg amputated. He is in a semiprivate room with another client who is receiving oxygen. What sign should be posted on the door?
1. "Amputee"
2. "No Visitors"
3. "No Smoking"
4. "Regular Diet"

2. A client, just admitted to the hospital, is overweight, unsteady on her feet, and visually impaired. Her two daughters enter the room as the nurse puts the side rails up on the bed. The client begins to cry. The daughters accuse her of being a baby. The best nursing intervention would be to:
1. tell the daughters to leave until their mother has calmed down.
2. explain to the daughters that they are making their mother feel worse.
3. explain to the client that side rails must be used to protect her from falling out of bed.
4. explain to the client and her daughters both the purpose of the side rails and the facility's alternate policy.

3. Hygiene is considered a safety measure because:
1. it changes a person's self-image.
2. the same thing is done for all clients.
3. it rids the body of all microorganisms.
4. it promotes the health of the body's first line of defense.

4. A 42-year-old client is admitted to the hospital with mental changes, a headache, and shakiness. The nurse knows that the priority for nursing care is:
1. safety.
2. timeliness.
3. one-to-one care.
4. the execution of procedures exactly as written.

5. The nurse's place of employment has recently conducted a seminar for all staff on the use of side rails. After attending the seminar, the nurse knows that the use of side rails:
1. is needed only at night.
2. is required for all clients.
3. has caused injury to clients.
4. relieves the nurse from checking on the client as frequently.

6. Nursing measures to prevent falls in elderly clients include: (Select all that apply.)
1. providing good lighting.
2. placing rugs on the floor to prevent client from slipping.
3. orienting client to the environment.
4. keeping bed in the lowest position.
5. not using restraints.
6. placing a call light within reach.

7. The nurse is teaching a client about safety and asks the client to identify four factors that affect client safety. Which of the following factors identified by the client indicates that further teaching is needed?
1. Age.
2. Body image.
3. Occupation.
4. Sensory changes.

8. Which nursing intervention is the most appropriate to utilize at night for a client who uses a walker and is taking diuretics?
1. Keep side rails up.
2. Check on client periodically.
3. Use a night-light.
4. Place commode at bedside.

9. The nurse is making rounds and discovers a fire in a client's room. Her first action would be to:
1. pull the nearest fire alarm.
2. extinguish the fire following the "PASS" method.
3. close doors on the unit to confine the fire.
4. evacuate clients in immediate danger.

10. A 55-year-old female client with cancer has recently received a radiation implant. The nurse knows that protection from radiation therapy involves all of the following except:
    1. using appropriate radiation shields.
    2. minimizing the time spent in contact with the client while the implant is in place.
    3. monitoring radiation exposure with a film badge.
    4. immediately placing the radiation implant into a lead-lined bag if it becomes dislodged.

REFERENCES/SUGGESTED READINGS

Association for Professionals in Infection Control and Epidemiology, Inc. (2003). *The use of hand sanitizers in the healthcare setting.* Available: http://www.apic.org/pdf/FINALHandSanitizers.pdf

Bulechek, G., Butcher, H., McCloskey, J., & Dochterman, J., eds. (2008). *Nursing Interventions Classification (NIC)* (5th ed.). St. Louis, MO: Mosby/Elsevier.

Carpenito-Moyet, L. N. (2007). *Handbook of nursing diagnosis* (12th ed). Philadelphia: Lippincott Williams & Wilkins.

Centers for Disease Control and Prevention. (2008). Falls among older adults: An overview. Retrieved November 16, 2008, from http://www.cdc.gov/ncipc/factsheets/adultfalls.htm

Centers for Disease Control and Prevention, National Center for Injury Prevention and Control. (2002a). The costs of fall injuries among older adults. Available: http://www.cdc.gov/ncipc/factsheets/fallcost.htm

Centers for Disease Control and Prevention, National Center for Injury Prevention and Control. (2002b). Preventing falls. Available: http://www.cdc.gov/ncipc/ duip/spotlite/falls.htm

Centers for Medicare and Medicaid Services. (2008). CMS guidance document: Revised interpretative guidelines for restraint or seclusion. Retrieved November 22, 2008, from http://cms.hhs.gov/EOG/downloads/EO%200306.pdf

Converso, A., DeMass Martin, S. L., & Markle-Elder, S. (2007). Health and safety: Is your hospital safe? *American Journal of Nursing, 107*(2), 37.

Guyton, A. C., & Hall, J. (2005). *Textbook of medical physiology* (11th ed.). Philadelphia: W. B. Saunders.

Jasniewski, J. (2006). Healthier aging: Take steps to protect your patient from falls. *Nursing2006, 36*(4), 24–25.

Joint Commission. (2001). *Comprehensive accreditation manual for hospitals.* Oakbrook Terrace, IL: Author.

Kimbell, S. (2001). Before the fall: Keeping your patient on his feet. *Nursing2001, 31*(8), 44–45.

Larson, E. (2002). The "hygiene hypothesis": How clean should we be? *American Journal of Nursing, 102*(1), 81–89.

Moorhead, S., Johnson, M., Maas, M. L., & Swanson, E. (2007). *Nursing Outcomes Classification (NOC)* (4th ed.). St. Louis, MO: Mosby.

Napierkowski, D. (2002). Using restraints with restraint. *Nursing2002, 32*(11), 58–62.

National Institute for Occupational Safety and Health. (2002). *About NIOSH research and services.* Available: http://www.cdc.gov/niosh/about.html

National Institute for Occupational Safety and Health. (2008). NIOSH safety and health topic: Traumatic occupational injuries. Retrieved November 16, 2008, from http://www.cdc.gov/niosh/injury/#data

North American Nursing Diagnosis Association International. (2010). *NANDA-I nursing diagnoses: Definitions and classification 2009-2011.* Ames, IA: Wiley-Blackwell.

Occupational Safety and Health Administration. (2009) Types of fire extinguishers. Retrieved May 16, 2009, from http://www.osha.gov/SLTC/etools/evacuation/portable_about.html#Types

Parini, S., & Myers, F. (2003). Keeping up with hand hygiene recommendations. *Nursing2003, 33*(92), 17.

Ramponi, D. (2001). Eye on contact lens removal. *Nursing2001, 31*(8), 56–57.

Schweon, S., & Novatnack, E. (2003). Don't underestimate Group A strep. *RN, 66*(8), 28–32.

Stanhope, M., & Knollmueller, R. (2000). *Handbook of community-based and home health nursing practice: Tools for assessment, intervention, and education* (3rd ed.). St. Louis, MO: Mosby.

Swauger, K., & Tomlin, C. (2002). Moving toward restraint free patient care. *Journal of Nursing Administration, 30*(6), 325–329.

Sweeney-Calciano, J., Solimene, A., & Forrester, D. (2003). Finding a way to avoid restraints. *Nursing2003, 33*(5), 32hn1–32hn4.

Talerico, K., & Capezuti, E. (2001). Myths and facts about side rails. *American Journal of Nursing, 101*(7), 43–48.

U.S. Department of Energy (Hanford Fire Department). (2001). HFD: All you ever wanted to know about fire extinguishers. Available: http://www.hanford.gov/fire/safety/extingrs.htm

U.S. Department of Labor. (2002). Workplace fire safety. Available: http://www.cdc.gov/nasd/docs/d000701-0000800/d000737/d000737.html

U.S. Food and Drug Administration. (1996). FDA safety alert: Entrapment hazards with hospital bed side rails. Available: http://www.fda.gov/cdrh/bedrails.html

U.S. Food and Drug Administration. (2008). A guide to bed safety bed rails in hospitals, nursing homes and home health care: The facts. Retrieved November 22, 2008, from http://www.fda.gov/cdrh/beds/bed_brochure.html

Walker, B. (1998). *Injury prevention for the elderly: Preventing falls.* Gaithersberg, MD: Aspen.

Walker, B. (1998). Preventing falls. *RN, 61*(5), 40–42.

Yoneyama, T., et al. (2002). Oral care reduces pneumonia in older patients in nursing homes. *Journal of the American Geriatric Society, 50*(3).

RESOURCES

Association for Professionals in Infection Control and Epidemiology, Inc., http://www.apic.org

Centers for Medicare and Medicaid Services, http://www.cms.hhs.gov

Environmental Protection Agency, http://www.epa.gov

Food and Drug Administration, http://www.fda.gov

Joint Commission, http://www.jointcommission.org

National Institute for Occupational Safety and Health, http://www.cdc.gov.niosh

U.S. Consumer Product Safety Commission, http://www.cpsc.gov

UNIT 6 Infection Control

CHAPTER 21
Infection Control/Asepsis

MAKING THE CONNECTION

Refer to the following chapters to increase your understanding of infection control/asepsis:

Basic Nursing
- ***Basic Nutrition***
- ***Safety/Hygiene***
- ***Standard Precautions and Isolation***
- ***Fluid, Electrolyte, and Acid–Base Balance***

Basic Procedures
- ***Hand Hygiene***
- ***Use of Protective Equipment***

Intermediate Procedures
- ***Surgical Asepsis: Preparing and Maintaining a Sterile Field***
- ***Performing Open Gloving***
- ***Applying a Dry Dressing***

LEARNING OBJECTIVES

Upon completion of this chapter, you should be able to:

- Define key terms.
- Describe the chain of infection.
- Discuss the body's nonspecific and specific immune defenses.
- Describe the stages of the inflammatory process.
- Discuss the stages of the infectious process.
- Identify the signs and symptoms of inflammation and infection.
- Explain the principles of medical and surgical asepsis.
- Provide client care maintaining the principles of medical and/or surgical asepsis.

KEY TERMS

acquired immunity
agent
airborne transmission
antibodies
asepsis
aseptic technique
bactericides
biological agents
carriers
chain of infection
chemical agents
clean objects

cleansing
colonization
communicable agents
communicable disease
compromised host
contact transmission
dirty objects
disinfectants
disinfection
edema
erythema
flora
fomites
germicide
hand hygiene
hospital-acquired infection
host
humoral immunity
immunization
infection
infectious agents
inflammation
localized infections
medical asepsis
mode of transmission
pathogens
pathogenicity
physical agents
portal of entry
portal of exit
purulent exudate
reservoir
resident flora
sterilization
surgical asepsis
susceptible host
systemic infection
transient flora
vaccination
vector-borne transmission
vehicle transmission
virulence

INTRODUCTION

Nurses are responsible for providing quality care that incorporates infection-control principles. These principles are a major component of a safe environment. This chapter discusses infection-control principles. including naturally occurring microorganisms, pathogens, infection and colonization, chain of infection, body defenses, stages of the infectious process, and hospital-acquired infections. Discussion of the nurse's role in controlling infections is emphasized.

FLORA

Flora are microorganisms that occur or have adapted to live in a specific environment, such as intestinal, skin, vaginal, or oral flora. There are two types of flora: resident and transient. **Resident** (normal) **flora** are microorganisms that are always present, usually without altering the client's health; an example would be *propionibacterium* on the skin. Resident flora prevent the overgrowth of harmful microorganisms; only when the balance is upset does disease result. **Transient flora** are microorganisms that are episodic (of limited duration); an example would be *staphylococcus aureus.* They attach to the skin for a brief period of time but do not continually live on the skin. Transient flora are usually acquired from direct contact with the microorganisms on environmental surfaces.

PATHOGENICITY AND VIRULENCE

Although most microorganisms found in the environment do not cause disease and infection, some do. Disease-producing microorganisms are called **pathogens**; **pathogenicity** refers to the ability of a microorganism to produce disease. **Virulence** refers to the frequency with which a pathogen causes disease. The factors affecting virulence are the strength of the pathogen to adhere to healthy cells, the ability of a pathogen to damage cells or interfere with the body's normal regulating systems, and the ability of a pathogen to evade the attack of white blood cells (WBCs).

Five types of microorganisms can be pathogenic: bacteria, viruses, fungi, protozoa, and *rickettsia*.

BACTERIA

Bacteria are small, one-celled microorganisms that lack a true nucleus or mechanism to provide metabolism. Therefore, bacteria need an environment that will provide food for survival. Bacteria can be spherical, rodlike, spiral, or curving in shape, usually appearing as single cells, pairs, chains, or groups. Although most bacteria multiply by simple cell division, some forms of bacteria produce spores, a resistant stage that withstands unfavorable environments. When proper environmental conditions return, spores germinate and form new cells. Spores are difficult to kill because of their resistance to heat, drying, and disinfectants. The growth rate of bacteria is affected by environmental factors such as changes in temperature and nutrition. The optimal temperature for pathogenic bacteria is 98.6°F.

Bacteria can be found in all environments, yet not all bacteria are harmful or cause disease. Only a small percentage of bacteria are actually pathogenic. Common bacterial infections include diarrhea, pneumonia, sinusitis, urinary tract infections, cellulitis, meningitis, gonorrhea, otitis media, and impetigo.

VIRUSES

Viruses are organisms that can live only inside cells. They cannot get nourishment or reproduce outside cells. Viruses contain a core of deoxyribonucleic acid (DNA) or ribonucleic acid (RNA) surrounded by a protein coating. Some viruses have the ability to create an additional coating called an envelope, which helps protect the cell from attack by the immune system. Viruses damage the cells they inhabit by blocking the normal protein synthesis of the cells and by using the cell's mechanism for metabolism to reproduce.

The same viral infection may cause different symptoms in different individuals, based on the individual's immune response to the invading virus. Some viruses will immediately trigger a disease response, whereas others may remain latent for many years. Common viral infections include influenza, measles, common cold, chickenpox, hepatitis B, genital herpes, and HIV.

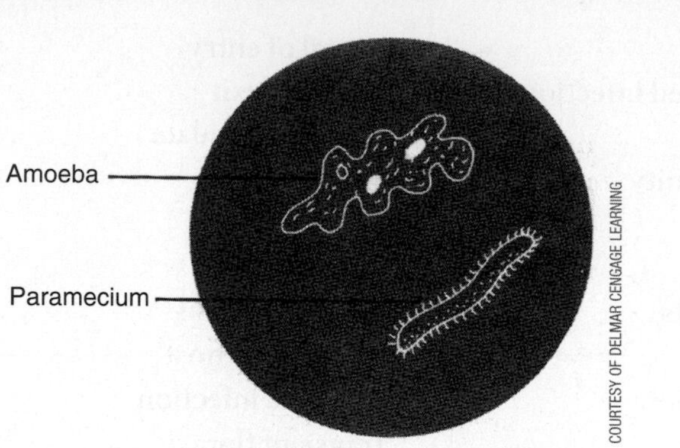

FIGURE 21-1 Protozoa

FUNGI

Fungi grow in single cells, as in yeast, or in colonies, as in molds. Fungi obtain food from dead organic matter or from living organisms. Most fungi are not pathogenic and make up many of the body's normal flora. Disease from fungi is found mainly in individuals who are immunologically impaired. Fungi can cause infections of the hair, skin, nails, and mucous membranes.

PROTOZOA

Protozoa are single-celled parasitic organisms with the ability to move (Figure 21-1). Most protozoa obtain their nourishment from dead or decaying organic matter. Infection is spread through ingestion of contaminated food or water or through insect bites. Common protozoan infections include malaria, gastroenteritis, and vaginal infections.

RICKETTSIA

Rickettsia are intracellular parasites that need to be in living cells to reproduce. Infection from *rickettsia* is spread through fleas, ticks, mites, and lice. Common *rickettsia* infections include typhus, Rocky Mountain spotted fever, and Lyme disease.

COLONIZATION AND INFECTION

Colonization is the multiplication of microorganisms on or within a host that does not result in cellular injury; an example of colonization is the normal flora (microorganisms) in the intestines. However, if host susceptibility increases or the microorganism's virulence increases, colonized microorganisms on a host may be a potential source of infection.

Infection is the invasion and multiplication of pathogenic microorganisms in body tissue that results in cellular injury; an example is strep throat. These microorganisms are called **infectious agents**. Infectious agents capable of being transmitted to a client by direct or indirect contact, through a vehicle (or vector) or airborne route are called **communicable agents**. Diseases produced by these agents are referred to as **communicable diseases**.

CHAIN OF INFECTION

Neither a susceptible host nor the presence of a pathogen means that an infectious process will occur. The **chain of infection** describes the development of an infectious process. An interactive process involving an agent, host, and environment is required. This interactive process involves several essential elements, or "links in the chain," for transmission of microorganisms to occur. Figure 21-2 identifies the six essential links (elements) in the chain of infection. An infectious process cannot occur without the transmission of microorganisms. Therefore, knowledge about the chain of infection facilitates control or elimination of microorganism transmission by breaking the links in the chain. Breaking the chain of infection is achieved by altering the interactive process of the agent, host, and environment. Each of the six links in the chain of infection is discussed following.

AGENT

An **agent** is an entity that is capable of causing disease. Agents that cause disease may be as follows:

- **Biological agents**: Living organisms that invade the host, causing disease, such as bacteria, viruses, fungi, protozoa, and rickettsia
- **Chemical agents**: Substances that can interact with the body, causing disease, such as food additives, medications, pesticides, and industrial chemicals
- **Physical agents**: Factors in the environment that are capable of causing disease, such as heat, light, noise, and radiation

In the chain of infection, the main concern is biological agents and their effect on the host.

RESERVOIR

The **reservoir** is a place where the agent can survive. Colonization and reproduction take place while the agent is in the reservoir. A reservoir that promotes growth of pathogens must contain the proper nutrients (such as oxygen and organic matter), maintain proper temperature, contain moisture, maintain a compatible pH level (neither too acidic nor too alkaline), and maintain the proper amount of light exposure. The most common reservoirs are:

- Humans
- Animals
- Environment
- **Fomites** (objects contaminated with an infectious agent, such as bedpans, urinals, bed linens, instruments, dressings, specimen containers, and other equipment)

Humans and animals can have symptoms of the infectious agents or can be strictly carriers of the agent. **Carriers** have the infectious agent but are symptom free. The agent can be spread to others in both instances.

PORTAL OF EXIT

The **portal of exit** is the route by which an infectious agent leaves the reservoir to be transferred to a susceptible host. The agent leaves the reservoir through body secretions including:

- Sputum, from the respiratory tract
- Semen, vaginal secretions, or urine, from the genitourinary tract
- Saliva and feces, from the gastrointestinal tract
- Blood
- Draining wounds
- Tears

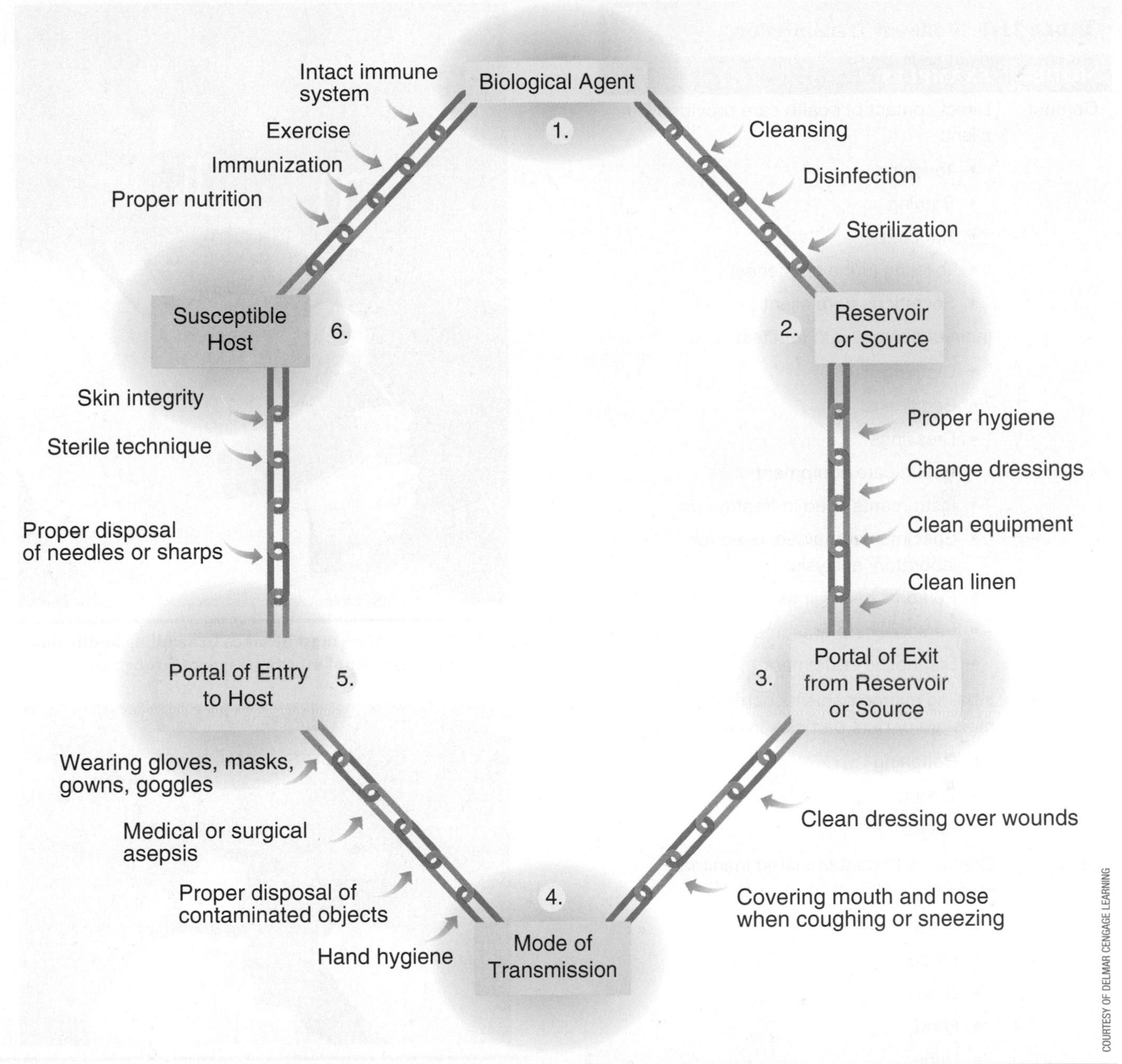

FIGURE 21-2 The Chain of Infection: Preventive Measures Follow Each Link of the Chain

Modes of Transmission

The **mode of transmission** is the process of the infectious agent moving from the reservoir or source through the portal of exit to the portal of entry of the susceptible "new" host. Most infectious agents have a usual or primary mode of transmission, but some microorganisms may be transmitted by more than one mode (Table 21-1). Depending on the agent, almost anything in the environment can become a potential mode of transmission.

Contact Transmission

The most important and frequent mode of transmission is **contact transmission**. This involves the transfer of an agent from an infected person to a host by direct contact with the infected person, indirect contact with the infected person through a fomite, or close contact with contaminated secretions (Figure 21-3). Sexually transmitted diseases are spread by direct contact. Common viral infections (cold, measles, flu) are spread by close contact with contaminated secretions.

Airborne Transmission

Airborne transmission occurs when a susceptible host contacts droplet nuclei or dust particles that are suspended in the air. Particle size influences the length of time that the organism can remain airborne. The longer the particle is suspended, the greater the chance it will find an available port of entry to the human host. A disease that relies on airborne transmission is measles. Contaminated droplets containing the measles virus are in the spray from sneezing. The droplet can find a portal of entry through the mucous membranes or conjunctiva.

Vehicle Transmission

Vehicle transmission occurs when an agent is transferred to a susceptible host by contaminated inanimate objects such as

Table 21-1 Modes of Transmission

MODE	EXAMPLES
Contact	Direct contact of health care provider with client: • Touching • Bathing • Rubbing • Toileting (urine and feces) • Secretions from client Indirect contact with fomites: • Clothing • Bed linens • Dressings • Health care equipment • Instruments used in treatments • Specimen containers used for laboratory analysis • Personal belongings • Personal care equipment • Diagnostic equipment
Airborne	Inhaling microorganisms carried by moisture or dust particles in air: • Coughing • Talking • Sneezing
Vehicle	Contact with contaminated inanimate objects: • Water • Blood • Drugs • Food • Urine
Vector-borne	Contact with contaminated animate hosts: • Animals • Insects

COURTESY OF DELMAR CENGAGE LEARNING

water, food, milk (Figure 21-4), drugs, and blood. Cholera is transmitted through contaminated drinking water, and salmonellosis is transmitted through contaminated meat.

Vector-Borne Transmission

Vector-borne transmission occurs when an agent is transferred to a susceptible host by animate means such as mosquitoes, fleas, ticks, lice, and other animals (Figure 21-5). Lyme disease, malaria, and West Nile virus are examples of diseases spread by vectors.

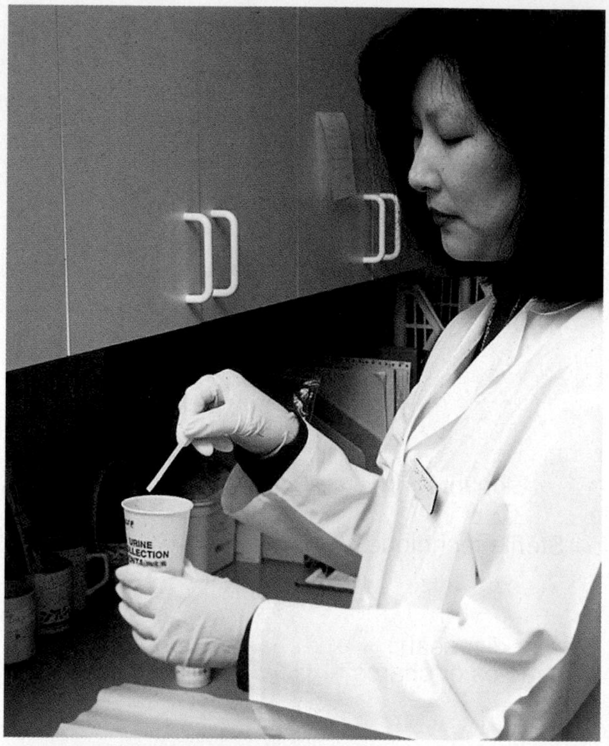

COURTESY OF DELMAR CENGAGE LEARNING

Figure 21-3 Care must be taken in handling bodily fluids to prevent the transfer of infectious agents through contact.

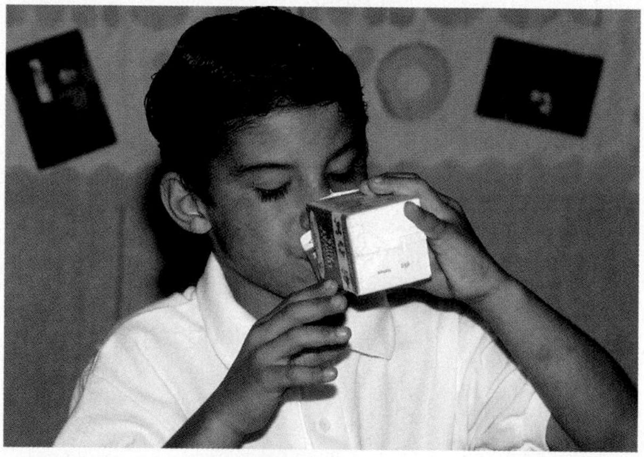

COURTESY OF DELMAR CENGAGE LEARNING

Figure 21-4 Vehicle transmission occurs through contamination of inanimate objects, such as milk.

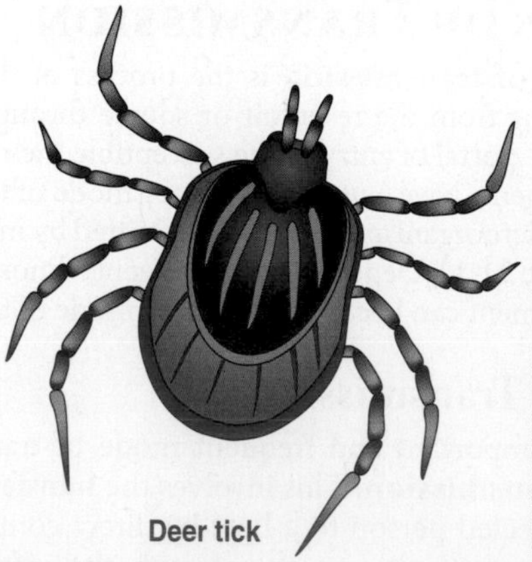

COURTESY OF DELMAR CENGAGE LEARNING

Figure 21-5 Lyme disease and other infections are caused by the bite of a tick.

Portal of Entry

A **portal of entry** is the route by which an infectious agent enters the host. Portals of entry include the following:

- *Integumentary system*, through a break in the integrity of the skin or mucous membranes (e.g., infections of surgical wounds)
- *Respiratory tract*, by inhaling contaminated droplets (such as cold, influenza, measles)
- *Genitourinary tract*, through contact with infected vaginal secretions or semen (as in sexually transmitted diseases)
- *Gastrointestinal tract*, by ingesting contaminated food or water (e.g., typhoid, hepatitis A)
- *Circulatory system*, through the bite of insects (such as mosquito bites resulting in malaria)
- *Transplacental*, through transfer of microorganisms from mother to fetus via the placenta and umbilical cord (including HIV, hepatitis B)

Host

A **host** is an organism that can be affected by an agent. A human being is usually considered a host. A **susceptible host** is a person who has no resistance to an agent and thus is vulnerable to disease. For example, an individual who has not received the measles vaccine is more likely to contract the infection because of the lack of immunity to the infectious agent. A **compromised host** is a person whose normal body defenses are impaired and is therefore susceptible to infection. For example, a person with a common cold or superficial burns is at greater risk for infection because of the impaired state of the body system mechanisms.

Characteristics of the host influence the susceptibility to and severity of infections. These include:

- *Age*. As a person ages, immunity declines, thus increasing susceptibility to infection.
- *Concurrent diseases*. The existence of comorbid diseases indicates an environment susceptible to infection.
- *Stress*. An individual experiencing a compromised emotional state may have altered or decreased immune system response.
- *Immunization/vaccination status*. Individuals who are not fully immunized are at greater risk for infection.
- *Lifestyle*. Lifestyle practices such as having multiple sex partners or sharing intravenous drug needles increase an individual's potential for illness.
- *Occupation*. Forms of employment that involve an increased exposure to pathogens might include dealing with chemical agents (such as asbestos) or handling sharp instruments (such as scalpels).
- *Nutritional status*. Individuals who maintain targeted weight for height and body frame are less prone to illness.
- *Heredity*. Some individuals are naturally more susceptible to infection than others.

Interaction between agent and host occurs in the environment, which is everything other than the agent and host. Many of the conditions promoting transmission of microorganisms reflect changes in the relationship between humans and their environments.

PROFESSIONAL TIP

Infectious Diseases

Berlinguer (1992) notes that the causes of most emerging infectious diseases are the same today as throughout recorded history: the transfer and dissemination of existing agents to new host populations (a process called "global microbial traffic"). For instance, cholera probably originated in Asia in ancient times; in the 19th century, it spread to Europe and the New World because of increased global travel. Cholera entered South America for the first time in 1992 through the possible contaminated bilge water released from a Chinese freighter. West Nile virus was unknown in the United States until 1999 (APIC, 2004). The causes of emerging infectious diseases and outbreaks require careful consideration of changes in relationship between humans and their environments.

BREAKING THE CHAIN OF INFECTION

Nurses focus on breaking the chain of infection by applying proper infection-control practices to interrupt the transmission of microorganisms. Specific strategies can be directed at breaking or blocking the transmission of infection from one link in the chain to the next. A discussion regarding each of the six links follows (refer back to Figure 21-2).

Between Agent and Reservoir

The first link in the chain of infection is between the agent and the reservoir. The keys to eliminating infection at this point in the chain are cleansing, disinfection, and sterilization. These practices prevent the formation of a reservoir where infectious agents can live and multiply.

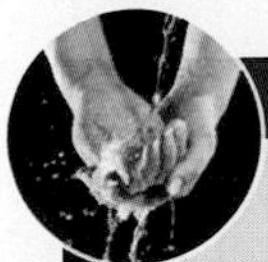

INFECTION CONTROL

First Line of Defense

Hand hygiene is the first line of defense against infection and is the single most important practice in preventing the spread of infection.

CRITICAL THINKING

Chain of Infection

How is the chain of infection applicable in everyday life in a person's home?

INFECTION CONTROL

Cleansing

Cleansing is a potential hazard to the nurse from the splashing of contaminated material onto the body. Nurses should wear gloves, masks, and goggles during cleansing.

Cleansing

Cleansing is the removal of soil or organic material from instruments and equipment used in providing client care. Nurses often cleanse instruments after assisting or performing invasive procedures. To reduce the amount of contamination and loosen the material on reusable objects, the objects are cleansed before sterilization or disinfection. Cleansing involves the use of water, mechanical action, and, sometimes, a detergent. Contaminated objects are cleansed using a soft-bristled brush to scrub the surface. The steps for proper cleansing are:

1. Wet the object with *cold* water; warm water coagulates the proteins in organic material and makes them stick.
2. Apply detergent and scrub the object under running water using a soft-bristled brush.
3. Rinse the object under warm running water.
4. Dry the object before sterilization or disinfection.

Disinfection

Disinfection is the elimination of pathogens, except spores, from inanimate objects. **Disinfectants** are chemical solutions used to clean inanimate objects. The U.S. Environmental Protection Agency (EPA) licenses intermediate and low-level disinfectants. The Food and Drug Administration (FDA) regulates high-level disinfectants. Common disinfectants are alcohol, sodium hypochlorite, quaternary ammonium, and phenolic solutions.

A **germicide** is a chemical that can be applied to both animate (living) and inanimate objects to eliminate pathogens. Antiseptic preparations such as alcohol and silver sulfadiazine are germicides.

Sterilization

Sterilization is destroying all microorganisms including spores. Equipment that enters normally sterile tissue or blood vessels must be sterilized. Methods of achieving sterilization are moist heat (steam), dry heat, and ethylene oxide gas. The method of sterilization depends on the object to be sterilized and the kind and amount of contamination.

COMMUNITY/HOME HEALTH CARE

Disinfection

In the home, Lysol and bleach are common disinfectants capable of eliminating some pathogens. The recommended concentration of bleach solution is one part bleach to nine parts water (CDC, 2007a).

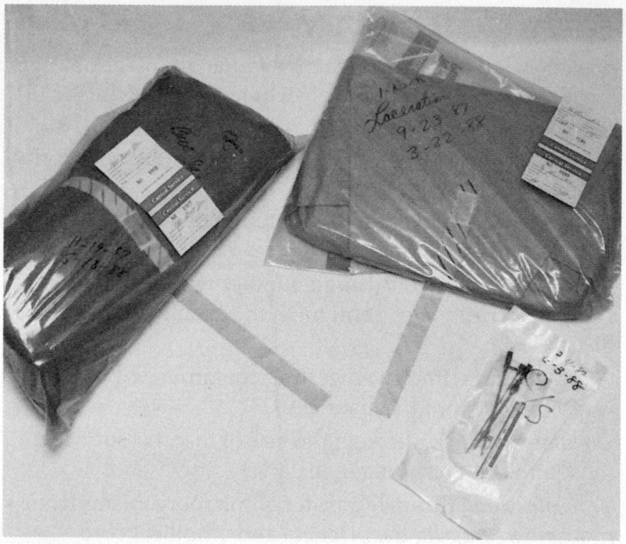

COURTESY OF DELMAR CENGAGE LEARNING

FIGURE 21-6 Sterilized packages. The strips below each package show the way they looked before sterilization. The strips on the packages have changed color because they have been sterilized.

Autoclaving sterilization, which uses moist heat or steam, is the most common sterilization technique used in the hospital setting (Figure 21-6). Boiling water is not an effective sterilization measure because some viruses and spores can survive boiling water.

BETWEEN RESERVOIR AND PORTAL OF EXIT

Promoting proper hygiene, changing dressings and linens, and ensuring that clean equipment is used in client care are ways to break the chain of infection between the reservoir and the portal of exit. The goal is to eliminate the reservoir for the microorganism before a pathogen can escape to a susceptible host.

Proper Hygiene

Educate clients on the importance of maintaining the cleanliness and integrity of the skin and the mucous membranes. Clean skin, hair, and nails maintain the body's normal flora and eliminate transient flora from the client's system. Bathing and hand hygiene are important ways to eliminate the potential for infection. Clients should be encouraged to practice daily bathing and teeth brushing. Clients who are unable to perform these activities independently should be assisted.

COMMUNITY/HOME HEALTH CARE

Sterilization at Home

The CDC (2008) recommends boiling water as the preferred way to kill harmful bacteria and parasites. Bringing water to a rolling boil for 1 full minute will kill most organisms. Chemical contaminants in water will not be removed by boiling.

PROFESSIONALTIP

The Client Who Is Bedridden

Be alert to the formation of pressure ulcers in clients who are bedridden. Open ulcers are a possible source for infection if left untreated.

Change Dressings

Any open injury or other break in skin integrity represents a potential reservoir for infectious agents and portal of exit for a pathogen to be transferred to another individual. Dressings on open or oozing wounds must be changed regularly. To protect both yourself and the client from infection, follow proper aseptic technique when changing dressings. This technique is discussed in detail later in this chapter.

Clean Linens

Bed linens, gowns, and towels are catchalls for bodily secretions. Infectious agents can be easily transferred from one individual to the next through contact with a client's linens. Linens must be changed regularly, and soiled linens must be properly disposed. When changing linens, take care to keep the soiled articles from contact with your uniform. This will prevent being infected from the soiled linens or passing the infection on to other clients.

Clean Equipment

All equipment used in the care of a client must be cleansed and disinfected after each use. Although many items such as disposable gowns can be discarded after use, items such as beds must be thoroughly cleansed after each use. Clients should be instructed never to share care items. Any nondisposable equipment used in an invasive procedure (such as equipment used in the operating room [OR]) must be sterilized before being used again. Wear gloves and masks when cleansing equipment to avoid being splashed with contaminated waste products or secretions.

Between Portal of Exit and Mode of Transmission

The goal in breaking the chain of infection between the portal of exit and the mode of transmission is to prevent the exit of the infectious agents. Clean dressings must be maintained on all wounds. Clients should be encouraged to cover their mouths and noses when sneezing or coughing, and the nurse must do so as well. Gloves must be worn when caring for a client who may have infectious secretions, and care must be taken to properly dispose of any contaminated article.

Between Mode of Transmission and Portal of Entry

To break the chain of infection between the mode of transmission and the portal of entry, asepsis must be ensured and barrier protection worn when the care of clients involves contact with body secretions. Gloves, masks, gowns, and goggles are barrier protection that can be used. Proper hand hygiene and proper disposal of contaminated equipment and linens are ways to prevent transmission of microorganisms to other clients and health care workers. A thorough discussion of asepsis and disposal of contaminated items is included later in this chapter.

Between Portal of Entry and Host

Maintaining skin integrity and using sterile technique for client contacts are methods of breaking the chain of infection between portal of entry and host. Avoiding needle sticks by properly disposing of sharps also reduces the potential for infection by denying a portal of entry. The goal at this point in the chain is to prevent the transmission of infection to a client or health care worker who is not infected.

Between Host and Agent

Breaking the chain of infection between host and agent means eliminating infection before it begins. There are many ways to reduce the risk of acquiring infection: Proper nutrition, exercise, adequate rest and sleep, and immunizations allow an individual to maintain an intact immune system, thus preventing infection.

Proper Nutrition

Proper nutrition assists the body's immune system to function properly. Clients need adequate amounts of protein in their diets to maintain and repair tissue as well as to produce the antibodies needed to fight infection. A balanced diet also allows the body to maintain appropriate acid–base balance.

Exercise

Exercise maintains the body's metabolic rate and, therefore, allows the body to maintain the antibodies and energy necessary to ward off infection.

Rest and Sleep

Rest and sleep are basic to a client's health and well-being. The quality of rest and sleep can have a significant impact on a person's health. Adequate levels of rest and sleep provide a restorative function needed for physiological and psychological healing.

Immunization

Immunization is the process of creating immunity, or resistance to infection, in an individual. Many immunizations are given in early childhood (e.g., measles, mumps, and rubella). Immunization for the flu must be given every year and for tetanus every 10 years.

BODY DEFENSES

A host's immune system is a defense against infectious agents. The immune system is able to recognize "self" and "nonself"; that is, the immune system recognizes what is not consistent with the genetic composition of the host (self). These agents are called antigens (nonself). An immune response against an antigen protects the body from infection.

CLIENT TEACHING

Inappropriate Use of Antibiotics

- Do not pressure the physician or nurse practitioner to prescribe antibiotics for every illness. Antibiotics are not always appropriate. They are not effective against viruses.
- When antibiotics are prescribed, the client should take all of the medication as directed.
- Antibiotics taken only until the client feels better allow the microorganisms to become resistant to the antibiotic, and the antibiotic will no longer be effective.
- Antibiotics also destroy normal flora microorganisms, and other illnesses may ensue.

Nonspecific Immune Defense

The nonspecific immune defense protects the host from all microorganisms; it does not depend on prior exposure to an antigen. Nonspecific immune defenses are skin and normal flora; mucous membranes; coughing, sneezing, and tearing reflexes; elimination and acidic environment; and inflammation.

Skin and Normal Flora

The skin, the first line of defense against infection, serves as a physical barrier to infectious agents. Skin cells, shed daily, remove potentially harmful microorganisms. Sebum, a substance produced by the skin, contains fatty acids that kill some bacteria. The normal flora residing on the skin and in the body compete with pathogenic flora for food and inhibit pathogen multiplication. The balance of normal flora may become disrupted, allowing pathogenic organisms to proliferate, causing infection or superinfection.

Mucous Membranes

Mucous membranes also are a physical barrier to infectious agents. Mucus produced by these membranes entraps infectious agents and inhibits bacterial growth. For example, the cilia of the respiratory tract trap and propel mucus and microorganisms away from the lungs, thereby reducing the potential for infection.

Coughing, Sneezing, and Tearing Reflexes

The cough and sneeze reflexes forcibly expel mucus and microorganisms from the respiratory tract. Tears protect the eyes by continually flushing away microorganisms. Tears also contain **bactericides**, which are bacteria-killing chemicals.

Elimination and Acidic Environment

Elimination and an acidic environment usually prevent growth of pathogenic organisms. Resident flora of the large intestines prevent the growth of pathogens. The mechanical process of defecation removes microorganisms with the feces. Urine acidity prevents microbial growth. Urination flushes and cleans the bladder neck and urethra of microorganisms and prevents microorganisms from ascending into the urinary tract.

Normal vaginal flora prevent growth of several pathogens. At puberty, lactobacilli ferment and produce sugars in the vagina that lower the pH to an acidic range. The acidic environment of the vagina prevents pathogenic growth.

Inflammation

Inflammation is a nonspecific cellular response to tissue injury. Tissue injury caused by bacteria, trauma, chemicals, heat, or any other occurrence releases substances, producing dramatic secondary changes in the injured tissue. This entire complex of tissue changes in response to injury is called the *inflammatory process* (Table 21-2). The body's response to injury produces characteristic local and systemic signs of inflammation.

Inflammation, while not necessarily the result of invading microorganisms, does have signs and symptoms similar to those of an infection. The primary signs of inflammation and infection are as follows:

- Redness (**erythema**) results from increased blood flow to the area.
- Heat results from increased blood flow and metabolism in the area.

Table 21-2 Stages of the Inflammatory Process

STAGE	DESCRIPTION	RESULT
1	Initial injury causes release of chemicals: histamine, bradykinin, serotonin, prostaglandins, and lymphokines.	Initiates the inflammation process
2	Blood flow increases to the injured area.	Produces characteristic redness and warmth
3	Increased capillary permeability leaks large amounts of plasma into the damaged tissue; tissue spaces and lymphatics are blocked by fibrinogen clots.	"Walls off" infection; results in nonpitting edema
4	Leukocytes infiltrate damaged tissue and engulf the bacteria and necrotic tissue. After several days, these leukocytes die and form a cavity of necrotic tissue and dead leukocytes.	Produces purulent exudate (pus)
5	Destroyed tissue cells are replaced by identical or similar structural and functioning cells and/or fibrous tissue.	Promotes tissue healing or the formation of fibrous (scar) tissue, which may reduce the functional capacity of the tissue

- Pain results from increased pressure on pain sensors in the area.
- Swelling (**edema**, a detectable accumulation of increased interstitial fluid) results from fluid and leukocytes entering the tissues from the circulatory system.
- Loss of function results from both pain and swelling and is the body's way of resting the injured part.
- Pus (**purulent exudate**), resulting from infection, is a secretion made up of white blood cells, dead cells, bacteria, and other debris.

The inflammatory process intensity is usually in proportion to the degree of tissue injury.

Specific Immune Defense

The specific immune defense is a response specific to the invading antigen. It is activated when phagocytes fail to completely destroy the antigen. This causes production of T lymphocytes (T cells), which regulate the immune response by activating other cells. The T cells move to the injured area and release chemical substances called lymphokines. Lymphokines attract other phagocytes and lymphocytes to the injured area and assist in antigen destruction.

The T cells also stimulate the production of B cells, which become plasma cells, producing antibodies specific to the antigen. **Antibodies** are protein substances that destroy the antigen. The stimulation of B cells and the production of antibodies are collectively known as **humoral immunity**.

Memory B cells are formed to remember the antigen and prepare the host for future antigen invasion. When the antigen enters the body again, the immune response occurs faster by rapidly producing antibodies. The formation of these antibodies is referred to as **acquired immunity**, which protects the individual against future invasions of already experienced antigens such as lethal bacteria, viruses, toxins, and even foreign tissues.

The process of **vaccination** (inoculation with a vaccine to produce immunity against specific diseases) provides acquired immunity. There are three types of vaccines:

1. Dead organisms that are no longer capable of causing disease but still have their chemical antigens, such as typhoid, whooping cough, and diphtheria
2. Toxins that have been chemically treated so their toxic nature is destroyed but their antigens are still intact, such as for tetanus and botulism
3. Live organisms that have been attenuated (rendered incapable of causing the disease yet still have the specific antigen), such as for poliomyelitis, yellow fever, measles, smallpox, and many other viral diseases (Guyton & Hall, 2005)

TYPES AND STAGES OF INFECTIONS

Infection is the result of tissue invasion and damage by an infectious agent. There are two types of infections:

1. **Localized infections** are limited to a defined area or single organ with symptoms that resemble inflammation (redness, tenderness, and swelling), such as a cold sore.
2. **Systemic infections** affect the entire body and involve multiple organs, such as AIDS.

All infections progress through four stages: incubation, prodromal, illness, and convalescence.

SAFETY

Incubation Period

Always verify the incubation period of a suspected infection. Remember that a client may be able to transmit the infection to another person before the onset of symptoms.

Incubation Stage

The incubation period is the time between entry of an infectious agent in the host and the onset of symptoms. During this time, the infectious agent invades the tissue and multiplies to produce an infection. The client is typically infectious to others during the latter part of this stage. For example, the incubation period for varicella (chickenpox) is 2 to 3 weeks; the infected person is contagious from 5 days before any skin eruptions to no more than 6 days after the skin eruptions appear.

Prodromal Stage

The prodromal stage is the time from the onset of nonspecific symptoms until specific symptoms begin to manifest. The infectious agent continues to invade and multiply in the host. A client may also be infectious to other persons during this time period. In the client with chickenpox, a slight elevation in temperature will occur during this stage, followed within 24 hours by eruptions on the skin.

Illness Stage

The illness stage is the time when the client has specific signs and symptoms of an infectious process. The client with chickenpox will experience a further rise in temperature and continued outbreaks of skin eruptions for at least 2 to 3 more days.

Convalescent Stage

The convalescent stage is from the beginning of the disappearance of acute symptoms until the client returns to the previous state of health. The client with chickenpox will see the skin eruptions and irritation begin to resolve during this stage.

HOSPITAL-ACQUIRED INFECTIONS

A **hospital-acquired infection** is an infection acquired in a hospital or other health care facility that was not present or incubating at the time of the client's admission. They also include those infections that become symptomatic after the client is discharged and infections passed among medical personnel. Hospital-acquired infections are also called *nosocomial infections* or health care–associated infections. These types of infections typically fall into four categories: urinary tract, surgical wounds, pneumonia, and septicemia.

Most hospital-acquired infections are transmitted by health care personnel who fail to practice proper hand hygiene or who fail to change gloves between client contacts.

PROFESSIONALTIP

Health Care–Associated Infections

Each year, 1.7 million health care–associated infections occur in the United States. Further, the client's length of stay is increased, costing nearly $20 billion annually for the associated extended care and treatment (Wright, 2008).

CRITICAL THINKING

Hospital-Acquired Infections

Why are hospital-acquired infections such a huge problem?

The hospital environment provides exposure to a variety of organisms to which the client has not typically been exposed in the past. Therefore, the client has no resistance to these organisms. Illness impairs the body's defenses.

NURSING PROCESS

Quality nursing care requires the reduction of microorganism transmission in the health care environment. Infection-control practices are directed at controlling or eliminating sources of infection in the health care agency or home. Nurses are responsible for protecting clients and themselves by using infection-control practices.

Assessment

Assessment data guides the prioritization of the client's problem and identification of appropriate nursing diagnoses. Clients at risk for infection require frequent reassessment followed by appropriate changes in the plan of care, goals, and nursing interventions.

The health history and physical examination data correlated with the laboratory results identify those clients at risk for infection. Appropriate risk appraisals may be incorporated into the nursing health history interview.

Subjective Data

Relevant data regarding the client at risk for infection are obtained in the health history. A comprehensive assessment also involves appraising the client's environment to detect potential hazards and the client's self-care abilities. Reviewing such factors as work environment, immunization status, and other health-related issues may help identify actual or possible infection risks.

Objective Data

Objective data are gathered through the physical examination and the diagnostic and laboratory findings.

Physical Examination A complete health assessment includes a systematic physical examination, generally conducted from head to toe, to obtain objective data relative to the client's health status and presenting problems. When assessing the client to determine the level of risk for infection, focus the physical examination on:

- Range of motion and mobility (A client with limited mobility is at risk for developing joint contractures, skin breakdown, and muscle atrophy)
- Localized redness, warmth, swelling, pain, and loss of use in a specific body part
- Fever with an increase in pulse and respirations; weakness; anorexia, nausea, vomiting, and/or diarrhea; enlarged and/or tender lymph nodes
- Secretions or exudate of the skin or mucous membranes; hydration status
- Auscultation of the lungs for crackles or wheezes

Diagnostic and Laboratory Data The laboratory indicators for an infection are:

- An elevated leukocyte (white blood cell [WBC]) and WBC differential:
  Neutrophils: Increased in acute, severe inflammation
  Lymphocytes: Increased in chronic bacterial and viral infections
  Monocytes: Increased in some protozoan and rickettsial infections and TB
  Eosinophils and basophils: Unaltered in an infectious process
- An elevated erythrocyte sedimentation rate (ESR): increased in the presence of inflammation
- An elevated pH of involved body fluids (gastric, urine, or vaginal secretions): indicative of microorganism presence
- Positive cultures of involved body fluids (blood, sputum, urine, or other drainage): indicative of microorganism growth (Guyton & Hall, 2005)

Nursing Diagnosis

After data collection and analysis, identify a nursing diagnosis. The North American Nursing Diagnosis Association International (NANDA-I) identifies one nursing diagnosis related to infection: *Risk for Infection.*

Risk for infection is an increased risk for being invaded by pathogenic organisms (NANDA-I, 2010). The risk factors that increase a client's susceptibility to infections are as follows:

- Inadequate primary defenses (broken skin, traumatized tissue, decrease in ciliary action, stasis of body fluids, change in pH of secretions, and altered peristalsis)

PROFESSIONALTIP

Questions Related to Infection Control

- What do you do to stay healthy?
- What health care concerns do you have?
- Have you recently been in contact with someone who has an infectious disease?
- When do you wash your hands?
- Have you traveled out of the country, especially to Third World countries, in the past 6 months?

MEMORYTRICK

Infection

A nurse can use the memory trick "**INFECTION**" to remember signs and symptoms of infection and important nursing assessment skills to use when assessing a client for an actual or potential infection:

I = Inflammation (swelling) is a sign of infection

N = Need to auscultate lungs for crackles or wheezes

F = Feels warm or hot (skin) to the touch

E = Erythema (redness) appears at the site of the infection

C = Check client's temperature for a fever

T = Tender (sore or painful) at the site of the infection

I = Inspect site of infection for secretions or exudates

O = Observe and practice proper hand hygiene protocol

N = Need to report abnormal lab values to the physician

- Inadequate secondary defenses (decreased hemoglobin, leukopenia, suppressed inflammatory response)
- Inadequate acquired immunity
- Immunosuppression
- Tissue destruction and increased environmental exposure
- Chronic disease
- Malnutrition
- Invasive procedures
- Pharmaceutical agents
- Trauma
- Rupture of amniotic membranes
- Insufficient knowledge to avoid exposure to pathogens (NANDA-I, 2010)

Clients who are at risk for infection may have other associated physiologic and psychological concerns. The common nursing diagnoses that often accompany *Risk for **I**nfection* include:

- *Imbalanced **N**utrition: Less Than Body Requirements* or *More Than Body Requirements*
- *Ineffective **P**rotection*
- *Impaired **T**issue Integrity*
- *Impaired **O**ral Mucous Membrane*
- *Impaired **S**kin Integrity*
- *Deficient **K**nowledge* (specify)

This list indicates several related problems that must be considered when planning care for the client at risk for infection.

COMMUNITY/HOME HEALTH CARE

Clients at Risk for Infection

Clients at risk for infection should have follow-up visits by the home health nurse to measure the effectiveness of client teaching and to assess resources in the home to prevent the transmission of infections.

Planning/Outcome Identification

The nurse collaborates with the client and other health care providers to determine goals, outcomes, and interventions to reduce the risk of infection. Outcomes provide direction for nursing care to reduce the risk of infection. Client and caregiver education about identifying potential hazards and health-promotion practices is another critical element of the care plan.

Implementation

Nurses are responsible for providing the client with a safe environment, including prevention of hospital-acquired infections. Nursing interventions to reduce the risk of infection center around ensuring asepsis and properly disposing of infectious materials to reduce or eliminate infectious agents. **Asepsis** refers to the absence of microorganisms. **Aseptic technique** is the infection-control practice used to prevent the transmission of pathogens. The use of aseptic technique decreases the risk and spread of hospital-acquired infections. There are two types of asepsis: medical and surgical.

Medical Asepsis

The term **medical asepsis** refers to those practices used to reduce the number, growth, and spread of microorganisms. It is also called *clean technique*. In medical asepsis, objects are generally referred to as "clean" or "dirty." **Clean objects** are considered to have the presence of some microorganisms that are usually not pathogenic. **Dirty** (soiled) **objects** are considered to have a high number of microorganisms, some being potentially pathogenic. Common medical aseptic measures used for clean or dirty objects are hand hygiene, daily changing of linens, and daily cleansing of floors and hospital furniture.

Hand Hygiene **Hand hygiene** is a general term that includes *hand washing* (using plain soap and water), *antiseptic hand wash* (using

INFECTION CONTROL

Hand Hygiene

- Wash hands before and after every client contact.
- The most common cause of hospital-acquired infections is contaminated hands of health care providers.
- When in doubt, *wash your hands.*

antimicrobial substances and water), *antiseptic hand rub* (using alcohol-based hand rub), and *surgical hand antisepsis* (using antiseptic hand wash or antiseptic hand rub preoperatively by surgical personnel to eliminate transient and reduce resident hand flora). Perform hand hygiene after arriving at work, before leaving work, before and after each client contact, after removing gloves, when hands are visibly soiled, before eating, after excretion of body waste (urination and defecation), after contact with body fluids, and after handling contaminated equipment. When hands are visibly dirty, wash hands with soap (plain or antimicrobial) and water. If hands are not visibly soiled, an alcohol-based hand rub may be used. If soap and water are not available, an alcohol-based wipe or hand gel may be used (Centers for Disease Control and Prevention [CDC], 2009a).

Hand washing is the rubbing together of all surfaces and crevices of the hands using plain soap and water, followed by rinsing in a flowing stream of water. Friction physically removes soil and transient flora, and a flowing stream of water rinses it all away. To remove transient flora from the hands, a washing time of 20 to 30 seconds is recommended. High-risk areas such as nurseries usually require a hand wash of approximately 2 minutes' duration. Soiled hands usually require more time. Hand washing is the most basic infection-control measure to prevent and control the transmission of infectious agents. According to the CDC (2009b), alcohol-based hand rubs (foam or gel) are more effective in killing bacteria than soap and water.

Antiseptic hand rub uses an alcohol-containing preparation designed to reduce the number of viable microorganisms on the hands. In the United States, these preparations usually contain 60% to 95% ethanol or isopropanol. Apply product to palm of one hand and rub hands together, covering all surfaces of hands and fingers, until hands are dry. Follow the manufacturer's recommendation for the amount of product to use.

Surgical Asepsis

Surgical asepsis, or sterile technique, consists of those practices that eliminate all microorganisms and spores from an object or area. Surgical asepsis relates to surgical hand washing, establishing and maintaining sterile fields, donning surgical attire (caps, masks, and eyewear), and sterile gloves, gowning, with closed gloving.

Surgical asepsis is practiced in the OR, in labor and delivery, and for many therapeutic and diagnostic interventions at the client's bedside. Common nursing procedures requiring sterile technique are:

- All invasive procedures, either entry into a bodily orifice (tracheobronchial suctioning, insertion of a urinary catheter) or intentional perforation of the skin (injections, insertion of intravenous needles or catheters)
- Nursing interventions when there is a disruption of skin surfaces (changing a surgical wound or intravenous site dressing) or destruction of skin layers (trauma and burns)

Surgical Hand Antisepsis Surgical hand antisepsis scrub removes soil and microorganisms from the skin. Workers in the OR do surgical hand antisepsis to minimize the client's risk for infection. The skin on the hands and arms should be intact (free of lesions). Agency policy determines the method and timing for the scrub.

Sterile Field and Equipment Establish and maintain a sterile field when performing procedures that require sterile technique, such as inserting a urinary catheter or changing wound dressings. Before preparing the sterile field, review the agency's policy and gather all the necessary supplies.

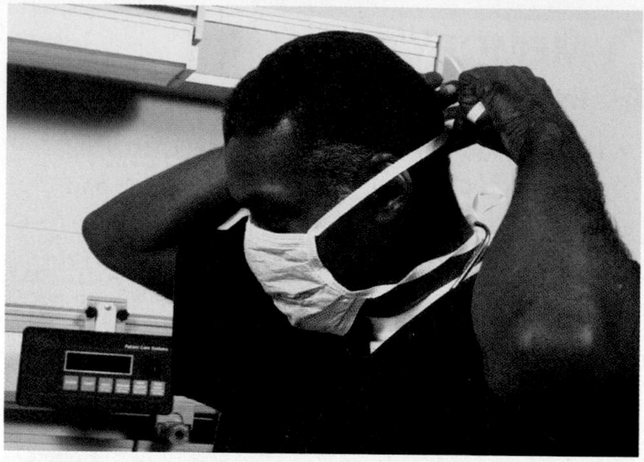

COURTESY OF DELMAR CENGAGE LEARNING

FIGURE 21-7 Putting on a Surgical Mask

Donning Surgical Attire Surgical nurses are required to wear a surgical mask (Figure 21-7) and a clean cap covering all of the hair. Protective eyewear (glasses or goggles) is worn during all procedures posing a threat of body fluids splashing into the eyes. Masks, caps, eyewear, gowns, and gloves are considered barrier precautions because they are a physical impediment to the spread of microorganisms.

Donning Sterile Gloves There are two methods of applying sterile gloves: open and closed. The open method is used when performing procedures requiring sterile technique, such as dressing changes. The closed method is used when the nurse wears a sterile gown, as in the OR.

Gowning with Closed Gloving When donning a sterile gown, nurses in the OR and special procedure areas such as cardiac cath labs use the closed gloved method. After the surgical scrub, don the sterile gown and gloves using the closed method. The sterile gown serves as a barrier to decrease the risk of wound contamination and also allows the nurse to move freely in the environment of sterile fields.

Disposal of Infectious Materials All health care facilities must have guidelines for the disposal of infectious-waste materials as required by the OSHA Act of 1991. The types of materials included are:

- Laboratory wastes
- All body fluids including blood, blood products
- Client care items (soiled bed linen and protection pads, urinals, and bedpans)
- Disposable instruments
- Medication and soiled treatment items
- Surgical wastes

All health care workers must be diligent in observing the biological hazard symbol and handling all infectious materials as hazardous.

CRITICAL THINKING

Medical and Surgical Asepsis

How are medical asepsis and surgical asepsis the same? How are they different?

When disposing of infectious waste, all personnel must be sure to:

- Wear gloves.
- Use the proper containers (red or one labeled with the biological hazard symbol as required by the facility), sharps containers for needles, scalpels, and other sharp instruments or devices; and leakproof plastic bags for waste from client areas (soiled dressings, gloves, linen).
- Ensure that all infectious waste is properly labeled.
- Carefully handle plastic bags to avoid punctures and tearing.
- Disinfect carts used to carry infectious waste.
- Dispose of waste only in designated areas.
- Wash hands after disposing of hazardous materials.

Containers for contaminated sharps should be readily accessible to personnel and maintained in an upright position.

The CDC (2003) reports that health care workers who have received the hepatitis B virus (HBV) vaccine and who have developed immunity to the virus are at virtually no risk for infection after an occupational exposure. For a health care worker who has not been immunized for HBV, the risk of infection after an occupational exposure ranges from 6% to 30%. The number of HBV occupational infections has decreased 95% since the HBV vaccine began being administered in 1982. The risk for a hepatitis C virus (HCV) infection after an occupation exposure is approximately 1.8%, and the risk for a human immunodeficiency virus (HIV) infection postexposure is 0.3% (CDC, 2003).

> **INFECTION CONTROL**
>
> **Needle Disposal**
>
> - Used needles should not be recapped, bent, or broken.
> - Needles should be placed in a puncture-resistant, marked or color-coded container close to the work site.
> - Correct disposal decreases the risk of needle punctures to caregivers.

EVALUATION

Evaluation of the effectiveness of nursing care is based on the achievement of goals and expected outcomes. Keeping the client free from infection requires frequent reassessment followed by timely adjustments made in the plan of care in order for nursing interventions to be effective. It is important for the client to remain free of infection during hospitalization as well as develop a true awareness of the factors that increase the risk for infection.

SAMPLE NURSING CARE PLAN

The Client at Risk for Infection

F.S., a 38-year-old homeless person, was struck and dragged by a speeding car as he crossed the street. He was taken to the hospital by ambulance. His left leg is broken, and there are lacerations and abrasions on his right side, arm, and leg. The left leg is in a cast and the lacerations have been sutured. F.S. grimaces when he tries to move his legs, but he does not verbalize pain. F.S. is very thin and says that he has not eaten for 2 days.

NURSING DIAGNOSIS 1 *Risk for Infection* related to inadequate primary defenses as evidenced by lacerations and abrasions

Nursing Outcomes Classification (NOC)
Tissue Integrity: Skin & Mucous Membranes
Nutritional Status

Nursing Interventions Classification (NIC)
Wound Care
Nutrition Management

PLANNING/OUTCOMES	NURSING INTERVENTIONS	RATIONALE
F.S. will not have developed an infection in the lacerations and abrasions at discharge.	Use proper hand hygiene before and after caring for F.S.	Reduces microorganisms on hands.
	Use sterile technique when caring for lacerations and abrasions.	Prevents introduction of microorganisms into lacerations and abrasions.
	Apply antibiotic ointment on abrasions, as ordered.	Promotes healing of abrasions.
	Keep bed linens clean and dry.	Removes any drainage that may harbor microorganisms.
	Administer oral antibiotics, as ordered.	Prevents or cures infection.

(Continues)

SAMPLE NURSING CARE PLAN (Continued)

EVALUATION

F.S. has some redness around one laceration.

NURSING DIAGNOSIS 2 *Acute **P**ain* related to physical injury as evidenced by facial grimacing

Nursing Outcomes Classification (NOC)
Pain Control
Symptom Severity
Memory

Nursing Interventions Classification (NIC)
Pain Management
Analgesic Administration
Hope Instillation

PLANNING/OUTCOMES	NURSING INTERVENTIONS	RATIONALE
F.S. will experience increased comfort and will verbalize that pain is under control within 24 hours.	Use pain scale to determine level of discomfort.	Provides objective measure of pain.
	Assist client to a position of comfort and elevate extremities.	Reduces pain and swelling by increasing blood return to the heart.
	Administer analgesics, as ordered.	Provides comfort.

EVALUATION

F.S. states that he is experiencing less discomfort by 16 hours but that he still desires pain medication.

NURSING DIAGNOSIS

*Imbalanced **N**utrition: Less Than Body Requirements* related to economic factors as evidenced by extreme thinness and not having eaten for 2 days.

NOC: *Nutritional Status: Nutrient Intake*

NIC: *Nutrition Management*

CLIENT GOAL

F.S. will eat balanced meals while hospitalized.

NURSING INTERVENTIONS

1. Assist F.S. to select foods high in protein, vitamins A and C, calcium, zinc, and copper.
2. Provide between-meal snacks, especially milk or milk products.

SCIENTIFIC RATIONALES

1. Wound healing depends on the availability of protein, vitamins, and minerals.
2. Snacks will increase overall caloric intake; increased protein will promote wound healing; increased calcium will promote bone healing.

EVALUATION

Is F.S. eating balanced meals while hospitalized?

CONCEPT CARE MAP 21-1

SUMMARY

- Flora are microorganisms that occur or have adapted to live in a specific environment.
- Pathogens are microorganisms that cause disease; they include bacteria, viruses, fungi, protozoa, and *rickettsia*.
- The elements of the chain of infection include the agent, the reservoir, the portal of exit, the modes of transmission, the portal of entry, and the host.
- The body has two primary defenses: the nonspecific immune defense, protecting the host from all microorganisms regardless of previous exposure, and the specific immune defense, reacting to a specific antigen that the body has previously experienced.
- Infections progress through four stages: incubation, prodromal, illness, and convalescence.
- Hand hygiene must be done before and after every client contact and after removing gloves. It is the most important procedure for preventing hospital-acquired infections.
- Other means of preventing the spread of infection include cleansing equipment, cleansing soiled linen, changing dressings over wounds, practicing barrier precautions, maintaining skin integrity, and receiving all appropriate immunizations.
- The OSHA regulations mandate that sharps be properly disposed of immediately after use.

REVIEW QUESTIONS

1. When caring for a client who is postoperative for a bowel resection, the nurse knows that which of the following procedures requires surgical aseptic technique?
   1. Administering PO medication.
   2. Removal of intravenous catheter.
   3. Insertion of Foley catheter.
   4. Disposal of surgical wound dressing.
2. The nurse is caring for a client with lower abdominal pain. Which of the following is the most effective infection-control measure to prevent and control the transmission of infectious agents?
   1. Sterilizing.
   2. Hand hygiene.
   3. Disinfecting.
   4. Use of bactericides.
3. A client with chickenpox will exhibit a slight elevation in body temperature followed within 24 hours by eruptions on the skin during which stage of infection?
   1. Incubation.
   2. Prodromal.
   3. Illness.
   4. Convalescent.
4. When disposing of infectious waste, all personnel must be sure to: (Select all that apply.)
   1. inform the Infectious Waste Department.
   2. write the client's name, room number, and allergies on the container.
   3. wear gloves.
   4. use proper biohazard containers.
   5. carefully handle biohazard plastic bags.
   6. disinfect carts used to carry infectious waste.
5. Which of the following is not a risk factor that increases a client's susceptibility to infection?
   1. Noninvasive procedure.
   2. Chronic disease.
   3. Malnutrition.
   4. Rupture of amniotic membranes.
6. A client is being discharged home, and prevention of infection is part of his treatment plan. Which of the following statements made by the client regarding prevention of infection indicates that further teaching is needed by the nurse?
   1. "I need to keep my bed linens clean and dry."
   2. "I need to take my antibiotic as ordered."
   3. "I need to wash my hands only before I change my dressings because I will be wearing gloves."
   4. "I need to keep my dressings clean and dry."
7. A client with an infected abdominal incision is brought to the primary care clinic. Which of the following assessments will the nurse be able to make?
   1. Pinpoint pupils, hypothermia, and elevated blood pressure.
   2. Decreased respirations, low blood pressure, and constricted pupils.
   3. Clammy skin, dilated pupils, slow pulse, and low blood pressure.
   4. Fever, localized redness, warmth, swelling, and pain.

8. The nursing care plan of a client who is at risk for an infection is likely to include:
   1. use clean gloves for all procedures.
   2. take a daily multivitamin.
   3. use proper hand hygiene before and after providing care.
   4. administer intravenous antibiotic.
9. A client with a sinus infection blows his nose in a facial tissue and asks the nurse to dispose of it. The nurse puts on gloves before touching the used facial tissue because she knows that the facial tissue is identified as which of the following links in the chain of infection?
   1. Portal of entry.
   2. Mode of transmission.
   3. Portal of exit.
   4. Susceptible host.
10. An AIDS client is admitted to the hospital with renal insufficiency, elevated liver enzymes, jaundice, pneumonia, elevated WBC, fever, and diarrhea. Which of the following types of infection is the client experiencing?
   1. Systemic infection.
   2. Humoral infection.
   3. Localized infection.
   4. Transient infection.

REFERENCES/SUGGESTED READINGS

Association for Professionals in Infection Control and Epidemiology. (2002a). Infection control—A few ounces of prevention. Available: http://www.apic.org/cons/icdesc.cfm

Association for Professionals in Infection Control and Epidemiology. (2002b). Infection control tips on handwashing. Available: http://www.apic.org/cons/washtips.cfm

Association for Professionals in Infection Control and Epidemiology. (2002c). West Nile virus: Consumer information. Available: http://www.apic.org/cons/westnile.cfm

Association for Professionals in Infection Control and Epidemiology. (2004). West Nile virus: General information. Retrieved October 20, 2008, from http://www.apic.org/Content/NavigationMenu/PracticeGuidance/Topics/WestNileVirus/West_Nile_Virus.htm#General_Information

Bender, K., & Thompson, F. (2003). West Nile Virus: A growing challenge. *American Journal of Nursing, 103*(6), 32–39.

Berlinguer, G. (1992). The interchange of disease and health between the old and new worlds. *American Journal of Public Health, 82*(10), 1407–1414.

Bulechek, G., Butcher, H., McCloskey, J., & Dochterman, J., eds. (2008). *Nursing Interventions Classification (NIC)* (5th ed.). St. Louis, MO: Mosby/Elsevier.

Centers for Disease Control and Prevention. (2003). *Exposure to blood: What healthcare personnel need to know* [Brochure], 1–10.

Centers for Disease Control and Prevention. (2007a). Appropriate disinfectants: Bleach. Retrieved October 20, 2008, from http://www.cdc.gov/healthyswimming/bodyfluidspill.htm

Centers for Disease Control and Prevention. (2007b). Preventing occupational HIV transmission to healthcare personnel. Retrieved October 5, 2008, from http://www.cdc.gov/hiv/resources/factsheets/hcwprev.htm

Centers for Disease Control and Prevention. (2008). Fact sheet: Keep food and water safe after a disaster or power outage. Retrieved October 20, 2008, from http://emergency.cdc.gov/disasters/foodwater/facts.asp

Centers for Disease Control and Prevention. (2009a). Hand hygiene interactive education. Retrieved May 9, 2009, from http://www.cdc.gov/handhygiene/training/interactiveEducation/frame.htm

Centers for Disease Control and Prevention. (2009b). An ounce of prevention keeps the germs away. Retrieved May 9, 2009, from http://www.cdc.gov/ounceofprevention/docs/oop_brochure_eng.pdf

Centers for Disease Control and Prevention/Hospital Infection Control Practices Advisory Committee. (2007). Type and duration of precautions recommended for selected infections and conditions. Retrieved October 8, 2008, from htp://www.cdc.gov/ncidod/dhqp/pdf/guidelines/Isolation2007.pdf

Czark, G., & Mattys, A. (2008). Nation's top healthcare organizations announce strategies to prevent deadly healthcare-associated infections. Retrieved October 12, 2008, from http://www.apic.org

Daniels, R. (2010). *Delmar's guide to laboratory and diagnostic tests,* 2nd edition. Clifton Park, NY: Delmar Cengage Learning.

Delahanty, K. M., & Myers, F. E., III. (2007). Nursing2007 infection control survey report. *Nursing2007, 37*(6), 28–36.

Dochterman, J., & Bulechek, G. (2004). *Nursing Interventions Classification (NIC)* (4th ed.). St. Louis, MO: Mosby.

Goldrick, B., & Goetz, A. (2003). Keeping West Nile Virus at bay. *Nursing2003, 33*(8), 44–47.

Guyton, A. & Hall, J. (2005). *Textbook of medical physiology* (11th ed.). Philadelphia: W. B. Saunders.

Hadaway, L. C. (2006). Keeping central line infections at bay. *Nursing2006, 36*(4), 58–63.

Hass, J. & Larson, E. (2008). Compliance with hand hygiene guidelines: Where are we in 2008? *American Journal of Nursing, 108*(8), 40–44.

Infection Control. (2002). "Hand hygiene" news. *Nursing2002,* 32(5), 32hn6.

Leung-Chen, P. (2008). Emerging infections: Everybody's crying MRSA. *American Journal of Nursing, 108*(8), 29.

Moorhead, S., Johnson, M., & Maas, M. (2008). *Nursing Outcomes Classification (NOC)* (4th ed.). St. Louis, MO: Mosby.

National Center for Infectious Disease. (2002). Sterilization or disinfection of medical devices: General principles. Available: http://www.cdc.gov/ncidod/hip/sterile/sterilgp.htm

National Foundation for Infectious Diseases. (2008). Call to action: Influenza immunization among health care personnel. Retrieved October 12, 2008, from http://www.nfid.org/pdf/publications/fluhealthcarecta08.pdf

North American Nursing Diagnosis Association International. (2010). *NANDA-I nursing diagnoses: Definitions and classification 2009-2011.* Ames, IA: Wiley-Blackwell.

Occupational Safety and Health Administration. (2001). Occupational exposure to bloodborne pathogens; needlestick and other sharps injuries; final rule, 29 CFR Part 1910 66:5317–5325. Retrieved

October 5, 2008, from http://www.osha.gov/pls/oshaweb/owadisp.show_document?p_table=FEDERAL_REGISTER&p_id=16265
Occupational Safety and Health Administration. (2003). Model plans and programs for the OSHA bloodborne pathogens and hazard communications standards. Retrieved October 5, 2008, from http://www.osha.gov/Publications/osha3186.html
Oriola, S. (2006). *C. difficile*: A menace in hospitals and homes alike. *Nursing2006, 36*(8), 14–15.
Schweon, S. (2003). West Nile virus: Get ready for its return. *RN, 66*(4), 56–60.
Siegel, J. Rhinehart, E., Jackson, M., Chiarello, L., & the Healthcare Infection Control Practices Advisary Committee. (2006). Management of multidrug-resistant organisms in healthcare settings, 2006. Retrieved on October 12, 2008, from http://www.cdc.gov/ncidod/dhqp/pdf/ar/mdroGuideline2006.pdf
Siegel, J. Rhinehart, E., Jackson, M., Chiarello, L., & the Healthcare Infection Control Practices Advisory Committee. (2007). Guideline for isolation precautions: preventing transmission of infectious agents in healthcare settings 2007. Retrieved on October 3, 2008, from http://www.cdc.gov/ncidod/dhqp/pdf/isolation2007.pdf
Wilson, M. (2003). The traveler and emerging infections: Sentinel, courier, transmitter. *Journal of Applied Microbiology, 94*(Suppl.), 1S–11S.
Wright, D. (2008). HHS efforts to reduce healthcare-associated infections. Retrieved October 20, 2008, from http://www.apic.org/AM/Template.cfm
Yokoe, D. & Classen, D. (2008). Supplement article: Introduction. Improving infection control: A new healthcare imperative. *Infection Control and Hospital Epidemiology, 29*, S3–S11.

RESOURCES

Association for Professionals in Infection Control and Epidemiology (APIC), http://www.apic.org
Centers for Disease Control and Prevention (CDC), http://www.cdc.gov
National Foundation for Infectious Diseases (NFID), http://www.nfid.org
Occupational Safety and Health Administration (OSHA), http://www.osha.gov
Society for Healthcare Epidemiology of America (SHEA), http://info@shea-online.org

CHAPTER 22
Standard Precautions and Isolation

MAKING THE CONNECTION

Refer to the following chapters to increase your understanding of Standard Precautions and isolation:

Basic Nursing
- ***Infection Control/Asepsis***

Basic Procedures
- ***Hand Hygiene***
- ***Initiating Strict Isolation Precautions***

Intermediate Procedures
- ***Performing Open Gloving***

LEARNING OBJECTIVES

Upon completion of this chapter, you should be able to:

- Define key terms.
- Describe each of the eleven aspects of Standard Precautions.
- Identify the three transmission-based precautions and when each is to be used.
- Apply Standard Precautions in providing appropriate client care.

KEY TERMS

Airborne Precautions
aseptic technique
barrier precautions
Contact Precautions
Droplet Precautions
endemic
epidemic
hospital-acquired infection
infection
isolation
nosocomial infections
reverse isolation
Standard Precautions
Transmission-Based Precautions

INTRODUCTION

For more than 120 years, health care facilities and their personnel have struggled to prevent the spread of infections among their clients. This chapter reviews some of the historical methods as well as the current methods used to prevent the spread of infection.

HISTORICAL PERSPECTIVE

A hospital handbook published in 1877 recommended placing clients with infectious diseases in a separate facility (Lynch, 1949). These facilities became known as infectious-disease hospitals. Yet, **hospital-acquired infections**, **infections** acquired in the hospital that were not present or incubating at the time of the client's admission (**nosocomial infections**), continued in these facilities because the infected clients were not separated according to disease, and **aseptic technique** (infection-control practices used to prevent the transmission of pathogens) was seldom, if ever, practiced. To combat the continuing problem of nosocomial infections in the infectious-disease hospitals, personnel began to set aside a floor or ward for clients with similar diseases (Gage, Landon, & Sider, 1959).

Nursing has always been at the forefront of preventing the spread of infections among clients and personnel. Infectious-disease hospital personnel began practicing aseptic technique as recommended in nursing textbooks published from 1890 to 1900 (Lynch, 1949). Isolation practices and the use of infectious-disease hospitals were altered in 1910 when the cubicle system of isolation was introduced in U.S. hospitals (Gage et al., 1959). The cubicle system of **isolation** (separation from other persons, especially those with infectious diseases) placed clients in multiple-bed wards, with hospital personnel using a separate gown when caring for each client, washing their hands in an antiseptic solution after contact with each client, and disinfecting objects contaminated by any client. These nursing procedures were known as *barrier nursing*. Barrier nursing was aimed at preventing transmission of pathogenic organisms to other clients and to health care personnel. The cubicle system of isolation, including the barrier nursing procedures, gave the clients the alternative of receiving care in general hospitals instead of the infectious-disease hospitals (Centers for Disease Control and Prevention [CDC]/Hospital Infection Control Practices Advisory Committee [HICPAC], 1997).

During the 1950s, infectious-disease hospitals closed, with the exception of the tuberculosis (TB) hospitals, which closed in the 1960s. Thus, by the end of the 1960s, clients with infectious diseases were cared for in general hospitals.

In 1970, the CDC published *Isolation Technique for Use in Hospitals*, a revised edition of which was released in 1975 (CDC, 1975). This manual introduced and recommended seven categories of isolation: Strict Isolation, Respiratory Isolation, Protective Isolation, Enteric Precautions, Wound and Skin Precautions, Discharge Precautions, and Blood Precautions. By the mid-1970s, 93% of U.S. hospitals had adopted the recommendations of this book (Haley & Shachtman, 1980).

By 1980, **endemic** (occurring continuously in a particular population and having low mortality) and **epidemic** (infecting many people at the same time, in the same geographic area) nosocomial infections were surfacing. Some of these infections were caused by multidrug-resistant (MDR) microorganisms, others by newly identified pathogens. Both types required isolation precautions different from those specified in any of the seven isolation categories. As Schaffner (1980) describes, isolation precautions needed to be directed more specifically at nosocomial transmission in special-care units rather than at community-acquired infectious diseases being spread within the hospital.

In 1983, the CDC replaced the 1975 isolation manual with the *Guideline for Isolation Precautions in Hospitals* (Garner & Simmons, 1983). One of the most important changes was the emphasis on decision making by the users as to which guideline was appropriate in a particular situation (Garner, 1984; Haley, Garner, & Simmons, 1985).

Another change was to rename Blood Precautions, primarily used for clients who were chronic carriers of hepatitis B virus (HBV), to Blood and Body Fluid Precautions, which now were to apply to clients with acquired immunodeficiency syndrome (AIDS); body fluids other than blood, such as semen and vaginal secretions; amniotic, cerebrospinal, pericardial, peritoneal, pleural, and synovial fluids; and any other body fluid visibly contaminated with blood. It did not apply to feces, nasal secretions, sputum, sweat, tears, urine, or vomitus unless blood was visible in them.

Until 1985, clients placed in isolation either had a confirmed diagnosis or were suspected of having an infectious disease. Mainly because of the human immunodeficiency virus (HIV) epidemic and those other blood-borne infections often yet unrecognized in a client, it was decided that Blood and Body Fluid Precautions were to be applied universally to all clients, regardless of their presumed infection status (CDC, 1985). Thus, the new name became Universal Precautions.

A new system of isolation called Body Substance Isolation (BSI) was proposed in 1987 as an alternative to the diagnosis-driven isolation system of the 1983 *Guideline for Isolation Precautions in Hospitals*. BSI focused on isolating all moist and potentially infectious body substances (blood, feces, urine, sputum, saliva, wound drainage, and other body fluids) from all clients. The use of gloves was the primary method of isolating infectious agents; however, BSI did not contain adequate provisions to prevent droplet transmission, direct or indirect contact transmission, or true airborne transmission of infections. Also, BSI recommended hand washing after removal of gloves only if the hands were soiled (Lynch, Jackson, Cummings, & Stamm, 1987), whereas Universal Precautions recommended hand washing after every removal of gloves (CDC, 1987, 1988).

In 1991, the HICPAC was established to provide advice and guidance to the secretary and assistant secretary of the U.S. Department of Health and Human Services (USDHHS), the director of the CDC, and the director of the National Center for Infectious Diseases (CDC/HICPAC, 1997). The committee also provides advice to the CDC about updating guidelines and other policy statements related to the prevention of nosocomial infections.

The CDC, with the assistance of HICPAC, revised the *Guideline for Isolation Precautions in Hospitals* in 1996. The new guideline combined the major features of Universal Precautions and Body Substance Isolation into a single set of Standard Precautions, and the specific isolation categories into three Transmission-Based Precautions.

The CDC recommendations are not subject to legal enforcement; however, regulations of the Occupational Safety and Health Administration (OSHA) must be followed by all health care facilities. These regulations, laws enforced through the Department of Labor (OSHA, 1991, 2001), ensure that Standard Precautions and Transmission-Based Precautions are followed. According to OSHA regulations, all health care facilities must:

- Determine which employees have occupational exposure
- Provide hepatitis B vaccine free of charge to all employees with occupational exposure
- Provide personal protective equipment (e.g., gowns, gloves, masks, goggles) for all employees with occupational exposure
- Provide adequate hand-washing facilities and supplies
- Provide training regarding these rules to all employees with occupational exposure, both at hire and then annually
- Provide evaluation and follow-up for any employee who experiences an exposure incident
- Provide appropriate, properly labeled containers for contaminated sharps
- Provide and prominently display an exposure control plan for staff to follow

STANDARD PRECAUTIONS

Standard Precautions, listed on the inside back cover of this book, are preventive practices to be used in the care of all clients in hospitals regardless of diagnosis or presumed infection status. These guidelines are designed to reduce the risk of microorganism transmission from both recognized and unrecognized sources of infection in hospitals.

Standard Precautions apply to:

- Blood
- All body fluids, secretions, and excretions except sweat, regardless of whether those fluids contain visible blood
- Nonintact skin
- Mucous membranes

PROFESSIONALTIP

Exposure Incident

- Immediately report all exposure incidents to the proper person in the health care facility.
- The OSHA regulations require initial screening and follow-up care.

INFECTION CONTROL

Standard Precautions

- Standard Precautions must be practiced with all clients.
- Standard Precautions represent the most effective means of decreasing the risk of infection among clients and caregivers.

CLIENTTEACHING

Standard Precautions

- Assist the client to understand that the techniques and procedures associated with Standard Precautions are designed to prevent the transmission of microorganisms and not to isolate the client.
- Explain why each technique and procedure is used.

Barrier precautions, used to minimize the risk of exposure to blood and body fluids, involve the use of personal protective equipment, such as masks, gowns, and gloves, to create a barrier between the person and the microorganism and thus prevent transmission of the microorganism. *Hand hygiene, however, is the most basic aspect of Standard Precautions.* The other aspects of Standard Precautions are gloves; mask, eye protection, and face shield; gown; client-care equipment; environmental control; linen; occupational health and blood-borne pathogens; and client placement.

HAND HYGIENE

Refer to hand hygiene in Chapter 21, "Infection Control/Asepsis." To prevent cross contamination of different body sites on one client, hand hygiene may be necessary between tasks and procedures on that client.

GLOVES

Clean, nonsterile gloves are to be worn when touching blood, body fluids, secretions, excretions, and contaminated items. Clean gloves should be put on just before touching mucous membranes and nonintact skin. Gloves must be changed between tasks and procedures being performed on one client if material that may contain microorganisms in high concentrations is touched. Gloves must be removed promptly after use, and hands must be cleansed immediately before touching uncontaminated items or providing care to another client.

SAFETY

Latex Allergies

- Standard Precautions include the use of gloves when there is a possibility of contact with client body fluids.
- Be alert that health care personnel or the client may be allergic to the latex gloves. Reactions range from an eczematous contact dermatitis to anaphylactic shock.
- Before touching clients when wearing latex gloves, ask whether they have a known allergy to latex products. If they do, use nonlatex gloves for those clients.

Mask, Eye Protection, Face Shield

A mask and eye protection or a face shield should be worn to protect the mucous membranes of the eyes, nose, and mouth when procedures and client-care activities are likely to generate splashes or sprays of blood, body fluids, secretions, or excretions.

Gown

A clean, nonsterile gown should be worn to protect the skin and prevent soiling of clothing during procedures and client-care activities that are likely to generate splashes or sprays of blood, body fluids, secretions, or excretions. A gown that is appropriate for the activity and potential amount of fluids should be selected. A soiled gown should be removed as promptly as possible and the hands cleansed to prevent transfer of microorganisms to other clients or environments.

Client-Care Equipment

Client-care equipment soiled with blood, body fluids, secretions, or excretions must be handled in a manner to prevent skin and mucous membrane exposure, clothing contamination, and microorganism transfer to other clients or environments. Reusable equipment must not be used in the care of another client until it has been cleansed and sterilized appropriately. All single-use items must be properly discarded.

Environmental Control

The hospital must have adequate procedures for the routine care, cleansing, and disinfection of environmental surfaces, beds, bed rails, bedside equipment, and other frequently touched surfaces. All personnel must ensure that these procedures are followed.

Linen

Linen that is soiled with blood, body fluids, secretions, or excretions must be handled, transported, and processed in a manner to prevent skin and mucous membrane exposure, clothing contamination, and microorganism transfer to other clients and environments. Follow agency policy.

Occupational Health and Blood-Borne Pathogens

Care must be taken to prevent injury when using needles, scalpels, and other sharp instruments and when handling, cleansing, and disposing of such items after use. The OSHA regulations state that "contaminated (used) sharps shall be discarded immediately or as soon as feasible in containers that are closable, puncture-resistant, leakproof on the sides and bottom and are labeled or color coded" (OSHA, 1991, 2001) (Figure 22-1).

Used needles should never be recapped by using both hands. A one-handed "scoop" method is acceptable. Used needles should never be removed from disposable syringes by hand, nor should they be bent, broken, or otherwise manipulated by hand. Disposable syringes and needles, scalpel blades, and other sharp items should be placed in designated puncture-resistant containers.

In areas where the need for resuscitation is predictable, mouth pieces, resuscitation bags, or other ventilation devices should be used instead of the direct mouth-to-mouth resuscitation method.

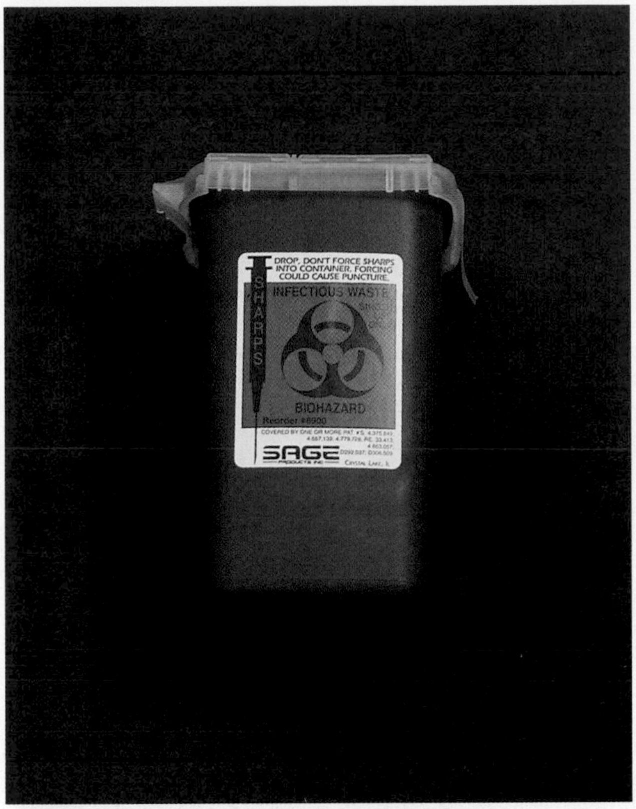

COURTESY OF DELMAR CENGAGE LEARNING

Figure 22-1 Sharps-Disposal Container

> **CRITICAL THINKING**
>
> **Standard Precautions**
>
> When, where, and why are Standard Precautions to be implemented?

Client Placement

Any client who contaminates the environment or who does not or cannot be expected to assist with maintaining appropriate hygiene or environment control should be placed in a private room. When a private room is unavailable, infection-control professionals must be consulted.

ISOLATION

The 1996 CDC guideline eliminated the previous category-specific isolation precautions and condensed the former disease-specific precautions into three sets of precautions based on the route of transmission: airborne (Figure 22-2), contact (Figure 22-3), or droplet (Figure 22-4). These new, Transmission-Based Precautions are to be used *in addition to* the Standard Precautions. **Transmission-Based Precautions** are practices designed for clients documented as or suspected of being infected with highly transmissible or epidemiologically important pathogens for which additional precautions beyond the Standard Precautions are required to interrupt transmission in hospitals (Table 22-1).

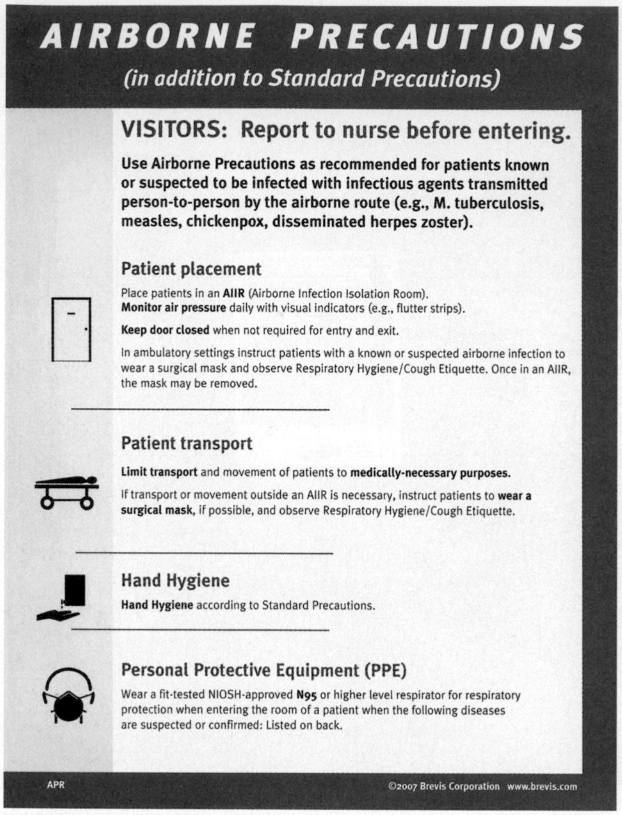

FIGURE 22-2 Transmission-Based Precautions: Airborne Precautions (© *2007. Reprinted with permission from Brevis Corporation, http://www.brevis.com.*)

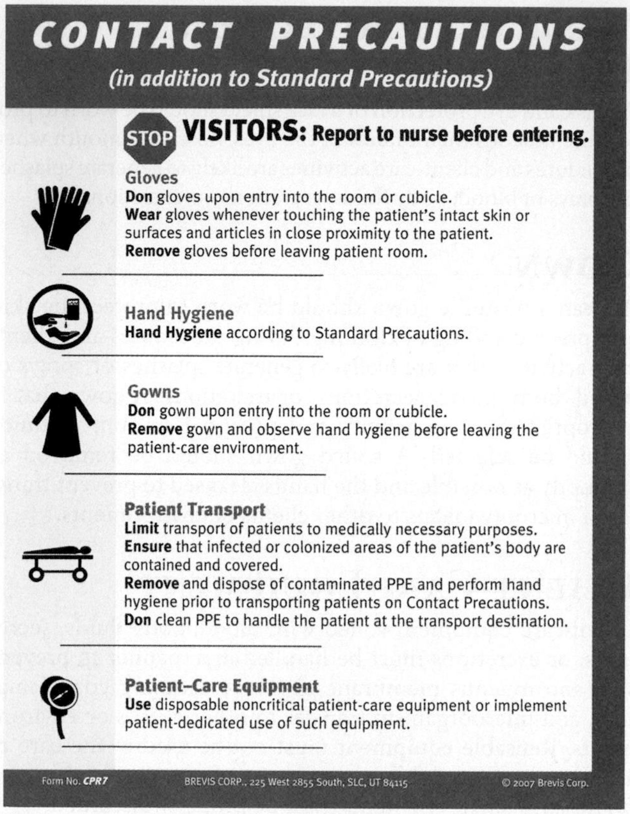

FIGURE 22-3 Transmission-Based Precautions: Contact Precautions (© *2007. Reprinted with permission from Brevis Corporation, http://www.brevis.com.*)

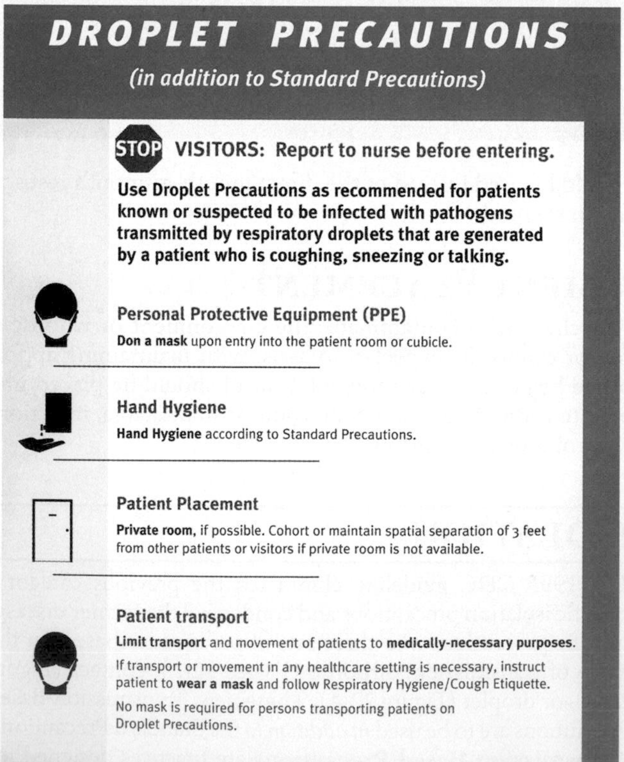

FIGURE 22-4 Transmission-Based Precautions: Droplet Precautions (© *2007. Reprinted with permission from Brevis Corporation, http://www.brevis.com.*)

CRITICAL THINKING

Transmission-Based Precautions

How are the three Transmission-Based Precautions the same? How are they different?

The Transmission-Based Precautions are also to be used in addition to the Standard Precautions in the event of suspicious infections and with clients who are immunosuppressed either from disease or chemotherapy. More than one of the transmission-based precautions is used at the same time for clients with certain infections or conditions.

Isolation precautions are usually ordered by the physician; however, nurses may initiate these precautions whenever a nursing diagnosis related to the infectious process is identified, for example, *Risk for Infection* related to decreased resistance of immune system. Most agencies require nurses to obtain a culture from a draining body area and to initiate isolation precautions when positive cultures are reported. After isolation precautions have been instituted, visitors and all personnel should comply with the agency's policy regarding isolation precautions. Signs should be posted in a prominent location outside the client's room. The signs should indicate the type of isolation precautions and preparation required before entering the room (Figure 22-5). The necessary supplies should be readily available.

Clients requiring isolation should be placed in a private room with adequate ventilation and should have their own supplies. Personal belongings should be kept to a minimum, and health care providers should use disposable supplies and

TABLE 22-1 Precautions Related to the Type of Disease

PRECAUTION	TYPE OF DISEASE
Standard Precautions	All clients, regardless of disease or condition
Airborne Precautions	In addition to Standard Precautions, used for clients known to have or suspected of having serious illnesses spread by airborne droplet nuclei, including: • Measles • Varicella • Tuberculosis
Contact Precautions	In addition to Standard Precautions, used for clients known to have or suspected of having serious illnesses easily spread by direct client contact or contact with fomites, including: • Wound infections • Gastrointestinal infections • Respiratory infections • Skin infections including: Herpes simplex Impetigo Major abscesses, cellulitis, or pressure ulcers Pediculosis Scabies Varicella (Zoster) • Viral hemorrhagic infections (Ebola)
Droplet Precautions	In addition to Standard Precautions, used for clients known to have or suspected of having illnesses spread by large particle droplets, including: • Meningitis • Adenovirus • Pneumonia • Influenza • Diphtheria • Mumps • Pertussis • Rubella • Scarlet fever • Parvovirus B19

From *Table I: Synopsis of Types of Precautions and Patients Requiring Precautions*, by Centers for Disease Control and Prevention (CDC)/Hospital Infection Control Practices Advisory Committee (HICPAC), 2002; *Guideline for Isolation Precautions: Preventing Transmission of Infectious Agents in Healthcare Settings 2007*, by CDC/HICPAC, 2007, available: http://www.cdc.gov/ncidod/dhqp/pdf/guidelines/Isolation2007.pdf.

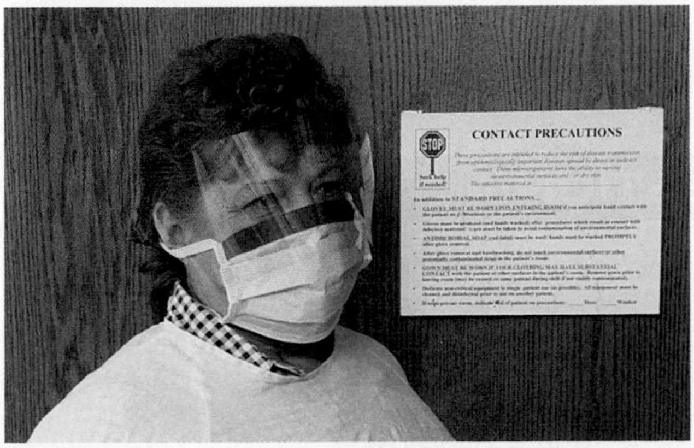

COURTESY OF DELMAR CENGAGE LEARNING

FIGURE 22-5 The sign on the door to the client's room indicates the type of isolation precaution and preparation needed before entering the room.

equipment whenever possible. All articles leaving the room, such as soiled linen and collected specimens, should be labeled and either placed in impermeable bags or double bagged.

Reverse isolation, also known as protective isolation, is a barrier protection designed to prevent infection in clients who are severely compromised and highly susceptible to infection. This includes clients who:

- are taking immunosuppressive medications
- are receiving chemotherapy or radiation therapy
- have diseases such as leukemia, which depress resistance to infectious organisms
- have extensive burns, dermatitis, or other skin impairments that prevent adequate coverage with dressings

These clients are at increased risk for infection from their own microorganisms, contact with health care workers whose hands have not been properly cleansed, and exposure to improperly disinfected and nonsterile items such as air, food, water, and equipment. Nursing responsibilities toward these clients include ensuring that everyone entering the client's room has completed meticulous hand hygiene and is properly attired in gown, gloves, and mask; ensuring that the client's environment is as clear of pathogens as possible; and knowing the institutional policy regarding caring for clients requiring reverse isolation.

COMMUNITY/HOME HEALTH CARE

Isolation

- Provide the client and family with appropriate written isolation instructions relative to the specific precautions.
- Provide necessary supplies or suggest a list of those things to buy and places to purchase the supplies.

MEMORYTRICK

ALONE

The nurse should use the memory trick "**ALONE**" when providing nursing care for a client in isolation:

A = Always post an isolation precaution sign on the client's door to notify individuals entering the room.

L = Listen to the client's feelings and concerns about being in isolation.

O = Observe isolation procedures to make sure they are accurately being followed.

N = Need to convey a sense of empathy, understanding, and support to the client.

E = Explain the pertinent isolation procedures to the client.

CLIENT RESPONSES TO ISOLATION

Isolation precautions are for the client's protection; however, clients who are placed on isolation precautions may experience psychological discomfort (Figure 22-6). Symptoms of anxiety, depression, rejection, guilt, or loneliness may be found in isolated clients. Clients should be educated on those isolation precautions that will be practiced and their purposes. Clients should be encouraged to verbalize their feelings regarding the isolation precautions and should be provided with intellectual stimulation and diversional activities such as paperback books, crossword puzzles, music, radio, or television. Visitors should be encouraged as a method to alleviate the client's feelings of isolation and loneliness. Wearing appropriate barrier precautions, visitors can safely enter an isolated client's room.

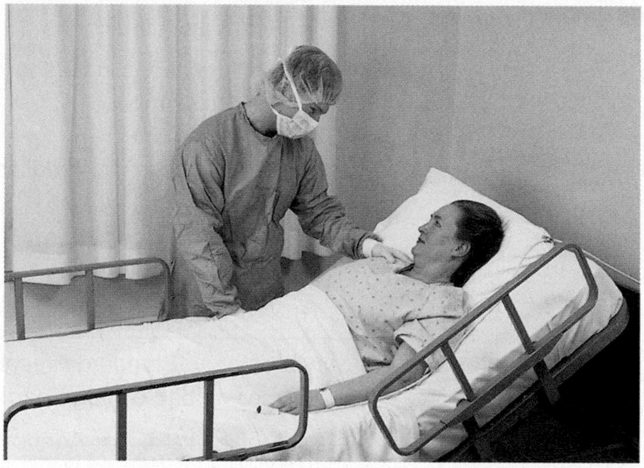

COURTESY OF DELMAR CENGAGE LEARNING

FIGURE 22-6 Nurse Interacting with Client Requiring Isolation Precautions

SUMMARY

- Standard Precautions are to be used when caring for *every* client.
- Airborne Precautions are to be used when caring for clients who have or may have serious illnesses spread by airborne droplet nuclei.
- Contact Precautions are to be used when caring for clients who have or may have serious illnesses spread by direct client contact or fomite contact.
- Droplet Precautions are to be used when caring for clients who have or may have serious illnesses spread by large-particle droplets.

REVIEW QUESTIONS

1. In 1996, the revised *Guideline for Isolation Precautions in Hospitals* combined Universal Precautions and Body Substance Isolation into:
   1. Barrier Precautions.
   2. Contact Precautions.
   3. Standard Precautions.
   4. Transmission-Based Precautions.
2. The use of masks, gowns, and gloves is termed:
   1. Droplet Precautions.
   2. Barrier Precautions.
   3. Contact Precautions.
   4. Standard Precautions.
3. The nursing action most basic to Standard Precautions is:
   1. gloving.
   2. gowning.
   3. hand hygiene.
   4. wearing a face mask.
4. Airborne Precautions require:
   1. paper masks.
   2. a private room.
   3. the wearing of gloves.
   4. the wearing of a gown.

5. Those precautions to be used in the care of all clients in hospitals regardless of diagnosis or presumed infection status are called:
   1. Standard Precautions.
   2. Airborne Precautions.
   3. Universal Precautions.
   4. Body Substance Isolation.
6. Nursing responsibilities for a client in reverse isolation include which of the following? (Select all that apply.)
   1. Ensuring that client's environment is as clear of pathogens as possible.
   2. Knowing institutional policies regarding caring for clients requiring reverse isolation.
   3. Discouraging visitation from family and friends.
   4. Observing that everyone entering the client's room is properly attired in gown, gloves, and mask.
   5. Encouraging the client to verbalize his or her feelings regarding isolation.
   6. Educating the client on the purpose of isolation.
7. A client has recently received a heart transplant and has been prescribed immunosuppressive medication. In which of the following types of isolation will the client be placed?
   1. Reverse.
   2. Institutional.
   3. Universal.
   4. Aseptic.
8. A nursing student is learning about clients placed in airborne precautions. Which of the following statements made by the student nurse indicates that further teaching is required?
   1. "The client needs to wear an N95 respirator mask when being transported to medically necessary purposes."
   2. "I need to keep the client's door closed when not required for entry and exit."
   3. "Visitors must report to the nurse before entering the client's room."
   4. "I need to wear a surgical mask when I enter the client's room."
9. Nursing responsibilities when caring for a client placed in contact isolation include:
   1. donning gloves when entering the client's room.
   2. hand hygiene according to standard precautions.
   3. removing gloves before leaving the client's room.
   4. all of the above.
10. The nurse observes a client in isolation crying. Which of the following responses made by the nurse is the most appropriate?
    1. "You will be alright. This will last only a week."
    2. "Don't worry. Lots of clients go through the same thing that you are."
    3. "You seem upset. Would you like to talk about it?"
    4. "Why are you crying? I can help you."

REFERENCES/SUGGESTED READINGS

Centers for Disease Control and Prevention. (1975). *Isolation techniques for use in hospitals* (2nd ed.) (HHS [CDC] Publication No. 80-8314). Washington, DC: U.S. Government Printing Office.

Centers for Disease Control and Prevention. (1985). Recommendations for preventing transmission of infection with human T-lymphotropic virus type III/lymphadenopathy-associated virus in the workplace. *Morbidity and Mortality Weekly Report, 34*, 681–686, 691–695.

Centers for Disease Control and Prevention. (1987). Recommendations for prevention of HIV transmission in health-care settings. *Morbidity and Mortality Weekly Report, 36*(2S), 1S–18S.

Centers for Disease Control and Prevention. (1988). Update: Universal precautions for prevention of transmission of human immunodeficiency virus, hepatitis B virus, and other blood borne pathogens in health-care settings. *Morbidity and Mortality Weekly Report, 37*(24), 377–382, 387–388. Available: http://www.cdc.gov/mmwr/preview/mmwrhtml/00000039.htm

Centers for Disease Control and Prevention. (2002). Guideline for hand hygiene in health care settings. Available: http://www.cdc.gov/mmwr/preview/mmwrhtml/rr5116a1.htm

Centers for Disease Control and Prevention. (2007a). Airborne precautions. Retrieved October 5, 2008, from http://www.cdc.gov/ncidod/dhqp/gl_isolation_airborne.html

Centers for Disease Control and Prevention. (2007b). Contact precautions. Retrieved October 5, 2008, from http://www.cdc.gov/ncidod/dhqp/gl_isolation_contact.html

Centers for Disease Control and Prevention. (2007c). Droplet precautions. Retrieved October 5, 2008, from http://www.cdc.gov/ncidod/dhqp/gl_isolation_droplet.html

Centers for Disease Control and Prevention. (2007d). Standard precautions. Retrieved October 5, 2008, from http://www.cdc.gov/ncidod/dhqp/gl_isolation_standard.html

Centers for Disease Control and Prevention. Preventing occupational HIV transmission to healthcare personnel. Retrieved October 5, 2008, from www.cdc.gov/hiv/resources/factsheets/hcwprev.htm

Centers for Disease Control and Prevention. (2009a). Hand hygiene interactive education. Retrieved May 9, 2009, from http://www.cdc.gov/handhygiene/training/interactiveEducation/frame.htm

Centers for Disease Control and Prevention. (2009b). An ounce of prevention keeps the germs away. Retrieved May 9, 2009, from http://www.cdc.gov/ounceofprevention/docs/oop_brochure_eng.pdf

Centers for Disease Control and Prevention/Hospital Infection Control Practices Advisory Committee (HICPAC). (1997). Part I: Evolution of isolation practices. Available: http://www.cdc.gov/ncidod/hip/isolat/isopart1.htm

Centers for Disease Control and Prevention/Hospital Infection Control Practices Advisory Committee. (2002). Table I. Synopsis of types of precautions and patients requiring precautions. Available: http://www.cdc.gov/ncidod/hip/isolat/isotab_1.htm

Centers for Disease Control and Prevention/Hospital Infection Control Practices Advisory Committee. (2007). Table 2. Clinical syndromes or conditions warranting empiric transmission-based precautions in addition to standard precautions in addition to standard precautions pending confirmation of diagnosis. Retrieved October 5, 2008, from http://www.cdc.gov/ncidod/dhqp/pdf/guidelines/Isolation2007.pdf

Centers for Disease Control and Prevention/Hospital Infection Control Practices Advisory Committeee. (2007a). Table 4. Recommendations for application of standard precautions for the care of all patients in all healthcare settings. Retrieved October 5, 2008, from http://www.cdc.gov/ncidod/dhqp/pdf/guidelines/Isolation2007.pdf

Centers for Disease Control and Prevention/Hospital Infection Control Practices Advisory Committeee. (2007b). Type and duration of precautions recommended for selected infections and conditions. Retrieved October 5, 2008, from http://www.cdc.gov/ncidod/dhqp/pdf/guidelines/Isolation2007.pdf

Delahanty, K. & Myers, F., III (2007). Nursing2007 infection control survey report. *Nursing2007, 37*(6), 28–36.

Gage, N. Landon, J. & Sider, M. (1959). *Communicable disease.* Philadelphia: F. A. Davis.

Garner, J. S. (1984). Comments on CDC guideline for isolation precautions in hospitals, 1984. *American Journal of Infection Control, 12,* 163.

Garner, J., & Simmons, B. (1983). *CDC Guideline for isolation precautions in hospitals* (HHS [CDC] Publication No. 83-8314). Atlanta: U.S. Department of Health and Human Services, Public Health Service, Centers for Disease Control. *Infection Control* (1983) 4:245–325; and *American Journal of Infection Control* (1984) 12:103–163.

Haley, R., & Shachtman, R. (1980). The emergence of infection surveillance and control programs in U.S. hospitals: An assessment, 1976. *American Journal of Epidemiology, 111,* 574–591.

Haley, R., Garner, J., & Simmons, B. (1985). A new approach to the isolation of patients with infectious diseases: Alternative systems. *Journal of Hospital Infection, 6,* 128–138.

Hass, J., & Larson, E. (2008). Compliance with hand hygiene guidelines: Where are we in 2008? *American Journal of Nursing, 108*(8), 40–44.

Hospital Infection Control Practices Advisory Committee. (1995). Recommendations for preventing the spread of Vancomycin resistance. *Infection Control and Hospital Epidemiology, 16*(2), 105–113.

Infection Control. (2002). "Hand hygiene" news. *Nursing2002, 32*(5), 32hn6.

Jagger, J. (2002). Avoiding blood and body fluid exposures. *Nursing2002, 32*(8), 68.

Jarvis, W. (2001). Infection control and changing health-care delivery systems. *Emerging Infectious Diseases,* 7(2). Available: http://www.cdc.gov/ncidod/eid/vol7no2/jarvis.htm

Lynch, P., Jackson, M. Cummings, J., & Stamm, W. (1987). Rethinking the role of isolation practices in the prevention of nosocomial infections. *Annals of Internal Medicine, 107,* 243–246.

Lynch, T. (1949). *Communicable disease nursing.* St. Louis, MO: Mosby.

Occupational Safety and Health Administration. (2001). Occupational exposure to bloodborne pathogens; needlestick and other sharps injuries; final rule, 29 CFR Part 1910 66:5317–5325. Retrieved October 5, 2008, from http://www.osha.gov

Occupational Safety and Health Administration. (2003). Model plans and programs for the OSHA Bloodborne Pathogens and Hazard Communications Standards. Retrieved October 5, 2008, from http://www.osha.gov

Perry, J. (2001). The bloodborne pathogens standard, 2001. *Nursing2001, 31*(6), 32hn16.

Porche, D. (1998). Nursing management of adults with immune disorders. In P. Beare & J. Myers (Eds.), *Adult health nursing* (3rd ed.). St. Louis, MO: Mosby.

Schaffner, W. (1980). Infection control: Old myths and new realities. *Infection Control, 1,* 330–334.

Siegel, J., Rhinehart, E., Jackson, M., Chiarello, L., & the Healthcare Infection Control Practices Advisory Committee. (2007). Guideline for isolation precautions: Preventing transmission of infectious agents in healthcare settings 2007. Retrieved October 3, 2008, from http://www.cdc.gov/ncidod/dhqp/pdf/isolation2007.pdf

RESOURCES

Association for Professionals in Infection Control and Epidemiology, Inc. (APIC), http://www.apic. org

Centers for Disease Control and Prevention (CDC), http://www.cdc.gov

Occupational Safety and Health Administration (OSHA), http://www. osha.gov

CHAPTER 23
Bioterrorism

MAKING THE CONNECTION

Refer to the following chapters to increase your understanding of the nursing process:

Basic Nursing

- ***Stress, Adaptation, and Anxiety***
- ***Infection Control/Asepsis***

LEARNING OBJECTIVES

Upon completion of this chapter, you should be able to:

- Identify and discuss major agents of bioterrorism.
- Define terminology pertinent to bioterrorism.
- Review the history of bioterrorism.
- Delineate the roles of each person in a potential or real terrorist attack.
- Delineate the roles of the various levels of government in a potential or real terrorist attack.
- Discuss protective measures, both prior to and following a terrorist attack.
- Describe the various components of the Centers for Disease Control and Prevention, including the Strategic National Stockpile, and its role in emergency preparedness.
- Describe the role of the nurse as a health care professional.
- List various agencies that have been designated as having a role in terrorist preparation or response.

KEY TERMS

anthrax
bioterrorism
Centers for Disease Control and Prevention (CDC)
Chemical, Biological, Radiological/Nuclear, and Explosive Enhanced Response Force Package (CEREPs)
chemical warfare agents
Expeditionary Medical Support (EMEDS)
first responders
nerve agents
plague
radiation sickness
ricin
sarin
smallpox
terrorism
zoonotic disease

INTRODUCTION

Terrorism consists of using any product or weapon or of the threat of using a harmful act or substance to kill or injure a large number of people. **Bioterrorism** is the purposeful use of a biological agent for the purposes of harming, killing, and/or instilling fear in large numbers of people. People who are intent on harming many others or causing death to large numbers of people at one time have used various bioterrorism methods for hundreds of years. Early humans used plants for bioterrorism attacks. Modern-day humans use substances manufactured in a laboratory, many of which have been adapted from the plants used hundreds or even thousands of years ago. Terrorism and bioterrorism are not new to the national or international scene. Sometimes the threat of an attack is all that is needed because a society becomes so afraid of what might happen that it becomes crippled and its members incapable of leading normal lives. Cities, counties, states, and the federal government, have plans in place to increase preparation and to deal with actual terrorism and bioterrorism attacks. Nurses and other health care professionals must also be prepared to respond.

UNDERSTANDING BIOTERRORISM

Following the World Trade Center attack on September 11, 2001, many terroristic and bioterroristic preparations were put into place, and *Bacillus anthracis* was one of the first threats against the American people. Anthrax spores were mailed to several locations around the country in a subsequent bioterroristic act causing illness and death. The spores were released into the air, resulting in the pulmonary form of anthrax. Five people lost their lives, at least 22 others were infected, and numerous postal workers were threatened (Centers for Disease Control and Prevention [CDC], 2007a). There were many reports of a mysterious white powder found in envelopes and packages in several areas of the country. This was assumed to be intentional bioterrorist activity. The public was instructed not to open any suspicious envelopes or packages but rather to take them to a safe place and notify the local police so that proper action could be taken. The packages were examined, and most were found to have an innocuous powder, but the perpetrators of these acts accomplished what they set out to do: instill fear in the people of the United States.

The **Centers for Disease Control and Prevention (CDC)** is an agency of the federal government whose goal is to promote health and quality of life by preventing and controlling disease, injury, and disability. Through programs of education and service, it has categorized infectious agents used by bioterrorists into three groups: biological, chemical, and nuclear radiation.

CRITICAL THINKING

September 11, 2001, Attack

Recall your feelings on September 11, 2001. Where were you when the planes crashed into the Twin Towers of the World Trade Center in New York City? What was your first thought? Feeling? Action?

BIOLOGICAL BIOTERRORISTIC AGENTS/DISEASES

Biological agents are bacteria, viruses, fungi, and toxins that are cultivated to cause harm to humans. These agents cause a variety of responses from mild, allergic reactions to serious infectious diseases resulting in death. The organisms in biologics are found in the natural environment, such as water, soil, plants, and animals. Specific agents may be plant or animal diseases that are readily available, highly virulent or lethal, and easy to aerosolize and disseminate without harming the terrorists themselves.

The CDC has three categories of biological agents classified as category A, category B, and category C (see columns titled "Category of Biological Agents" and "Examples" in Table 23-1 for categorized biological agents). The biological agents in these categories produce serious infectious diseases. The CDC divided the infectious diseases on the basis of their ability to disseminate or be disseminated to large numbers of persons. See Table 23-1 for an adaptation of that information. More complete information on emerging infectious diseases can be obtained at http://www.cdc.gov.

Biologics have certain advantages over other substances when used as a weapon. They are easy to obtain, are inexpensive to produce, do not need a large area for production, and do not need specialized equipment. The potential for widespread dissemination exists. In addition, it is easy to create mass public panic because biologics are colorless and odorless and people cannot be certain if they were exposed. Just the threat of a biologic being released into the air will cause large numbers of persons to panic. Biologics can easily overwhelm available medical services when large groups of persons have been exposed to a biological substance in a short period of time. These persons do not have to demonstrate symptoms but will seek medical care because they have been exposed or believe they have been exposed. The final advantage is that the person who released the substance can easily escape detection. It is not necessary to have a large quantity of the substance, so no one would be suspicious of someone transporting a large package. It would take no special equipment to disseminate the substance, so again suspicion would not be aroused. Knowing which agents bioterrorists are most likely to use helps plan appropriate action for public health preparedness. Several biologic bioterrorism agents exist, but the four potential biologic agents are anthrax (bacterial), botulism (toxin), plague (bacteria), and smallpox (virus). All these are lethal biologic weapons. The untreated mortality of anthrax is more than 90%, for pneumonic plague more than 90%, and for bubonic plague more than 60% (Ohio Department of Health [ODH], 2005). Any of the following bacteria or viruses can cause infectious diseases and could conceivably be used to unleash a massive bioterrorist attack on the people of the world.

ANTHRAX

Anthrax is an acute infectious disease caused by a spore-forming gram-positive bacterium, *Bacillus anthracis*. It normally affects domestic animals, mainly cattle, goats, and sheep. Horses,

TABLE 23-1 Categories of Biological Agents and Infectious Diseases

CATEGORY OF BIOLOGICAL AGENTS	DISSEMINATION	MORTALITY/ MORBIDITY RATES	IMPACT ON PUBLIC	ACTION NEEDED	EXAMPLES
A	Agents that can be easily disseminated person to person	High mortality	Potential for major public health impact with public panic and social disruption	Special, for public health preparedness	Anthrax (*Bacillus anthracis*) Smallpox (*Variola major*) Plague (*Yersinia pestis*) Botulism (*Clostridium botulinum* toxin) Viral hemorrhagic fevers (filoviruses [e.g., Ebola, Marburg] and arenaviruses [e.g., Lassa, Machupo]) Tularemia (*Francisells tularensis*)
B	Moderately easy to disseminate	Moderate morbidity; low mortality	Potential for major health impacts	Enhancement of CDC's diagnostic capacity and disease surveillance	Brucellosis (*Brucella* species) Glanders (*Burkolderia mallei*) Psittiacosis (*Chlamydia psittaci*) Ricin toxin from *Ricinus communis* (castor beans) Epsiolon toxin of *Clostridium perfringens* Food safety threats (e.g., *Salmonella* species, *Escherichia coli* O157:H7, *Shigella*) *Staphylococcal enterotoxin B* Typhus fever (*Rickettsia prowazekii*) Viral encephalitis (*Alphaviruses* [e.g., Venezuelan equine encephalitis, eastern equine encephalitis, western equine encephalitis]) Water safety threats (e.g., *Vibio cholerae*, *Crytosporidium parvum*) Melioidosis (*Burkholderia pseudomallei*) Q fever (*Coxiella burnetii*)
C	Could be specifically engineered for mass dissemination	Potential for high morbidity and high mortality	Potential for major health impacts	Watchfulness; awareness of possibility; vigilance for new infectious agents	Hantavirus (*Sin Nombre* virus) Yellow fever Tick-borne encephalitis viruses (TBEV) Multi-drug-resistant tuberculosis (MDR TB)

From Biological and chemical terrorism: Strategic plan for preparedness and response. By CDC, 2000a, *Morbidity and Mortality Weekly Report, 49*(RR04), 1–14; Bioterrorism. By CDC, 2008a, retrieved November 5, 2008, from http://emergency.cdc.gov/agent/agentlist-category.asp; Public health preparedness report—Appendix 6. By CDC, 2008e, retrieved November 5, 2008, from http://emergency.cdc.gov/publications/feb08phprep/appendix/appendix6.asp.

donkeys, and pigs are also affected. Wild animals, such as elephants, lions, antelopes, and the American bison, can become infected. Three forms of human anthrax infection exist: pulmonary, cutaneous, and gastrointestinal. The infection depends on the route of exposure. *Bacillus anthracis* enters the human body through contaminated food, by inhalation, or through an open wound. Person-to-person transmission of inhalation type anthrax does not occur, but inhalation of the anthrax bacterium causes a serious form of the disease in humans. Bioterrorists use the spores as an inhalant (ODH, 2005). However, anthrax is usually acquired when a break in the skin comes into direct contact with infected animals and their hides. Direct contact with secretions from cutaneous anthrax lesions may cause a cutaneous infection.

A real problem surrounding *B. anthracis* is that it has the ability to form spores, which can remain viable in soil for at hundreds, perhaps thousands, of years. These spores appear to be resistant to heat, drying, and some harsh chemicals. The spores pose a public health problem because they are responsible for producing inhalation anthrax. If treatment is not immediate and aggressive, the infected person will die. The person may develop tissue necrosis, hemorrhage, edema, or meningitis. Anthrax spores also can be made into a fine powder that is difficult to detect and then spread onto almost any surface.

Diagnosis

Pulmonary or inhalation anthrax is diagnosed with a chest x-ray. If the x-ray shows mediastinal widening, indicating hemorrhaging in the mediastinum, mortality is 90% (ODH, 2005) (Figure 23-1). A blood culture shows the presence of gram-positive bacilli. Enzyme-linked immunosorbent assay

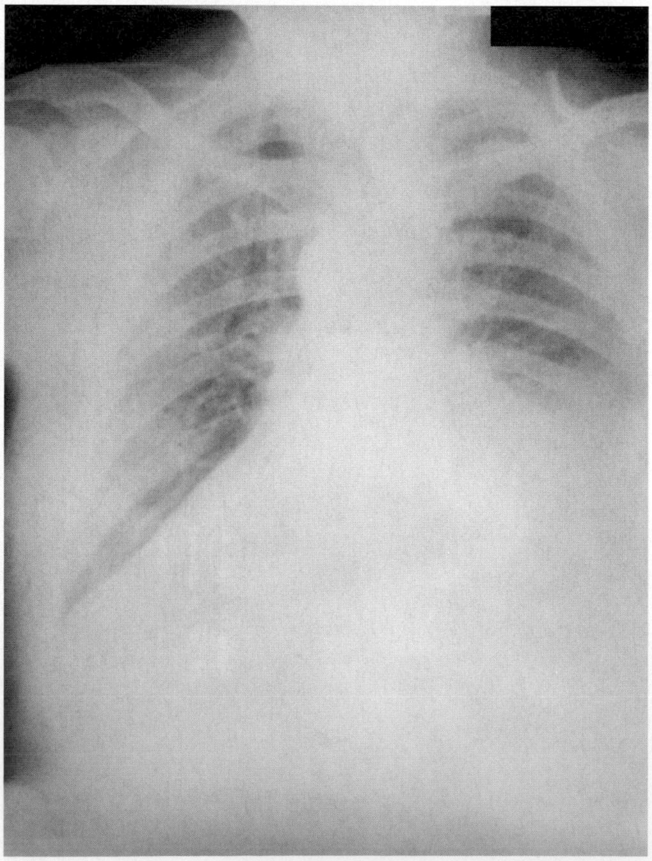

FIGURE 23-1 PA Chest Radiograph of Anthrax, Fourth Day of Illness (*Courtesy of Centers for Disease Control and Prevention.*)

(ELISA) and polymerase chain reaction (PCR) tests determine the presence of anthrax.

Symptoms of Exposure

The incubation period for pulmonary anthrax is 1 to 5 days, but it can last up to 60 days (CDC, 2006b). Pulmonary anthrax disease has two phases. The first phase presents with flu-like symptoms of sore throat, low-grade fever, nonproductive cough, malaise, fatigue, profound sweats, chest discomfort, and muscle aches. One to 3 days of improvement may follow this phase of symptoms. The second phase, 1 to 5 days after the onset of initial symptoms, is an acute phase of respiratory failure and toxemia. The serious symptoms are pulmonary flu-like symptoms (dyspnea, stridor, and cyanosis) and acute hemorrhagic mediastinitis (CDC, 2006b; ODH, 2005). Shock and death may occur within 24 to 36 hours of the later symptoms.

The incubation period for skin or cutaneous anthrax is 1 to 7 days following exposure. Cutaneous anthrax occurs when skin comes into direct contact with spores or bacilli. The first symptoms of cutaneous anthrax are localized itching followed by skin reactions resembling ulcerated papular lesions that become vesicular, which then forms a dark scab within 7 to 10 days surrounded by brawny edema.

Preventing Exposure

A vaccination for anthrax has been available in the United States for more than 30 years. It has not been widely used because anthrax was not a problem in this country prior to 2001. Controversy surrounds the issue of how protective and how safe the vaccine is. The CDC does not recommend widespread vaccination programs for anthrax. The only persons it recommends get the anthrax vaccination are military members who travel to high-risk areas, laboratory workers who come into contact with anthrax, and persons who deal with animal products imported from high-risk areas (CDC, 2000b, 2002b).

Medical Treatment

Only two antibiotics have been proven to be effective in treating anthrax: doxycycline hydrochloride (Doxylin) and ciprofloxacin (Cipro). Doxylin is approved by the Food and Drug Administration for naturally occurring anthrax (ODH, 2005). However, Cipro is recommended for a bioterrorist attack because a penicillin-resistant strain of anthrax is used.

Nursing Care

After exposure, remove contaminated clothing with minimal handling and place them in a labeled plastic bag. Decrease contamination by having the client shower with soap and water. Postexposure prophylactic treatment is antibiotic therapy for 8 weeks. The exposed person can also receive a vaccination of three doses. One dose is given on exposure followed with other doses in 2- and 4-week intervals. Antibiotic therapy is reduced to 4 weeks with a vaccination. Environmental surfaces or fomites are washed with an Environmental Protection Agency–registered, facility-approved sporicidal/germicidal agent or 0.5% hypochlorite solution (1:9 ratio of household bleach to water) (CDC, 1999).

When a client is diagnosed with anthrax, care is initiated as soon as possible to save his life. Treatment includes medication, supportive care, and prevention of spreading cutaneous anthrax to other persons, including health care workers. Health care personnel should maintain standard precautions (ODH,

2005). When the client is discharged, stress the importance of client adherence to antibiotic therapy.

Smallpox

Smallpox, or variola (a highly contagious viral disease in which humans are the only reservoir for the virus), is considered to be a potential biohazard. Even though the CDC and other governmental agencies throughout the world consider naturally occurring smallpox as eradicated, it was discovered that the virus is stored in some research laboratories in various countries (CDC, 2007a). The last known case of smallpox in the United States was in 1949 (CDC, 2007b), and the last known case of smallpox in the world was in 1977 in Somalia (CDC, 2007b). The occurrence of smallpox is well known throughout history.

Routine immunizations of American citizens stopped in 1972 because smallpox was eradicated in the United States (CDC, 2007c). In 1980, the World Health Organization stated that smallpox was eradicated because of a worldwide vaccination program (Casey et al., 2005). Individuals immunized prior to these dates may retain some degree of immunity, but the population as a whole is susceptible to smallpox. The Advisory Committee on Immunization Practices recommends that states establish and maintain immunized smallpox response teams and that acute care facilities identify and vaccinate designated health care workers to provide screening for or direct medical care to suspected smallpox clients in the event of a terrorist attack (CDC, 2002a).

Smallpox is highly contagious and potentially fatal. Two varieties exist: variola minor and variola major. Variola minor is a mild disease and is less common, with a 1% mortality rate [CDC, 2007b]. Variola major occurs in 90% of smallpox cases and has approximately a 30% mortality rate [CDC, 2007b]. Infection occurs when a very small amount of virus is inhaled and then travels from lungs to regional lymph nodes, where the virus replicates.

LIFE SPAN CONSIDERATIONS

Immunization Protection

Each of us must make a proactive choice to be as protected as possible against biological attack. The only way to do this is for children and adults to become immunized and keep all immunizations up to date. The adult population is the group that is the least protected against some diseases. We refer to diseases that can be protected against by immunizations as diseases of childhood and forget that adults can also contract them. The CDC publishes recommended immunization schedules and updates them annually (see Appendix B: Recommended Childhood and Adolescent Immunization Schedule [CDC, 2009b] and Appendix C: Recommended Adult Immunization Schedule [CDC,2009a]). Each of us must keep abreast of new developments and see to it that we and our children, relatives, and acquaintances are protected. This is the only way that we can be active in protecting ourselves against the illnesses and possible death following a terrorist attack.

Transmission

Smallpox is spread person to person as an aerosol or a droplet or by contact with contaminated objects, such as clothing or bedding. Only a very small amount of viral particles is needed to cause infection. Animals or plants are not a reservoir for the smallpox virus. It is estimated that as many as one-third of persons could die if the virus is unleashed into an unvaccinated population (ODH, 2005).

Symptoms of Exposure

The symptoms of smallpox include fever, prostration, and a vesicular, pustular rash. A papular rash appears on the face 2 to 3 days later, spreading to the extremities, including the palms of the hands and soles of the feet. The rash then becomes vesicular, painful, and pustular (Figure 23-2). A person experiences the onset of headache, high fever, and myalgias 10 to 17 days following airborne or droplet virus inhalation or contact with an infected person who has bleeding lesions. Death may follow the appearance of symptoms. The patient is contagious from the onset of the rash until the scabs separate, about a 3-week period.

Preventing Exposure

The U.S. government has stockpiled an adequate supply of smallpox vaccine to vaccinate every person in the United States.

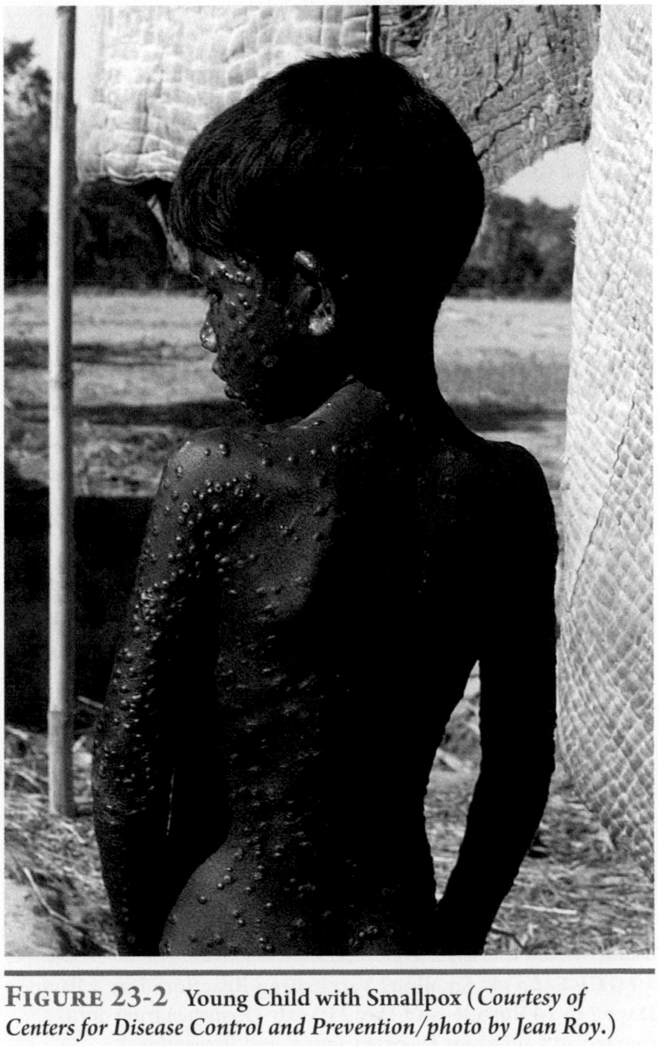

FIGURE 23-2 Young Child with Smallpox (*Courtesy of Centers for Disease Control and Prevention/photo by Jean Roy.*)

INFECTION CONTROL

Notification of the CDC and the Health Department

One identified case of smallpox is considered to be a public health emergency, secondary to the highly contagious nature and mortality associated with the disease. As soon as smallpox is suspected, both the CDC and the local health department must be notified.

The vaccine will protect an individual if given prior to exposure or up to 3 days following exposure. The U.S. government has been reluctant to order mass vaccination programs because of the side effects associated with the smallpox vaccination, including death (CDC, 2007c).

Medical Treatment

No effective treatments for smallpox exist. The only recommendations are vaccinations within 2 to 3 days of exposure and immediate initiation of airborne isolation procedures. Figure 23-3 shows a smallpox vaccination reaction.

Nursing Care

Nursing care must begin as soon as a diagnosis of smallpox is suspected. Standard contact and airborne precautions must be initiated for any patient with a vesicular rash. Supportive care is provided to the patient, and symptoms are treated accordingly. Nurses and other personnel caring for the patient with suspected or confirmed smallpox must be extremely careful to avoid contact with the organism while providing care to the patient. This includes wearing protective clothing, including gown, gloves, and a special mask.

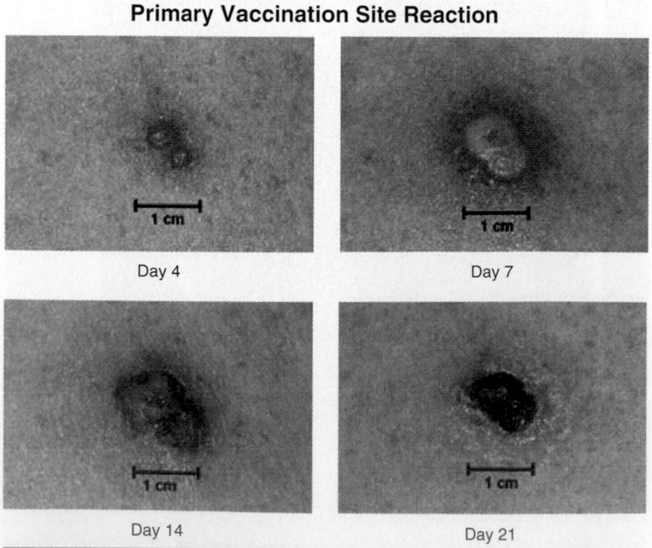

FIGURE 23-3 Smallpox Vaccination Reaction: Day 1 Papule, Days 7 to 14 Pustule, and Day 21 Scab (*Redrawn from data courtesy of Centers for Disease Control and Prevention.*)

PLAGUE

Plague is a disease caused by the bacterium *Yersinia pestis*. It is a **zoonotic disease**, a disease of animals that can be directly transmitted to humans by the animals that have the disease. Two types of plague exist: bubonic plague and pneumonic plague. The transmission and symptoms of the two types of plague are different. Humans acquire bubonic plague from the bite of a flea feeding on a rat or other rodent infected with *Y. pestis* or when an open wound is exposed to the bacterium. If bubonic plague is not treated, the bacterium enters the bloodstream and invades the lungs, causing pneumonic plague. A person can also acquire pneumonic plague by breathing in *Y. pestis* particles from the air. Pneumonic plague is less common but highly contagious and frequently fatal. Pneumonic plague is transmitted from person to person by droplets containing the plague bacterium. Bubonic plague is not transmitted from person to person. Bioterrorists could release *Y. pestis* as an aerosol weapon, causing many people to develop pneumonic plague within 1 to 6 days. The plague could also spread to those who come in close contact with those first exposed. One exposure advantage of *Y. pestis* is that it is destroyed by sunlight and drying and survives up to 1 hour when released into the air.

Diagnosis

Bubonic plague is diagnosed by blood cultures and lymph gland samples. Pneumonic plague is diagnosed by blood cultures and sputum specimens. If plague is present, all cultures and samples contain *Y. pestis.*

Symptoms of Exposure

A client becomes ill within 2 to 6 days of exposure. The main symptom of bubonic plague is a painful, swollen, tender lymph gland in the groin, armpit, or neck. The swollen gland is called a "bubo" (thus "bubonic plague"). Other symptoms are fever, chills, headache, malaise, and extreme exhaustion. Bubonic plague can progress to septicemia (septicemic plague), shock and death, or pneumonic plague.

The incubation period for pneumonic plague, if the client is exposed by intentional aerosol release or by close or direct contact, is 1 to 6 days (CDC, 2005). The first signs of pneumonic plague are fever, headache, weakness, chest pain, cough, and sometimes bloody or watery sputum. Pneumonia develops quickly with shortness of breath (CDC, 2004). Other symptoms that may occur are nausea, vomiting, and abdominal pain. If antibiotic treatment is not started within 24 hours after symptom onset, the disease progresses to respiratory failure, shock, and rapid death.

DRUGS

Antibiotics for Pneumonic Plague

The antibiotics of choice for pneumonic plague are streptomycin sulfate (Streptomycin), gentamicin sulfate (Garamycin), tetracyclines, and chloramphenicol (Chloromycetin). Antibiotics must be given within 24 hours of the first symptoms to prevent respiratory failure, shock, and death. Do not start antibiotic therapy until all cultures and specimens are obtained.

Preventing Exposure

Researchers are working on developing an oral vaccine to protect against plague, cholera, and anthrax, but it will not be available for several more years. Military personnel will be the first ones to receive this vaccine when it becomes available. Immunity is expected to occur in a matter of days (Fox, 2008). Persons in contact with infected clients are placed on antibiotics for 7 days. Caregivers should also wear a close-fitting surgical mask to prevent inhalation of the *Y. pestis* bacterium (CDC, 2004).

Medical Treatment

The treatment for bubonic plague includes antibiotics, supportive care, isolation, and surgical drainage of any lesions in the neck, groin, or axilla. The most important treatment component is preventing the spread of disease to others. With pneumonic plague as well, preventing its spread to others is of prime importance. Since pneumonic plague results in bronchopneumonia, the patient is treated as any patient with bronchopneumonia, with the addition of isolation being instituted immediately on suspicion of the disease.

The antibiotic of choice for bubonic plague is streptomycin. Gentamicin is used if streptomycin is contraindicated. Tetracyclines and chloramphenicol can also be used.

If a client acquires pneumonic plague by close contact with an infected person, antibiotics should be started within 7 days of exposure and taken for at least 7 days. To prevent death from intentional aerosol release, start antibiotics within 24 hours of the first symptoms. Effective oral antibiotics are doxycycline (Vibramycin) and ciprofloxacin (Cipro) and, for injection or intravenous use, streptomycin sulfate or gentamicin sulfate (Garamycin).

Nursing Care

Nursing care of the client with plague includes droplet precautions until 72 hours after initiating antibiotic therapy. Contact precautions are necessary until decontamination is complete, especially if many people are suspected or known to have been contaminated. Standard precautions are recommended if the patient has lesions that have been incised.

CHEMICAL BIOTERRORIST AGENTS

Bioterrorists could also use **chemical warfare agents**, including gases, liquids, or solids that cause injury or death to people, animals, and plants. The extent of injury depends on the chemical and the amount and length of exposure. The chemical categories are nerve, blood, choking or vomiting, and blister or vesicant agents. Chemical agents include nerve agents, blood agents, choking or vomiting agents, and blister or vesicant agents. The most common chemical agents are sulfur mustard (mustard gas), sarin, and VX (nerve agents). **Nerve agents** are powerful acetylcholinesterase inhibitors, altering cholinergic synaptic transmission at neuroeffector junctions (muscarinic effects), at skeletal myoneural junctions and autonomic ganglia (nicotinic effects), and in the central nervous system. Death can occur within 15 minutes if one drop to a few milliliters of a nerve agent come in contact with the skin (Agency for Toxic Substances and Disease Registry [ATSDR], 2008). Table 23-2 provides examples of each category of chemical bioterrorist agent.

Chemical agents have been available since World War I. Most chemical agents were designed to create one of two situations: to kill as many persons as possible or to make the soldiers and others so sick that they would be unable to continue fighting.

MEMORY TRICK

Antibiotic Therapy for Pneumonic Plague

For close contact acquired pneumonic plague, give antibiotics 7/7—within 7 days of exposure and for at least 7 days.

COMMUNITY/HOME HEALTH CARE

Plans for a Terrorist Attack

The United States is now focused on how to recognize possible terrorist attacks and how to treat those who have been exposed regardless of the form of the attack—biological, chemical, or nuclear. Researchers are attempting to develop antidotes and vaccinations against biological agents. Possible chemical and nuclear agents are being identified and studied. Government agencies have banded together to plan for the aftermath of terrorist attacks. Not only have plans been made, but mock attacks are routinely held so that each person is aware of his role following an attack. Each person is given information on how to protect himself, one's family, and also one's role in the community should an attack occur. It is far better to be prepared and never need to put the plans into action than to be attacked and not have a well-planned response.

RICIN

Ricin is one of the newest chemicals identified as a nerve agent. It is a poison made from the waste products of processing castor beans into castor oil. According to the CDC (2008b), ricin has some potential medical uses, such as bone marrow transplants and as a treatment to kill cancer cells. Accidental exposure is extremely unlikely. It would take a deliberate act of terrorism to make ricin and use it as a poison. Ricin can be a powder, a mist, a pellet, or a weak acid preparation. Humans are poisoned by breathing in ricin as a mist or powder. Ricin can also be put into food or dissolved in water and then swallowed. A final way to poison someone with ricin is to dissolve it and then inject it into a person's body. Ricin poisoning is not contagious and cannot be spread from person to person through casual contact.

Ricin enters the cells of a human body and prevents the cells from making necessary proteins. Without these proteins, the cells die. Eventually, this is harmful to the entire body, and death may occur.

TABLE 23-2 Examples of Each Category of Chemical Agent

CATEGORY OF CHEMICAL AGENT	EXAMPLES	FORM(S)	SYMPTOMS OF EXPOSURE
Nerve agents	Sarin (GB) Soman (GD) Tabun (GA) VX	Gaseous liquid	Runny nose, sweating, blurred vision, headache, difficulty breathing, drooling, nausea, vomiting, muscle cramps and twitching, confusion, convulsions, paralysis, coma, and death
Blood agents	Hydrogen cyanide	Liquid	Headache, dizziness, confusion, nausea, shortness of breath, convulsions, vomiting, weakness, anxiety, irregular heartbeat, tightness in chest, and unconsciousness
	Cyanogen chloride	Gas	Rhinorrhea, sore throat, drowsiness, confusion, nausea, vomiting, cough, unconsciousness, and edema
Choking/vomiting agents	Phosgene	Gas	Coughing, burning sensation in throat and eyes, tearing, blurred vision, difficulty breathing, nausea, vomiting Skin contact: frostbite or burn-type lesions Pulmonary edema occurs within 2 to 6 hours of exposure.
	Adamsite—vomiting agent	Crystalline dispensed in aerosol	Rapid onset; irritation of the eyes, skin, and upper airway; nausea; vomiting; spasmodic blinking; corneal necrosis; burning in throat; chest tightness and pain; uncontrollable and violent coughing and sneezing; increased nasal secretions; abdominal cramps; diarrhea; malaise; headache; mental depression; and chills
Blister/vesicant agents	Distilled mustard (HD) Mustard gas (H) Lewisite Mustard/lewisite Mustard/T Nitrogen mustard Phosgene oxime Sesqui mustard Sulfur mustard	Liquid or crystalline	**Respiratory exposure:** rhinorrhea, nasal irritation and pain, sore throat, cough, dyspnea, chest tightness, tachypnea, and hemoptysis **Skin exposure:** itching and erythema Immediate blanching with phosgene oxime Blisters (within 1 hour with phosgene oxime, 2 to 12 hours with lewisite, and 2 to 24 hours with mustards) Necrosis and eschar in 7 to 10 days **Eye exposure:** conjunctivitis, lacrimation, eye burning and pain, photophobia, blurred vision, eyelid edema, corneal ulceration, and blindness **Gastrointestinal ingestion exposure:** abdominal pain, nausea and vomiting, hematemesis, and diarrhea (possibly bloody) **High-dose exposure:** hypotension, atrioventricular block with cardiac arrest, tremors, convulsions, ataxia, and coma

From Medical management guidelines for nerve agents: Tuban (GA); sarin (GB); soman (GD); and VX. By Agency for Toxic Substances and Disease Registry, 2008, Department of Health and Human Services, retrieved September 9, 2008, from http://www.atsdr.cdc.gov/MHMI/mmg166.html; NIOSH emergency response card: Cyanogen chloride (ERC506-77-4). By CDC, 2005, retrieved November 14, 2008, from http://emergency.cdc.gov/agent/cyanide/erc506-77-4.pr.asp; Facts about Phosgene. By CDC, 2006a, retrieved November 14, 2008, from http://emergency.cdc.gov/agent/phosgene/basics/facts.asp; NIOSH emergency response card: Hydrogen cyanide (ERC74-90-8). By CDC, 2006c, retrieved November 14, 2008, from http://emergency.cdc.gov/agent/cyanide/erc74-90-8.asp; Toxic syndrome description: Vesicant/blister agent poisoning. By CDC, 2006e, retrieved November 13, 2008, from http://www.bt.cdc.gov/agent/vesicants/tsd.asp

Symptoms of Exposure

The symptoms of ricin poisoning depend on whether ricin was inhaled, ingested, or injected. A large dose may affect many organs. Symptoms begin to appear within 8 hours after ricin inhalation. Following inhalation, symptoms include respiratory distress, fever, cough, nausea, and tightness in the chest. Diaphoresis and pulmonary edema follow. Cyanosis becomes apparent. Severe hypotension and respiratory failure occur, leading to death. Powder or mist forms of ricin cause redness and pain of the skin and eyes. Symptoms usually appear within 6 hours of ingesting ricin. The symptoms include vomiting and diarrhea (that may become bloody) and severe dehydration, followed by hypotension. Hallucinations, seizures, and hematuria occur. Within several days, kidney, hepatic, and spleen failure also occur; if this happens, the person will likely die. Death may occur within 36 to 72 hours following exposure to ricin, depending on the route and the amount of exposure. If the person is still alive after 3 to 5 days, recovery is likely.

Preventing Exposure

The most important preventive factor is avoiding exposure to ricin. No antidote is available, only supportive care. If exposure occurred, it is important to get the ricin out of or off of the body as quickly as possible.

Medical Treatment

If exposed to ricin, get away from the area of exposure or get outside. Remove clothing, wash the entire body with large amounts of soap and lukewarm (not hot) water, and then seek medical attention. Do not let soap get into the eyes during the shower. Do not remove clothing by taking it over the victim's head and re-exposing them to ricin; instead, cut the clothing off the person. Clothing and anything that comes into contact with the clothing is double bagged. Notify emergency health care personnel of bagged items so that they can properly dispose of the bag. Eyeglasses are washed with soap and water, dried, and then put back on. Contacts must be disposed of with the contaminated clothing and not put back into the eyes. Client care may be as simple as rinsing out the eyes or as complicated as ventilatory assistance and administering medications to raise the blood pressure or control seizures.

Nursing Care

A nurse or **first responder**, the first people who will spring into action when a terrorist attack occurs, must be extremely careful to avoid contact with anything that may have been exposed to ricin when assisting a client. The health care provider wears rubber gloves and does not handle clothing and other articles with bare hands. Other nursing care is based on the needs of the patient and the medical orders given. Much emotional support is needed both for the patient and for the family members. Education is also important since ricin exposure is a new and previously unknown condition to most people.

> **MEMORYTRICK**
>
> **Ricin Exposure**
>
> If a person is exposed to ricin, remember "**GROWS**":
>
> **G** = Get away from the exposed area.
>
> **R** = Remove clothing and all personal items (i.e., eyeglasses, contacts).
>
> **O** = Over the head; cut it **O**ff.
>
> **W** = Wash eyes with water.
>
> **S** = Seek medical help.

> **CRITICAL THINKING**
>
> **First Responders**
>
> Why is it of major importance to protect the first responders in a bioterrorist attack?

SARIN

Sarin GB (O-isopropyl methylphosphonofluoridate) is a dangerous nerve agent that has been available since World War II (CDC, 2006d). During the rush hour on March 20, 1995, a Japanese cult, Aum Shinrikyo, released a liquid form of sarin in five cars of three different Tokyo subway lines that joined at the Kasumigaseki station, the location of several government ministries. Twelve people were killed, and approximately 6,000 sought medical care. This attack shows how easy it is for a small terrorist group to plan and launch a chemical warfare terrorist attack (Council on Foreign Relations, 2008; Salmon, 2008).

Sarin is a clear, colorless, odorless, and tasteless gas and is the most toxic and fastest acting of all the chemical agents. Sarin is also the most volatile nerve agent, meaning that it can easily and rapidly evaporate from a liquid form into a vapor and spread rapidly through the environment. Extremely small amounts (0.01 mg/kg) of sarin can kill a person. Food and water can also be contaminated; sarin mixes easily with water. Sarin is slightly heavier than air, and it hovers close to the ground when released. People are exposed to liquid forms of sarin through skin or eye contact or by breathing air containing sarin vapors. Sarin vapors are absorbed through the skin only at very high concentrations. It is not necessary to come into contact with the liquid form of the agent. Exposure to sarin vapor can and does cause serious symptoms of exposure. Sarin is released from clothing in approximately half an hour after it comes in contact with sarin vapor.

Symptoms of Exposure

Sarin is a powerful acetylcholinesterase inhibitor, producing muscarinic and nicotinic effects. Sarin exposure symptoms include loss of consciousness, seizures, paralysis, and respiratory failure, leading to death within seconds to minutes of exposure. Three factors determine the amount of poisoning caused by exposure to sarin: the amount of sarin to which a person was exposed, how the exposure occurred, and the length of time the exposure lasted. For specific symptoms of exposure to small amounts of sarin, see Table 23-3.

Preventing Exposure

The best prevention is to avoid exposure to sarin. If exposure cannot be prevented, then treatment must be started as soon as possible following exposure.

Table 23-3 Symptoms of Sarin and Other Nerve Agent Exposure

MUSCARINIC EFFECTS	NICOTINIC EFFECTS
Pinpoint pupils	Skeletal muscle twitching, cramping, and weakness
Blurred or dim vision	
Conjunctivitis	Tachycardia
Eye and head pain	Hypertension
Hypersecretion of salivary, lacrimal, sweat, and bronchial glands	
Bronchial restriction	
Nausea	
Vomiting	
Diarrhea	
Abdominal cramping	
Urinary and fecal incontinence	
Bradycardia	

Medical Treatment

Treatment of sarin exposure and other nerve agents involves removing the sarin from the body as soon as possible and providing supportive care.

Nursing Care

After exposure to sarin, if possible, move to an area where there is fresh air; this action is effective in decreasing the possibility of death from sarin exposure. Move to the highest ground available since the sarin vapor will stay in low-lying areas. If the sarin was released indoors, then the persons exposed should move outside as quickly as possible. Any clothing that has liquid sarin on it must be removed and double bagged in plastic bags. If the nurse is assisting other people to remove contaminated clothing, avoid touching any areas contaminated with liquid sarin. If the person complains of any burning of the eyes or blurred vision, assist in rinsing the eyes with plain water for 10 to 15 minutes. Immediately wash liquid sarin from the body with copious amounts of soap and water. If sarin has been swallowed, do not induce vomiting or give any fluids by mouth. Atropine sulfate, an acetylcholine inhibitor, and pralidoxime chloride (pyridine-2-aldoxime methochloride and 2-PAM chloride) are the only known antidotes for sarin poisoning. Persons with mild or moderate exposure to sarin usually recover completely. Persons with severe exposure are not expected to survive. Neurological problems should not last longer than 1 to 2 weeks. As soon as the previously mentioned measures have been completed and emergency personnel notified, take the client to the emergency room. Emergency

CRITICAL THINKING

Sarin

Why is sarin so dangerous as a biological weapon?

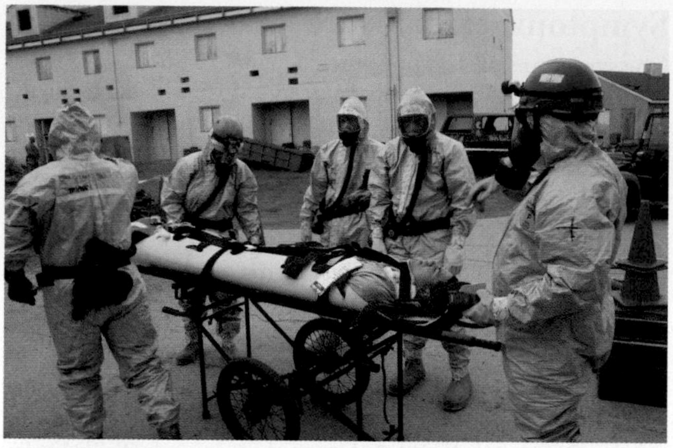

Figure 23-4 First responders and emergency personnel must take appropriate precautions to protect themselves during an attack. (*Courtesy U.S. Army/photo by Lt. Col. Richard Goldenberg.*)

personnel must protect themselves against exposure before getting near the client (Figure 23-4).

Specific care depends on the client's symptoms. A patent airway must be established and maintained. Administer antidotes of atropine sulfate and pralidoxime chloride (Protopam Chloride) as soon as possible. If seizures are present, administer diazepam (Valium) as needed. Cardiac manifestations are treated as they appear.

Nuclear Radiation Bioterrorist Agent

Radiation sickness, or, more properly, acute radiation syndrome (an abnormal condition resulting from exposure to ionizing radiation), is dependent primarily on the dose of radiation that a person receives. Radiation sickness can occur hours or days after high doses of radiation exposure.

Symptoms of Exposure

The first symptoms are nausea, vomiting, and diarrhea. Later symptoms include anorexia, fatigue, weight loss, and bone marrow suppression. Persons who live through the acute exposure are at high risk for developing certain cancers, especially leukemia, secondary to bone marrow suppression.

Preventing Exposure

Unfortunately, exposure to nuclear radiation cannot be prevented. One is not aware of potential exposure until a bomb is dropped and exposure has already occurred. If a person is working with nuclear radiation, prevent accidents that lead to exposure.

Medical Treatment

Little to no effective treatments exist for radiation exposure. The best treatment available is to treat the symptoms. Administration of potassium iodide (KI) tablets following radiation exposure prevents up to 100% of the radioactive iodine released by a nuclear explosion from entering the thyroid gland and damaging the thyroid cells. KI should be taken prior to or immediately following exposure to radiation but is effective if taken as long as 3 to 4 hours following exposure. KI protects only the thyroid gland; it does not protect any other body structures.

Nursing Care

Initial care of external radiation exposure involves removing all clothing and properly disposing of it, cleansing the skin, and initiating isolation procedures to protect others. Initial care of a person who has inhaled or ingested radioactive material should follow protocols for anyone who has been exposed to chemical poisons. Body wastes are checked for radiation levels. If a wound is present, extra care is taken to prevent cross contamination of exposed surfaces. Any and all emergency lifesaving techniques must be done at the same time to avoid the spread of the radiation effects. Nursing staff and others caring for the patient must wear surgical gowns, gloves, and caps.

BIOTERRORISM PREPAREDNESS

In the event of a covert bioterrorist attack, nurses and other health care professionals will be the first ones to see the victims after the first responders. Victims appear in emergency rooms, physician offices, clinics, or school health settings. Since nurses staff these areas and are the first persons who see and evaluate potential clients, they must be able to identify symptoms, unusual happenings, trends in client symptoms, and other significant events.

Nurses must be aware of the emergency response system at local, state, and federal levels. They also are aware of their role in emergency response and emergency preparations. Nurses are vital committee members in developing, maintaining, and evaluating emergency response plans for health care facilities and communities. Hospitals have emergency plans in place to care for clients involved in bioterrorism acts and other emergency situations.

Government Agency Involvement

Many government agencies are available to assist with planning for disasters. Two of the older agencies are the U.S. Department of Defense and the CDC. Although their primary functions are very different, they join in efforts to combat terrorism. Their common goals are to inform, educate, and prepare U.S. citizens for unusual disease outbreaks.

Department of Health and Human Services

The Department of Health and Human Services is the main agency of the U.S. government tasked with protecting the health of all Americans and providing essential human services, especially to those who are least able to provide for themselves. This department works closely with state and local governments.

One of the branches of the Department of Health and Human Services is the Coordinating Office for Terrorism Preparedness and Emergency Response. The mission of this branch is to protect the health and enhance the potential for living at the highest possible level across the life span of all people in all communities related to community preparedness and response. It works with the CDC and maintains response operations, including the Strategic National Stockpile (SNS). The SNS is a program managed by the CDC that is designed to ensure that essential medical supplies are sent immediately to a community that has sustained a large-scale chemical or biological attack.

Federal Emergency Management Agency

The Federal Emergency Management Agency (FEMA) was established by a law passed in 1974, PL 93-288, the Disaster Relief Act. FEMA's mission is to decrease the loss of life and property and to protect the United States from all hazards, including natural disasters, acts of terrorism, and other man-made disasters.

The intent of Congress was to provide an orderly and continuing means of assistance by the federal government to state and local governments in carrying out their responsibilities to citizens, specifically to alleviate suffering and damage resulting from disasters. The Stafford Act expanded the scope of existing disaster relief programs. Among its provisions are encouraging the development of comprehensive disaster preparedness and assistance plans and programs by state and local governments, encouraging all entities to obtain insurance coverage that would supplement or replace government assistance, and providing federal assistance programs for both private and public losses incurred as a result of disasters.

The administrator of FEMA is appointed by the president and reports directly to the secretary of Homeland Security. The administrator may be called on by the president to serve as a member of the cabinet in the event of a disaster or an act of terrorism.

CDC

The CDC expanded its programs to inform all Americans of the new threats against health and life. One of its functions is managing the SNS, which ensures that a community that has experienced a massive chemical or biological attack will have immediate necessary supplies. Some of the materials included are antibiotics, vaccines, chemical antidotes, antitoxins, bandages, airways, and intravenous equipment. The SNS has two divisions. One division consists of large prepackaged emergency supplies that are stored in various places throughout the country. Each storage site was chosen so that no site is more than 12 hours away from every community in the country. The 50-ton packaged supplies are stored in a climate-controlled warehouse.

The second division of the SNS is a vendor-managed inventory (VMI), which consists of materials that are more specific to certain biological preparations. They arrive at a site that has experienced a bioterroristic attack after the agent used is identified and within 24 to 36 hours after the attack occurs. Because of the SNS, individuals or even individual communities should not attempt to store materials in preparation for an attack because the materials would most likely become outdated before the need would arise.

National Guard Medical Services Branch

The National Guard established two programs to promptly provide supplies to emergency situations: the **Expeditionary Medical Support (EMEDS)** and the **Chemical, Biological, Radiological/Nuclear, and Explosive Enhanced Response Force Package (CERFPs)**. The EMEDS is a total package that includes everything necessary to screen and treat clients who need outpatient care. It also releases clients that need more than outpatient care to other facilities for longer-term care. EMEDS used in civilian settings provides emergency care while local facilities gear up to provide necessary care. EMEDS has enhanced packages, called EMEDS + 10 or EMEDS + 25, that include up to 25 critical care beds.

A medical component to CERFP is similar to an EMEDS and can be expanded to the same contents and capabilities of an EMEDS. This component can be deployed alone without the rest of the CERFP. It can also include a surgical suite if needed. The CERFP can respond rapidly following a call by the governor to a state adjutant general and be at the scene of a disaster, ready to function in 6 hours (Figure 23-5). It can also respond to disasters outside the home state, but the governor can deny the request if an emergency exists in that state.

The Joint Commission

The Joint Commission, previously known as the Joint Commission on the Accreditation of Healthcare Organizations, has had emergency preparedness as part of its core components for many years. Until recently, the Joint Commission focused on preparing for natural disasters, such as floods and tornados, rather than man-made ones. In today's world, facilities prepare to handle natural disasters as well as man-made situations. Facilities must have written plans for dealing with the situation at hand, for being sure that their usual functions are completed, and for returning to normal functioning once the situation has been resolved. All employees must be aware of these plans and know where the written plans are located.

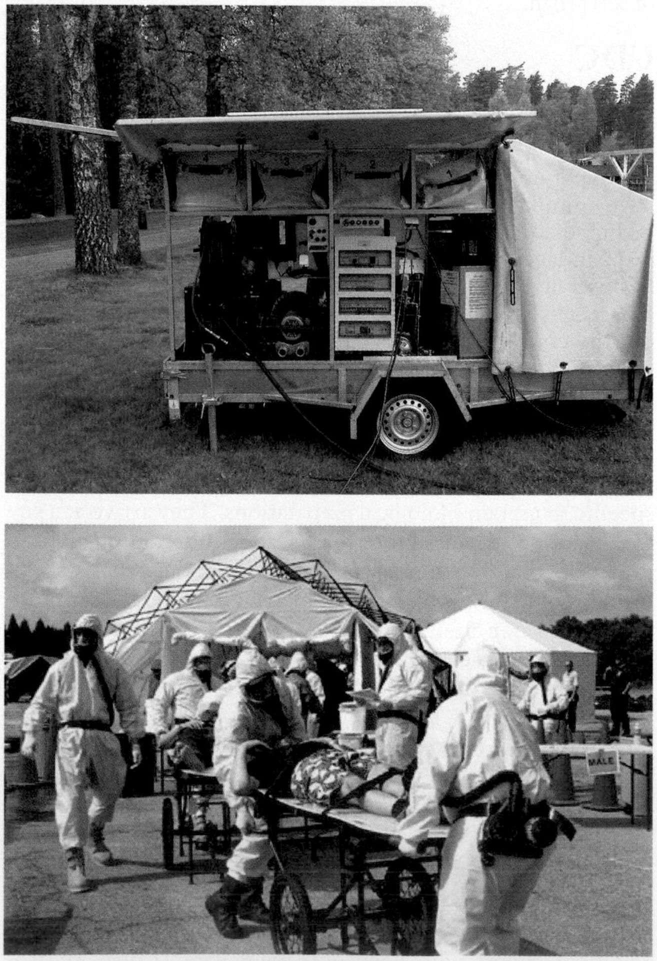

FIGURE 23-5 EMEDS and CERFP respond to bioterrorist sites with trailers, vehicles, and tents to treat emergency situations. *(Images courtesy of SEDAB and National Guard.)*

The Joint Commission sets standards ensuring that health care facilities provide a safe environment for both clients and health care workers. Disaster planning falls under these standards in the section titled "Environment of Care" (Joint Commission, 2007).

Each facility should have an emergency operations plan (EOP). The EOP contains information on when to activate a response and who will be notified first, both internally and within the community. Once the emergency plan has been activated, protection of the facility environment takes priority. This will most likely be accomplished by security personnel. Persons already within the facility, such as employees, clients, and other people, are protected from infection or contamination by suspected victims. These victims are kept in an area away from the general occupants of the facility. If a bioterrorism attack occurs or is suspected to have occurred, standard precautions in addition to disease-specific precautions are instituted. If the agent is unknown, efforts are made to identify it so that disease-specific precautions can be instituted.

After the previous steps are completed, a decontamination protocol is followed. The published protocol for decontamination includes guidelines for handling contaminated clients, facilities availability, and specific measures to complete, depending on the type of contamination that occurred.

An agency has an EOP to prevent chaos in the event of a disaster. Practice drills are conducted on a regular basis so that everyone knows their expected role.

EMERGENCY RESPONSE TEAMS

A group of persons are identified as those who will be **first responders** in case of a terrorist attack. They are nurses, emergency room personnel, EMS personnel, public health personnel, primary care providers, and other persons, such as law enforcement, animal control officers, firefighters, and veterinarians. Communities around the country are asked to identify and train persons who are designated as first responders should the need for them arise.

PROFESSIONAL TIP

Terrorist Attack

The possibility of a terrorist attack exists on a day-to-day basis in the United States. Nurses, especially those employed in an emergency room setting, must be aware of the symptoms of exposure to chemical agents. They recognize the symptoms and are prepared to take immediate steps to protect themselves, other persons who are nearby, and the client. It is better to err on the side of caution and to institute actions if the client's symptoms indicate exposure to a chemical agent than to ignore such symptoms or deny that an attack can happen.
A bioterrorist attack can occur, and health care personnel must be prepared to act competently and quickly.

Nurse need to understand the rationale for preparing for the possible consequences of any disaster or attack. Many thousands of people could be injured or killed and many more people could suffer long-term effects following the occurrence, both physical and psychological. Nurses have a responsibility to get involved in disaster planning and disaster awareness programs. Part of this involvement is knowing which agents may be used, effects of various agents, emergency care needed by the victims, and personal protection precautions. Many web sites sponsored by the CDC and other official groups provide information about biological warfare and bioterrorism preparation. The web sites provided in the "Resources" section at the end of the chapter are informative resources for the nurse to use professionally and as a resource for clients.

CASE STUDY

A licensed practical nurse works for a physician who is employed by the Indian Health Service at a Navajo reservation. The nurse and physician are not Native American but have worked in the clinic for 8 years and know most of the residents. They have a trusting relationship with the tribal elders and, through them, with the people, many of whom are elderly. Within the past 36 hours, 37 persons have come into the clinic with the following symptoms: vomiting, diarrhea that has become bloody in some cases, dehydration, hallucinations, and fainting. The persons who initially showed symptoms now have hematuria. Two of the first persons who demonstrated symptoms died. The elders are concerned because their people are generally healthy and not had any flu outbreaks or other mass illness in many years. The nurse suspects ricin poisoning.

1. What symptoms led the nurse to her conclusion?
2. What assessment questions would the nurse ask the clients and elders?
3. What precautions would the nurse, physician, and other health care personnel take in caring for the clients?
4. What interventions would the nurse and physician continue for those who are ill?
5. What interventions can be done to prevent others (including health care workers) from becoming ill with the same symptoms?
6. What reassurances could the nurse give to the tribal elders?

SUMMARY

- The three forms of terrorist attacks are biological, chemical, and nuclear.
- Government agencies have expanded and new agencies formed in planning and preparing for the possibility of terrorist attacks.
- Agencies from the federal government to a community hospital prepare for bioterrorists attacks.
- The CDC is one of the major agencies involved in bioterrorist attack preparedness.
- The Joint Commission incorporated terrorist attack preparedness in its survey criteria for health care facilities.
- The major biologic substances expected in terroristic attacks are variola (smallpox), plague, sarin, and ricin.
- Nurses are aware of the symptoms of bioterroristic agents and the emergency care for clients exposed to agents.
- First responders are well trained and know how to protect themselves against contamination and care for the victims of an attack.

REVIEW QUESTIONS

1. The top priority for a first responder following a terrorist attack is:
   1. protecting oneself from contamination.
   2. identifying the agent that was used.
   3. removing uncontaminated persons from the site.
   4. cordoning off the immediate area.
2. The federal agency designated to lead the overall planning effort to upgrade the ability of the United States to respond in a bioterrorist attack is the:
   1. Center for Domestic Preparedness.
   2. U.S. Department of Health and Human Services.
   3. Centers for Disease Control and Prevention.
   4. U.S. Army Corps of Engineers.
3. Biologic agents may be more successful than other types of agents in a terrorist attack because they:
   1. are very effective in small quantities.
   2. are readily available.
   3. are manufactured of volatile ingredients.
   4. provide no protection with immunizations.
4. Clients who receive priority care immediately following a terrorist act are those clients who:
   1. are important to the local governmental structure.
   2. are most seriously injured.
   3. have the greatest chance for survival.
   4. have jobs and contribute positively to society as a whole.

5. The first priority action when a person is exposed to ricin vapors is to:
   1. rinse eyes with plain water.
   2. remove all clothing.
   3. move away from the exposed area.
   4. seek medical assistance.
6. An agency's emergency operations plan must include information about: (Select all that apply.)
   1. who will notify the community agencies involved.
   2. what agent was used in the attack.
   3. notifying family members of a relative's deaths.
   4. how people will be prevented from leaving or entering the agency.
   5. decontamination of any staff needing it.
   6. managing the Strategic National Stockpile.
7. The first priority action when a person is exposed to sarin is to:
   1. remove all clothing and double bag them in a plastic bag.
   2. wash the body with copious amounts of soap and water.
   3. notify the emergency personnel and take the victim to an emergency room.
   4. move to the highest ground where there is fresh air.
8. A bioterrorist released an aerosol in a Chicago subway. Two days later, a client enters the emergency room with a fever and a pustular rash on his face, hands, and soles of the feet. The nurse suspects that the client has smallpox. Her first action is to:
   1. don protective clothing, including gown, gloves, and a special mask.
   2. obtain an order for atropine sulfate.
   3. remove the clothing and wash the client with soap and water.
   4. request an order for smallpox vaccine.
9. A sheep rancher came to the emergency room with a cut on his hand that he received while shearing his sheep 5 days ago. The man stated that the area around the cut has "itched awfully" for the past 3 days. He states that the cut has changed in appearance today. When the nurse exams the cut, he notices that the cut is an ulcerated papular lesion. He suspects the man has:
   1. plague.
   2. been exposed to ricin.
   3. smallpox.
   4. anthrax.
10. The local hospital does not need to stock up on supplies in case of a bioterrorist attack because:
   1. EMEDS is a total package that includes everything necessary to screen and treat clients who need outpatient care.
   2. each facility has an emergency operations plan that would immediately be put into effect to cover the emergency situation.
   3. the Strategic National Stockpile has prepackaged emergency supplies that are stored 12 hours away from every community in the country.
   4. a bioterrorist attack will not occur in the United States with all the security precautions presently in place.

REFERENCES/SUGGESTED READINGS

Agency for Toxic Substances and Disease Registry. (2008) Medical management guidelines for nerve agents: Tuban (GA); sarin (GB); soman (GD); and VX. Department of Health and Human Services. Retrieved September 9, 2008, from http://www.atsdr.cdc.gov/MHMI/mmg166.html

Casey, C., Iskander, J., Roper, M., Mast, E., Wen, X., Torok, T., et al. (2005). Adverse events associated with smallpox vaccination in the United States, January–October 2003. *Journal of the American Medical Association, 294*(21), 2734–2743.

Cava, M., Fay, K., Beanlands, H., McCay, E., & Wignall, R. (2005). Risk perception and compliance with quarantine during the SARS outbreak. *Journal of Nursing Scholarship, 37*(4), 343–347.

Centers for Disease Control and Prevention. (1999). Bioterrorism readiness plan: A template for healthcare facilities. Retrieved November 6, 2008, from http://www.cdc.gov/ncidod/dhqp/pdf/bt/13apr99APIC-CDCBioterrorism.PDF

Centers for Disease Control and Prevention. (2000a, April 21). Biological and chemical terrorism: Strategic plan for preparedness and response. *Morbidity and Mortality Weekly Report, 49*(RR04), 1–14.

Centers for Disease Control and Prevention. (2000b, December 15). Use of anthrax vaccine in the United States. *Morbidity and Mortality Weekly Report, 49*(RR15), 1–20.

Centers for Disease Control and Prevention. (2002a). Message from HHS: Smallpox vaccination. Retrieved November 7, 2008, from http://www.bt.cdc.gov/training/smallpoxvaccine/reactions/message.htm

Centers for Disease Control and Prevention. (2002b, November 15). Notice to readers: Use of anthrax vaccine in response to terrorism: Supplemental recommendations of the advisory committee on immunization practices. *Morbidity and Mortality Weekly Report, 51*(45), 1024–1026.

Centers for Disease Control and Prevention. (2004). Facts about pneumonic plague. Retrieved August 25, 2008, from http://emergency.cdc.gov/agent/plague/factsheet.asp

Centers for Disease Control and Prevention. (2005). NIOSH emergency response card: Cyanogen chloride (ERC506-77-4). Retrieved November 14, 2008, from http://emergency.cdc.gov/agent/cyanide/erc506-77-4pr.asp

Centers for Disease Control and Prevention. (2006a). Facts about Phosgene. Retrieved November 14, 2008, from http://emergency.cdc.gov/agent/phosgene/basics/facts.asp

Centers for Disease Control and Prevention. (2006b). Fact sheet: Anthrax information for health care providers. Retrieved November 8, 2008, from http://www.bt.cdc.gov/agent/anthrax/anthrax-hcp-factsheet.asp

Centers for Disease Control and Prevention. (2006c). NIOSH emergency response card: Hydrogen cyanide (ERC74-90-8). Retrieved November 14, 2008, from http://emergency.cdc.gov/agent/cyanide/erc74-90-8.asp

Centers for Disease Control and Prevention. (2006d). Sarin (GB). Retrieved January 20, 2007, from http://www.bt.cdc.gov/agent/sarin

Centers for Disease Control and Prevention. (2006e). Toxic syndrome description: Vesicant/blister agent poisoning. Retrieved November 13, 2008, from http://www.bt.cdc.gov/agent/vesicants/tsd.asp

Centers for Disease Control and Prevention. (2007a). The history of bioterrorism [Video]. Retrieved November 7, 2008, from http://emergency.cdc.gov/training/historyofbt

Centers for Disease Control and Prevention. (2007b). Smallpox fact sheet: Smallpox disease overview. Retrieved November 7, 2008, from http://emergency.cdc.gov/agent/smallpox/overview/disease-facts.asp

Centers for Disease Control and Prevention. (2007c). Smallpox fact sheet: Vaccine overview. Retrieved November 7, 2008, from http://emergency.cdc.gov/agent/smallpox/vaccination/facts.asp

Centers for Disease Control and Prevention. (2008a). Bioterrorism agents/diseases. Retrieved November 5, 2008, from http://emergency.cdc.gov/agent/agentlist-category.asp

Centers for Disease Control and Prevention. (2008b, March 3). CDC fact sheet: Facts about ricin. Retrieved August 25, 2008, from http://www.bt.cdc.gov/agent/ricin/facts.asp

Centers for Disease Control and Prevention. (2008c). MMWR quick guide: Recommended adult immunization schedule—United States, October 2007–September 2008. Retrieved August 21, 2008, from http://www.cdc.gov/mmwr/pdf/wk/mm5641-Immunization.pdf

Centers for Disease Control and Prevention. (2008d, February 29). Official CDC health advisory: CDC alert on ricin. Retrieved April 24, 2008, from http://www.cdcinfo@cdc.gov

Centers for Disease Control and Prevention. (2008e). Public health preparedness report—Appendix 6. Retrieved November 5, 2008, from http://emergency.cdc.gov/publications/feb08phprep/appendix/appendix6.asp

Center for Disease Control and Prevention. (2009a). Adult immunization schedule. Retrieved June 8, 2009 from http://www. cdc.gov/vaccines/recs/schedules/adult-schedule.htm

Center for Disease Control and Prevention. (2009b). Child and adolescent immunization schedules. Retrieved June 8, 2009 from http://www.cdc.gov/vaccines/recs/schedules/child-schedule.htm#printable

Chettle, C. (2007). Are you prepared for a flu pandemic? *NurseWeek; South Central edition*, 16–19.

Council on Foreign Relations. (2008). Aum Shinrikyo. Retrieved November 13, 2008, from http://www.cfr.org/publication/9238

Department of Homeland Security. (2007, October 9). Fact sheet: National strategy for homeland security. Retrieved April 23, 2008, from http://www.whitehouse.gov/deptofhomeland/analysis

Desenclos, J., & Guillemot, D. (2004, April 23). Consequences of bacterial resistance to antimicrobial. Retrieved August 25, 2008, from http://www.cdc.gov/nicod/EID/index.htm

Eckert, S. (2006). Preparing for disaster: How to plan for the unthinkable. *American Nurse Today, 1*(1), 34–37.

Fauci, A. (2005) Emerging and re-emerging infections diseases: The perpetual challenge. *Academic Medicine, 80*, 1079–1085.

Fox, M. (2008, January 22). Avant works on oral vaccine for plague, anthrax. Retrieved August 25, 2008, from http://www.ph.ucla.edu/epi/bioter/avantoralvaccine.html

Guillemin, J. (2005). *Biological weapons: From the invention of state-sponsored programs to contemporary bioterrorism.* New York: Columbia University Press.

Ignatavicius, D., & Workman, M. (2006). *Medical-surgical nursing: Critical thinking for collaborative care* (5th ed.). St. Louis, MO: Elsevier/Saunders.

Johnson, C. (2003, December 3). Emergency preparedness and bioterrorism fact sheets: Sarin as a chemical terrorist agent. Retrieved August 25, 2008, from http://webserver.health.state.pa.us/health/cwp/view.asp%3Fa%3D171%26Q%3D233572

Joint Commission. (2007). Joint Commission Resources: Environment of Care, Inc. Retrieved August 26, 2008, from http://www.jcrinc.com/26632

Nursing World. (2002, June 30). ANA, HHS establish national nurses response team. Retrieved August 25, 2008, from http://nursingworld.org/Functional MenuCategories/MediaResources/PressReleases/2006

Ohio Department of Health. (2005). Health care facilities and bioterrorism preparedness. Retrieved November 5, 2008, from http://www.odh.ohio.gov/search/search.asp?SearchString=bioterrorism

Pilch, R., & Zilinskas, R. (Eds.). (2005). *Encyclopedia of bioterrorism defense.* Hoboken, NJ: Wiley-Liss.

Salmon, A. (2008). *1995:* Aum Shinrikyo Tokyo subway gas attack. Retrieved November 9, 2008, from http://terrorism.about.com/od/originshistory/a/AumShinrikyo.htm

U.S. Department of Labor. (2008). Biological agents. Retrieved November 5, 2008, from http://www.osha.gov/SLTC/biologicalagents/index.html

Washington State Department of Health. (2008) Chemical agents (DOH Publication No. 821-019). Olympia: Author. Retrieved November 9, 2008, from http://www.doh.wa.gov/phepr/handbook/hbk_pdf/chemical.pdf

RESOURCES

American Nurses Association, http://www.nursingworld.org
American Red Cross, http://www.redcross.org
Centers for Disease Control and Prevention, http://www.cdc.gov
Department of Defense, http://www.defenselink.mil
Department of Homeland Security, http://www.whitehouse.gov/deptofhomeland
Federal Emergency Management Agency, http://www.fema.gov
National Disaster Medical System, http://ndms.dhhs.gov
National Institutes of Health, http://www.nih.gov
National Nurses Response Team, http://nursingworld.org
U.S. Army Medical Research Institute of Chemical Defense, http://chemdef.apgea.army.mil
U.S. Army Surgeon General, http://www.surgeongeneral.gov
U.S. Department of Health and Human Services, http://www.dhhs.gov

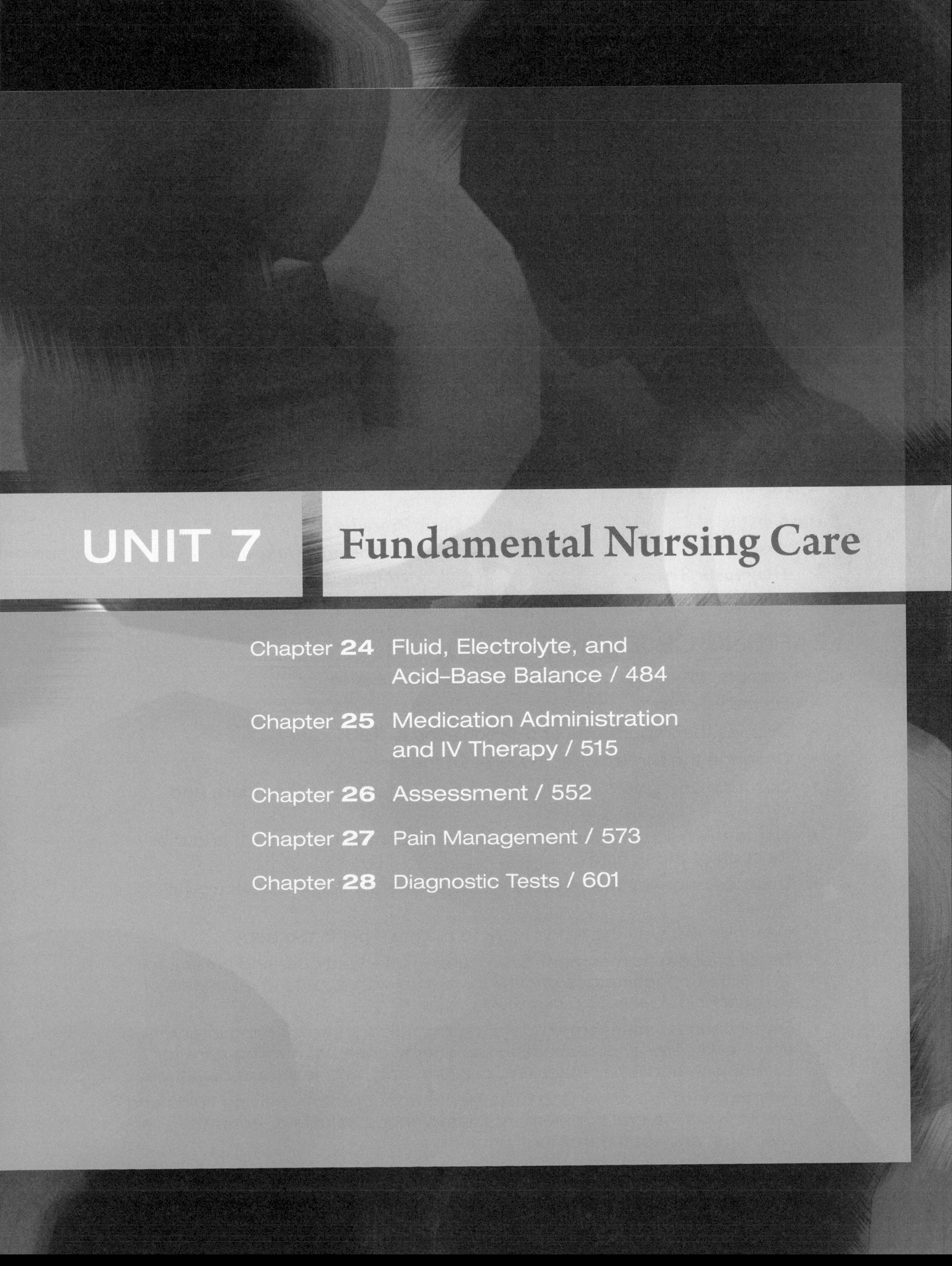

UNIT 7 Fundamental Nursing Care

CHAPTER 24
Fluid, Electrolyte, and Acid–Base Balance

MAKING THE CONNECTION

Refer to the following chapters to increase your understanding of fluid, electrolyte, and acid–base balance:

Basic Nursing
- ***Assessment***
- ***Diagnostic Tests***

Basic Procedures
- ***Measuring Intake and Output***

LEARNING OBJECTIVES

Upon completion of this chapter, you should be able to:

- Define key terms.
- Discuss the importance of pH regulation in the body.
- Describe the three buffer systems of the body.
- Describe and give examples in the body of diffusion, osmosis, and filtration.
- Name the fluid compartments, the fluids contained in them, and the function of those fluids.
- Describe the way the kidneys work to maintain fluid and electrolyte balance.
- Describe the way the lungs work to maintain pH in the body.
- Detail causes, assessment data, nursing interventions, and criteria for evaluating effectiveness of care for clients with a nursing diagnosis of *Deficient Fluid Volume* or *Excess Fluid Volume*.
- Detail causes, assessment data, nursing diagnoses, nursing interventions, and criteria for evaluating the effectiveness of nursing care for clients with sodium, potassium, calcium, and magnesium imbalances.
- Relate principles of nursing management for clients receiving fluids and electrolytes via oral supplements, intravenous solutions, enteral feedings, and total parenteral nutrition.

- Differentiate the causes, assessment data, and nursing management of metabolic and respiratory acidosis and alkalosis.
- Use the nursing process to plan care for a client experiencing a fluid, electrolyte, and/or acid–base imbalance.

KEY TERMS

acid
acidosis
alkalosis
anion
arterial blood gases
atom
base
buffer
cation
compound
crenation
decomposition
dehydration
dialysis
diffusion
edema
electrolyte
element
extracellular fluid
filtration
hemolysis
homeostasis
hydrostatic pressure
hypertonic solution
hypotonic solution
hypoxemia
infiltration
interstitial fluid
intracellular fluid
intravascular fluid
intravenous therapy
ion
isotonic solution
isotope
matter
mixture
molecule
osmolality
osmolarity
osmosis
osmotic pressure
oxidized
permeability
potential hydrogen (pH)
salt
selectively permeable membrane
semipermeable membrane
synthesis
turgor

INTRODUCTION

The external environment within which we live undergoes continual changes, both small and large. For example, the daily and seasonal temperatures may fluctuate over a wide range. The light intensity is bright on sunny days and less so on cloudy days. The humidity may be either high or low. These are just a few of the many factors that constantly change in the external environment. Our bodies must continually adjust to such changes in the external environment. In order for life to continue, however, our internal environment—the one inside our bodies—must remain relatively constant, varying only slightly within narrow ranges. This internal environment consists of the various body fluids such as the fluid inside cells, the blood, tissue fluids that bathe the cells, and other fluids. Maintenance of the internal environment within very narrow limits is termed **homeostasis** (equilibrium).

HOMEOSTASIS

Homeostasis is an ongoing process; that is, the body simply does not reach a state of equilibrium and remain there. Small changes constantly occur in response to physiologic processes. The body must therefore continuously make subtle adjustments to maintain the constancy of the internal environment within a normal range.

Homeostasis is accomplished by various physiologic processes and the coordinated activities of the organ systems. Some examples are as follows:

- The gastrointestinal (GI) system changes large, complex molecules of ingested food to simpler, less complex molecules that can be utilized by the cells of the body to produce the energy necessary for life.
- The respiratory system supplies the cells with the constant source of oxygen required to release the energy from the products of digestion. It also eliminates carbon dioxide, the waste product produced by the cells as a result of energy production.
- The blood acts as a transport mechanism, carrying the products of digestion along with hormones and oxygen to the cells, where these substances are utilized.
- It also transports carbon dioxide from the energy-releasing processes of the cells to the lungs, where it will be eliminated.
- All the activities of the various organ systems are integrated and coordinated through the nervous system and the endocrine system.

When the body loses the ability to maintain homeostasis and the internal environment changes, the physiologic processes can be interrupted or changed, leading to disease, disorder, or death. In essence, then, maintaining homeostasis is essential to life. Because the processes of homeostasis involve many chemical and physical processes, it is necessary to examine some of these before studying homeostasis in more detail.

CHEMICAL ORGANIZATION

The human body is highly organized. This organization exists in increasing levels of complexity. Most basic is the chemical level. To understand the higher levels of organization, it is necessary to know something about basic chemical and physical principles.

ELEMENTS

The cell consists of living matter. **Matter** is anything that occupies space and possesses mass. All matter has certain physical properties such as color, odor, hardness, and density. Matter also has extensive properties such as size, shape, and weight. Matter is composed of basic substances called **elements**. Elements are made of tiny units called atoms. Atoms of each element are alike. Different elements have different kinds of atoms. Presently, 112 elements are recognized. Some examples are iron, gold, carbon, hydrogen, oxygen, nitrogen, and copper. Many of the elements occur in the human body in varying amounts. Some are present in large amounts, and others are found in only trace amounts. The four elements oxygen, carbon, hydrogen, and nitrogen constitute more than 95% of the total body weight of the elements. Some of the elements and their function in the body are presented in Table 24-1.

TABLE 24-1 Elements Occurring in the Human Body

ELEMENT	APPROXIMATE % OF BODY WEIGHT	FUNCTION
Major Elements		
Oxygen (O)	65.0	Found in both organic and inorganic compounds; as a gas, is necessary in metabolizing glucose and other chemical compounds into energy
Carbon (C)	18.5	Found in all organic compounds such as carbohydrates, protein, lipids, and nucleic acids; necessary for cellular respiration
Hydrogen (H)	9.5	Found in many organic and inorganic compounds; in ionic form, involved in pH; component of water; necessary for life
Nitrogen (N)	3.2	Important in proteins, which are the body's building blocks, an energy source, and a component of hormones
Calcium (Ca)	1.5	Important element in bone and tooth composition; involved in nerve conduction, muscle contraction, and blood clotting
Phosphorus (P)	1.0	Found in bones, teeth, the high-energy carrying compound adenosine triphosphatase (ATP), some proteins, and nucleic acid
Potassium (K)	0.4	Major electrolyte in intracellular fluid; important in muscle contraction and transmission of nerve impulses; activates enzymes; influences cellular osmotic pressure; involved in kidney function and acid–base balance
Sulfur (S)	0.3	Found in some proteins, nucleic acids, and some vitamins and hormones
Sodium (Na)	0.2	Constitutes major electrolyte in extracellular fluid; important in osmoregulation and acid–base balance; necessary for nerve transmission and muscle contraction
Chlorine (Cl)	0.2	Found in extracellular fluid; important in water balance, acid–base balance, and production of hydrochloric acid in the stomach
Magnesium (Mg)	0.1	Important to muscle and nerve function and bone formation and in some coenzymes
Essential Trace Elements		
Present in the human body in minimal amounts, constituting approximately 0.1% of body weight; have known functions		
Cobalt (Co)		Important component of vitamin B_{12}
Copper (Cu)		Necessary for formation of hemoglobin and for bone development
Chromium (Cr)		A cofactor involved with enzymes for fat, cholesterol, and glucose metabolism
Fluorine (F)		Gives hardness to teeth and bones
Iodine (I)		Necessary for synthesis of thyroid hormone
Iron (Fe)		Necessary for transportation of oxygen by hemoglobin
Manganese (Mn)		Necessary in activating some enzymes
Selenium (Se)		Acts with vitamin E as an antioxidant; component of teeth
Zinc (Zn)		Found in some enzymes; needed for protein metabolism and carbon dioxide transport
Other Trace Elements		
Have probable, but as yet undetected, functions		
Aluminum (Al) Nickel (Ni) Arsenic (As) Tin (Sn) Boron (B) Silicon (Si) Cadmium (Cd) Vanadium (V)		

ATOMS

An **atom** is the smallest unit of chemical structure, and no chemical change can alter it. Atoms are made up of three basic particles: protons, neutrons, and electrons. Protons and neutrons are similar in size, but whereas protons have a positive electrical charge, neutrons have no charge. Together, they form the nucleus of the atom. Because the protons have a positive charge and the neutrons are neutral, the nucleus of an atom has a positive charge. The electrons have a negative charge and move in an orbit around the nucleus. There are as many electrons as protons, rendering the overall atom neutral. The number of protons in an atom is called its atomic number. The simplest element is hydrogen. It has an atomic number of 1. One proton with a positive charge forms the nucleus, and one electron moves in an orbit around the nucleus. Hydrogen atoms may or may not have a neutron. A hydrogen atom is illustrated in Figure 24-1.

Depending on the element, other atoms may have more than one proton and one electron and may have neutrons. The number of protons and neutrons in the nucleus is approximately equal to the atomic weight. Thus, hydrogen has an atomic weight of 1.

Isotopes

The number of protons in the nucleus is the same for all atoms of a given element, but the number of neutrons may vary in atoms of the same element. For instance, all hydrogen atoms have one proton and one electron; however, some hydrogen atoms have one neutron in the nucleus, while others have two (Figure 24-2). Atoms of the same element that have different atomic weights (i.e., have a different number of neutrons) are called **isotopes**. All the isotopes of a given element react the same way chemically.

Some isotopes, called radioactive isotopes, have an unstable nucleus, which decomposes and gives off energy in the form of radiation. This radiation can be in the form of alpha, beta, or gamma rays. All are damaging to cells. Alpha radiation is the least harmful, and gamma radiation is the most harmful. Iodine, oxygen, and cobalt are examples of elements having radioactive isotopes. Some of the radioactive isotopes are useful as biological markers and can be used to track metabolic pathways of food. Others such as iodine^{131} can be injected into the body and used to track the circulation of blood. Still others such as cobalt^{60} are used in cancer treatment.

MOLECULES AND COMPOUNDS

Atoms of the same element can unite with each other to form a **molecule**. For example, atoms of hydrogen unite to form a

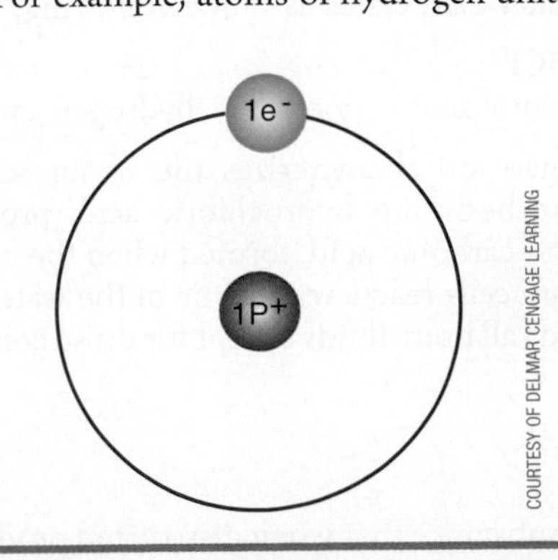

FIGURE 24-1 Hydrogen Atom Showing Positively Charged Proton in the Nucleus and Negatively Charged Electron in Orbit

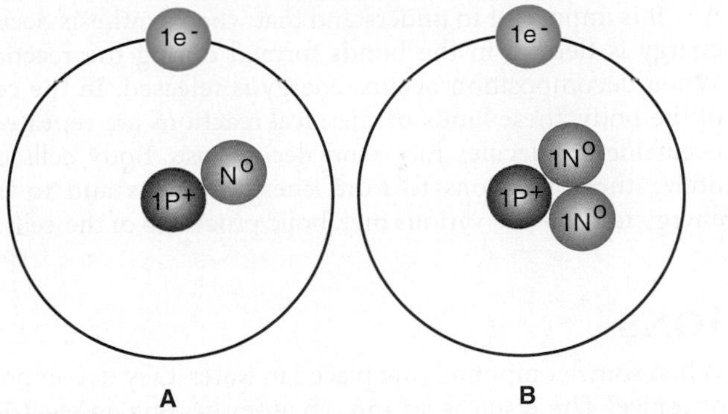

FIGURE 24-2 Isotopes of Hydrogen; *A*, Deuteridium has one positively charged proton and one neutron in the nucleus and one electron in orbit; *B*, Tritium has one positively charged proton and two neutrons in the nucleus and one electron in orbit.

hydrogen molecule. This can be expressed in a chemical equation using the chemical symbol for hydrogen:

$$H + H \rightarrow H_2$$

In this reaction, the atoms on the left are the reactants, the arrow is read as "yield," and the last symbol is the product—a molecule of hydrogen. A chemical equation uses the chemical symbols of elements and shows the ratios by which they combine. Because atoms of elements always combine in the same ratio under similar conditions, it is possible to predict the nature of a chemical change.

When atoms of two or more different elements combine (react), they form a **compound**. For example, if one atom of sodium (Na) and one atom of chlorine (Cl) react, they form a molecule of the compound called sodium chloride. This is expressed in the following equation:

$$Na + Cl \rightarrow NaCl$$

Compounds can be divided into two groups. Those without carbon are inorganic compounds, and those with carbon are organic compounds. By using chemical equations, chemical changes, called reactions, can be shown. Sometimes, different substances are combined in no specific way, and the components do not have a definite ratio every time. For instance, water, sugar, and table salt mixed without being measured will yield different results depending on the ratio of each substance. Such a combination is called a **mixture**. Its composition may vary each time the components are mixed.

Chemical reactions occur whenever atoms join together or separate. They join together by forming bonds, and they separate by breaking bonds. Either way, new combinations result. When two or more atoms (reactants) bond and form a more complex molecular product, the reaction is called **synthesis**. A sample equation would be as follows:

$$\underset{\text{hydrogen and}}{2H} + \underset{\text{oxygen}}{O} \underset{\text{yields}}{\rightarrow} \underset{\text{water}}{H_2O}$$

When the bonding between the atoms in a molecule is broken and simpler products are formed, the reaction is called **decomposition**. If a molecule of sodium chloride is decomposed, it forms sodium and chlorine. This can be expressed as follows:

$$\underset{\text{sodium chloride}}{NaCl} \underset{\text{yields}}{\rightarrow} \underset{\text{sodium and}}{Na} + \underset{\text{chloride}}{Cl}$$

(decomposition)

It is important to understand that when synthesis occurs, energy is tied up in the bonds formed during the reaction. When decomposition occurs, energy is released. In the cells of the body, these kinds of chemical reactions are repeatedly occurring: Molecules form and decompose. Body cells can utilize these reactions to form energy sources and to free energy to drive the various metabolic processes of the cells.

IONS

When some compounds are placed in water, they decompose, or ionize. The result is an **ion**, an atom bearing an electrical charge. An ion with a positive charge is called a **cation**; an ion with a negative charge is termed an **anion**. For example, sodium chloride in water dissociates to form sodium ions bearing a positive charge and chloride ions bearing a negative charge (Figure 24-3). Because the atoms in this combination are charged, they will conduct electricity. The reaction can be shown as follows:

NaCl	$\rightarrow$	Na^+ + Cl^-
sodium chloride	yields	sodium (cation) and chloride (anion)

A compound that dissociates into ions in water is called an **electrolyte**. Many electrolytes are extremely important in body chemistry.

WATER

Water constitutes approximately 60% of the total body weight of an adult and is involved in many of the physical and physiological processes of the body. Because water is so integral to the body's processes, fluctuations in the amount of water in the body can have harmful or even fatal consequences.

Water is the major component of blood. Approximately 92% of the body's organic and inorganic compounds dissolve in this water into less complex molecules and atoms and then are transported throughout the body. Necessary substances such as oxygen and nutrients from the GI system are carried to the cells, where they are utilized. Cellular waste products such as carbon dioxide, urea, and excessive minerals are carried by water to sites of elimination: carbon dioxide to the lungs and urea and minerals to the kidneys.

Water also absorbs heat resulting from muscle contractions and distributes this heat over the body. Water in the form of perspiration released from sweat glands in the skin can cool the body by evaporation. Water also can break apart the bonds in large molecules such as starches to form smaller molecules in the digestive process. This type of reaction is called *hydration*.

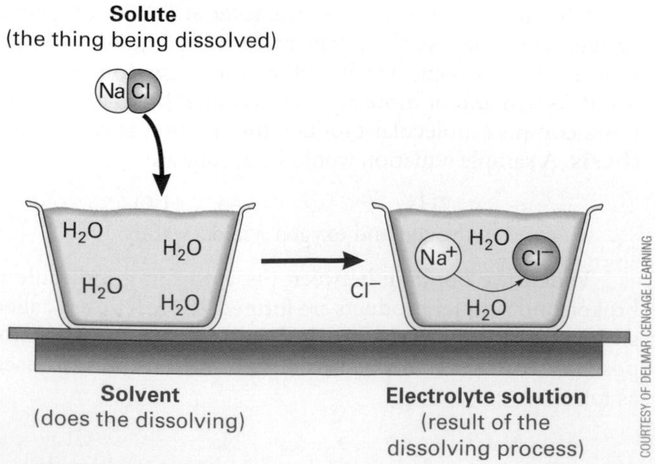

FIGURE 24-3 Dissociation of Electrolytes

LIFE SPAN CONSIDERATIONS

Body Water and Body Size

The amount of body water is inversely proportional to body size. The smaller the body, the higher the water content:

Embryo:	97%
Infant:	70% to 80%
Child:	60% to 77%
Adult:	60%
Older Adult:	45% to 55%

Body water diminishment in older adults is related to tissue loss.

GASES

Two important gases in the body are oxygen (O_2) and carbon dioxide (CO_2). Because these elements are gases, their molecules are free and can move swiftly in all directions. Oxygen enters the body through the lungs and is transported by the red blood cells throughout the body to the cells. The cells use oxygen in the release of energy from glucose and other molecules. This energy is needed by the cells to carry out their activities. As a result of the energy-releasing processes, carbon dioxide is produced by the cells and transported in the blood to the lungs, where it is eliminated.

ACIDS, BASES, SALTS, AND pH

Other chemical substances important for life are acids, bases, and salts; pH is the measure of acid and base strength.

ACIDS

An **acid** is any substance that in solution yields hydrogen ions bearing a positive charge. As an example, hydrochloric acid (HCl) in water dissociates as shown following:

HCl	$\rightarrow$	H^+ + Cl^-
hydrochloric acid	yields	hydrogen and chloride

The hydrogen ion characterizes this as an acid. Important acids in the body are hydrochloric acid, produced in the stomach, and carbonic acid, formed when the carbon dioxide released from cells reacts with some of the water in the extracellular fluid (all body fluids except for those contained within the cells).

BASES

A **base** is a substance that when dissociated produces ions that will combine with hydrogen ions. For example, when sodium hydroxide dissociates in water, it forms a sodium ion bearing a positive charge and a hydroxyl ion bearing a negative charge as shown following:

NaOH	$\rightarrow$	Na^+	+	OH^-
sodium hydroxide	yields	sodium	and	hydroxyl

The hydroxyl ion is capable of combining with a hydrogen ion to form water. Sodium bicarbonate is an example of a base found in the body.

Salts

A **salt** is formed when an acid and a base react with each other. Salts result from the neutralization of an acid by a base, as illustrated by the following reaction:

HCl	+	NaOH	$\rightarrow$	H_2O	+	NaCl
hydrochloric acid	and	sodium hydroxide	yields	water	and	sodium chloride

The hydrochloric acid reacts with the sodium hydroxide to form a molecule of water and a molecule of a salt—sodium chloride. When salts are placed in water, they dissociate into a cation and an anion. For instance, in water, the sodium chloride would dissociate into Na^+ and Cl^-. One reason salts are of great biological importance is that many of the compounds that dissociate into ions in living cells are salts. For example, sodium and chlorine ions are present in great amounts in body fluids. Many other salts occur in lesser amounts.

pH

Acid and bases are classified as either strong or weak by the number of hydrogen ions or hydroxyl ions they produce when they dissociate. Strong acids release many hydrogen ions; weak acids release relatively few. The same is true of hydroxyl ions in strong and weak bases. The acidity or alkalinity of a solution is determined by the concentration of hydrogen ions in the solution. **Potential hydrogen (pH)** indicates the hydrogen ion concentration in a solution, expressed as a number from 0 to 14. A solution with a pH of 7 is neutral (i.e., it is neither an acid nor a base). A solution with a pH greater than 7 is a base, or alkaline. A solution with a pH less than 7 is an acid. The higher above 7 the pH, the more alkaline the solution; the lower below 7 the pH, the more acid the solution. pH is of great biological importance. The human body can tolerate only very slight changes in pH. For example, the pH of human blood ranges from 7.35 to 7.45 (Figure 24-4). Blood pH above or below this range can cause severe or even fatal physiological problems.

Although small amounts of acids may enter the body through food intake, the greatest source of acids—and thus H^+ ions—is cellular metabolism, resulting in products including lactic acid, phosphoric acid, pyruvic acid, and many fatty acids. When blood pH falls below 7.35 as a result of an elevated concentration of H^+ ions, **acidosis** occurs. Rarely does blood pH fall to 7 or become acidic because death will usually occur first. As acidosis increases, the central nervous system (CNS) becomes involved, and the client may become unconscious. The heartbeat may become weak and irregular, and blood pressure may decrease or even disappear.

When blood pH increases above 7.45, **alkalosis** occurs. Alkalosis is a condition characterized by an excessive loss of hydrogen ions. This happens less often than does acidosis. Symptoms of alkalosis include a heightened state of nervous system activity, resulting in spasmodic muscle contractions, convulsions, and even death.

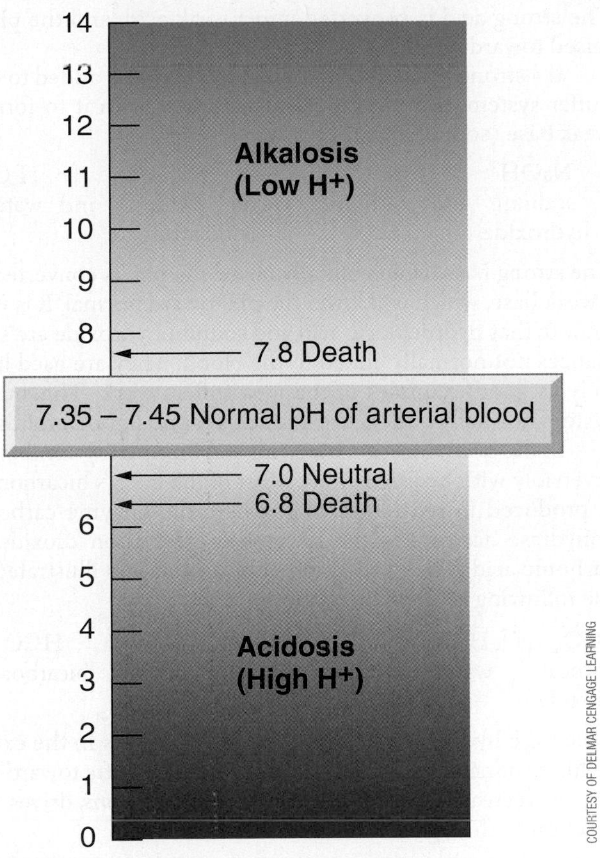

FIGURE 24-4 The pH of human blood ranges from 7.35 to 7.45.

BUFFERS

Buffers are substances that attempt to maintain pH range, or H^+ ion concentration, in the presence of added acids or bases. Buffers usually occur in pairs in the body fluids. They act to keep the pH of body fluids within normal range. If body fluids become acidic, buffers in the body fluids combine with the excess hydrogen ions and restore normal pH. Likewise, if the body fluids become alkaline, other buffers in the blood combine with the strong bases, converting them to weak bases and restoring normal pH.

Three important buffer systems occur in body fluids: the bicarbonate buffer system, the phosphate buffer system, and the protein buffer system. Because a change in pH of one fluid may bring corresponding changes in the pH of other fluids, an interplay between buffer systems acts to maintain the body's pH. The buffer systems react quickly to prevent excessive changes in the hydrogen ion concentration.

Bicarbonate Buffer System

The bicarbonate buffer system is found in both the extracellular and intracellular fluids and is the body's primary buffer system. It has two components: carbonic acid (H_2CO_3) and sodium bicarbonate ($NaHCO_3$). When a strong acid such as hydrochloric acid is added to this buffer system, the acid will react with the sodium bicarbonate and form a weaker acid (carbonic acid) and a salt (sodium chloride).

HCl	+	$NaHCO_3$	$\rightarrow$	H_2CO_3	+	NaCl
hydrochloric acid	and	sodium bicarbonate	yields	carbonic acid	and	sodium chloride

The strong acid is converted into a weak acid, and the pH is raised toward normal.

If a strong base such as sodium hydroxide is added to this buffer system, the carbonic acid will react with it to form a weak base (sodium bicarbonate) and water.

NaOH	+	H_2CO_3	$\rightarrow$	$NaHCO_3$	+	H_2O
sodium hydroxide	and	carbonic acid	yields	sodium bicarbonate	and	water

The strong base, which initially raised the pH, is converted to a weak base, which will lower the pH toward normal. It is vital to note that hydrochloric acid and sodium hydroxide are substances not normally added to the blood. They are used here only as good examples of the way buffers work. This buffer system normally buffers organic acids found in body fluids.

In the body, bicarbonate helps stabilize pH by combining reversibly with hydrogen ions. Most of the body's bicarbonate is produced in red blood cells, where the enzyme carbonic anhydrase accelerates the conversion of carbon dioxide to carbonic acid. The production of bicarbonate is illustrated in the following reversible equation:

CO_2	+	H_2O	$\leftrightarrow$	H_2CO_3	$\leftrightarrow$	H^+	+	HCO_3^-
carbon dioxide		water		carbonic acid		hydrogen		bicarbonate

When the hydrogen ion concentration increases in the extracellular (outside the cell) space, the reaction shifts toward the left. A decreased concentration of hydrogen ions drives the reaction to the right.

PHOSPHATE BUFFER SYSTEM

The phosphate buffer system is involved in regulating the pH of intracellular fluid and the fluid of the kidney tubules. It has two phosphate compounds: sodium monohydrogen phosphate ($NaHPO_4$) and sodium dihydrogen phosphate (NaH_2PO_4). In the presence of a strong acid such as hydrochloric acid, the sodium monohydrogen phosphate reacts with the acid to form a weak acid (sodium dihydrogen phosphate) and a salt (sodium chloride), thus raising the pH.

HCl	+	$NaHPO_4$	$\rightarrow$	NaH_2PO_4	+	NaCl
hydrochloric acid	and	sodium monohydrogen phosphate	yields	sodium dihydrogen phosphate	and	sodium chloride

When sodium dihydrogen phosphate encounters a strong base such as sodium hydroxide, a weak base (sodium monohydrogen phosphate) and water are formed.

NaOH	+	NaH_2PO_4	$\rightarrow$	$NaHPO_4$	+	H_2O
sodium hydroxide	and	sodium dihydrogen phosphate	yields	sodium monohydrogen phosphate	and	water

PROTEIN BUFFERS

Proteins are complex substances formed when amino acids bond. Each amino acid contains a carboxyl group (COOH) and an amino group (NH_2). The carboxyl group can ionize and release hydrogen, thus acting as an acid. The amino group can accept hydrogen, thus acting as a base. This ability allows proteins to act as a buffer system. The protein buffer system is found inside cells, especially in the hemoglobin of red blood cells, where the proteins can act to maintain the pH inside the cell. They are also found in the plasma.

SUBSTANCE MOVEMENT

Substances must be able to both enter and leave cells. For example, oxygen and various end products of digestion must enter a cell through the cell membrane for use by the cell. Waste products from cellular processes must be eliminated from the cell. Various ions must also both enter and leave cells. Everything that enters and leaves the cell must pass through the cell membrane. Thus, the cell membrane serves not only as an envelope around the cell but also as a gatekeeper, regulating which substances can enter and leave the cell. The cell membrane is a very thin and delicate, but complex and living, elastic covering around each cell. It consists of an inner and outer layer of phospholipids in which protein molecules are embedded. Many small channels pass through the membrane. These channels allow some water molecules and some water-soluble substances to pass through the membrane. The ability of a membrane to permit substances to pass through it is called **permeability**. Because a cell membrane allows passage of only certain substances, it is called a **selectively permeable membrane**. An artificial membrane such as cellophane is known as a **semipermeable membrane** (Kee, Paulanka, & Polek, 2010).

Some substances can pass through the cell membrane without energy expenditure on the part of the cell. This is called passive transport. The passage of other substances requires an expenditure of energy by the cell. This is called active transport.

PASSIVE TRANSPORT

There are several types of passive transport: diffusion, osmosis, and filtration.

Diffusion

Diffusion is the tendency of molecules of either gases, liquids, or solids to move from a region of higher molecular concentration to a region of lower molecular concentration until an equilibrium is reached. This movement is caused by the kinetic energy in molecules. Kinetic energy causes the molecules to move constantly, colliding with one another and knocking each other about, thus causing them to move farther apart. An example is a drop of black ink placed in a glass of water; over time, the glass of water will turn a uniform black color because of diffusion, as shown in Figure 24-5.

In the body, oxygen moves by diffusion from the lungs to the bloodstream because the oxygen concentration is higher in the lungs and lower in the blood. Carbon dioxide moves by diffusion from the bloodstream, where the concentration of carbon dioxide is higher, to the lungs, for elimination. The size of

CRITICAL THINKING

Substance Movement: Class Activity

During class, place a tea bag into a glass of warm water. Allow time for the students to record their observations. Ask the students to write an explanation of which type(s) of substance movement occurred using the correct terminology (Science Spot, 2009). For more class activity ideas, visit http://sciencespot.net/index.html.

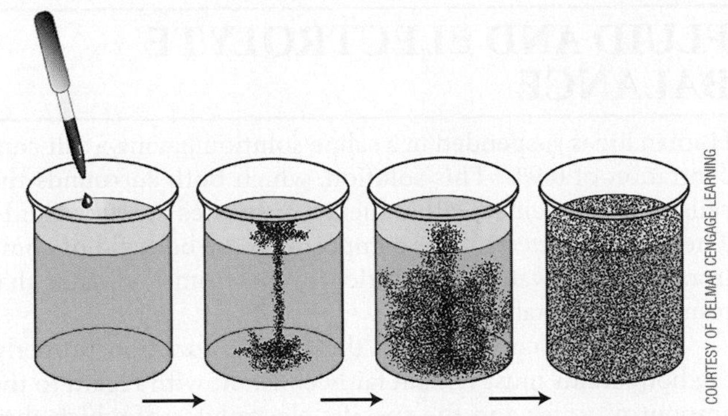

FIGURE 24-5 Diffusion is the spreading of particles from an area of greater concentration to an area of lesser concentration. Dye put into a beaker of water gradually spreads throughout the water.

the channels in the cell membrane can prevent large molecules from passing through the membrane. Some substances, such as glucose molecules, combine with carrier molecules, which carry them into the interior of the cell, where they are released.

The term **dialysis** is used when diffusion is employed to separate molecules out of a solution by passing them through a semipermeable membrane. Dialysis is the process used in the artificial kidney. As blood from a client circulates through a machine, small, toxic waste molecules such as urea leave the blood and pass through the semipermeable membrane by diffusion and out into the surrounding fluid. The blood, thus cleaned, is then returned to the body.

Osmosis

Osmosis is the diffusion of water through a semipermeable membrane from a region of higher water concentration to a region of lower water concentration. In a solution undergoing osmosis, only the water (solvent) molecules move through the membrane; the dissolved molecules do not (Figure 24-6).

If a cell, having both a membrane that will not allow sodium chloride to pass through and a molecular concentration of 10% sodium chloride, were placed in a container with a 5% sodium chloride solution, the cell would contain 10% sodium chloride and 90% water, and the 5% solution in which it was placed would contain 5% dissolved sodium chloride and 95% water. There would be more water outside than inside the cell; thus, water would pass through the membrane into the cell. Because the cell membrane is elastic, the cell would increase in size as a result of the water accumulation within it facilitated by the process of osmosis. The pressure exerted against the cell membrane by the water inside the cell is called **osmotic pressure**.

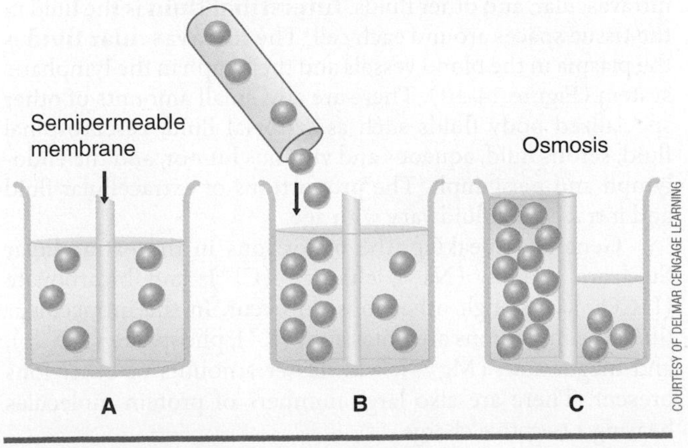

FIGURE 24-6 The process of osmosis.

A solution that has the same molecular concentration as the cell is called an **isotonic solution**. It neither increases nor decreases the size of the cell. A solution that has a lower molecular concentration than the cell is called a **hypotonic solution**. Placing cells in a hypotonic solution causes them to swell, possibly to the point of eventual rupture. The rupture of red blood cells due to osmosis is called **hemolysis**. As red blood cells swell, the hemoglobin contained within passes to the outside of the cell and into the solution surrounding the cell, rendering the blood cells no longer capable of carrying oxygen. A solution that has a higher molecular concentration than the cell is called a **hypertonic solution**. When placed in such a solution, water leaves the cell, and the cell decreases in size. In the case of red blood cells, they shrivel and become wrinkled. This shrinkage, called **crenation**, leaves the cells incapable of functioning.

In persons who have lost large volumes of blood, it is sometimes necessary to administer additional fluids to maintain blood pressure. Generally, normal saline can be used. This 0.9% sodium chloride solution has approximately the same osmotic concentration as blood. Because it is isotonic, it will not damage the cells. Figure 24-7 shows osmosis in cells with different solution concentrations.

Filtration

In **filtration**, fluids and the substances dissolved in them are forced through cell membranes by **hydrostatic pressure**—the pressure the fluid exerts against the membrane. The molecules passing through the membrane are determined by

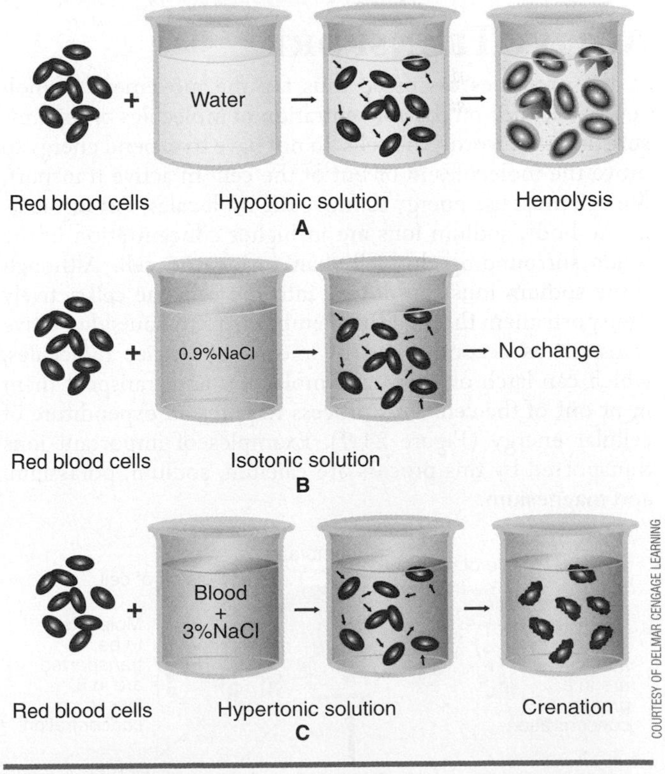

FIGURE 24-7 Osmosis is the movement of water through a membrane from an area of lower concentration to one of higher concentration. *A,* In a hypotonic solution, the water moves into the cells, causing them to swell and burst. *B,* In an isotonic solution, cells are normal in size and shape because the same amount of water is entering and leaving the cells. *C,* In a hypertonic solution, cells are losing water because water moves from an area of lower concentration (inside the cell) to an area of higher concentration (outside the cell).

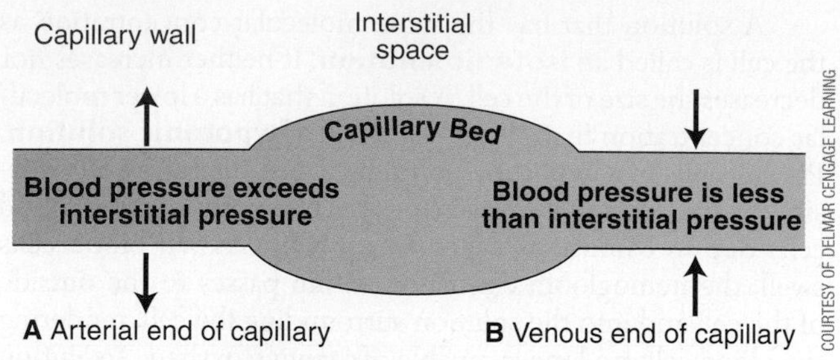

FIGURE 24-8 Filtration; *A*, Pressure in the arteriole is greater then interstitial (between the cells) pressure, causing fluid with dissolved substances to move out of capillaries. *B*, Pressure in venules is less than interstitial fluid pressure, causing fluid and waste products to move back into the capillaries.

the size of the pores in the membrane. Tissue fluids are formed by filtration. As blood passes through the capillaries, hydrostatic pressure exerted by the pumping action of the heart causes some of the liquid fraction of the blood (but not the cells) to pass out of the capillaries, resulting in formation of the tissue fluid (Figure 24-8). As the blood circulates through the capillaries of the kidneys, the hydrostatic pressure of the blood causes many materials to leave the blood through the filtration process. These materials pass into the tubules of the kidneys, where the toxic waste products are removed to form urine. The urine is then eliminated from the body.

ACTIVE TRANSPORT

In the processes discussed thus far, the movement of molecules depends on the concentration of molecules or on pressure. In other words, the cells do not have to expend energy to move the molecules in or out of the cell. In active transport, the cell must use energy to move the molecules. For instance, in the body, sodium ions are in higher concentration in the fluids surrounding the cell than inside the cell. Although some sodium ions can diffuse into the cell, the cell actively transports them through the membrane to the outside. Active transport is accomplished by means of carrier molecules, which can latch onto specific molecules and transport them in or out of the cell. This process requires an expenditure of cellular energy (Figure 24-9). Examples of important ions transported by this process are calcium, sodium, potassium, and magnesium.

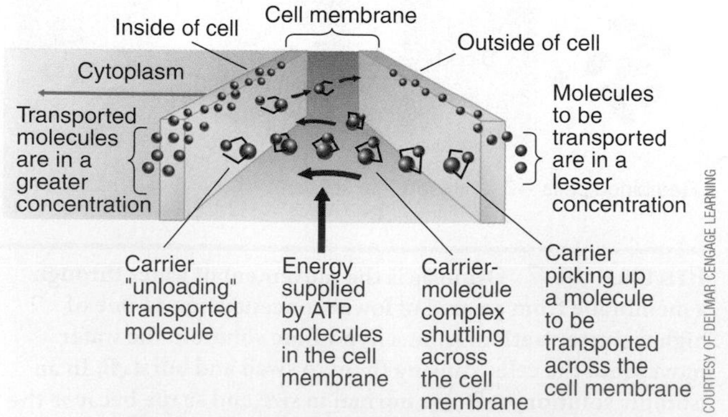

FIGURE 24-9 Active Transport of Molecules from an Area of Lesser Concentration to an Area of Greater Concentration

FLUID AND ELECTROLYTE BALANCE

Human life is suspended in a saline solution having a salt concentration of 0.9%. This solution, which both surrounds the cells and is contained within them, constitutes the body fluids. The water and electrolytes composing these body fluids come from ingested water and nutrients, and from the water that results from metabolism.

For life to continue and the cells to function properly, the body fluids must remain fairly constant with regard to the amount of water and the specific electrolytes of which they are composed. Water is essential because it is the basic component of all the body fluids. Water is involved in many of the metabolic processes in the body and is a by-product of some of these reactions. The various electrolytes all have essential roles in cellular physiological processes. If some of either is lost, it must be replaced, and if either water or an electrolyte is in excess, it must be removed. Maintaining the consistency of this fluid environment is homeostasis.

For cells to survive and carry out their multitude of physiologic functions, they need both a continuing source of water, nutrients, and oxygen and a mechanism to remove cellular wastes. These physiologic processes affect the amount of water, the pH, and the ions both inside and outside the cells. A balance must be maintained between the components of the fluids inside and outside the cell. Because the ions are dissolved in water, these two components are tied together: Anything affecting the amount of water in the body will affect the ion concentration.

BODY FLUIDS

Much of the body weight of an average adult is due to the water in the body fluids surrounding the cells and contained within them. The fluid around the cells cushions them and serves as the medium of exchange. Everything that enters or leaves the cells must pass through this fluid layer.

There are two kinds of body fluids. They can be thought of as being contained within two separate containers, called compartments. The **intracellular fluid** (ICF) compartment contains all the water and ions inside the cells. By far the largest amount of water in the body, approximately 65%, is found within this compartment.

The extracellular fluid compartment contains the remaining body fluids, called **extracellular fluid** (ECF), or fluid outside the cells. These can be further subdivided into interstitial, intravascular, and other fluids. **Interstitial fluid** is the fluid in the tissue spaces around each cell. The **intravascular fluid** is the plasma in the blood vessels and the lymph in the lymphatic system (Figure 24-10). There are also small amounts of other specialized body fluids such as synovial fluid, cerebrospinal fluid, serous fluid, aqueous and vitreous humor, and the endolymph and perilymph. The proportions of extracellular fluid and intracellular fluid vary with age.

Generally speaking, the major ions in the extracellular fluid are sodium (Na^+), chloride (Cl^-), and bicarbonate (HCO_3^-), although other ions do occur. In the intracellular fluid, the major ions are potassium (K^+), phosphate (PO_4^{--}), and magnesium (Mg^{++}), with lesser amounts of other ions present. There are also large numbers of protein molecules bearing a negative charge.

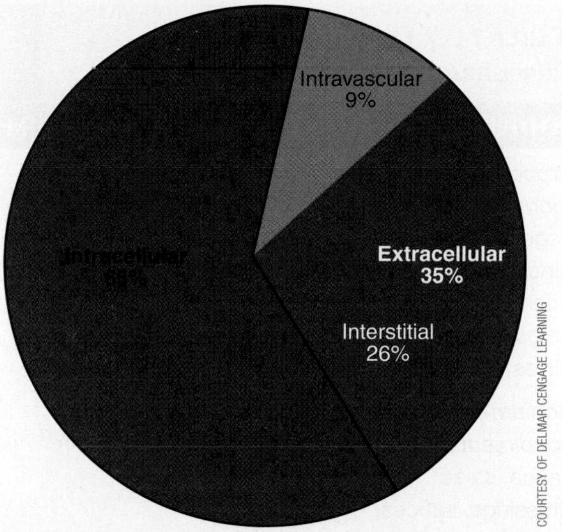

FIGURE 24-10 Body Fluid Compartments of an Adult

EXCHANGE BETWEEN THE EXTRACELLULAR AND INTRACELLULAR FLUIDS

Water and ions moving between the extracellular and intracellular fluids must first pass through the selectively permeable cell membrane. This movement is governed primarily by osmosis. Diffusion and active transport also play a role.

The difference in the ion concentration inside the cell and outside the cell is due primarily to the cell's ability to pump some ions inside and pump others out. If the intracellular fluid becomes hypertonic to the extracellular fluid, water from the extracellular fluid will move by osmosis into the cell to restore the balance and vice versa.

A fluid balance also occurs between the interstitial fluid and the plasma. This balance is regulated primarily by hydrostatic pressure (blood pressure) and osmotic pressure. When the circulating blood passes from the arterioles into the capillaries, the pressure in the capillaries is higher than that in the interstitial fluid. This forces some of the water from the plasma out of the capillaries and into the interstitial fluid. Because of osmotic pressure, some of the water in the interstitial fluid is forced back into the capillaries in the area where they join the venules. Some water is also returned to the bloodstream through the lymphatic system. If the amount of interstitial fluid returned to the circulatory system lessens and the fluid accumulates in the tissue spaces, the tissues become swollen. This condition is called **edema**. Several conditions can cause edema, including kidney or liver disease and heart disorders. Many of these conditions can have serious consequences.

When more water is lost from the body than is replaced, **dehydration** occurs. Among the various causes of dehydration are water deprivation, excessive urine production, profuse sweating, diarrhea, and extended periods of vomiting. As water is lost, the amount of water in the interstitial fluid decreases. Water then moves from the cells to the tissue spaces by osmosis, causing an electrolyte imbalance. Circulatory impairment occurs, which in turn affects the kidney's ability to function normally. This condition is corrected by supplying water and the appropriate electrolytes.

REGULATORS OF FLUID AND ELECTROLYTE BALANCE

There must be a balance in the amounts of fluids and electrolytes consumed and lost daily. Under typical conditions, the average adult loses some water through the skin, lungs, and GI tract and loses the largest amount of water through urine production. This can amount to a per-day fluid loss of approximately 2,500 mL, depending on conditions.

Skin

In the average adult, an estimated water loss of 300 to 500 mL per day occurs by diffusion through the skin. Because the person is not aware of this water loss, it is called *insensible loss*. Water is also lost through the skin by perspiration. The total amount of water lost through perspiration varies depending on environmental factors and body temperature.

Lungs

In the average adult, an estimated insensible water loss of 400 to 500 mL per day occurs with expired air, which is saturated with water vapor. This amount varies with the rate and depth of respirations.

Gastrointestinal Tract

Although a large amount of fluid—approximately 8,000 mL per day in the average adult—is secreted into the gastrointestinal tract, almost all of this fluid is reabsorbed by the body. In adults, approximately 200 mL of water are lost per day in feces. Severe diarrhea can cause a fluid and electrolyte deficit because the GI fluids contain a large amount of electrolytes.

Kidneys

The kidneys play a major role in maintaining fluid balance by excreting 1,000 to 1,500 mL of water per day in the average adult. The excretion of water by healthy kidneys is proportional to the fluid ingested and the amount of waste or solutes excreted.

When an extracellular fluid volume deficit occurs, hormones play a key role in restoring the extracellular fluid volume. Release of the following hormones into circulation causes the kidneys to conserve water:

- *Antidiuretic hormone (ADH)*. Released by the posterior pituitary gland; acts on the distal tubules of the kidneys to reabsorb water.
- *Aldosterone*. Produced in the adrenal cortex; causes the reabsorption of sodium from the renal tubules, leading to water retention in the extracellular fluid, thereby increasing its volume.
- *Renin*. Released by the juxtaglomerular cells of the kidneys; promotes vasoconstriction and the release of aldosterone.

The interaction of these hormones with regard to renal functions serves as the body's compensatory mechanism to maintain homeostasis.

Sodium is the main electrolyte that promotes the retention of water. An intravascular water deficit causes the renal tubules to reabsorb more sodium into circulation. Because water molecules go with the sodium ions, the intravascular water deficit is corrected by this action of the renal tubules.

TABLE 24-2 Average Fluid Losses and Gains in 24 Hours

INTAKE		OUTPUT	
Oral liquids	1,300 mL	Urine	1,000 mL – 1,500 mL
Water in food	1,000 mL	Stool	200 mL
Water from metabolism	300 mL	Insensible losses	
		Lungs	400–500 mL
		Skin	300–500 mL
Total	2,600 mL	Total	2,600 mL (average)

Adapted from: Roth, R. (2007). *Nutrition and Diet Theray* (9th ed.). Clifton Park, New York: Delmar Cengage Learning.

TABLE 24-3 Foods Rich in Sodium, Potassium, and Calcium

SODIUM	POTASSIUM	CALCIUM
Processed/prepared foods: canned vegetables, soups, luncheon meats, frozen foods, potato chips, snack foods, olives, pickles	Banana	Milk
	Orange	Yogurt
	Apricot	Cheese
	Cantaloupe	Tofu/soybeans
	Dried fruit	Almonds
	Avocado	Broccoli
Sodium-containing condiments: soy sauce, salad dressings, sauces, dips, ketchup, mustard, relishes	Raw carrots	Spinach
	Baked potato	
	Spinach	
	Milk	
Natural foods: meat, poultry, dairy, vegetables	Yogurt	
	Meat	
	Fish	

COURTESY OF DELMAR CENGAGE LEARNING

Fluid and Food Intake

Fluids must be replaced in the amounts lost. The primary source of fluid replacement is water consumption. Approximately 60% may be obtained in this way, with an additional 30% being obtained from foods and 8% to 10% being a product of metabolism (metabolic water), for a total of 2,600 mL. Table 24-2 illustrates fluid balance.

Thirst

Water consumption usually occurs in response to the sensation of thirst. This mechanism is poorly understood. It is generally believed to be brought about by the loss of body fluids, which in turn causes a dryness in the mouth and the thirst sensation. Replacing the lost fluids by water consumption causes the sensation to diminish. The thirst mechanism appears to be regulated by the hypothalamus in the brain.

Dehydration is one of the most common and most serious fluid imbalances that can result from poor monitoring of fluid intake. One nursing goal is to ensure that all clients understand both the role that water plays in health and the way to maintain adequate hydration.

DISTURBANCES IN ELECTROLYTE BALANCE

In health, normal homeostatic mechanisms function to maintain electrolyte balance. In illness, one or more of the regulating mechanisms may be affected, or an imbalance may become too great for the body to correct without treatment. Electrolytes are measured by laboratory analysis of a blood sample. Table 24-3 lists foods rich in sodium, potassium, and calcium. Table 24-4 lists the types, causes, signs and symptoms, and nursing interventions for electrolyte imbalances.

SODIUM

Sodium (Na^+) is the major electrolyte in extracellular fluid. It regulates fluid balance through osmotic pressure that results from water following sodium in the body. Sodium stimulates conduction of nerve impulses and helps maintain neuromuscular activity. Excretion occurs primarily via the kidneys. The normal serum sodium for an adult is 135 to 145 mEq/L. Critical values are $<$130 or $>$160 mEq/L (Daniels, 2010; Daniels, Nosek, & Nicoll, 2007).

Hyponatremia

A subnormal serum sodium value indicates hyponatremia. The cause is either a sodium deficit or a water excess. A hypo-osmotic state exists: The water moves out of the vascular space, into the interstitial space, and then into the intracellular space, causing edema. Hyponatremia may be caused by prolonged vomiting, diarrhea, or gastric or intestinal suctioning. This can be life threatening.

Hypernatremia

An elevated serum sodium level indicates hypernatremia. Excess sodium or a loss of water causes a rise in the extracellular osmotic pressure and pulls water out of the cells and into the extracellular space.

POTASSIUM

Potassium (K^+) is the major electrolyte in intracellular fluid. Its concentration inside cells is approximately 150 mEq/L. The normal value range of extracellular (serum) potassium is narrow: 3.5 to 5.3 mEq/L. Critical values are $<$3.5 or $>$5.3 mEq/L (Kee et al., 2010). Consequently, the slightest changes can dramatically affect physiological functions. Potassium maintains normal nerve and muscle activity, especially of the heart, and osmotic pressure within the cells. It also assists in the cellular metabolism of carbohydrates and proteins. The kidneys prefer to retain sodium and excrete potassium, even when both electrolytes are depleted. When potassium is lost from cells, sodium and hydrogen move into the cells. This aids

Table 24-4 Electrolyte Imbalances

ELECTROLYTE AND TYPE OF IMBALANCE	CAUSES OF IMBALANCE	SIGNS AND SYMPTOMS	NURSING INTERVENTIONS
Sodium			
Hyponatremia *(serum sodium level <135 mEq/L)*	• Sodium deficit • Water excess • Prolonged vomiting, diarrhea, excessive perspiration, burns, or gastric or intestinal suctioning • Syndrome of inappropriate ADH (SIADH) • Diuretics	Hypotension, tachycardia, edema, headache, lethargy, confusion, muscle weakness and twitching, abdominal cramps, dry mucous membranes, dry skin	Monitor serum sodium lab results. Assess for physical manifestations. Encourage foods and fluids high in sodium if ordered. Monitor I&O. Teach the client about sodium rich foods. Administer IV solution as ordered.
Hypernatremia *(serum sodium level >145 mEq/L)*	• Excess sodium • Loss of water • Decreased renal function	Muscle twitching, tremor, hyperreflexia, agitation, restlessness, stupor, increased body temperature, tachycardia	Monitor serum sodium lab results. Limit foods and fluids high in sodium if ordered. Assess for physical manifestations. Monitor I&O.
Potassium			
Hypokalemia *(serum potassium level <3.5 mEq/L)*	• Excessive loss of gastric fluids • Use of diuretics	Muscle weakness, paralytic ileus, polyuria, polydipsia, EKG changes, elevated blood glucose level	Teach the client about potassium rich foods. Administer oral potassium replacement as ordered. Administer IV potassium as ordered. Monitor and assess heart rate, rhythm, and EKG readings. Monitor serum potassium lab results. Monitor I&O. Assess for physical manifestations. Encourage foods and fluids high in potassium if ordered.
Hyperkalemia *(serum potassium level >5.3 mEq/L)*	• Renal disease • Extensive trauma • Insulin deficiency	Anxiety, irritability, diarrhea, abdominal cramping, EKG changes, cardiac arrest	Be prepared to administer IV calcium gluconate. May need to prepare client for dialysis and/or the administration of Kayexalate. Monitor serum potassium lab results. Monitor I&O. Assess for physical manifestations. Monitor and assess heart rate, rhythm, and EKG readings.
Calcium			
Hypocalcemia *(total serum calcium <8.5 mg/dL)*	• Hypoalbuminemia • Renal failure • Chronic diarrhea • Hormonal and electrolyte influence	Anxiety, irritability, tetany, abdominal and muscle cramps, positive Chvostek's sign, positive Trousseau's sign, weak heart contractions, fractures	Teach the client about calcium-rich foods. Monitor serum calcium lab results. Monitor I&O. Assess for physical manifestations. Monitor and assess heart rate, rhythm, and EKG readings. Administer oral calcium replacement as ordered. Encourage foods and fluids high in calcium if ordered.

(Continues)

Table 24-4 Electrolyte Imbalances (Continued)

ELECTROLYTE AND TYPE OF IMBALANCE	CAUSES OF IMBALANCE	SIGNS AND SYMPTOMS	NURSING INTERVENTIONS
Hypercalcemia *(total serum calcium >10.5 mg/dL)*	• Increased use of calcium supplements • Renal dysfunction • Diuretics • Use of steroids • Hyperparathyroidism	Depression, signs of heart block, pathological fractures, kidney stones	Monitor serum calcium lab results. Monitor I&O. Assess for physical manifestations. Monitor and assess heart rate, rhythm, and EKG readings.
Magnesium			
Hypomagnesemia *(serum magnesium level <1.5 mEq/L)*	• Diarrhea, • Steatorrhea • Chronic alcoholism • Diabetes mellitus malnutrition • Chronic use of laxatives acute renal failure • Acute myocardial infarction	Hyperirritability, tetany-like symptoms, increased tendon reflexes, hypertension, cardiac dysrhythmias	Monitor serum magnesium lab results. Monitor I&O. Assess for physical manifestations.
Hypermagnesemia *(serum magnesium level >2.5 mEq/L)*	• Renal insufficiency • Laxatives and antacids with magnesium • Severe dehydration • Diabetic ketoacidosis	Bradycardia, cardiac arrest, hypotension, EKG changes, muscle weakness, paralysis, CNS depression, confusion, flushing	Monitor serum magnesium lab results. Monitor I&O. Assess for physical manifestations. Monitor and assess heart rate, rhythm, and EKG readings.
Phosphate			
Hypophosphatemia *(serum phosphorus level <2.5 mg/dL)*	• Malnutrition • Chronic alcoholism • TPN administration vomiting • Chronic diarrhea • Hyperparathyroidism • Burns • Diuretics • Aluminum-containing antacids • Respiratory alkalosis	Muscle weakness, fatigue, tremors, bone pain, seizures, coma, weak pulse, anorexia, bone changes	Use safety precautions to prevent falls or injury. Monitor serum phosphorus lab results. Monitor I&O. Assess for physical manifestations.
Hyperphosphatemia *(serum phosphorus level >4.5 mg/dL)*	• Chemotherapy • Renal insufficiency • Hypoparathyroidism • Metabolic and respiratory acidosis	Tetany, hyperreflexia, flaccid paralysis, muscle weakness, tachycardia, abdominal cramps	Monitor serum phosphorus lab results. Monitor I&O. Assess for physical manifestations.

TABLE 24-4 Electrolyte Imbalances (Continued)

ELECTROLYTE AND TYPE OF IMBALANCE	CAUSES OF IMBALANCE	SIGNS AND SYMPTOMS	NURSING INTERVENTIONS
Chloride			
Hypochloremia *(serum chloride level <95 mEq/L)*	• Prolonged diarrhea or diaphoresis • Vomiting • Gastric surgery • Gastric suctioning	Tremors, twitching, hypotension, slow, shallow breathing	Monitor serum chloride lab results. Monitor I&O. Assess for physical manifestations.
Hyperchloremia *(serum chloride level >108 mEq/L)*	• Dehydration • Hypernatremia • Metabolic acidosis	Weakness, deep and rapid breathing, lethargy	Monitor serum chloride lab results. Monitor I&O. Assess for physical manifestations.

PROFESSIONALTIP

Hypokalemia

Hypokalemia can cause cardiac arrest when:
- The potassium level is <2.5 mEq/L.
- The client is taking digitalis (a drug that strengthens the contraction of the myocardium and slows down the heart rate). *Hypokalemia enhances the action of digitalis, causing toxicity.*

in regulating acid–base balance. Intracellular potassium deficit may coexist with an excess of extracellular potassium.

Hypokalemia

A low serum potassium level indicates hypokalemia. Excessive loss of gastric fluids and the use of diuretics can place the client at risk for hypokalemia and an acid–base imbalance (metabolic alkalosis). Potassium-wasting diuretics, such as furosemide (Lasix) or chlorothiazide (Diuril) can cause hypokalemia.

SAFETY

Potassium Chloride

- Use IV route only when hypokalemia is life threatening or when oral replacement is not feasible.
- Always dilute potassium chloride in a large amount of IV solution.
- Never administer more than 10 mEq/L of IV potassium chloride (KCl) per hour; the normal dose of IV KCl is 20 to 40 mEq/L infused over an 8-hour period.
- Never give KCl intramuscularly (IM) or as an IV bolus; potentially fatal hyperkalemia may result.
- Monitor the IV site frequently for early signs of infiltration, as potassium is caustic to the tissues.

Hyperkalemia

An elevated serum potassium level indicates hyperkalemia. Clients with renal disease develop hyperkalemia because potassium cannot be excreted adequately by the kidneys. Extensive trauma causes potassium to be released from the cells and enter the bloodstream, leading to hyperkalemia. Hyperkalemia inhibits the action of digitalis. This condition is much more critical than is hypokalemia.

CALCIUM

Calcium (Ca^{++}) plays an essential role in bone and teeth integrity, blood clotting, muscle functioning, and nerve impulse transmission. Vitamin D is required for absorption of calcium from the GI tract. Only 1% of the body's calcium is found in the blood plasma (serum). Normally, 50% of the serum calcium is ionized (physiologically active), with the remaining 50% being bound to protein. Free, ionized calcium is needed for cell membrane permeability. The calcium that is bound to plasma protein cannot pass through the capillary wall and, therefore, cannot leave the intravascular compartment. Total serum calcium concentration measures both the ionized calcium and the calcium bound to albumin. The normal value range of total serum calcium concentration for an adult is 8.5 to 10.5 mg/dL. Critical values are <7.0 or >12 mg/dL. Values for the older adult are slightly lower (Daniels, 2010; Daniels et al., 2007).

PROFESSIONALTIP

Serum Calcium

Approximately 50% of serum calcium is bound to protein. When evaluating laboratory results, correlate the serum calcium level with the serum albumin level. *Any change in serum protein will result in a change in the total serum calcium.*

CLIENT TEACHING

Calcium and Vitamin D

Vitamin D is necessary for the absorption of calcium from the GI tract. Clients who do not get adequate exposure to the sun or who use sunscreen (which is needed to prevent skin cancer) may not make enough vitamin D to support adequate calcium absorption. Advise these clients to consult their physicians regarding a vitamin D supplement.

Hypocalcemia

Hypocalcemia is indicated by a low serum calcium level. Alkalosis, elevated serum albumin, and the rapid administration of citrated blood increase the activity of calcium binders, thereby decreasing the amount of free calcium.

Hypercalcemia

An elevated total serum calcium level indicates hypercalcemia. Generally, three separate evaluations of either total serum calcium or ionized serum calcium are performed before a diagnosis of hypercalcemia is made. Hypercalcemia is often a symptom of an underlying disease such as metastatic bone tumors, Paget's disease, acromegaly, and hyperparathyroidism, which all increase bone reabsorption and, thereby, foster the release of calcium into circulating blood. Calcium-containing antacids and excess calcium from the diet may also cause hypercalcemia.

MAGNESIUM

Most magnesium (Mg^{++}) is found in intracellular fluid and in combination with calcium and phosphorus in bone, muscle, and soft tissue. Blood serum contains only approximately 1%. Magnesium plays an important role as a coenzyme, in the metabolism of carbohydrates and proteins, and as a mediator, in neuromuscular activity. It is the only cation that is found in higher concentration in cerebrospinal fluid than in extracellular fluid. When a magnesium deficiency develops, the body conserves magnesium at the expense of excreting potassium. A close relationship exists between magnesium, calcium, and potassium in the intracellular fluid: A low level of one results in low levels of the other two. The normal serum magnesium level for an adult is 1.5 to 2.5 mEq/L (Kee et al., 2010).

HYPOMAGNESEMIA

A serum magnesium level of $<$1.5 mEq/L indicates hypomagnesemia (Daniels, 2010), which most commonly results from chronic alcoholism. Increased renal excretion is associated with prolonged diuretic therapy or use of gentamicin (Garamycin), cyclosporin (Sandimmune), or cisplatin (Platinol).

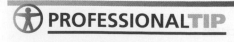

PROFESSIONAL TIP

Hyperalimentation

Total parenteral nutrition (TPN) provided continuously (hyperalimentation) and without a magnesium supplement can cause hypomagnesemia.

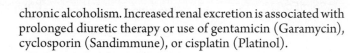

SAFETY

Magnesium Level

When the serum magnesium level reaches 10 to 15 mEq/L, respiratory paralysis may occur.

HYPERMAGNESEMIA

A serum magnesium level of $>$2.5 mEq/L indicates hypermagnesemia (Daniels, 2010). This condition rarely occurs if kidney function is normal. An increased magnesium level is associated with uncontrolled diabetes (ketoacidosis), renal failure, and ingestion of magnesium antacids (Maalox, Mylanta) or laxatives (milk of magnesia [MOM], magnesium citrate [Citromal]).

PHOSPHATE

Phosphate (PO_4^{--}) is the main intracellular anion. It appears as phosphorus in the serum, where the normal value range is 2.5 to 4.5 mg/dL (Kee et al., 2010). Phosphorus is critical for normal cell functioning. Most phosphorus is found combined with calcium in teeth and bones. Phosphate and calcium exist in an inverse relationship (i.e., as one increases the other decreases).

Hypophosphatemia

A client with a low serum phosphorus level has hypophosphatemia. Rarely does this condition result from decreased dietary intake. More commonly, it stems from respiratory alkalosis. Intense, prolonged hyperventilation can cause severe hypophosphatemia.

Hyperphosphatemia

A client with an elevated serum phosphorus level has hyperphosphatemia. This condition most commonly results from renal failure with resultant decreased renal phosphorus excretion. Excessive use of phosphate-containing laxatives or phosphate enemas may cause hyperphosphatemia.

CHLORIDE

Chloride (Cl^-) is the major anion in extracellular fluid. Chloride functions in combination with sodium to maintain

PROFESSIONAL TIP

Hyperphosphatemia

A client with hyperphosphatemia generally remains asymptomatic unless hypocalcemia results, in which case the client may describe both tingling sensations around the mouth and in the fingertips as well as muscle cramps.

CRITICAL THINKING

Vomiting

A client has been vomiting for 3 days and is unable to keep anything down. Besides fluid volume deficit, what other problems would you expect to find?

osmotic pressure. It also assists in maintaining acid–base balance. When the carbon dioxide level increases, bicarbonate shifts from the intracellular compartment to the extracellular compartment. Chloride, in an effort to maintain homeostasis, then moves into the intracellular compartment. The kidneys selectively excrete chloride or bicarbonate ions depending on the acid–base balance. The normal serum chloride range is 95 to 108 mEq/L (Kee et al., 2010).

Hypochloremia

A low serum chloride level indicates hypochloremia. Excess losses of chloride may result from prolonged diarrhea or diaphoresis. Loss of hydrochloric acid related to vomiting, gastric suctioning, or gastric surgery may cause hypochloremia.

Hyperchloremia

An elevated serum chloride level indicates hyperchloremia, which usually occurs in conjunction with dehydration, hypernatremia, or metabolic acidosis.

ACID–BASE BALANCE

As described earlier, the body maintains a normal pH within the relatively narrow range of 7.35 to 7.45. Body pH is maintained by the buffer systems, the respiratory system, and the kidneys. A pH below 7.35 is termed acidosis, and a pH above 7.45 is termed alkalosis. Either of these conditions can be brought about by respiratory or metabolic changes.

Regulators of Acid–Base Balance

The body has three main control systems that regulate acid–base balance to counter acidosis or alkalosis: the buffer systems, respirations, and renal control of hydrogen ion concentration. These systems vary in their reaction times in regulating and restoring balance to the hydrogen ion concentration.

Buffer Systems

The buffer systems bicarbonate, phosphate, and protein were previously discussed. They react quickly to prevent excessive changes in the hydrogen ion concentration.

Respiratory Regulation of Acid–Base Balance

The respiratory system helps maintain acid–base balance by controlling the content of carbon dioxide in extracellular fluid. The *rate of metabolism* determines the formation of carbon dioxide. Various intracellular metabolic processes continuously form carbon dioxide in the body. The carbon in foods is **oxidized** (joined with oxygen) to form carbon dioxide.

It takes the respiratory regulatory mechanism several minutes to respond to changes in the carbon dioxide concentration of extracellular fluid. With the increase of carbon dioxide in extracellular fluid, respiration increases in rate and depth so that more carbon dioxide is exhaled. As the respiratory system removes carbon dioxide, less carbon dioxide is present in the blood to combine with water to form carbonic acid. Likewise, if the blood level of carbon dioxide is low, respirations decrease to maintain a normal ratio between carbonic acid and basic bicarbonate.

Renal Control of Hydrogen Ion Concentration

The kidneys control extracellular fluid pH by eliminating either hydrogen ions or bicarbonate ions from body fluids. If the bicarbonate concentration in the extracellular fluid is greater than normal, the kidneys excrete more bicarbonate ions, making the urine more alkaline. Conversely, if more hydrogen ions are excreted in the urine, the urine becomes more acidic. The renal mechanism for regulating acid–base balance cannot readjust the pH within seconds, as can the extracellular fluid buffer system, nor within minutes, as can the respiratory compensatory mechanism, but it can function over a period of several hours or days to correct acid–base imbalance.

Diagnostic and Laboratory Data

The biochemical indicators of acid–base balance are assessed by measuring the **arterial blood gases** (ABGs). The arterial blood gas test measures the levels of oxygen and carbon dioxide in arterial blood. The test assesses pH, partial pressure of oxygen (PO_2 or PaO_2), partial pressure of carbon dioxide (PCO_2 or $PaCO_2$), saturation of oxygen (SaO_2), and bicarbonate (HCO_3). pH has already been discussed.

The PO_2 or PaO_2 expresses the amount of oxygen that can combine with hemoglobin to form oxyhemoglobin, the form in which oxygen is transported through the body. At sea level, the normal range is 80 to 100 millimeters of mercury (mm Hg). The rate at which the oxygen/hemoglobin reaction occurs is influenced by pH. The rate decreases as the pH value decreases.

The PCO_2 or $PaCO_2$ in the blood is a reflection of the efficiency of gaseous exchange in the lungs. At sea level, the normal range is 35 to 45 mm Hg. If the alveoli are obstructed or damaged by disease, carbon dioxide cannot be eliminated and will combine with water to form carbonic acid, which in turn causes acidosis. Conversely, in a person who

PROFESSIONAL TIP

Pulse Oximeter Reading

Warming a client's cold hand will provide more accurate results from a pulse oximeter.

is hyperventilating, too much carbon dioxide is eliminated, which may trigger alkalosis.

The SaO_2 is the percentage of oxygen that combines with hemoglobin in the blood. The normal range is 95% to 100% saturation. This value, along with the PO_2 and hemoglobin levels, indicates the degree to which the tissues are receiving oxygen. Oxygen saturation can also be measured with a pulse oximeter, a noninvasive technique.

Determining the amount of bicarbonate (HCO_3) in the blood is important because, along with carbonic acid, bicarbonate is a major buffer in the blood. The two substances occur in a ratio of 20 parts bicarbonate to 1 part carbonic acid. Regardless of the carbonic acid and bicarbonate values, the pH of the blood will remain in the normal range as long as the ratio remains 20:1. The normal range for HCO_3 at sea level is 24 to 28 mEq/L. The carbonic acid level is always 3% of the PCO_2 level.

DISTURBANCES IN ACID–BASE BALANCE

The acid–base imbalances are respiratory acidosis and alkalosis and metabolic acidosis and alkalosis. In determining whether the acid–base imbalance is caused by a respiratory or a metabolic alteration, the key indicators are bicarbonate and carbonic acid levels (Figure 24-11). Table 24-5 lists those changes in laboratory values that indicate the various acid–base imbalances.

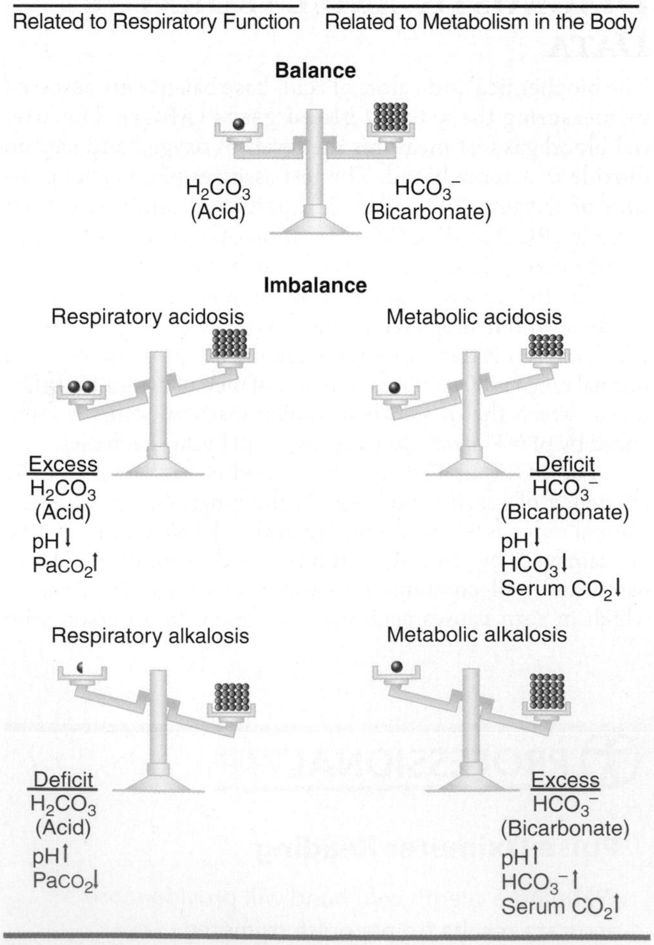

FIGURE 24-11 Acid-Base Balance and Imbalance

TABLE 24-5 Laboratory Values in Acid–Base Imbalances

SITUATION	pH	PCO_2	HCO_3
Normal parameters	7.35 to 7.45	35 to 45 mm Hg	24 to 28 mEq/L
Respiratory acidosis			
Acute	<7.35	>45 mm Hg	Normal
Chronic	<7.35	>45 mm Hg	>28 mEq/L
Respiratory alkalosis	>7.45	<35 mm Hg	Normal
Metabolic acidosis	<7.35	Normal	<24 mEq/L
Metabolic Alkalosis	>7.45	Normal	>28 mEq/L

RESPIRATORY ACIDOSIS

When carbon dioxide is not eliminated by the lungs as fast as it is produced by cellular metabolism, the amount of carbon dioxide increases in the blood. It then reacts with water and forms excess hydrogen ions, as shown in the following reaction:

$$CO_2 + H_2O \rightarrow H^+ + HCO_3$$

In respiratory acidosis, there is an increased concentration of hydrogen ions (a blood pH below 7.35), an increased PCO_2 level (greater than 45 mm Hg), and an excess of carbonic acid. It is caused by hypoventilation or any condition that depresses ventilation. Hypoventilation can be caused by brain injury, chest injuries, emphysema, and chronic obstructive pulmonary disease (COPD). When the respiratory rate and the amount of oxygen supplied to the lungs suddenly lessen, acute respiratory acidosis can occur. This condition can be life threatening, and it must be recognized and corrected quickly. Chronic respiratory acidosis occurs when the respiratory rate is continually depressed.

Clients with respiratory acidosis experience neurological changes as a result of the cerebrospinal fluid and brain cells acidity. Hypoventilation causes **hypoxemia** (decreased oxygen in the blood), which in turn causes further neurological impairment. Hyperkalemia may accompany acidosis.

PROFESSIONALTIP

Electrolyte Shift

An electrolyte shift occurs in metabolic acidosis. Hydrogen and sodium ions move into the cells, and potassium moves into the extracellular fluid. Hyperkalemia may cause ventricular fibrillation and death.

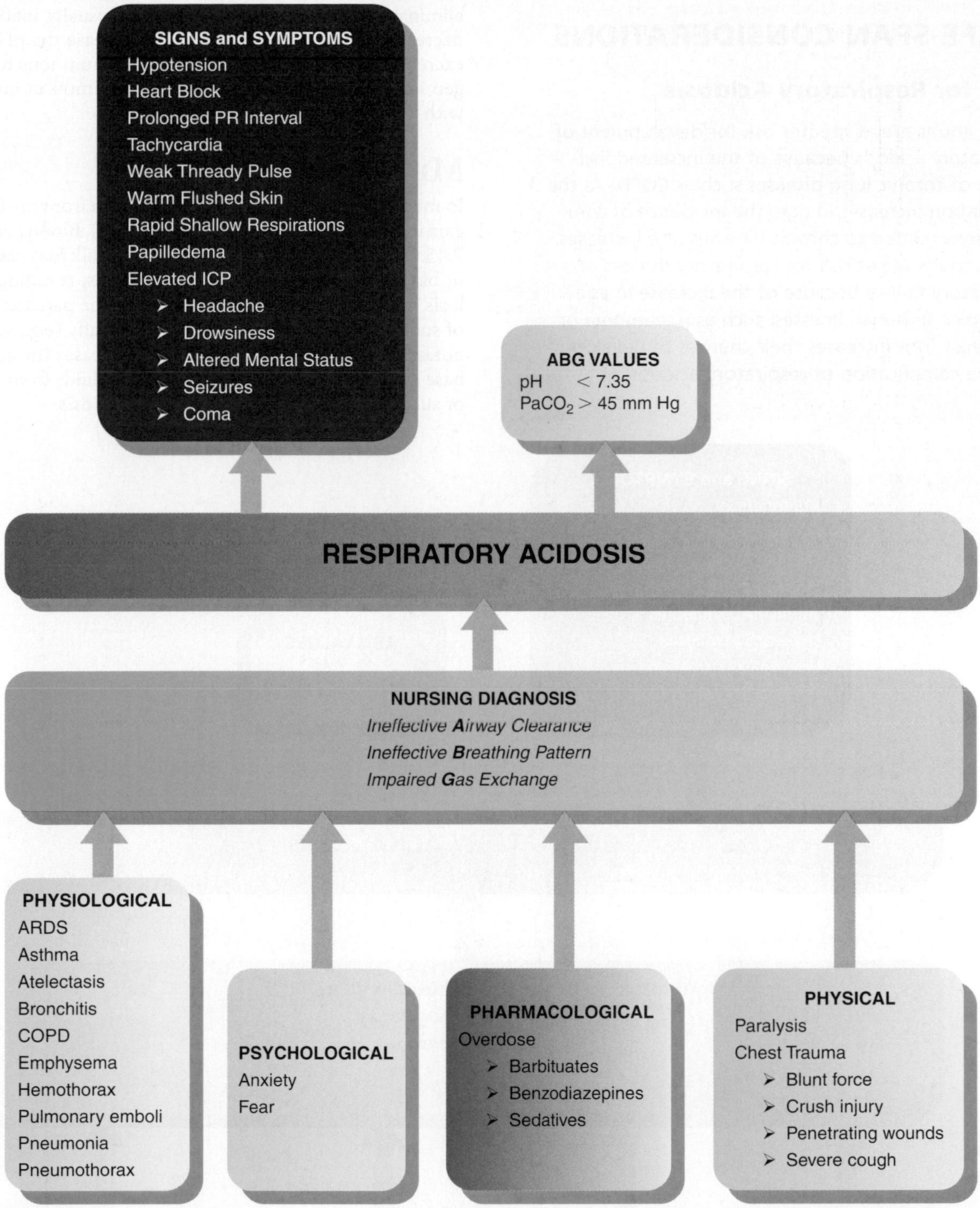

CONCEPT MAP: Respiratory Acidosis (*Courtesy of Leon Klopfenstein and Eric Mason: Lima, Ohio.*)

RESPIRATORY ALKALOSIS

In respiratory alkalosis, there is a decreased concentration of hydrogen ions (a blood pH above 7.45) and a below-normal PCO_2 level (lower than 35 mm Hg). It is caused by hyperventilation (excessive exhalation of carbon dioxide) resulting in hypocapnia (decreased arterial carbon dioxide concentration). As the breathing rate increases, the amount of carbon dioxide in the blood decreases, which in turn increases the pH of the blood.

Hyperventilation can be triggered by anxiety, fear, fever, pain, rapid mechanical ventilation, and hypoxia at high altitudes. This condition is usually self-correcting. As the breathing returns to normal, the carbon dioxide level in the blood increases, and the normal pH is restored. Other causes of hyperventilation, which involves overstimulation of the respiratory center, include salicylate poisoning, brain tumors, meningitis, encephalitis, and pulmonary embolus.

METABOLIC ACIDOSIS

In metabolic acidosis there is an increased concentration of hydrogen ions (blood pH below 7.35) or a decrease in bicarbonate concentration. Such a change may be brought about by kidney disease when the mechanism to excrete excess hydrogen ions is compromised. Diarrhea, diabetes mellitus, and, sometimes, diuretics may also be responsible. The lungs

LIFE SPAN CONSIDERATIONS

Risk for Respiratory Acidosis

Older adults are at greater risk for development of respiratory acidosis because of the increased incidence of chronic lung diseases such as COPD. As the population increases in age, the incidence of complications related to chronic illnesses also increases. Older adults are at risk for respiratory distress or respiratory failure because of the increase in age-related or seasonal illnesses, such as pneumonia or influenza. This increases their chances of developing the complication of respiratory acidosis.

eliminate more carbon dioxide but are usually ineffective in decreasing acids. The kidneys try to increase the pH and the excretion of hydrogen by exchanging sodium ions for hydrogen ions. Metabolic acidosis is most common in individuals with kidney disease or diabetes mellitus.

METABOLIC ALKALOSIS

In metabolic alkalosis there is a loss of acid from the body or a gain in base (increased level of bicarbonate). Blood pH is above 7.45. Excessive ingestion of antacids and milk may cause a gain in base. These substances neutralize acids, resulting in alkalosis and hypercalcemia. Excessive oral or parenteral intake of sodium bicarbonate or other alkaline salts (e.g., sodium or potassium acetate, lactate, or citrate) increases the amount of base in extracellular fluid. Loss of gastric fluids from vomiting or suctioning may result in metabolic alkalosis.

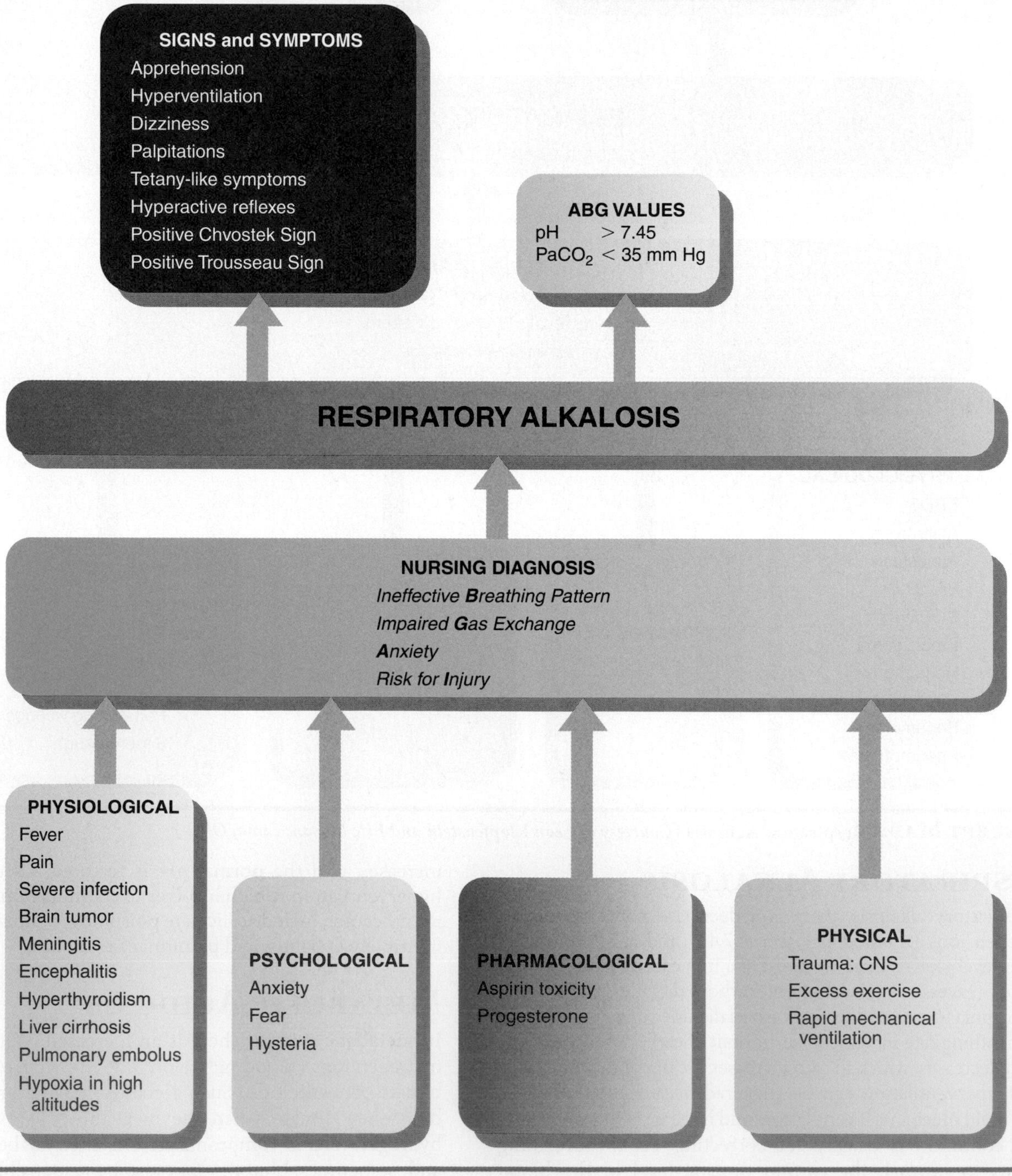

CONCEPT MAP: Respiratory Alkalosis

PROFESSIONALTIP

Metabolic Alkalosis

The following clinical conditions can place clients at risk for metabolic alkalosis:

- Vomiting and nasogastric suctioning or lavage cause a loss of hydrochloric acid and chloride. With the loss of the hydrogen and chloride ions, bicarbonate ions are absorbed, unneutralized, into the bloodstream, and the pH of the extracellular fluid rises (alkalosis).
- Diarrhea and steroid or diuretic therapy can cause excessive loss of potassium, chloride, and other electrolytes. The potassium deficit causes the kidneys to exchange hydrogen ions (instead of potassium ions) for sodium ions, which promotes the loss of hydrogen, thereby increasing bicarbonate level.

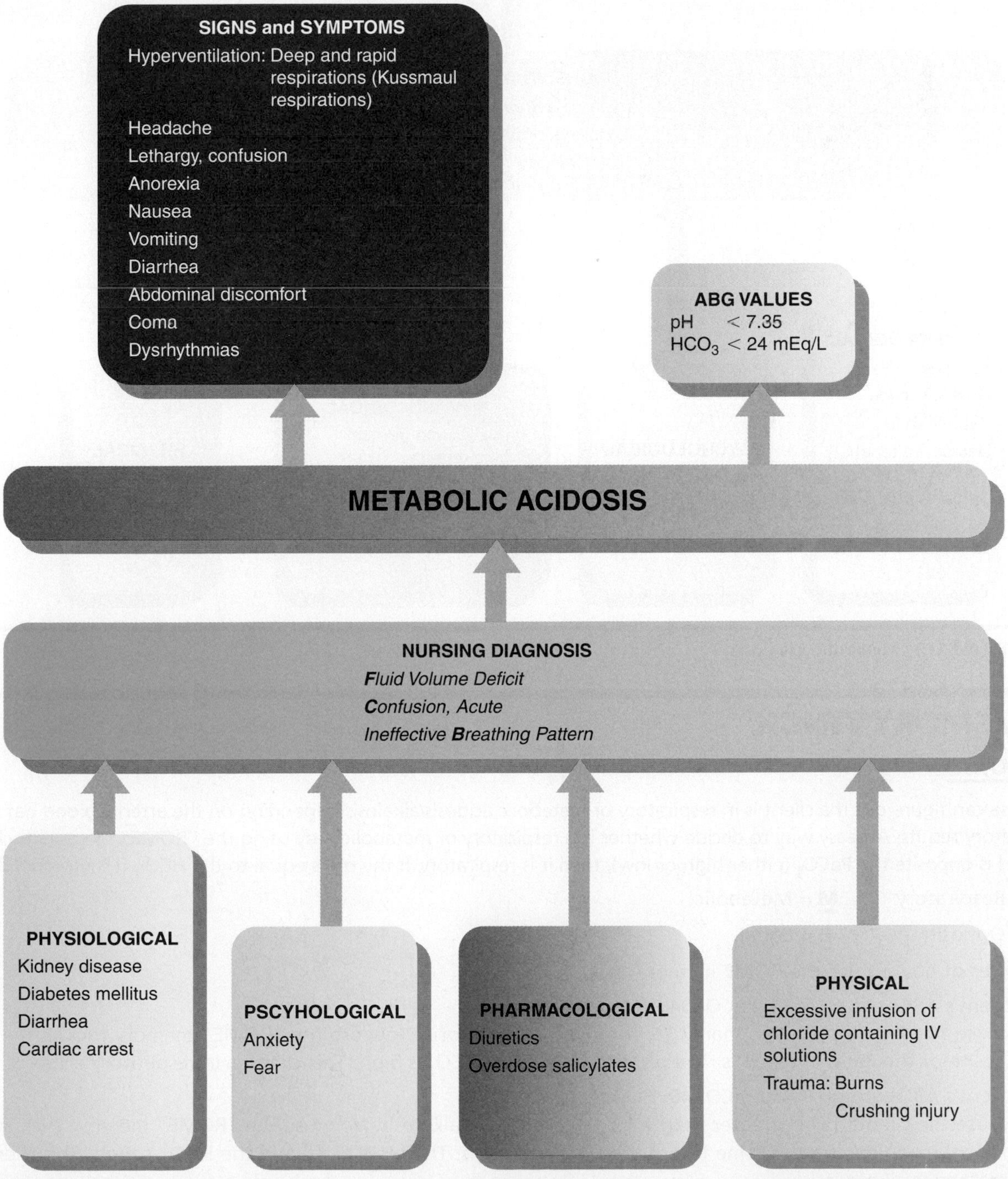

CONCEPT MAP: Metabolic Acidosis (*Courtesy of Kami L. Fox, MS, CNP.*)

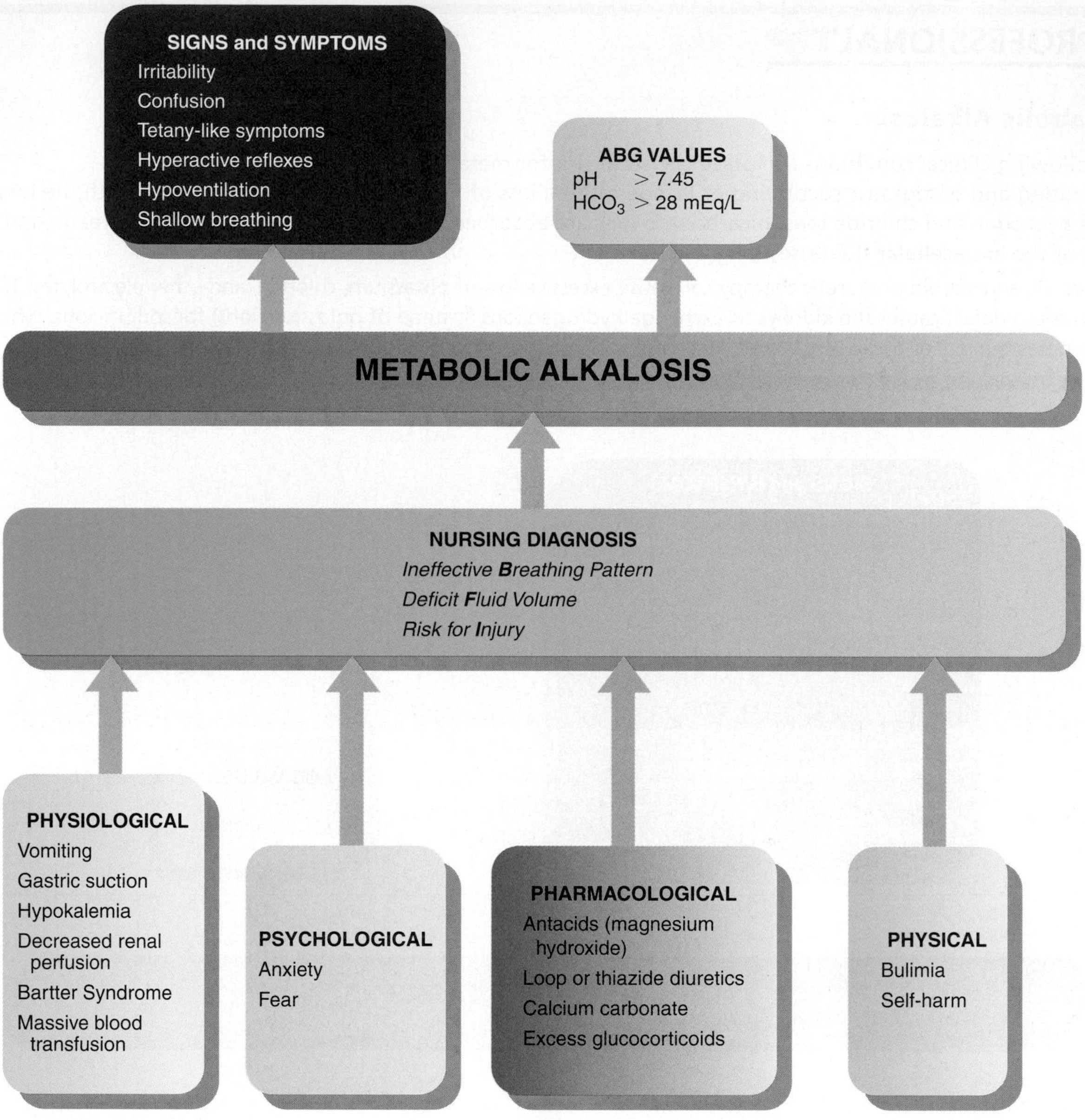

Concept Map: Metabolic Alkalosis

MEMORY**TRICK**

ROME

A nurse can figure out if a client is in respiratory or metabolic acidosis/alkalosis depending on the arterial blood gas (ABG) laboratory results. An easy way to decide whether it is respiratory or metabolic is by using the "ROME" memory trick. If the pH is opposite the $PaCO_2$ (either high or low), then it is respiratory. If the pH is equal to the HCO_3, it is metabolic.

R = Respiratory   **M** = Metabolic

O = Opposite   **E** = Equal

Examples of how to use the ROME memory trick:

1. A client's ABGs are pH 7.31, $PaCO_2$ 54, HCO_3 24, PaO_2 62
   Because the client's pH is less than 7.35, the client is in acidosis. Now use the "ROME" memory trick. Is the pH opposite of the $PaCO_2$? Yes, it is. The pH is low, and the $PaCO_2$ is high. This client is in respiratory acidosis.
2. A client's ABGs are pH 7.49, $PaCO_2$ 40, HCO_3 42, PaO_2 80
   Because the client's pH is greater than 7.45, the client is in alkalosis. Now use the "ROME" memory trick. Is the pH equal to (following the same trend) the HCO_3? Yes, it is. The pH is high, and the HCO_3 is high. This client is in metabolic alkalosis.

The renal and respiratory compensatory mechanisms respond to an increased bicarbonate/carbonic acid ratio. In an effort to retain carbon dioxide, the rate and depth of respirations decreases. To counter the pH imbalance of metabolic alkalosis, the arterial carbon dioxide concentration rises, creating respiratory acidosis.

A normal serum potassium level is necessary for renal compensation. When potassium ions enter the cells in exchange for hydrogen ions, in alkalosis hypokalemia results. The kidneys cannot function as a compensatory mechanism when hypokalemia is present; they continue to excrete hydrogen, and bicarbonate excess continues.

NURSING PROCESS

The nursing process assists the nurse in planning client care.

ASSESSMENT

Assessment data are used to identify clients who have potential or actual alterations in fluid volume. Electrolyte and acid-base imbalances are identified primarily with laboratory data, while fluid balances are identified primarily with the health history and physical examination.

Health History

The nursing history should elicit data in the following areas:

- Lifestyle (sociocultural and economic factors, stress, exercise)
- Dietary intake (recent changes in the amount and types of fluid and food, increased thirst)
- Weight (sudden gain or loss)
- Fluid output (recent changes in the frequency or amount of urine output)
- Gastrointestinal disturbances (prolonged vomiting, diarrhea, anorexia, ulcer, hemorrhage)
- Fever and diaphoresis
- Burns, trauma, draining wounds
- Disease conditions that can upset homeostasis (renal disease, endocrine disorders, neural malfunction, pulmonary disease)
- Therapeutic programs that can produce imbalances (special diets, medications, chemotherapy, IV fluid or total parenteral nutrition [TPN] administration, gastric or intestinal suction)

Table 24-6 lists health history assessment questions to ask a client experiencing a fluid, electrolyte, and/or acid–base imbalance.

TABLE 24-6 Health History Assessment Questions

- What recent illnesses have you experienced?
- What prescription medications are you currently taking?
- Do you have any chronic illnesses which affect the way you breathe? If so, please describe the illnesses.
- What over-the-counter medications including herbs are you currently taking?
- Have you recently traveled outside of the continental United States? If so, where?
- What type of work do you do regularly?
- What types of environmental allergies do you have?
- Have you been diagnosed with diabetes? If so, what are your last several blood glucose readings?
- Have you or anyone else noticed a difference in the odor of your breath?
- Have you had any recent changes in your kidney function?
- What types of respiratory illnesses have you experienced recently?
- Have you experienced any changes in your appetite recently?
- What types of foods including fruits do you eat on a regular basis?
- Have you noticed any difference in the way your heart feels?
- Have you experienced any unusual muscle weakness or loss of strength?
- Have you recently experienced diarrhea, vomiting, headache, or dehydration?

Physical Examination

Because fluid alterations may affect any body system, the nurse performs a complete physical examination and identifies all abnormalities.

Daily Weight Changes in the body's total fluid volume are reflected in body weight. For instance, each liter (1,000 mL) of fluid gained or lost is equivalent to 1 kilogram (2.2 lb) of weight.

Vital Signs The client with an elevated temperature is at risk for dehydration related to an increased loss of body fluid. Changes in the pulse rate, strength, and rhythm may indicate fluid alterations. Fluid volume changes may cause the following pulse changes:

- *Fluid volume deficit.* Increased pulse rate and weak pulse strength
- *Fluid volume excess.* Increased pulse strength and third heart sound

Inspect chest wall movement, count the respiratory rate, and auscultate the lungs to assess respiratory changes. Rate and depth changes may cause respiratory acid–base imbalances or may indicate a compensatory response to metabolic acidosis or alkalosis.

The degree of fluid volume deficit can be assessed by blood pressure measurements. Fluid volume deficit can lower the blood pressure. A narrow pulse pressure (lower than 20 mm Hg) may indicate severe hypovolemia (fluid volume deficit).

Intake and Output The client's I&O should be measured and recorded for a 24-hour period to assess for an actual or potential imbalance. A minimum intake of 1,500 mL is essential to balance urinary output and the body's insensible water loss. All liquids taken by mouth (e.g., soup, ice cream, gelatin, juice, and water) and liquids administered through tube feedings (nasogastric or jejunostomy) and parenterally (IV fluids and

SAFETY

Fluid Measurements

To protect both the nurse and the client from transfer of microorganisms, Standard Precautions are always followed during fluid administration and output measurement.

blood or its components) are included. Output includes urine, vomitus, diarrhea, and drainage from tubes such as gastric suction or surgical drains.

Thirst Thirst is the most common indicator of fluid volume deficit. The hypothalamus triggers a thirst response when there is a decrease in extracellular fluid volume or an increase in plasma osmolality.

Food Intake Ingested food also helps maintain extracellular fluid volume. One-third of the body's fluid needs are met

Skin Edema and skin turgor are two important indicators of fluid, electrolyte, and acid–base balances.

Edema The main symptom of fluid volume excess is edema. It may be confined to a specific area (localized) or occur throughout the body (generalized). The skin is taut, shiny, smooth, and pale in localized edema. Assess and palpate edematous areas for color, tenderness, and temperature. Firmly press your thumb against the edematous area or a dependent portion of the client's body (hands, arms, feet, ankles, legs, or sacrum) for 5 seconds. Release pressure and observe for indentation on the skin (Estes, 2010). Edema is not normally present (Daniels et al., 2007). Pitting edema is rated on a 4-point scale, as follows:

+0: no pitting
+1: 0 to ¼ inch pitting (mild)
+2: ¼ to ½ inch pitting (moderate)
+3: ½ to 1 inch pitting (severe)
+4: greater than 1 inch pitting (severe)

Turgor Skin **turgor** refers to the normal resiliency of the skin, a reflection of hydration status. When skin is pinched and released, it springs back to a normal position because the cells and interstitial fluid exert outward pressure. To measure the client's skin turgor, use the thumb and forefinger to grasp and raise and then release a small section of skin (Figure 24-12). Dehydration is the main cause of decreased skin turgor, which manifests as lax skin that returns slowly to the normal position. Increased

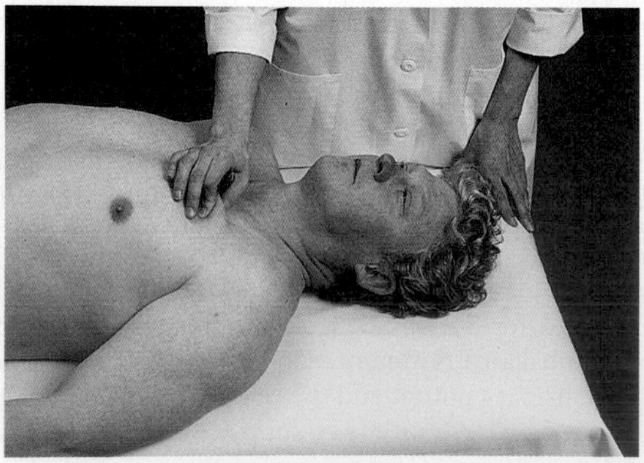

COURTESY OF DELMAR CENGAGE LEARNING

FIGURE 24-12 Assessing Skin Turgor

CRITICAL THINKING

Pitting Edema

Nursing assessment reveals a client with new onset (+2) pitting edema of both hands and (+4) pitting edema of both ankles. What nursing action is warranted for (+2) pitting edema? What nursing action is warranted for (+4) pitting edema?

skin turgor, which occurs in conjunction with edema, manifests as smooth, taut, shiny skin that cannot be grasped and raised.

Buccal (Oral) Cavity The nurse should inspect the buccal cavity. With fluid volume deficit, saliva decreases, causing sticky, dry mucous membranes and dry, cracked lips. The tongue has longitudinal furrows.

Eyes The eyes should be inspected for sunkenness, dry conjunctiva, and decreased or absent tearing, all signs of fluid volume deficit. Puffy eyelids (periorbital edema or papilledema) are signs of fluid volume excess. The client may have a history of blurred vision.

Jugular and Hand Veins Circulatory volume is assessed by measuring venous filling of the jugular and hand veins. With the client in a low Fowler's position:

1. Palpate the jugular (neck) veins. Fluid volume excess causes a distention in the jugular veins (Figure 24-13).
2. Place the client's hand below heart level and palpate the hand veins. Fluid volume deficit causes decreased venous filling (flat hand veins).

Neuromuscular System Fluid and electrolyte imbalances may cause neuromuscular alterations. The muscles lose tone, becoming soft and flabby, and reflexes diminish. Calcium and magnesium imbalances cause an increase in neuromuscular irritability. To assess for neuromuscular irritability, the tests for Chvostek's sign and Trousseau's sign are performed. Other neurological signs of fluid, electrolyte, and acid–base imbalances include inability to concentrate, confusion, and emotional lability.

Diagnostic and Laboratory Data

Laboratory tests can reveal imbalances before clinical symptoms are evident in the client; however, unless clients are having the tests for some other reason, symptoms are detected first.

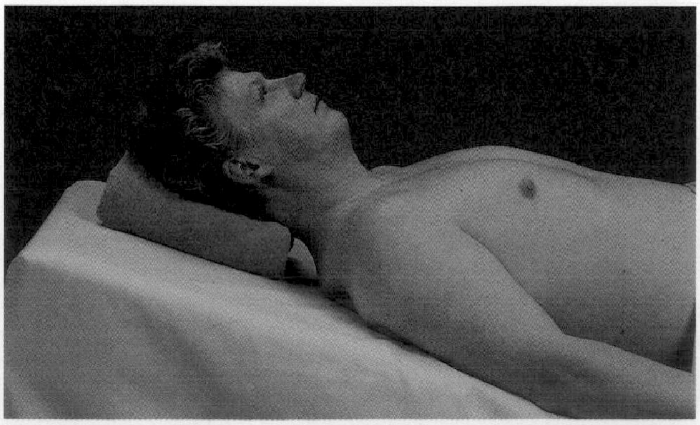

COURTESY OF DELMAR CENGAGE LEARNING

FIGURE 24-13 Client Position when Assessing Jugular Vein Distention

Hemoglobin and Hematocrit Indices The hemoglobin (Hgb) level decreases in the event of severe hemorrhage. Hematocrit (Hct) is affected by changes in plasma volume. For instance, with severe dehydration and hypovolemic shock, hematocrit increases. Conversely, overhydration decreases hematocrit.

Osmolality **Osmolality** is a measurement of the total concentration of dissolved particles (solutes) per kilogram of water. Osmolality measurements are performed on both serum and urine samples to identify changes in fluid and electrolyte balance.

Serum Osmolality Serum osmolality is a measurement of the total concentration of dissolved particles per kilogram of water in serum, recorded in milliosmoles per kilogram (mOsm/kg). The particles measured in serum osmolality include electrolyte ions (i.e., sodium and potassium), and electrically inactive substances (i.e., glucose and urea). Water and sodium are the main entities controlling the osmolality of body fluids. Serum sodium is responsible for 90% of the serum osmolality (Daniels, 2010). The normal range of serum osmolality is 280 to 300 mOsm/Kg (Daniels, 2010). The value increases with dehydration and decreases with water excess.

In clinical practice, the terms *osmolality* and **osmolarity** (the concentration of solutes per liter of cellular fluid) are often used interchangeably to refer to the concentration of body fluid; however, these terms actually have different meanings, in that osmolality refers to the concentration of solutes in the total body water rather than in cellular fluid. The appropriate term to use in conjunction with IV fluid therapy is *osmolarity*.

Urine Osmolality Urine osmolality measures the number of solute particles in a defined amount of solution. The particles measured are nitrogenous waste (creatinine, urea, and uric acid), with urea being predominant. Urine osmolality varies greatly with diet and fluid intake and reflects the kidney's ability to concentrate urine. The normal range of urine osmolality is 500 to 800 mOsm/kg (Daniels, 2010).

Urine pH The measurement of urine pH reveals the hydrogen ion concentration in the urine, indicating the urine's acidity or alkalinity. The pH of the urine should be within normal range (4.5 to 8.0) when the kidney buffering system is compensating for either metabolic acidosis or alkalosis. This is considered a sign of normal function; however, when the renal compensatory function fails to respond to the blood pH, the urine pH will either increase, with acidosis, or decrease, with alkalosis.

NURSING DIAGNOSIS

The North American Nursing Diagnosis Association-International (NANDA-I, 2010) identifies the primary nursing diagnoses for clients with fluid imbalances as *Deficient **Fluid** Volume, Excess **Fluid** Volume, Risk for Deficient **Fluid** Volume,* and *Risk for Imbalanced **Fluid** Volume.* Numerous secondary nursing diagnoses may also apply.

> **PROFESSIONALTIP**
>
> **Urine Osmolality**
>
> Urine osmolality is more accurate than urine specific gravity as an indicator of hydration. Some medications and the presence of glucose and protein solutes in urine can give a false high specific gravity reading.

Deficient Fluid Volume

*Deficient **Fluid** Volume* is defined as "decreased intravascular, interstitial, and/or intracellular fluid. This refers to dehydration, water loss alone without change in sodium" (NANDA-I, 2010). The many causes of fluid volume deficit include:

- Excessive fluid loss resulting from diaphoresis, vomiting, diarrhea, hemorrhage, burns, ascites, wound drainage, indwelling tubes, or suction
- Diabetes insipidus
- Diabetes mellitus
- Addison's disease (adrenal insufficiency)
- Gastrointestinal fistula or draining abscess
- Intestinal obstruction

Assessment findings in the client with fluid volume deficit include thirst and weight loss of an amount consistent with the degree of dehydration. Marked dehydration manifests as dry mucous membranes and skin; poor skin turgor; low-grade temperature elevation; tachycardia; respirations of 28 or greater; decreased (10 to 15 mm Hg) systolic blood pressure; slowed venous filling; decreased urine output (less than 25 mL/hr); concentrated urine; elevated Hct, Hgb, and BUN; and acidic blood pH (less than 7.4).

Severe dehydration is characterized by the symptoms of marked dehydration plus a flushing of the skin. Systolic blood pressure continues to drop (60 mm Hg or below), and behavioral changes (restlessness, irritability, disorientation, and delirium) occur. The signs of fatal dehydration are anuria and coma, leading to death.

Excess Fluid Volume

*Excess **Fluid** Volume* is defined as "increased isotonic fluid retention" (NANDA-I, 2010). Fluid volume excess is related to excess fluid in either the tissues or the extremities (peripheral edema) or the lung tissues (pulmonary edema). The several causes of excess fluid volume include:

- Excessive fluid intake (e.g., IV therapy, sodium)
- Excessive loss or decreased intake of protein (chronic diarrhea, burns, kidney disease, malnutrition)
- Compromised regulatory mechanisms (kidney failure)
- Decreased intravascular movement (impaired myocardial contractility)
- Lymphatic obstruction (cancer, surgical removal of lymph nodes, obesity)
- Medications (steroid excess)
- Allergic reactions

The client with fluid volume excess will exhibit acute weight gain; decreased serum osmolality (lower than 275 mOsm/Kg), Hgb, Hct; protein and albumin, blood urea nitrogen (BUN); increased central venous pressure (greater than 12 to 15 cm H2O); and signs and symptoms of edema. The clinical expressions of edema are relative to the area of involvement, either pulmonary or peripheral (Table 24-7).

Risk for Deficient Fluid Volume

*Risk for Deficient **Fluid** Volume* is defined as "at risk for experiencing vascular, cellular, or intracellular dehydration" (NANDA-I, 2010). The many factors that place a client at risk for fluid volume deficit were listed previously.

TABLE 24-7 Clinical Manifestations of Edema

PULMONARY EDEMA	PERIPHERAL EDEMA
Cough	Pitting edema in extremities
Pink, frothy sputum	Edematous area: tight, smooth, dry
Dyspnea	Shiny, pale, cool skin
Cold, clammy skin	Puffy eyelids
Engorged neck and hand veins	Weight gain
Crackles and wheezes in lungs	
Tachypnea	
Tachycardia	

Risk for Imbalanced Fluid Volume

*Risk for Imbalanced **Fluid** Volume* is defined as "at risk for a decrease, increase, or rapid shift from one to the other of intravascular, interstitial, and/or intracellular fluid. This refers to body fluid loss, gain, or both" (NANDA-I, 2010). The greatest risk factor is a client undergoing a major invasive procedure.

Other Nursing Diagnoses

In clients with a fluid imbalance, the relationship between the primary nursing diagnoses previously discussed and the secondary nursing diagnoses is reciprocal: The primary nursing diagnoses influence and are influenced by the secondary nursing diagnoses. Some commonly identified secondary nursing diagnoses include:

- *Impaired **Gas** Exchange*
- *Decreased **Cardiac** Output*
- *Ineffective **Breathing** Pattern*
- ***Anxiety***
- *Disturbed **Thought** Processes*
- *Risk for **Injury***
- *Risk for **Infection***
- *Impaired **Oral** Mucous Membrane*
- *Deficient **Knowledge*** (specify)

PLANNING/OUTCOME IDENTIFICATION

Holistic nursing care requires collaborating with each client to identify goals for each nursing diagnosis. These individualized goals should reflect the client's abilities and limitations.

PROFESSIONAL TIP

Loss of Gastric Juices

Clients who lose excessive amounts of gastric juices, either through vomiting or suctioning, are prone to not only fluid volume deficit but also metabolic alkalosis, hypokalemia, and hyponatremia. Gastric juices contain hydrochloric acid, pepsinogen, potassium, and sodium.

CRITICAL THINKING

Student Activity

Review the chart of a client who has been receiving IV fluids for at least 48 hours for the following information: vital signs, subjective and objective assessment findings, intake and output records, lab results, and medications administered. What conclusions can you make about the client's fluid, electrolyte, and acid–base balance?

Nursing interventions are selected and prioritized to support the client's achievement of expected outcomes based on the goals. For example, if vomiting and diarrhea along with dry mucous membranes and a 5% weight loss led to a nursing diagnosis of *Deficient **Fluid** Volume*, the goals might include to relieve vomiting and diarrhea and achieve the proper balance of intake and output.

IMPLEMENTATION

The nurse has a responsibility to collaborate with and advocate for clients to ensure they receive appropriate and ethical care based on practice standards. The data obtained from the history serve as the basis for formulating expected outcomes and selecting nursing interventions appropriate to the client's natural patterns as revealed in their history.

Interventions related to changes in fluid, electrolyte, or acid–base balance are based on the goal of maintaining homeostasis and regulating and maintaining essential fluids and nutrients. Clients' adaptive capabilities are kept in mind when selecting interventions based on the clients' perceptions of their support systems, strengths, and options.

The nurse is responsible for performing frequent assessments and monitoring for adverse effects of fluid and electrolyte therapy to prevent complications.

Nursing activities related to assessment and implementation often involve the same measurements (e.g., weight and vital signs). Common interventions that promote reaching expected outcomes for restoring and maintaining homeostasis are discussed following.

Monitor Daily Weight

One of the main indicators of fluid and electrolyte balance is weight. The accurate measuring and recording of the client's daily weight is a vital responsibility. This information along with other clinical findings determine fluid therapy requirements for the client.

Measure Vital Signs

The client's acuity level and clinical situation determine the frequency of vital sign measurement. For example, vital signs are taken every 15 minutes until stable on the typical postoperative client, whereas vital signs should be monitored continuously on the client in shock or hemorrhaging. Vital signs and other clinical data are used to determine the amount and type of fluid therapy.

Measure Intake and Output

Intake and output (I&O) measurements monitor the client's fluid status over a 24-hour period. Agency policy for I&O may vary regarding:

- Times for charting (e.g., every 8 hours versus every 12 hours)
- Time when 24-hour totals are calculated
- Definition of "strict" I&O

PROFESSIONALTIP

"Strict" I&O

- "Strict" I&O measurement usually involves accounting for incontinent urine, emesis, and diaphoresis and might require weighing soiled bed linens.
- *Gloves should always be worn when handling soiled linen.*

Review the client's 24-hour I&O calculations to evaluate fluid status. Intake should exceed output by 500 mL to offset insensible fluid loss. Intake and output and daily weight are critical interventions because they are used to evaluate the effectiveness of rehydration or diuretic therapy.

Having an accurate I&O requires the efforts of the client and family. The client and family must be taught how to measure and record the I&O.

Provide Oral Hygiene

Providing oral hygiene that promotes both client comfort and the integrity of the buccal cavity is an important responsibility. The condition of the client's buccal cavity and the type of fluid imbalance dictates the frequency of oral hygiene.

Initiate Oral Fluid Therapy

Depending on the client's clinical situation, oral fluids may be totally restricted, commonly referred to as *nothing by mouth* (NPO, which is from the Latin *non per os*), or they may be restricted or forced.

COMMUNITY/HOME HEALTH CARE

Considerations for Measuring I&O

- Ask for client and family input to select household items for intake measurement.
- Provide containers for measuring output, adapting the urinary container to home facilities, and teach client and family about proper washing and storage of the containers.
- Teach proper hand hygiene.
- Provide written instructions on what is to be measured.
- Leave sufficient I&O forms to last until the nurse's next visit.
- Identify the parameters for evaluating a discrepancy between the intake and the output and for notifying the nurse or physician.

SAFETY

Remove Gloves Before Charting

To prevent the transfer of microorganisms when the I&O form is removed from the client's room, remove gloves and wash hands before recording the amount of drainage on the form.

PROFESSIONALTIP

Mouthwashes

Mouthwashes with alcohol or glycerin and swabs with lemon or glycerin may feel refreshing, but these ingredients dry the mucous membranes.

Nothing by Mouth Clients are designated NPO as prescribed by the physician. Based on agency policy and clarification from the physician, the client may be allowed small amounts of ice chips when designated NPO. The NPO status may be required to:

- Avoid aspiration in unconscious, perioperative, and preprocedural clients who will receive anesthesia or conscious sedation
- Rest and heal the GI tract when there is severe vomiting or diarrhea or a GI disorder (inflammation or obstruction)
- Prevent more loss of gastric juices in clients on nasogastric suctioning

Clients who are NPO should receive oral hygiene every 1 to 2 hours or as needed to prevent alterations of the mucous membranes and for comfort

Restricted Fluids Fluid intake is commonly restricted when treating fluid volume excess related to heart and renal failure. Intake may be restricted to 200 mL in a 24-hour period.

The way fluids are limited should be determined in collaboration with the client. For example:

- Half of the allowed fluid might be divided between breakfast and lunch, and
- The remaining half might be divided between the evening meal and before bedtime, unless the client must be awakened during the night for medication.

Forced Fluids "Forcing" or encouraging the intake of oral fluids, mainly water, is sometimes done when treating clients who are at risk for dehydration or who have renal and urinary problems (kidney stones). Compliance is obtained through client education and honoring client preferences of timing and type of liquids. A client might, for example, be requested to consume 2,000 mL over a 24-hour period. Explain that this is only eight glasses or one glass every 2 hours. Also tell the client that ice, gelatin, soups, and ice cream all count as liquid.

Maintain Tube Feeding

The client who cannot ingest oral fluids but has a normal GI tract can have fluids and nutrients administered through a feeding tube as prescribed by a physician.

PROFESSIONALTIP

Temperature of Fluids

Clients should drink room-temperature fluids. Hot or cold fluids may increase peristalsis and abdominal cramping.

PROFESSIONALTIP

Fluid Replacement

Fluid replacement is based on weight loss. A 2.2-pound (1 kg) weight loss is equivalent to 1 liter (1,000 mL) of fluid loss.

Monitor Intravenous Therapy

Fluid volume is replaced parenterally when fluid loss is severe or the client cannot tolerate oral or tube feedings. **Intravenous** (IV) **therapy** is the administration of fluids, electrolytes, nutrients, or medications by the venous route. The physician prescribes IV therapy to prevent or treat fluid, electrolyte, or nutritional imbalances. There are specific nursing responsibilities during IV therapy. Specifically, the nurse must:

- Know why the IV fluid is prescribed
- Document client understanding
- Select, according to agency policy, the appropriate equipment
- Obtain the correct prescribed solution
- Assess the client for allergies to iodine, tape, ointment, or antibiotic preparations used for skin preparation of the venipuncture site
- Administer the fluid at the prescribed rate
- Observe for signs of **infiltration** (seepage of the fluid into the interstitial tissue as a result of accidental dislodgement of the needle from the vein) and other complications that are fluid specific
- Document in the client's medical record the implementation of the prescribed IV therapy

EVALUATION

Evaluation is an ongoing process. When evaluating whether the time frames and expected outcomes are realistic (such as whether the intake and output are within 200 to 300 mL of each other), the focus should be on the client's responses such as vital signs within normal limits, the IV infusion rate maintains the client's hydration, and the IV site remains free from erythema, edema, and purulent drainage. The nursing care plan should be modified as necessary to support the client's expected outcomes.

CASE STUDY

J.M. is a 71 year old man diagnosed with type II diabetes 10 years ago with an average blood sugar of 220 mg/dl. In addition, J.M. was diagnosed with congestive heart failure 15 years after his 5 vessel coronary artery bypass grafts (CABG). The cardiac history is a result of the untreated hypertension he suffered from for 12 years before his bypass surgery. Physical assessment data reveals: oral temperature 98.4 F, respiratory rate 10 bpm, apical pulse 128 bpm, blood pressure 186/96 mm Hg, and pulse oximetry is 80%, and crackles scattered throughout all lung fields. J.M. complains of shortness of breath (SOB) with activity, denies pain, is able to perform ADLs, states problems with swallowing thin liquids, and requests to be placed in high Flower's position. Respiratory pattern is irregular and shallow. J.M. is alert and oriented to person and place, and skin is cool, moist, and pale. Bowel sounds are active in all 4 quadrants, and the abdomen is semi hard and slightly distended. J.M. has (+2) pitting edema to the lower extremities

The following questions will guide your development of a nursing care plan for the case study.

1. List subjective and objective assessment data.
2. What acid-base imbalance does the nurse suspect?
3. Select 3 priority nursing diagnoses for J.M.'s acid-base imbalance.
4. Choose the priority nursing diagnosis and develop an appropriate client centered goal.
5. What nursing interventions should the nurse implement to assist J.M.?

SAMPLE NURSING CARE PLAN

The Client with Excess Fluid Volume

When brought to the emergency department by his granddaughter, R.W., a 68-year-old widower, stated, "I can't breathe." R.W. has a history of hypertension and heart disease, and he is obese. The practitioner ordered a stat chest x-ray, CBC, and electrolytes, which revealed pulmonary congestion (X-ray), decreased Hct, and decreased Hgb. The physical assessment results were as follows: Wt 162; TPR 97.6, 98, 30 (labored); BP 186/114; shortness of breath, crackles; constant cough; pitting edema (ankles); and engorged neck veins. R.W. stated, "I thought I could stop taking the heart medication and eat what I wanted when I felt good again."

NURSING DIAGNOSIS 1 *Excess Fluid Volume* related to a compromised regulatory mechanism as evidenced by edema, shortness of breath, crackles, decreased Hgb and Hct, and jugular vein distention

Nursing Outcomes Classification (NOC)	Nursing Interventions Classification (NIC)
Cardiac Pump Effectiveness	*Fluid Management*
Respiratory Status: Ventilation	*Medication Management*
Fluid Balance	*Fluid Monitoring*

SAMPLE NURSING CARE PLAN (Continued)

PLANNING/OUTCOMES	NURSING INTERVENTIONS	RATIONALE
R.W. will have a balanced I&O for 2 days.	Measure and document hourly I&O; restrict fluids as ordered.	Monitors fluid status.
	Administer diuretics as ordered and document response.	Increases excretion of fluids and electrolytes.
R.W. will identify a specific amount of weight to lose over the next 6 months.	Weigh daily at the same time, with the same scale, and with R.W. wearing the same clothing.	Allows weight to be compared from one day to another.
	Discuss with R.W. the need for weight loss.	Allows R.W. to voice his thoughts about weight loss and provides an avenue to determine number of pounds to be lost.
R.W. will show normal hydration status before discharge.	Measure and document vital signs every hour until shortness of breath subsides, then every 2 hours.	Monitors R.W.'s response to therapy.
	Hourly assess heart sounds; breath sounds; rate, rhythm, and depth of respirations; and the position R.W. takes to relieve the shortness of breath.	Provides information for use in modifying the plan of care.

EVALUATION

Output for the first 3 hours was 2,020 mL; on day 2, I&O indicated fluid balance. R.W. identified the need to lose 30 pounds over the next 6 months. R.W. demonstrated normal hydration status, as shown by normal levels of Hct and Hgb, BP 156/92, normal breath sounds, and absence of shortness of breath, jugular engorgement, and peripheral edema.

NURSING DIAGNOSIS 2 *Deficient **K**nowledge* related to information misinterpretation as evidenced by R.W.'s statement "I thought I could stop taking the heart medication and eat what I wanted when I felt good again."

Nursing Outcomes Classification (NOC)
Knowledge: Disease Process
Communication: Receptive Ability
Memory

Nursing Interventions Classification (NIC)
Teaching: Disease Process
Teaching: Prescribed Medication
Medication Management

PLANNING/OUTCOMES	NURSING INTERVENTIONS	RATIONALE
R.W. will demonstrate an understanding of the causes of fluid excess and the role of heart medications, foods, and exercise in assisting with weight reduction.	Assess R.W.'s knowledge of hypertension; decreased cardiac output; digitalis; the effects of a large abdominal girth on breathing; and foods low in sodium, fats, and carbohydrates.	Provides a basis for educating R.W. about causes, aggravating and alleviating factors, and effects of fluid excess.

EVALUATION

R.W. was unable to verbalize understanding of how weight, high-sodium diet, and failure to take his heart medications caused the fluid excess. He was referred to home health for client teaching.

(Continues)

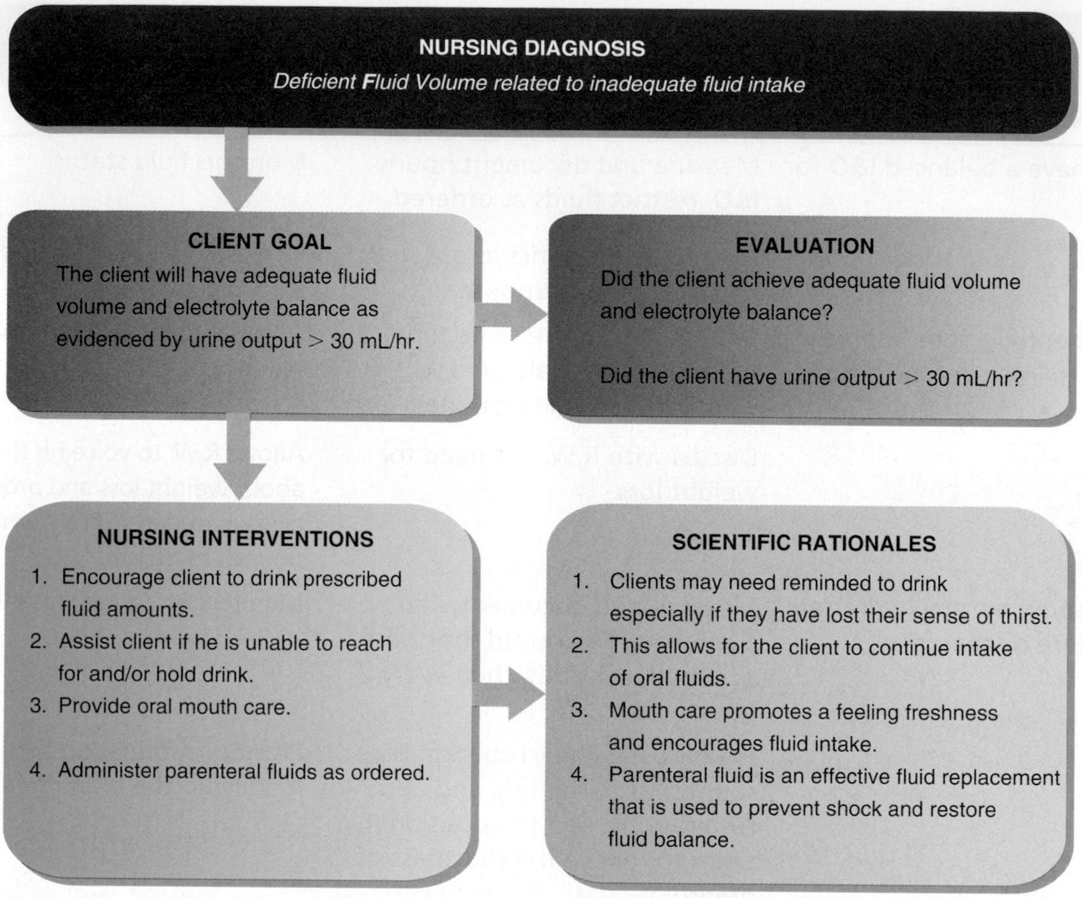

NURSING DIAGNOSIS
Deficient Fluid Volume related to inadequate fluid intake
CLIENT GOAL
The client will have adequate fluid volume and electrolyte balance as evidenced by urine output > 30 mL/hr.
EVALUATION
Did the client achieve adequate fluid volume and electrolyte balance?
Did the client have urine output > 30 mL/hr?
NURSING INTERVENTIONS
1. Encourage client to drink prescribed fluid amounts.
2. Assist client if he is unable to reach for and/or hold drink.
3. Provide oral mouth care.
4. Administer parenteral fluids as ordered.
SCIENTIFIC RATIONALES
1. Clients may need reminded to drink especially if they have lost their sense of thirst.
2. This allows for the client to continue intake of oral fluids.
3. Mouth care promotes a feeling freshness and encourages fluid intake.
4. Parenteral fluid is an effective fluid replacement that is used to prevent shock and restore fluid balance.

CONCEPT CARE MAP 24-1 Deficit Fluid Volume (*Courtesy of Janice Eilerman, RN, MSN, Lima, Ohio.*)

SUMMARY

- Homeostasis is the maintenance of the body's internal environment within a narrow range of normal values. It is an ongoing process, with changes constantly occurring in the body.
- Compounds that ionize in water are called electrolytes.
- The normal range of blood pH is 7.35 to 7.45. A decrease or increase beyond this range can cause severe or even fatal physiologic problems.
- The bicarbonate buffer system works to regulate pH in both intracellular and extracellular fluids.
- The phosphate buffer system works to regulate the pH of intracellular fluid and fluid in kidney tubules.
- Protein buffers work to regulate pH inside cells, especially red blood cells.
- Substances move in and out of cells by the passive transport methods of diffusion, osmosis, and filtration and by active transport.
- The kidneys regulate fluid and electrolyte balance.
- Sodium is the main electrolyte that promotes the retention of water.
- The slightest decrease or increase in electrolyte levels can cause serious, adverse, or life-threatening effects on physiologic functions.
- Hospitalized clients, especially elderly clients, are at risk for developing dehydration.
- Clients receiving IV therapy require constant monitoring for complications.

REVIEW QUESTIONS

1. A nurse is assessing a 77-year-old postoperative client using a morphine sulfate PCA pump for pain control. The assessment data reveals a respiratory rate of 8 bpm and irregular. The client is lethargic and confused. The nurse is updating the client's care plan and selects which nursing diagnosis as top priority?
   1. Risk for injury related to regulatory function.
   2. Impaired gas exchange related to inadequate ventilation.

3. Ineffective airway clearance related to viscosity of secretions.
4. Rest and sleep disturbance related to ineffective breathing pattern.

2. The nurse determines that which of the following clients is at greatest risk for developing a decrease in pH?
   1. 39-year-old client diagnosed with pneumonia.
   2. 89-year-old client prescribed Vasotec 5mg, IV push.
   3. 45-year-old client diagnosed with asthma
   4. 64-year-old client diagnosed with irritable bowel syndrome
3. A nurse is caring for a client receiving mechanical ventilation treatment for respiratory failure. The nurse suspects that the ventilator rate is set too high, causing hyperventilation. What acid–base problem could result from the ventilator rate being set too high?
   1. Metabolic acidosis
   2. Respiratory acidosis
   3. Metabolic alkalosis
   4. Respiratory alkalosis
4. Acidosis and alkalosis are identified by changes in the pH. Which of the following statements is true?
   1. A pH above 7.45 is called acidosis.
   2. A pH above 7.45 is called alkalosis.
   3. A pH increase caused by an increase of bicarbonate in the blood is metabolic acidosis.
   4. A pH decrease caused by an accumulation of carbonic acid results in respiratory alkalosis.
5. A nurse is taking a health history from a client who admits to using an excessive amount of base-containing antacids every day. The nurse's best response to client is:
   1. "Antacids can decrease the risk of alkalosis."
   2. "The more antacids you take, the greater risk you have for developing alkalosis."
   3. "You should not take antacids."
   4. "Acidosis is increased when an excessive amount of antacids are used."
6. Which client is at greatest risk for developing metabolic acidosis?
   1. 29-year-old client with broken ribs.
   2. 41-year-old client with hypertension.
   3. 63-year-old client positive for ketones.
   4. 58-year-old client with hypokalemia.
7. The nurse is teaching a client with a serum potassium level of 3.2 mEq/L about foods that are rich in potassium. The client correctly identifies all the following foods as potassium rich except:
   1. dinner roll.
   2. raw carrots.
   3. baked potato.
   4. apricot.
8. A client experiencing fever, pain, and rapid, shallow respirations is brought to the emergency department for treatment. Assessment findings include hyperactive reflexes, a positive Chvostek's sign, and muscle tremors. The ABG results are pH 7.50 and $PaCO_2$ 28 mm Hg. This client is at risk for:
   1. respiratory acidosis.
   2. respiratory alkalosis.
   3. metabolic acidosis.
   4. metabolic alkalosis.
9. Which of the following arterial blood gas values would the nurse document as respiratory acidosis?
   1. pH = 7.31; $PaCO_2$ = 50; HCO_3 = 30
   2. pH = 7.32; $PaCO_2$ = 39; HCO_3 = 25
   3. pH = 7.42; $PaCO_2$ = 29; HCO_3 = 19
   4. pH = 7.50; $PaCO_2$ = 35; HCO_3 = 22
10. When the intracellular fluid (ICF) compartment develops an osmolality greater than the extracellular fluid (ECF) compartment, water shifts from the ECF into the ICF compartment. This fluid shift is known as:
    1. active transport.
    2. osmosis.
    3. diffusion.
    4. filtration.

REFERENCES/SUGGESTED READINGS

Bulechek, G., Butcher, H., McCloskey, J., & Dochterman, J., eds. (2008). *Nursing Interventions Classification (NIC)* (5th ed.). St. Louis, MO: Mosby/Elsevier.

Chernecky, C., Macklin, D., & Murphy-Ende, K. (2001). *Fluids and electrolytes.* Philadelphia: W. B. Saunders.

Daniels, R. (2010). *Delmar's guide to laboratory and diagnostic tests* (2nd ed.) Clifton Park, NY: Delmar Cengage Learning.

Daniels, R., Nosek, L. J., & Nicoll, L. H. (2007). *Contemporary medical-surgical nursing.* Clifton Park, NY: Delmar Cengage Learning.

Eilerman, J. (2009). *Concept care map: Deficient Fluid Volume.* Lima, OH.

Estes, M. E. Z. (2010). *Health assessment and physical examination* (4th ed.). Clifton Park, NY: Delmar Cengage Learning.

Fox, K. (2009). *Concept map: Metabolic acidosis.* Lima, OH.

Hadaway, L. (2002). I.V. infiltration: Not just a peripheral problem. *Nursing2002, 32*(8), 36–42.

Hamilton, S. (2001). Detecting dehydration and malnutrition in the elderly. *Nursing2001, 31*(12), 56–57.

Hogstel, M. (2001). *Nursing care of the older adult* (4th ed.). Clifton Park, NY: Delmar Cengage Learning.

Incredibly Easy! (2002). Understanding hypokalemia. *Nursing2002,* 32(3), 56.

Incredibly Easy! Understanding hypokalemia. (2000) *Nursing2000, 30*(11), 74–76.

Josephson, D. L. (2004). *Intravenous infusion therapy for nurses: Principles and practice* (2nd ed.). Clifton Park, NY: Delmar Cengage Learning.

Kee, J. L., Paulanka, B. J., & Polek, C. (2010). *Fluids and electrolytes with clinical applications: A programmed approach* (8th ed.). Clifton Park, NY: Delmar Cengage Learning.

Klopfenstein, L. (2009). *Concept map: Respiratory acidosis.* Lima, OH.

Krueger, D., & Tasota, F. (2003). Keeping an eye on calcium levels. *Nursing2003, 33*(6), 68.

Mader, S. (2001). *Understanding human anatomy and physiology* (4th ed.). Boston: McGraw-Hill College Division.

Marieb, E. (2002). *Essentials of human anatomy and physiology* (7th ed.). Redwood City, CA: Cummings.

Martini, F., & Welch, K. (2001). *Fundamentals of anatomy and physiology* (5th ed.). Englewood Cliffs, NJ: Prentice Hall.

Mason, E. (2009). *Caring for clients with acid-base imbalances.* Manuscript submitted for publication.

McConnell, E. (2002). Measuring fluid intake and output. *Nursing2002, 32*(7), 17.

Moorhead, S., Johnson, M., Maas, M., & Swanson, E. (2007). *Nursing Outcomes Classification (NOC)* (4th ed.). St. Louis, MO: Mosby.

North American Nursing Diagnosis Association International. (2010). *NANDA-I nursing diagnoses: Definitions and classification 2009-2011.* Ames, IA: Wiley-Blackwell.

Scanlon, V., & Sanders, T. (2003). *Essentials of anatomy and physiology* (4th ed.). Philadelphia: F. A. Davis.

Schmidt, T. C., & Williams-Evans, S. A. (2000). How to recognize hypokalemia. *Nursing2000, 30*(2), 22.

Science Spot. (2009). *Biology lesson plans.* Retrieved June 26, 2009, from http://sciencespot.net/Pages/classbio.html

Senisi-Scott, A., & Fong, E. (2009). *Body structures and functions* (11th ed.). Clifton Park, NY: Delmar Cengage Learning.

White, L., & Duncan, G. (2002). *Medical-surgical nursing: An integrated approach* (2nd ed.). New York: Delmar Cengage Learning.

RESOURCE

Infusion Nurses Society, http://www.ins1.org

CHAPTER 25
Medication Administration and IV Therapy

MAKING THE CONNECTION

Refer to the following chapters to increase your understanding of medication administration and IV therapy:

Basic Nursing
- ***Legal and Ethical Responsibilities***
- ***Nursing Process/Documentation/ Informatics***
- ***Basic Nutrition***
- ***Infection Control/Asepsis***
- ***Standard Precautions and Isolation***
- ***Diagnostic Tests***

Basic Procedures
- ***Administering an Enema***
- ***Measuring Intake and Output***

Intermediate Procedures
- ***Administering an Oral, Sublingual, and Buccal Medication***
- ***Withdrawing Medication from an Ampule***
- ***Withdrawing Medication from a Vial***
- ***Administering an Intradermal Injection***
- ***Administering a Subcutaneous Injection***
- ***Administering Intramuscular Injections***
- ***Administering Eye and Ear Medications***

Advanced Procedures
- ***Performing Venipuncture (Blood Drawing)***
- ***Preparing an IV Solution and Starting an IV***
- ***Setting the IV Flow Rate***
- ***Administering Medications via IV Piggyback***
- ***Assessing and Maintaining an IV Insertion Site***

LEARNING OBJECTIVES

Upon completion of this chapter, you should be able to:

- Define key terms.
- Describe how drug standards and legislation influence medication administration.
- Explain pharmacokinetics, including absorption, distribution, metabolism, and excretion of drugs.

- Describe factors that can affect a drug's action.
- Explain the different types of medication orders, when each is used, and the nurse's responsibilities for each type.
- Identify principles of safe medication administration.
- Discuss potential liabilities for the nurse administering medications.
- Develop teaching guidelines for clients regarding medication administration in the home.
- Explain procedures for the various methods of medication administration, including the choice of route and site.

KEY TERMS

absorption
angiocatheter
aspiration
bioavailability
butterfly needles
chemical name
distribution
drug allergy
drug incompatibilities
drug interaction
drug tolerance
enteral instillation
excretion
extravasation
flashback
flow rate
generic name
half-life
hypervolemia
idiosyncratic reaction
implantable port
infiltration
intracath
intradermal (ID)
intramuscular (IM)
intravenous (IV)
IV push (bolus)
metabolism
onset of action
parenteral
patency
peak plasma level
pharmacokinetics
phlebitis
piggybacked
plateau
stock supplied
subcutaneous
toxic effect
trade (brand) name
unit dose
vesicant

INTRODUCTION

Managing medications requires collaboration of many health care providers. Medications are prescribed by a physician, dentist, or other authorized prescriber such as advanced practice registered nurses as determined by individual state licensing boards. Medications are prepared and dispensed by pharmacists. Nurses are responsible for administering medications. Dietitians may be involved in identifying possible food–drug interactions.

Medication administration requires specialized knowledge, judgment, and nursing skills based on the principles of pharmacology. This chapter focuses on assisting students to apply knowledge of pharmacology and to acquire safe administration of medications skills. The nursing process directs nursing decisions about safe drug administration and ensures compliance with standards of practice.

DRUG STANDARDS AND LEGISLATION

A drug is a chemical substance intended to have a specific effect. Nurses assume, before administering any medication, that the drug will be safe for the client if the dose, route, and frequency are within the therapeutic range for that drug. This assumption is implied by standards ensuring drug uniformity in strength, purity, efficacy, safety, and **bioavailability** (readiness to produce a drug effect).

STANDARDS

Standards ensure drug uniformity for predictable effects. The *United States Pharmacopeia* and the *National Formulary* (USP and NF) are books of drug standards used in the United States. The USP and NF list drugs recognized for compliance with legal standards of purity, quality, and strength.

The USP has been providing standards for pharmaceutical preparations since its first edition was published in 1851. The American Pharmaceutical Association first published the NF in 1898 to provide a list of drugs complying with established standards.

LEGISLATION

The USP and the NF were designated by the Pure Food and Drug Act of 1906 as the official bodies to establish drug standards. The authority to enforce these standards was given to the federal government. The federal Food, Drug, and Cosmetic Act of 1938 authorized the Food and Drug Administration (FDA) to test all new drugs for toxicity before giving approval to market a drug. In 1952, the federal Food, Drug, and Cosmetic Act of 1938 was amended to differentiate prescription (legend) drugs from nonprescription (over-the-counter) drugs and to regulate prescription dispensing. Drug effectiveness testing came with the Kefauver-Harris Act of 1962 (Lehne, 2006).

In 1914, the Harrison Narcotic Act classified habit-forming drugs as narcotics and began regulating them. This law and other drug abuse laws were replaced with the Comprehensive Drug Abuse Prevention and Control Act (Controlled Substance Act) in 1970. This act defines a *drug-dependent person* in terms of physical and psychological dependence and provides for strict regulation of narcotics and other controlled drugs such as barbiturates with the five categories of scheduled drugs (Table 25-1). Records must be kept by the dispensing pharmacist for all controlled substances. Pharmacists employed by the Drug Enforcement Agency (DEA) inspect records and prescriptions to discover illicit distribution of these substances.

All states must adhere to the schedule of controlled substances as minimum standards; however, individual states can pass stricter controls of these substances. For example, the Controlled Substance Act has antitussives with codeine as a schedule V drug, but an individual state may place this drug in the more restrictive schedule II category.

DRUG NOMENCLATURE

The terms *medication, medicine,* and *drug* are used interchangeably by laypersons and health care providers.

Drugs are identified by a chemical, generic, official, or trade name. The **chemical name** is a precise description of the drug's chemical formula. The **generic name** (*nonproprietary*) in the United States is the name assigned by the U.S. Adopted Names Council to the manufacturer who first develops the drug. When a drug is approved, it is given an *official name,* which may be the same as the nonproprietary name (Lehne, 2006). Drugs with proven therapeutic value are listed by their official name in the USP and NF. Pharmaceutical companies assign a *proprietary name,* also called a **trade (brand) name,** when they market a drug. One generic drug may have several trade names depending on how many companies market the drug. For example, ibuprofen is a generic name; trade names for this drug include Advil, Motrin, Excedrin IB, and Nuprin. *Generic names are not capitalized, but trade names are always capitalized.*

DRUG ACTION

Drug action refers to a drug's ability to combine with a cellular receptor. Depending on the location of cellular receptors affected by a given drug, a drug can have a local effect, a systemic effect, or both. For example, when diphenhydramine hydrochloride (Benadryl) cream is applied to the skin, it has only a local effect; however, when administered

TABLE 25-1 Controlled Substances

Schedule (C-I): Includes substances for which there is a high abuse potential and no current approved medical use (e.g., heroin, marijuana, LSD, other hallucinogens, certain opiates and opium derivatives).
Schedule (C-II): Includes drugs that have a high abuse potential and a high ability to produce physical and/or psychological dependence and for which there is a current approved or acceptable medical use (e.g., narcotics, amphetamines, dronabinol, and some barbiturates).
Schedule (C-III): Includes drugs for which there is less potential for abuse than drugs in Schedule II and for which there is a current approved medical use (e.g., nonbarbiturate sedatives, nonamphetamine stimulants, and limited amounts of certain narcotics). Also, anabolic steroids are classified in Schedule III.
Schedule (C-IV): Includes drugs for which there is a relatively low abuse potential and for which there is a current approved medical use (e.g., sedatives, antianxiety agents, and nonnarcotic analgesics).
Schedule (C-V): Drugs in this category consist mainly of preparations containing limited amounts of certain narcotic drugs (e.g., codeine used as antitussive and antidiarrheals). Federal law provides that limited quantities of these drugs may be bought without a prescription by an individual at least 18 years of age. The product must be purchased from a pharmacist, who must keep appropriate records. However, state laws vary, and in many states such products require a prescription.

From *2010 Delmar Nurse's Drug Handbook* by G. Spratto & A. Woods, 2010, Clifton Park, NY: Delmar Cengage Learning; *Nursing Fundamentals: Caring and Clinical Decision Making* by R. Daniels, R. Grendell, & F. Wilkins, 2010, Clifton Park, NY: Delmar Cengage Learning.

in a tablet or injectable form, it has both a systemic and a local effect.

Pharmacology

The study of drug effects on living organisms is called pharmacology. This section discusses the pharmacological activities of drug action as related to medication management, drug classification, and routes of administration.

Medication Management

Medication management is to produce the desired drug action by maintaining a constant drug level. Drug action is based on the half-life of a drug. A drug's **half-life** is the time it takes the body to eliminate half of the blood concentration level of the original drug dose. For example, if a drug has a half-life of 8 hours, 50% of the drug's original dose is present in the blood 8 hours after administration, and 25% of the drug is present 16 hours after administration. Because of a drug's half-life, repeated doses are given to maintain a therapeutic drug level over a 24-hour interval. Maintaining a therapeutic drug level ensures antibiotic effectiveness against bacteria within the body, and pain medication provides an effective pain threshold.

Other terms describing drug action include onset, peak plasma level, and plateau. **Onset of action** is the time for the body to respond to a drug after administration. **Peak plasma level** is the highest blood concentration of a single drug dose before the elimination rate equals the rate of absorption. The blood concentration level will decrease steadily once the peak plasma level is reached, unless another dose is given. When a series of scheduled drug doses is administered, the blood concentration level is maintained and is called a **plateau**.

Classification

Drugs are generally classified by the body system with which they interact (e.g., cardiovascular) or by the drug's approved therapeutic usage (e.g., antihypertensive). Drugs with several therapeutic uses are usually classified by their most common use.

Routes

Drugs are prepared in many forms for administration by a specific route (Table 25-2). The route is how the drug is absorbed: oral, buccal, sublingual, parenteral, topical, and respiratory.

SAFETY

Do Not Substitute Drug Forms

Drugs prepared for administration by one route cannot be substituted by the drug prepared for another route. For example, when a client has difficulty swallowing a large tablet or capsule, an oral solution or elixir of the same drug cannot be administered without first consulting the physician. A liquid may be more easily and completely absorbed, producing a higher blood level than a tablet.

Oral Route Most drugs are administered by the oral route because it is the most convenient, least expensive, and safest method, but it acts more slowly than the other routes. Drugs are not given orally to clients with GI intolerance, those on NPO (nothing by mouth) status, or those in a coma.

The buccal or sublingual route is used when small amounts of drugs are required. Buccal and sublingual drugs act quickly because of the oral mucosa's thin epithelium and large vascular system, allowing the drug to be quickly absorbed.

Buccal drugs are placed in the buccal pocket (superior-posterior aspect of the internal cheek next to the molars) for absorption by the mucous membrane. Sublingual medications are made to dissolve quickly when placed under the tongue. For example, nitroglycerin (Nitrostat), an antianginal drug, can be given either sublingually or buccally as prescribed, whereas isoproterenol hydrochloride (Isuprel), a bronchodilator, is given only sublingually, and methyltesterone (Testred), an androgen, is given only buccally.

Parenteral Route **Parenteral** drugs are administered by injection using sterile technique. By definition, parenteral route refers to any route other than the oral-gastrointestinal tract; however, the medical usage of the term excludes topical and respiratory routes. The four routes that nurses use to administer medications parenterally are:

- **Intradermal (ID)**, an injection into the dermis
- **Subcutaneous**, an injection into the subcutaneous tissue
- **Intramuscular (IM)**, an injection into the muscle
- **Intravenous (IV)**, an injection into a vein

Other parenteral routes, such as intrathecal or intraspinal, intrapleural, intracardiac, intra-arterial, and intra-articular, are used by physicians and sometimes by advanced-practice registered nurses.

Topical Route Most topical drugs are given to deliver a drug at or immediately beneath the point of application. Many topical drugs are applied to the skin, but other topical drugs include eye, nose and throat, ear, rectal, and vaginal preparations. Drugs directly applied to the skin are absorbed into the dermis, where they have a local effect or are absorbed into the bloodstream. The vascularity of the skin varies the drug action. Usually several applications over a 24-hour period are required for the desired therapeutic effect.

Transdermal patches are used to deliver medications such as nitroglycerin (Transdermal-NTG), an antianginal, and some supplemental hormone replacements for absorption to produce systemic effects. Some topical drugs, such as eye

PROFESSIONAL TIP

Special Considerations for Oral Route

- Chewable tablets are chewed before swallowing; chewing enhances gastric absorption.
- Buccal and sublingual medications must dissolve completely before the client drinks or eats.
- Suspensions and emulsions are administered immediately after shaking and pouring from the bottle.

TABLE 25-2 Types of Drug Preparations

TYPE	DESCRIPTION
Oral Solids	• Tablets: compressed or molded substances, to be swallowed whole, chewed before swallowing, or placed in the buccal pocket or under the tongue (sublingual) • Capsules: substances encased in a hard or a soft soluble cover or gelatin shell that dissolves in the stomach • Caplets: gelatin-coated tablets that dissolve in the stomach • Powders and granules: finely ground substances • Troches, lozenges, and pastilles: designed to dissolve in the mouth • Enteric-coated tablets: coated tablets that dissolve in the intestines • Time-release capsules: encased substances that are further enclosed in smaller casings that deliver a drug dose over an extended period • Sustained-release: compounded substances that release a drug slowly to maintain a steady plasma level
Topicals	• Liniments: substances mixed with an alcohol, oil, or soapy emollient; applied to the skin • Ointments: semisolid substances for topical use • Pastes: semisolid substances, thicker than ointments, absorbed slowly through the skin • Suppositories: gelatin substances designed to dissolve when inserted in the rectum, urethra, or vagina
Inhalants	• Inhalations: drugs or dilutions of drugs administered by the nasal or oral respiratory route for a local or systemic effect
Solutions	• Solutions: contain one or more soluble chemical substances dissolved in water • Enemas: aqueous solutions for rectal instillation • Douches: aqueous solutions that function as a cleansing or antiseptic agent that may be dispensed in the form of a powder with directions for dissolving in a specific quantity of warm water • Suspensions: particles or powder substances that must be mixed with, not dissolved in, a liquid by shaking vigorously before administration • Emulsions: two-phase systems in which one liquid is dispersed in the form of small droplets throughout another liquid • Syrups: substances dissolved in a sugar liquid • Gargles: aqueous solutions • Mouthwashes: aqueous solutions that may contain alcohol, glycerin, and synthetic sweeteners • Nasal solutions: aqueous solutions instilled as drops or sprays • Optic (eye) and otic (ear) solutions: aqueous solutions instilled as drops • Elixirs: solutions that contain water, varying amounts of alcohol, and sweeteners

and nasal drops and vaginal and rectal suppositories, applied directly to the mucous membranes, are absorbed quickly and, depending on the drug's dose (strength and quantity), may cause systemic effects.

Respiratory Route Inhalants such as oxygen and most general anesthetics deliver gaseous or volatile substances that are almost immediately absorbed into systemic circulation. The inhalants, delivered into the alveoli of the lungs, promote fast absorption due to:

- Permeability of the alveolar and vascular epithelium
- Abundant blood flow
- Very large surface area for absorption

Oropharyngeal handheld inhalers deliver topical drugs to the respiratory tract to create local and systemic effects. The three types of inhalers—the metered-dose inhaler, or nebulizer; the turbo-inhaler; and the nasal inhaler—are explained later in this chapter.

PHARMACOKINETICS

Pharmacokinetics is the study of the absorption, distribution, metabolism, and excretion of drugs to determine the relationship between the dose of a drug and the drug's concentration in biological fluids. This knowledge is used by health care providers in medication management.

The physician is concerned mainly with the dose and route that will produce the most therapeutic effects. Pharmacists, physicians, and nurses work together to identify appropriate times for drug administration and to avoid interactions with other substances that might alter the drug's actions. Nurses and physicians monitor the client's response to the drug's action. Drug actions are dependent on four properties: absorption, distribution, metabolism, and excretion.

Absorption

The degree and rate of **absorption**, or movement of a drug from administration site into the bloodstream, depend on several factors: the drug's physicochemical effects, its dosage, its route of administration, its interactions with other substances, and various client characteristics such as age (Blanchard & Loeb, 2006). After ingestion, oral preparations, such as tablets and capsules, disintegrate into smaller particles so that gastric juices can dissolve and prepare the drug for absorption in the small intestines.

Intramuscularly administered drugs are absorbed through the muscle into the bloodstream. Suppositories are absorbed through the mucous membranes into the blood. Intravenous drugs are immediately bioavailable because they are directly injected into the blood.

Distribution

Distribution is the movement of medications from the blood into various body tissues and fluids. Drug distribution in the body is affected by cardiac output, cell membrane permeability, protein-binding capacity of the medication, and body fat. A client's cardiac output can increase or decrease blood flow, and peripheral vascular disease decreases circulation to body tissues. The blood–brain barrier allows only fat-soluble medications through the membrane. A malnourished client or one with liver disease has decreased albumin or protein circulating in the blood, allowing a higher concentration of the medication in the blood. Drug duration is increased in obese clients, resulting in slower drug distribution (Daniels, 2010).

Metabolism

Metabolism is the physical and chemical processing of a drug by the body. Most drugs are metabolized in the liver. The presence of enzymes in the liver that detoxify the drugs determine the rate of metabolism. Some drugs can increase the rate of metabolism.

Excretion

Excretion is the elimination of drugs from the body. This occurs mainly through hepatic metabolism and renal excretion, but the lungs, exocrine glands, skin, and intestinal tract can eliminate some drugs.

Drug Interaction

Drug interaction is the effect one drug can have on another drug. Drug interactions may occur when two drugs are administered at the same time or within a short time interval. Drugs can be purposely combined for a positive effect; for example, hydrochlorothiazide (HydroDIURIL), a potassium-depleting diuretic, and spironolactone (Aldactone), a potassium-sparing diuretic, when combined maintain a normal blood level of potassium. When one drug is purposely given to potentiate the action of another drug, as in preoperative medications, a positive drug interaction occurs.

Not all drug interactions are therapeutic. Some interactions can interfere with the absorption, effect, or excretion of other drugs. For example, calcium products and magnesium-containing antacids can cause inadequate absorption of tetracycline (Tetracyn), an antibiotic, in the digestive tract.

Side Effects and Adverse Reactions

Drug effects other than those therapeutically intended and expected are called *adverse reactions*. A nontherapeutic effect may be mild and predictable (side effect) or unexpected and potentially dangerous (adverse reaction). There are several types of adverse reactions: drug allergy, drug tolerance, toxic effect, and idiosyncratic reactions.

A **drug allergy** (hypersensitivity to a drug) is an antigen–antibody immune reaction occurring when an individual previously exposed to a drug has developed antibodies against the drug. The type of reaction may be mild (skin rash, urticaria, headache, nausea, or vomiting) or severe (anaphylaxis). Drug reactions are often seen on the skin because of its abundant blood supply.

Anaphylaxis is an immediate, life-threatening reaction to a drug, such as penicillin, marked by respiratory distress, sudden severe bronchospasm, and cardiovascular collapse. Anaphylaxis can be fatal if emergency measures are not begun immediately (administration of epinephrine, bronchodilators, and antihistamines).

Drug tolerance occurs when the body is so accustomed to a specific drug that larger doses are needed to produce the desired therapeutic effect. For example, clients with cancer experiencing severe pain may require larger and larger doses of morphine (a narcotic analgesic) to control the pain.

A **toxic effect** occurs when the body cannot metabolize a drug and the drug accumulates in the blood. Digoxin, a cardiac drug, has a narrow margin of safety between an effective therapeutic dose and a toxic dose (Spratto & Woods, 2009).

An **idiosyncratic reaction** is a very unpredictable response that may be an overresponse, an underresponse, or an atypical response. For example, 1 of 40,000 clients will develop aplastic anemia after receiving chloramphenicol (Chloromycetin), an antibiotic (Blanchard & Loeb, 2006).

Food–Drug Interactions

Medication management works to avoid possible food–drug interactions. There are three main types of food–drug interactions:

1. Some drugs interfere with the absorption, excretion, or use in the body of one or more nutrients.
2. Some foods increase or decrease the absorption of a drug into the body.
3. Some foods alter the chemical actions of drugs, preventing the therapeutic effect on the body.

Most interaction problems occur with the use of oral antibiotics, diuretics, anticoagulant, and antihypertensive drugs. Clients on sodium-restricted diets should consult with a pharmacist about the sodium content of prescription and over-the-counter drugs. Some drugs contain almost half the total daily allowance of sodium. Alcohol interacts with many drugs, such as antihistamines, antibiotics, anticoagulants, and sleeping pills. Food–drug interactions vary depending on the dose and the form of the drug taken and the client's age, gender, nutritional status, body weight, and specific medical condition.

Many herbals interact with drugs to change their effect, such as with digoxin, a cardiac drug. Herbal teas such as Woodruff, tonka bean, and melitot contain natural coumarins

LIFE SPAN CONSIDERATIONS

Age-Related Factors Influence Drug Action and Dosing

- Neonates and infants have underdeveloped gastrointestinal systems, muscle mass, and metabolic enzyme systems and inadequate renal function.
- Elderly clients often experience decreased hepatic or renal function and diminished muscle mass.

that can potentiate the effects of Coumadin, an anticoagulant (Spratto & Woods, 2009).

FACTORS INFLUENCING DRUG ACTION

Individual client characteristics such as genetic factors, age, height, weight, and physical and mental conditions can influence drug actions on the body. Genetic factors can interfere with drug metabolism, producing an abnormal sensitivity to certain drugs.

The physician often correlates the client's age, height, and weight to determine the dosage for many drugs. This information must be accurately recorded in the client's medical record. The amount of body fat may also alter drug distribution.

The client's physical condition can also alter the effects of drugs. For example, in an edematous client, the drug must be distributed to a larger volume of body fluids than in a nonedematous client; therefore, the edematous client may require a larger dose to produce the desired action, whereas a dehydrated client may require a smaller dosage. Diseases affecting liver and renal functioning can alter the metabolism and elimination of most drugs.

MEDICATION ORDERS

In health care facilities, medication orders are written on a physician's order form in each client's medical record.

All orders must be written clearly and legibly. A drug order should contain seven parts:

1. Client's name
2. Date and time when the order is written
3. Name of the drug to be administered
4. Dosage
5. Route for administration and special directives about its administration
6. Time of administration and frequency
7. Signature of the person writing the order, such as the physician or advanced-practice registered nurse

Drug prescriptions outside acute care facilities may also specify whether the generic or trade name drug is to be used, the quantity to be given, and how many times the prescription can be refilled.

If, in the nurse's judgment, a drug order is in error, the nurse is responsible and held accountable for questioning that order. The error may be in any part of the drug order, and the nurse should clarify the order with the prescriber. The conversation must be documented in the client's medical record (Smith, 2003). A drug error has serious legal implications if the nurse involved could have been expected, on the basis of experience and knowledge, to have noted the error.

Most agencies have policies relative to medication administration, such as stop dates for certain types of drugs, regularly scheduled times to administer medications as specified in the drug order, and a listing of abbreviations officially accepted for use in the agency. The agency's medical records department maintains the official listing of abbreviations adopted by the medical staff of that agency. Only abbreviations from the official list can be used in any part of the client's medical record at that agency (see appendices).

TYPES OF ORDERS

Medications are prescribed differently, depending on their purpose. Medications can be prescribed as stat, single-dose, scheduled, and prn orders.

Stat Orders

Stat medication orders are those that should be administered immediately, not an hour or two later. Stat orders are often encountered in emergency situations, such as a stat dose of nitroglycerin for a client experiencing chest pain. The client's response to all stat medications must be assessed and documented.

Single-Dose Orders

Single-dose orders are one-time medications. They should be administered either at a time specified by the prescriber or at the earliest convenient time. These orders are often used in preparation for a diagnostic or therapeutic procedure; for example, a laxative may be ordered to prepare a client for a lower GI x-ray.

Scheduled Orders

Scheduled orders are administered as specified until the order is changed or canceled by another order or until the specified number of days has elapsed as set by agency policy. Scheduled orders are used to maintain the desired blood level of the medication.

Agency policy sets the actual times for administering medications over a 24-hour time interval. For example, t.i.d. drugs may be administered at 0800, 1400, and 2000 or at 0900, 1500, and 2100. Medications ordered daily may have a time specified in the order, such as Isophane (NPH) Insulin 10 units subcutaneous daily at 0630, or they will be given at the agency's designated time; for example, Lanoxin 0.25 mg po daily would be given at 0900.

An order specifying the number of days or dosages the client is to receive has an automatic stop date for the drug. For example, an order for tetracycline 250 mg po q6h for 5 days would provide tetracycline 250 mg orally every 6 hours for 5 days, a total of 20 doses. Day 1 begins with the administration of the first dose.

PRN Orders

A prn (as needed) drug is administered when, in the nurse's judgment, the client's condition requires it. This type of order is generally written for laxatives, analgesics, and antiemetics.

For example, a client may have an order for oxycodone hydrochloride (OxyContin), a narcotic analgesic, 5 to 10 mg qid prn. The pain medication is given based on the assessment of the client's pain and as specified in the order.

SYSTEMS OF WEIGHT AND MEASURE

Medication administration requires a knowledge of weight and volume measurement systems. In the United States three different systems of measurement are used in medication management: metric, apothecary, and household.

Metric System

In 1890, the USP adopted the metric system of weights and measures exclusively except for equivalent dosages. In 1944, the Council on Pharmacy and Chemistry of the American Medical Association adopted the metric system exclusively. The metric system is used in every major country of the world except the United States but is used almost exclusively in U.S. health care facilities.

The metric (decimal system) is a simple system based on units of 10. Move the decimal point to the right to change from a larger unit to a smaller unit and move the decimal point to the left to change from a smaller unit to a larger unit. For example:

5 g = 5,000 mg	0.5 mg = 500 mcg
5 mcg = 0.005 mg	1.25 L = 1,250 milliliters (mL)
0.25 g = 250 mg	2.45 kg = 2,450 g

The basic measurement units are the meter (linear), the liter (volume), and the gram (mass, or weight). Important abbreviations and equivalents to remember are:

- Volume (liquid)
  1,000 milliliters = 1 liter (L)
- Weight
  1,000 micrograms (mcg) = 1 milligram (mg)
  1,000 milligrams = 1 gram (g)
  1,000 grams = 1 kilogram (kg)

The metric system uses Latin prefixes to designate subdivisions of the basic units and Greek prefixes to designate multiples of the basic units (Table 25-3).

TABLE 25-3 Metric System Prefixes

PREFIX	EXAMPLE
Latin Prefixes—Subdivisions of the basic unit	deci (1/10, or 0.1)
	centi (1/100, or 0.01)
	milli (1/1,000, or 0.001)
	micro (1/1,000,000 or 0.000001)
Greek Prefixes—Multiples of the basic unit	deka (10)
	hecto (100)
	kilo (1,000)

COURTESY OF DELMAR CENGAGE LEARNING

SAFETY

Metric System

A zero is *not* written after a decimal point (1, *not* 1.0), and a zero is always placed in front of the decimal for values less than 1 (0.5) to prevent errors.

Apothecary System

The apothecary system originated in England and is based on the weight of one grain of wheat. The grain (gr) is the basic unit of weight and the minim (the approximate volume of water that weighs a grain) is the basic unit of volume. Important equivalents and abbreviations are:

- Volume (liquid)
  60 minums (♏) = 1 fluid dram (fl dr, or ʒ)
  8 fluid drams = 1 fluid ounce (fl oz, or ℥)
  16 fluid ounces = 1 pint (pt)
- Weight
  60 grains (gr) = 1 dram (dr, or ʒ)
  8 drams = 1 ounce (oz, or ℥)
  12 ounces = 1 pound (lb)

Household System

The household system of measurement is the least accurate of the three systems. It is not ordinarily used to calculate dosage but only as a reference to help the client. The units of liquid measure are drop (gtt), teaspoon (tsp), tablespoon (Tbsp), ounce (oz), and cup (Figure 25-1). The 16-ounce pound of

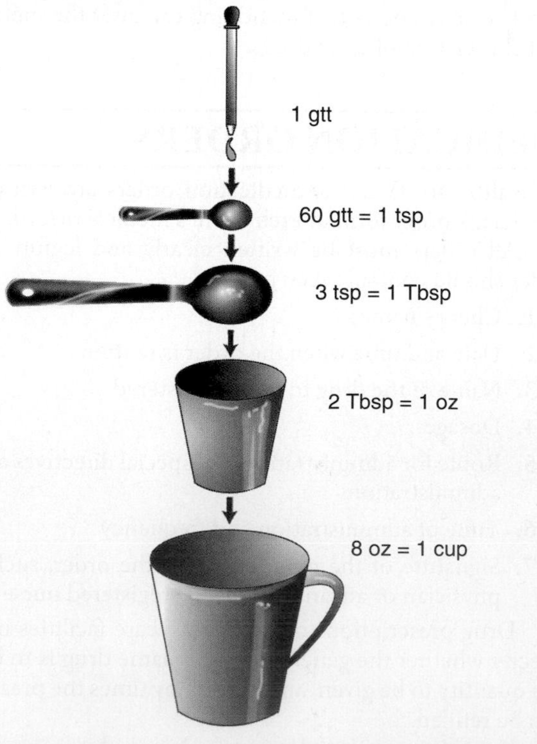

COURTESY OF DELMAR CENGAGE LEARNING

FIGURE 25-1 Relationship Between Household Measures

the household system is used to calculate dosage, with 2.2 lb equal to 1 kg.

The USP recognizes the teaspoon for household medication administration and states that the teaspoon may be regarded as representing 5 mL (American Society of Health-System Pharmacists, 2008). Household spoons are not accurate (varying sizes) for measuring a liquid medication; therefore, the USP recommends using a calibrated oral syringe or dropper for accurate measurement of liquid drug doses.

Household units are generally used in calculating a client's intake and output. Important household equivalents and abbreviations to remember are:

- Volume (liquid)

60 drops (gtt)	= 1 teaspoon (tsp)
3 tsp	= 1 tablespoon (Tbsp)
2 Tbsp	= 1 ounce (oz)
8 oz	= 1 cup (c)
2 cups	= 1 pint (pt)
2 pints	= 1 quart (qt)

- Weight

16 ounces	= 1 pound (lb)

APPROXIMATE EQUIVALENTS

The conversion of metric with the apothecary and household systems are *approximate equivalents* (Table 25-4). The approximate equivalents represent quantities usually ordered by physicians using either the metric or apothecary system of weights and volumes for drug doses (American Society of Health-System Pharmacists, 2008). When a dosage is prescribed in the metric system, the pharmacist may dispense the corresponding approximate equivalent in the apothecary system and vice versa. For example, if the physician prescribes magnesium hydroxide (milk of magnesia, MOM) 30 mL, the pharmacist may dispense MOM 1 ounce. The USP and NF reference *exact equivalents* that must be used to calculate quantities in pharmaceutical formularies and prescription compounding.

CONVERTING UNITS OF WEIGHT AND VOLUME

Knowledge of measurement systems and their conversions must be applied when a drug dosage is prescribed in one system and the pharmacy dispenses the equivalent dose in another. The conversions may be accomplished with either a proportion or a ratio. For example:

Proportion

Means

$$2 : 4 = 6 : 12$$

Extremes

Ratio

$$\frac{2}{4} = \frac{6}{12}$$

In a proportion, the product (multiplication) of the means equals the product of the extremes. In a ratio, the products of cross-multiplication are equal.

$$4 \times 6 = 24 \qquad 2 \times 12 = 24$$
$$2 \times 12 = 24 \qquad 4 \times 6 = 24$$

If one of the terms is unknown, it can be determined by substituting *x* for the number. The letter *x* denotes the unknown or unknown equation. It does not matter if the unknown *x* is on the right or left when setting up the problem, but when calculating the problem and at the end of the problem, the unknown equation or the unknown *x* is always put on the left.

$$2{:}x = 6{:}12 \qquad \frac{2}{x} = \frac{6}{12}$$

$$6x = 24 \qquad 6x = 24$$
$$x = 4 \qquad x = 24$$

Proof that the answer is correct can be determined by substituting the answer for the *x* and multiplying.

Proportion can be used when converting units of weight and volume, conversions within the metric system, conversions between systems, and in drug dosage calculations. When the physician orders morphine gr ¼ and the pharmacist dispenses morphine 15 mg, the nurse is responsible for ensuring the correct dose. The nurse knows that 1 grain equals 60 milligrams;

TABLE 25-4 Approximate Equivalents to the Metric System

METRIC		APOTHECARY		HOUSEHOLD		
Liquid (Volume)						
Liquid	*Weight*	*Liquid*	*Weight*		*Weight*	
0.06 mL	= 60 mg	= 1 ♏	= 1 gr	= 1 gtt	0.4 mg (400 mcg)	= 1/150 gr
1 mL	= 1 g	= 15–16 ♏	= 15 gr	= 15 gtt	1 mg (1,000 mcg)	= 1/60 gr
5 mL	= 5 g	= 1 fl dr	= 1 dr	= 1 tsp	4 mg	= 1/15 gr
15 mL	= 15 g	= 4 fl dr	= 4 dr	= 1 Tbsp	10 mg	= 1/6 gr
30 mL	= 30 g	= 1 fl oz	= 1 oz	= 1 oz	15 mg	= 1/4 gr
240 mL	= 240 g	= 8 fl oz	= 8 oz	= 8 oz	30 mg	= 1/2 gr
380 mL	= 380 g	= 12 fl oz	= 1 lb	= 16 oz	1000 g (1 kg)	= 2.2 lb
500 mL	= 500 g	= 1 pt	= 16 oz	= 1 pt		
1,000 mL	= 1,000 g	= 1 qt	= 32 oz	= 1 qt		

SAFETY

Know What Is Being Calculated

Label all terms (gr, mg, mL, and so on) to avoid errors.

COMMUNITY/HOME HEALTH CARE

Converting a Liquid Dose to an Approximate Household Unit

A common error in household units is to equate one drop to one minim. Use a calibrated dropper to administer medications because drops vary in size.

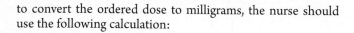

to convert the ordered dose to milligrams, the nurse should use the following calculation:

Proportion	Ratio
1 gr: 60 mg = 1/4 gr: x	$\frac{1 \text{ gr}}{4 \text{ gr}} \times \frac{x \text{ mg}}{60 \text{ mg}}$
(the grains cancel out)	
$1x = (60 \text{ mg})(1/4)$	60 ÷ 4= x or 15 mg
(divide 60 by 4)	
$x = 15$ mg	

Conversions Within the Metric System

Dose equivalents within the metric system are computed by either dividing or multiplying. For example, to change milligrams to grams (1,000 mg equals 1 g) or milliliters to liters (1,000 mL equals 1 L), divide the number by 1,000:

250 mg = x g
(move the decimal point three places to the left)
$x = 0.25$ g

or

500 mL = x L
(move the decimal point three places to the left)
$x = 0.5$ L

To convert grams to milligrams or liters to milliliters, multiply the number by 1000:

0.005 g = x mg
(move the decimal point three places to the right)
$x = 5$ mg

or

0.725 L = x mL
(move the decimal point three places to the right)
$x = 725$ mL

Converting the volume of liters and milliliters may be necessary for enemas and irrigating solutions for bladder and wound irrigations. Intravenous solutions are prepackaged, sterile solutions dispensed in volumes as ordered by the physician, such as 50 mL, 100 mL, 250 mL, 500 mL, or 1,000 mL (1 liter).

Conversions between Systems

Converting between systems is necessary when the physician orders nitroglycerin (an antianginal drug) gr 1/150 po for chest pain and the dispensed dose is 0.4 mg:

1 gr: 60 mg = 1/150 gr: x
1 gr x = (60 mg)(1/150 gr)
(the grains cancel out)
1 x = 60/150 mg
(divide 60 by 150)
$x = 0.4$ mg

The nurse can use proportion when converting pounds to kilograms (2.2 lb = 1 kg). For example, if the client weighs 154 lb, what is the weight in kilograms?

2.2 lb:1 kg = 154 lb: x
(the pounds cancel out)
2.2 x = 154
(divide 154 by 2.2)
$x = 70$ kg

Dosage Calculations

Several formulas may be used by the nurse when calculating drug doses. One formula uses ratios based on the *desired dose* and the *dose on hand*. For example, cephalexin hydrochloride (Keftab), an anti-infective cephalosporin, 500 mg po q.i.d. (dose desired) is ordered by the physician; the dose on hand is 250 mg/5 mL. The formula is as follows:

$$\frac{500 \text{ mg (desired dose)}}{250 \text{ mg (dose on hand)}} \times \frac{x \text{ (quantity desired)}}{5 \text{ mL (quantity on hand)}}$$

(cross-multiply)
(milligrams cancel out)
250 x = 500 × 5
250 x = 2,500
(divide 2,500 by 250)
$x = 10$ mL

In another example, the physician orders heparin (an anticoagulant) 10,000 units subcutaneous; the dose on hand is 40,000 units/mL:

$$\frac{10{,}000 \text{ units}}{40{,}000 \text{ units}} \times \frac{x}{1 \text{ mL}}$$

(cross-multiply)
(units cancel out)
40,000 x = 10,000
(zeros cancel out)
$x = 0.25$ mL

Pediatric Dosages

There are several rules to calculate infants' and children's dosages, such as *Young's Rule, Clark's Rule,* and *Fried's Rule.* Another method, body surface area (BSA), is considered to be one of the most accurate methods of calculating medication dosages for infants and children up to 12 years of age (Rice, 2002). No matter which method is used in calculating pediatric drug dosages, the dosages are approximate and, depending on the child's response, may need adjustment.

PROFESSIONAL TIP

Reasonable Answer

- *The final step in figuring dosage is to ask whether the answer is reasonable.*
- Seldom are more than 2 or 3 tablets or capsules given of one medication or more than 2 or 3 ounces of a liquid medication.
- Seldom is a parenteral injection, except for IV, given of more than 3 mL.
- If your calculations are outside these parameters, recheck your calculations and have a colleague check the calculations too.

Body surface area refers to the square meter surface area method of relating the surface area of individuals to drug dosage. The BSA based on height and weight gives an approximate dose using the following formula:

$$\frac{\text{Body surface area of child}}{\text{Body surface area of adult}} \times \text{Usual adult dose} = \text{Child's dose}$$

The BSA of an adult is 1.73 square meters (m^2); the 1.73 m^2 is based on an adult weighing 150 pounds.

A nomogram is used to compute the child's BSA (Figure 25-2). Draw a straight line from the child's height in the left column to the child's weight in the right column. The point where this line intersects the body surface area column (designated SA) is the child's BSA. For example: A 3-year-old child is 38 inches tall and weighs 36 pounds. The physician orders meperidine (Demerol) for pain. The average adult dose is 50 mg. How much Demerol should the child receive? From the nomogram the child's BSA is 0.66 m^2.

$$\frac{0.66\ (m^2)}{1.73\ (m^2)} \times 50\text{ mg}$$

(square meters cancel out)

$$\frac{33}{1.73}$$

(divide 33 by 1.73)

$$= 19.07\text{ mg} = 19\text{ mg}$$

Now use the desired dose/dose on hand formula to determine how much to give.

$$\frac{19\text{ mg}}{50\text{ mg}} = \frac{x}{1\text{ mL}}$$

(milligrams cancel out)

(cross-multiply)

$$50x = 19\text{ mL}$$

$$x = 0.32\text{ mL}$$

This will have to be given in a tuberculin syringe. Nomograms are used primarily in calculating pediatric drug dosages; however, they are also used when calculating some adult drug dosages such as aminoglycosides and antineoplastic agents.

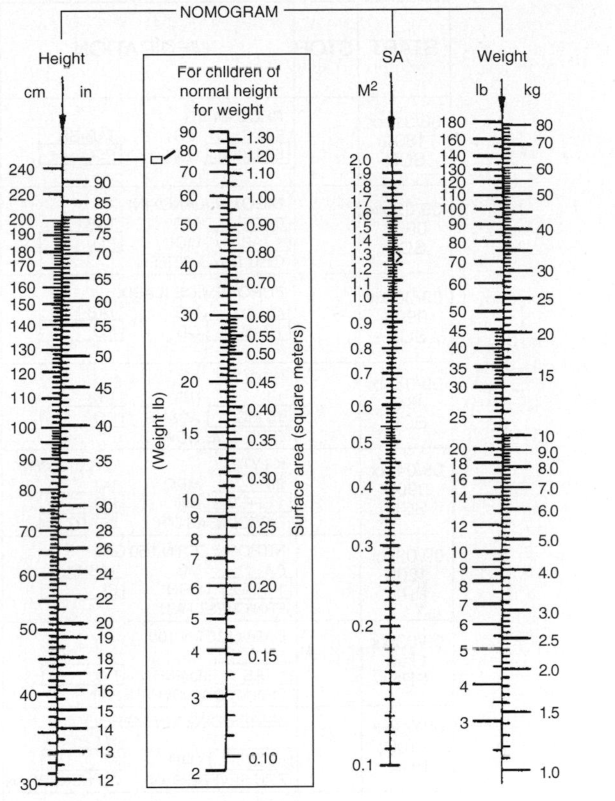

Directions for use: (1) Determine client height. (2) Determine client weight. (3) Draw a straight line to connect the height and weight. Where the line intersects on the SA line is the derived body surface area (M^2).

FIGURE 25-2 Nomogram for Estimating Body Surface Area (*From Nelson Textbook of Pediatrics, 17th Edition, by R. E. Behrman, R. Kliegman, & HY.B. Jenson, 2004, Philadelphia: Saunders. Copyright 2000 by Elsevier. Reprinted with permission.*)

DRUG ADMINISTRATION SAFETY

Many drugs must be administered in an efficient and safe manner according to nursing standards of practice and agency policy. Other responsibilities of the nurse include safe storage and maintaining an adequate supply of drugs.

The nurse documents the actual administration of medications on the medication administration record (MAR). The MAR contains the drug's name, dose, route, and frequency of administration. Drug data are entered either by the pharmacist when dispensing the order (computer-generated form; Figure 25-3) or by the nurse when transcribing the order (handwritten onto the form).

GUIDELINES FOR MEDICATION ADMINISTRATION

Nurses use the "seven rights" of drug administration as a guideline to protect clients from medication errors (see Memory Trick on the following page).

1. Right client
2. Right drug
3. Right dose
4. Right route
5. Right time
6. Right documentation
7. Right to refuse

START	STOP	MEDICATION	SCHEDULED TIMES	OK'D BY	0001 HRS. to 1200 HRS.	1201 HRS. to 2400 HRS.
08/31/xx 1800 SCH		PROCAN SR 500 MG TAB-SR 500 MG Q6H PO	0600 1200 1800 2400	WB	0600 LW 1200 LW	1800 GD 2400 WB
09/03/xx 0900 SCH		DIGOXIN (LANOXIN) 0.125 MG TAB 1 TAB QOD PO ODD DAYS-SEPT.	0900	WB	0900 LW	
09/03/xx 0900 SCH		FUROSEMIDE (LASIX) 40 MG TAB 1 TAB QD PO	0900	WB	0900 LW	
09/03/xx 0845 SCH		REGLAN 10 MG TAB 10 MG AC&HS PO GIVE ONE NOW!	0730 1130 1630 2100	WB	0730 LW 1130 LW	1630 GD 2100 GD
09/04/xx 0900 SCH		K-LYTE 25 MEQ EFFERVESCENT TAB 1 EFF.TAB BID PO DISSOLVE AS DIR. START 9-4	0900 1700	WB	0900 LW	1700 GD
09/03/xx 1500 PRN		NITROGLYCERIN 1/50 GR 0.4 MG TAB-SL 1 TABLET PRN* SL PRN CHEST PAIN		WB		
09/03/xx 1700 PRN		DARVOCET-N 100* 1 TAB Q4-6H PO PRN MILD-MODERATE PAIN		WB		
09/03/xx 2100 PRN		MEPERIDINE*(DEMEROL) INJ 50 MG Q4H IM PRN SEVERE PAIN W PHENERGAN		WB		2200 (H) GD
09/03/xx 2100 PRN		PROMETHAZINE (PHENERGAN) INJ 50 MG Q4H IM PRN SEVERE PAIN W DEMEROL		WB		2200 (H) GD

Gluteus	Thigh	Nurse's Signature	Initial
A. Right	H. Right		
B. Left	I. Left	7-3 L. White, R.N.	LW
Ventro Gluteal			
C. Right	J. Right	3-11 G. Duncan, R.N.	GD
D. Left	K. Left		
E. Abdomen	1 2 / 3 4	11-7 W. Baumle, R.N.	WB

Allergies: NKA

Diagnosis: CHF

Patient: Patient, John D.

Patient #: 3-81512-3

Admitted: 08/31/xx

Physician: J. Physician, MD

Room: PCU-14 PCU

COURTESY OF DELMAR CENGAGE LEARNING

FIGURE 25-3 Computerized Medication Administration Record (MAR)

The nurse is legally responsible for knowing the usual dose, the expected action, the side effects, the adverse reactions, and any interactions with other drugs or food of every drug administered. Without this knowledge, the nurse should not administer any medication.

MEMORY TRICK

The seven rights of drug administration are as listed. They can be remembered by memorizing "**CDDRTRD**":

C = Right **C**lient
D = Right **D**rug
D = Right **D**ose
R = Right **R**oute
T = Right **T**ime
R = Right to **R**efuse
D = Right **D**ocumentation

Right Client

Never identify a client by calling the person's name because confused clients may answer to any name. Correctly identify the client by checking the client's identification band and by asking the client to state his or her full name. Many institutions ask the nurse to verify the client's name and date of birth (DOB) on the client's name band. Some facilities request nurses to ask the client's birthday, the last four numbers of the Social Security number, or the middle name.

When medications are dispensed with a computer-controlled system, the client is identified by scanning the bar code on the client's wrist band. The unit dose medication bar code is also scanned (Figure 25-4). The two bar codes have to agree before the computer affirms the medication, medication dose, and time.

Right Drug

The medications listed on the electronic medical record, MAR, or, less frequently, medication card are checked against the physician's order before any medication is administered. When procuring a medication, check the label on the container

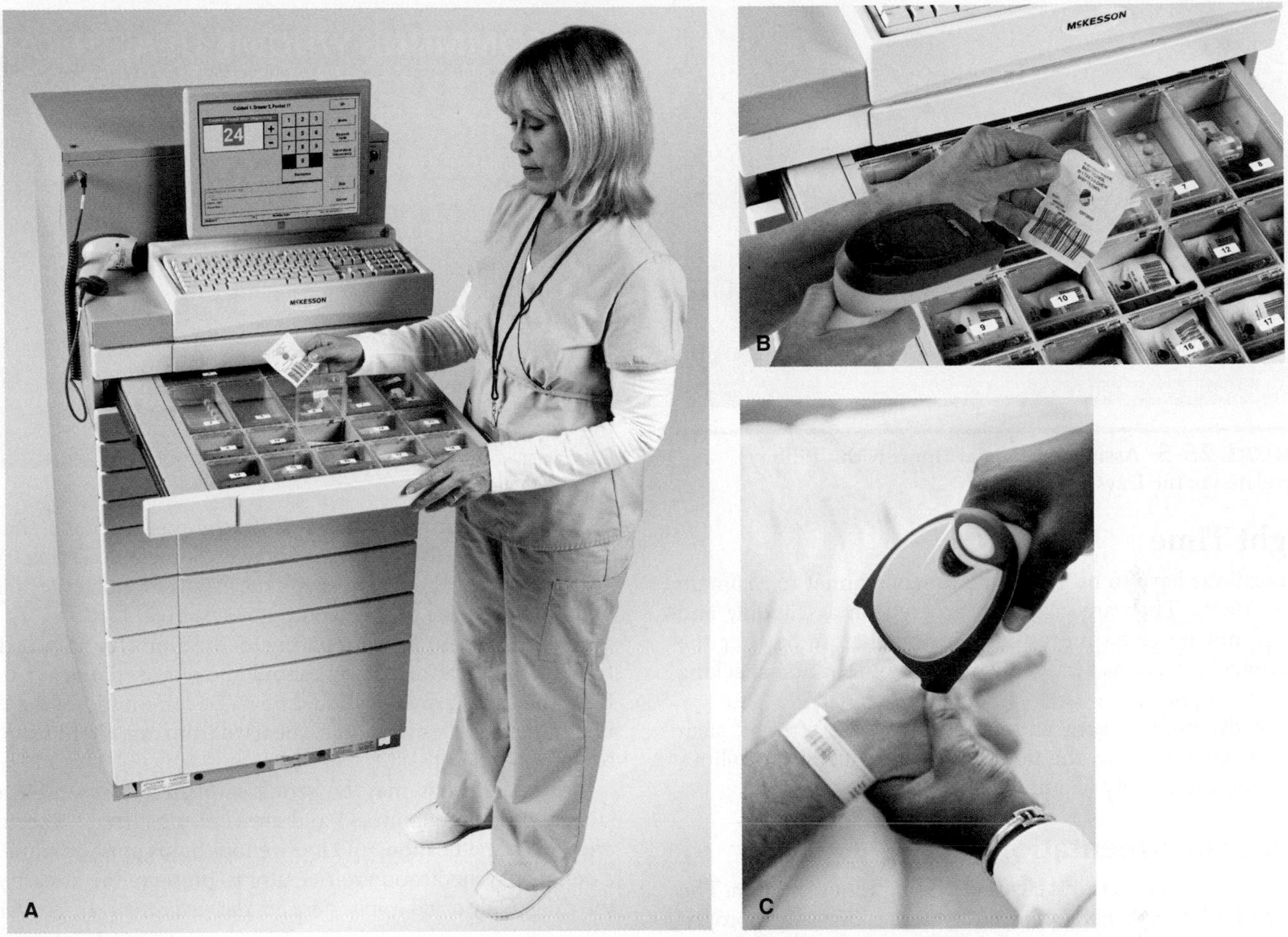

FIGURE 25-4 *A*, **Computer-Controlled Medication Dispensing System;** *B*, **Nurse Scans the Bar Code of a Unit Dose Medication;** *C*, **Nurse Scans the Bar Code on the Client's Wrist Identification Band** (*All images courtesy of McKesson Corporation.*)

against the electronic medical record or MAR at least three times:

1. When removing the drug container from the client's medication drawer
2. When removing the drug from the container
3. Before returning it to the client's medication drawer

Right Dose

Know how to correctly calculate dosages and have them checked before administration. Policy in some facilities requires two nurses to check insulin and heparin dosages to ensure accuracy.

Scored tablets are seldom broken, but if they are, make sure the tablets are broken evenly with tablet scorer. This prevents overdosage or underdosage. After crushing pills with a mortar and pestle, thoroughly cleanse the mortar and pestle to avoid mixing different medications.

Right Route

The route for giving the medication is specified in the written order. If a route is not identified in the order, the route ordered differs from the recommended one, or the route prescribed is questioned, the prescriber should be consulted. For example, the nurse should never substitute an oral medication for an intramuscular medication simply because the oral medication is available.

▼ SAFETY ▼

Medication Administration

- *Never administer medications prepared by another nurse.* You are responsible for a medication error if you administer a medication that was inaccurately prepared by another nurse.
- Listen carefully to the client questioning the addition or deletion of a medication and recheck the order.
- When circumstances prevent giving prescribed medications to the client, the exact reason must be documented in the client's record.
- *Do not leave medications at the client's bedside.*
- Document on the electronic medical record or initial the MAR only for those medications you actually have administered.
- Advise clients not to offer their medications to others and not to take medications belonging to others.

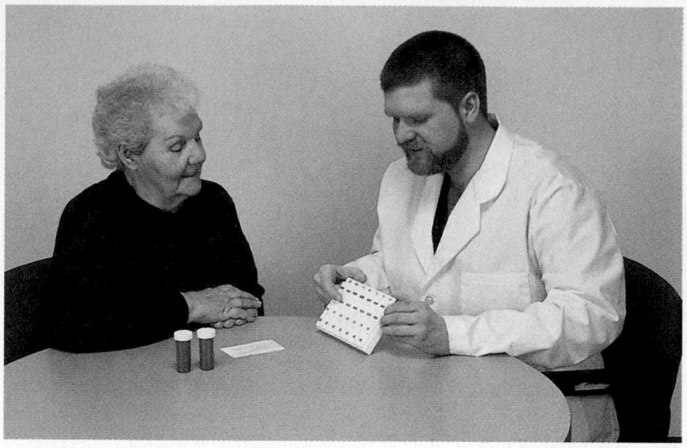

FIGURE 25-5 Assisting Client at Home with a Pillbox Correlated to the Days of the Month

COMMUNITY/HOME HEALTH CARE

Considerations for Drug Safety

- Encourage and assist the client in removing outdated prescriptions and over-the-counter drugs from medication cabinets.
- Encourage the client or caregivers to maintain drug refills to decrease the risk of missing scheduled medications.
- Use a pillbox or reminder calendar (Figure 25-5) to help the client or caregiver remember to take or administer medications as scheduled.

Right Time

Medications have to be given in a timely manner to maintain their effects. They are generally ordered on a schedule and should not be given more than an hour before or after the scheduled time, or as per agency policy, without first checking with the physician.

In the home health and community care settings, such as a retirement home, the nurse has different responsibilities regarding drug safety (Figure 25-5).

Right Documentation

Documentation is a critical element of drug administration. The standard is *"if it was not documented, it was not done."* Appropriate documentation can prevent many drug errors. The nurse administering a medication must initial the medication on the electronic medical record or MAR for the time the drug was given. Usually space is available for a full signature on the MAR record. Documentation should be done *after* the client has received the drug. Medication times are rescheduled for clients having various diagnostic tests or treatments at the time the medication is to be administered and the change documented.

Right to Refuse

If a client refuses to take a medication, document that a dose was missed, why the dose was missed, and notify the physician. Clients do have the right to refuse a medication, but most will be willing to take it if they understand the actions of the medication.

DRUG SUPPLY AND STORAGE

Drugs are dispensed by the pharmacy to nursing units by various methods, accommodating the facility's medication system. After the pharmacy delivers drugs to a nursing unit, the nurse is responsible for their safe storage.

Scheduled drugs are usually dispensed in a unit dose form for each client. **Unit dose** is a system of packaging and labeling each dose of medication by the pharmacy, usually to supply the scheduled drugs for a 24-hour time period. Unit dose drugs are usually stored in a mobile medication dispensing computer system, a medication cart containing individual drawers for each client's medications, or a medication room in separate containers for each client. The unit dose system makes it easy to administer the correct dose, thereby minimizing the number of medication errors.

At the beginning of each shift, the nurse usually checks the medications in each client's drawer. Some medication carts are locked and the nurse keeps the key. The nurse keys in a code to access the mobile computer system.

When the nurse is preparing medications for administration, the medication drawers should be removed one at a time from the cart. A drawer should never be left on top of the cart unattended. Drugs should not be used from one client's supply for another client.

Certain drugs may be **stock supplied** (dispensed and labeled in large quantities) and are kept together in a secured area. Some medications and intravenous fluids must be stored in a designated medication refrigerator to preserve the integrity of the drug. *Only drugs can be stored in the medication refrigerator.*

Narcotics and Controlled Substances

Health care facilities have special forms to record the supply on hand and the administration of narcotics and controlled substances according to federal regulations. These forms usually require the following information for each drug administered:

- Name of the client receiving the drug
- Amount of the drug dispensed
- Time the drug was administered
- Name of the prescribing physician
- Name of the nurse administering the drug

Nurses are required to count the narcotics and controlled substances at specified times, usually at the change of shifts. One nurse going off duty counts the drugs with a nurse coming on duty. Each drug dose must be accounted for on the narcotic record. When the narcotic count does not check, the discrepancy must be reported immediately. Narcotics and controlled substances are kept in a double-locked drawer, box, room, or medication-dispensing cart, such as a computer-controlled dispensing system, as shown in Figure 25-4. The law requires these safety precautions for narcotics and controlled substances.

MEDICATION COMPLIANCE

When clients do not take their prescribed medications consistently or when they adjust the scheduling or dose of the medication, they are *noncompliant.*

Clients may have several reasons why they choose not to take ordered medications. They may not understand the need to take prescribed medications, medications may cost too much for the client on a fixed income, the medication may not provide prompt relief, or the medication may cause undesirable side effects.

Compliance can be enhanced by the nurse teaching the client information on the medications to take at home. Large print or illustrations should be used if the client is elderly. When the nurse teaches the client, include the caregiver. Compliance may be enhanced by giving the client a telephone number to call if questions arise.

LEGAL ASPECTS OF MEDICATION ADMINISTRATION

Remember the "seven rights" for safe administration of medications. Giving the wrong medicine to the client is an error; giving the right medicine but wrong dose or wrong route is an error; giving a medication at the wrong time is an error. The physician must be informed of all errors and needs accurate information to make appropriate decisions. Medications given in error must be documented on the electronic medical record or MAR.

Medication errors must be reported in a timely manner. Incident reports are generally required for medication errors. An incident report, also known as an occurrence or variance report, is documentation of any occurrence or accident that, during the delivery of care, harmed or could have harmed the client. The purpose of an incident report is to provide safety to the client and not to punish the caregiver. Ethically, it is the responsibility of the nurse to complete the incident report so the client's safety is ensured. The report must include the name of the medication, dose given, route, time administered, specific error, time the physician was contacted about the error, what countermeasures were taken, and the clients' response. The nurse includes only accurate and objective facts; no opinions, judgments, assumptions, blame, or incident prevention methods are written in the report. The incident report is not mentioned in the client's medical record. Sometimes nurses discover errors made by other nurses. These must also be reported and documented.

The two purposes of the incident report are to notify the facilities' Risk Management or Continuous Quality Control committee of the incident so that another occurrence of the incident is prevented and to notify the facilities' insurance company of a potential claim and further needed research into the situation. Prompt Risk Management committee review of the incident may prevent litigation. The incident report does not become part of the medical record but may be used if litigation occurs (Daniels, Grendell, & Wilkins, 2010).

Health care institutions should have a national tracking system for medication errors. The USP collects and shares data about actual and potential medication errors. It shares the occurrence of medication errors and methods to prevent the errors with the FDA, the Institute for Safe Medication Practices, and health care professionals (DeLaune & Ladner, 2006). To report medication errors, call 1-800-23-ERROR or go online at http://www.usp.org.

NURSING PROCESS

The nursing process is vital in planning client care and in ensuring safe and accurate medication administration.

ASSESSMENT

The subjective data include medication history and medical history. Objective data include a physical examination and diagnostic and laboratory data.

Medication History

A medication history obtained when a client is admitted to a health care facility should contain information about the client's medication background, including allergies, and use of prescription and over-the-counter drugs.

Allergies Inquire about all medication and food allergies. The nurse asks the client who has had an allergic reaction to a drug to describe the details of the reaction: name of the drug; dosage, route, and number of times the drug was taken before the reaction; onset of the reaction; and evidences of the reaction. Ask about possible contributing factors to the allergic reaction, such as concurrent use of stimulants or depressants (tobacco, alcohol, or illegal drugs) or significant changes in nutritional status.

Allergies to foods should also be discussed because drugs may contain the same substances that cause allergic reactions to some foods. For example, clients who are allergic to shellfish may have a reaction to drugs containing iodine. Vaccines are commonly derived from chick embryos and would be contraindicated for clients with allergies to eggs. If a client has a history of allergies, the nurse may want to obtain an order for an EpiPen® (epinephrine) and oxygen if a new medication is administered.

Prescription Drugs The client should identify all current prescription drugs and describe the following:

- The reason the drug was prescribed and by whom
- The drug's dosage, route, and frequency
- The client's knowledge of the drug's action: side and adverse effects, when to notify the physician, and special administration considerations such as with or without foods

Over-the-Counter Drugs Ask specifically about nonprescription drugs taken by the client. For example, determine if the client takes aspirin, laxatives, or antacids routinely, along with the dosage, route, and frequency of these drugs. Also ask about the use of creams, ointments, patches, or sprays.

Medical History

Gather information about chronic diseases and disorders and correlate these data with the prescription drugs.

Sensory and Cognitive Status Assess for and inquire about sensory deficits such as vision or hearing impairments. Assess the client's cognitive abilities during the history interview by noting if the client is alert and oriented and interacts appropriately.

CRITICAL THINKING

Incorrect Drug

You discover that a similar but incorrect drug (not the drug ordered) is being given IV to a client. What is the first thing you should do? What is your next course of action? How do you feel about the nurse who made the medication error and did not recognize it?

Physical Examination

The client's condition is assessed before administering any drug to establish the client's baseline, or normal, health status. For example, the nurse assesses the client's apical pulse for 1 full minute before administering digoxin (Lanoxin), a cardiac glycoside with positive inotropic effects, to determine that the pulse is above 60 and to assess the heart rhythm. After the client receives the drug, the heart rate is compared with the baseline measurement.

Diagnostic and Laboratory Data

Common laboratory values, such as electrolytes, blood urea nitrogen, creatinine, glucose, complete blood count, and a white blood cell count, are usually monitored over a period to identify trends and to measure the body's response to medications.

Nursing Diagnosis

Once the actual or potential problems are identified, relevant nursing diagnoses can be identified. The North American Nursing Diagnosis Association International (NANDA-I) (2010) nursing diagnoses commonly related to medication administration include:

- *Ineffective **H**ealth Maintenance*
- *Deficient **K**nowledge* (specify)
- *Ineffective **T**herapeutic Regimen Management*
- *Impaired Physical **M**obility*
- *Disturbed **S**ensory Perception*
- *Impaired **S**wallowing*

Planning/Outcome Identification

The care plan and goals are developed based on the nursing diagnoses. For example, the client with a knowledge deficit related to a newly prescribed drug may have the following expected outcomes:

Before discharge the client will:

- Correctly state the actions of the drug in the body
- Prepare the correct dose of the drug
- List the possible side effects of and possible adverse reactions to the drug
- Correctly identify special considerations (i.e., take with food, no alcohol)

Implementation

The main nursing interventions related to medication management are assessment, administration, and teaching. Use the time spent when administering medications to assess the client's knowledge of and response to the drug.

Medication administration requires implementing safety guidelines, following the "seven rights." Medications are administered according to set procedures based on the prescribed route. This section presents information for medication administration by the following routes: oral, including sublingual and buccal; parenteral; site-specific topical applications; and inhalation.

Drug teaching usually takes place in two phases. The first phase is usually a formal teaching session, when the drug's action, route, side and adverse effects, and the specific signs of a drug reaction that require physician notification are explained. Clients may need assistance developing a drug schedule that fits their lifestyle. Teaching the client and/or support person specific procedural techniques, such as subcutaneous injection, may be necessary.

The second phase of client teaching occurs whenever a drug is administered. At each interaction, assess and reinforce the client's knowledge of drugs. When a client is taught self-administration, the teaching plan should identify dates for teaching and a date for achievement of goals.

> **CLIENT TEACHING**
>
> **Written Medication Information**
>
> Written medication information for clients should be accurate, specific, comprehensive, and presented in a legible and understandable format. It should:
>
> - Include generic and trade names.
> - State indications for use, contraindications, precautions, adverse reactions, risks, and storage.
> - Provide straightforward instructions.
> - Have conspicuous drug warnings.
> - Have print size appropriate to client's visual abilities.
> - Be appropriate for client literacy level.

Oral Drugs

Oral administration of drugs is the most common route; however, potential risk factors must be considered. Assess the client's ability to take the medication before administering oral drugs by assessing the client's state of consciousness, gag reflex, and presence of nausea and vomiting. These assessments assist in protecting the client from aspiration. **Aspiration** is the inhalation of secretions or fluids into the pulmonary system.

Liquid medications are measured out in a calibrated medicine cup. Doses, smaller than 1 dr, 1 tsp, or 5 mL, are measured in a syringe for accuracy. Solid oral medications are put into a medicine cup or small paper (soufflé) cup, depending on agency policy. Individually wrapped medications should be opened at the bedside.

Remain with the client when administering oral drugs, until all medications have been swallowed. When in doubt that the client has swallowed a pill, don a nonsterile glove and visually inspect the client's mouth using a tongue depressor (Figure 25-6).

Sublingual and Buccal Assess the integrity of the mucous membranes by inspecting under the client's tongue and in the buccal cavity before administering sublingual and buccal drugs. When oral membranes are excoriated or painful, withhold the medication and notify the physician. For buccal drugs that irritate the mucosa, alternate sides of the mouth. Drugs given by these routes are quickly absorbed by the mucosa's abundant blood supply and the thin epithelium.

Enteral **Enteral instillation** is the delivery of drugs through a gastrointestinal tube. Enteral tubes provide a way to directly

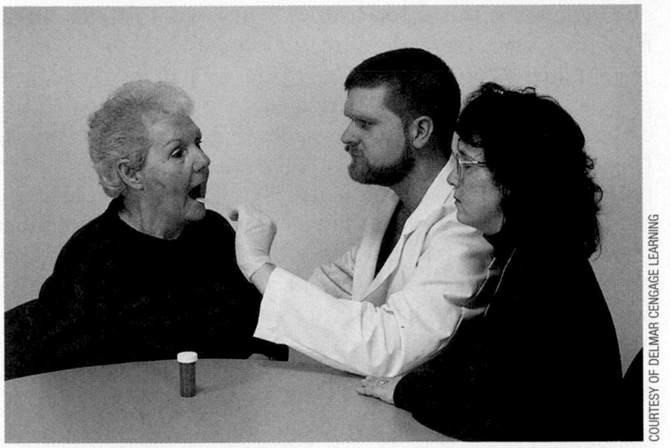

FIGURE 25-6 Check the client's mouth if you are unsure that medications have been swallowed.

instill medications into the gastrointestinal system of clients who cannot take them orally.

There are several types of enteral tubes. A nasogastric tube (NG) is a soft rubber or plastic tube inserted through a nostril and into the stomach. The gastrostomy tube is surgically inserted into the stomach through the abdomen.

Check the tube for **patency** and placement and assess the client for the presence of bowel sounds before administering a medication. Patency is being freely open. When the tube is obstructed or improperly placed, the client is vomiting, or bowel sounds are absent, the instillation of drugs is contraindicated.

Once the patency and placement of the tube are determined, prepare the medication for instillation as prescribed by the physician. When the physician orders a drug in tablet form, crush the tablet into minute particles and dissolve the crushed tablet in 15 to 30 mL of warm water before instillation. Do not dissolve all medications and give at one time. Instead, dissolve each medication in a separate cup in 15 to 30 mL of water and give each medication separately. To clear the tubing, instill 30 mL of water between each medication and at the end of the medication administration. Contact the physician or nurse practitioner to clarify medication administration orders if the client is on a fluid restricted diet. Cold water may cause abdominal cramps when instilled. Open capsules and empty the contents into a liquid.

CLIENT TEACHING

Sublingual and Buccal Drugs

Sublingual Drugs:

- Keep the medication under the tongue until completely dissolved to ensure absorption.
- To prevent accidental swallowing, avoid chewing the tablet or moving it with the tongue.
- Nicotine has a vasoconstrictive effect that slows absorption; therefore, do not smoke until the drug is completely dissolved.

Buccal Drugs:

- Keep the medication in place until completely dissolved to ensure absorption.
- Some tablets take up to an hour to dissolve; therefore, do not drink liquids for an hour.
- Nicotine has a vasoconstriction effect that slows absorption; therefore, do not smoke until the drug is completely dissolved.

PROFESSIONAL TIP

Special Considerations for Enteral Tube Management

- When a client is receiving intermittent tube feedings, schedule medications to prevent the two solutions from being given together.
- An adult client should not receive more than 400 mL of liquid at one time. If feeding and medication administration coincide, give the medication first to ensure that the client receives the prescribed dosage on time; the feeding may not be given in its entirety.
- When the client is receiving a continuous feeding, stop the feeding and aspirate the gastric contents. If the gastric contents are greater than 150 mL, withhold the medication and notify the physician.
- *Never put tablets into tube-feeding bags.*
- For clients who have an NG tube for decompression (removal) of gastric contents, turn off the suction for 20 to 30 minutes after instillation of the medication to allow time for the gastric contents to be emptied into the intestines, where most drugs are absorbed.

Parenteral Drugs

Parenteral medications are given through a route other than the alimentary canal; these routes are intradermal, subcutaneous, intramuscular, or intravenous. The insertion angle of the needle and the depth of penetration indicate the type of injection (Figure 25-7).

Equipment To administer parenteral medications, special equipment such as syringes, needles, ampules, and vials are used.

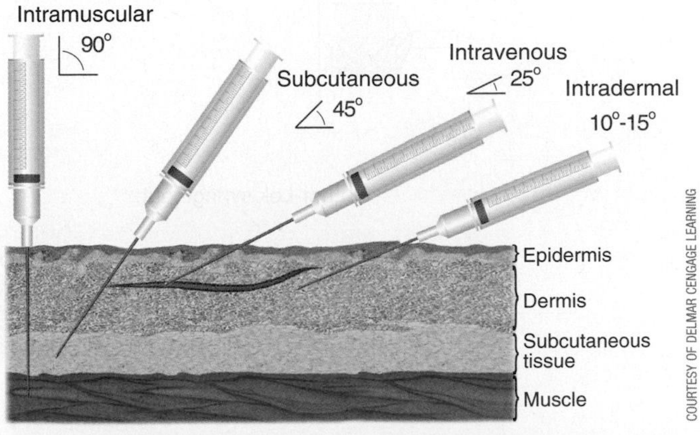

FIGURE 25-7 Angle of Insertion for Parenteral Injections

Syringes A syringe has three basic parts: the hub, which connects with the needle; the barrel, or outside part, which has measurement calibrations; and the plunger, which fits inside the barrel and has a rubber tip (Figure 25-8). The hub, the inside of the barrel, and the shaft and rubber plunger tip must be kept sterile. When handling a syringe, touch only the outside of the barrel and the plunger's handle.

Two designs for syringe hubs are the Luer-Lok tip and the slip tip (see Figure 25-8). The hub of a needle twists into the threaded Luer-Lok tip so that the needle cannot slip off of the syringe. The needle easily slides on and off the slip tip. The choice of syringe type depends on the situation of use and the preference of the user.

Most syringes are disposable, made of plastic, and individually packaged. There are hypodermic, insulin, and tuberculin syringes (Figure 25-9). When a medication is incompatible with plastic, it is usually prefilled into a single-dose glass syringe. Syringes are often packaged with the size and gauge needle commonly used.

The *hypodermic syringe* comes in 2-, 2.5-, and 3-mL sizes. The measurement calibrations are usually in mL, and some syringes have minims. The hypodermic syringe is used most often when a medication is ordered in milliliters. When the order is written in minims, it is safer to use a tuberculin syringe.

The *insulin syringe* is designed especially for use with insulin. For example, if the physician writes the order for 30 units of U-100 insulin, use an insulin syringe calibrated on the 100-unit scale. Always compare the size of the insulin syringe and the strength indicated on the insulin bottle with the physician's order; all three units must be the same. There are three sizes of U-100 insulin syringes: 1 mL, ½ mL, and 3/10 mL (see Figure 25-9). The ½- and 3/10-mL sizes are called low-dose insulin syringes.

The *tuberculin syringe* is a narrow syringe, calibrated in tenths and hundredths of a milliliter (up to 1 mL) on one scale and in sixteenths of a minim (up to 1 minim) on the other scale. This syringe is generally used to administer small or precise doses (i.e., pediatric dosages). The tuberculin syringe should be used for doses 0.5 mL or less.

Prefilled single-dose syringes should not be confused with a unit dose. The prescribed dose must be checked against that in the prefilled syringe and the excess discarded. For example, if the physician orders diazepam (Valium) 5 mg IM as a preoperative sedative and the prefilled single-dose contains 10 mg/2 mL, the dosage must be calculated (5 mg/1 mL) and 1 mL discarded from the syringe before administration.

Needles Most needles are made of stainless steel, disposable, and individually packaged. A prefilled single-dose cartridge is inserted into a reusable injection system holder (Figure 25-10) to give the medication. Depending on the type of holder, the cartridge is usually slid into the holder and tightened in place and the plunger twisted onto the rubber plunger. The reusable holders are called a Tubex are Carpuject, depending on the manufacturer. A needle has three aspects: the hub, which fits onto the syringe hub; the cannula, or shaft; and the bevel, which is the slanted part at the tip of the shaft (Figure 25-11). Needles come in many sizes, from ¼ to 5 inches long, with gauges from 32 to 14. The *gauge* refers to the diameter of the shaft; the larger the number, the smaller the diameter of the shaft. Smaller needles (larger gauge) produce less trauma to the body's tissue; however, the viscosity of a solution must be considered when selecting the gauge.

The *shaft* of the needle indicates its length. The length of the needle is selected based on the client's muscle development and weight and the type of injection, such as intravenous versus intramuscular.

Needles may have a short or a long *bevel*. The bevel length is selected based on the type of injection. Long bevels are sharp and produce less pain when inserted into the subcutaneous or muscle tissues. A short bevel is used for intradermal and intravenous injections to prevent the tissue or blood vessel wall from occluding the bevel.

The hub of the needle should be immediately attached to the hub of the syringe when removed from its sterile wrapper to prevent contamination. The protective cover should remain on the needle until it is ready to be used.

Most syringes come with a protective system to cover needles after giving an injection. Some have an outside shield that slides down over the needle as shown in Figure 25-9A and Figure 25-9D. Another syringe is designed with a plastic hinge as shown in Figure 25-9E. After giving the injection, the nurse slides the plastic hinge over the needle locking it in place. Some syringes automatically retract the needle after the injection is given. Go to the following Web site for an example of this syringe and search for BD Integra retracting syringe: http://www.bd.com.

Used needles must be disposed of in the proper receptacles, such as a sharps container, to prevent needlesticks. All client care areas have sharps containers in most facilities.

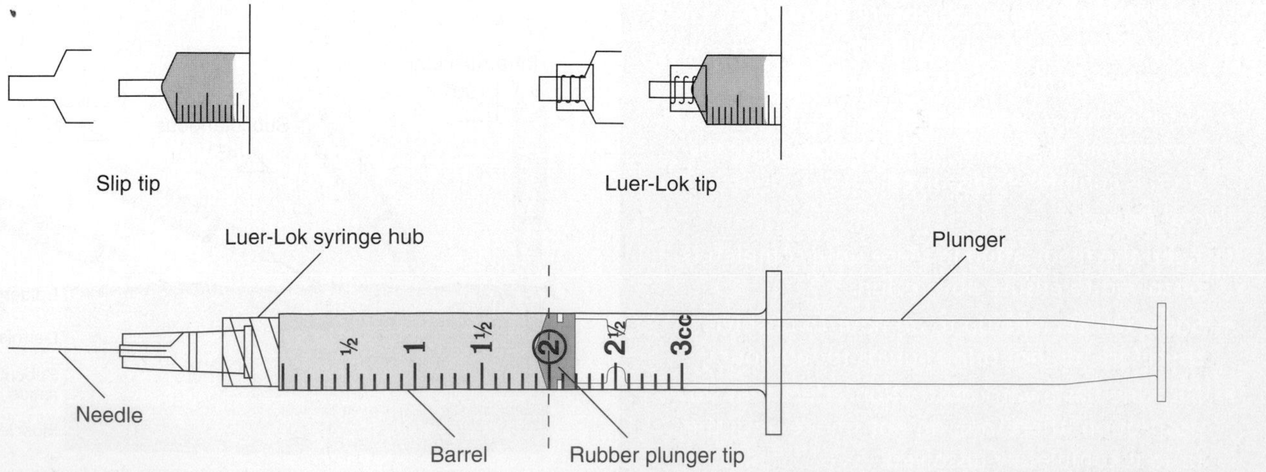

FIGURE 25-8 The Parts of a Syringe with Syringe Tip Options of Slip Tip or Luer-Lok

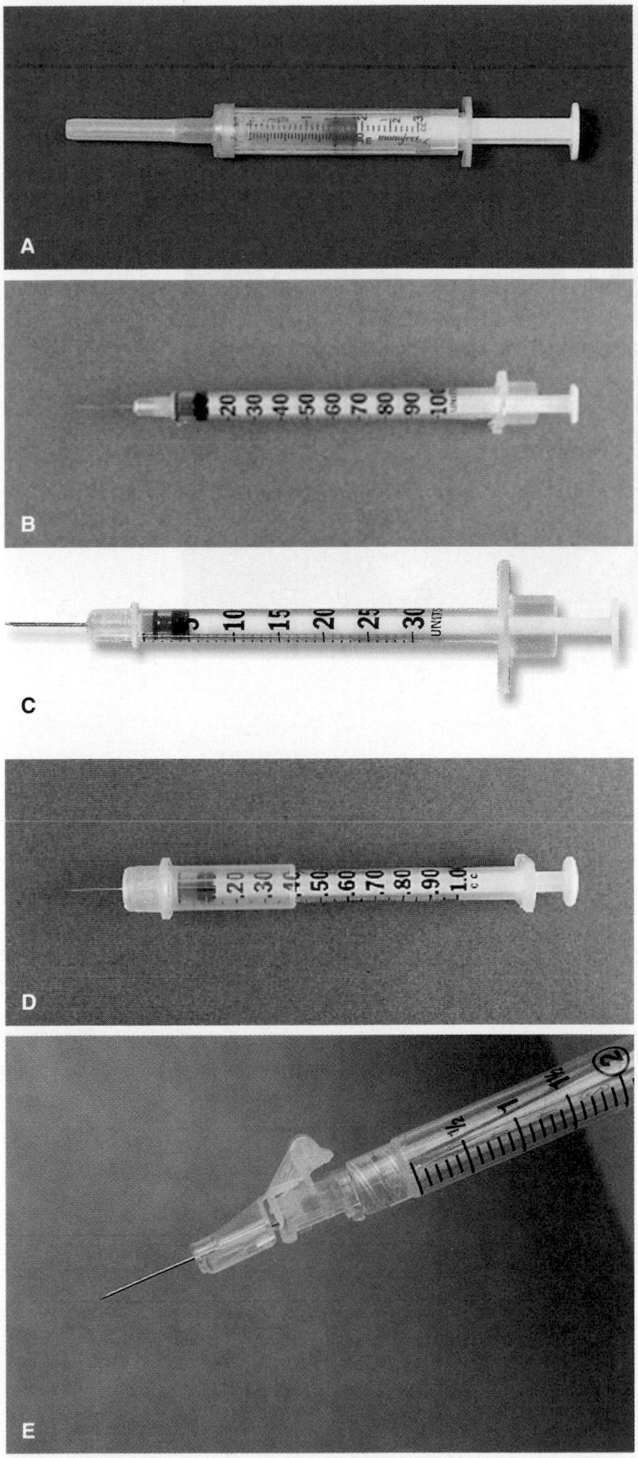

FIGURE 25-9 Types of Syringes; *A,* 3 mL Hypodermic with Plastic Needle Guard; *B,* Standard U-100 Insulin Syringe; *C,* Insulin 3/10 mL; *D,* 1 mL Tuberculin with Plastic Needle Guard; *E,* Syringe with Plastic Hinge that Slides Over the Needle (*Images A, B, C, and D courtesy and copyright Becton, Dickinson and Company. Image E courtesy of Delmar Cengage Learning.*)

Discussion of the needleless system is found under IV therapy later in this chapter.

Ampules and Vials Drugs for parenteral injections must be sterile. Those that deteriorate in solution are dispensed as tablets or powders to be dissolved in a solution immediately before injection. Drugs remaining stable in solution are dispensed in ampules and vials in an aqueous or an oily solution or suspension.

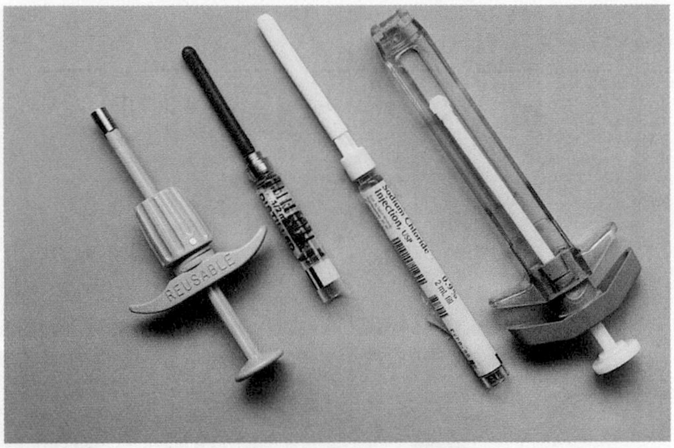

COURTESY OF DELMAR CENGAGE LEARNING

FIGURE 25-10 Prefilled Single-Dose Cartridges with Reusable Injection System Holders

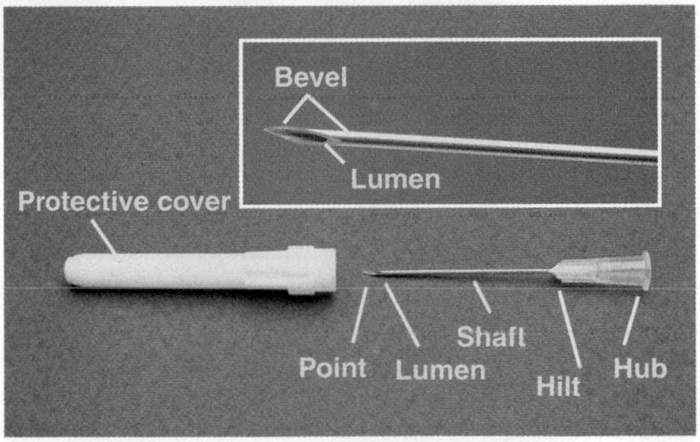

COURTESY OF DELMAR CENGAGE LEARNING

FIGURE 25-11 Parts of a Needle

Ampules are glass containers of single-dose drugs (Figure 25-12A). The glass container has a constriction in the stem to facilitate opening the ampule. When opening an ampule, the nurse slides a plastic shield over the tip to assist in breaking it and to prevent a finger cut (Figure 25-12B). Drugs may be irritating to the subcutaneous tissue, so the needle should be changed after withdrawing a drug from an ampule.

Glass, single- or multiple-dose rubber-capped drug containers are called vials (Figure 25-12D). A vial usually has an easily removed soft metal or plastic cap. The needle should be changed after withdrawing a drug from a vial.

Intradermal Injection Intradermal (ID) or intracutaneous injections are used to administer local anesthetics, identify allergens, and diagnose tuberculosis. An ID injection is administered below the epidermis; drugs are absorbed slowly from this site. Commonly used sites for ID injection are the inner aspect of the forearm, upper back, and upper chest.

The drug's dosage for an ID injection is usually a small amount of solution (0.01 to 0.1 mL). To provide accurate measurement, use a 1-mL tuberculin syringe with a short bevel, 25 to 27 gauge, 3/8- to 1/2-inch needle. For repeated doses, the sites are rotated. Intradermal injections are administered into the epidermis by angling the needle 10 to 15 degrees to the skin.

Subcutaneous Injection Subcutaneous injections are used to administer insulin and heparin because they are absorbed

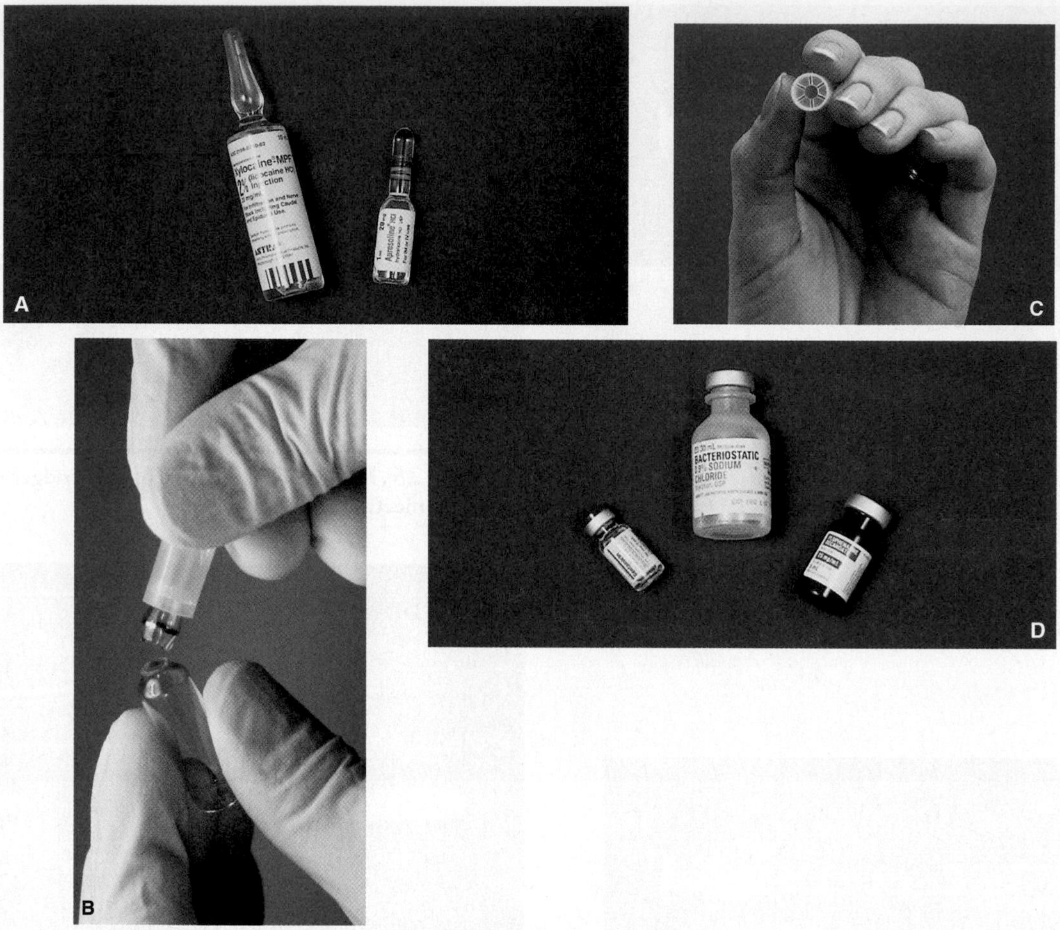

FIGURE 25-12 ***A,*** **Ampules;** ***B,*** **Using Safety Cap to Break Ampule;** ***C,*** **Safety Cap to Slide Over the Tip of the Ampule When Breaking;** ***D,*** **Vials** *(Images A and D courtesy of Delmar Cengage Learning. Images B and C courtesy of Sigma-Aldrich.)*

PROFESSIONALTIP

Expiration Date

- Laws require manufacturers to put expiration dates on all drugs.
- To ensure a drug is current, check the expiration date.
- Return outdated drugs to the pharmacy for proper disposal.

PROFESSIONALTIP

Heparin Administration

- Heparin is given in the abdomen 2 inches away from the umbilicus and above the iliac crests.
- When giving heparin subcutaneously, do not aspirate on the plunger; doing so may cause tissue damage and bruising.
- Do not massage the heparin injection site because it may cause the drug to absorb more quickly.
- Give heparin at a 90-degree angle with a 3/8-inch needle, unless the client is lean, then give the injection at a 45-degree angle (Berman, Snyder, Kozier, & Erb, 2008).

slowly, creating a sustained effect. Subcutaneous injections put the medication between the dermis and the muscle into the subcutaneous tissue. The amount of medication given varies but seldom exceeds 1.5 mL. For repeated doses the site should be rotated.

Common sites for subcutaneous injections include the abdomen, the lateral aspect of the upper arm or the anterior aspect of the upper thigh, the scapular area on the back, and the upper ventrodorsal gluteal area. Select a sterile 0.5- to 3-mL syringe with a 25 to 27 gauge and a 3/8- to 5/8-inch needle. The medication is administered by angling the needle 45 to 90 degrees to the skin.

Intramuscular Injection Intramuscular (IM) injections promote rapid drug absorption and provide another route for drugs that are irritating to subcutaneous tissue. The absorption rate is greater because there are more blood vessels in the muscles than in subcutaneous tissue; however, the client's circulatory status may affect the absorption rate.

The four common sites for administering IM injections are the dorsogluteal and ventrogluteal (gluteus maximus muscle), the anterolateral aspect of the thigh (vastus lateralis muscle), and the upper arm (deltoid muscle). These sites are identified by using appropriate anatomic landmarks. An IM injection is administered at a 90-degree angle to the skin, injecting only up to 3 mL into well-developed muscle tissue. See Table 25-5 for amounts of solution to inject in various types of tissue.

Z-Track Injection A Z-track (zigzag) injection is a method for administering IM injections, most commonly in the ventrogluteal and dorsogluteal muscles.

For administration of a Z-track injection, the client is placed in the prone position; the skin is pulled to one side, the needle is inserted at a 90-degree angle, and the medication is administered. After 10 seconds the needle is withdrawn and then the skin is released. Do not massage the site; it may cause tissue irritation. Never inject more than 3 mL in a single site.

IV Therapy The LPN/VN role in IV therapy varies widely from state to state and facility to facility. It is the responsibility of the LPN/VN to know the standards of practice for the state in which one practices. IV therapy requires parenteral fluids (solutions) and special equipment: administration set, IV pole, filter, regulators to control IV flow rate, and an established venous route.

Parenteral Fluids Read the physician's order in the client's medical record to confirm the type and amount of IV solution. Intravenous solutions are sterile and usually packaged in plastic bags. Solutions incompatible with plastic are in glass containers.

Plastic IV solution bags collapse under atmospheric pressure, allowing the solution to enter the infusion set. Plastic solution bags are packaged with an outer plastic bag, which should remain intact until the solution is prepared for administration. The solution bag should be dry when removed from its outer wrapper. If it is wet, the solution should not be used. Moisture on the bag shows that the integrity of the bag has been compromised, and the solution cannot be considered sterile. Return the bag to the department that issued the solution. Glass containers are discussed in the section on equipment.

Parenteral fluids are classified based on their relationship to normal blood plasma. Solutions may be hypotonic, isotonic, or hypertonic. The solution prescribed is based on the client's diagnosis and the goal of therapy. The solution's effect is:

- *Hypotonic fluid.* Lowers osmotic pressure and makes fluid move into the cells. Water intoxication may result if fluid is infused beyond the client's tolerance.
- *Isotonic fluid.* Increases only extracellular fluid volume. Cardiac overload may result if fluid is infused beyond the client's tolerance.
- *Hypertonic fluid.* Increases osmotic pressure and draws fluid from the cells. Cellular dehydration may result if fluid is infused beyond the client's tolerance (Bulechek & McCloskey, 2000).

Common intravenous solutions are shown in Table 25-6.

LIFE SPAN CONSIDERATIONS

Choosing IV Equipment

Neonates, infants, and children are at risk for *Excess Fluid Volume* related to rehydration. A microdrip and special volume-control chamber are used to regulate the fluid amount administered in a specific time.

TABLE 25-5 Summary of Intradermal, Subcutaneous, and Intramuscular Injections

TYPE OF INJECTION	PURPOSE	SITE	NEEDLE SIZE	MAXIMUM DOSE	ANGLE OF INSERTION
Intradermal	Injects medication below the epidermis; drugs are absorbed slowly; typically used for diagnosis of tuberculosis and allergens	Inner aspect of forearm; upper chest; upper back	Syringe with short bevel; 25–27-gauge; 3/8 to 1/2-inch	0.01–0.1 mL	10° to 15° 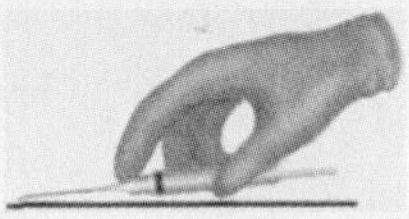
Subcutaneous	Injects medication between dermis and muscle; absorbed slowly; typically used for insulin and anticoagulants	Abdomen; lateral and anterior aspects of upper arm and thigh; scapular area on back; ventrogluteal area	25-27-gauge, 3/8-5/8-inch needle (varies by size of person)	0.5–1mL	45° to 90° 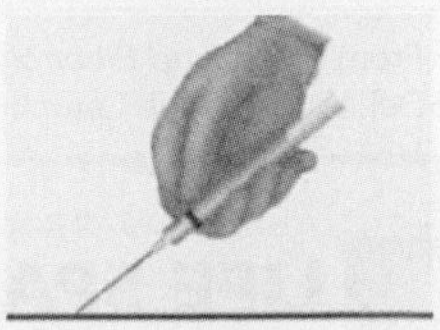
Intramuscular	Used to promote rapid drug absorption and to provide an alternative route when drug is irritating to subcutaneous tissue	Ventrogluteal; dorsogluteal; anterolateral aspect of thigh (vastus lateralis); upper arm (deltoid)	The gauge and length of needle are selected on the basis of medication volume and viscosity and client's body size	Well-developed adult: 3 mL in a large muscle; infant and small child: 0.5–1 mL; children and elderly: 1–2 mL; deltoid muscle: 0.5–1 mL	90° 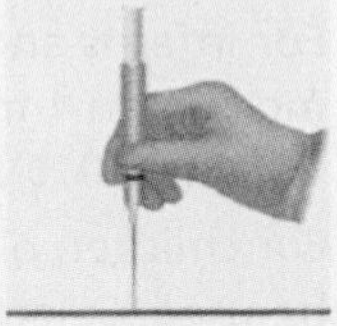

COURTESY OF DELMAR CENGAGE LEARNING

TABLE 25-6 Common Intravenous Solutions

TONICITY	SOLUTION	CONTENTS (MEQ/L)	CLINICAL IMPLICATIONS
Hypotonic	Sodium chloride 0.45%	77 Na^+, 77 Cl^-	Daily maintenance of body fluid and establishment of renal function.
Isotonic	Dextrose 2.5% in 0.45% saline	77 Na^+, 77 Cl^-	Promotes renal function and urine output.
	Dextrose 5% in 0.2% saline	77 Na^+, 77 Cl^-	Daily maintenance of body fluids when less Na^+ and Cl^- are required.
	Dextrose 5% in water (D_5W)	38 Na^+, 38 Cl^-	Promotes rehydration and elimination; may cause urinary Na^+ loss; good vehicle for K^+.
	Ringer's lactate	130 Na^+, 4 K^+, Ca^{2+}, 109 Cl^-, 28 lactate	Resembles the normal composition of blood serum and plasma; K^+ level below body's daily requirement.
	Normal saline (NS), 0.9%	154 Na^+, 154 Cl^-	Restores sodium chloride deficit and extracellular fluid volume.
	Dextran 40 10% in NS (0.9%) or D_5W		A colloidal solution used to increase plasma volume of clients in early shock; it should not be given to severely dehydrated clients and clients with renal disease, thrombocytopenia, or active hemorrhaging.
	Dextran 70% in NS		A long-lived (20 hours) plasma volume expander; used to treat shock or impending shock caused by hemorrhage, surgery, or burns. *It can prolong bleeding and coats the RBCs (draw type and cross match before administering).*
Hypertonic	Dextrose 5% in 0.45% saline	77 Na^+, 77 Cl^-	Daily maintenance of body fluid and nutrition; treatment of fluid volume deficit (FVD).
	Dextrose 5% in saline 0.9%	154 Na^+, 154 Cl^-	Fluid replacement of sodium, chloride, and calories (170).
	Dextrose 10% in saline 0.9%	154 Na^+, 154 Cl^-	Fluid replacement of sodium, chloride, and calories (340).
	Dextrose 5% in lactated Ringer's	130 Na^+, 4 K^+, 3 Ca^{2+}, 109 Cl^-, 28 lactate	Resembles the normal composition of blood serum and plasma; K^+ level below body's daily requirement; caloric value 180.
	Hyperosmolar saline 3% and 5% NaCl	856 Na^+, 865 Cl^-	Treatment of hyponatremia; raises the Na osmolarity of the blood, and reduces intracellular fluid excess.
	Ionosol B with dextrose 5%	57 Na^+, 25 K^+, 49 Cl^-, 25 lact., 5 Mg^{2+}, 7 PO^{4-}	Treatment of polyionic parenteral replacement caused by vomiting-induced alkalosis, diabetic acidosis, fluid loss from burns, and postoperative FVD.

From *Fluids and Electrolytes with Clinical Applications: A Programmed Approach* (7th ed.), by J. Kee, B. Paulanka, and C. Polek, 2009, Clifton Park, NY: Delmar Cengage Learning.

LIFE SPAN CONSIDERATIONS

Site for Administering an IM Injection

- For infants and toddlers, use the vastus lateralis site. Select a 22- to 25-gauge needle, 5/8 to 1 inch long. No more than 1 mL is injected into the muscle of a small child and 0.5 mL in an infant (Daniels, Grendell, & Wilkins, 2010). Obtain assistance to hold the infant and child still during an injection.
- For children older than 3 years of age and for adults, the deltoid, dorsogluteal area, or ventrogluteal area may be used. Select a 22 to 25 gauge needle ½ to 1½ inches long (Pope, 2002).
- An older client may have less muscle mass and require a shorter needle (Daniels, Grendell, & Wilkins, 2010).

Equipment Intravenous equipment is disposable, sterile, and prepackaged with user instructions. The user instructions, including a schematic labeling the parts, are usually placed on the outside of the package, which allows the user to read the package before opening. IV equipment requires sterile technique when handling because it is in direct contact with fluids to be infused into the bloodstream.

The administration (infusion) set includes an insertion spike with a protective cap, a drip chamber, tubing with a slide clamp and regulating (roller) clamp, a rubber injection port, and a protective cap over the needle adapter (Figure 25-13). Protective caps keep both ends of the set sterile and are removed only when used. The insertion spike is inserted into the port of the IV solution container.

There are two types of drip chambers: a macrodrip, which releases 10 to 20 drops per milliliter of solution, and a microdrip, which releases 60 drops per milliliter. The drop rate, which varies with the manufacturer, is indicated on the package.

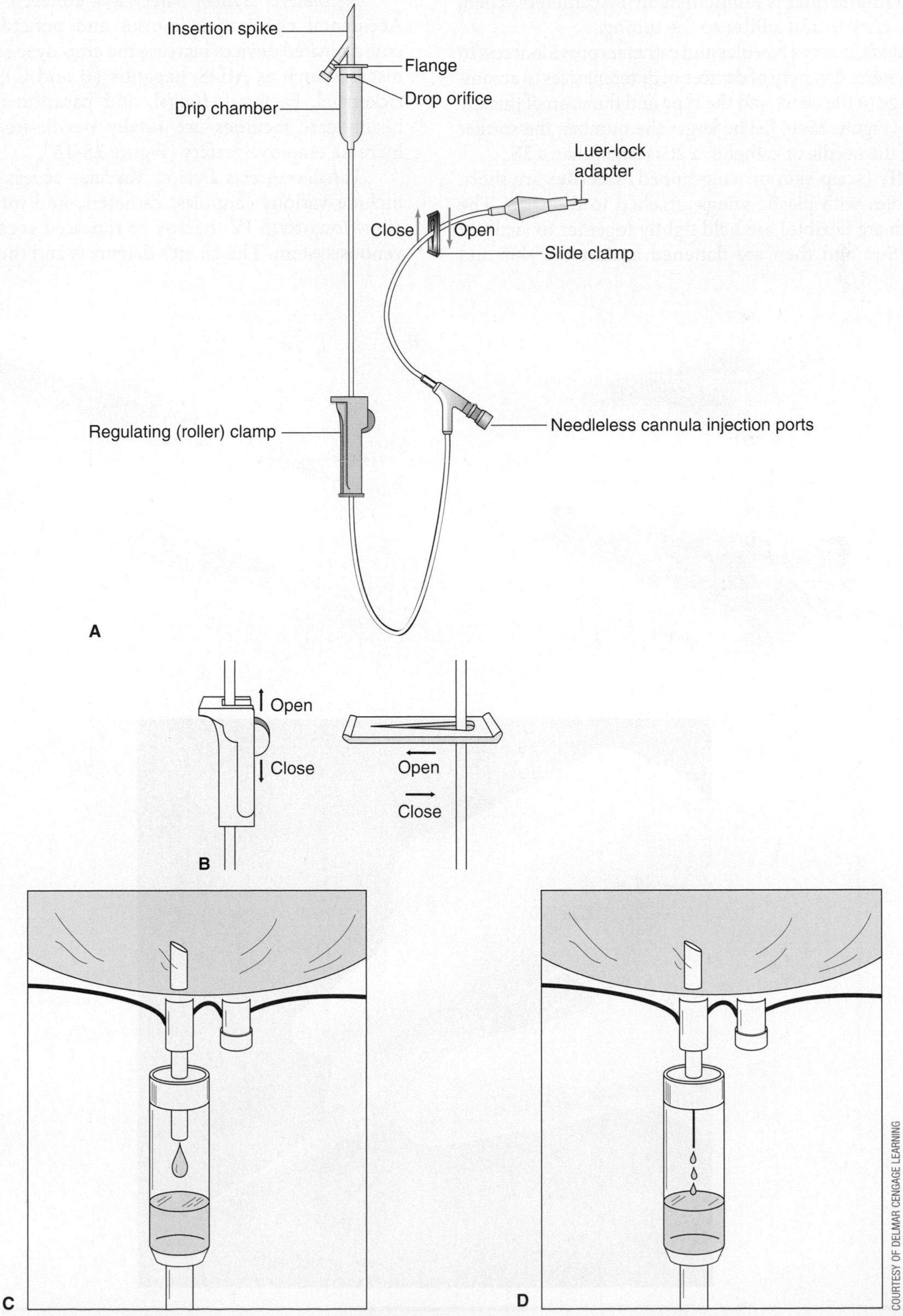

FIGURE 25-13 ***A,*** **Basic IV Administration Set;** ***B,*** **Regulating Roller Clamp and Slide Clamp;** ***C,*** **Macrodrip Chamber;** ***D,*** **Microdrip Chamber**

The roller clamp compresses the plastic tubing to control the flow rate. At the end of the IV tubing is a needle adapter that connects to a sterile injection device inserted into the client's vein. Extension tubing may be used to lengthen the primary tubing or provide additional Y-injection ports for administering additional solutions.

Intravenous Filters Intravenous filters remove particulate matter that may cause irritation and **phlebitis** (inflammation of a vein) from the solution. Intravenous filters come in various sizes. An in-line filter is found in many IV catheters. Then, it is not necessary to add a filter to the tubing.

Needles and Catheters Needles and catheters provide access to the venous system. A variety of devices of different sizes to accommodate the age of the client and the type and duration of therapy are available (Figure 25-14). The larger the number, the smaller the lumen of the needle or catheter; a 20 is larger than a 28.

Butterfly (scalp vein or wing-tipped) **needles** are short, beveled needles with plastic wings attached to the shaft. The wings (which are flexible) are held tightly together to facilitate needle insertion and then are flattened against the skin and taped to prevent dislodgment. These are generally used for short-term or intermittent therapy and for infants and children.

Several types of catheters are used to access peripheral veins. Some of these catheters are threaded over a needle, and others are threaded inside a needle during insertion. **Intracath** refers to a plastic tube inserted into a vein. An **angiocatheter** (angiocath, for short) is a type of intracath with a metal stylet to pierce the skin and vein, then the plastic catheter is threaded into the vein and the metal stylet removed.

Needle-Free System Safety is a concern with IV therapy. Accidental needlestick injuries and puncture wounds with contaminated devices increase the employee's risk for infectious diseases such as AIDS, hepatitis (B and C), and other viral, rickettsial, bacterial, fungal, and parasitic infections. Many health care facilities use totally needle-free IV systems to increase employee safety (Figure 25-15).

Vascular Access Devices Vascular access devices (VADs) include various cannulas, catheters, and infusion ports that allow long-term IV therapy or repeated access to the central venous system. The client's diagnosis and the type and length

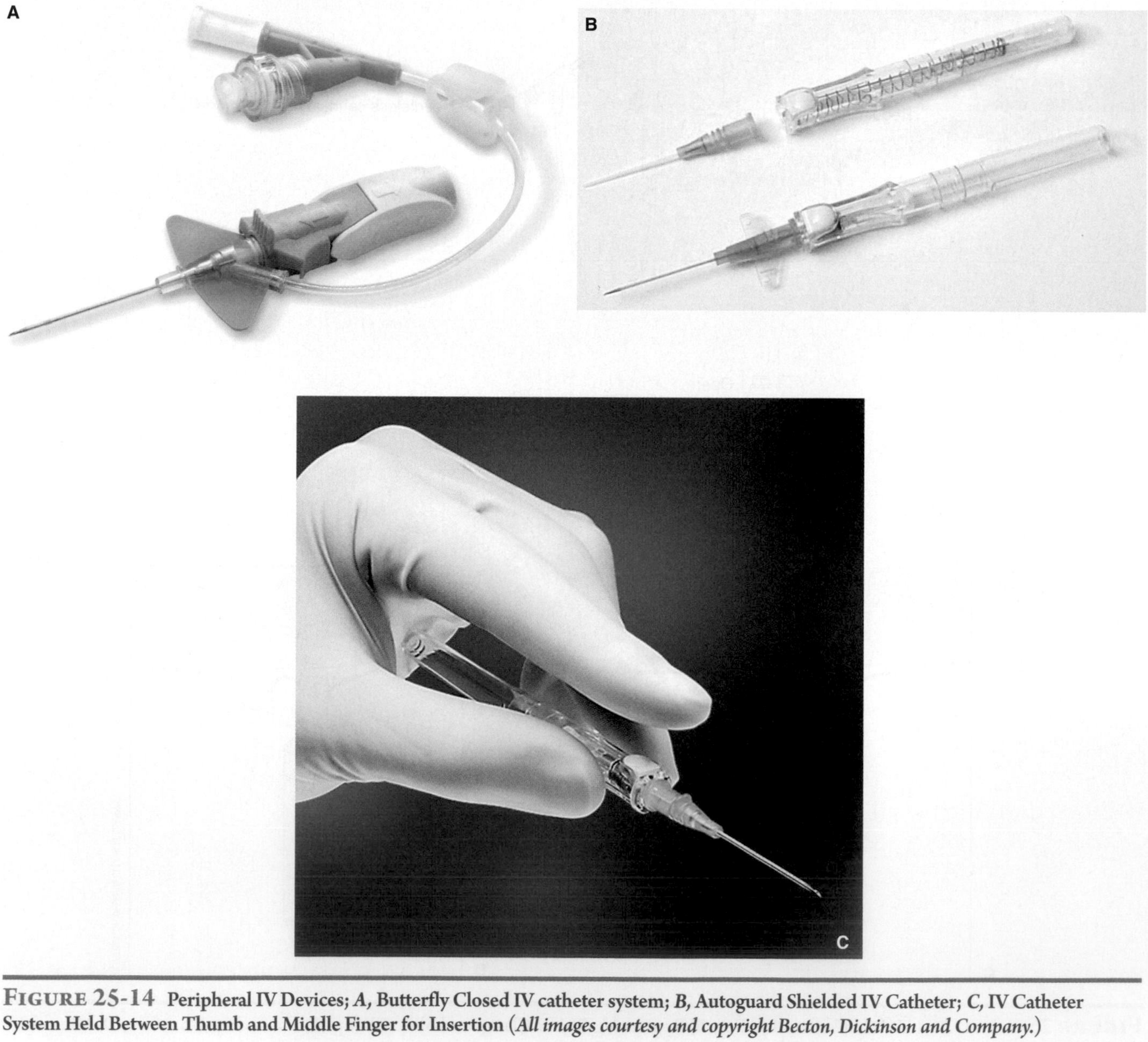

FIGURE 25-14 Peripheral IV Devices; *A*, Butterfly Closed IV catheter system; *B*, Autoguard Shielded IV Catheter; *C*, IV Catheter System Held Between Thumb and Middle Finger for Insertion (*All images courtesy and copyright Becton, Dickinson and Company.*)

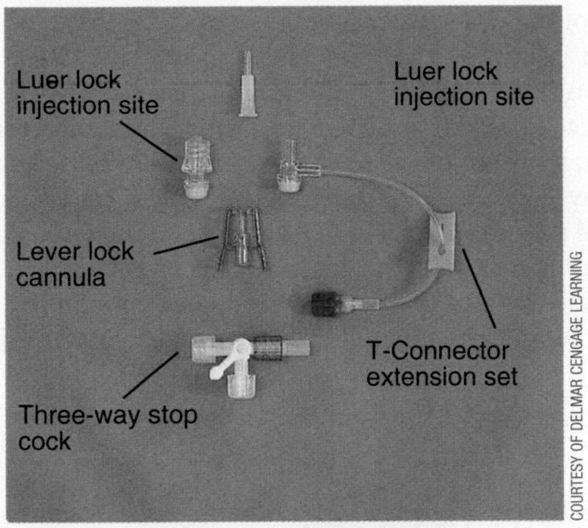

FIGURE 25-15 Needle-Free IV Systems

of treatment determine the kind of VAD used. Central venous catheters (CVCs) are inserted by a physician or an intravenous infusion nurse.

The **implantable port** (a device made of a radiopaque silicone catheter and a plastic or stainless steel injection port with a self-sealing silicone-rubber septum) is another type of VAD. *Only nurses who are specially trained are allowed to access an implanted port because of the risk of infiltration into the tissue if needle placement is incorrect.*

Preparing an Intravenous Solution Before preparing an IV solution, first read the physician's order and the agency's protocol, then gather necessary equipment. Because IV solutions and equipment are sterile, the package expiration date should be checked before use. The IV can be prepared in the client's room or in a nurses' work area.

The IV infusion rate is generally regulated by an infusion pump. Sometimes a time strip is applied to the IV solution bag as a safety check for the infusion pump or to monitor that the infusion rate is the rate prescribed by the physician if an infusion pump is not used (Figure 25-16). Tag the IV tubing

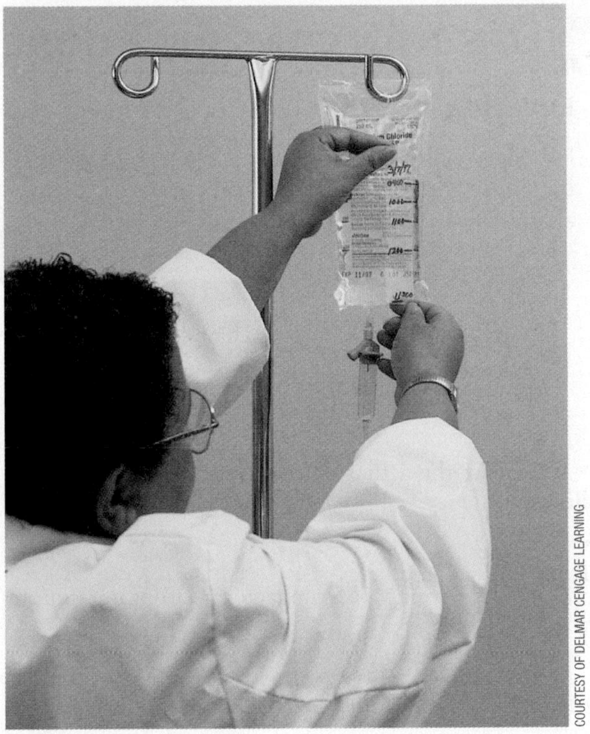

FIGURE 25-16 Applying a Time Strip to the IV Container

with the date and time to notify when the tubing needs to be replaced. Intravenous tubing is changed every 24 to 48 hours according to agency policy. The time strip and the IV tubing tag should be initiated by the nurse.

Initiating IV Therapy Before starting IV therapy, consider the type of fluid to be infused, calculate the flow rate, and assess for a venipuncture site. Altman (2009) suggests that the smallest gauge and shortest needle appropriate be selected (20 to 22 gauge for maintenance fluids and routine antibiotics, 18 to 19 gauge for blood products).

Calculating Flow Rate The physician prescribes the **flow rate**, the volume of fluid to infuse over a set period. For example, 125 mL per hour or 1,000 mL over an 8-hour period. The hourly infusion rate is calculated as follows:

$$\frac{\text{Total volume}}{\text{Number of hours to infuse}} = \text{mL/hour infusion rate}$$

LIFE SPAN CONSIDERATIONS

Selecting Needle Gauge

Consider the client's age and body size and the type of solution to be administered when selecting the gauge of the needle or catheter.

- Infants and small children, 24 gauge
- Preschool through preteen, 24 or 22 gauge
- Teenagers and adults, 22 or 20 gauge
- Elderly, 24 or 22 gauge

SAFETY

Marking an IV Bag

The ink from a felt-tip pen can leak through the plastic and contaminate the solution. Do not use such a pen.

PROFESSIONALTIP

Inserting a CVC

When assisting with the insertion of a long-line central catheter, observe the client for symptoms of a pneumothorax:

- sudden shortness of breath or sharp chest pain
- increased anxiety
- a weak, rapid pulse
- hypotension
- pallor or cyanosis

These symptoms indicate accidental puncture of the pleural membrane.

LIFE SPAN CONSIDERATIONS

Locating a Vein

For clients who are elderly or have fragile veins, eliminate the tourniquet or apply it very loosely if a vein can be palpated.

For example, if 1,000 mL is to be infused over 8 hours:

$$\frac{1{,}000}{8} = 125 \text{ mL/hour}$$

Calculate the actual infusion rate (drops per minute) as follows:

$$\frac{\text{Total fluid volume}}{\text{Total time (minutes)}} \times \text{Drop factor} = \text{Drops per minute}$$

For example, if 1,000 mL is to be infused over 8 hours with a tubing drop factor of 10 drops per milliliter:

$$\frac{1{,}000 \text{ mL}}{8(60)\text{min}} \times 10 \text{ drops/mL} = \frac{10{,}000 \text{ drops}}{480 \text{ min}} = \begin{array}{c}20.8 \text{ or } 21\\ \text{drops/min}\end{array}$$

Another way to calculate the actual infusion rate is to use the hourly infusion rate; for the first example:

$$\frac{125 \text{ mL} \times 10 \text{ drops/mL}}{60 \text{ min}} = 20.8 \text{ or } 21 \text{ drops/min}$$

Consider body size, age, skin condition, clinical status, and impairments when assessing for a potential IV site. Venipuncture site contraindications are as follows:

- Any signs of infection, infiltration, or thrombosis
- Affected arm of a postmastectomy client
- Arm with a functioning arteriovenous fistula (dialysis)
- A paralyzed arm
- Arm with circulatory or neurological impairments

Because venous blood flows upward toward the heart, select a vein for an IV at its most distal end to maintain the integrity of the vein. When a vein is punctured with a needle, fluids can infiltrate (leak from the vein into the tissue at the site of puncture). When IV therapy is discontinued for infiltration, it can only be restarted above the initial puncture site. Generally, it is best to begin with the hand and advance up the arm if new sites are needed. Figure 25-17 illustrates common peripheral sites for initiating IV therapy.

Locating a Vein With the client's arm extended on a firm surface, place a tourniquet on the arm, tight enough to impede venous flow yet loose enough that a radial pulse can still be pal-

PROFESSIONALTIP

Setting Volume to Be Infused

When setting the volume to be infused (e.g., 1,000 mL), set it slightly lower (e.g., 950 mL) so that the alarm goes off before the fluids are completely gone. This practice provides time to have the next bag of fluids ready when all 1,000 mL have been infused. This is especially helpful when having to warm refrigerated fluids. Report to the next shift that the alarm is set to go off early.

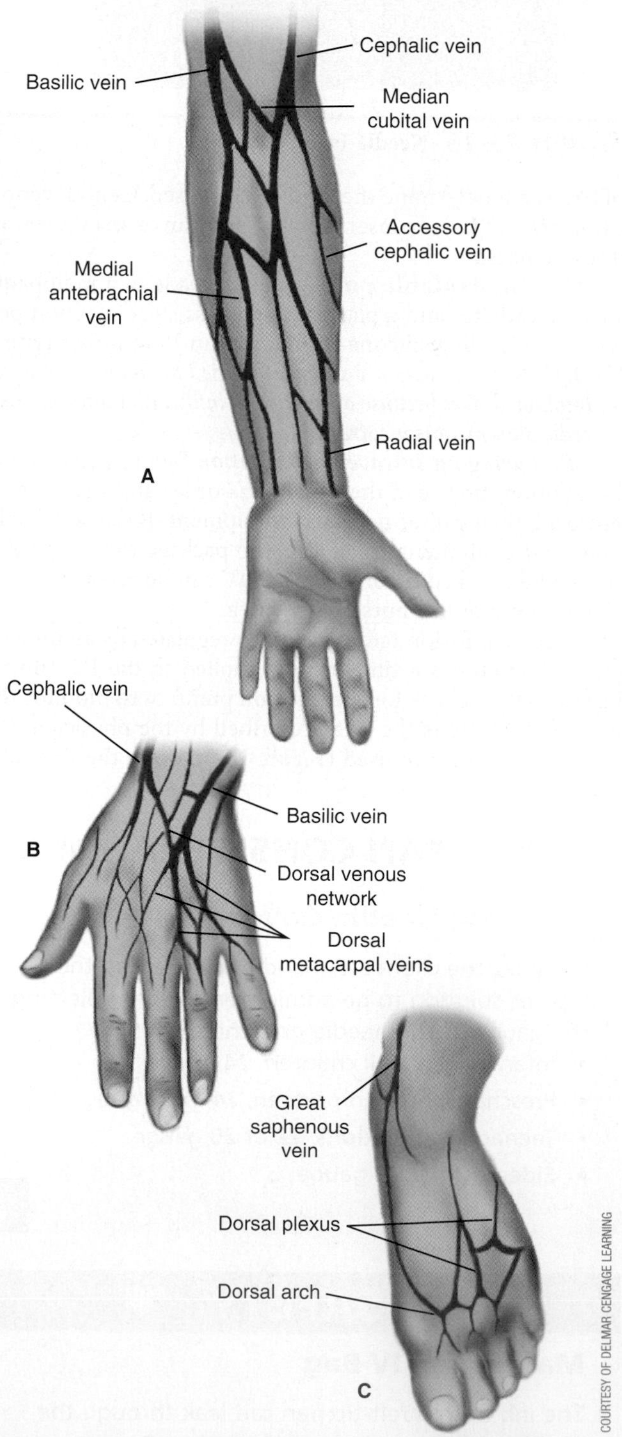

FIGURE 25-17 Peripheral Veins Used in Intravenous Therapy; *A*, Foreman; *B*, Dorsum of the Hand; *C*, Dorsal Plexus of the Foot

INFECTION CONTROL

Venipuncture

Standard Precautions must be followed when performing a venipuncture.

pated. Next, the index and middle fingers of the nondominant hand are used to palpate a vein. It should feel soft and resilient and not have a pulse. If no vein can be seen or felt, a warm, moist compress may be applied for 10 to 20 minutes, the area may be massaged toward the heart, or the client may open and close the fist (Berman, Snyder, Kozier, & Erb, 2008; Jensen, 2008a).

Placing the Needle After hand hygiene and gloving is completed, prepare the selected site according to agency policy. Without touching the prepared site, stabilize the vein by placing the thumb of the nondominant hand beside the vein and pulling down, making the skin taut. This technique also makes the needle insertion less painful. Hold the needle at a 10- to 30-degree angle, bevel up to puncture the skin, then lessen the angle to prevent puncturing the back of the vein (Berman et al., 2008; Ellenberger, 1999; Jensen, 2008a). Secure the needle in place according to agency policy.

Administering IV Therapy When the solution has been prepared and the rate calculated, explain the procedure to the client. Administration may be continuous over a 24-hour period, or intermittent, 1,000 mL once in a 24-hour period. Although fluids may be continuous, the type of fluids can change over a 24-hour period. For example, a physician's order might read for the pharmacy to: *Add 40 mEq of KCl to first bag of 1,000 mL of normal saline.*

Intravenous medications may be **piggybacked**, connected to an existing IV to infuse concurrently. Refrigerated solutions and medications should be warmed to room temperature before administration (usually for 30 minutes) for client comfort.

Regulating IV Solution Flow Rate The flow rate for IV solutions can be regulated by calculating the drops per minute and adjusting the drip rate to that number or by the use of volume controllers and pumps (Figure 25-18).

Volume Controllers and Pumps Controllers are devices dependent on gravity to maintain a preselected flow but do not add pressure to overcome resistance (e.g., Dial-a-Flo or

PROFESSIONALTIP

IV-Related Sepsis

If a client has chills and fever, check how long the IV solution has been hanging and the needle or catheter has been in place. Assess the client's vital signs and for other symptoms of pyrogenic reactions, such as backache, malaise, headache, nausea, and vomiting. If IV-related sepsis occurs, the pulse rate increases, and temperature is usually above 100°F. Stop the infusion, notify the physician, and obtain blood specimens if ordered.

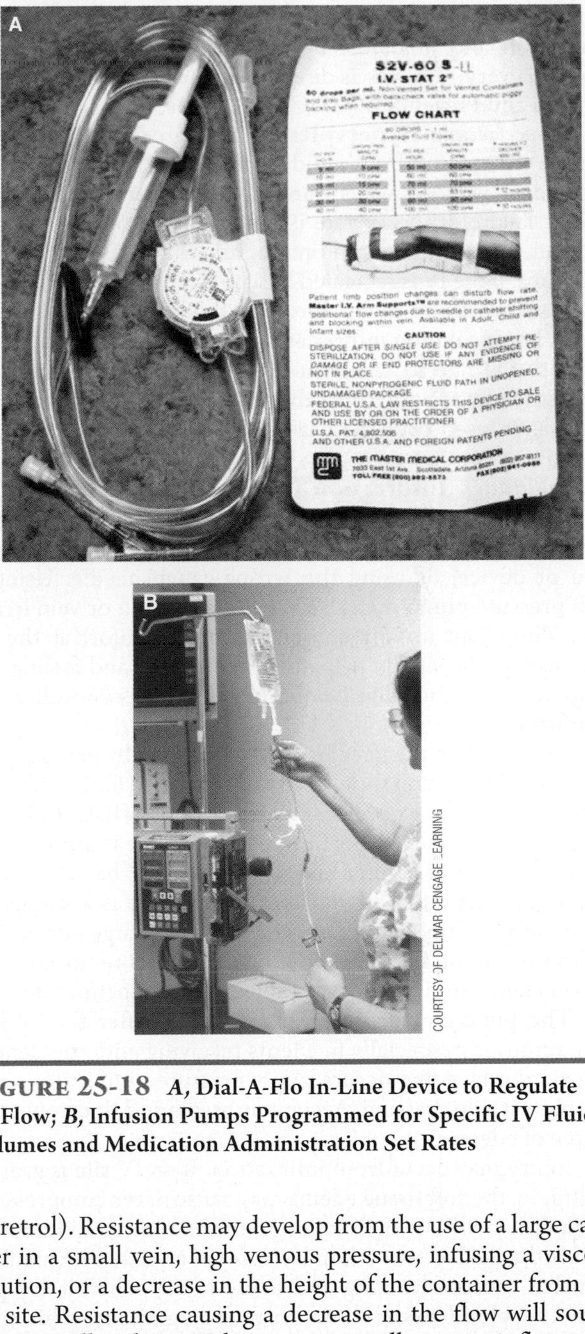

COURTESY OF DELMAR CENGAGE LEARNING

FIGURE 25-18 ***A,*** **Dial-A-Flo In-Line Device to Regulate IV Flow;** ***B,*** **Infusion Pumps Programmed for Specific IV Fluid Volumes and Medication Administration Set Rates**

Buretrol). Resistance may develop from the use of a large catheter in a small vein, high venous pressure, infusing a viscous solution, or a decrease in the height of the container from the IV site. Resistance causing a decrease in the flow will sound the controller alarm. Volumetric controllers permit flow rates to be set in milliliters per hour.

Pumps maintain a preselected volume delivery by adding pressure when needed. Pumps may be used when large volumes must be delivered in a short period and for viscous fluids. Pumps have maximum pressure limits that sound an alarm when reached. When a drug or solution is administered under high pressure, clients have a greater risk for complications.

Managing IV Therapy Intravenous therapy requires frequent client monitoring to ensure an accurate flow rate. Other nursing actions are to ensure client comfort and position; check the IV solution to ensure that the solution, amount, and timing are correct; monitor expiration dates of the IV system (tubing, venipuncture site, dressing) and change as necessary; and be aware of safety factors.

Client care is coordinated with the maintenance of IV lines. If the facility does not have snaps or Velcro on the gown sleeves, changing the gown and IV tubing when doing site care decreases the number of times the access device is manipulated. This client care action decreases the risk for infiltration and phlebitis. Peripherally inserted devices are changed every 72 hours as directed by the Centers for Disease Control and Prevention (CDC) guidelines.

Hypervolemia **Hypervolemia** (increased circulating fluid volume) may result from rapid IV infusion of solutions, causing cardiac overload, which can lead to pulmonary edema and cardiac failure. If the IV rate is not regulated by a pump, the infusion rate must be monitored hourly to prevent these complications. If the IV is regulated by a pump, check that the rate is flowing correctly on clients at risk for fluid volume overload.

When a solution infuses at a rate greater than prescribed, decrease the rate to *keep vein open* (KVO) and immediately notify the physician. Report the amount and type of solution that was infused over the exact time period and the client's response.

Infiltration **Infiltration** (inadvertent administration of a nonvesicant solution into surrounding tissue) may result from dislodging the device from the vein, inserting the wrong type of device, or using the wrong-gauge needle. Using a high pressure pump may also cause infiltration or vein irritation. The client usually complains of discomfort at the IV site. Inspect the site by palpating for swelling and feeling the temperature of the skin. Cool and pale skin is an indication of infiltration.

Confirm that the needle is still in the vein by pinching the IV tubing. This action should cause **flashback** (blood will rush into the tubing if the needle is still in the vein). If flashback does not occur, the injection port nearest the device is aspirated by an RN. If the port cannot be aspirated, the IV has infiltrated. Follow the institution's guidelines when there is a suspected infiltration, such as notifying an IV nurse or charge nurse. If an infiltration occurred, the needle or catheter is removed from the vein and a sterile dressing applied to the puncture site.

The puncture site may ooze or bleed after the IV has been removed (especially in clients receiving anticoagulants). If oozing or bleeding occurs, apply pressure until it stops and reapply a sterile dressing. Accurately assess and document the degree of edema.

Injury may occur from infiltration. If an IV site is grossly infiltrated, the soft tissue edema may cause nerve compression with permanent loss of function to the extremity. **Extravasation** is the inadvertent administration of a **vesicant** (medication that causes blistering and tissue injury when it escapes from the blood vessel) into surrounding tissue. This may cause significant tissue loss with permanent disfigurement and loss of function (Hadaway, 2002a).

Phlebitis Phlebitis may result from either mechanical or chemical trauma. Inserting a device with too large a gauge, using a vein that is too small or fragile, or leaving the device in place for too long may cause mechanical trauma. Chemical trauma may result from infusing too rapidly or from an acidic solution, hypertonic solution, a solution containing electrolytes (especially potassium and magnesium) or other medications.

Phlebitis may be a precursor of sepsis. Client descriptions of tenderness are usually the first indication of an inflammation. The IV site must be inspected for changes in skin color and temperature (a reddened area or a pink or red stripe along the vein, warmth, and swelling are indications of phlebitis).

If phlebitis is present, the IV infusion must be discontinued. Before removing and discarding the venous device, check the facility's protocol to see whether the tip of the device is to be cultured. If so, it is sent to the laboratory for a culture and sensitivity test. After removing the device, apply a sterile dressing to the site and wet, warm compresses to the affected area. Document the time, symptoms, and nursing interventions.

Intravenous Dressing Change Standard Precautions and aseptic technique are followed for intravenous dressing changes. The frequency of care is determined by institutional protocol and the type of intravenous access device and dressing. Persistent drainage at the IV site may require more frequent dressing changes or may necessitate changing the IV site.

Intravenous Drug Therapy When a rapid drug effect is desired or a medication is irritating to tissue, the IV route is used. Intravenous administration immediately releases medication into the bloodstream; therefore, it can be dangerous. Intravenous medications are administered by one of the following modes:

- Intravenous fluid container
- Volume-control administration set
- Intermittent infusion by piggyback or partial fill
- Intravenous push (IVP or bolus)

Adding Drugs to an Intravenous Fluid Container Before administering IV medications, assess the patency of the infusion system and the condition of the injection site for signs of infiltration and phlebitis. Some IV medications or solutions with high or low pH or high osmolarity are irritating to veins and can cause phlebitis. Also note the client's allergies, drug or solution incompatibilities, the amount and type of diluent needed to mix the medication, and the client's general condition to establish a baseline before administering medication. **Drug incompatibilities** are an undesired chemical or physical reaction between a drug and a solution, between a drug and the container or tubing, or between two drugs. For example, diazepam (Valium) and chlordiazepoxide hydrochloride (Librium) are not compatible with a saline solution; insulin sticks to the inside of the solution bag, so use glass bottles.

Adding Drugs to a Volume-Control Administration Set

A volume-control set is used to administer small volumes of IV solution. They have various names, such as Soluset, Metriset, VoluTrol, or Buretrol. To use this method, do the following:

- Withdraw the prescribed amount of medication into a syringe
- Cleanse the injection port of a partially filled volume-control set with an alcohol swab
- Inject the prepared medication through the port of the volume-control set
- Gently mix the solution in the volume-control chamber
- Check the infusion rate and adjust as necessary

Administering Medications by Intermittent Infusion A common method of administering IV medications is by using a secondary, or partial-fill additive bag, often called IV piggyback (IVPB). The secondary line is a complete IV set (fluid container and tubing with either a microdrip or a macrodrip system) connected to a Y-port of a primary line. The primary line maintains venous access. The IVPB is used for medication administration. When the IVPB medication is incompatible with the primary IV solution, flush the primary IV tubing with normal saline before and after administering the medication. Another method of infusing a medication that is incompatible with the primary line is to disconnect the primary line from the IV catheter, flush the catheter, connect the secondary set IV tubing to the IV catheter and infuse the medication.

Intermittent Infusion Devices When the client requires only IV medications without a quantity of solution, an intermittent infusion device is attached to a peripheral needle or catheter in the client's vein. This device is commonly referred to as a heparin or saline lock, depending on the facility's policy of heparin or saline maintenance. A lock provides continuous venous access, eliminating the need for a continuous IV and increasing the client's mobility.

The device is used to infuse intermittent IVPB or IV push (also called bolus) medications, or it can be converted to a primary IV. An **IV push (bolus)** is the administration of a large dose of medication in a relatively short time, usually 1 to 30 minutes. A saline lock device provides venous access in case of an emergency and is routinely used with cardiac clients.

Administering IV Push Medications An IV push medication can be injected into a saline or a heparin lock (Figure 25-19A) or into a continuous infusion line. When giving an IV push medication into a continuous infusion line, stop the fluids in the primary line by pinching the IV tubing closed while injecting the drug (Figure 25-19B). This technique is safe and prevents having to recalculate the drip rate of the primary infusion line.

PROFESSIONALTIP

New Process for Blood Transfusions

A new process developed by a team of researchers produces an enzyme that strips the A and B antigens from the red blood cell, making the blood useful for all blood types. Commercial production of these enzymes will help make blood transfusion safer by reducing the need for stringent blood typing and matching procedures, eliminating the risk of hemolytic transfusion reactions. The blood supply could be distributed more efficiently and less blood wasted; persons with rare blood types would be able to receive any blood type after the enzyme antigen stripping process (Liu et al., 2007).

Documentation

When IV therapy is begun, the date, time, venipuncture site, number of attempts made, amount and type of fluid, and equipment used must be documented. Each time the insertion site, venipuncture device, or IV tubing is changed, the reason for the change must be documented (e.g., routine, infiltration). The condition of the insertion site and the fluid type, amount, and flow rate are documented each shift and at intervals specified by agency policy. Any complications are precisely documented along with the nurse's actions.

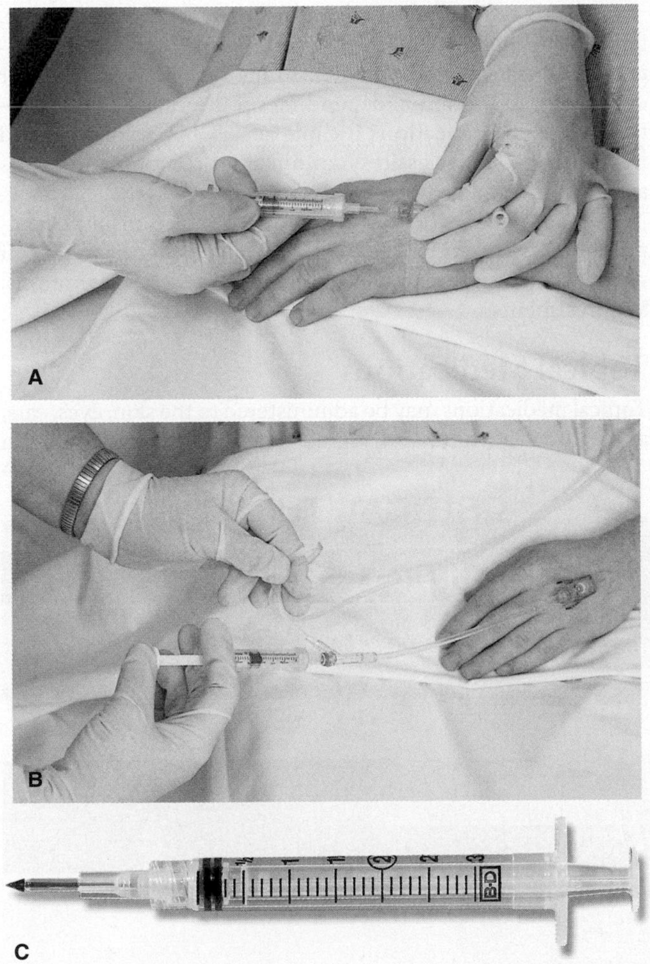

FIGURE 25-19 Injecting an IV Push (Bolus) Medication; *A,* Into a peripheral saline lock; *B,* Into a primary infusion line. The IV tubing must be pinched closed first; *C,* A needleless syringe to give intravenous medications. (*Images A and B courtesy of Delmar Cengage Learning. Image C courtesy and copyright Becton, Dickson and Company.*)

Blood Transfusion

A blood transfusion is given to replace blood loss (deficit) with whole blood or blood components. Based on the client's unique needs, the physician determines the type of transfusion, either whole blood or a component of whole blood.

Whole Blood and Blood Products Whole blood contains red blood cells (RBCs) and plasma components of blood. It is used when all the components of blood are needed to restore blood volume and to restore the oxygen-carrying capacity of the blood.

When the physician prescribes whole blood or a blood product, the client's blood is typed and cross matched. If time and the client's condition permit, the family may arrange for donors. The blood is stored in the blood bank after typing and cross matching.

Whole blood has a refrigerated shelf life of 35 days, but platelets must be administered within 3 days after extracted from whole blood. If the RBCs and plasma are frozen, their shelf life is up to 3 years (Kee & Paulanka, 2009).

Initial Assessment and Preparation Perform an initial assessment before administering blood that includes the following:

- Verify that the client has signed a blood administration consent form and that this consent matches what the physician has prescribed.
- Identify the gauge of needle or catheter used if IV in place. The viscosity of whole blood usually requires an 18-gauge needle or catheter to prevent red blood cell damage. If blood is to be infused quickly, a 14- or 15-gauge device must be used.
- Ensure patency of the existing IV site.

LIFE SPAN CONSIDERATIONS

Initial Assessment

If pediatric, elderly, or clients with congestive heart failure or malnutrition are at risk for circulatory overload, notify the blood bank to divide the 500-mL bag of blood into two 250-mL bags or discuss with the physician other alternatives, such as packed RBCs rather than whole blood.

PROFESSIONALTIP

Transfusion Reaction

Transfusion reaction severity is related to the time of onset. Severe reactions usually occur shortly after the blood begins to infuse. At the first sign of a reaction, stop the blood infusion immediately.

- Establish vital signs baseline data, especially temperature, and assess skin for eruptions or rashes.
- Verify label on the whole blood or blood component with the client's blood type before administration, to ensure compatibility. Some facilities require two nurses to verify that the client's name and blood type match the name and blood type on the transfusion bag.
- Assess the client's age and state of nutrition.

Scheduled IV medications should be infused before blood administration to prevent a medication reaction while blood is infusing. If a reaction were to occur, it would not be known whether the medication or the blood was causing the reaction.

Administering Whole Blood or a Blood Component A facility's blood protocol may require that a licensed person sign a release for blood from the blood bank and that two licensed personnel check blood products before infusion. Information that must be on the blood bag label and verified for accuracy includes the client's name and identification number, ABO group and Rh factor, donor number, type of product ordered, and expiration date.

SAFETY

Blood Transfusion Incompatibilities

Only 0.9% normal saline can be used with a blood product. Blood transfusions are incompatible with dextrose and with Ringer's solution.

To maintain RBC integrity and decrease the chance of infection, blood administration should begin within 30 minutes after it is received from the bank. Whole blood should not be unrefrigerated for more than 4 hours. Room temperature causes RBC lysis, releasing potassium and causing hyperkalemia.

Safety Measures Observe the client for the initial 15 minutes for a transfusion reaction. Take vital signs every 15 minutes for the first hour, then every hour while the blood is infusing.

The three basic types of transfusion reactions are allergic, febrile, and hemolytic and may be mild or severe, depending on the cause. Hemolytic reactions may be immediate or delayed up to 96 hours, depending on the cause of the reaction. Other complications include sepsis, hypervolemia, and hypothermia. The classic symptoms of a reaction and sepsis are fever and chills.

The nursing actions for all types of reactions and complications are given in Table 25-7. Table 25-8 gives details of several transfusion reactions, etiologies, signs and symptoms, and treatments.

Topical Medications

Topical medications may be administered to the skin, eyes, ears, nose, throat, rectum, and vagina. The medication provides a

CRITICAL THINKING

Transfusion Reactions

How can transfusion reactions be differentiated?

TABLE 25-7 Nursing Actions for Blood Reactions

IMMEDIATE NURSING ACTION	OTHER MEASURES
• Stop transfusion.	• Monitor client's vital signs every 15 minutes for 4 hours or until stable.
• Keep vein open with 0.9% normal saline.	• Monitor I&O.
• Notify the physician.	• Send IV tubing and bag of blood back to the blood bank.
	• Obtain a blood and urine specimen.
	• Label specimen "Blood Transfusion Reaction."
	• Process a transfusion reaction report.

TABLE 25-8 Transfusion Reactions, Etiologies, Signs and Symptoms, and Treatments

REACTION	ETIOLOGY	SIGN AND SYMPTOMS	TREATMENTS
ACUTE			
Acute hemolytic transfusion reaction (intravascular hemolysis)	Incompatible blood product transfused because of errors during processing the blood products and the type and cross match	Fever, low back pain, pain at IV site, hypotension, tachycardia, abdominal pain, dyspnea, nausea/vomiting, rash/hives, headache, anxiety, renal failure	Stop the transfusion immediately Keep the vein open with a 0.9% normal saline IV Contact physician stat Support vital functions—may require hemodialysis Complete lab tests necessary to determine if blood reaction occurred
Nonhemolytic transfusion reaction	Reaction to donor leukocytes in the blood products	Fever, anemia, increased bilirubin levels	Give premedications to reduce reaction: acetaminophen, diphenydramine, hydrocortisone
Allergic reactions	Recipient antibodies against donor antigens (foreign proteins)	Itching to rashes to anaphylaxis and shock	Stop the transfusion, treat with antihistamines, may resume slowly when symptoms resolved
Transfusion-related acute lung injury (TRALI)	Anti-HLA antibodies and neutrophil antibodies	Acute respiratory insufficiency, chills, fever, cyanosis, hypotension	Support respiratory function, IV steroids
Bacterial contamination of blood product	Endotoxins from gram-negative and gram-positive bacteria	Fever, shock, disseminated intravascular coagulation (DIC), renal failure	High-dose antibiotics, vital organ support, steroids
Circulatory overload	Too rapid a flow rate for client's cardiovascular system	Dyspnea, cough, frothy sputum	Support respiratory system, administer diuretic between units, slower infusion rates for clients with known cardiovascular compromise
Citrate toxicity	Hypocalcemia resulting from citrate binding with calcium in the recipient's bloodstream	Tetany	Monitor for signs and symptoms, monitor calcium level, transfuse extra calcium, if warranted
DELAYED			
Graft-versus-host disease	Lymphocytes infused with blood product into an immunosuppressed recipient	Fever, hepatitis, bone marrow suppression, overwhelming infection, 90% to 100% mortality rate	Pretransfusion radiation of blood products containing lymphocytes preventing replication of donor lymphocytes and the engrafting process
Disease transmitted with the blood product: bacterial, syphilis, protozoal, viral	Contamination during processing, preexisting donor infection, contamination during donation	Depends on disease transmitted	Careful aseptic technique through all portions of donation and transfusion, careful screening of donors and testing blood products for viruses
Delayed hemolytic reaction	Reaction to donor antibodies	None to fever, mild jaundice and anemia	Conduct additional antibody testing prior to additional blood transfusions
Iron overload	Repeated blood transfusions for chronic anemic conditions, such as sickle cell anemia	Liver failure Cardiac toxicities	Infuse chelation treatment, Desferal®, to bind to iron and remove from system, monitor iron level routinely

local effect but may also have systemic effects. Drugs applied directly to the skin for a local effect include lotions, pastes, creams, ointments, powders, and aerosol sprays. The vascularity of the area determines the rate and degree of the drug's absorption.

Topical drugs provide continuous absorption to produce various effects: to relieve pruritus (itching), to prevent or treat an infection, to provide local anesthesia, to protect the skin, or to create a systemic effect. Topical medications are usually applied two or three times a day to achieve their therapeutic effect.

Before applying a topical preparation, the condition of the skin is assessed for any rashes, open lesions, or areas of erythema and skin breakdown. The nurse checks with the client and the medical record for any known allergies.

Cleanse the area by washing it with soap and warm water, unless contraindicated by a specific order. Allow the skin to thoroughly dry before applying a topical medication. Open wounds require the use of aseptic technique.

When the skin is dry, the medication is applied. To apply a paste, cream, or an ointment, follow Standard Precautions. To prevent cross contamination, use a sterile tongue depressor for removing the medication from the container. Transfer the medication from the tongue blade to a gloved hand for application. Apply the medication in long, smooth strokes in the direction of the hair follicles to prevent the medication from entering the hair follicles. When more medication is removed from the container, a new sterile tongue depressor is used. Assess the area for signs of an allergic reaction 2 to 4 hours after the application.

Eye Medications Eye medications are in the form of drops, ointments, or disks. These drugs are used for diagnostic and therapeutic purposes, to lubricate the eye or socket for a prosthetic eye, and to treat or prevent eye conditions such as glaucoma (elevated pressure within the eye) and infection. Diagnostically, eyedrops are used to dilate the pupil, anesthetize the eye, or stain the cornea to identify abrasions and scars.

Medication disks are inserted at bedtime because they usually cause blurred vision. Follow Standard Precautions when administering eye care and medications; there is a potential for contact with bodily secretions.

Ear Medications Solutions ordered for the ear are often called *otic* (pertaining to the ear) drops or irrigations. Eardrops are instilled to soften ear wax, treat infection or inflammation, produce anesthesia, or facilitate removal of a foreign body.

SAFETY

Prevent Cross Contamination

- Never share a bottle of eyedrops between clients.
- After instillation, discard any solution remaining in the dropper.
- Discard the dropper if the tip is accidentally contaminated (i.e., touching the bottle or any part of the client's eye).

PROFESSIONALTIP

Preventing Systemic Effects of Eyedrops

- Apply pressure to the inner canthus when instilling eyedrops that have potential systemic effects, such as atropine and timolol maleate (Timoptic).
- Gentle pressure over the inner canthus prevents the medication from flowing into the tear duct, thereby decreasing the absorption rate of the drug.

External auditory canal irrigations are usually performed for cleansing purposes.

Inspect the ear for signs of drainage (an indication of a perforated tympanic membrane) before instilling a solution into the ear. Eardrops are usually contraindicated with a perforated tympanic membrane. Aseptic technique must be used if the tympanic membrane is damaged. Otherwise, medical asepsis is used for ear medications.

Nasal Instillations Nasal instillations can be either drops or nebulizers (atomizer or aerosol). Nasal drugs produce one or more of the following effects: shrink swollen mucous membranes, loosen secretions and facilitate drainage, or treat infections of the nasal cavity or sinuses. Because the nose is connected with the sinuses, medical asepsis is used when performing nasal instillations.

COMMUNITY/HOME HEALTH CARE

Considerations for Use of Nasal Inhalers

- The client should have the manufacturer's directions for the specific type of inhaler, such as how to replace a medication cartridge for a nasal aerosol.
- Inhalers are kept at room temperature.
- Aerosols are prepared under pressure, so do not puncture or place in an incinerator.
- No one but the client should use the inhaler.
- Caution that overuse can cause a rebound effect, making the condition worse.
- Ensure that the client knows the expected and adverse effects of the drug. Some of these drugs take several days to 2 weeks of continuous use for the effects to appear.
- Provide the client with a telephone number to call if assistance is needed.

Many of these products are nonprescription drugs, so clients should be taught their correct usage. Nasal decongestants are common over-the-counter drugs to shrink swollen mucous membranes; however, they may have a reverse or rebound effect by increasing nasal congestion when used in excess.

Nebulizers (inhalers) deliver a fine mist containing medication droplets. The client who is discharged with a nasal inhaler must be taught how to store and use the device. Assist clients in the use of atomizers and aerosols:

- Have the client clear the nostrils by blowing the nose.
- Client should be in an upright position with head tilted back slightly.

For atomizers:

- Occlude one nostril to prevent air from entering the nasal cavity and allow the medication to flow freely into the open nostril.
- Insert the atomizer tip into the open nostril and ask the client to inhale, while the atomizer is squeezed once, then ask the client to exhale.

For aerosols:

- Shake the aerosol well before each use.
- Grasp between thumb and index finger and insert the adapter tip into one nostril while occluding the other nostril with a finger, then press the adapter cartridge firmly to release one measured dose of medication.
- Repeat the above steps for the other nostril.
- Have the client keep the head tilted backward for 2 to 3 minutes and breathe through the nose while the medication is being absorbed.

Respiratory Inhalants Respiratory inhalants are delivered by devices that produce fine droplets to be inhaled deep into the respiratory tract. They are absorbed very quickly through the alveolar epithelium into the bloodstream. This section discusses only oropharyngeal handheld inhalers.

Oropharyngeal handheld inhalers deliver medications, such as bronchodilators and mucolytics, that produce both local and systemic effects. Bronchodilators (drugs that dilate the bronchi) improve airway patency and prevent or treat asthma, bronchospasms, and allergic reactions. Mucolytics liquify tenacious (thick) bronchial secretions.

Clients must be able to assemble the turbo-inhaler and form an airtight seal around the inhaling devices. This requirement prevents some clients from using these devices. Bronchodilators are contraindicated for clients with a history of tachycardia.

Rectal Instillations Rectal instillations are in the form of suppositories, ointments, or enemas. Rectal ointments treat local conditions and hemorrhoid symptoms of pain, inflammation, and itching. Rectal suppositories are cone-shaped medications designed to melt at body temperature and be absorbed at a slow and steady rate.

Suppositories are a convenient and safe route for administering drugs that interact poorly with digestive enzymes or have a bad taste or odor. They are used to provide temporary relief for clients who cannot tolerate oral preparations (e.g., to relieve nausea and vomiting). They are also used to reduce fever, relieve pain and local irritation, and stimulate peristalsis and defecation in clients who are constipated.

The rectum should be assessed for irritation or bleeding and sphincter control checked. Some clients may have a problem retaining the suppository. Ask those clients to remain in Sims' position for at least 15 minutes or have the client lie on the abdomen, if allowed, and hold the buttocks closed. When the client is unable to retain a suppository, notify the physician so that another route can be ordered.

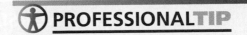

PROFESSIONALTIP

Contraindications for Rectal Suppositories

- Cardiac clients because insertion may stimulate the vagus nerve, causing cardiac dysrhythmias (abnormal heart patterns).
- Clients recovering from rectal or prostate surgery because suppositories may cause pain on insertion and trauma to the tissues.

Vaginal Instillations Medications inserted into the vagina are suppositories, creams, ointments, gels, foams, or douches. They treat infections, inflammation, and discomfort or as a contraceptive measure.

Vaginal creams, gels, ointments, and foams usually come with a disposable applicator with a plunger to insert the drug. Suppositories are usually inserted with the index finger of a gloved hand; however, small suppositories may come with an applicator. After insertion of these preparations, the client may notice drainage and is told to expect this. To prevent soiling of the underpants, tell the client to wear a perineal pad.

Agency policy usually requires sterile technique when administering a vaginal douche (irrigation). Check that the client does not have an allergy to iodine because many vaginal preparations contain povidone-iodine.

EVALUATION

Administering medications according to the "seven rights" requires the nurse to verify that safe nursing care was provided. Evaluation includes that each client knows the effects, side effects, adverse reactions, special considerations, and when to call the physician for each drug.

A nurse identifying a potential medication risk and initiating actions to prevent client injury is performing another form of evaluation.

CLIENTTEACHING

Tampon Use

Clients should not use tampons after the insertion of vaginal medications because the tampon can absorb the medication and decrease the drug's effect.

SAMPLE NURSING CARE PLAN

The Client with Deep Vein Thrombosis

M.L., a 45-year-old, was admitted to your floor with a diagnosis of deep vein thrombosis. She noticed swelling of her left leg about a week ago but decided to treat it at home. Four days later the lower leg was very edematous, warm, and painful to move. After an office visit, M.L. was admitted to the hospital. This is her first hospitalization. On examination the left leg is warmer than the right. The left thigh circumference is 3 inches larger than the right. The physician ordered a heparin IV drip after a loading dose bolus was given. The drip contained 10,000 units heparin in 500 mL of D_5W at 10 mL/hour (200 units/hour). The physician anticipates that M.L. will be weaned off the heparin drip and started on subcutaneous heparin within 5 days. At the time of discharge she will be given Coumadin.

NURSING DIAGNOSIS 1 *Ineffective Tissue Perfusion (peripheral)* related to the development of venous thrombi in the deep femoral vein as evidenced by left leg being warmer than right leg and left thigh circumference being 3 inches larger than right thigh circumference

Nursing Outcomes Classification (NOC)
Tissue Perfusion: Peripheral
Tissue Integrity

Nursing Interventions Classification (NIC)
Peripheral Sensation Management
Circulatory Care: Venous Insufficiency

PLANNING/OUTCOMES	NURSING INTERVENTIONS	RATIONALE
M.L. will report an absence of pain.	Maintain on bed rest.	Reduces the possibility of embolus; may decrease the pain and swelling.
	Apply moist heat to the affected extremity.	Provides an analgesic effect; it decreases venospasms and pain.
M.L. will have a decrease of edema.	Elevate the legs above the heart.	Facilitates venous return and decreases the edema.
	Measure the circumference of the left thigh and compare with that of the right thigh.	Provides a quantitative reference point that can be used to evaluate the swelling.
M.L. will experience the same degree of skin temperature in both legs.	Administer the heparin drip at 200 units/hour.	Prevents the conversion of fibrinogen to fibrin and prothrombin to thrombin, thereby limiting the extension of the thrombus.
	Monitor the partial thromboplastin time (PTT).	Monitors heparin therapy because heparin, a short-acting anticoagulant, increases the PTT.

EVALUATION

M.L. is able to ambulate without difficulty or pain. M.L.'s left thigh is only 1/2 inch larger than her right thigh. M.L.'s legs are the same temperature to touch.

SAMPLE NURSING CARE PLAN (Continued)

NURSING DIAGNOSIS 2 *Risk for Injury (bleeding)* related to the administration of an anticoagulant

Nursing Outcomes Classification (NOC)	Nursing Interventions Classification (NIC)
Risk Control	*Health Education*
Safety Behavior: Personal	*Medication Management*

PLANNING/OUTCOMES	NURSING INTERVENTIONS	RATIONALE
M.L. will not demonstrate evidence of bleeding from gums or nose, in urine or stool, or under the skin.	Withhold the medication in the event that bleeding occurs and to notify the physician immediately.	The dose may need to be adjusted.
	Encourage the client to discontinue smoking.	May increase the metabolism of the medication, necessitating an increase in the dose.
M.L. will maintain her prothrombin time (PT) or international normalized ratio (INR) within therapeutic range.	Advise the client to watch food intake.	Foods high in fat and foods rich in vitamin K can interfere with the PT.
	Warn against taking oral contraceptive medication.	Decreases anticoagulant effect.
	Warn against taking aspirin and other over-the-counter medications.	May increase the risk of bleeding; it inhibits platelet formation.

EVALUATION

M.L. has had no bleeding episodes. M.L. still has many questions about taking the oral anticoagulant on discharge. Discharge follow-up will be needed to monitor the client's progress on the oral anticoagulant.

SUMMARY

- The *United States Pharmacopeia* and the *National Formulary* list drug standards for use in the United States.
- The Food and Drug Administration tests all drugs before granting a company the right to market a drug.
- Drugs are usually referred to by their generic name (not capitalized) or by their trade name (always capitalized).
- The safest and least expensive administration route is the oral route, although it is also the slowest to act.
- Parenteral drugs are injected through intradermal (ID), subcutaneous, intramuscular (IM), or intravenous (IV) routes and are typically fast acting.
- The pharmacokinetics of drugs includes absorption, distribution, metabolism, and excretion.
- The "seven rights" of safe drug administration are right client, right drug, right dose, right route, right time, right documentation, and right to refuse.
- Nurses are legally and morally responsible for correct administration of medications.
- Although the physician determines the dose and route of a parenteral drug, the nurse chooses the correct gauge and length of the needle to be used.
- Always monitor client reactions to medications and ensure that clients know the actions, side effects, and contraindications of all medications they take.
- Clients receiving intravenous therapy or blood transfusions require constant monitoring for complications.

REVIEW QUESTIONS

1. A client is unable to swallow the pills ordered by the physician. The best action for the nurse is to:
   1. tell the client to chew the pills.
   2. crush the pills and give them to the client.
   3. call the physician for a change in the orders.
   4. ask the pharmacy to send the medications in liquid form.
2. The client is in the bathroom when the nurse brings the medications. The best action for the nurse is to:
   1. return with the medications when the client is finished in the bathroom.
   2. leave the medications for the client to take when finished in the bathroom.
   3. knock on the bathroom door and give the medications to the client at this time.
   4. ask the nursing assistant to see that the client takes the medications when finished in the bathroom.
3. The best time for the nurse to document medication administration is:
   1. whenever the nurse has time.
   2. before the client receives the medication.
   3. only after the client has received the medication.
   4. toward the end of the shift so all medications can be charted at one time.
4. Standard Precautions are required with: (Select all that apply.)
   1. venipuncture.
   2. IM injections.
   3. oral medications.
   4. nasal instillation.
   5. rectal instillations.
5. A client receiving a blood transfusion tells the nurse, who is taking the first set of 15-minute vital signs, that she is cold (chills) and her chest hurts. The first thing the nurse should do is:
   1. stop the transfusion.
   2. get a warm blanket for the client.
   3. call the blood bank to come and check the blood.
   4. stay with the client and talk quietly to her to help her relax.
6. A 76-year-old client has a peripheral IV infusing in her left arm. The nurse discovers all the following findings in her assessment. To what should the nurse react and treat immediately?
   1. The IV site is bruised without edema.
   2. The patient reports tingling in her hands and muscle cramping.
   3. The patient has a moist cough and distended neck veins.
   4. The patient's urine output was 150 mL for the past 8 hours.
7. The client is complaining of pain at her IV site. The nurse assesses the site and notes that there is a hard cord along the vein, diffuse redness, and slight edema. The nurse opts to remove the IV and does which nursing intervention?
   1. Cleanse the site carefully with chlorhexidine.
   2. Apply warm soaks.
   3. Culture the IV site.
   4. Elevate the extremity.
8. The healthcare provider orders benzylpencillin potassium (Penicillin G Potassium) 2.4 million units IM. The nurse chooses the equipment to administer the medication. The appropriate equipment is a:
   1. 3 mL syringe, a 22 gauge 2 inch long needle, gloves, and an antiseptic cleansing pad.
   2. 3 mL syringe, an 18 gauge 1 inch long needle, gloves, and an antiseptic cleansing pad.
   3. 3 mL syringe, a 22 gauge 5/8 inch long needle, gloves, and an antiseptic cleansing pad.
   4. 3 mL syringe, a 20 gauge short bevel needle, gloves, and an antiseptic cleansing pad.
9. A health care provider orders 2,000 mL D_5W over 24 hours. Drop factor is 10 gtts/mL. The IV should run at how many Run IV at gtts/minute?
   1. 1.4 gtts/min.
   2. 14 gtts/min.
   3. 83 gtts/min.
   4. 833 gtts/min.
10. A nurse gives a client her medications. The client states, "I usually only take 3 pills at 10 AM. Is there a reason I have 4 pills today?" The nurse's best response is:
    1. to state she has the correct number of pills for the client and request she take the pills.
    2. ask the client to wait one moment while she checks the orders again.
    3. to state that orders in the hospital are not always the same as when she is home and request the client take the medication.
    4. to check the orders and, after determining the client is to have 4 pills, explain the reason for the additional pill.

REFERENCES/SUGGESTED READINGS

About BD Integra™ Retracting Syringes. (2008). Retrieved September, 22, 2008, from http://www.bd.com/injection/products/integra

American Society of Health-System Pharmacists. (2008). *AHFS drug information 2008*. Bethesda, MD: Author.

Ampule Breaker/Collar. (2008). Retrieved September, 22, 2008, from http://www.sigmaaldrich.com/catalog/search/ProductDetail/ALDRICH/Z122904

Behrman, R., Kliegman, R., & Jenson, H. (Eds.). (2004). *Nelson textbook of pediatrics* (17th ed.). Philadelphia: W. B. Saunders.

Berman, A., Snyder, S., Kozier, B., & Erb, G. (2008). *Kozier and Erb's fundamental of nursing: Concepts, process, and practice* (8th ed.). Upper Saddle River, NJ: Pearson Prentice Hall.

Blanchard & Loeb. (2006). *Nurse's drug handbook 2006*. Philadelphia: Blanchard & Loeb Publishers, LLC.

Bulechek, G., Butcher, H., McCloskey, J., & Dochterman, J., eds. (2008). *Nursing Interventions Classification (NIC)* (5th ed.). St. Louis, MO: Mosby/Elsevier.

Carroll, P. (2003). Medication errors: The bigger picture. *RN, 66*(1), 52–57.

Charting Tips. (2000a). Documenting IV therapy, part I. *Nursing2000, 30*(2), 73.

Charting Tips. (2000b). Documenting IV therapy, part II. *Nursing2000, 30*(3), 83.

Daniels, R., Grendell, R., & Wilkins, F. (2010). *Nursing fundamentals: Caring and Clinical Decision Making* (2nd ed.). Clifton Park, NY: Delmar Cengage Learning.

Daniels, J., & Smith, L. (1999). *Clinical calculations* (4th ed.). Clifton Park, NY: Delmar Cengage Learning.

DeLaune, S., & Ladner, P. (2006). *Fundamentals of nursing* (3rd ed.). Clifton Park, NY: Delmar Cengage Learning.

Ellenberger, A. (1999). Starting an IV line. *Nursing99, 29*(3), 56–59.

Fitzpatrick, L., & Fitzpatrick, T. (1997). Blood transfusion: Keeping your patient safe. *Nursing97, 27*(8), 34–41

Giving Z-track injections. (2002). *Nursing2002, 32*(9), 81.

Goldy, D. (1998). Circulatory overload secondary to blood transfusion. *American Journal of Nursing, 98*(7), 33.

Hadaway, L. (1999a). Choosing the right vascular access device, part I. *Nursing99, 29*(2), 18.

Hadaway, L. (1999b). Choosing the right vascular access device, part II. *Nursing99, 29*(7), 28–29.

Hadaway, L. (2002a). IV infiltration: Not just a peripheral problem. *Nursing2002, 32*(8), 36–42.

Hadaway, L. (2002b). What you can do to decrease catheter-related infections. *Nursing2002, 32*(9), 46–48.

Hadaway, L. (2003). Infusing without infecting. *Nursing2003, 33*(10), 58–63.

Hrouda, B. (2002). Warming up to IV infusion. *Nursing2002, 32*(3), 54–55.

Jensen, B. (2008a). *Managing peripheral venous access.* Manuscript submitted for publication.

Jensen, B. (2008b). *Transfusing blood and blood products.* Manuscript submitted for publication.

Joint Commission. (2008). Official "do not use" list. Retrieved September 19, 2008, from http://www.jointommission.org/patientsafety/donotuselist

Josephson, D. (1999). *Intravenous infusion therapy for nurses: Principles and practice.* Clifton Park, NY: Delmar Cengage Learning.

Karch, A., & Karch, F. (2002). Double dosing. *American Journal of Nursing, 102*(10), 23.

Karch, A., & Karch, F. (2003). Not so fast. *American Journal of Nursing, 103*(8), 71.

Kee, J., Paulanka, B, & Polek, C. (2009). *Fluids and electrolytes with clinical applications* (7th ed.). Clifton Park, NY: Delmar Cengage Learning.

Larouere, E. (1999). Deaccessing an implanted port. *Nursing99, 29*(6), 60–61.

Lehne, R. (2006). *Pharmacology for nursing care* (6th ed.). St. Louis, MO: Elsevier, Health Sciences Division.

Liu, Q., Sulzenbacher, G., Yuan, H., Bennett, E., Pietz, G., Saunders, K., et al. (2007). Bacterial glycosidases for the production of universal red blood cells. *Nature Biotechnology, 25*(4), 454–464.

Macklin, D. (2000). Removing a PICC. *American Journal of Nursing, 100*(1), 52–54.

Masoorli, S. (2002). How to accurately document IV insertion. *Nursing2002, 32*(6), 65.

Matheny, N., Wehrle, M., Wiersema, L., & Clark, J. (1998). Testing feeding tube placement: Auscultation vs. pH method. *American Journal of Nursing, 98*(5), 37–42.

McConnell, E. (1998). Giving medications through an enteral feeding tube. *Nursing98, 28*(3), 6.

McConnell, E. (1999). Administering a Z-track IM injection. *Nursing99, 29*(1), 26.

McConnell, E. (2001). Instilling ear drops. *Nursing2001, 31*(4), 17.

McConnell, E. (2002). Administering medication through a gastrostomy tube. *Nursing2002, 32*(12), 22.

Metheny, N., & Titler, M. (2001). Assessing placement of feeding tubes, *American Journal of Nursing, 101*(5), 36–45.

Millam, D. (original manuscript), Hadaway, L. (revised manuscript). (2003). On the road to successful I.V. starts. A supplement to *Nursing2003, 33*(5 Suppl.), between pages 64 and 65.

Moorhead, S., Johnson, M., & Maas, M. (2004). *Nursing Outcomes Classification (NOC)* (3rd ed.). St. Louis, MO: Mosby.

North American Nursing Diagnosis Association International. (2010). *NANDA-I nursing diagnoses: Definitions and classification 2009–2011*. Ames, IA: Wiley-Blackwell.

Obenour, P. (1998). Administering an S.C. medication continuously. *Nursing98, 28*(6), 20.

Pickar, G. (2004). *Dosage calculation* (7th ed.). Clifton Park, NY: Delmar Cengage Learning.

Pope, B. (2002). How to administer subcutaneous and intramuscular injections. *Nursing2002, 32*(1), 50–51.

Przybylek, C. (2002). Two ways to avoid a "sticky" IV situation. *Nursing2002, 32*(11), 47–49.

Rice, J. (2002). *Medications and mathematics for the nurse* (9th ed.). Clifton Park, NY: Delmar Cengage Learning.

Royer, T. (2001). Looking for a vein? Stick with venous ultrasound. *Nursing2001, 31*(11), 72–73.

Saxton, D., & O'Neill, N. (1998). *Math and meds for nurses.* Clifton Park, NY: Delmar Cengage Learning.

Schatzlein, K. (2003). Hold tight: Keeping catheters secure. *Nursing2003, 33*(3), 20–21.

Smetzer, J. (2001). Take 10 giant steps to medication safety. *Nursing2001, 31*(11), 49–53.

Smith, L. (2003). Clarifying a medication order. *Nursing2003, 33*(5), 26.

Spratto, G., & Woods, A. (2010). *Delmar nurse's drug handbook.* Clifton Park, NY: Delmar Cengage Learning.

Togger, D., & Brenner, P. (2001). Metered dose inhalers. *American Journal of Nursing, 101*(10), 26–32.

Trimble, T. (2003a). Peripheral IV starts: Insertion tips. *Nursing2003, 33*(8), 17.

Trimble, T. (2003b). Starting peripheral IVs: Tips for planning ahead. *Nursing2003, 33*(4), 30.

RESOURCES

Infusion Nurses Society, http://www.ins1.org

Institute for Safe Medication Practices, http://www.ismp.org

National Coordinating Council for Medication Error Reporting and Prevention, http://www.nccmerp.org

U.S. Pharmacopeia, http://www.usp.gov

CHAPTER 26
Assessment

MAKING THE CONNECTION

Refer to the following chapters to increase your understanding of health assessment:

Basic Nursing

- ***Communication***
- ***Cultural Considerations***
- ***End-of-Life Care***
- ***Complementary/Alternative Therapies***
- ***Fluid, Electrolyte, and Acid–Base Balance***
- ***Pain Management***

Basic Procedures

- ***Hand Hygiene***
- ***Taking a Temperature***
- ***Taking a Pulse***
- ***Counting Respirations***
- ***Taking Blood Pressure***
- ***Weighing A Client, Mobile and Immobile***

LEARNING OBJECTIVES

Upon completion of this chapter, you should be able to:

- Define key terms.
- Identify the components of functional health patterns.
- Utilize the framework of functional health to facilitate a holistic assessment process.
- Analyze the components of the head-to-toe assessment.
- Incorporate the four assessment techniques within the head-to-toe assessment.
- Utilize the head-to-toe assessment in clinical situations.

KEY TERMS

adventitious breath sounds
affect
auscultation
borborygmi
bradycardia
bradypnea
bronchial sounds
bronchovesicular sounds
crackles
cyanosis
dyspnea
eupnea
health history
hyperventilation
hypoventilation
inspection
orthostatic hypotension
palpation
percussion
pleural friction rub
pulse amplitude

pulse deficit
pulse rate
pulse rhythm
review of systems (ROS)
sibilant wheezes
Snellen chart
sonorous wheeze
stridor
tachycardia
tachypnea
vesicular sounds

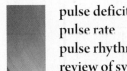

INTRODUCTION

Within the scope of the nursing profession, a complete nursing assessment is necessary to analyze each client's needs in a holistic manner. Nursing assessment includes both physical and psychosocial aspects to evaluate a client's condition. Caring, respect, and concern are demonstrated for each client when doing a nursing assessment.

A thorough nursing assessment includes both a health history and a physical examination. For a health history, the client is interviewed to identify how the client adjusts to or lives within the environment. This is subjective data, or information based on client self-report. The physical examination, objective data, includes observations made by the nurse while utilizing the assessment techniques of inspection, palpation, percussion, and auscultation. Other sources of objective data are laboratory tests, x-rays, and measurements of the client's vital signs, height, and weight.

The initial nursing assessment generally occurs within 8 hours of a client's admission to a health care facility and continues throughout the stay. In a physician's office or health care clinic, the nursing assessment would be completed immediately. Most institutions have a standard assessment form (Figure 26-1).

Usually a health history is completed before the physical examination, but in emergency situations or when performing care in a health care facility after the initial admitting assessment, it will be necessary to incorporate history taking into the physical examination. When incorporating a health history into the head-to-toe assessment, the nurse must remember to incorporate questions about the client's habits or usual patterns along with the physical data collected in the head-to-toe assessment. Functional assessment is best done within the framework of the physical assessment because the environment in which each client resides and participates becomes a part of the physical assessment. The functional assessment brings the environment in which the client lives and the physical needs of that client together to establish a holistic picture.

HEALTH HISTORY

A primary focus of the data collection interview is the health history. The **health history** is a review of the client's functional health patterns before the current contact with a health care agency. Whereas the medical history concentrates on symptoms and the progression of disease, the nursing health history focuses on the client's functional health patterns, responses to changes in health status, and alterations in lifestyle. The health history is also used in developing the plan of care.

Demographic Information

Personal data including name, address, date of birth, gender, religion, race/ethnic origin, occupation, and type of health plan/insurance should be included. This information may be useful in understanding a client's perspective.

Reason for Seeking Health Care

The client's reason for seeking health care should be described in the client's own words. For example, the statement "fell off four-foot ladder and landed on right shoulder; unable to move right arm" is the client's actual report of the event that precipitated a need for health care. The client's perspective is important because it explains what is significant about the event from the client's point of view. It is also important to know the time of the onset of symptoms.

Perception of Health Status

Perception of health status refers to the client's opinion of his or her general health. It may be useful to ask clients to rate their health on a scale of 1 to 10 (with 10 being ideal and 1 being poor), along with the client's rationale for the rating score. For example, the nurse may record a statement such as the following to represent the client's perception of health: "Rates health a 7 on a scale of 1 (poor) to 10 (ideal) because he must take medication regularly to maintain mobility, but the medication sometimes upsets his stomach."

Previous Illnesses, Hospitalizations, and Surgeries

The history and timing of any previous experiences with illness, surgery, or hospitalization are helpful in order to assess recurrent conditions and to anticipate responses to illness because prior experiences often affect current responses.

Client/Family Medical History

Ascertain any family history (blood relative) of acute and chronic illnesses that tend to be familial. Health history forms often include checklists of various illnesses that can be used as the basis for questions. It is also helpful to indicate the relative's relationship to the client (e.g., mother, father, sister).

Immunizations/Exposure to Communicable Diseases

A record of current immunizations should be obtained. This is particularly important with children; however, records of immunizations for tetanus, influenza, pneumonia, and hepatitis B are important for adults. A history of childhood or other communicable diseases should be noted. If the client has traveled out of the country, the time frame should be noted in order to determine incubation periods for relevant diseases. Also ask about potential exposure to communicable diseases such as tuberculosis or human immunodeficiency virus (HIV).

DATE:
TIME:

REASON FOR HOSPITALIZATION (E.R. TRIAGE/DIAGNOSIS)

MODE OF ARRIVAL
- Ambulance ☐
- Wheelchair ☐
- Stretcher ☐
- Ambulatory ☐

ONSET OF SYMPTOMS (E.R. TRIAGE)

PAST HISTORY: (Past Surgeries / Hospitalization) (E.R. TRIAGE)

COMMENTS:

VITAL SIGNS		HEALTH HISTORY				PERSON TO NOTIFY IN CASE OF EMERGENCY
		✓ Only those conditions that patient has history or current condition				
TEMP						
PULSE		GLAUCOMA	☐	GASTRIC ULCERS	☐	NAME
RESP		CANCER	☐	HEPATITIS	☐	
BP		LUNG DISEASE	☐	HIV DISEASE	☐	
HEIGHT	STATED	ASTHMA	☐	DIABETIC # OF YRS		RELATIONSHIP
	ACTUAL	KIDNEY DISEASE	☐	ANESTHESIA REACTION	☐	
WEIGHT	STATED	HEART DISEASE	☐	STROKE	☐	
	ACTUAL	PACEMAKER	☐	SEIZURE	☐	HAS POWER OF ATTORNEY
ALLERGIES		HYPERTENSION	☐	TUBERCULOSIS	☐	FOR HEALTH CARE?
FOOD		ALCOHOL	☐	PSYCHIATRIC DX	☐	☐ YES ☐ NO
LATEX ☐		SMOKING	☐	BLOOD TRANSFUSION	☐	TELEPHONE #
OTHER		DRUGS	☐	IN PAST 10 YEARS		

DRUG ALLERGIES	REACTION	DATE
1.		
2.		
3.		
4.		
5.		

MEDICATIONS (E.R. MEDS)

Name	Dose	Freq	Reason	Last Dose

Meds Sent Home: YES ☐ NO ☐ N/A ☐

ORGAN DONATION

Do you want information on organ donation?

YES ☐ NO ☐

Referred to: ☐ Organ Transplant Alliance 887-6189

PATIENT RIGHTS

☐ Received copy of Patient Rights
☐ Verbalizes understanding and ability to implement

SIGNATURES:

Completed by: ______
Entered by: ______

CHRISTUS SPOHN HEALTH SYSTEM

PATIENT ADMISSION DATA BASE

4013

2705318

NEW: 06/95
REVISED: 02/99.F10

FUNCTIONAL SCREENING (ADULT)

*Physical Therapy:
- 0 pts = complete independence
- 1 pt = recent onset of neurological problem
- 1 pt = recent onset of orthopedic problem
- 1 pt = recent onset of problem with impaired mobility (ambulation, stair climbing, bed mobility, transferring)
- 2 pts = open wound or an acute burn

______ TOTAL POINTS

* **A Score of 2 or More Points Requires a Physical Therapy Screening.**
Physical Therapy Screening Requested ☐ Yes ☐ No

*Occupational Therapy
- 0 pts = complete independence
- 1 pt = acute decline in upper extremity function
- 1 pt = recent onset of a neurological or orthopedic problem
- 1 pt = recent onset of a problem causing a decrease in ADL function (Bathing, Dressing, Feeding Toileting)

______ TOTAL POINTS

* **A Score of 2 or More Points Requires an Occupational Therapy Screen.**
Occupational Therapy Screening Requested ☐ Yes ☐ No

*Speech Therapy
- 0 pts = no identified problems
- 2 pt = recent onset of swallowing problems
- 2 pt = recent onset of speech difficulty
- 1 pt = recent neurological problem affecting ability to follow commands
- 2 pt = radical ENT surgery

______ TOTAL POINTS

* **A Score of 2 or More Points Requires a Speech Therapy Screen.**
Speech Therapy Screening Requested ☐ Yes ☐ No

PASTORAL CARE SCREEN

[ ] Would you like a special request sent for a visit from our chaplain?
[ ] Yes [ ] No
[ ] If Yes, Send Request to Pastoral Care

PATIENT INSTRUCTION CHECKLIST

☐ Signal Light	☐ Telephone	☐ Shower	☐ Dentures/Hearing Aid
☐ Bed Controls	☐ Brochure	☐ T.V.	
☐ Light Controls	☐ Visiting Privileges	☐ I.D./Allergy Band On	
☐ Bathroom	☐ Safety Precautions	☐ Pillow Speaker Placement	

PSYCHOSOCIAL/DISCHARGE PLANNING SCREEN

PSYCHOSOCIAL STATUS
(circle all that apply)

History of non-compliance impacting medical treatment	1
History alcohol/chemical abuse needing treatment	1
Suspected neglect/abuse	4
Unsafe home environment (domestic violence/self-neglect)	4
Prolonged confusion/disorientation	1
Illness related anxiety impacting care	1
Ineffective family coping patterns	1
Recent loss of body limb	1
Terminal illness	4
Suicide attempt/Ideation	4
Significant Grief impacting care/treatment	1
Teen Pregnancy (with high risk social factors)	2
Birth Anomalies or retardation	4
Loss of Infant (fetal demise)	4
Adoption	4
Other: ______	

LIVING ARRANGEMENT:

Family Unable to help/no known friends	2
Age > 70 years lives alone	1
Patient admitted from other institution:	1
__ SNF __ NH	
__Rehab __ Other Hospital	
Patient is disabled	1
Homeless or no address available	3

ADMISSION STATUS:

Readmitted within 1 -30 days	1
Admitted through ER	1

TOTAL OF ALL ______

Low Risk = 0-2
Moderate Risk = 3 pts
High Risk = 4 or > pts
*HIGH RISK requires Social Services consult. Social Services notified ☐ Yes ☐ No

Current Resource Being Utilized:	Yes	No
Home Health	☐	☐
Provider	☐	☐
Private Sitter	☐	☐
Meals on wheels	☐	☐
Hospice	☐	☐
MHMR	☐	☐
Adult Day Program	☐	☐
WIC Program	☐	☐

DME AT HOME
☐ Oxygen ☐ Walker
☐ Wheelchair ☐ Trapeze
☐ Hospital Bed
☐ Bedside commode
Living with______

VALUABLES BROUGHT WITH PATIENT TO HOSPITAL (SECURITY TAG)

Date: ______

☐ **Cane/Walker**	☐ **Bridgework no. of pieces** ______	☐ **Prothesis type** ______	☐ **Money (purse)**	☐ **Electric Razor**
☐ **Clocks**	☐ **Eyeglasses**	☐ **Hearing Aids L/R**	☐ **Wheelchair**	☐ **Clothing** ______
☐ **Dentures U/L**	☐ **Contact Lens**	☐ **Jewelry**	☐ **Radio**	☐ **Other** ______
☐ **Partial U/L**	☐ **Watches**	☐ **Money (billfold)**	☐ **T.V.**	

I take entire responsibility for keeping in my possession the articles listed above. I am holding nothing in my possession which I have not declared here. I understand and agree that Christus Spohn Health System shall not be liable for the loss or damage to any money, jewelry, eyeglasses, dentures, hearing aids or otther articles of value left in the care, custody and control of the patient or family/significant other.
It is understood and agreed that Christus Spohn Health System maintains a locked safe for money and valuables. The hospital shall not be liable for any of the patient's personal property that is not secured in the valuables storage envelope or in the hospital locked safe.

SIGNATURE OF PATIENT______
I have fully explained to this patient that Christus Spohn Health System takes no responsibility for articles retained by the patient.
SIGNATURE OF EMPLOYEE RECORDING ARTICLES______

Valuables given to: ______
VALUABLES STORAGE ENVELOPE: When valuables storage envelope is used, record the following information:
Valuables Storage Envelope Number ______ Date property received ______
Employee taking envelope to cashier ______

2705318-2.F10 02/25/99

FIGURE 26-1 Patient Admission Database (*Courtesy of CHRISTUS Spohn Health System, Corpus Christi, TX.*)

RN ASSESSMENT: DATE: TIME: SIGNATURE: ____________, RN

INSTRUCTION:
1. Complete physical assessment
2. Identify problems/nursing diagnosis for each system as appropriate
3. Prioritize Problems
4. Enter problems for problem list in computer

SYSTEMS	YES	NO	COMMENTS	PROBLEM
NEUROLOGICAL L.O.C. • Alert • Drowsy • Comatose • Disoriented • Cooperative • Agitated				☐ Thought processes, alteration in ☐ Coping, ineffective ☐ Communication, impaired
EYES • Pearl • Vision Normal • Prosthesis				☐ Injury potential ☐ Vision, impaired
MOUTH • Moist • Lesions • Teeth • Other				☐ Sensory, perception ☐ Other
EARS • Responds to normal voice tone • Drainage				
SPEECH • Clear • Slurred • Hoarse / raspy • Aphasic				
RESPIRATORY				
RESPIRATIONS • Rate • Labored				☐ Airway clearance, ineffective ☐ Breathing pattern ineffective
BREATH SOUNDS • Clear • Wheezes • Rales / Rhonchi				☐ Gas exchange; impaired ☐ IF PROBLEM IDENTIFIED SEND RESPIRATORY CONSULT
COUGH • Present • Sputum				☐ Other
MUSCLE / SKELETAL				
EXTREMITIES • Moves all on command WEAKNESS (specify) RA___ LA___ RL___ LL___ • Edema • Normal ambulation • Prosthesis (specify)				☐ Self Care deficit ☐ Mobility impaired, physical ☐ Activity intolerance comfort, alterations in ACUTE ☐ CHRONIC ☐ ☐ Tissue perfusion; alterations in

27053183.F10 02/12/99

SYSTEMS	YES	NO	COMMENTS	PROBLEM
CARDIOVASCULAR Apical Rate ☐ Rhythm (circle one) Regular Irregular On Cardiac Monitor: Yes ☐ No ☐ If Yes: Rhythm ________ Peripheral Pulses: Right / Left Carotid ☐ ☐ Radial ☐ ☐ Popliteal ☐ ☐ Femoral ☐ ☐ Pedal ☐ ☐				☐ Tissue perfusion alterations in ☐ Comfort, alterations in pain: ACUTE ☐ CHRONIC ☐ Post Operative ☐ Other ☐
Pacemaker Peripheral Edema Chest Pain Jugular Vein Distention Extremity Discoloration Rt. Arm/Hand Lt. Arm/Hand Rt. Leg/Foot Lt. Leg/Foot				
GENITOURINARY				
VOIDING • Normal • Frequency • Burning				☐ Urinary Elimination, alterations in pattern
Decreased Force of urinary stream INCONTINENCE: • Stress • Nocturia				☐ Urinary Retention ☐ Incontinence, Total
UROSTOMY DIALYSIS If Yes: Hemo Peritoneal Routine schedule Date of last Dialysis Catheter insertion Date Date of last menstrual period				☐ Incontinence, Stress ☐ Comfort, alterations in ACUTE ☐ CHRONIC ☐

GASTROINTESTINAL	YES	NO	COMMENT	PROBLEM
ABDOMEN • Soft • Distended • Tenderness ELIMINATION • Bowel Sounds • Diarrhea • Constipation • Incontinence • Ostomy Last B.M. Date:				Bowel elimination alterations in ☐ Diarrhea ☐ Constipation ☐ Incontinence, ☐ Comfort altered pain ACUTE ☐ CHRONIC ☐

SAFETY ASSESSMENT

☐ (5) Age greater than 60
☐ (5) History of previous falls
☐ (3) From nursing home
☐ (3) Has had sitter / companion at home
STATUS: MENTAL/PHYSICAL
☐ (5) Confused / Judgement Impaired
☐ (5) Sensory impairment
☐ (5) Combative/Aggressive
☐ (5) "Sundowners" Syndrome
☐ (5) Noncompliance/uncooperativeness
☐ (5) Paralysis / amputee
☐ (5) Weakness / debilitation
☐ (5) Urgent/frequent elimination needs
________ TOTAL

MEDICATIONS
☐ (5) Diuretics
☐ (5) Laxatives / G.I. preps
☐ (3) Antihypertensives
☐ (3) Antiseizures
☐ (5) Sedative / hypnotics
☐ (3) Analgesics
☐ (3) Antipsychotics / antidepressants

☐ LEVEL 1 (0-17)
☐ LEVEL 2 (18-24)
☐ LEVEL 3 (25 or greater)

☐ Safety precautions implemented
☐ Restraints per protocol
☐ Patient/family instructed
☐ Color coded band on

INTEGUMENTARY SKIN	YES	NO	COMMENT	PROBLEM
• Color Normal • Warm, dry • Turgor good • Bruises abrasions, lacerations Color, Size, Location			☐ Referral to Social Service (screen for neglect / abuse)	☐ Other: ______ ☐ Tissue perfusion, alterations in ☐ Skin integrity impairment of: actual
• Poor hygiene • Rash, lesions • Scars • Dressing • Pressure points intact • coccyx • heels • elbows • hips • ankles • cast edges • Other______ E-Z graph • Vascular access				☐ Skin integrity impairment of: potential ☐ Tissue integrity, comfort, alterations in pain ACUTE ☐ CHRONIC ☐ WOUND CARE ☐

Type________ Insertion Date:________
Site:________ Purpose________

NUTRITIONAL SCREENING

Indicate as appropriate for patient Previous diet ________
☐ (8) TPN/Parental Nutrition
☐ (8) Tube Feeding
☐ (2) Unplanned weight loss or gain > 20 lbs in 3 months
☐ Referral to S.S. screen for neglect/abuse?
☐ (1) Loss of appetite/Eats less than 50% of meal
☐ (1) Nausea, vomiting or diarrhea
☐ (1) Difficulty chewing
☐ (1) Difficulty swallowing
*Diagnosis of:
☐ (2) Heart disease, hypertension, CHF, gestational diabetic, hepatic or renal failure, diabetic, anemia, cancer other than ENT, geriatric surgery
☐ (5) AIDS, malnutrition, DKA, decubitus ulcer, septic condition requiring ICU, burn patient, ENT cancer
☐ (1) modified diet, NPO for 48 hrs.
☐ (1) age > 65 years
*LAB VALUES: Albumin ☐ (1) 2.5 - 3.0 ☐ (2) < 2.5; Glucose ☐ (1) <60 or > 300; Hgb ☐ (1) male < 13 ☐ (1) female < 11
________ TOTAL SCORE
High Risk - 8 pts or >
Moderate Risk - 5-7 pts
Low Risk - 0-4 pts
☐ SEND NUTRITION SCREEN CONSULT WITH TOTAL SCORE OF 5 OR ABOVE AND IDENTIFY SCORE OF PATIENT IN ORDER

SKIN BREAKDOWN POTENTIAL CHECKLIST

________ (1) Fair: Major underlying disease, controlled
________ (2) Poor: Uncontrolled underlying disease
MENTAL STATUS
________ (1) Lethargic: Listless
________ (2) Confused: Inappropriate communication
________ (4) Comatose: Unresponsive
MOBILITY / ACTIVITY
________ (2) Minor Deficit: Some limitation in movement Needs assistance w / ADL's
________ (4) Major Deficit: Movement requires assistance
________ (6) Immobile: No voluntary movement
INCONTINENCE
________ (1) Mild: Stress incontinence, 1 BM / day
________ (4) Frequent: No bladder control, BMs > 2-4 /day
________ (6) Total: No bladder control, frequent / continuous BM
NUTRITION
________ (2) Fair: Intake < body requirements, eats 75% or less
________ (3) Poor: Eats 50% or less, started on TPN or tube feeding
________ (4) Compromised: No intake, dehydrated
SKIN INTEGRITY
________ (2) Fair: Single stage I or II
________ (4) Poor: More than one break in skin integrity
________ TOTAL SCORE OF 8 OR ABOVE, ENTER SKIN INTEGRITY POTENTIAL ON PCP PROBLEM LIST, INITIATE PREVENTATIVE ADL's

PATIENT / SIGNIFICANT OTHER PARTICIPATION IN ADMISSION PROCESS

1. Answered question Yes ____ No ____
2. Volunteered information Yes ____ No ____
3. Family/significant other present Yes ____ No ____
4. Plan of care reviewed with: Patient ____ Family / Significant other____
5. Comments:

2705318-4.F10

FIGURE 26-1 (Continued)

▼ SAFETY ▼

Assessment for Allergies

It is essential to explore possible allergies before administering any medications. Allergic reactions can be life threatening and can occur with very low dosages of medications. A client's sensitivity to a drug can also change over time, resulting in severe reactions even though the client has successfully taken the drug during prior illnesses or experienced only mild reactions to the drug in the past.

Allergies

Any drug, food, or environmental allergies are noted in the health history, along with the type of reaction to the substance. For example, a client may report that a rash or shortness of breath developed after taking penicillin. This reaction is recorded. Clients may report an "allergy" to a medication because their stomach was upset after ingesting it. This is a side effect that would not preclude administration of the drug in the future.

Current Medications

All medications currently taken, both prescription and over-the-counter, are recorded by name, frequency, and dosage. Ask about birth control pills, laxatives, nonprescription pain relief medications, herbal remedies, and vitamin and mineral supplements. Clients may be hesitant to share herb use with the nurse and medical staff. Ask the client, in an accepting manner, if she is taking any herbal supplements. Sometimes herbal therapies interact with other medications, causing serious side effects.

Developmental Level

Knowledge of developmental level is essential for considering appropriate norms of behavior and for appraising the achievement of relevant developmental tasks. Any recognized theory of growth and development can be applied in order to determine if clients are functioning within the parameters expected for their age-group. For example, if Erikson's stages of psychosocial development are used, validation of an adult client's attainment of the developmental task of generativity versus stagnation can be made by a statement such as "client prefers to spend time with his family; very involved in children's school activities." (Refer to Erickson's Stages of Psychosocial Development in Chapter 10.)

PROFESSIONALTIP

Expired Medications

Remind clients to check all medications for expiration dates before use.

Psychosocial History

Psychosocial history refers to assessment of self-concept and self-esteem as well as usual sources of stress and the client's ability to cope. Sources of support for clients in crisis, such as family, significant others, religion, or support groups, are explored.

Sociocultural History

The client's sociocultural history includes the home environment, family situation, and client's role in the family. For example, the client could be the parent of three children and the sole provider in a single-parent family. The responsibilities of the client are important data through which the impact of changes in health status and the most beneficial care plan for the client are determined. Caffeine and alcohol intake and use of tobacco or recreational drugs also are explored.

Complementary/Alternative Therapy Use

Alternative therapy and complementary therapy are often used interchangeably but are not the same. Alternative therapy supplants (replaces) traditional medical treatment, and complementary therapy complements or enhances medical practices. Complementary methods are used alongside medical practices to improve the client's health status (Gecsedi & Decker, 2001).

The University of Maryland Medicine (2002) reports that nearly 70% of U.S. citizens have used at least one complementary/alternative therapy in their lifetime. According to a study in a Brooklyn, New York, hospital, one in four clients seen in the emergency department had taken an herbal supplement but did not share their use of herbs with the medical staff (Gulla & Singer, 2000). Herbal use without health care practitioner notification can have serious consequences since some herbs interact with medications and cause serious side effects. The nursing staff can prevent herbal related issues by developing a trusting relationship with clients and asking if they take herbs or do anything to improve their health. As clients share alternative and complementary therapy choices, the nurse enhances a trust relationship by being knowledgeable about the various therapies and genuinely accepting the client's personal choices.

Activities of Daily Living

The activities of daily living (ADLs) is a description of the client's lifestyle and capacity for self-care and is useful both as baseline information and as a source of insight into usual health behaviors. This baseline should include information on nutritional intake and eating habits, elimination patterns, rest/sleep patterns, and activity/exercise.

Review of Systems

The **review of systems (ROS)** is a brief account from the client of any recent signs or symptoms associated with any of the body systems. This can most effectively be obtained as the physical examination is performed. The ROS relies on subjective information provided by the client rather than on the physical examination. When a symptom is encountered, either while eliciting the health history or during the physical examination of the client, as much information as possible about the symptom is obtained. Relevant data include:

- *Location:* The area of the body in which the symptom (such as pain) is felt

- *Character:* The quality of the feeling or sensation (e.g., sharp, dull, stabbing)
- *Intensity:* The severity or quantity of the feeling or sensation and its interference with functional abilities. The sensation can be rated on a scale of 1 (very little) to 10 (very intense)
- *Timing:* The onset, duration, frequency, and precipitating factors of the symptom
- *Aggravating/alleviating factors:* The activities or actions that make the symptom worse or better

PHYSICAL EXAMINATION

A physical examination is performed for all age-groups in all health care settings (home, outpatient facilities, extended care institutions, and acute care facilities) to gather comprehensive, pertinent client data. The physical examination, a picture of the client's physiological functioning, combined with a health and psychosocial assessment, forms a database for decision making. The examination is performed according to the agency's policy, which may vary from one agency to another.

To ensure a thorough assessment of each system, the physical examination is done in a sequential, head-to-toe fashion. This method decreases the number of times the nurse and the client have to change positions and prevents forgetting to examine an area.

The physical or the head-to-toe assessment is performed by using the specific assessment techniques of inspection, palpation, percussion, and auscultation.

INSPECTION

Inspection consists of a thorough visual observation of the client, providing a picture of the body's outward response to its internal functioning. Inspection of the skin, for example, can assist in identifying signs of a fever by the client's flushed face. The skin can also be an indicator of a decreased oxygen supply when **cyanosis**, a bluish or dark purple coloration, is noted in the client's lips, skin, or nail beds. Sharing observations with the client during inspection enhances the holistic data collected. For example, when mentioning the observation of visible scars, the client may discuss previous surgeries or hospitalizations. Instruments such as a penlight and otoscope are often used to enhance visualization.

Effective inspection requires adequate lighting and exposure of the body parts being observed. Show sensitivity to the client's feelings of embarrassment by discussing the technique with the client and using appropriate draping.

PALPATION

Palpation uses the sense of touch to assess texture, temperature, moisture, organ location and size, vibrations, pulsations, swelling, masses, and tenderness. The finger pads are placed flat against the client's skin, exerting slight pressure for light palpation, as seen in Figure 26-2. Assessment of the kidneys, liver, spleen, bowel, and fundal height may be accomplished through deep palpation, in which more pressure is exerted. Pulses are also palpated. The abdomen is palpated for distention, softness, firmness, rigidity, or tenderness.

Palpation requires a calm, gentle approach and is used systematically, with light palpation preceding deep palpation and palpation of tender areas performed last.

> **▼ SAFETY ▼**
>
> **Palpation**
>
> Deep palpation is a technique requiring significant expertise and beginning nursing students do not perform this procedure without supervision.

PERCUSSION

Percussion uses short, tapping strokes on the surface of the skin to create vibrations of underlying organs. It is used to assess the density of structures or determine the location and size of organs. The fingertips are used to tap the client's body to produce sounds and vibrations. Place the middle finger of the nondominant hand on the client's skin in the area to be percussed, then tap lightly with the middle finger of the dominant hand on the distal phalanx of the middle finger positioned on the body surface (Figure 26-3). Tap twice in

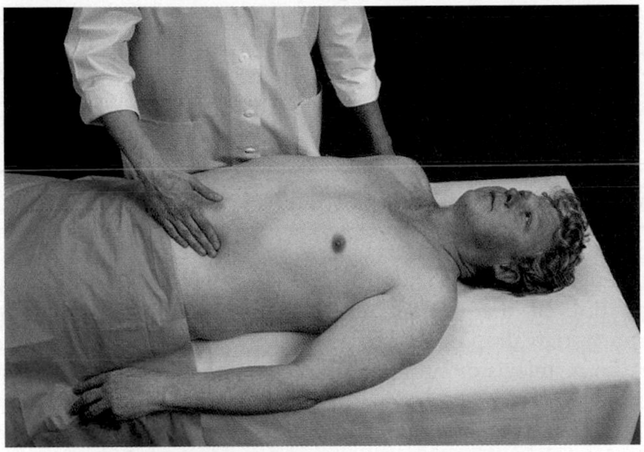

FIGURE 26-2 Light Palpation

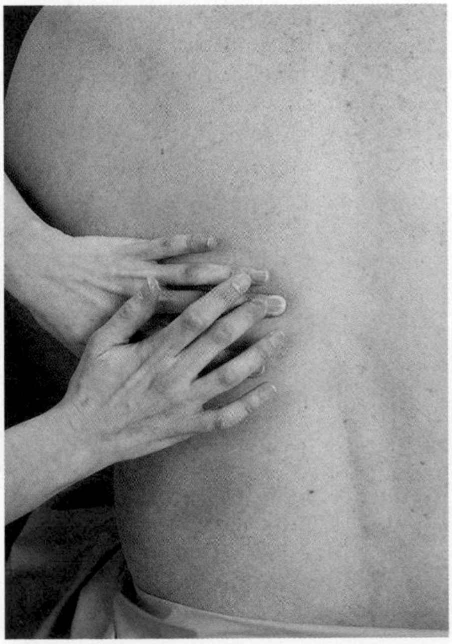

FIGURE 26-3 Percussion

Table 26-1 Description of Percussion Tones

TONE	INTENSITY	PITCH	DURATION	QUALITY	NORMAL LOCATION
Dullness	Medium	High	Medium	Thudlike	Liver
Flatness	Soft	High	Short	Extreme dullness	Muscle
Hyperresonance	Very loud	Very low	Long	Booming	Child's lung
Resonance	Loud	Low	Long	Hollow	Peripheral lung
Tympany	Loud	High	Medium	Drumlike	Stomach

one place before moving to a new area. Percussion should not be painful to the client. If it is painful, the percussion should be discontinued and the response documented.

Percussion requires much practice to master, and it is important to be familiar with the sounds produced when percussion is used. Table 26-1 describes the various percussion tones.

Auscultation

Auscultation involves listening to sounds in the body that are created by movement of air or fluid. Areas most often auscultated include the lungs, heart, abdomen, and blood vessels. A stethoscope is used to channel the sound (Figure 26-4).

HEAD-TO-TOE ASSESSMENT

Some important concepts are kept in mind and utilized throughout the examination. The client's privacy is respected by pulling the curtain, closing the door, and providing appropriate draping. When possible, distracting noises such as radio or television and people talking are eliminated. Assessment is performed under natural light because fluorescent light can change the color tones of the skin. All procedures are explained to the client and confidentiality of data acquired during the examination maintained.

The client is positioned to ensure accessibility to the body part being assessed. Figure 26-5 illustrates positions used in conducting a physical examination.

Draping the client prevents unnecessary exposure during the examination. Embarrassment causes tension and restlessness and decreases the client's ability to cooperate. Draping also prevents the client from being chilled.

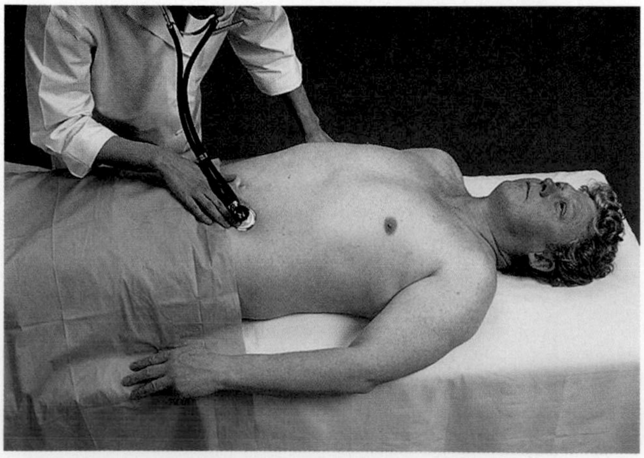

Figure 26-4 Auscultation

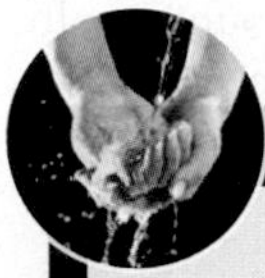

INFECTION CONTROL

Standard Precautions

Remember to utilize Standard Precautions when in contact with any body fluids by using gloves, gown, or mask as appropriate.

General Survey

During the introductory time, use inspection to make a general assessment of the client. This overview is the first impression of the client and is the beginning point of the head-to-toe assessment. Such aspects as the general state of health and any signs of distress, such as pain or breathing difficulties, the client's awareness of the surroundings, body type and posture, facial expressions, and mood are noted.

Document the general survey data to portray an overall picture of the client. The elderly, disabled, and abused clients will require special consideration during the physical examination.

Elderly

Before assessing elderly clients, it is important to know the normal changes of aging. Aging may reduce the body's tolerance of stress, resistance to illness, and ability to recuperate from illness. Be sure the client understands and can follow instructions and allow extra time for the client having difficulty changing positions.

Disabled Clients

When assessing disabled clients, adapt the process to the client's ability; for example, give a hearing-impaired client

CRITICAL THINKING

Performing a Physical Assessment

Do you feel comfortable performing a complete physical assessment on a client? Identify the areas that are of concern. What could you do to be more confident in performing physical assessments?

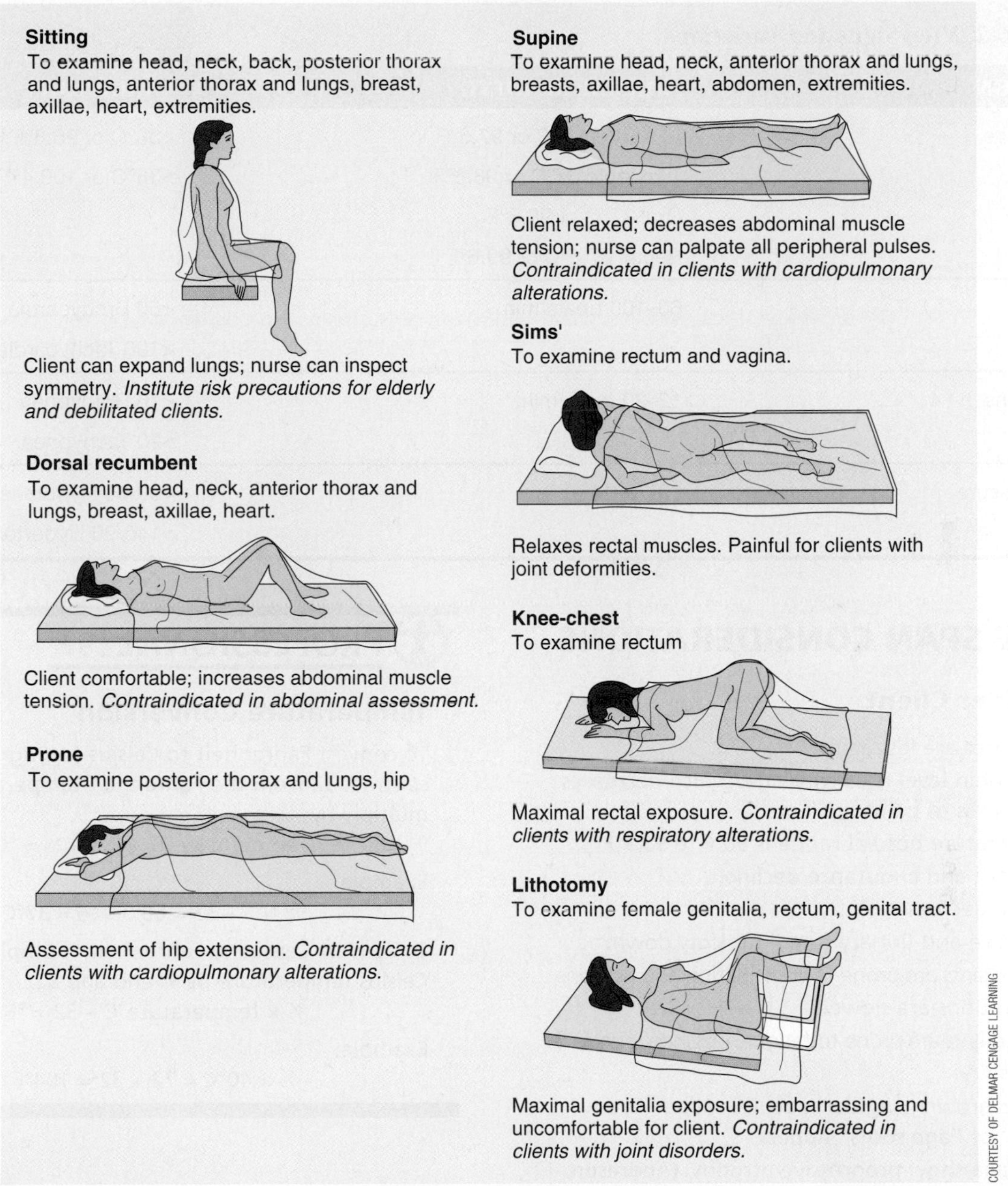
Sitting
To examine head, neck, back, posterior thorax and lungs, anterior thorax and lungs, breast, axillae, heart, extremities.
Client can expand lungs; nurse can inspect symmetry. *Institute risk precautions for elderly and debilitated clients.*
Dorsal recumbent
To examine head, neck, anterior thorax and lungs, breast, axillae, heart.
Client comfortable; increases abdominal muscle tension. *Contraindicated in abdominal assessment.*
Prone
To examine posterior thorax and lungs, hip
Assessment of hip extension. *Contraindicated in clients with cardiopulmonary alterations.*
Supine
To examine head, neck, anterior thorax and lungs, breasts, axillae, heart, abdomen, extremities.
Client relaxed; decreases abdominal muscle tension; nurse can palpate all peripheral pulses. *Contraindicated in clients with cardiopulmonary alterations.*
Sims'
To examine rectum and vagina.
Relaxes rectal muscles. Painful for clients with joint deformities.
Knee-chest
To examine rectum
Maximal rectal exposure. *Contraindicated in clients with respiratory alterations.*
Lithotomy
To examine female genitalia, rectum, genital tract.
Maximal genitalia exposure; embarrassing and uncomfortable for client. *Contraindicated in clients with joint disorders.*
COURTESY OF DELMAR CENGAGE LEARNING

FIGURE 26-5 Various Positions for Physical Examination

a written questionnaire. Simple, direct sentences and questions or pictures might be required for an intellectually impaired client. It is best to determine the client's ability to participate before conducting the examination. To allay the disabled client's fears and anxiety, encourage a family member to remain with the client during the examination. The client's level of independence and feelings about the disability are noted.

Abused Clients

Observe for signs of abuse, especially in children and the elderly. Symptoms may be psychological as well as physical; for example, refusal to be touched, inability to maintain eye contact, or unwillingness to talk about bruises, burns, or other injuries may indicate abuse. Bruises or lacerations most typically appear on breasts, buttocks, thighs, or genitalia. Inspect for healed scarring or burns and know state laws and agency policies for reporting possible abuse.

VITAL SIGNS

After establishing rapport with the client through introductions, measurement of vital signs is the next step in an assessment. Vital signs are the "signs of life," providing a way of connecting the external inspection with the internal functioning of the client's organs. When checking vital signs, obtain the temperature (T), pulse (P), respirations (R), blood pressure (BP), and pain assessment of the client. See Table 26-2 for normal values and variations.

Temperature

When assessing the client's temperature (T), an electronic, chemical, mercury-free, tympanic, or temporal artery

Table 26-2 Vital Signs and Variations

VITAL SIGN	NORMAL READING	VARIATIONS
Temperature	Axillary 36.5°C or 97.6°F Tympanic 37°C or 98.6°F Oral 37°C or 98.6°F Rectal 37.5°C or 99.6°F	<36°C or 96.8°F Hypothermia >38°C or 100.4°F Pyrexia
Pulse	60–100 beats/min.	<60 Bradycardia <100 Tachycardia
Respirations	12–20 resp./min.	<16 Bradypnea >20 Tachypnea
Blood pressure	90/60–140/90	<90/60 Hypotension >140/90 Hypertension

LIFE SPAN CONSIDERATIONS

The Older Client

- All senses are less acute.
- Endorphin level rises with age, which decreases awareness of painful events.
- Temperature normal range is 96°F to 98.9°F.
- Strength and endurance decline.
- Height decreases.
- Digestive and urinary functions slow down.
- Older clients are prone to constipation and nocturia.
- Respirations are slowed.
- Older clients are prone to fatigue, dizziness, and falls.
- Skin is dry.
- Tan to brown irregular macules called "liver spots" or "age spots" appear.
- Genitalia show progressive atrophy. (Andresen, 1998; Scott, 2008; Williams & Keen, 2007)

CULTURAL CONSIDERATIONS

Cultural Values and Assessment

Although cleanliness is highly valued by mainstream American society, in some cultures, a daily bath is not believed necessary or desirable. In fact, some cultures do not interpret natural body odors as offensive. Consider the client in the context of cultural beliefs. The terms *dirty*, *unkempt*, or *foul smelling* are value laden and can cloud the assessment process and care provided to a client.

PROFESSIONAL TIP

Temperature Conversion

To convert Fahrenheit to Celsius (centigrade), subtract 32 from the Fahrenheit temperature and multiply by $\frac{5}{9}$:

$$(\text{Temperature °F} - 32) \times \frac{5}{9} = \text{°C}$$

Example:

$$98.6\text{°F} - 32 = 66.6 \times \frac{5}{9} = 37\text{°C}$$

To convert Celsius to Fahrenheit, multiply the Celsius temperature by $\frac{9}{5}$ and add 32:

$$\frac{9}{5} \times \text{temperature°C} + 32 = \text{°F}$$

Example:

$$\frac{9}{5} \times 40\text{°C} = 72 + 32 = 104\text{°F}$$

thermometer can be used (see Figure 26-6). Body temperature can be taken by five routes: oral, rectal, axillary, skin, or tympanic membrane. The route chosen depends on the client's age and physical condition. Factors such as age, gender, physical activity, and environment affects a person's temperature. Craig, Lancaster, Taylor, Williamson, and Smyth (2002) found ear temperatures in children to be inaccurate. Consumption of hot or cold food or beverage and smoking 15 to 30 minutes before taking an oral temperature can affect the results.

Pulse

Pulse assessment measures a pressure pulsation created when the heart contracts and ejects blood into the aorta. Assessment of pulse characteristics provides clinical data regarding the heart's pumping action and the adequacy of peripheral artery blood flow.

There are many pulse points (Figure 26-7). The most accessible are the radial and carotid sites. The body diverts blood to the brain when a cardiovascular emergency such

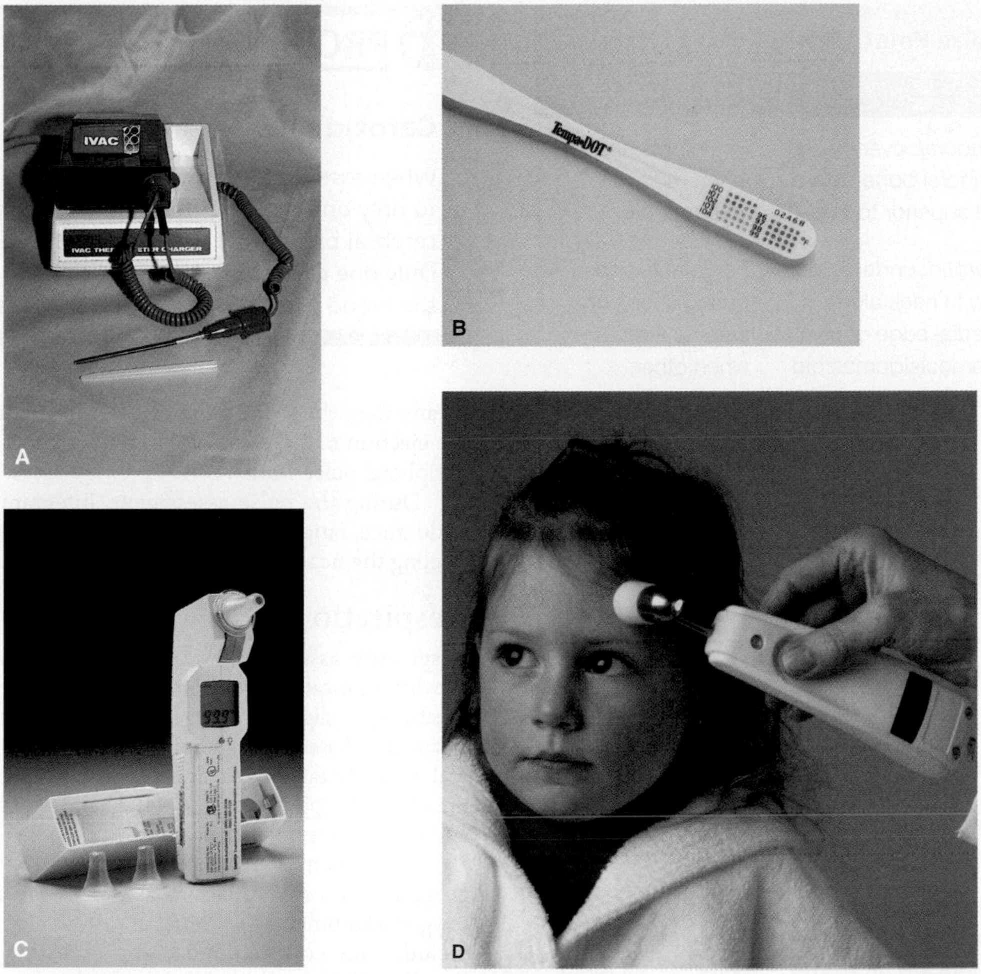

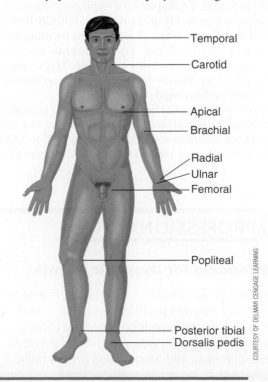

FIGURE 26-6 Different Types of Thermometers for Taking a Client's Temperature: *A,* Electronic Thermometer with a Probe (Red Color Indicates Rectal Thermometer Probe); *B,* Disposable Chemical Thermometer; *C,* Tympanic Thermometer with Disposable Speculums and Infrared-Sensing Electronics; *D,* Temporal Artery Thermometer *(Images A and B courtesy of Delmar Cengage Learning; image C courtesy of The Gilette Company; and image D courtesy of Exergen Corporation, Watertown, MA.)*

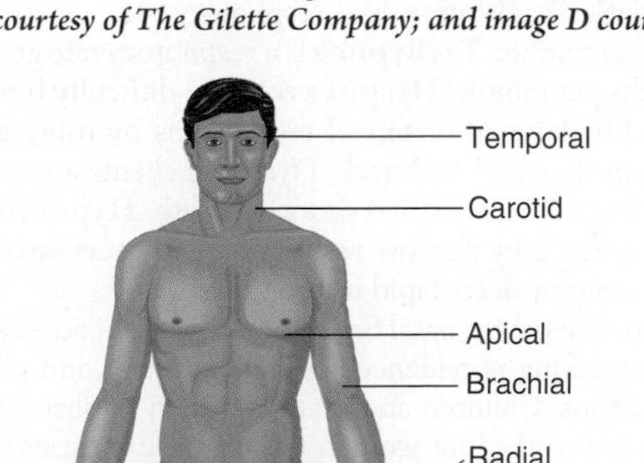

FIGURE 26-7 Pulse Points

as hemorrhage occurs, so in these situations the carotid site should always be used to assess the pulse. Specific pulse sites are shown and pulse point assessments described in Table 26-3.

Pulse rate is an indirect measurement of cardiac output obtained by counting the number of peripheral pulse waves over a pulse point. Assessment of the client's pulse (P) includes the rate, rhythm, and amplitude. A normal pulse rate for adults is between 60 and 100 beats per minute. **Bradycardia** is a heart rate less than 60 beats per minute in an adult. **Tachycardia** is a heart rate greater than 100 beats per minute in an adult.

Pulse rhythm is the regularity of the heartbeat. It indicates how evenly the heart is beating—regular (the beats are evenly spaced) or irregular (the beats are not evenly spaced)—and is also called dysrhythmia.

Pulse amplitude is a measurement of the strength or force exerted by the blood against the arterial wall with each heart contraction. It is described as normal (full, easily palpable), weak (thready and usually rapid), or strong (bounding).

Usual assessment of the radial pulse occurs for 30 seconds, and the number of beats is doubled for documentation. If the pulse rhythm is irregular, the nurse listens to the apical pulse (point of maximum impulse or PMI) for 1 full minute to obtain an accurate pulse rate. In addition, the nurse must assess for a **pulse deficit** (condition in which the apical pulse rate is

TABLE 26-3 Pulse Point Uses

PULSE POINT		USE
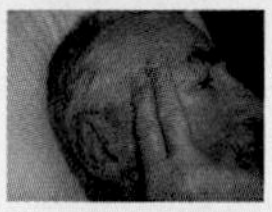	*Temporal:* over temporal bone, lateral and superior to eye	For infants and when radial is inaccessible
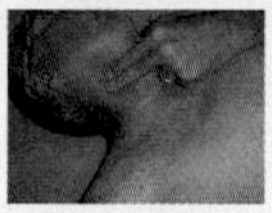	*Carotid:* under lower jaw in neck along medial edge of sternocleidomastoid muscle	For infants and during shock or cardiac arrest when other peripheral pulses are too weak to palpate; also to assess cranial circulation
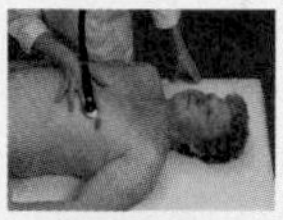	*Apical:* left midclavicular line at fourth to fifth intercostal space	To auscultate heart sounds and assess apical-radial deficit
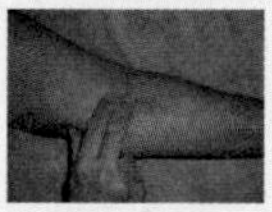	*Brachial:* between groove of biceps and triceps muscles at antecubital fossa	In cardiac arrest for infants, to assess lower arm circulation, and to auscultate blood pressure
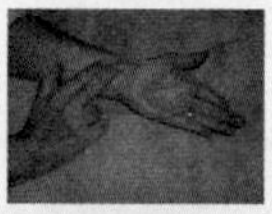	*Radial:* inner aspect of forearm on thumb side of wrist	To routinely assess pulse
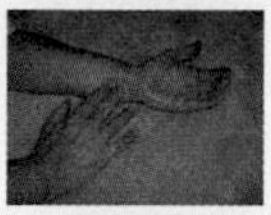	*Ulnar:* outer aspect of forearm on finger side of wrist	To assess circulation to ulnar side of hand
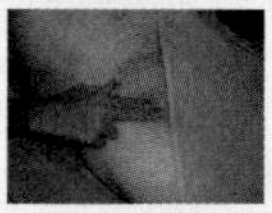	*Femoral:* in groin, below inguinal ligament (midpoint between symphysis pubis and anterosuperior iliac spine)	To assess circulation to legs and during cardiac arrest
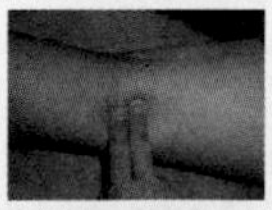	*Popliteal:* behind knee, at center in popliteal fossa	To assess circulation to legs and to auscultate leg blood pressure
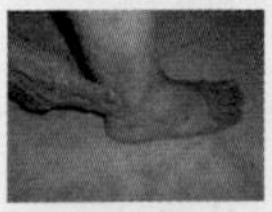	*Posterior tibial:* inner aspect of ankle between Achilles tendon and tibia	To assess circulation to feet
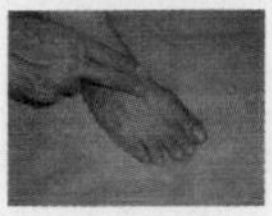	*Dorsalis pedis:* over instep, midway between extension tendons of great and second toe	To assess circulation to feet

COURTESY OF DELMAR CENGAGE LEARNING

PROFESSIONALTIP

Carotid Pulse Assessment

When assessing a carotid pulse, apply light pressure to only one carotid artery to avoid disruption of cerebral blood flow. Then assess the other one. Only one carotid artery is checked at a time so that the blood supply to the brain is not restricted.

greater than the radial pulse rate). A pulse deficit results from the ejection of a volume of blood that is too small to initiate a peripheral pulse wave.

During the pulse assessment, integrate questions about endurance, fatigue, and any possible episodes of palpitations, "feeling the heart beating," over the chest area.

Respirations

Respiratory assessment measures the breathing pattern. This provides clinical data regarding the pH of arterial blood. Normal breathing is slightly observable, quiet, effortless, regular, and automatic. Assess by observing chest wall expansion and bilateral symmetrical movement of the thorax. Another way to assess breathing is to place the back of the hand next to the client's nose and mouth to feel the expired air.

Assessment of external respirations (R) includes specific characteristics of respirations as well as the use of any type of oxygen equipment, the route, and flow rate. Each respiration includes one complete inhalation (breathing in) and exhalation (breathing out) by the client. When identifying the characteristics of respirations, the rate, depth, and rhythm of each breath is determined.

Eupnea refers to easy respirations with a rate that is age appropriate. **Bradypnea** is a respiratory rate of 10 or fewer breaths per minute. **Tachypnea** is a respiratory rate greater than 24 breaths per minute. **Dyspnea** refers to difficulty breathing as observed by labored or forced respirations by using accessory muscles in the chest and neck. Dyspneic clients are very aware of their respirations and feel short of breath. **Hypoventilation** is characterized by shallow respirations. **Hyperventilation** is characterized by deep, rapid respirations.

Also observe for nasal flaring and the use of accessory muscles for breathing as evidenced by sternal, costal, and subclavicular retractions. Children and males typically utilize abdominal muscles to breathe, but women use thoracic muscles (Fuller &

PROFESSIONALTIP

Positioning for Dyspneic Clients

Dyspneic clients should be maintained in a semi-Fowler's or Fowler's position, never flat in bed. For maximal lung expansion, have the client leaning forward over a padded, raised over-bed table with head and arms resting on the table.

Schaller-Ayers, 2000). During respiration assessment, determine functional ability by asking about any shortness of breath, difficulty in breathing with increased exercise, or problems completing activities of daily living.

Blood Pressure

After checking a client's respirations, assess the client's blood pressure (BP). The most common site for indirect blood pressure measurement is the client's arm over the brachial artery.

When pressure measurements in the upper extremities are not accessible, the popliteal artery, located behind the knee, is the site of choice. Blood pressure can also be assessed in other sites, such as the radial artery in the forearm and the posterior tibial or dorsalis pedis artery in the lower leg. The extremity should be at the level of the heart when blood pressure is measured. Because it is difficult to auscultate sounds over the radial, tibial, and dorsalis pedis arteries, these sites are usually palpated to obtain a systolic reading.

A person's blood pressure is the result of the interaction of cardiac output and peripheral resistance and depends on the speed with which the arterial blood flows, the volume of blood supplied, and the elasticity of the walls of the artery. The force exerted by the blood against the wall of the artery as the heart contracts and relaxes is called the *arterial pressure.* When the ventricles contract and blood is forced into the aorta and pulmonary arteries, the *systolic pressure* is measured. This is the first sound heard. When the heart is in the filling or relaxed stage, the force is described as the *diastolic pressure.* This is when the last sound is heard. The difference between the systolic and diastolic blood pressures is called the *pulse pressure.* A pulse pressure is usually between 30 and 40 mm Hg. Refer to Table 26-4 for normal age-related variations in vital signs.

According to the U.S. Department of Health and Human Services (2003), the client should sit for 5 minutes in a chair rather than on an exam table, with both feet on the floor and the arm supported at heart level. An accurate reading requires the correct width of blood pressure cuff, determined by the circumference of the client's extremity. The cuff bladder encircles 80% of the arm to obtain an accurate blood pressure, and obtaining two measurements ensures accuracy. A falsely elevated reading results if the bladder is too narrow, and a falsely low reading results if it is too wide.

PROFESSIONALTIP

Contraindications for Brachial Artery Blood Pressure Measurement

When the client has any of the following, *do not* measure blood pressure on the involved side:

- Venous access devices, such as an intravenous infusion or arteriovenous fistula for renal dialysis
- Surgery involving the breast, axilla, shoulder, arm, or hand
- Injury or disease to the shoulder, arm, or hand, such as trauma, burns, or application of a cast or bandage

TABLE 26-4 Normal Age-Related Variations in Temperature, Pulse, Respiration, and Blood Pressure

AGE	MEASUREMENT ROUTE	NORMAL RANGE	
		Celsius	**Fahrenheit**
Newborn	Axillary	35-5–39.5° C	96.0–99.5°F
1 yr	Oral	37.7°C	99.7°F
3 yr	Oral	37.2°C	99.0°F
5 yr	Oral	37.0°C	98.6°F
Adult	Oral	37.0°C	98.6°F
	Axillary	36.4°C	97.6°F
	Rectal	37.6°C	99.6°F
70+ yr	Oral	36.0°C	96.8°F

RESTING PULSE

AGE	NORMAL RANGE	AVERAGE RATE/MIN
Newborn	100–170	140
1 yr	80–170	120
3 yr	80–130	110
6 yr	75–120	100
10 yr	70–110	90
14 yr	60–110	90
Adult	60–100	80

RESTING RESPIRATION

AGE	NORMAL RANGE	AVERAGE RATE/MIN
Newborn	30–50	40
1 yr	20–40	30
3 yr	20–30	25
6 yr	16–22	19
14 yr	14–20	17
Adult	12–20	18

BLOOD PRESSURE

AGE	SYSTOLIC (MM HG)	DIASTOLIC (MM HG)	AVERAGE
Newborn	65–95	30–60	80/60
Infant	65–115	42–80	90/61
3 yr	76–122	46–84	99/65
6 yr	85–115	48–64	100/56
10 yr	93–125	46–68	109/58
14 yr	99–137	51–71	118/61
Adult	100–140	60-90	120/80
Elderly	100–160	60-90	130/80

COMMUNITY/HOME HEALTH CARE

Electronic Sphygmomanometers

Electronic sphygmomanometers are useful for clients who must monitor their own pressure at home. The device electronically inflates and deflates the cuff and displays the systolic and diastolic pressures. They must be recalibrated routinely to ensure an accurate reading.

This is an appropriate time to ask if the client ever becomes light-headed or dizzy when moving from a reclining position to a sitting or standing position. This may occur as a result of an abnormally low blood pressure caused by the inability of the peripheral blood vessels to compensate quickly for the change in position and is referred to as **orthostatic hypotension**.

Pain

According to the Joint Commission standards for ambulatory care, behavioral health care, home care, hospital, health care network, long-term care, and long-term care pharmacy, pain is considered the fifth vital sign. Pain is assessed and recorded along with the client's temperature, pulse, respirations, and blood pressure (JCAHO, 2000a, 2000b; Joint Commission, 2004, 2008). The pain assessment includes pain intensity and quality (character, frequency, location, and duration). Regular assessment and follow-up are according to agency policy. This statement on pain management, "All patients have a right to pain relief," is to be posted in all client care areas (e.g., client rooms, clinic rooms, waiting rooms) (JCAHO, 2000a).

HEIGHT AND WEIGHT MEASUREMENT

Height and weight measurements are as important as the client's vital signs. Routine measurement provides data about growth and development in infants and children. Alterations may indicate illness at any age. Height and weight are routinely taken on visits to physicians' offices, to clinics, on admission to acute care facilities, and in other health care settings.

Height

A height-measuring rod, calibrated in either inches or centimeters, is usually found on a standing weight scale. The client stands erect on the scale's platform and the metal arm, attached to the back of the scale, is extended to gently rest on the top of the client's head. The measurement is read at eye level.

Weight

When a client has an order for "daily weight," the weight should be obtained at the same time of day on the same scale, with the client wearing the same type of clothing. The scale should be balanced before each client is weighed.

INFECTION CONTROL

Measuring Weight

When standing on a scale, the client wears some type of light foot covering, such as socks or disposable operating room slippers, to prevent the transmission of infection and to enhance comfort.

HEAD AND NECK ASSESSMENT

Assessment of the head and neck determines the client's mental and neurological status and the client's overall **affect** (outward expression of mood or emotion).

Hair and Scalp

The hair and scalp of a client is inspected. Note hair distribution, quantity, texture, and color. The scalp should be smooth and free of any debris or infestations.

Eyes

Examine the eyes to determine if they are symmetrical. Look at the eyebrows and eyelids to see if there is any drooping, which may be a sign of muscle weakness or neurological impairment. Note the color of the sclera and conjunctiva as well as the presence of any drainage.

Assess the pupils to determine their size, shape, and reaction to light. This is accomplished by darkening the room and asking the client to gaze into the distance. Move a light in from the side and notice if the pupil constricts; this is called the *direct light reflex*. Note the pupil size in millimeters both before and after the light response (Figure 26-8). Accommodation is tested by asking the client to focus on an object in the distance; this will dilate the pupils. The client is then asked to move his or her gaze to a near object such as a pen or finger held approximately 3 inches from the nose. The pupils should constrict as they focus on the near object, and the eyes will converge or move in toward midline. This normal response is documented as Pupils Equal, Round, Reactive to Light and Accommodation (PERRLA).

Ask if the client wears glasses and for what reason. Check if any eye problems, such as blurry vision, diplopia (double vision), or difficulty seeing at night, are experienced.

Visual acuity is assessed by a simple, noninvasive procedure using a **Snellen chart** (a chart that contains various-sized letters with standardized numbers at the end of each line of letters). The standardized numbers (called the denominator)

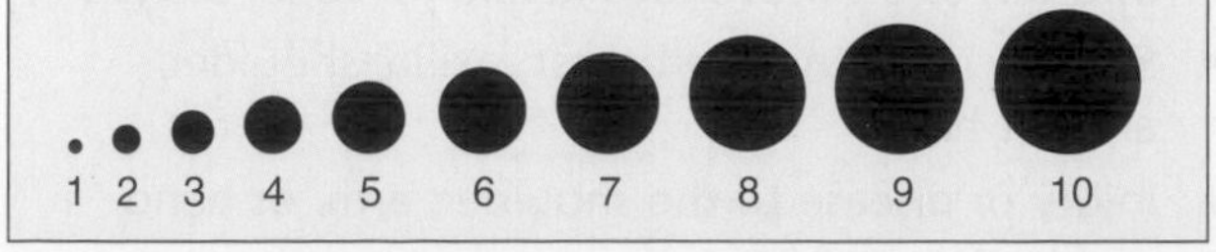

COURTESY OF DELMAR CENGAGE LEARNING

FIGURE 26-8 Scale Used to Measure Pupil Size in Millimeters

PROFESSIONALTIP

Common Abnormal Breath Odors

- Acetone breath ("fruity" smell) is common in malnourished or diabetic clients with ketoacidosis.
- Musty smell is caused by the breakdown of nitrogen and presence of liver disease.
- Ammonia smell occurs during the end stage of renal failure from a buildup of urea.

indicate the degree of visual acuity when the client is able to read that line of letters at a distance of 20 feet.

Nose

The nose should be symmetrical, midline, and in proportion to other features. Note any deformity, inflammation, or prior trauma. The patency of the nostrils is tested by asking the client to sniff inward while closing off each nostril. Ask the client if the following are ever experienced: nosebleeds, dryness, or decrease in sense of smell.

Lips and Mouth

The lips and mucous membranes of the mouth are observed for color, symmetry, moisture, or lesions. Ask the client with dentures or partial plates to remove them for a more thorough inspection of the mouth. Unusual breath odors are noted. Inspect the oral mucosa by inserting a tongue depressor between the teeth and the cheek. The mucous membranes and gums should be pink, moist, smooth, and free of lesions. Inspection of the tongue assists in determining the client's hydration. The tongue should be pink with a slightly rough texture. During the examination, determine if the client is able to enunciate words appropriately and if there are any voice changes such as hoarseness. Discuss usual dental hygiene practices and obtain the client's history of tobacco usage.

Neck

The neck is assessed for full range of motion. The accessory neck muscles should be symmetrical. As the client moves the head, note any enlargement of the lymph nodes or thyroid gland. Observe for any pulsations in the neck. The carotid pulsation, seen just below the angle of the jaw, normally is the only visible pulsation while the client is in the sitting position.

Mental and Neurological Status and Affect

A head-to-toe assessment incorporates an assessment of the client's mental and neurological status and affect. A client's mental status includes the level of orientation to person, place, and time and the client's responsiveness to the environment. When assessing, observe for responsiveness, the client's ability to follow directions and to respond appropriately to comments and to her name when called.

Neurological assessment of the client focuses on the level of consciousness (LOC), pupil response, hand grasps, and foot pushes. Each of these assessments is discussed in the area of the head-to-toe assessment in which it is observed. The LOC is the client's degree of wakefulness. For example, a client who is alert is fully awake with eyes open and responds to environmental stimuli. The client who is less awake will be drowsy and slow responding to environmental stimuli.

When documenting the client's affect, judgmental words such as *pleasant, happy, cooperative, uncooperative, angry, depressed,* or *hostile* should not be used. Focus specifically on the behaviors exhibited by the client, such as facial expression and verbal and nonverbal behaviors. In doing this, the accuracy of the conversation or the behaviors observed is maintained as well as the legal appropriateness of the assessment.

Skin Assessment

Skin assessment is performed as each area of the body is assessed. Note the color of the skin as well as its moisture or dryness. Inspect and palpate the client's skin, assessing temperature, turgor, edema, and integrity. Palpation of the skin with the dorsal aspect of the hand on the right and left sides of the body provides a comparison of the client's skin temperature. Ask the client if any pain or discomfort in relation to the skin and/or mucous membranes has occurred. Identification of the skin's turgor is best accomplished by gently pinching the skin of the anterior chest and observing the speed of skin return to its previous position. If the skin stays pinched, it may indicate dehydration, and further assessment is needed.

Edema is the visible accumulation of excess interstitial fluid (Daniels, Grendell, & Wilkins, 2010) and is present in overhydration, increased capillary permeability, heart failure, renal failure, cirrhosis of the liver, incompetent lymph system, and varicosities. Vasodilators, calcium antagonists, and nonsteroidal anti-inflammatory drugs (NSAIDS) also cause edema. A client gains 5 to 10 pounds before edema is detected. Assess the weight of clients with congestive heart failure and renal failure on a daily basis. The client is weighed on the same scale, at the same time each day, and with the same amount of clothing so an accurate accounting is made of fluid retention.

Palpate dependent areas (hands, sacrum, legs, ankles, and feet) for edema and assess by firmly applying pressure with a thumb or finger for 5 seconds, noting the amount of indentation (Figure 26-9a). Pitting edema is when an indentation remains after pressure is applied. The degree of edema is based on the depth of indentation and how long it remains. Evaluate pitting edema according to the following rating scale (Assessment Technologies Institute, 2007; Estes, 2010; Gehring, 2002):

+0 no edema

+1 indentation of 2 mm (0–¼ inches), disappears rapidly (trace)

+2 pitting of 4 mm (¼–½ inch), disappears in 10 to 15 seconds (mild)

+3 pitting of 6 mm (½–1 inch), lasts 1 to 2 minutes (moderate)

+4 pitting of 8 mm or more (greater than 1 inch), lasts 2 to 5 minutes (severe) (Figure 26-9b)

Note the location, size, distribution, and appearance of skin lesions throughout the body. Document any breaks or changes in the skin integrity, such as scratches, bruises, skin tears, cuts, and scars from previous injuries or surgeries. Note the general hygiene of the skin and ask the client about usual skin care routines.

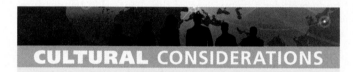

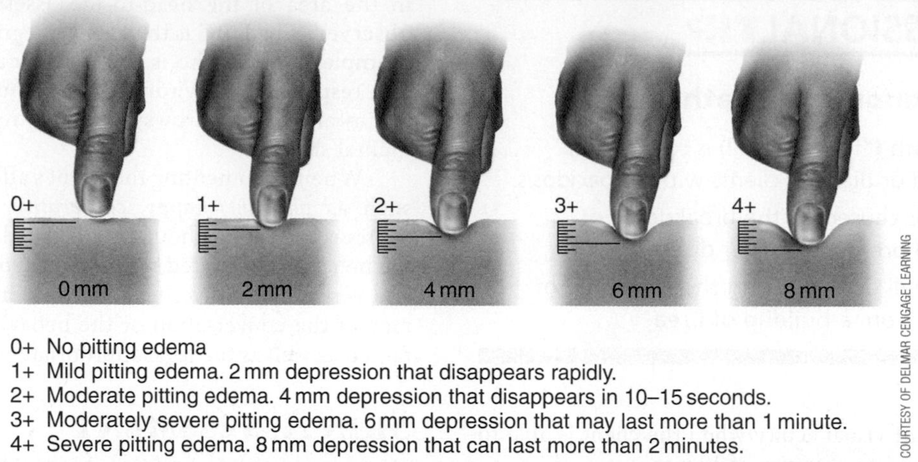

0+
1+
2+
3+
4+
0 mm
2 mm
4 mm
6 mm
8 mm
0+ No pitting edema
1+ Mild pitting edema. 2 mm depression that disappears rapidly.
2+ Moderate pitting edema. 4 mm depression that disappears in 10–15 seconds.
3+ Moderately severe pitting edema. 6 mm depression that may last more than 1 minute.
4+ Severe pitting edema. 8 mm depression that can last more than 2 minutes.
COURTESY OF DELMAR CENGAGE LEARNING

FIGURE 26-9 **Assessing edema. Palpate for edema in the lower extremities on the tibia, the dorsal aspect of the foot, and behind the medial malleolus and Assess edema according to the rating scale.**

CULTURAL CONSIDERATIONS

Skin, Mouth, and Eye Color

- The darker the client's skin, the more difficult it is to assess changes in color.
- Establish a baseline skin color by observing the least pigmented skin surfaces, which include the volar surfaces of the forearms, the palms of the hands, the soles of the feet, the abdomen, and the buttocks. There should be an underlying red tone in these areas. Absence of this red tone may indicate pallor.
- African American oral mucosa has a bluish hue. Caucasians have pink mucosa (Estes, 2010).
- Oral hyperpigmentation often is found in dark-skinned persons. If the hard palate is not hyperpigmented, it has a yellow discoloration in the presence of jaundice.
- The lips may be used to assess jaundice and cyanosis, and the sclera may be used to assess jaundice if a baseline color has been established for each.
- The conjunctiva reflect color changes of cyanosis or pallor.
- Nail beds are used to note how quickly the color returns after pressure has been released from the free edge of the nail, regardless of the nail bed color.

THORACIC ASSESSMENT

During thoracic assessment, the condition of the client's cardiovascular and respiratory systems along with assessment of the breasts are determined.

Cardiovascular Status

Assessment of the client's cardiovascular status by the LP/VN focuses specifically on listening to the apical pulse, identifying heart tones, and checking the nail beds. The apical pulse (point of maximum impulse or PMI) is determined by using auscultation and palpation. To assess the apical pulse, palpate over the apex of the heart at the fifth left intercostal space at the midclavicular line. A slight, short duration tap against the fingers will be felt, and this is where the apical pulse is auscultated (Figure 26-10). Listening to the apical pulse is the most accurate assessment of the heart rate and should occur for 60 seconds. The apical pulse is assessed first with the diaphragm of the stethoscope for the regularity or irregularity of its rhythm. Second, the bell of the stethoscope is used to differentiate the loudness or tones of the heart. Along with the apical pulse, the other pulse points may be assessed now or when the extremities are assessed.

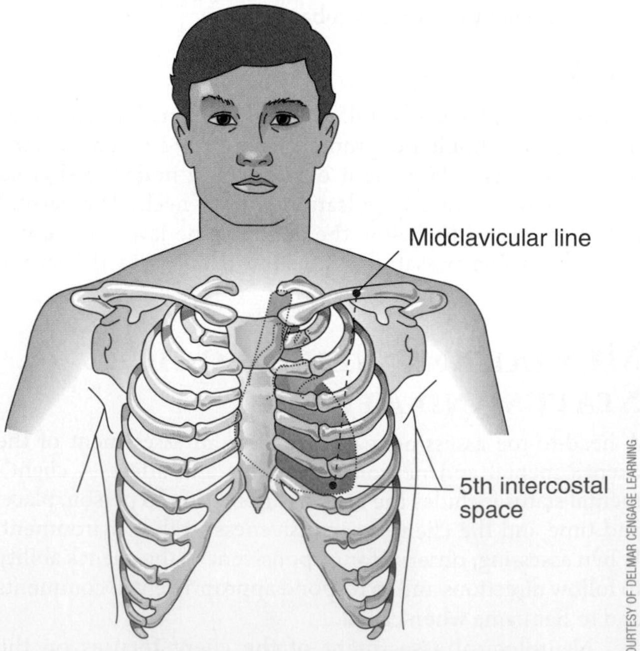

FIGURE 26-10 **Assessing the Apical Pulse**

To assess blood perfusion of peripheral vessels and skin, note changes in skin temperature, color, and sensation and changes in the pulses and feel the toes for warmth and color. Because the position of the extremities can affect the skin temperature and appearance, extremities must always be assessed at heart level and at normal room and body temperature. Compare peripheral pulses bilaterally and note changes in strength and quality. The nurse checks the degree to which the tissues are perfused by measuring the SaO_2 with a pulse oximeter. The normal range is 95% to 100% saturation.

The focus of the functional assessment includes personal habits contributing to or preventing cardiovascular disease. Ask about the client's personal exercise habits and elicit information regarding past chest pain or shortness of breath. The client should describe any pain; its location, duration, and precipitating factors; and what is done to alleviate the pain. Also ask if the client has ever fainted or felt dizzy. Any lower leg swelling and its cause should also be noted.

Respiratory Status

Breath sound assessment is performed after assessing the apical pulse rate. The presence of normal and abnormal breath sounds is revealed by respiratory auscultation. Ask the client to breathe only through the mouth during auscultation because mouth breathing decreases air turbulence, which interferes with an accurate assessment.

There are three types of normal breath sounds, each having a unique pitch, quality, intensity, location, and duration in the inspiratory and expiratory phases of respiration:

- **Bronchial sounds**. Loud, high-pitched sounds with a hollow quality heard longer on expiration than inspiration from air moving through the trachea
- **Bronchovesicular sounds**. Medium-pitched, blowing sounds heard equally on inspiration and expiration from air moving through the large airways, posteriorly between the scapula and anteriorly over bronchioles lateral to the sternum at the first and second intercostal spaces
- **Vesicular sounds**. Soft, breezy, low-pitched sounds heard longer on inspiration than expiration resulting from air moving through the smaller airways over the lung's periphery, with the exception of the scapular area

Nonnormal breath sounds are described as either abnormal or **adventitious breath sounds**. Adventitious breath sounds include sibilant wheeze (formerly wheeze), sonorous wheeze (formerly rhonchi), fine and coarse crackle (formerly rales), pleural friction rub, and stridor. **Sibilant wheezes** are high-pitched, whistling sounds heard during inhalation and exhalation. A **sonorous wheeze** is a low-pitched snoring sound that is louder on exhalation. Coughing may alter the sound if caused by mucus. **Crackles** are popping sounds heard on inhalation or exhalation, not cleared by coughing. A **pleural friction rub** is a low-pitched grating sound on inhalation and exhalation. **Stridor** is a high-pitched, harsh sound heard on inspiration when the trachea or larynx is obstructed. Assess breath sounds of the anterior, posterior, and lateral chest wall for normal as well as adventitious breath sounds. Monitor adventitious breath sounds consistently. The lungs are assessed from side to side so the two sides can be compared, as shown in Figure 26-11.

The functional assessment information to be obtained when assessing the respiratory status includes any difficulty breathing or the presence of a cough. Ask the client if the cough is nonproductive or productive and to describe the secretions produced. Terms used to describe secretions expectorated are *thick, thin, yellow, green*. The client's occupational or home environment may affect breathing patterns; exposure to dust, chemicals, vapors, tobacco, smoke, or paint fumes, and irritants such as asbestos are noted.

CRITICAL THINKING

Assessing Breath Sounds

When listening to your client's breath sounds, you hear a sound that you think is a pleural friction rub. How do you determine if the sound you heard is really a friction rub?

Wounds, Scars, Drains, Tubes, Dressings

When assessing the thorax, note any type of wounds, scars, drains, tubes, or dressings. Documentation of these include the location, size, and amount of drainage or discharge and, if present, signs of inflammation.

Breasts

Assessment of the breasts is done for both male and female clients. Begin by inspecting the breasts for size and symmetry. It is common to have a slight difference in size of breasts. Note any obvious masses, dimpling (a depression in the surface skin), or inflammation. The skin normally is smooth and even in color. Determine if the nipples and areola are symmetrical in size, shape, and color and note any discharge from the nipples.

Any abnormal area should be palpated for size, consistency, mobility, tenderness, and location of the lesion. Another area to include in breast assessment is the axillary lymph nodes that drain the breasts. Palpate the axilla for enlarged or inflamed lymph nodes, ask if there is any tenderness, and determine if and when the client performs breast self-exams. Note if the client has had a mammogram and when the last one was taken.

PROFESSIONALTIP

Assessment of the Abdomen

Although the usual sequence for implementing assessment techniques is inspection, palpation, percussion, and auscultation, assessment of the abdomen entails a different sequence. Because palpation can affect sounds heard on auscultation, the sequence for abdominal assessment is as follows:

- Inspection
- Auscultation
- Percussion
- Palpation

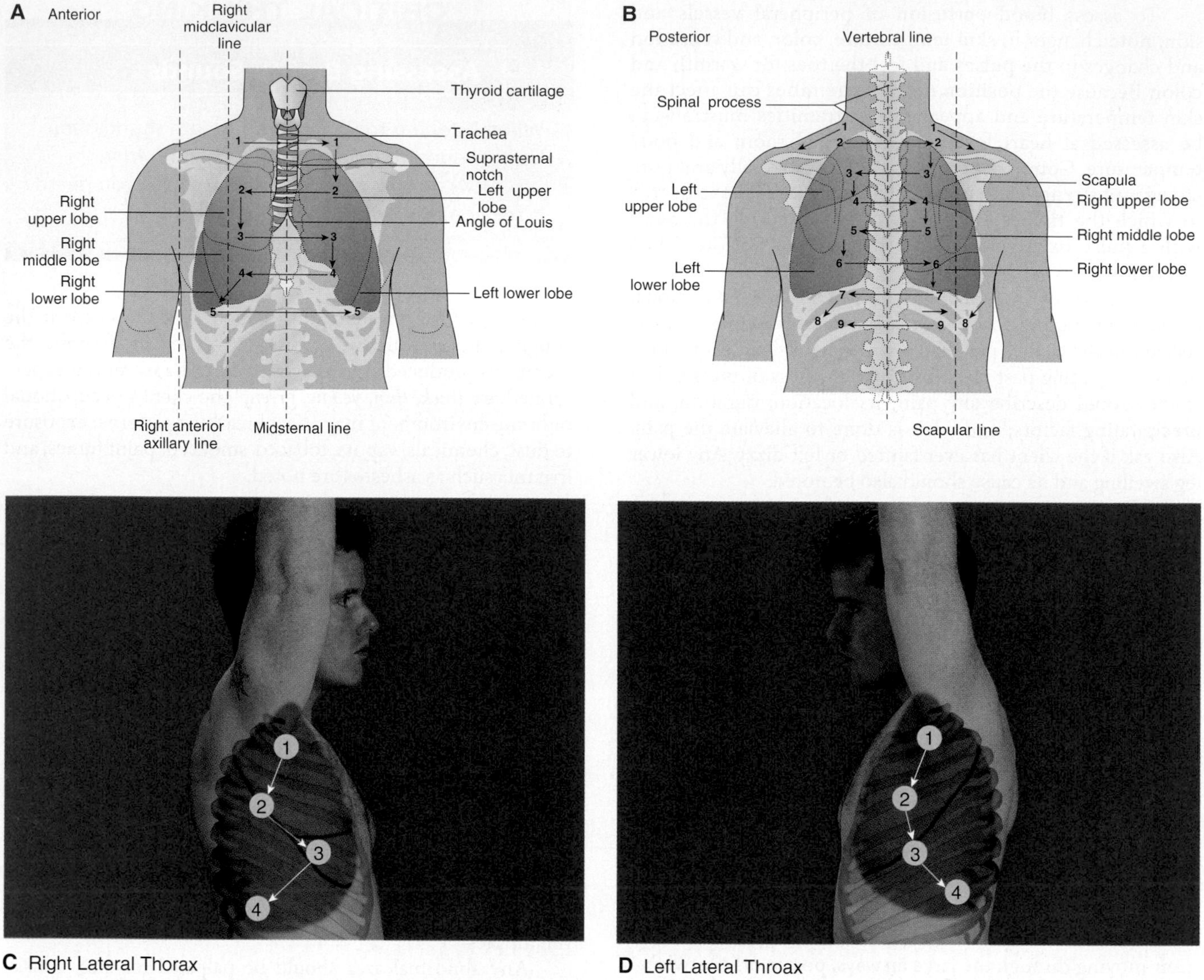

FIGURE 26-11 Symmetrical Assessment of Breath Sounds; *A,* Anterior; *B,* Posterior; *C,* Right lateral; *D,* Left lateral. A method of assessing breath sounds is to move the bell of the stethoscope as directed by the arrows in pictures A and B. It is important to find a system that covers all areas of the lungs for thorough lung assessment.

ABDOMINAL ASSESSMENT

Abdominal assessment determines the status of the client's gastrointestinal and genitourinary systems. Note any type of wounds, scars, drains, tubes, dressings, or ostomies. Documentation of these must include the location, size, and amount of drainage or discharge, and if present, signs of inflammation.

Gastrointestinal Status

The abdomen is first inspected for rashes and scars. Assess if the abdomen is flat, rounded, or distended and observe the abdomen for symmetry and visible signs of peristalsis or pulsations. If the abdomen is distended, ask the client questions pertaining to bowel movements and urinary status.

Auscultation is the second component of the abdominal assessment of a client's bowel status. A "bubbly-gurgly" sound, caused by peristalsis and movement of the intestinal contents, can be heard by placing the stethoscope on each quadrant of the abdomen and listening for approximately 1 minute. These sounds should be present in all four quadrants of the abdomen, beginning in the right lower quadrant (RLQ) and moving clockwise around the four quadrants, as shown in Figure 26-12. When approximately 5 to 20 bowel sounds are heard per minute, or one at least every 5 to 15 seconds, the bowel sounds are considered active.

The absence of bowel sounds during 1 minute of auscultation in each quadrant is documented as absent bowel sounds. Bowel sounds of less than five per minute are described as hypoactive, while an excess of 20 or more bowel sounds per minute is defined as hyperactive. High-pitched, loud, rushing sounds heard with or without a stethoscope are termed **borborygmi**. This is caused by the passage of gas through the liquid contents of the intestine.

Percussion of the abdomen is done in all four quadrants. The predominant abdominal percussion sound is tympany caused by percussing over the air-filled stomach and intestines.

Light palpation of the abdomen is done to assess for muscle tone, masses, pulsations, or any signs of tenderness or discomfort. Abdominal muscles may be palpated and should feel relaxed on light palpation, not tightly contracted or

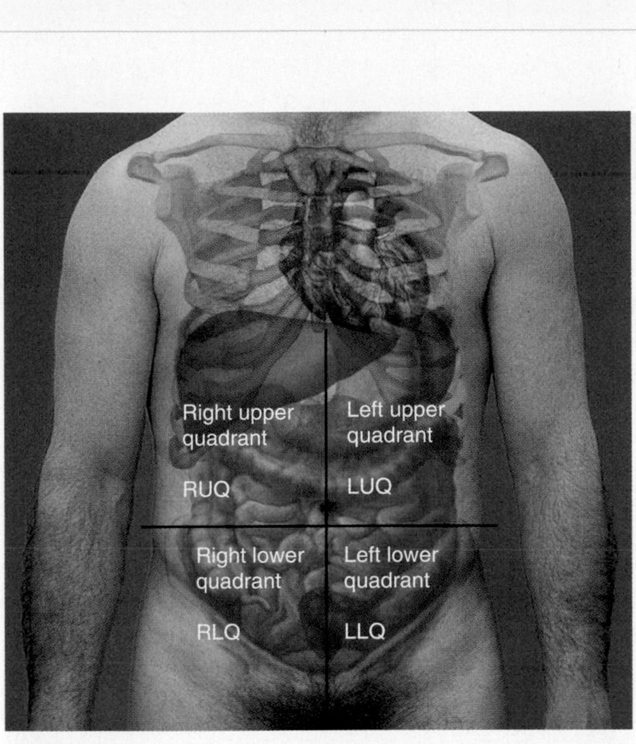

FIGURE 26-12 The Four Quadrants of the Abdomen

spastic. If the client is anxious, muscle contraction may be evident. Palpation of a separation of the rectus abdominis muscle may be felt, especially in clients who are obese or pregnant. The rectus abdominis muscle includes two large, midline muscles that extend from the xiphoid process to the symphysis pubis and can be palpated midline as the client raises his or her head. Rebound tenderness, indicating possible inflammation of the appendix, may be elicited by depressing the abdomen in the right lower quadrant and quickly withdrawing the fingers. This examination is done at the end of the abdominal assessment because of the possibility of increasing the client's level of pain. If any of the abdominal organs can be felt with light palpation, this is abnormal and should be reported to the nursing supervisor. After assessment of bowel sounds, question the client about diet, usual bowel patterns, appetite, weight changes, indigestion, heartburn, nausea, pain, and use of enemas or laxatives.

Genitourinary Status

Assessment of the client's urinary and reproductive status is accomplished mainly by inspection and use of interview skills. Genitourinary assessment includes examination of the abdomen, urinary meatus and genitalia, and assessment of the client's urine.

Inspect the abdomen for any enlargement or fullness. In the normal adult, the abdomen is smooth, flat, and symmetrical. The urinary meatus is inspected for any abnormalities such as inflammation and discharge, which may signal a urethral infection.

In females, observe the appearance of the genitalia (labia, clitoris, vaginal opening). Questions to ask the client that focus on the reproductive history include pregnancies, use of birth control, menstrual cycle history, present sexual activity, use of protection during intercourse, date of the last Pap test, and determination of how any present illness has or will affect sexual activity.

In males, inspect the penis, urethral meatus, foreskin (if uncircumcized), and scrotum. Questions to ask the client that focus on the reproductive history include present sexual activity, use of protection during intercourse, and how the present illness has or will affect sexual activity. Ask if the client performs testicular self-examinations.

Note any lesions or ulcerations that may indicate sexually transmitted disease. The usual voiding pattern and any recent changes should be determined if the client has had any history of urinary tract infections, kidney stones, change in the urinary stream, or painful urination or nocturia.

CULTURAL CONSIDERATIONS

Genitourinary Assessment

Middle Eastern women often will remain veiled during this assessment.

Musculoskeletal and Extremity Assessment

Assess symmetry and strength of major muscle groups throughout the head-to-toe assessment. Any time during the assessment when the client is repositioned, observe the range of movement the client utilizes to make that position change. Ask the client to walk across the room and observe the client's movements and posture when sitting up in bed to assess gross motor movement and posture. Assessment of the client's handshake gives an estimate of muscle strength. Palpating muscles lightly identifies swelling, tone, or any specific changes in the shape of the muscles.

Hand grasps and foot pushes assess the strength and equality of the client's extremities. Upper extremity strength is assessed by having the client grasp the nurse's index and middle fingers of each hand. The grasp should be equal in both hands. Foot pushes assess the lower extremities. The nurse's hands are placed on the soles of the client's feet and the client is asked to push both feet against the nurse's hands. The push should be equal in both feet. Ask the client to touch the tip of her nose with a finger and then the tip of the nurse's finger as it is moved to different locations to test the client's coordination skills.

Assess strength and symmetry of some of the major muscle groups by watching gait and postural movements. Note any aids to ambulation. Examine muscles, first in one extremity and then the other; note equality of size, contour, tone, and strength.

Carefully assess the skin of the lower extremities to determine color changes, loss of feeling or hair, change in temperature within the extremity and from one extremity to the other, and presence of varicose veins, ulcers, and edema. Ask if the client experiences any leg pain or cramps or if muscle weakness is experienced or if difficulty or pain when walking or performing routine daily activities occurs. The functional assessment includes asking the client about routine activities such as cooking, shopping, exercise, yard work, and hobbies. Tolerance limitations can be identified by observing for stiffness, crepitus, or fatigue during ambulation. Determine if the client can safely and appropriately perform functions essential for home life and ADLs.

CASE STUDY

K.J., a 17-year-old male, was in a motorcycle accident and sustained fractures of the lower jaw, right humerus, left femur, and right tibia and a dislocated shoulder. His mouth is wired shut, and he has a long arm cast on his right arm, a sling on the left arm, a short leg case on the right lower leg, and skeletal traction on the left leg. He is assigned to you, and you are to complete an assessment on him.

1. You do not have a temporal artery thermometer on your unit. How would you obtain a temperature on K.J.?
2. What would you include when completing the neurological assessment? Why is the neurological assessment so important to this client?
3. When listening to heart tones, you notice a different sound than the usual lubb-dubb. What would you do with this information?
4. Describe how you would listen to breath sounds on K.J. Why is it so important to assess breath sounds on K.J.?
5. Describe how you would assess bowel sounds. Why is it so important to assess bowel sounds on K.J.?
6. K.J. has a catheter inserted. Practice your documentation skills by writing a normal urine finding as if you were charting on K.J.
7. How would you assess for edema? According to the edema rating scale, how would you document pitting edema of 4 mm?
8. Describe how you would assess K.J.'s musculoskeletal system and extremities.

SUMMARY

- Psychosocial needs of clients are identified within the scope of a functional assessment.
- The health history and the physical examination used together present a holistic view of client needs.
- Collection of vital signs is the foundation of each head-to-toe assessment and includes temperature, pulse, respirations, blood pressure, and pain.
- Assessment of a client's mental and neurological status is determined by obtaining information about the client's level of consciousness, pupil response, as well as hand grip and foot push capabilities.
- When describing a client's affect, utilize terms that are descriptive of the specific behavior observed, not a judgment about the behavior.
- Assessing the cardiovascular status of each client includes palpation of specific pulse points.
- Auscultation of lung fields assists in collection of data regarding the breath sounds of the client.
- An abdominal assessment includes use of inspection, auscultation, percussion, and palpation within the four quadrants of the abdomen to establish bowel status and function.
- Through observation of client gait and overall range of movement, some knowledge of the symmetry and strength of muscles is obtained.
- During the assessment of wounds, drains, dressings, and other external devices, maintain accurate documentation of the amount of drainage, color, or other changes.

REVIEW QUESTIONS

1. S.J. is 54 years old. While performing the assessment overview, S.J. states, "I just get so lightheaded when I first get up in the morning." S.J. most likely has:
   1. cyanosis.
   2. hypertension.
   3. orthostatic hypertension.
   4. orthostatic hypotension.

2. During the physical head-to-toe assessment of the client, the nurse checks the pulse and blood pressure. Which of the four assessment techniques did the nurse utilize?
   1. Auscultation, palpation, and inspection.
   2. Auscultation, percussion, and inspection.
   3. Auscultation and palpation.
   4. Palpation and inspection.

3. On admission to your unit, the client verbalizes increased pain in her left leg. What would be the pertinent assessment information to collect about this client?
   1. Listen to the client's bowel sounds.
   2. Check circulation in the right leg.
   3. Assess both of the client's legs.
   4. Ask the client about her current diet.

4. How often a nurse assesses a client's vital signs depends on the:
   1. availability of personnel.
   2. doctor's orders.
   3. nurse's discretion.
   4. client's condition.

5. The nurse checks the radial pulse for 30 seconds and multiplies by 2. She notices an irregularity in the beat. What is the next action the nurse should take?
   1. Check the radial pulse for 60 seconds
   2. Listen to the apical pulse for 60 seconds
   3. Listen to the apical for 30 seconds and multiply by 2
   4. Continue with the rest of the assessment
6. In what order would a nurse assess a client's abdomen?
   1. Inspection, palpation, percussion, auscultation
   2. Inspection, auscultation, palpation, percussion
   3. Auscultation, palpation, percussion, inspection
   4. Palpation, percussion, inspection, auscultation
7. The best way for a nurse to conduct a physical assessment of the lungs is to: (Select all that apply.)
   1. Ask the client to breathe through the nose
   2. Ask the client to breathe through the mouth
   3. Listen to breath sounds on the anterior and posterior chest wall
   4. Listen to breath sounds on the anterior, posterior, and lateral chest wall
   5. Listen to the lung sounds from side to side
   6. Ask the client if the cough is productive or nonproductive
8. In what position is a client placed in preparation for a rectal exam?
   1. Supine
   2. Prone
   3. Sims'
   4. Right lateral
9. A 72-year-old woman was recently admitted to a nursing home because of confusion, disorientation, and self-destructive behaviors. She was accompanied by her daughter, who says that she does not have a history of these behaviors. The woman asks the nurse, "Where am I?" The best response for the nurse to make is:
   1. "Don't worry. You're safe here."
   2. "Tell me where you think you are."
   3. "What did your daughter tell you?"
   4. "You're at the community nursing home."
10. The nurse is preparing the client for a physical assessment. The first thing he should do is:
    1. shut the door for privacy.
    2. turn down the sound on the television.
    3. explain the procedure to the client.
    4. listen to lung sounds.

REFERENCES/SUGGESTED READING

Andresen, G. (1998). Assessing the older patient. *RN, 61*(3), 46–55.

Assessment Technologies Institute. (2007). *Fundamentals of nursing content mastery series review module.* Stillwell, KS: Author.

Barkauskas, V., Bauman, L., & Darling-Fisher, C. (2002). *Health and physical assessment* (3rd ed.). St. Louis, MO: Mosby.

Bickley, L. S., & Sailagyi, P. (2002). *Bates' guide to physical examination and history taking* (8th ed.). Philadelphia: Lippincott Williams & Wilkins.

Clayton, M. (2006). Communication: An important part of nursing care. *American Journal of Nursing, 106*(11), 70–71.

Craig, J., Lancaster, G., Taylor, S., Williamson, P., & Smyth, R. (2002). Now, hear this: Ear temps in children found to be inaccurate. *Lancet, 360*(9333), 603–609.

Crow, S. (1997). Your guide to gloves. *Nursing97, 27*(3), 26–28.

Daniels, R., Grendell, R., & Wilkins, F. (2010). Nursing fundamentals: Caring and clinical decision making (2nd ed.). Clifton Park, NY: Delmar Cengage Learning.

Estes, M. (2010). *Health assessment and physical examination* (4th ed.). Clifton Park, NY: Delmar Cengage Learning.

Finesilver, C. (2001, April). Perfecting your skills: Respiratory assessment. *RN's Travel Nursing Today*, 16–26.

Fuller, J., & Schaller-Ayers, J. (2000). *Health assessment: A nursing approach.* (3rd ed.). Philadelphia: Lippincott Williams & Wilkins.

Gallauresi, B. (1998). Pulse oximeters. *Nursing98, 28*(9), 31.

Gecsedi, R., & Decker, G. (2001). Incorporating alternative therapies into pain management: More patients are considering complementary approaches. *American Journal of Nursing, 101*(4), 35–39.

Gehring, P. (2002, April). Perfecting your skills: Vascular assessment. *RN's Travel Nursing Today*, 16–24.

Gulla, J., & Singer, A. (2000). Over half of ED patients use alternative therapy. *American Journal of Nursing, 100*(8), 24J.

Heery, K. (2000). Straight talk about the patient interview. *Nursing2000, 30*(6), 66–67.

Hodge, P., & Ullrich, S. (1999). Does your assessment include alternative therapies? *RN, 62*(6), 47–49.

Husain, M., & Coleman, R. (2002). Should you treat a fever? *Nursing2002, 32*(10), 66–70.

Joint Commission. (2004). Nutritional, functional, and pain assessments and screens. Retrieved October 29, 2008, from http://www.jointcommission.org/AccreditationPrograms/Hospitals/Standards/FAWs/Provi

Joint Commission. (2008). Joint Commission urges patients to "speak up" about pain. Retrieved October 29, 2008, from http://www.jointcommission.org/Library/TM_Physicians/tmp_10_08.htm

Joint Commission on Accreditation of Healthcare Organizations. (2000a). Comprehensive accreditation manual for hospitals (CAMH) revised pain management standards. Available: http://www.jcaho.org/standard/pm_hap.html

Joint Commission on Accreditation of Healthcare Organizations. (2000b). Pain assessment and management standards. Available: http://www.jcaho.org/standard/pm_coll.html

Karch, A., & Karch, F. (2000). When a blood pressure isn't routine. *American Journal of Nursing, 100*(3), 23.

Kirton, C. (1997). Assessing bowel sounds. *Nursing97, 27*(3), 64.

Klingman, L. (1999a). Assessing the female reproductive system. *American Journal of Nursing, 99*(8), 37–43.

Klingman, L. (1999b). Assessing the male genitalia. *American Journal of Nursing, 99*(7), 47–50.
Lower, J. (2002). Facing neuro assessment fearlessly. *Nursing2002, 32*(2), 58–64.
Mehta, M. (2003a). Assessing the abdomen. *Nursing2003, 33*(5), 54–55.
Mehta, M. (2003b). Assessing cardiovascular status. *Nursing2003, 33*(2), 56–58.
Mehta, M. (2003c). Assessing respiratory status. *Nursing2003, 33*(2), 54–56.
Murray, R., Zentner, J., & Yakimo, R. (2008). *Health promotion strategies through the lifespan* (8th ed.). Norwalk, CT: Prentice Hall.
O'Hanlon-Nichols, T. (1997). Basic assessment series: The adult cardiovascular system. *American Journal of Nursing, 97*(12), 34–40.
O'Hanlon-Nichols, T. (1998). Basic assessment series: Gastrointestinal system. *American Journal of Nursing, 98*(4), 48–53.
O'Hanlon-Nichols, T. (1998a). Basic assessment series: Musculoskeletal system. *American Journal of Nursing, 98*(6), 48–52.
O'Hanlon-Nichols, T. (1998c). Basic assessment series: The adult pulmonary system. *American Journal of Nursing, 98*(2), 39–45.
O'Hanlon-Nichols, T. (1999). Neurologic assessment. *American Journal of Nursing, 99*(6), 44–50.
Owen, A. (1998). Respiratory assessment revisited. *Nursing98, 28*(4), 48–49.
Pullen, R. (2003). Using an ear thermometer. *Nursing2003, 33*(5), 24.
Rice, K. (1998). Sounding out blood flow with a Doppler device. *Nursing98, 28*(9), 56–57.
Rice, K. (1999). Measuring thigh BP. *Nursing99, 29*(8), 58–59.
Scott, T. (2008). How do I differentiate normal aging of the skin from pathologic conditions? Retrieved October 29, 2008, from http://www.medscape.com/viewarticle/575293_print
Stanley, W. (2003). Nailing a key assessment. *Nursing2003, 33*(8), 50–51.
Thomas, J., & Feliciano, C. (2003). Measuring BP with a Doppler device. *Nursing2003, 33*(7), 52–53.
University of Maryland Medicine. (2002). An introduction to CAM. Available: http://www.umm.edu/altmed/ConsModalities/AnIntroductionToCAMcm.html
U.S. Department of Health and Human Services, National Institutes of Health. (2003). The seventh report of the Joint National Committee on Prevention, Detection, Evaluation, and Treatment of High Blood Pressure JNC 7 Express (NIH Publication No. 03-5233). Washington, DC: Author. Retrieved October 28, 2008, from http://www.nhlbi.nih.gov/guidelines/hypertension/express.pdf
Warner, P., Rowe, T., & Whipple, B. (1999). Shedding light on the sexual history. *American Journal of Nursing, 99*(6), 34–40.
Weber, J., & Kelley, J. (2006). *Health assessment in nursing* (3rd ed.). Philadelphia: Lippincott Williams & Wilkins.
Williams, M., & Keen, P. (2007). Gynecologic assessment of the elderly patient. Retrieved October 28, 2008, from http://www.medscape.com/viewprogram/6881_pnt

CHAPTER 27

Pain Management

MAKING THE CONNECTION

Refer to the following chapters to increase your understanding of pain management:

Basic Nursing

- ***Communication***
- ***Cultural Considerations***
- ***End-of-Life Care***
- ***Complementary/Alternative Therapies***

Intermediate Procedures

- ***Administering Oral, Sublingual, and Buccal Medication***
- ***Withdrawing Medication from an Ampule***
- ***Withdrawing Medication from a Vial***
- ***Administering an Intradermal Injection***
- ***Administering a Subcutaneous Injection***
- ***Administering an Intramuscular Injection***

LEARNING OBJECTIVES

Upon completion of this chapter, you should be able to:

- Define key terms.
- Identify the four components of pain conduction.
- Discuss the gate control theory of pain.
- Describe the types of pain.
- List three guidelines that should be included in a thorough pain assessment.
- Identify three general principles of pain management.
- List the nurse's responsibilities in administration of analgesics.
- Identify site of action of both nonopioid and opioid analgesics.
- Describe three examples of nonpharmacological measures for pain relief.
- List nursing diagnosis for pain.
- Discuss nursing interventions that promote comfort.
- Evaluate client's pain relief.

KEY TERMS

acupuncture
acute pain
adjuvant medications
afferent pain pathway
analgesia
analgesics
ceiling effect
chronic acute pain
chronic nonmalignant pain
chronic pain
colic
cryotherapy
cutaneous pain
distraction
efferent pain pathway
endorphins
epidural analgesia
gate control pain theory
hypnosis
intrathecal analgesia
ischemic pain
mixed agonist-antagonist
modulation
myofascial pain syndromes
neuralgia
nociceptors
noxious stimulus
pain
pain threshold
pain tolerance
patient-controlled analgesia (PCA)
perception
phantom limb pain
progressive muscle relaxation
recurrent acute pain
referred pain
reframing
relaxation techniques
somatic pain
tolerance
transcutaneous electrical nerve stimulation (TENS)
transduction
transmission
visceral pain

INTRODUCTION

Pain is a phenomenon found in all specialties of nursing. No matter the setting, including neonatal intensive care, intraoperative, home care, or clinics, there are challenges in pain management. While other health care team members address pain management with clients, the nurse spends the most time with the client experiencing pain. For example, in an acute care setting, the physician orders the **analgesics** (substances that relieve pain) for the client but may spend only 10 to 15 minutes a day with that client. Nurses are present 24 hours a day, administer the medications, assess the client's response, and report the response to the physician. The nurse's role can be pivotal in relieving the client's pain.

The experience of pain can have a significant impact on a client's health. It is a personal experience affecting all aspects of an individual's health, including physical well-being, mental status, and effectiveness of coping mechanisms. This chapter provides an overview of the complex phenomenon of pain, including pain definitions, pain physiology, and pain assessment. Strategies to control pain are also discussed, including pharmacological, noninvasive, and invasive techniques.

DEFINITIONS OF PAIN

The phenomenon of pain is referenced as far back as the Babylonian clay tablets. Aristotle (4th century B.C.) described pain as an emotion, being the opposite of pleasure. Although emotions certainly play an important role in pain perception, there is much more to the experience than the feelings involved.

In the Middle Ages, pain had religious connotations. Pain was seen as God's punishment for sins or as evidence that an individual was possessed by demons. This definition of pain is still embraced by some clients who might tell the nurse that the suffering is their "cross to bear." Pain relief may not be the goal for those individuals who believe in this definition of pain. Spiritual counseling may need to be implemented before this person is willing to work toward relief.

The most widely accepted definition of **pain** is one developed by the International Association for the Study of Pain (IASP). This organization defines pain as "an unpleasant sensory and emotional experience associated with actual or potential tissue damage or described in terms of such damage" (IASP, 2008). This definition incorporates both the sensory and the emotional components of pain. It also acknowledges that evidence of actual tissue damage is not required in order for the pain to be considered real.

Many pain experts emphasize the subjective nature of pain. Unlike a blood pressure or a blood glucose measurement, the intensity of discomfort the client is feeling cannot be measured with an instrument. McCaffery and Pasero (1999) say it best by defining pain as "whatever the person experiencing it says it is, existing whenever he says it does" (p. 17). All nursing actions are based on what pain means to the client. The first and most important step in assessing a client's pain is to believe the client. The client's description of the pain experience, or self-report, should be the basis of all care decisions. Without it, care will be ineffective (Teeter & Kemper, 2008a).

Because of widespread undertreatment of pain, in 1995 the American Pain Society launched an international campaign to raise awareness about the problem and to promote the routine assessment of pain by health care providers. This quickly led to the incorporation of pain assessment into the daily activities of clinicians as the "fifth vital sign" after the Joint Commission initiated pain management quality standards of care in 2001. However, research conducted by the U.S. Veterans Administration showed no improvement in pain management after adopting this strategy (Mularski et al., 2006). Assessment itself is not enough to ensure adequate pain management for clients. Health care providers must act on the assessment findings (Teeter & Kemper, 2008a).

Although pain has had many definitions throughout history, research in pain physiology shows that pain is a complex phenomenon. Pain is often difficult for clients to describe and nurses to understand, yet it is among the most common complaints leading individuals to seek health care. Until recently, pain was viewed as a symptom that required diagnosis and treatment of the underlying cause. It is now clear that pain itself can be detrimental to the health and healing of clients. Pain control, not just relief from pain once it occurs, must be recognized as a priority in the care of clients in all settings.

NATURE OF PAIN

Pain experience is a signal of tissue damage, as in the pain of cancer and chronic illness. Pain can also be a protective mechanism to prevent further injury, as when a client guards or protects an injured body part. Pain, as a warning of potential tissue damage, may be absent in people with hereditary sensory neuropathies, congenital nerve or spinal cord abnormalities, multiple sclerosis, diabetic neuropathy, alcoholism, leprosy, and nerve or spinal cord injury.

COMMON MYTHS ABOUT PAIN

Pain is often misunderstood and misjudged because it is subjective (depends on the client's perception) and cannot be objectively measured through a laboratory test or diagnostic data. A client's report of the level of pain varies based on cultural and experiential background. The nurse's interpretation of a client's pain is filtered through the nurse's biases and expectations. Some common myths related to pain are discussed in Table 27-1.

TYPES OF PAIN

Pain can be described by its origin or cause and by its nature or description. Pain categorized by its origin is either cutaneous, somatic, or visceral; by its nature, it is either acute or chronic.

PAIN CATEGORIZED BY ORIGIN

Cutaneous pain is caused by stimulating the cutaneous nerve endings in the skin and results in a well-localized "burning" or "prickling" sensation; tangled hair that is pulled during combing causes cutaneous pain. **Somatic pain** is nonlocalized and originates in support structures such as tendons, ligaments, and nerves; twisting an ankle results in somatic pain. **Visceral pain** is discomfort in the internal organs, is less localized, and is more slowly transmitted than cutaneous pain. Pain originating from the abdominal organs is often called **referred pain** because pain is not felt in the organ but instead is perceived at the spot where the organs were located during fetal development, making it difficult to assess (Figure 27-1).

PAIN CATEGORIZED BY NATURE

It is important to understand the difference between acute and chronic pain because they each present a different clinical picture.

Acute Pain

Acute pain has a sudden onset, relatively short duration, mild to severe intensity, with a steady decrease in intensity over a period of days to weeks. Once the **noxious stimulus** (underlying pathology) is resolved, the pain usually disappears (Table 27-2). It is usually associated with a specific condition, injury, or tissue damage caused by disease. As healing occurs, acute pain should diminish. Everyone has experienced acute

TABLE 27-1 Common Myths About Pain

MYTH	FACT
• The nurse is the best judge of a client's pain.	• Pain is a subjective experience; only the client can judge the level and severity of pain.
• If pain is ignored, it will go away.	• Pain is a real experience that is appropriately treated with nursing and medical intervention.
• Clients should not take any measures to relieve their pain until the pain is unbearable.	• Pain control and relief measures are effective in lowering the pain level, which will help clients function more normally and comfortably.
• Most complaints of pain are purely psychological (e.g., "it's all in your head"); only "real" pain manifests in obvious physical signs such as moaning or grimacing.	• Most clients honestly report their perception of pain, both physical and emotional, and need effective intervention and teaching; physical responses vary greatly depending on experience and cultural norms, and visible expressions of pain are not always reliable indicators of its severity.
• Clients taking pain medications will become addicted to the drug.	• Addiction is unlikely when analgesics are carefully administered and closely monitored.
• Clients with severe tissue damage will experience significant pain; those with lesser damage will feel less pain.	• Individuals' perceptions of pain are subjective; the extent of tissue damage is not necessarily proportional to the extent of pain experienced.
• Clients ask for pain medication when they need it.	• Many clients do not ask for medication because they are afraid of side effects, do not want to bother the nurse, have cultural norms and beliefs against it, or believe pain is inevitable and untreatable.

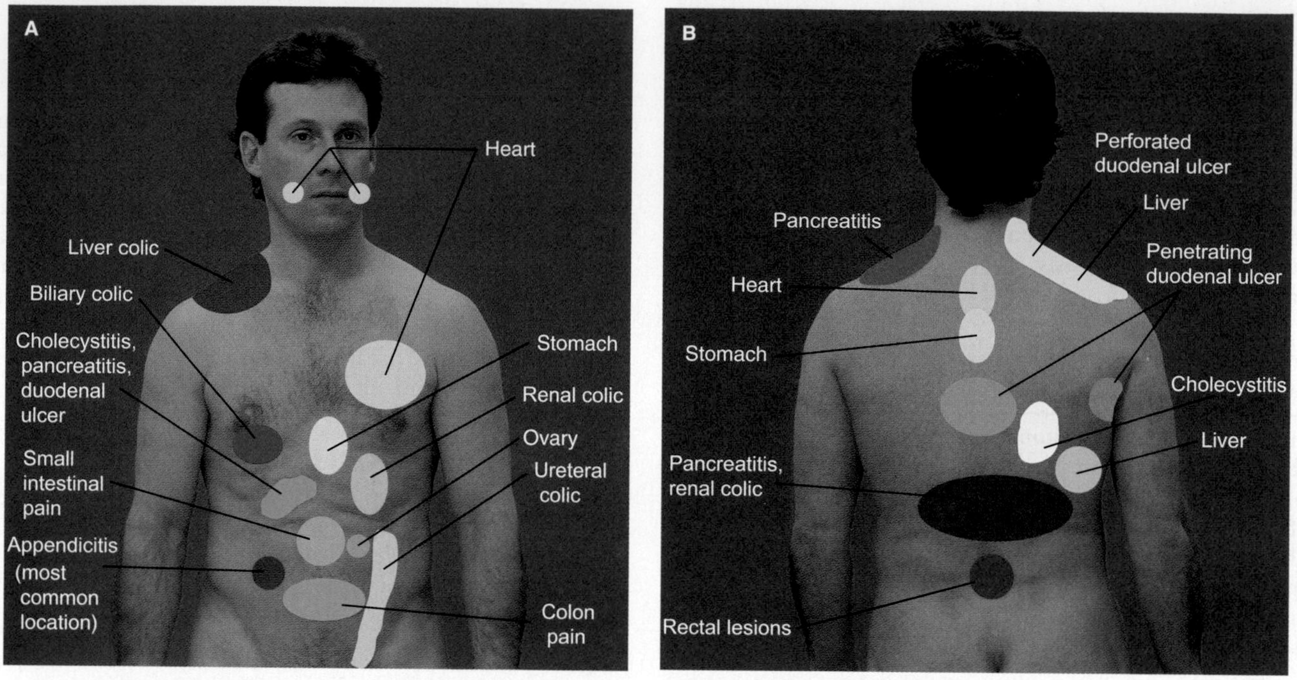

FIGURE 27-1 Areas of Referred Pain; *A*, Anterior View; *B*, Posterior View

pain (e.g., toothaches, headaches, needlesticks, skinned knees, burns, muscle pain, childbirth, postoperative pain, a sprained ankle, and fractures). The client is usually able to pinpoint the hurt. Acute pain is often described as sharp, although deep pain may be described as dull and aching. The client will exhibit elevated heart rate, respiratory rate, and blood pressure and may become diaphoretic and have dilated pupils. These signs resemble those of anxiety, which often accompanies acute pain. Behaviors may include crying and moaning, rubbing the site of pain, guarding, frowning, grimacing, and verbal complaints of the discomfort.

Recurrent acute pain is repetitive painful episodes that recur over a prolonged period or throughout the client's lifetime. Pain-free intervals alternate with painful episodes.

TABLE 27-2 Acute Versus Chronic Pain

	ACUTE	CHRONIC
Time Span	Less than 6 months	More than 6 months
Location	Localized, associated with a specific injury, condition, or disease	Difficult to pinpoint
Characteristics	Often described as sharp, diminishes as healing occurs	Often described as dull, diffuse, and aching
Physiologic Signs	• Elevated heart rate • Elevated BP • Elevated respirations • May be diaphoretic • Dilated pupils	• Normal vital signs • Normal pupils • No diaphoresis • May have loss of weight
Behavioral Signs	• Crying and moaning • Rubbing site • Guarding • Frowning • Grimacing • Complains of pain	• Physical immobility • Hopelessness • Listlessness • Loss of libido • Exhaustion and fatigue • Complains of pain only when asked

COURTESY OF DELMAR CENGAGE LEARNING

Examples of recurrent pain seen in children include recurrent abdominal, chest, limb pain, and headaches. In adults, recurrent pain experience includes migraine headaches, sickle cell crises pain, and angina.

Chronic Pain

Chronic pain is usually defined as long-term (lasting 6 months or longer), persistent, nearly constant, or recurrent pain producing significant negative changes in the client's life. Chronic pain may last long after the pathology is resolved. Although some infants, children, and adolescents experience chronic pain, it is more common in adults. In the United States, one in four individuals lives with chronic pain. Chronic pain is the reason for more than 80% of all physician visits (National Pain Foundation, 2009).

Chronic acute pain occurs almost daily over a long period, months or years, and may never stop. Cancer and severe burns are examples of pathophysiology leading to chronic acute pain. Sometimes the pain ends only at the time of death, as in terminal cancer clients (McCaffery & Pasero, 1999). This type of pain is also called *progressive pain.*

Chronic nonmalignant pain, also called *chronic benign pain*, occurs almost daily and lasts for at least 6 months, ranging from mild to severe intensity. Three critical characteristics of chronic nonmalignant pain are identified by McCaffery and Pasero (1999):

- Caused by non–life-threatening causes
- Not responsive to currently available pain relief methods
- May continue for the rest of the client's life

Examples of pathophysiology leading to chronic nonmalignant pain include the following:

- Many forms of **neuralgia** (paroxysmal pain that extends along the course of one or more nerves)
- Low-back pain
- Rheumatoid arthritis
- Ankylosing spondylitis
- **Phantom limb pain** (a form of neuropathic pain that occurs after amputation with pain sensations referred to an area in the missing portion of the limb)
- **Myofascial pain syndromes** (a group of muscle disorders characterized by pain, muscle spasm, tenderness, stiffness, and limited motion)

When chronic nonmalignant pain is severe enough to disable the client, it is identified as *chronic intractable nonmalignant pain syndrome.*

Signs and Symptoms The signs and symptoms of chronic pain can look very different from those of acute pain. The body cannot tolerate the sympathetic nervous system signs for a long period and, therefore, adapts. Vital signs will often be normal, with no accompanying pupil dilatation or perspiration. Lack of these signs may prompt some health care workers to question the client's description of pain.

The hopelessness, listlessness, and loss of libido (sex drive) and weight of chronic pain are similar to those of depression. The client often describes exhaustion and fatigue. Behaviors include no complaint of pain unless asked and physical inactivity or immobility leading to functional disability. The crying, moaning, guarding, and grimacing that most clinicians associate with pain are absent. Treatment of chronic pain is more complex than that of acute pain. Chronic pain is viewed by pain experts as a disease state rather than a symptom. Management includes identifying the cause of pain, recognizing emotional and environmental factors contributing to the pain, and rehabilitation to improve the client's functional abilities.

PURPOSE OF PAIN

Pain serves as a protective mechanism. If a person touches a hot stove, the pain signal causes the person to pull the hand away immediately. The skin would be seriously burned if this did not happen.

Pain can be a diagnostic tool. The quality and duration of the pain give important clues in determining a client's medical diagnosis. For example, in acute appendicitis, the clinician looks for rebound tenderness (the pain increases after applying firm pressure for several seconds and then quickly releasing the pressure) when palpating the abdomen. This particular type of pain helps confirm the diagnosis of appendicitis rather than other gastrointestinal disorders.

PHYSIOLOGY OF PAIN

When pain occurs, sensory input from injured tissue causes peripheral **nociceptors** (receptive neurons for painful sensations) and central nervous system (CNS) pain pathways to enhance future responses to pain stimuli. Long-lasting changes in cells within the spinal cord **afferent** (ascending) and **efferent** (descending) **pain pathways** may thus occur after a brief noxious stimulus.

Physiological responses (such as elevated blood pressure, respiratory rate, and pulse rate; dilated pupils; perspiration; and pallor) to even a brief acute pain episode will show adaptation within minutes to a few hours. The body cannot sustain the extreme stress response physiologically for more than short periods. The body conserves its resources by physiological adaptation: a return to normal or near normal blood pressure, respiratory rate, and pulse rate; pupil size; and dry skin with little evidence of poor perfusion, *even with continuing pain of the same intensity.*

Stimulation of Pain

The specific action of pain depends on the type of pain. Cutaneous pain rapidly travels through a simple reflex arc from the nerve ending (point of pain) to the spinal cord at approximately 300 feet per second, with a reflex response evoking an almost immediate reaction. This is why, when a hot stove is touched, the person's hand jerks back *before* there is conscious awareness of damage (Figure 27-2). After a hot stove is touched, a sensory nerve ending in the finger skin initiates nerve transmission that travels through the dorsal root ganglion to the dorsal horn in the gray matter of the spinal cord. The impulse then travels though an interneuron that synapses with a motor neuron at the same level in the spinal cord. This motor neuron stimulating the muscle is responsible for the swift movement of the hand away from the hot stove.

In the case of the hot stove, the sensory neuron also synapses with an afferent sensory neuron. The impulse travels up the spinal cord to the thalamus, where a synapse sends the impulse to the brain cortex. Once the impulse is interpreted, the information is consciously available. Then the person is aware of the location, intensity, and quality of pain. Previous experience adds the affective feature to the pain experience.

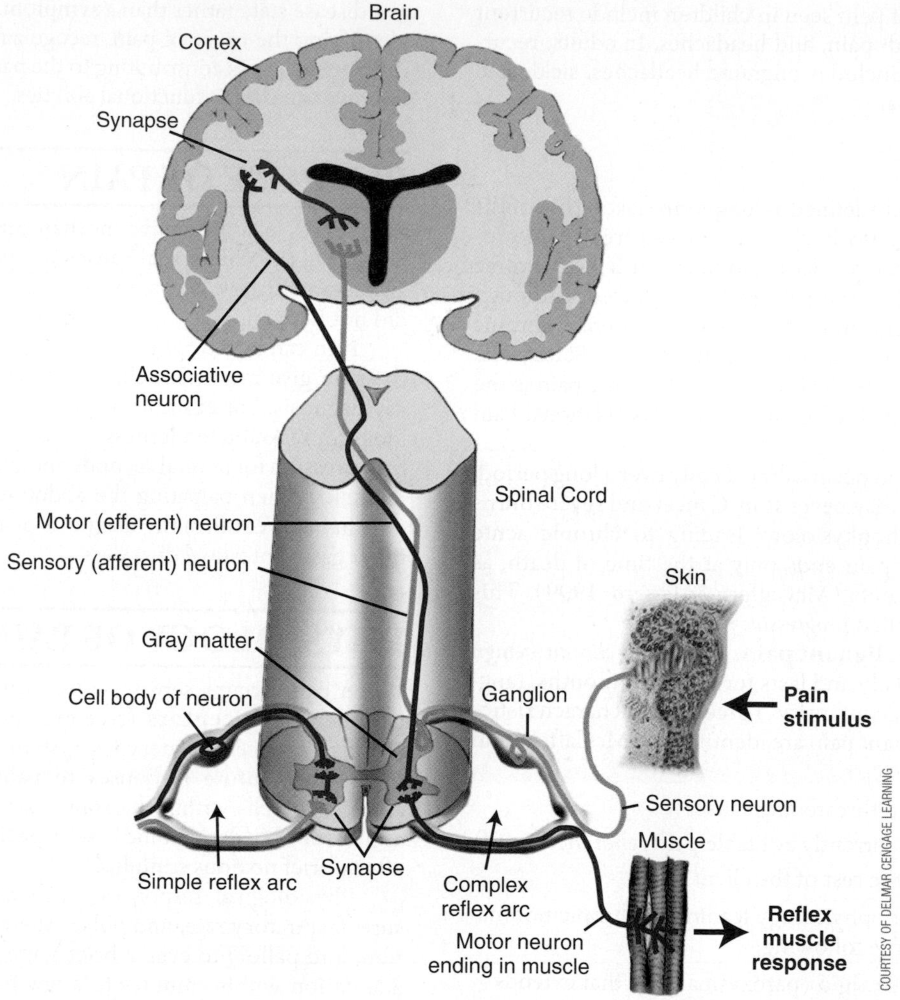

FIGURE 27-2 Reflex Arcs

Descending or efferent motor neuron response moves from the brain through the spinal cord, synapsing with a motor neuron in the spinal cord, and innervates the muscle.

The transmission of visceral pain impulses is slower and less localized than cutaneous pain. Internal organs (including the gastrointestinal tract) have few nociceptors, which is why visceral pain is poorly localized and is felt as a throbbing sensation or dull ache; however, internal organs are very sensitive to distension. The cramping pain of **colic** (acute abdominal pain) results when:

- Constipation or flatus distends the stomach or intestines
- There is hyperperistalsis, as in gastroenteritis
- Something tries to pass through an opening that is too small

The physiology of **ischemic pain**, or pain occurring when the blood supply to an area is restricted or cut off completely, also differs. Blood flow restriction causes inadequate oxygenation of the tissue supplied by those vessels and inadequate removal of metabolic wastes. The onset of ischemic pain is most rapid in an active muscle and much slower in a

PROFESSIONALTIP

Pain in Americans

According to statistics compiled by the American Pain Foundation in 2007, pain impacts the everyday lives of more Americans than cancer, diabetes, and heart disease *combined*—an estimated 76.5 million Americans per day. Adults between the ages of 45 and 64 were the most likely to report pain; adults over age 65 were least likely. This may reflect age-related changes in pain perception or the underassessment of pain in the elderly.

CRITICAL THINKING

Types of Pain

What are the differences among somatic, cutaneous, visceral, referred, ischemic, acute, chronic, and phantom limb pain?

SAFETY

Ischemic Pain

Administer supplemental oxygen and pain medication quickly to clients with ischemic pain to minimize oxygen deprivation and prevent infarction (tissue death).

passive muscle. Examples of ischemic pain are muscle cramps, myocardial infarction, angina pectoris, and sickle cell crisis. When ischemic pain occurs in a muscle that continues to work, a muscle spasm (cramp) occurs. If the blood supply to the heart is completely cut off or severely restricted and not restored quickly, a myocardial infarction occurs.

Substances released from injured tissue in acute pain episodes lead to stress hormone responses. There is an increase in metabolic rate, enhanced breakdown of body tissue, increased blood clotting, impaired immune function, and water retention. The fight-or-flight reaction is triggered, leading to tachycardia and negative emotions.

The Gate Control Theory

Pain transmission and interpretation theories try to describe and explain the pain experience. Early pain theorists focused on the neuroanatomical and neurophysiological mechanisms.

Melzack and Wall (1965) proposed the **gate control pain theory**, which was the first one recognizing that psychological aspects of pain are as important as physiological aspects. The gate control theory combined cognitive, sensory, and emotional components—in addition to the physiological aspects—and proposed that they can act on a gate control system to block the individual's perception of pain. The basic premise is that transmission of potentially painful nerve impulses to the cortex is modulated by a spinal cord gating mechanism and by CNS activity. As a result, the level of conscious awareness of painful sensation is altered.

The theory suggests that nerve fibers that contribute to pain transmission come together at a site in the dorsal horn of the spinal cord. This site is thought to act as a gating mechanism that determines which impulses will be blocked and which will be transmitted to the thalamus. The image of a gate is useful in teaching clients and their families about pain relief measures. If the "gate" is closed, the signal is stopped before it reaches the brain, where awareness of pain occurs. If the gate is open, the signal will continue on through the spinothalamic tract to the cortex, and the client will feel the pain (Figure 27-3). Whether the gate is opened or closed is influenced by impulses from peripheral nerves (the sensory components) and nerve signals that descend from the brain (motivational-affective and cognitive components). For example, stimulation of some types of peripheral nerves by cutaneous stimulation such as massage can close the gate, whereas stimulation of the nociceptors will open the gate.

If a person is anxious, the gate can be opened by signals sent from the brain down to the mechanism in the dorsal horn of the spinal cord. On the other hand, if the person has had positive experiences with pain control in the past, the cognitive influence can send signals down to the gating mechanism and close it. The gate theory offered a great benefit by suggesting new approaches to relieving both acute and chronic pain. Pain could be relieved by blocking the transmission of pain impulses to the brain by both physical modalities and by altering the individual's thought processes, emotions, or other behaviors.

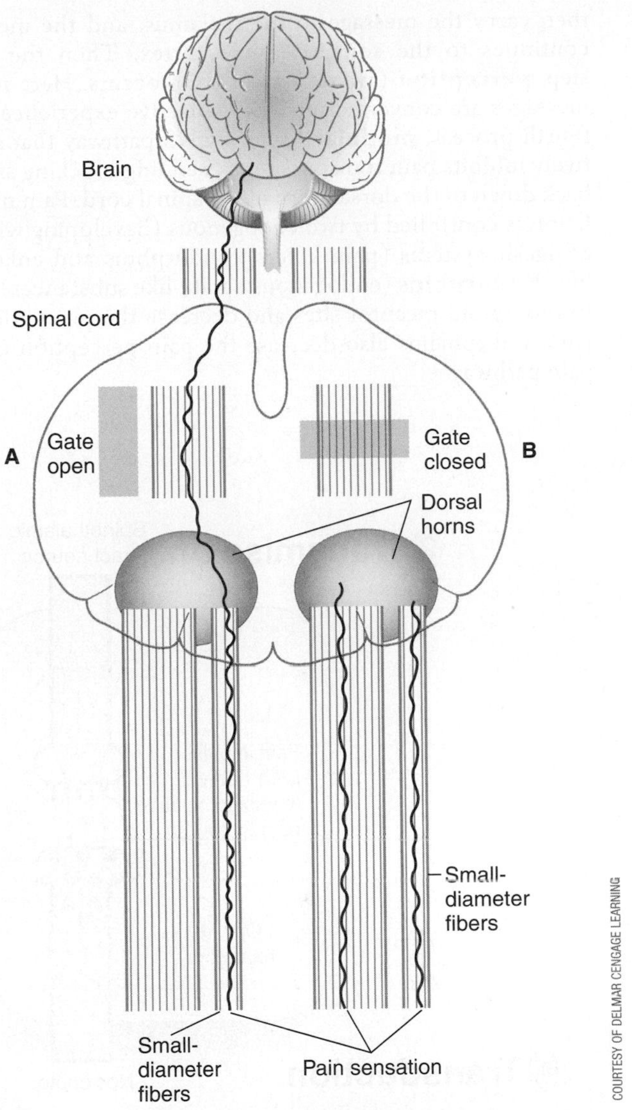

FIGURE 27-3 Gate Control Theory; *A*, An "open gate" allows nerves to transmit pain sensation to the brain; *B*, A "closed gate" stops nerve transmission of pain sensation to the brain.

Conduction of Pain Impulses

Conduction of pain impulses refers to the physiologic processes that occur from the initiation of the pain signal to the realization of pain by the individual. Four processes are involved in the conduction of this signal, as illustrated in Figure 27-4. The first, **transduction**, is when a noxious stimulus triggers electrical activity in the endings of afferent nerve fibers (nociceptors). Once the signal is triggered, **transmission** occurs. The impulse travels from the receiving nociceptors to the spinal cord. Projection neurons then carry the message to the thalamus, and the message continues to the somatosensory cortex. Then the third step, **perception** (awareness) of pain, occurs. Here neural messages are converted into the subjective experience. The fourth process, **modulation**, is a CNS pathway that selectively inhibits pain transmission by sending blocking signals back down to the dorsal horn of the spinal cord. Pain modulation is controlled by two endogenous (developing within) analgesic systems (pain killers): endorphins and enkephalins. **Endorphins** (endogenous opiate-like substances) bind to the opioid receptor sites and decrease the perception of pain. Enkephalins also decrease the pain perception in the pain pathway.

FACTORS AFFECTING THE PAIN EXPERIENCE

According to McCaffery and Pasero (1999), the client is the only authority on the existence and nature of his or her pain. Age, previous experience with pain, drug abuse, and cultural norms account for the differences in clients' individual responses to pain.

AGE

Age can greatly influence clients' perception of pain. Individuals may continue pain behaviors learned as children and may

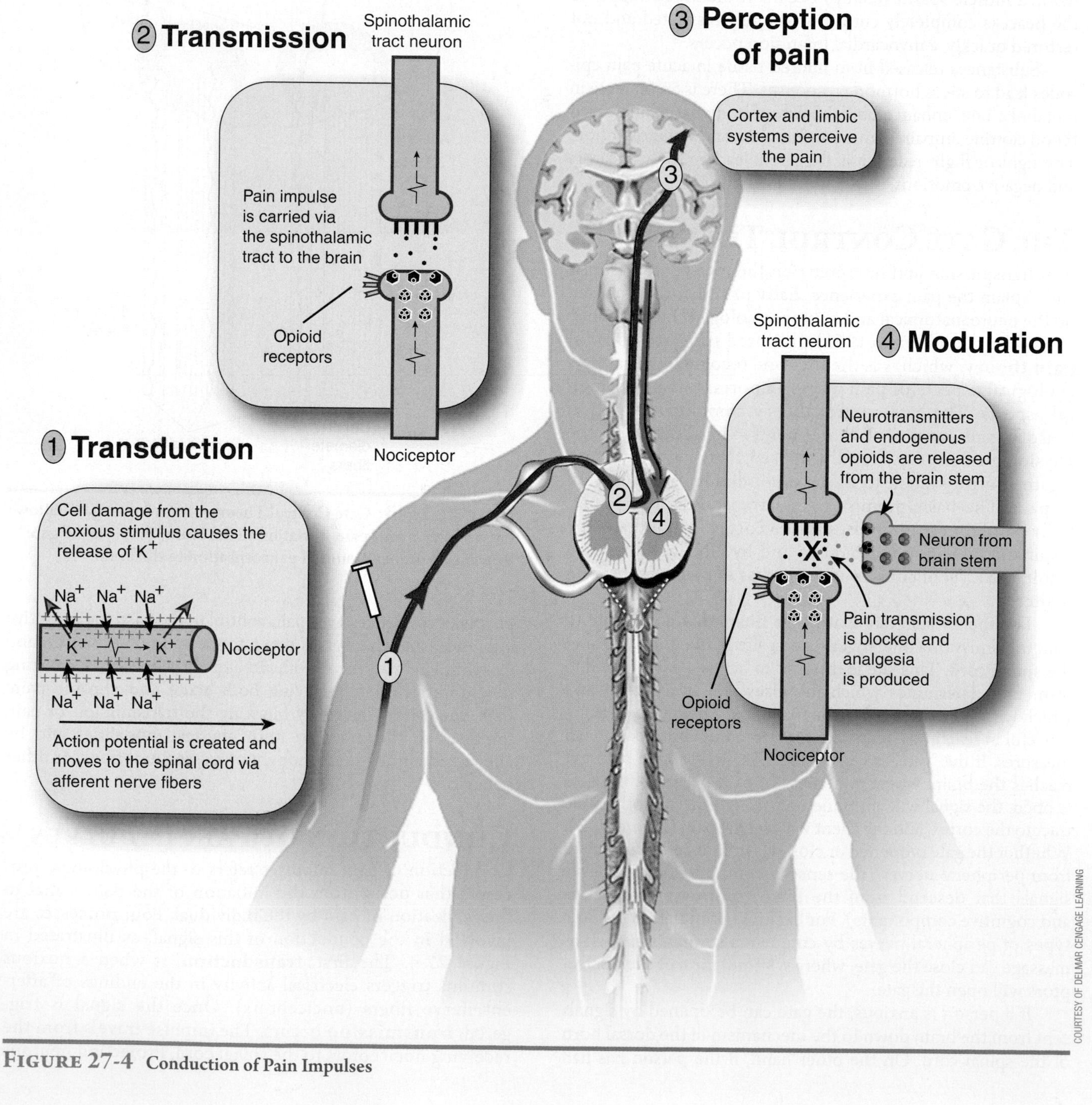

FIGURE 27-4 Conduction of Pain Impulses

LIFE SPAN CONSIDERATIONS

Elders and Pain

Older clients often live with pain, believing that nothing can be done. Pain often is not reported by older clients for fear of being labeled a "bother" or "complainer." Encourage the client to request pain relief as needed.

be reluctant to admit pain or seek medical care because they fear the unknown or fear how treatment may impact their lifestyle. Older adults may ignore their pain, believing it is a consequence of aging. Family and health care members may thoughtlessly support this idea and be less responsive to an older client's complaints of pain.

Previous Pain Experiences

Previous experience with pain often influences clients' reactions. Past coping mechanisms may affect clients' judgments about how pain will affect their lives and which measures they can use to successfully manage the pain on their own. Teaching clients about pain expectations and management methods can often allay their fears and lead to successful pain management.

Drug Abuse

According to Compton (1999), a drug abuser is likely to be *less* tolerant of pain than someone who does not use drugs. Drug abuse may cause changes in the central nervous system, resulting in an exaggerated neurophysiologic response to painful stimuli. To keep a drug abuser comfortable, withdrawal must be prevented.

Cultural Norms

Cultural differences in pain responses can lead to pain management problems. Studies on subjects of various cultures found no significant difference among the groups in the intensity level at which pain becomes perceptible. The same studies showed that the intensity level or duration of pain the client was willing to endure differed significantly. Cultural values guide the expression of pain. Some cultures tolerate pain and "suffering in silence," whereas others fully express pain, including physical and emotional responses. Be careful not to equate the level of pain expression with the level of actual pain experienced but consider cultural and other influences that affect the expression of pain.

JOINT COMMISSION STANDARDS

Each institution should have clearly defined standards for pain management. The Joint Commission Pain Management Standards of Care has made pain management a priority and requires that pain be assessed on admission and throughout the client's stay in an institution. Relating to pain management, the health care organizations are expected to:

- Recognize the right of clients to appropriate assessment and management of their pain
- Assess pain in all clients
- Record the results of the assessment in a way that facilitates regular reassessment and follow-up
- Educate relevant providers in pain assessment and management
- Determine competency in pain assessment and management
- Establish policies and procedures that support appropriate prescription or ordering of pain medications
- Ensure that pain does not interfere with participation in rehabilitation
- Educate clients and their families about the importance of effective pain management
- Include clients' needs for symptom management in the discharge planning process
- Collect data to monitor the appropriateness and effectiveness of pain management (Integrative Pain Center of Arizona, 2003; Joint Commission, 2009; Teeter & Kemper, 2008b)

NURSING PROCESS

The nursing process provides the framework for managing a client's pain.

Assessment

Assessment of the client's pain is a crucial nursing function. During the assessment process, be aware of your own values and expectations about pain behaviors. Just as the client's experience and cultural background help determine how pain is demonstrated, nurses' cultures and experiences help determine which pain behaviors are viewed as acceptable. Be aware of these values and avoid biases when assessing client pain and planning client care. Once a self-assessment about pain has been conducted, the nurse is ready to assess the client.

Pain as the fifth vital sign is assessed and recorded along with the client's temperature, pulse, respiration, and blood pressure. Pain assessment tools are the most effective method to

MEMORY**TRICK**

Pain Assessment PQRST

P = What Provokes the pain (aggravating factors) and palliative measures (alleviating factors)

Q = Quality of pain (gnawing, pounding, burning, stabbing, pinching, aching, throbbing, and crushing)

R = Region (location) and radiation to other body sites

S = Severity (quantity of pain on 0–10 scale: 0 = no pain and 10 = worst pain experienced) and setting (what causes the pain)

T = Timing (onset, duration, frequency)

(Adapted from Estes, 2010.)

COMPLETE WITH 1ST DOSE OF PAIN MEDICATION

1. Onset and frequency (When did it start?) (How often) ________
2. Provokes (What makes it worse?) ________
3. Radiates? ________
4. Severity/Intensity (What is an acceptable level of pain [0–10]) ________
5. Timing/Duration (How long does it last?) ________
6. Past & Current analgesic/alternative modalities that make it better. ________
7. Does your pain affect: sleep__ appetite__ physical activity__ emotions__ social relationships__

COMMENTS:

INITIALS	SIGNATURE

Source of Information	Side Effects:	Safety:
1=Patient	1=Nausa/Vomiting	1=Bed low
2=Child	2=Resp. Depression	2=Call bell in reach
3=Parent	3=Pruritis	3=Side rails ×2
4=Nurse	4=Urinary Retention	4=Side rails ×4
5=Family	5=Altered Mental Status	5=Bed alert
6=Other	6=None	6=Family/Sitter

Pediatrics/Noncommunicative Clients (0–10)

A. Verbal/Vocal	B. Body Movements	C. Facial	D. Touching (localizing pain)
0=positive	0=moves easily	0=smiling	0=no touching
1=other complaint, whimper	1=neutral shifting	1=neutral	1=reaching, patting
2=pain, crying	2=tense, flailing arms & legs	2=frown, grimace	2=grabbing
3=screaming		3=clenched teeth	

Nonpharmacological Interventions		Pediatrics	Mode of Administration		
1=Cold	7=Massage				
2=Distractions	8=Music	13=Holding	PCA	SQ	Rectal (R)
3=Environmental Control	9=Positioning	14=Rocking	IV	PO	Nasal (N)
4=Exercises	10=Relaxation	15=Pacifier	IM	SL	
5=Heat	11=TENS	16=Security object	Epidural (EP)		
6=Imagery	12=Spiritual Care		Transdermal (TD)		

LEVEL OF CONSCIOUSNESS KEY (LOC)*

1. Alert, engages in conversation; puposefully travels with eyes, if mute
2. Lethargic, drowsy, sedate—focuses on personal interchange—but unable to maintain focus
3. Responds only to maximal stimulation (shaking). Response only a grunt or moan—not a clear sentance.
4. Coma—unable to respond at all.

Date/ Time	Location of Pain	Character: Dull, Stabbing, Pressure, Sharp, Throbbing	Severity Rating 0–10	Pharmacologic// (Med Name)/ Nonpharmacologic	Mode of Adminis-tration	Source of Information	B	P	R	LOC / Side Effects	Safety	Time of Evaluation	Evaluation of Interventions/ Frequency Rating 0–10 Response/ Comments	Initails

2006

CHRISTUS SPOHN HEALTH SYSTEM

PAIN MANAGEMENT FLOW SHEET
PATIENT CARE SERVICES

2763751

NEW: 07/99
REVISED: 05/30/2001
FM15

FIGURE 27-5 Pain Assessment and Management *(Courtesy of CHRISTUS Spohn Health System, Corpus Christi, TX.)*

PROFESSIONALTIP

Location of Pain

During intershift report on a postoperative client recovering from abdominal surgery, the nurse reported that the client had stated she had pain and had been medicated with IM Demerol. When greeting her client, the nurse asked the client about the pain she had experienced during the night. The client replied, "Oh, it is fine now, I only had a headache." The night nurse had assumed the client's pain was in her surgical site and chose the medication accordingly. The headache probably could have been relieved with a milder medication. All reports of pain must be thoroughly assessed before implementing any interventions.

identify the presence and intensity of pain in clients. Good nursing practice uses pain assessment tools and accepts the results of the tools (Figure 27-5). Using the "PQRST" mnemonic is an ideal way for a nurse to assess a client's pain. This method is described in the Memory Trick "Pain Assessment PQRST."

Subjective Data

The first step in pain assessment is gathering subjective information regarding the client's pain. A client's pain threshold and pain tolerance level is determined. **Pain threshold** is the intensity level where a person feels pain. It varies with each individual and with each type of pain. **Pain tolerance** is the intensity level or duration of pain the client is able or willing to endure.

The client's description of the pain covers several qualifiers, including its location, onset and duration, quality, intensity, aggravating factors (variables that worsen the pain, such as exercise, certain foods, or stress), alleviating factors (measures the client can take that lessen the effect of the pain, such as lying down, avoiding certain foods, or taking medication), associated manifestations (factors that often accompany the pain, such as nausea, constipation, or dizziness), and what pain means to the client.

Whenever subjective and objective data conflict, the subjective reports of pain are to be considered the primary source.

Location The client can point to the location of the pain on the client's own body or locate it on a body diagram on a pain assessment tool. Ask the client if there is more than one site of pain; if the pain radiates and, if so, to where; and if the pain is deep or superficial.

Onset and Duration Ask the client how long the pain has existed; what, if anything, triggers its onset; and if there are any patterns to the pain (e.g., whether it is worse at certain times of the day or night).

Quality Ask the client what the pain feels like, and record the words used to describe the pain. Clients may use sensory-type words, such as "pricking," "radiating," "burning," or "throbbing." Other clients use words that have an affective connotation, such as "fearful," "sickening," or "punishing." Other words used may be evaluative, such as "miserable" or "unbearable." The quality of pain provides information that may be useful in diagnosing the cause of the pain. For example, pain described as "burning" or "freezing" is usually neuropathic in origin.

Intensity The client may have difficulty in judging the intensity of pain; however, it is important to obtain an estimate of the severity of the pain. This information allows the clinician to evaluate the effectiveness of pain relief measures tried by comparing intensity before and after the interventions.

Pain intensity scales are an effective method for clients to rate the intensity of their pain (Figure 27-6). The simple descriptive pain-intensity scale and the visual analog scale (VAS) are best used by showing the scale to the client and asking the client to point to the spot on the scale that corresponds to the present pain. The pain scale most frequently used with adolescent and adult clients is the verbal 0-to-10 scale. It needs no equipment or supplies and requires only one question: "On a scale of 0 to 10, with 0 being no pain at all and 10 being the worst pain possible, how much do you hurt right now?" If there are multiple painful areas, this question can be asked regarding each area. A study by Twycross et al. (1996) showed that pain ratings of 4 or higher on a 0-to-10 scale interfered with client activities and that scores of 6 and 7 markedly interfered with client quality of life. This study with other studies (Cleeland & Syrjala, 1992) and clinical experience have brought clinicians to believe that a pain level of

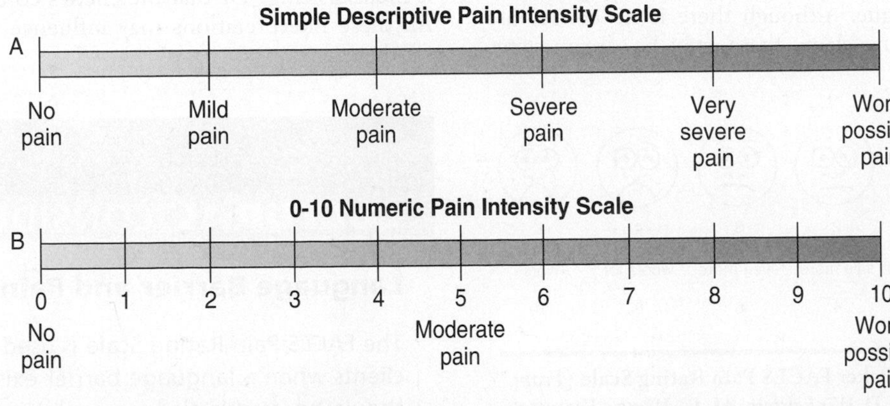

FIGURE 27-6 **Pain Intensity Scales; *A*, Simple Descriptive Pain Intensity Scale; *B*, 0-10 Numeric Pain Intensity Scale** *(Courtesy of Acute Pain Management: Operative or Medical Procedures and Trauma. Clinical Practice Guideline [AHCPR Publication No. 92-0032].)*

CLIENT TEACHING

Pain at Night

Teach the client that pain is commonly worse at night, when there are fewer distractions. If the client knows this fact, he will not attribute the increased pain to complications.

3 indicates a need to change the pain intervention plan with an increase in analgesics, and/or other medications, or interventions (Office of Quality and Performance, U.S. Department of Veterans Affairs, 2008). Clients must be taught how to correctly use the pain intensity scale.

Although developed for use with children, the FACES Pain Rating Scale (Figure 27-7) can be used effectively with clients when a language barrier exists. A translator is used initially to explain what the faces represent.

Another pain assessment tool is the "Painometer" developed by Dr. Gaston-Johansson (Mattson, 2000). The client positions a pointer between "no pain" and "worst possible pain." Quantifying numbers are on the back. The client also indicates the quality of pain by selecting sensory and affective descriptors from a list.

Aggravating and Alleviating Factors Ask the client about what makes the pain worse and what makes the pain better, including behaviors or activities that influence the pain. This information helps develop the plan of care for the client in pain. If specific activities relieve the pain, incorporate them into the care plan. Being aware of activities that increase the pain can allow for interventions that may prevent the pain. For example, if physical therapy exercises trigger an increase in pain, administer an analgesic according to physician's or nurse practitioner's orders before the treatment.

Associated Manifestations The initial pain assessment includes the impact of pain on the activities of daily living. Pain may cause changes in sleep patterns or the ability to work and carry out the many roles in a client's life. Pain may affect appetite, mood, sexual functioning, or the ability to participate in recreational activities. If pain is interfering with daily life, the client's quality of life is greatly affected.

Pain is fatiguing. It requires a significant amount of energy to deal with pain. The longer a person has pain, the greater the level of fatigue. Although there is no conscious awareness of pain during sleep, there may be dream-state awareness (McCaffery & Pasero, 1999). The stress response (which can be seen even in clients under general anesthesia) continues, and the body physiologically pays the price. Clients also wake up with more pain than they had going to sleep, thereby requiring even more intervention (pharmacologic and nonpharmacologic) to reduce the pain.

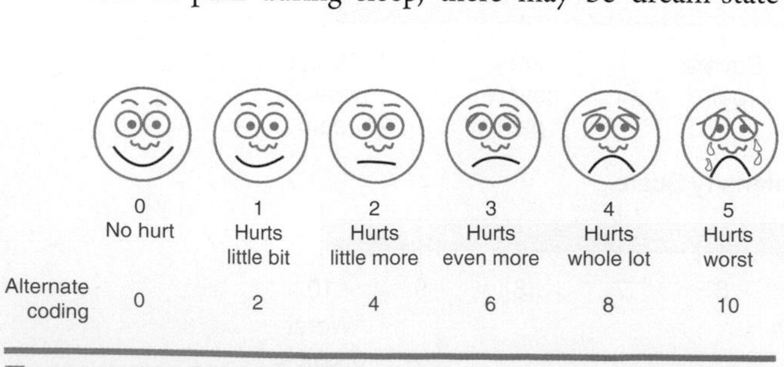

FIGURE 27-7 Wong/Baker FACES Pain Rating Scale *(From Hockenberry, M. J., Wilson, D. Winkelstein, M. L., Wong's Essentials of Pediatric Nursing, ed 7, St. Louis, 2005, p. 1259. Used with permission. Copyright Mosby.)*

LIFE SPAN CONSIDERATIONS

Children and Pain Assessment

Children provide a special challenge in pain assessment. Two useful tools for assessing pain in children are the Wong/Baker FACES Pain Rating Scale and the Oucher scale.

- The Wong/Baker FACES Pain Rating Scale can be used with children as young as 3 years. It helps children express their level of pain by pointing to a cartoon face that most closely resembles how they are feeling (Figure 27-7).
- The Oucher pediatric pain intensity scale (Figure 27-8) consists of two scales: a 0-to-10 numeric scale and a 6-point facial scale. If the child can count from 1 to 10, the numeric scale is used; if not, the facial scale is used. The facial scale has been successfully used in children as young as 3 to 4 years.

Meaning of Pain Because of the motivational-affective components of the pain experience, the meaning of pain can have a great impact on how the client perceives the pain. A frequently cited classic study on this phenomenon was conducted by Beecher (1956), who compared the pain perceived by soldiers wounded in battle to pain perceived by civilians with similar surgical wounds. He found that only 32% of the soldiers required narcotics for pain relief, whereas 85% of the civilians needed the narcotics. This was interpreted that for the soldiers, the wound represented a ticket away from the battlefield; for the civilians, the surgical wound was a depressing event.

Explore with the client what implications the pain may have for the individual. Does it mean that the client's cancer is metastasizing? Or that the client's condition is worsening? All these interpretations may influence the pain experience for the client.

CULTURAL CONSIDERATIONS

Language Barrier and Pain

The FACES Pain Rating Scale is used effectively with clients when a language barrier exists. A translator should be used initially to explain what the faces represent.

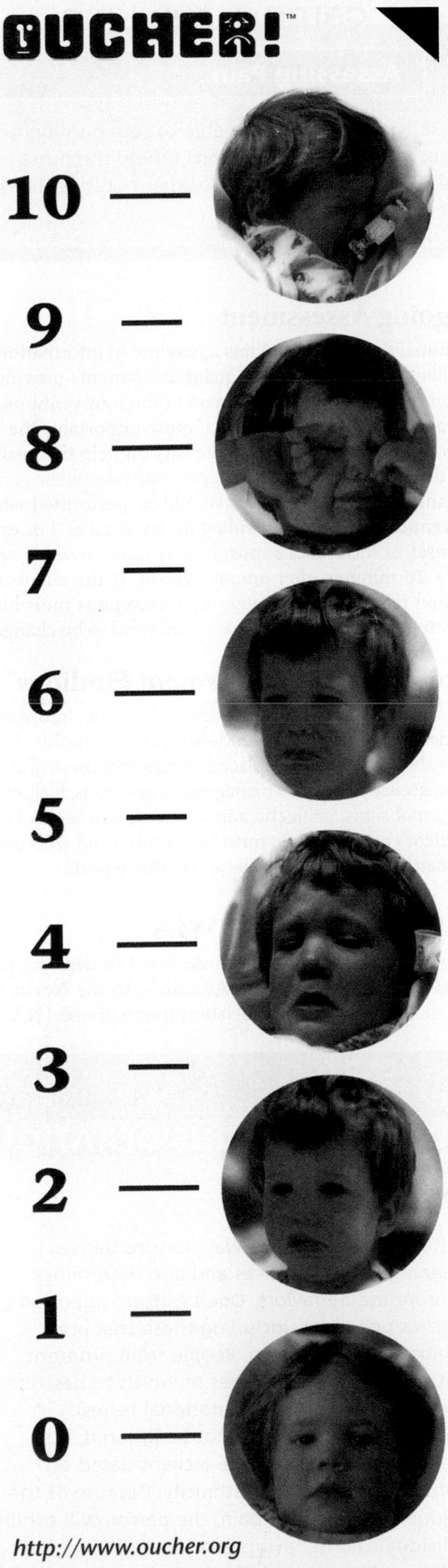

THE OUCHER: A SUMMARY

What is the OUCHER?

The OUCHER is a poster developed for children to help them communicate how much pain or hurt they feel. There are two scales on the OUCHER: A number scale for older children and a picture scale for younger children.

Which scale should be used?

Children who are able to count to 100 by ones or tens and who understand, for example, that 71 is greater than 43, can use the numerical scale. Children who do not understand numbers should use the picture scale. Some children who are able to use the number scale might prefer to use the picture scale. Ask the child which scale he or she would prefer.

How do I use the OUCHER?

Picture scale: The following is an example of how to explain the picture scale to a younger child. The words can be changed when using the picture scale with an older child.

This is a poster called the OUCHER. It helps children tell others how much hurt they have. (For younger children, it might be useful to ask: Do you know what I mean by hurt? If the child is not sure, then an explanation should be provided.) Here's how this works. This picture shows not hurt (point to the bottom picture), this picture shows just a little bit of hurt (point to the 2nd picture), this picture shows a little more hurt (point to the 3rd picture), this picture shows even more hurt (point to the 4th picture), this picture shows a lot of hurt (point to the 5th picture), and this picture shows the biggest hurt you could ever have (point to the 6th picture). Can you point to the picture that shows how much hurt you are having right now?

Once a child selects a picture, their picture selection is changed to a number score from 0-10.

10 – Picture at the top of the scale
8 – Second picture from the top
6 – Third picture from the top
4 – Fourth picture from the top
2 – Fifth picture from the top
0 – Picture at the bottom of the scale

Number scale: The following is an example of how to explain the number scale.

This is a poster called the OUCHER. It helps children tell others how much hurt they have. Here's how it works. 0 means no hurt. Here (point to the lower third of the scale, about 1 to 3), this means you have little hurts; here (point to the middle third of the scale, about 3 to 6) it means you have middle hurts. If your hurt is about here (point to the upper third of the scale, about 6 to 9), it means you have big hurts. But if you point to 10, it means you have the biggest hurt you could ever have. Can you point to the number (or tell me which number) that is like the hurt you are having right now?

The pain score for the number scale is the exact number from 0 to 10 that the child gives you.

What does the score mean? How should it be used?

The person who has pain is the expert or the one who knows best how the pain feels. The OUCHER score gives parents, teachers, nurses, and doctors some idea of how much pain the child is feeling. OUCHER scores can be used as a means to see if certain actions used to relieve pain, such as rest, applying heat or cold, eating or drinking, and medicine make a difference in how much pain the child feels. OUCHER scores can be recorded over a period of hours or days and would be useful information to share with nurses and doctors.

Remember, OUCHER scores only communicate how much pain the child is feeling. Other observations, such as changes in activity, location of the pain, what it feels like, and how long it lasts, are important. If you, as a parent or teacher, are concerned about the child's pain, you should contact your health care provider.

For information about the Oucher, write to: Dr. Judith E. Beyer, P.O. Box 411714, Kansas City, MO 64141 or go to the www.OUCHER.com website.

FIGURE 27-8 **The Oucher Pain Assessment Tool: For Use with Children 3-12 Years of Age. Caucasian, Hispanic, and African American versions are available.** *(The Caucasian version of the Oucher, developed and copyrighted by Judith E. Beyer, RN, PhD, 1983.)*

Objective Data

As discussed when addressing acute versus chronic pain, the objective data often present a different picture depending on the type of pain the client is experiencing.

Physiologic Acute pain activates the sympathetic nervous system, and the client may exhibit elevated heart rate, elevated respiratory rate, elevated blood pressure, diaphoresis, pallor, muscle tension, and dilated pupils. These signs resemble those of anxiety, which often accompanies acute pain. The signs and symptoms of chronic pain show adaptation and, therefore, are different from those of acute pain, with vital signs being normal and no accompanying pupil dilation or perspiration.

Behavioral Acute pain behaviors may include crying and moaning, rubbing the site of pain, restlessness, a distorted posture, clenched fists, guarding the painful area, frowning, and grimacing. The client usually speaks of the discomfort and may be restless or afraid to move.

The client in chronic pain may demonstrate behaviors similar to those of depression, such as hopelessness, listlessness, and loss of libido and weight. Chronic pain often leads to physical inactivity or immobility, which can lead to functional disability. **Distraction** (focusing attention on stimuli other than pain) may also be used by clients. According to McCaffery and Pasero (1999), clients often minimize the pain behaviors they are able to control for several reasons, including:

- To be a "good" client and avoid making demands
- To maintain a positive self-image by not being a "sissy"
- Distraction makes pain more bearable (young children are particularly adept at this)
- Exhaustion

Client pain behaviors include splinting of the painful area, distorted posture, impaired mobility, anxiety, insomnia, attention seeking, and depression. Occasionally, a discrepancy exists between pain behaviors observed by the nurse (objective data) and the client's self-report of pain. Discrepancies between behaviors and the client's self-report can result from good coping skills (e.g., relaxation techniques or distraction), anxiety, stoicism, or cultural differences in pain behaviors. Whenever these discrepancies occur, they should be addressed with the client and the pain management plan renegotiated accordingly.

PROFESSIONALTIP

Assessing the Effect of Pain on Sleep

Questioning clients about the effect pain has on their sleep habits will help clarify the intensity of the pain and its effect on the clients' patterns of daily living. Ask the client whether the pain:

- Prevents the client from falling asleep
- Makes it difficult to find a comfortable sleeping position
- Wakes the client from a sound sleep
- Prevents the client from falling back to sleep
- Leaves the client feeling tired and unrefreshed after sleeping

CRITICAL THINKING

Assessing Pain

A 38-year-old client is unable to rate his pain on a 0-to-10 scale. What actions should the nurse take to perform a pain assessment on this client? (Teeter & Kemper, 2008a).

Ongoing Assessment

The initial assessment obtains a baseline of information about the client's pain, while subsequent assessments provide information regarding the effectiveness of the interventions. Physiologic and behavioral signs and, most important, the client's subjective pain ratings of the intensity all help the health care team determine whether the interventions should be continued or changed. Pain assessments should be performed when the intervention should be providing the most relief. For example, the onset of intravenous morphine is rapid, peaking approximately 20 minutes after administration. If the client has not obtained relief by 20 minutes, the intravenous morphine was ineffective, and the plan of care would need to be changed.

Recording Pain Assessment Findings

Pain assessment is of little value unless the information is recorded in a manner easily understood by the health care team. A flow sheet provides one place to document most of the information used to make pain management decisions, including pain rating, vital signs, analgesic administered, and level of arousal. The client's report of pain must be accepted and recorded, with pain management decisions based on that report.

Nursing Diagnoses

The two primary nursing diagnoses used to describe pain are *Acute **Pain*** and *Chronic **Pain***. According to the North American Nursing Diagnosis Association-International (NANDA-I,

CULTURAL CONSIDERATIONS

Perception of Pain

Culture determines the way persons derive meaning from their lives and also determines appropriate behaviors. One's cultural upbringing teaches behaviors, including those that are exhibited when in pain. People from different cultures use different types of words to describe pain (e.g., in sensory or emotional terms). These differences should not be ignored, but be careful not to prejudge a client based on cultural background or ethnicity. Because of the unique experience of pain, the person will exhibit individualized behaviors even though they are influenced by cultural upbringing.

2010), *Acute* ***P****ain* is defined as "an unpleasant sensory and emotional experience arising from actual or potential tissue damage or described in terms of such damage . . . [with] sudden or slow onset of any intensity from mild to severe, with an anticipated or predictable end and a duration of less than 6 months." *Chronic* ***P****ain* is defined the same as *Acute* ***P****ain*, with the last phrase replaced by "constant or recurring without an anticipated or predictable end and a duration of greater than 6 months."

Pain may be the etiology (cause) of other problems (e.g., *Impaired Physical* ***M****obility*, related to arthritic hip pain). Whether the pain is addressed in the problem statement or the etiology is determined by the client's primary problem. Many diagnoses can be related to the client in pain depending on the effects of the pain:

- *Activity* ***I****ntolerance*
- ***A****nxiety*
- ***C****onstipation*
- *Deficient* ***K****nowledge (specify)*
- *Disturbed* ***B****ody Image*
- *Disturbed* ***S****leep Pattern*
- ***F****atigue*
- ***F****ear*
- ***H****opelessness*
- *Impaired* ***S****ocial Interaction*
- *Ineffective* ***B****reathing Pattern*
- *Ineffective* ***C****oping*
- *Ineffective* ***R****ole Performance*
- *Ineffective* ***S****elf-Health Management*
- ***P****owerlessness*

PLANNING/OUTCOME IDENTIFICATION

When planning care, mutual goal setting with the client experiencing pain is of utmost importance. The nurse and client work together to develop realistic outcomes. Consider both nonpharmacologic and pharmacologic interventions.

Often, several approaches must be combined for adequate relief to be obtained. No matter which type of intervention is being utilized, general principles apply: individualization, prevention, and utilization of a multidisciplinary approach.

Individualize the Approach

A variety of pain relief measures can be tried in many combinations until the goal of pain relief is reached. This often means some trial-and-error of interventions until the right combination is found. It is important to include measures that the client believes will be effective. The cognitive component of pain perception can have a powerful influence on the effectiveness of interventions. This may mean including folk remedies or nonscientific relief measures. It is important to keep an open mind. This comes with the caution to avoid those remedies that may harm the client.

Use a Preventive Approach

Pain is much easier to control if it is treated before it gets severe. Interventions should be implemented when pain is mild or when it is anticipated. For example, medicate a client before a painful dressing change or treatment rather than waiting for the pain to occur.

Use a Multidisciplinary Approach

Pain relief is a complex phenomenon requiring input from various members of the health care team. The nurse's role is pivotal in managing a client's pain. The physician also plays a key role, diagnosing and treating the medical cause of the pain, which includes prescribing appropriate medications. In complex cases, other professionals, such as physical therapists, psychologists, social workers, or chaplains, may be needed. The multidisciplinary team approach is the most successful way to manage chronic pain and improve the quality of a client's life.

IMPLEMENTATION

Pharmacologic and nonpharmacologic interventions can both be effective in caring for clients in pain. Nonpharmacologic techniques may be the primary intervention in some cases of mild pain, with medication available as "backup." Cases of moderate to severe pain may use nonpharmacologic techniques as effective adjunctive, or complementary, treatment.

There are three categories of pain control interventions: pharmacological, noninvasive, and invasive. Each category is discussed separately, but these methods are often used in combination.

Pharmacological Interventions

Caring for a client experiencing pain is a collaborative process. Drug therapy is the mainstay of treatment for pain control. The American Pain Society (APS) provides pain management guidelines that can be used as a framework for providing drug therapy in pain control (APS, 2006; Gordon et al., 2005). These guidelines are based on pain management research and thus are termed *evidence-based*. These guidelines represent concise information that can help nurses, physicians, and other health care workers effectively administer medications for pain relief. The word *action* incorporates these principles of pain management and can be recalled by using the acronym in the "ACTION" Memory Trick (Teeter & Kemper, 2008b).

MEMORYTRICK

Principles of Pain Management

Use the acronym "ACTION" to recall the principles of pain management:

A = Assess clients for pain at regular intervals
C = Choose a variety of interventions for pain
T = Treat pain promptly to avoid escalation of pain
I = Include client-specific cultural, spiritual, and developmental considerations in the pain management plan
O = Optimize the pain management plan through ongoing evaluation
N = Negotiate pain interventions and goals with the client to enhance adherence to the plan

(APS, 2006; Gordon et al., 2005; Teeter and Kemper, 2008b)

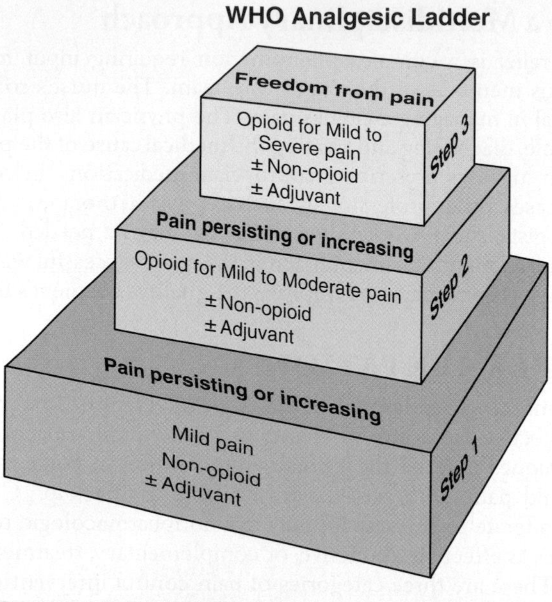

FIGURE 27-9 The WHO analgesic ladder gives guidelines for choosing analgesic therapy for cancer pain based on the level of pain the client is experiencing *(Courtesy of World Health Organization, 2008, Used with permission.)*

The World Health Organization (WHO, 1990) has made worldwide relief of cancer pain one of its primary goals. In order to help meet this goal, it developed an analgesic ladder to help the clinician determine which analgesic to prescribe (Figure 27-9). Step 1 is for mild pain and includes a nonopioid with or without an adjuvant medication. If pain persists or increases, an opioid for mild to moderate pain can be added (step 2). Step 3, for pain that continues or increases despite step 2 treatments, recommends an opioid for moderate to severe pain with or without a nonopioid or an adjuvant.

All the nonopioids have ceiling doses; that is, if the dose is increased above a certain level, no additional pain relief is provided, only an increase in adverse or toxic effects. This is important to remember for clients who are receiving several medications that contain a nonopioid. For example, a client may be prescribed both acetaminophen for fever and Percocet (a combination drug containing acetaminophen and oxycodone) for pain. Be sure to consider both sources of acetaminophen to ensure that the client does not exceed the 24-hour ceiling dose of 4 grams. Liver necrosis can result from acetaminophen overdose (Lehne, 2004).

Opioids are recommended on step 2 and step 3 of the WHO Pain Relief Ladder. Weak opioids (step 2) include codeine, hydrocodone, and oxycodone. Most often, these drugs are administered orally in combination products containing acetaminophen. As noted previously, dosing of combination products is limited by the ceiling dose of nonopioids. Strong opioids (step 3), such as morphine, hydromorphone, and fentanyl, are given for severe pain (Teeter & Kemper, 2008b). Combining analgesics and the use of adjuvant medication provides effective pharmacologic intervention for clients with pain. **Adjuvant medications** are those drugs used to enhance the analgesic efficacy of opioids, to treat concurrent symptoms that exacerbate pain, and to provide independent analgesia for specific types of pain. The ladder recommends that the analgesic, plus or minus an adjuvant, is chosen based on the level of pain the client is experiencing. This ladder gives health care workers guidelines in determining if the drug regimen is appropriate for the client with cancer pain.

Nurses' Role in Administration of Analgesics The nurse spends the most time with the client in pain and is the team member who most often assesses the effectiveness of pain control interventions. When analgesics are prescribed, the nurse often has choices of drug, route, and interval. For example, the postoperative client may have the following orders:

- Morphine 2.5 to 15 mg IV every 2 to 4 hours prn severe pain
- Vicodin one to two tabs every 3 to 4 hours prn moderate pain

When this client complains of pain, which analgesic should the nurse administer? Which route? Which dose? How frequently? The nurse has a large responsibility in making these decisions but also has autonomy in making these decisions.

McCaffery and Pasero (1999) identify the following as the responsibilities of the nurse in administering analgesics:

- Determine whether to give the analgesic, and if more than one is ordered, which one.
- Assess the client's response to the analgesic, including assessing the effectiveness in pain relief and occurrence of any side effects.
- Report to the physician when a change is needed, including making suggestions for changes based on the nurse's knowledge of the client and pharmacology.
- Teach the client and family regarding the use of analgesics.

Principles of Administering Analgesics "How an analgesic is used is probably more important than which one is used" (McCaffery & Pasero, 1999). Principles should be applied in the administration of analgesics, no matter which one is given.

Establishing and maintaining a therapeutic serum level is important. Peaks and valleys often occur when analgesics are administered in the traditional PRN (as needed) manner. When the dose is administered on an intermittent schedule, a larger dose is often required, causing the client to have a peak serum drug level in the sedation range. The client must wait for the return of pain before requesting the next dose of analgesic. Depending on the length of time it takes to obtain the medication and, once taken, to reestablish an adequate blood level, there could be a period of up to an hour or so without adequate pain control.

Preventive Approach Pain is much easier to control if treated when it is anticipated or at a mild intensity. Once pain becomes severe, the analgesics ordered may not be effective enough to relieve it. Many clinicians still teach their clients to wait to take medication until they are sure they really need it. This practice leads to uncontrolled pain. There are two ways the preventive approach may be implemented:

- ATC (around the clock). When pain is predictable, for example, the first few days following surgery or with

CLIENT TEACHING

Timed-Release Tablets

Emphasize that the extended-release tablets become immediate release if crushed (e.g., for a client who has difficulty swallowing the tablet).

CLIENT TEACHING

Pain Management

- It is import to take or request pain medication before the pain becomes severe and more difficult to control.
- Numerous nonpharmacologic approaches can be used to augment pharmacologic pain management.
- Pain management is individual. (The client may be taking different medications or dosages than other individuals.)

chronic cancer pain, the medication is administered on a scheduled basis. This prevents the peaks and valleys of serum drug level that can lead to oversedation or toxicity and recurrence of pain, respectively. If the analgesics are ordered by the physician to be given PRN, it can still be a nursing measure to administer the drugs ATC, as long as they are given within the time constraints of the order.

- PRN (Latin for *pro re nata*, which means "as required"). Pain is not always predictable; therefore PRN dosing may be required. For some clients this may be used in addition to scheduled dosing for "breakthrough" pain (pain that surpasses the level of **analgesia**, or pain relief without anesthesia, that the steady level of analgesics is providing). Examples of this include a cancer client on prolonged-release morphine who needs extra analgesics to participate in activities such as shopping or receiving visitors. Another example would be the orthopedic client who is receiving regularly scheduled analgesics for postoperative pain who needs additional pain relief for therapy sessions. In order to implement the preventive approach with PRN dosing, the medications are given as soon as the pain appears, or when it is anticipated to begin.

Titrate to Effect Because of the unique nature of the pain experience, the analgesic regimen needs to be titrated until the desired effect is achieved. This involves adjusting the following:

- *Dosage*. Some clients may require more or less than the standard dose. Many factors may influence the pharmacokinetics in an individual client. The individual's response is assessed, and the dosage of the analgesic is regulated accordingly. In clients with chronic cancer pain, opioid analgesics are increased until pain relief is obtained or unacceptable side effects occur. This may be done because of the lack of a **ceiling effect** (the dosage beyond which no further analgesia occurs) in pure opioids. The lack of a ceiling effect means there is no limit to the dose that can be given. For example, cancer clients have been known to receive more than 1 gram per hour intravenously. Because the dosage is gradually increased, the client develops a **tolerance** (requiring larger and larger doses of an analgesic to achieve the same level of pain relief) to the side effects of the opioid.
- *Interval*. Some clients metabolize the analgesics faster than others. For example, young adults tend to metabolize opioids faster; therefore, they may need more frequent doses. Older clients tend to metabolize them slower, so they require a longer interval between doses.
- *Route*. The appropriate route is chosen depending on how rapidly pain relief is required, the client's ability to take medications orally, the client's diagnosis, and assessment of the client's response to the current route. Intravenous administration provides the most rapid onset of pain relief. All other routes require a lag time for absorption of the analgesic into the circulation. In postoperative pain, IV is the preferred route for opioids when the oral route is not appropriate. If IV access is not available, sublingual, rectal, or transdermal routes are considered.

With cancer pain, the oral route is preferred. If the client is unable to take oral medications, rectal and transdermal routes are preferred because they are less invasive than other routes (Agency for Healthcare Research and Quality, 2007). In addition, tolerance develops at a slower rate with the oral route compared to the more invasive routes.

- *Choice of drug*. If one drug is not providing relief or has unacceptable side effects, another analgesic is tried.

The key to administering an analgesic is to monitor the client's response to it. This includes assessing the effectiveness of pain relief and the occurrence of side effects.

Classes of Analgesics Three classes of drugs are used for pain relief: (a) nonopioid analgesics, (b) opioid analgesics, and (c) analgesic adjuvants already discussed (WHO, 2008).

Nonopioids The medications in this category are useful for a variety of painful conditions, including surgery, trauma, and cancer (APS, 1999). The indications include mild to moderate pain, and they are used in conjunction with opioids. These drugs differ from opioids in several ways in that they:

- Are subject to the ceiling effect.
- Do not produce the effect of tolerance or physical dependence.
- Are antipyretic and should not be given in cases where they may mask an infection.

Ketorolac tromethamine (Toradol) is the only nonsteroidal anti-inflammatory drug (NSAID) available in parenteral form and has proven useful in clients on NPO status who would benefit from a NSAID. Even when administered intramuscularly or intravenously, ketorolac produces significant gastric irritation and the potential for gastric bleeding. The most frequent use of ketorolac is orally or intramuscularly in adults, but some pediatric centers have used it intravenously under strict supervision for a limited course (less than 5 days) in children and adolescents with great success.

Action Action of these drugs is thought to inhibit prostaglandin formation. If prostaglandins are inhibited, the sensory neurons are less likely to receive the pain signal. Thus, this class of analgesics works in the peripheral nervous system.

Opioids The opioid analgesics fall into three classes: pure opioid agonists, partial agonists, and **mixed agonist-antagonists** (a compound that blocks opioid effects on one receptor type while producing opioid effects on a second receptor type). Pure agonists produce a maximal response from cells when they bind to the cells' opioid receptor sites. Morphine (the gold standard against which all other opioids are measured), fentanyl, methadone (Dolophine), hydromorphone hydrochloride (Dilaudid), and codeine are pure agonists. Meperidine (Demerol), although classified as a pure agonist, is not recommended except in clients with a true allergy to all other narcotics because of its neurotoxicity. Meperidine produces clinical analgesia for only 2.5 to 3.5 hours when given intramuscularly in adults.

PROFESSIONALTIP

Ketorolac tromethamine (Toradol)

Ketorolac should not be given to a client with any history of renal dysfunction, gastric irritation, bleeding problems, low platelet count, or allergy to aspirin or other NSAIDs.

Unlike the NSAIDs, pure agonist opioids are not subject to the ceiling effect. As the dosage is increased, pain relief increases.

Action Opioids act in the CNS by binding to opiate receptor sites on afferent neurons. The pain signal is stopped at the spinal cord level and does not reach the cortex where pain is perceived.

Side Effects The only limiting factor in the use of pure agonist opioids is the degree of side effects, particularly respiratory depression and constipation. Other side effects include pruritus and nausea, but the degree to which they are present from each medication varies among individuals. Clients must be instructed regarding these normal responses to opioids and informed that it does not mean that they are allergic to them. A true allergy to opioids would be indicated by a rash or hives that starts after receiving the opioid, a local histamine release at the site of infusion, or anaphylaxis. Clients also need to know that the pruritus and nausea generally subside after 4 to 5 days of opioid therapy. In the meantime, an antihistamine such as diphenhydramine hydrochloride (Benadryl) or hydroxyzine hydrochloride (Atarax, Vistaril) may be used for pruritus, and an antiemetic such as metoclopramide hydrochloride (Clopra) or trimethobenzamide hydrochloride (Tigan) can be used to treat the nausea.

PROFESSIONALTIP

Types of Nonopioid Drugs

- *Salicylates.* These include aspirin and other salicylate salts. Common side effects of aspirin include gastric disturbances and bleeding caused by the antiplatelet effect. Some of the salicylate salts, such as choline magnesium trisalicylate (Trilisate) and salsalate (Salgesic), have fewer gastrointestinal and bleeding effects than aspirin.
- *Acetaminophen.* This nonsalicylate is similar to aspirin in its analgesic action but has no anti-inflammatory effect. Its mechanism of action for pain relief is not known.
- *NSAIDs.* The effectiveness of these drugs varies, with some being close to the effectiveness of aspirin and acetaminophen, whereas others are much stronger. Clients tend to vary in response, so once the maximum recommended dose has been tried with ineffective results, it would be worth trying another NSAID. The drugs in this group inhibit platelet aggregation and are contraindicated in clients with coagulation disorders or on anticoagulation therapy.

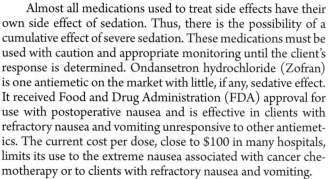

LIFE SPAN CONSIDERATIONS

Effects of Meperidine (Demerol)

- In the elderly, most of whom show decreased glomerular filtration rates, there is generally a higher peak and longer duration of action because it takes longer to excrete the opioid as well as its toxic metabolite, normeperidine.
- In pediatric clients receiving intravenous meperidine, analgesia may last for only 1.5 to 2 hours.

Almost all medications used to treat side effects have their own side effect of sedation. Thus, there is the possibility of a cumulative effect of severe sedation. These medications must be used with caution and appropriate monitoring until the client's response is determined. Ondansetron hydrochloride (Zofran) is one antiemetic on the market with little, if any, sedative effect. It received Food and Drug Administration (FDA) approval for use with postoperative nausea and is effective in clients with refractory nausea and vomiting unresponsive to other antiemetics. The current cost per dose, close to $100 in many hospitals, limits its use to the extreme nausea associated with cancer chemotherapy or to clients with refractory nausea and vomiting.

Mixed agonist-antagonist opioids are believed to be subject to the ceiling effect for pain relief, as well as a ceiling effect for respiratory depression. Mixed agonist-antagonist opioids activate one opioid receptor type while simultaneously blocking another type. Butorphanol tartrate (Stadol), pentazocine hydrochloride (Talwin), and nalbuphine hydrochloride (Nubain) are the most frequently used in pain management.

Opioid antagonists include naloxone (Narcan) and naltrexone (Trexal), with the most commonly used being naloxone (Narcan). They work by blocking opioid stimulation of receptor sites. Naloxone effectively reverses opioid side effects of sedation, respiratory depression, and nausea, and *it completely reverses any pain control.*

Alternative Delivery Systems Opioids are administered in more than just the traditional oral, subcutaneous, intramuscular, intravenous, and rectal routes.

Patient-Controlled Analgesia **Patient-controlled analgesia (PCA)** is most often delivered by a device that allows the client to control the delivery of intravenous, epidural, or subcutaneous pain medication in a safe, effective manner through

PROFESSIONALTIP

Constipation and Opioids

Clients who are expected to require opioid analgesics for more than 1 or 2 days should be administered a stool softener as soon as they are taking fluids orally. While they are still NPO, a glycerin or bisacodyl (Dulcolax) suppository should be administered if the client has not had a bowel movement in 1 or 2 days.

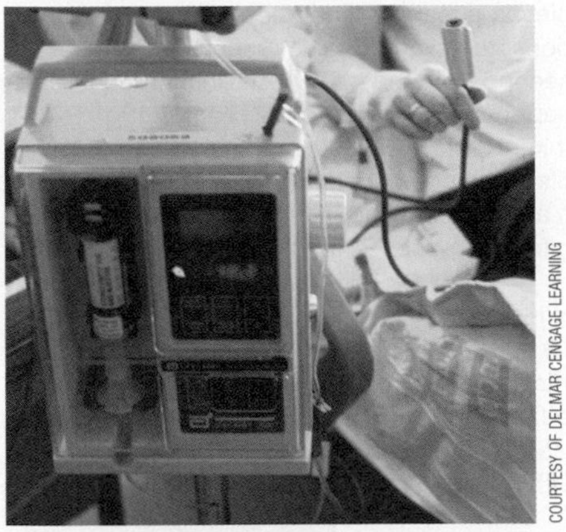

FIGURE 27-10 **Client on IV Patient-Controlled Analgesia (PCA)**

a programmable pump (Figure 27-10). This system helps eliminate the time required for the nurse to draw up the medication and allows the client control over the pain. The pump has the safety feature of locking out once a maximum dose is reached. This prevents the client from overdosing. The PCA has been successfully used with many types of pain and in many settings, including postoperative, pediatrics, and home health.

Requirements for using a PCA are the cognitive ability to understand how to use the pump and the physical ability to push the button. The nurse teaches the client and family about the PCA pump and pain medication, how to activate the pump, and that the client is the only one to activate the pump. The nurse explains the pain rating scale to the client and continues to regularly monitor the client's pain even when the client is using the pump. Teach the client to "push the button" only when medication for pain is needed. The client or family notifies the nurse if the medication is not controlling the pain so that alternative measures can be taken.

Oral PCA is relatively new in hospitals and is becoming increasingly popular (Rosati et al., 2007). Client teaching is the key for success. The client must understand how pain, pain medication, and pain relief are related and how to maintain a pain-relief diary. A Velcro®-sealed wrist pouch is applied to the client with one or two doses of the prescribed oral analgesic, even controlled substances, in the pouch. The client notifies the nurse when a dose is taken so that it can be replaced. If the client does not comply with the oral PCA policy, it is discontinued.

Medication on demand (MOD®) is another method of oral PCA. The facility pharmacy places eight doses of oral medication in the medication tray, which is then loaded into the device. The cover is closed, locking the medication securely inside. The MOD® locks to an IV pole for easy client access as shown in Figure 27-11A. The client accesses the MOD® with his radio-frequency identification (RFID) wristband, dials in his pain level from 0 to 10 by touching the pad on the front of the device, and receives the prescribed medication. The device is programmed to respond only to a specific client's RFID wristband. Once the client accepts the medication, the device has a lockout interval so the client cannot receive more than the prescribed dose. At the end of the lockout time, a light on the MOD® illuminates, indicating that the client can have medication when needed. Nurses may access the device with a programmed RFID card. The device stores the information for reference, printing, or inclusion in the client's electronic medical record. (Figure 27-11B).

Epidural/Intrathecal Analgesia **Epidural analgesia** refers to administering the opioid via a catheter that terminates in the epidural space, the space outside the dura mater that protects the spinal cord. **Intrathecal analgesia** refers to administering the drug directly into the subarachnoid space. These may be administered as a one-time injection by the anesthesiologist or via a catheter that has been placed. Both of these routes are occasionally referred to as *intraspinal anesthesia*. Because the opioid is delivered close to the site of action, these routes require much lower doses of opioid (usually morphine [Duramorph] or fentanyl [Sublimaze] are used) for pain relief. The incidence of systemic side effects is also much lower with these routes. Duration is longer than systemic routes (e.g., the duration of one dose of intrathecal morphine can last 24 hours).

Transdermal Analgesia Another route of opioid administration is the transdermal patch. The only opioid drug currently available via this route is fentanyl (Duragesic). This medication is on an adhesive patch that attaches to the skin. It is available in 25, 50, 75, and 100 mcg/hour dosages. The fentanyl transdermal patch allows slow infusion of the drug through the skin. The fentanyl patch is indicated for continuous pain with high dosage requirements. The advantage of this route is that it is simple to apply and effective for 72 hours. The disadvantage is that dosage adjustments are difficult to make because of the slow infusion rate. In addition, side effects may not be reversed as rapidly as when opiates are administered via the oral route.

Local Anesthesia Local anesthetics are effective for pain management in a variety of settings. Topical anesthetics are available for teething, sore throats, denture pain, laceration repair, and intravenous catheter insertions. One topical anesthetic, EMLA cream, is a mixture of local anesthetics, combining prilocaine (Citanest) and lidocaine (Xylocaine). It produces complete anesthesia for at least 60 minutes when topically applied on intact skin. Another topical anesthetic, TAC, is available for anesthesia during closure of lacerations. It is a combination of tetracaine hydrochloride (Pontocaine) 0.5%, adrenaline (epinephrine) 1:2000, and cocaine 11.8% in a normal saline solution that can be applied directly to the open wound surface in place of local anesthetic infiltration with a needle. This allows pain-free cleansing of the laceration as well as suturing. Because both adrenaline

LIFE SPAN CONSIDERATIONS

Opioid Analgesia in the Elderly

- Cheyne-Stokes respiratory patterns are not unusual during sleep in the elderly and should not be used as a reason to restrict appropriate opioid pain relief unless accompanied by unacceptable degrees of arterial desaturation (less than 85%).
- The elderly are more sensitive to sedation and respiratory depressant effects and experience a higher peak and longer duration of effect from opioid medications.
- Opioid dose titration must be based on analgesic effects and degree of side effects, such as sedation, urinary retention, constipation, respiratory depression, or exacerbation of Parkinson's disease.

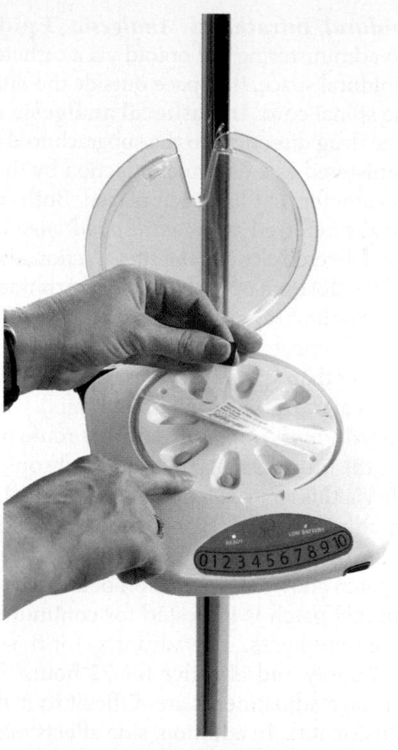

A

After completing a teaching module with hands-on instructions, the client obtains oral pain medication as needed from the MOD®. An illuminated ready light appears indicating to the client that the lockout interval has passed and medication is now available when needed. The client obtains medication as needed without requesting the medication from a nurse. To get the medication, the client:

1. Indicates his pain level from 0-10 on the pain scale. This activates the radio frequency identification (RFID) reader within the MOD® device.
2. Swipes the RFID wristband across the MOD®'s faceplate.
3. Removes the prescribed dose of pain medication and self administers the medication.

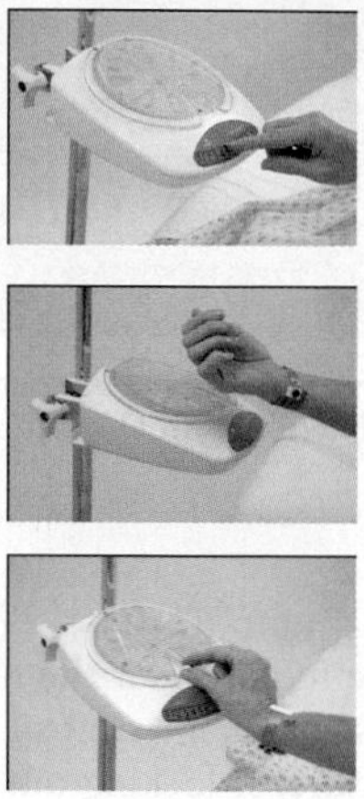

B

FIGURE 27-11 Oral Patient-Controlled Analgesia Device called Medication on Demand (MOD®); *A*, MOD® is locked to an IV pole for client accessibility. The facility pharmacy places oral medication in the medication tray which is then loaded into the device; *B*, Guidelines for obtaining medication for the MOD®. *(Images courtesy of AVANCEN)*.

(epinephrine) and cocaine cause vasoconstriction, TAC cannot be used in areas supplied by end-arteriolar blood supply such as a client's digits, ear, or nose. It also is contraindicated on burned or abraded skin because this could lead to increased systemic absorption of cocaine and tetracaine, thus placing the client at risk for seizures.

Noninvasive Interventions

Noninvasive relief measures consist of cognitive-behavioral strategies and physical modalities that use cutaneous stimulation. These treatments can be used to supplement pharmacological therapy and other modalities to control pain. Clients and their families can also be instructed to utilize these treatments at home and in inpatient settings.

Cognitive-Behavioral Interventions The cognitive-behavioral interventions influence the cognitive and the motivational-affective components of pain perception. These methods can not only help influence the level of pain, but also help the client gain a sense of self-control.

Trusting Nurse–Client Relationship Establishing a therapeutic relationship is the foundation for effective nursing care. The clients most likely to be comfortable are those who trust their nurses to be there, to listen, and to act.

Relaxation **Relaxation techniques** (a variety of methods used to decrease anxiety and muscle tension) result in decreased heart rate and respiratory rate and decreased muscle tension. The body's response to pain is almost "tricked" into reversing itself when relaxation exercises are implemented.

Relaxation exercises help reduce pain by decreasing anxiety and decreasing reflex muscular contraction. There are a wide variety of relaxation techniques, including focused breathing, progressive muscle relaxation, and meditation. Simple techniques should be used during episodes of brief pain (e.g., during procedures) or when pain is so severe that the client is unable to concentrate on complicated instructions.

To teach simple relaxation techniques, the nurse can instruct the client to (a) take a deep breath and hold it, (b) exhale slowly and concentrate on going limp; and (c) start yawning (McCaffery & Pasero, 1999). The yawning triggers a conditioned response in the client (i.e., the body associates yawning with relaxation and will relax when the client yawns). The technique can be enhanced if the nurse starts yawning. It is so contagious that even the client compromised by severe pain will usually start yawning with the nurse.

A more complex technique is **progressive muscle relaxation**, a strategy in which muscles are alternately tensed and relaxed. This type of technique is especially useful for clients who do not know what muscle relaxation feels like. By purposely contracting and releasing the muscle groups, the client is able to compare the difference and identify feelings of relaxation. Meditative relaxation techniques are also available, including audiotapes sold in most bookstores.

LIFE SPAN CONSIDERATIONS

Injections and Children

Children lack the cognitive ability to weigh the pain of injection against the pain relief from the medication, so oral and rectal routes are preferred over injections.

PROFESSIONALTIP

Using Distraction

Distraction should never be the *only* pain management intervention used, but it can be very helpful while waiting for other techniques to take effect.

CLIENTTEACHING

Hot or Cold Applications

Teach the client or family that hot or cold applications:

- Must have at least one layer of towel between the heating or cooling device and the skin.
- Should not exceed 20 minutes when placed on the skin (Department of Health, NSW, 2005).
- Should not be applied to tissue that has been exposed to radiation therapy (Agency for Health Care Policy and Research, 1994).

Relaxation is a learned response. The more frequently the client practices these techniques, the more skilled the body will be in learning to relax. Ideally, the best time to teach the client these methods is when pain is controlled or before the pain occurs (e.g., in the preoperative period).

Reframing **Reframing** is a technique that teaches clients to monitor their negative thoughts and replace them with more positive ones. For example, teach a client to replace an expression such as "I can't stand this pain, it's never going away" with one such as "I've had similar pain before, and it's gotten better."

Distraction Distraction focuses one's attention on something other than the pain, therefore placing pain on the periphery of awareness. Successful use of distraction does not eliminate the pain; it makes it less troublesome. The main disadvantage of distraction is that as soon as the distractive stimuli stop, the pain returns in full force. For this reason, the most appropriate use of distraction techniques is for the relief of brief, episodic pain. It can be effective for procedural pain or the period between administration of an analgesic and the onset of the drug. Examples of distraction include the following:

- Active listening to recorded music (have the client tap fingers in rhythm to the beat)
- Reciting a poem or rhyme (children do this well)
- Describe a plot of a novel or movie
- Describe a series of pictures

Guided Imagery Guided imagery uses one's imagination to provide a pleasant substitute for the pain. It incorporates features of both relaxation and distraction. The client imagines a pleasant experience, such as going to the beach or the mountains. The experience should use all five senses to fully involve the client in the image.

The images chosen need to be ones that are pleasant for the client. Describing an ocean cruise would not be appropriate for a person who becomes seasick.

Humor The old saying, "Laughter is the best medicine," carries some truth to it. Although there is nothing very funny about pain, laughing has been shown to provide pain relief. The act of laughing can cause distraction from the pain, induce relaxation by taking deep breaths and releasing tension, release endorphins, and provide a pleasant substitute for pain. Norman Cousins (1991) relates obtaining 2 hours of pain relief from watching episodes of the *Candid Camera* television show and Marx Brothers films. This technique can be implemented by encouraging the client to watch humorous movies, read funny books, or listen to comedy routines. Because different people see humor in different types of situations, be sensitive to what the client views as funny.

Biofeedback Biofeedback is a method that may help the client in pain to relax and relieve tension. Individuals learn to influence their physiological responses to stimuli and thus alter their pain experience.

Cutaneous Stimulation The technique of cutaneous stimulation involves stimulating the skin to control pain. It is theorized that this technique provides relief by stimulating nerve fibers that send signals to the dorsal horn of the spinal cord to "close the gate." The main advantage of these therapies is that many techniques are easy for the nurse to implement and easy to teach the client and family to perform. They are not usually meant to replace analgesic therapy, but to complement it.

Hot and Cold Application In addition to stimulating nerves that can block pain transmission, superficial heat application increases circulation to the area, which promotes oxygenation and nutrient delivery to the injured tissues. It also decreases joint and muscle stiffness. Heat is contraindicated in cases of acute injury because it can increase the initial response of edema. It is also contraindicated in rheumatoid arthritis flare-ups and over topical applications of mentholated ointments. Heat treatments should be limited to 20- to 30-minute intervals because maximum vasodilatation occurs in that time.

Cryotherapy (cold applications) induces local vasoconstriction and numbness, therefore altering the pain sensations. It is contraindicated in any condition where vasoconstriction might increase symptoms (e.g., peripheral vascular disease). For best results, cold therapy should be limited to 20- to 30-minute intervals. Either heat or cold can be used as cutaneous stimulation unless one is specifically contraindicated. Cold often provides faster relief (McCaffery & Pasero, 1999). If the client has used heat or cold before, incorporate the modality that the client believes will be the most effective. Combining the two might provide better relief. An example of this would be to apply a hot pack for 4 minutes, followed by an ice pack for 2 minutes, repeated four times. In a hospital setting, a physician order is required for this therapy.

Acupressure and Massage One of the first responses to pain is to rub the painful part. People seem to instinctively understand the pain-relieving aspects of this intervention. In addition to blocking the pain transmission through nerve stimulation, massage can also promote relaxation. Acupressure is a type of massage that consists of continuous pressure on or the rubbing of acupuncture points. Massage is based on the same principles as acupuncture, but needles are not used. Massage also provides a form of nonverbal communication that can be therapeutic on its own.

Mentholated Rubs Ointments or lotions containing menthol are thought to provide relief by providing a counterirritation to the skin. The menthol gives the client the perception that the temperature of the skin has changed (becoming either warmer or cooler). This alters the sensation of pain or provides a distraction from the pain. Client response varies to mentholated rubs; some gain effective relief, but others have

SAFETY

TENS Contraindications

- No electrodes are placed in the area over or surrounding demand cardiac pacemakers.
- No electrodes are placed over the uterus of a pregnant woman.

poor results. Their use is contraindicated on broken skin, on mucous membranes, or if pain increases.

Transcutaneous Electrical Nerve Stimulation **Transcutaneous electrical nerve stimulation (TENS)** is the process of applying a low-voltage electrical current to the skin through cutaneous electrodes. This modulates pain transmission, as do other cutaneous stimulation methods, but also distracts the client from pain. Research supports the effectiveness of using TENS for the relief of postoperative pain (Agency for Health Care Policy and Research, 1992; Rakel & Frantz, 2003). It has also been used successfully in many pain syndromes (e.g., chronic low-back pain, menstrual cramps, temporomandibular joint [TMJ] syndrome, phantom limb pain, and others). It is administered by specially trained health professionals, usually a physical therapist. Other modalities of pain management should not be abandoned while a trial of TENS occurs.

Exercise Exercise is an important treatment for chronic pain because it helps mobilize joints, strengthens weak muscles, and helps restore balance and coordination. Do not use passive range of motion if it increases discomfort or pain. Immobilization is frequently used to stabilize fractures or for clients with episodes of acute pain. Prolonged immobilization can lead to muscle atrophy and cardiovascular deconditioning.

Psychotherapy Psychotherapy may be beneficial to some clients, particularly those:

- Who are clinically depressed
- Who have a history of psychiatric problems
- Whose pain is difficult to control

Some psychotherapists use **hypnosis** (altered state of consciousness when a person is more receptive to suggestion) to help clients alter pain perception. Hypnosis can be effective but should be used only by specially trained professionals.

Positioning The final noninvasive technique is proper positioning and body alignment. Moving the client with the least possible stress on joints and skin will minimize exposure to painful stimuli. This includes supporting joints appropriately and maintaining wrinkle-free sheets.

Invasive Interventions

Invasive interventions are meant to complement behavioral, physical, and pharmacological therapies in those clients who do not obtain relief from those measures alone. Invasive measures are indicated primarily for chronic cancer pain and in some cases of chronic benign pain. These procedures are usually tried only when noninvasive measures have been attempted first with poor results.

CRITICAL THINKING

Noninvasive Intervention

How would you decide which noninvasive intervention to use with a client?

Nerve Block Neural blockade is the process of injecting a local anesthetic or neurolytic agent into the nerve. An anesthetic agent may be injected to act as a diagnostic tool in order to identify the nerves involved in a pain syndrome. A neurolytic agent is a chemical agent that causes destruction of the nerve and, therefore, creates an interruption in the pain signal.

Neurosurgery Neurosurgical measures for pain control include neurostimulation procedures and destructive or ablative procedures. Neurostimulation procedures involve the implantation of electrical stimulation devices that send impulses to different parts of the nervous system. Some of these devices stimulate areas of the brain; others stimulate the spinal cord. Relief is thought to be provided by blocking the afferent fiber input at the spinal cord level or by stimulating release of endorphins using the body's ability to modulate pain.

Destructive or ablative procedures are used to destroy part of the nervous system that conducts pain. By interrupting the pain signal, it is prevented from reaching the cortex where realization of pain occurs. These procedures are reserved for clients with terminal illness.

Radiation Therapy Radiation can be used as a palliative measure for pain relief in clients with cancer. It can relieve both metastatic pain and pain caused by tumors at the primary cancer site. It enhances other pain management strategies, such as analgesic therapy, because it is aimed specifically at the cause of the client's pain. When administered for pain relief, the smallest dose of radiation is utilized to minimize side effects.

Acupuncture **Acupuncture** is the insertion of small needles into the skin at specific (hoku) sites. The sites are chosen after the practitioner takes a detailed history and uses traditional Asian diagnostic techniques. The needles used for acupuncture have rounded ends that enter the skin without cutting the tissue. The practitioner may twirl or vibrate the needles manually or electrically. It is important that the nurse keep an open mind when the client chooses this therapy, or the client may be reluctant to discuss its use.

Evaluation

Evaluating pain management interventions is ongoing, focusing primarily on the client's subjective reports. Objective data to evaluate pain management include the following:

- Continuing use of pain assessment tools
- Client's facial expression and posture
- Presence (or absence) of restlessness
- Vital sign monitoring

CASE STUDY

C.S. is a 76-year-old male with arthritis. He and his wife are residents of a nursing home. His wife is bedridden because of a cardiac disorder. Each day, C.S. sits at his wife's bedside and talks to her. Today, C.S. is agitated and short with his wife. He is moving slowly, his knees are edematous, and he winces when he walks.

1. List factors that may indicate that C.S. is experiencing pain.
2. Identify factors that may be impacting C.S.'s pain experience.
3. Describe the nursing actions necessary to perform a comprehensive pain assessment of C.S.

Adapted from *Caring for Clients with Pain*, by M. Teeter and D. Kemper, 2008b, manuscript submitted for publication.

SAMPLE NURSING CARE PLAN

The Client With Chronic Pain

S.J., a 48-year-old woman, injured her back 3 years ago while lifting some boxes of paper at work. Since that time, she has had four epidural steroidal injections for the pain associated with two ruptured discs. Her pain has been intermittent, with some alleviation from the epidural injections. Her last epidural was 3 months ago. She arrives at the clinic stating, "I just don't know how I can go on like this. The pain has been tolerable until last night. I'm hurting so bad!" She is tearful and pacing, saying, "It hurts too much when I sit down." Verbalizes pain is "9" on a 1-to-10 pain intensity scale. Blood pressure is 148/90. Pulse is strong and regular at 92. She has guarded movements.

NURSING DIAGNOSIS 1 *Chronic **Pain***, related to muscle spasm and lower back pain as evidenced by back injury 3 years ago and client statement "I just don't know how I can go on like this. The pain has been tolerable until last night. I'm hurting so bad!"

Nursing Outcomes Classification (NOC)
Comfort Level
Pain Control

Nursing Interventions Classification (NIC)
Pain Management
Medication Management
Coping Enhancement

PLANNING/OUTCOMES	NURSING INTERVENTIONS	RATIONALE
S.J. will verbalize a decrease in pain.	Assess S.J.'s level of pain, determining the intensity at its best and worst.	Determines a baseline for future assessment.
	Listen to S.J. while she discusses the pain; acknowledge the presence of pain.	Decreases anxiety by communicating acceptance and validating her perceptions.
	Discuss reasons why pain may be increased or decreased.	Helps S.J. understand her pain.
S.J. will practice selected noninvasive pain relief measures.	Teach relaxation techniques such as deep breathing, progressive muscle relaxation, and imagery.	Reduces skeletal muscle tension and anxiety, which potentiates the perception of pain.
	Teach S.J. about the use of medication for pain relief. Provide accurate information to reduce fear of addiction.	Lack of knowledge and fear may prohibit S.J. from taking analgesic medications as prescribed.
	Encourage S.J. to rest during the day.	Fatigue increases the perception of pain.

EVALUATION

After practicing relaxation techniques, S.J. rates her pain as a 2 to 3 on the pain intensity scale. S.J. demonstrates the use of deep breathing and progressive muscle relaxation.

(Continues)

SAMPLE NURSING CARE PLAN (Continued)

NURSING DIAGNOSIS 2

Anxiety related to chronic pain as evidenced by pacing and tears.

NOC: *Coping; Anxiety Reduction*
NIC: *Anxiety Reduction; Anticipatory Guidance*

CLIENT GOALS

1. S.J. will verbalize an increase in psychological and physiological comfort level.
2. S.J. will demonstrate ability to cope with anxiety as evidenced by normal vital signs and a verbalized reduction in pain intensity.

NURSING INTERVENTIONS	SCIENTIFIC RATIONALES
1-1. Assess S.J.'s level of anxiety.	1-1. Determines baseline for future assessment.
2-1. Encourage S.J. to verbalize angry feelings.	2-1. Provides an outlet for her anger.
2-1. Speak slowly and calmly.	2-2. Avoids escalating S.J.'s anxiety level and increases the likelihood of her comprehension.

EVALUATION

After practicing relaxation techniques, how does S.J. rate her pain on a pain intensity scale?
Is S.J. verbalizing decreased pain intensity?
After a relaxation session, are S.J.'s vital signs within normal ranges?

SUMMARY

- Pain may be defined as "an unpleasant sensory and emotional experience associated with actual or potential tissue damage" (IASP, 2008) and "whatever the client says it is, existing whenever the client says it does" (McCaffery & Pasero, 1999).
- The gate control theory proposes that several processes (sensory, motivational-affective, and cognitive) combine to determine how a person perceives pain.
- Assessment of pain helps establish a baseline of data and helps evaluate the effectiveness of interventions.
- Factors influencing pain perception include age, previous experience with pain, and cultural norms.
- The subjective data to gather include location of pain, onset and duration, quality, intensity (on a scale of 0 to 10), aggravating and relieving factors, and how pain affects the activities of daily living.
- The three general principles to follow with pain relief measures are (a) individualize the approach, (b) use a preventive approach, and (c) use a multidisciplinary approach.

- The nurse carries a great deal of autonomy in administering analgesics, which leads to specific responsibilities for which the nurse is accountable.
- Pharmacologic agents can be therapeutic for clients experiencing pain; however, the medications should not be the only interventions used.
- Noninvasive treatments for pain relief are measures that can supplement pharmacological and invasive treatments for pain relief.
- Invasive techniques are interventions used when the noninvasive and pharmacological measures do not provide adequate relief. Methods include nerve blocks, neurosurgery, radiation therapy, and acupuncture.

REVIEW QUESTIONS

1. According to McCaffery and Pasero, pain may be defined as:
1. discomfort resulting from identifiable physiologic or iatrogenic sources.
2. a syndrome of behavioral and physical manifestations that can be objectively identified by the nurse.
3. whatever the patient says it is, existing whenever and wherever the patient says it does.
4. a sensory response to noxious stimuli.

2. Which of the following is a useful tool for assessing the intensity of pain that is easy to use?
1. The gate control scale.
2. Acute pain monitor.
3. Numeric pain scale.
4. Pressure pain monitor.

3. B.L., 45, has experienced chronic low-back pain since a fall 8 years ago. He describes his pain as "a gnawing, constant dull pain" that makes him feel tired. The nurse caring for him recognizes that one of the differences between acute and chronic pain characteristics is:
1. acute pain is more severe.
2. chronic pain is often described as dull and is difficult to localize.
3. chronic back pain is often not real.
4. acute pain is more diffuse and difficult to describe.

4. N.J., 84 years old, is recuperating from a total hip replacement. Morphine, 8 mg IV q4h PRN, is prescribed for N.J. Her respiratory rate is 18, her pulse rate is 96 beats per minute, and her blood pressure is elevated slightly above her normal level. She is complaining of severe pain, 8 on a scale of 0 to 10. The most appropriate initial nursing intervention is:
1. question the physician regarding the dosage amount for a client this age.
2. turn her and then reevaluate her need for opioid analgesia.
3. administer the medication as ordered.
4. advise N.J. to cough and breathe deeply since you are unable to give her anything for pain until her respiratory rate is 20.

5. O.R., 55 years old, is hospitalized with an exacerbation of rheumatoid arthritis. She has a favorite television show she watches every afternoon. She reports feeling comfortable during this show and seldom requests pain medication when she is watching it. The nurse's assessment of this phenomenon is that:
1. the assessment of pain that prompted hospitalization is inaccurate.
2. O.R. is bored and the boredom usually makes her pain seem worse.
3. inactivity is the best approach to O.R.'s pain.
4. distraction is an effective modifier of the pain experience for O.R.

6. Which of the following Joint Commission pain management standards apply to the bedside nurse? (Select all that apply.)
1. Identify symptoms of pain in the client.
2. Understand the institutional standards of pain management.
3. Assess factors impacting the pain experience.
4. Order the appropriate pain medication for the client.
5. Implement pain management techniques.
6. Evaluate the effectiveness of pain management techniques.

7. The client's family expresses concern that the client could overdose with a PCA. The most appropriate response by the nurse is:
1. "Overdose is not possible with PCA."
2. "The client receives extensive teaching prior to PCA use, which should prevent overdose."
3. "The client can stop drug administration but not initiate it, so it is unlikely he will get too much medication."
4. "The PCA pump is programmed with specific dose limits, reducing the chances of overmedication."

8. A client with terminal cancer is receiving morphine via PCA. The client is grimacing and moaning occasionally but sleeping for short intervals. Respiratory rate is 20, heart rate is 100, and blood pressure is 140/90. What is the most accurate assessment of this client's pain?
1. The client is able to sleep, so the pain is manageable.
2. The client is exhibiting respiratory depression and should not receive more medication.
3. The client may need additional pain medication or an increase in dosage.
4. The client can be assumed to be comfortable.

9. The nurse is providing preoperative teaching to a client who will most likely receive PCA after surgery. The nurse tells the client that the primary reason for utilizing PCA is that it:
   1. is cost effective.
   2. results in use of less medication.
   3. is convenient for nursing staff.
   4. allows the client control of pain relief.

10. Which factor is most important when determining whether PCA should be used for a client's pain management?
    1. The client's developmental and cognitive abilities.
    2. The client's weight.
    3. The length of the surgical procedure.
    4. The preferences of the surgeon.

REFERENCES/SUGGESTED READING

Acello, B. (2000a). Facing fears about opioid addiction. *Nursing2000, 30*(5), 72.

Acello, B. (2000b). Meeting JCAHO standards for pain control. *Nursing2000, 30*(3), 52–54.

Adler, P., Good, M., Roberts, B., & Snyder, S. (2000). The effects of tai chi on older adults with chronic arthritis pain. *Journal of Nursing Scholarship, 32*(4), 377.

Agency for Health Care Policy and Research. (1992). *Clinical practice guideline: Acute pain management: Operative or medical procedures and trauma* (AHCPR Publication No. 92-0032). Rockville, MD: U.S. Department of Health and Human Services.

Agency for Health Care Policy and Research. (1994). *Clinical practice guideline: Management of cancer pain* (AHCPR Publication No. 94-0592). Rockville, MD: U.S. Department of Health and Human Services.

Agency for Healthcare Research and Quality. (2007). Clinical practice guidelines: Major recommendations. Rockville, MD: Author. Available: http://wwwguideline.gov/summary/summary.aspx?doc_id=3748&nbr=002974&string=p

American Pain Society. (1999). *Principles of analgesic use in the treatment of acute pain and cancer pain* (4th ed.). Glenview, IL: Author.

American Pain Society. (2006). Pain: Current understanding of assessment, management, and treatments. Retrieved July 25, 2006, from http://www.ampainsoc.org/ce/downloads/npc/npc.pdf

American Pain Foundation. (2007). *Pain facts and figures.* Retrieved March 28, 2008, from http://www.painfoundatoin.org/page.asp?file=Newsroom/PainReference.htm.

AVANCEN, LLC. (2008). *A physician introduction to the MOD an oral PCA device for your patients.* Retrieved December 16, 2008, from http://www.avancen.com/news_files/Physician_Information_Flyer.pdf

Beecher, H. (1956). Relationship of significance of wound to pain experienced. *Journal of the American Medical Association, 161,* 1609–1613.

Brand, P., & Yancey, P. (1993). *Pain: The gift nobody wants.* New York: HarperCollins.

Brown, J., Horn, J., Calbert, J., & Nolan-Goslin, K. (1999). A question of pain. *Nursing99, 29*(10), 48–51.

Bulechek, G., Butcher, H., McCloskey, J., & Dochterman, J., eds. (2008). *Nursing Interventions Classification (NIC)* (5th ed.). St. Louis, MO: Mosby/Elsevier.

Chapman, G. (1999). Documenting a pain assessment. *Nursing99, 29*(11), 25.

Choiniere, M. (2001). Burn pain: A unique challenge. *Pain: Clinical Updates, 9*(1). Retrieved January 1, 2009, from http://www.iasp-pain.org/AM/AMTemplate.cfm?Section=Home&CONTENTID=7606&TEMPLATE=/CM/ContentDisplay.cfm

Cleeland, C., & Syrjala, K. (1992). How to assess cancer pain. In D. Turk & R. Melzack (Eds.), *Pain assessment.* New York: Guilford Press.

Collins, P., Auclair, M., Butler, E., Hush, M., Bernstein, B., Aguirre, F., et al. (2000). Educating staff about pain management. *American Journal of Nursing, 100*(1), 59.

Compton, P. (1999). Managing a drug abuser's pain. *Nursing99, 29*(5), 26–28.

Controlling Pain. (2001). Taming pain with TENS. *Nursing2001, 31*(11), 84.

D'Arcy, Y. (2002). How to treat arthritis pain. *Nursing2002, 32*(7), 30–31.

Department of Health, NSW. (2005). Hot or cold packs application (GL2005_015). Retrieved January 30, 2008, from http://www.health.nsw.gov.au/policies/GL/2005/pdf/GL2005_015.pdf

Derby, S. (1999). Opioid conversion guidelines for managing adult cancer pain. *American Journal of Nursing, 99*(10), 62–65.

Dillard, J., & Hirschman, L. (2002). *The chronic pain solution: The comprehensive, step-by-step guide to choosing the best alternative and conventional medicine.* Philadelphia: Bantam Doubleday Dell.

Estes, M. (2010). *Health assessment and physical examination* (4th ed.). Clifton Park, NY: Delmar Cengage Learning.

Faries, J. (1998a). Easing your patient's postoperative pain. *Nursing98, 28*(6), 58–60.

Faries, J. (1998b). Making a smooth switch from IV analgesia. *Nursing98, 28*(7), 26.

Feinberg, S. (2000). Complex regional pain syndrome. *American Journal of Nursing, 100*(12), 23–24.

Flor, H. Birbaumer, N., & Sherman, R. (2000). Phantom limb pain. *Pain: Clinical Updates, 8*(3). Available: http://www.iasp-pain.org/AM/AMTemplate.cfm?Section=Home&TEMPLATE=/CM/ContentDisplay.cfm&CONTENTID=7591

Gordon, D., Dahl, J., Miaskowski, C., McCarberg, B., Todd, K., Paice, J., et al. (2005). American Pain Society recommendations for improving the quality of acute and cancer pain management. *Archives of Internal Medicine, 165,* 1574–1579.

Haddad, A. (2000). Ethics in action: Treating pain in substance abusers. *RN, 63*(1), 21–24.

Hockenberry-Eaton, M., Wilson, D., & Winkelstein, M. L. (2003). *Wong's nursing care of infants and children* (7th ed.). New York: Elsevier Science.

Integrative Pain Center of Arizona. (2003). New JCAHO pain care treatment standards. Retrieved July 20, 2008, from http://www.ipcaz.org/pages/new.html

International Association for the Study of Pain. (2008). IASP pain terminology. Retrieved December 30, 2008, from http://www.iasp-pain.org/AM/Template.cfm?Section=Pain_Definitions&Template=/CM/HTMLDisplay.cfm&ContentID=1728

Joint Commission. (2009). Setting the standard: The Joint Commission and health care safety and quality. Retrieved July 9, 2009, from http://www.jointcommission.org/NR/rdonlyres/6C33FEDB-BB50-4CEE-950B-A6246DA4911E/0/setting_the_standard.pdf

Kedziera, P. (1998). The two faces of pain. *RN, 61*(2), 45–46.

Loeb, J. (1999). Pain management in long-term care. *American Journal of Nursing, 99*(2), 48–52.

Lehne, R. (2004). *Pharmacology for nursing care* (5th ed.). St. Louis, MO: Saunders.

Mattson, J. (2000). The language of pain. *Reflections on Nursing LEADERSHIP, 26*(4), 10–14.

Mayer, D., Torma, L., Byoch, I., & Norris, K. (2001). Speaking the language of pain. *American Journal of Nursing, 101*(2), 44–49.

McCaffery, M. (1979). *Nursing management of the patient with pain* (2nd ed.). Philadelphia: Lippincott Williams & Wilkins.

McCaffery, M. (1999a). Pain control. *American Journal of Nursing, 99*(8), 18.

McCaffery, M. (1999b). Understanding your patient's pain tolerance. *Nursing99, 29*(12), 17.

McCaffery, M. (2001). Using the 0-to-1 pain rating scale. *American Journal of Nursing, 101*(10), 81–82.

McCaffery, M. (2002). Choosing a faces pain scale. *Nursing2002, 32*(5), 68.

McCaffery, M. (2003). Switching from IV to PO: Maintaining pain relief in the transition. *American Journal of Nursing, 103*(5), 62–63.

McCaffery, M. & Ferrell, B. (1999). Opioids and pain management. *Nursing 99, 29*(3), 48–52.

McCaffery, M., & Pasero, C. (1999). *Pain: Clinical manual* (2nd ed.). St. Louis, MO: Mosby.

McCaffery, M., & Robinson, E. (2002). Your patient is in pain: Here's how you respond. *Nursing2002, 32*(10), 36–45.

Melzack, R., & Wall, P. (1965). Pain mechanisms: A new theory. *Science, 150,* 971–979.

Merskey, J., & Bogduk, N. (Eds.). (1994). *Classification of chronic pain* (2nd ed.)., WA: IASP.

Moorhead, S., Johnson, M., Maas, M., & Swanson, E. (2007). *Nursing Outcomes Classification (NOC)* (4th ed). St. Louis, MO: Elsevier, Health Sciences Division.

Morris, D. (2001). Ethnicity and pain. *Pain: Clinical Updates.* Retrieved January 1, 2009, from http://www.iasp-pain.org/AM/AMTemplate.cfm?Section=Home&CONTENTID=7617&TEMPLATE=/CM/ContentDisplay.cfm

Morrison, C. (2000). Fear of addiction: Balancing the facts and concerns about opioid use. *American Journal of Nursing, 100*(7), 81.

Mularski, R. White-Chu, F., Overbay, D., Miller, L., Asch, S. M., & Ganzini, L. (2006). Measuring pain as the 5th vital sign does not improve quality of pain management. *Journal of General Internal Medicine, 21,* 607–612.

National Pain Foundation. (2009). Untying the knot. *National Pain Awareness.* Retrieved January 2, 20009, from http://www.nationalpainfoundation.org/NationalPainAwareness/QA_on_Pain.pdf

North American Nursing Diagnosis Association International. (2010). *NANDA-I nursing diagnoses: Definitions and classification 2009–2011.* Ames, IA: Wiley-Blackwell.

Nichols, R. (2003). Pain management in patients with addictive disease, *American Journal of Nursing, 103*(3), 87–90.

Office of Quality and Performance, U.S. Department of Veterans Affairs. (2008). *Management of postoperative pain—Annotation L: Did the intervention produce adequate and tolerable pain relief?* Retrieved December 15, 2008, from http://www.opq.med.va.gov/cpg/PAIN/pain_cpg/content/algann_1_anno.htm

Pace, J. (2002). Understanding nociceptive pain. *Nursing2002, 32*(3), 74–75.

Panke, J. (2002). Difficulties in managing pain at the end of life. *American Journal of Nursing, 102*(7), 26.

Pasero, C. (1999). Using superficial cooling for pain relief. *American Journal of Nursing, 99*(3), 48–52.

Pasero, C. (2000a). Continuous local anesthetics. *American Journal of Nursing, 100*(8), 22–23.

Pasero, C. (2000b). Oral patient-controlled analgesia. *American Journal of Nursing, 100*(3), 24.

Pasero, C., & McCaffery, M. (2000a). Reversing respiratory depression with naloxone. *American Journal of Nursing, 100*(2), 26.

Pasero, C., & McCaffery, M. (2000b). When patients can't report pain. *American Journal of Nursing, 100*(9), 22–23.

Pasero, C., & McCaffery, M. (2001). The patient's report of pain. *American Journal of Nursing, 101*(12), 73–74.

Pasero, C., & Montgomery, R. (2002). Intravenous fentanyl. *American Journal of Nursing, 102*(4), 73–76.

Perkins, E. (2002). Less morphine, or more? *RN, 65*(11), 51–54.

Portenoy, R., Payne, R., et al. (1999). Oral transmucosal fentanyl citrate (OTFC) for the treatment of breakthrough pain in cancer patients: A controlled dose titration study. *Pain, 79,* 303.

Poulain, P., Langlade, A., & Goldberg, J. (1997). Cancer pain management in the home. *Pain Clinical Updates, 5*(1). Available: http://www.iasp-pain.org/PCU97a.html

Rakel, B., & Frantz, R. (2003). Effectiveness of transcutaneous electrical nerve stimulation on postoperative pain with movement. *Journal of Pain.* 4, 455–464.

Reiff, P., & Niziolek, M. (2001). Troubleshooting TIPS for PCA. *RN, 64*(4), 33–37.

Rosati, J., Gallagher, M., Shook, B., Luwisch, E., Favis, G., Deveras, R., et al. (2007). Evaluation of an oral patient-controlled analgesia device for pain management in oncology inpatients. *Journal of Supportive Oncology, 5*(9), 443–448.

Scholz, M. (2000). Managing constipation that's opioid-induced. *RN, 63*(6), 103.

Slaughter, A., & Pasero, C. (2002). Unacceptable pain levels. *American Journal of Nursing, 102*(5), 75–76.

Smith-Stoner, M. (2003). How Buddhism influences pain control choices. *Nursing2003, 33*(4), 17.

Spratto, G., & Woods, A. (2009). *Delmar's nurses drug handbook.* Clifton Park, NY: Delmar Cengage Learning.

Strevy, S. (1998). Myths and facts about pain. *RN, 61*(2), 42–45.

Teeter, M., & Kemper, D. (2008a). *Assessing pain.* Manuscript submitted for publication.

Teeter, M., & Kemper, D. (2008b). *Caring for clients with pain.* Manuscript submitted for publication.

Thomas, M., & Lundeberg, T. (1996). Does acupuncture work? *Pain Clinical Updates, 4*(3). Available: http://www.iasp-pain. org/PCU96c.html.

Travell, J., & Simons, D. (1983, 1999). *Travell & Simon's myofascial pain and dysfunction: The trigger point manual* (2nd ed., Vols. 1 & 2). Baltimore: Lippincott Williams & Wilkins.

Twycross, R. et al. (1996). A survey of pain in patients with advanced cancer. *Journal of Pain Symptom Management, 12*(5), 273–282.

Vasudevan, S. (1993). *Pain: A four letter word you can live with.* Milwaukee, WI: Montgomery Media.

Victor, K. (2001). Properly assessing pain in the elderly. *RN, 64*(5), 45–49.

Wentz, J. (2003). Understanding neuropathic pain. *Nursing 2003, 33*(1), 22.

Wong, D. (2003). Topical local anesthetics. *American Journal of Nursing, 103*(6), 42–45.

World Health Organization. (1986). *Cancer pain relief.* Geneva: Author.

World Health Organization. (1990). *Cancer pain relief and palliative care* (World Health Organization Technical Report Series, 804). Geneva: Author.

World Health Organization. (2007). *New guide on palliative care services for people living with advanced cancer.* Retrieved December 16, 2008, from http://www.who.int/mediacentre/news/notes/2007/np31/en

World Health Organization. (2008). *WHO's pain relief ladder.* Retrieved December 16, 2008, from http://www.who.int/cancer/palliative/painladder/en

Young, D., Mentes, J., & Titler, M. (1999). Acute pain management protocol. *Journal of Gerontological Nursing, 26*(5), 10.

RESOURCES

Agency for Healthcare Research and Quality (AHRQ), http://www.ahrq.gov

American Chronic Pain Association, http://www.theacpa.org

American Pain Society (APS), http://www.ampainsoc.org

American Society of Pain Management Nurses, http://www.aspmn.org

City of Hope, http://www.cityofhope.org

International Association for the Study of Pain (IASP), http://www.iasp-pain.org

Joint Commission, http://www.jointcommission.org

National Chronic Pain Outreach Association, http://www.medhelp.org

National Foundation for the Treatment of Pain, http://www.paincare.org

National Guidelines Clearinghouse, http://www.guideline.gov

National Headache Foundation, http://www.headaches.org

National Hospice and Palliative Care Organization, http://www.nhpco.org

National Pain Foundation, http://www.nationalpainfoundation.org

CHAPTER 28
Diagnostic Tests

MAKING THE CONNECTION

Refer to the following chapters to increase your understanding of diagnostic tests:

Basic Nursing
- ***Complementary/Alternative Therapies***
- ***Assessment***
- ***Safety/Hygiene***
- ***Standard Precautions and Isolation***

Basic Procedures
- ***Urine Collection: Closed Drainage System***
- ***Urine Collection: Clean Catch, Female/Male***

Intermediate Procedures
- ***Performing Urinary Catheterization: Female/Male***
- ***Performing a Skin Puncture***

Advanced Procedures
- ***Performing Venipuncture (Blood Drawing)***

LEARNING OBJECTIVES

Upon completion of this chapter, you should be able to:

- Define key terms.
- Discuss the care of the client before, during, and after diagnostic testing.
- Describe the methods of specimen collection.
- Describe common noninvasive and invasive diagnostic procedures.
- Demonstrate the nursing responsibilities for common diagnostic procedures.

KEY TERMS

agglutination
agglutinin
agglutinogen
analyte
aneurysm
angiography
antibody
antigen
arteriography
ascites
aspiration
bacteremia
barium
biopsy
central line
computed tomography
contrast medium
culture
cytology
electrocardiogram
electroencephalogram
electrolyte
endoscopy
enzyme
fluoroscopy
hematuria
invasive
ketone
lipoprotein
lumbar puncture
magnetic resonance imaging (MRI)
necrosis
noninvasive
occult blood
oliguria

papanicolaou test	radiography	trocar
paracentesis	sensitivity	type and crossmatch
phlebotomist	stable	ultrasound
pneumothorax	stress test	urobilinogen
port-a-cath	thoracentesis	venipuncture
procedural sedation	transducer	void

INTRODUCTION

Information from a thorough history and physical examination determines the need for diagnostic testing. Results of diagnostic procedures are used to formulate a medical diagnosis and to plan a course of treatment. The challenge of cost-effective health care encourages practitioners to rely on basic assessment and to be selective about expensive diagnostic tests. The emphasis on cost containment has changed the nurse's role from doing for the client to teaching clients to do for themselves. The nurse teaches the client, family, and significant others about the diagnostic testing, how to prepare for the specific test(s), and the care required after the test. Although the primary focus is on teaching, the nurse may assist in performing various diagnostic tests. To deliver appropriate care to the client, nurses must know the implications of diagnostic tests and must know anatomy and physiology to understand the nature of diagnostic tests. Nurses can then relate diagnostic tests to specific disease processes and understand the test results.

This chapter discusses common diagnostic tests. The terms *test* and *procedure* are used interchangeably. The term *practitioner* is used to refer to either the physician or an advanced-practice registered nurse. Most state boards of nursing allow advanced-practice registered nurses to order and perform certain diagnostic tests.

DIAGNOSTIC TESTING

Diagnostic tests are either noninvasive or invasive. **Noninvasive** means that the body is not entered with any type of instrument; the skin and other body tissues, organs, and cavities remain intact. **Invasive** means that the body's tissues, organs, or cavities are accessed through some type of instrument.

Client Care

Diagnostic testing is a critical element of assessment. In collaboration with the client, assessment data are used to formulate nursing diagnoses, outcome measures, and a plan of care. Evaluation of the client's expected outcomes requires the incorporation of diagnostic findings.

▼ SAFETY ▼

Diagnostic Testing

To protect your health and safety, as well as that of other health care providers and the client, use Standard Precautions whenever performing invasive or noninvasive procedures.

Preparing the Client for Diagnostic Testing

The nurse plays a key role in scheduling and preparing the client for diagnostic testing. Tests not scheduled correctly inconvenience the client and delay interventions, which may place the client's health at risk. The institution is also at risk to lose money. Table 28-1 outlines a sample protocol of nursing care to prepare a client for diagnostic testing.

Ensure that the client is wearing an identification band and understands those things to be done. Also see that needed consent forms have been signed (Figure 28-1).

Nursing measures to ensure client safety are establish baseline vital signs, identify known allergies, and assess teaching effectiveness. In ambulatory and outpatient centers, there might be only one opportunity to assess and record vital signs. It is important to confirm that the vital signs are normal values for the client. Compare the vital signs taken during and after the procedure to those obtained before as baseline data to accurately assess the client's response to anesthetic agents and the procedure performed.

Advise the client of those things to expect during the procedure. Such teaching can both increase the level of cooperation and decrease the degree of anxiety. The client's family should also be informed of what will happen during the procedure and approximately how long the procedure should last. Know the facility's specific protocols and procedures because these are not standardized.

Care of the Client during Diagnostic Testing

Although client care must be individualized according to the specific procedure, general guidelines for client care during a procedure are outlined in Table 28-2. Protocols are used to assist with client care.

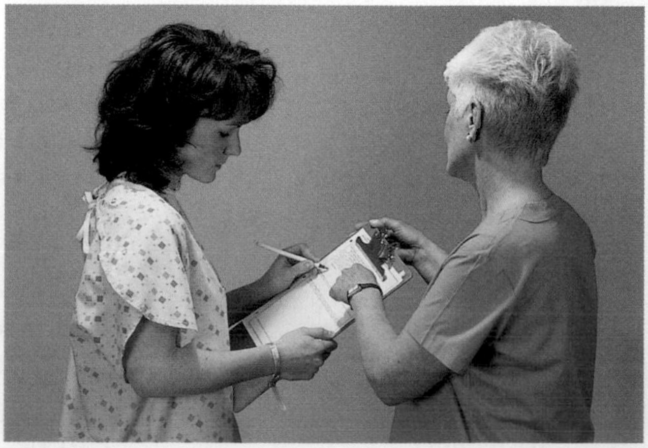

COURTESY OF DELMAR CENGAGE LEARNING

FIGURE 28-1 Preparing a Client for Diagnostic Testing

TABLE 28-1 Protocol: Preparing the Client for Diagnostic Testing

Purpose	To increase the reliability of the test by providing client teaching on the reason the test is being performed, those things the client can expect during the test, and the outcomes and side effects of the test To decrease the client's anxiety about the test and the associated risks
Supportive Data	Increase the client's knowledge, thereby promoting cooperation and enhancing the quality of the testing Decrease the time required to perform the tests, thereby increasing cost effectiveness Prevent delays by ensuring proper physical preparation
Assessment	Ensure that the client is wearing an identification band Review the medical record for allergies and previous adverse reactions to dyes and other contrast media; a signed consent form; and the recorded findings of diagnostic tests relative to the procedure Assess for the presence, location, and characteristics of physical and communicative limitations or preexisting conditions Monitor the client's knowledge of the reasons for the test and things to expect during and after testing Monitor vital signs, including pain, of the client scheduled for invasive testing, to establish baseline data Assess client outcome measures relative to the practitioner's preferences for preprocedure preparations Monitor level of hydration and weakness for clients who are designated nothing by mouth (NPO)
Report to Practitioner	Notify practitioner of allergy, previous adverse reaction, or suspected adverse reaction following the administration of drugs Notify practitioner of any client or family concerns not alleviated by discussions with nurse
Interventions	Clarify with practitioner whether regularly scheduled medications are to be administered Implement NPO status, as determined by the type of test Administer cathartics or laxatives as noted on the test's protocol; instruct clients who are weak to call for assistance to the bathroom Teach relaxation techniques, such as deep breathing and imagery Establish intravenous (IV) access if necessary for the procedure
Evaluation	Evaluate the client's knowledge of those things to expect Evaluate the client's anxiety level Evaluate the client's level of safety and comfort

Client Teaching	Discuss the following with the client and family, as appropriate to the specific test:
	• The reason for the test and those things to expect
	• An estimate of how long the test will take
	• Specifics of NPO status, including amount of water to drink if oral medication is to be taken
	• Cathartics or laxative: amount, frequency
	• Sputum: cough deeply, do not clear throat
	• Urine: voided, clean-catch specimen; timing of collection
	• Removal of objects (e.g., jewelry or hair clips) that will obscure x-ray film
	• Contrast medium:
	    • Barium: taste, consistency, after-effects (lightly colored stools for 24 to 72 hours; possibly, obstruction/impaction)
	    • Iodine: metallic taste, delayed allergic reaction (itching, rashes, hives, wheezing and breathing difficulties)
	• Positioning during the test
	• Positioning posttest (e.g., immobilize limb after angiography)
	• Posttest (encourage fluid intake if not contraindicated)

Documentation	Record in the client's medical record: • Practitioner notification of allergies or suspected adverse reaction to contrast media • Presence, location, and characteristics of symptoms • Teaching and the client's response to teaching • Responses to interventions (client outcomes)

TABLE 28-2 Protocol: Care of the Client during Diagnostic Testing

Purpose	To increase cooperation and participation by allaying the client's anxiety To provide the maximum level of safety and comfort during a procedure
Supportive Data	Encourage relaxation of the muscles and thus facilitate instrumentation by increasing the client's participation and comfort Ensure efficient use of time during the test and reliable results from the test with proper client preparation
Assessment	Check the client's identification band to ensure the correct client Review the medical record for allergies Assess the client's reaction to the preprocedure sedatives administered prior to the induction of anesthesia during the procedure Assess airway maintenance and gag reflex, if a local anesthetic is sprayed into the client's throat Assess vital signs, including pain, throughout the procedure and compare to baseline data Assess the client's ability to maintain and tolerate the prescribed position Assess the client's comfort level (pain) to ensure the effectiveness of the anesthetic agent Assess for related symptoms indicating complications specific to the procedure (e.g., accidental perforation of an organ)
Report to Practitioner	Notify the practitioner of any client concerns or questions not answered in discussions with the nurse Notify the practitioner of any family members present and their location during the procedure Notify the practitioner when the client is positioned properly and the anesthetic agent has been administered to the client
Interventions	Institute Standard Precautions or appropriate aseptic technique for the specific test Report to all personnel involved in the test any known client allergies Place the client in the correct position, drape, and monitor to ensure that breathing is not compromised Remain with the client during induction and maintenance of anesthesia If the procedure requires the administration of a dye, ensure that the client is not allergic to the dye; if the client has not received the dye before, perform the skin allergy test according to the manufacturer's instructions that accompany the medication Monitor the client's airway and keep resuscitative equipment available Assist the client to relax during insertion of the instrument by telling the client to breathe through the mouth and to concentrate on relaxing the involved muscles Explain what the practitioner is doing so that the client knows what to expect Label and handle the specimen according to the type of materials obtained and the testing to be done Report to the practitioner any symptoms of complications Secure client transport from the diagnostic area Posttest in the diagnostic area: • Assist the client to a comfortable, safe position • Provide oral hygiene and water to clients who were designated NPO for the test, if they are alert and able to swallow • Remain with the client awaiting transport to another area
Evaluation	Evaluate the client's ventilatory status and tolerance to the procedure Evaluate the client's need for assistance Evaluate the client's understanding of what was performed during the procedure Evaluate the client's understanding of findings identified during the procedure Evaluate the client's knowledge of what to expect after the procedure
Client Teaching	Discuss the following with the client and family, as appropriate to the specific test: • Those things that occurred during the procedure • Questions and concerns of the client or family member • Those things to expect during the immediate recovery phase • Those things to report to the nurse during the immediate recovery phase

TABLE 28-2 Protocol: Care of the Client during Diagnostic Testing (Continued)

Documentation	Record in the client's medical record: • Person who performed the procedure • Reason for the procedure • Type of anesthetic, dye, or other medications administered • Type of specimen obtained and where it was sent • Vital signs and other assessment data such as client's tolerance of the procedure or pain/discomfort level • Any symptoms of complications • Person who transported the client to another area (designate the names of persons who provided transport and the destination)

Standard Precautions are used when possible exposure to body fluids may occur. Protective barriers, such as gown, gloves, and goggles, should be used during invasive procedures.

Label all specimens with the client's name and room number (for hospitalized clients) and the date, time, and specimen source. Some specimens may need to be taken immediately to the laboratory or placed on ice (e.g., arterial blood gases [ABGs]).

Ongoing assessment of the client is required during any procedure. The patency of the client's airway should be continuously assessed because it may be compromised by the client's position, by anesthesia, or by the procedure itself. During an invasive procedure, monitor for signs and symptoms of accidental perforation of an organ (e.g., sudden changes in vital signs).

The nurse has the following additional responsibilities:

- Prepare the procedure room (e.g., ensure adequate lighting)
- Gather and charge for supplies to be used during the procedure
- Test the equipment to ensure it is functional and safe
- Secure proper containers for specimen collection

Practitioners usually have preference cards within the diagnostic testing area that specify the type of equipment to be used, the position in which to place the client, and the type of sedative or anesthetic agent to be used.

Some diagnostic tests are performed with the RN administering IV sedation, also called procedural sedation. **Procedural sedation** is a minimally depressed level of consciousness during which the client retains the ability to maintain a continuously patent airway and respond appropriately to physical stimulation or verbal commands. The nurse managing procedural sedation functions in an expanded role that requires additional education and demonstrated ability beyond the basic education.

CARE OF THE CLIENT AFTER DIAGNOSTIC TESTING

Postprocedure nursing care is directed toward restoring the client's prediagnostic level of functioning (Table 28-3). Nursing assessment and interventions are based mainly on the nature of the test and whether the client received anesthesia.

The client is closely monitored for signs of respiratory distress and bleeding. Some diagnostic tests require vital signs measurement every 15 minutes for the first hour and then at gradually longer intervals until the client is **stable** (alert and with vital signs within the client's normal range).

Some diagnostic tests use medications that are excreted through the kidneys. The client's intake and output (I&O) is monitored for 24 hours. The client is taught to monitor I&O and to report **hematuria** (presence of blood in the urine).

Clients should receive written instructions when discharged after diagnostic testing. Most agencies have discharge forms on which teaching regarding medications, dietary and activity restrictions, and signs and symptoms to be reported immediately to the practitioner are documented.

LABORATORY TESTS

Common laboratory studies are usually simple measurements to determine the amount or number of **analytes** (i.e., measured substances) present in a specimen. Laboratory tests are ordered by the practitioner to:

- Detect and quantify future disease risk
- Establish or exclude diagnoses
- Assess the disease process severity and formulate a prognosis
- Guide intervention selection
- Monitor the progress of the disorder
- Monitor treatment effectiveness

SPECIMEN COLLECTION

The scheduling and sequencing of laboratory tests are important. All tests requiring **venipuncture** (the use of a needle to puncture a vein to aspirate blood) should be grouped together so the client has only one venipuncture. Fasting laboratory

SAFETY

Radioactive Iodine and Urine Collection

Clients receiving radioactive iodine must have their urine collected and properly discarded in a special container, according to agency policy for handling radioactive medical wastes.

and radiological studies should be scheduled on the same day so that the client is only required to fast for 1 day. The client's comfort level and satisfaction increases with appropriate scheduling.

PROFESSIONALTIP

Documentation of Specimen-Collection Difficulties

Document on the laboratory requisition slip and in the nurses' notes any difficulty experienced during collection. Such problems may indicate adverse effects related to the nature of the test and thus must be reported and treated immediately.

Accuracy in laboratory testing requires that:

- The correct requisition form is used
- All requested information is written on the form (e.g., the client's full name and medical number)
- Pertinent data that could influence the test's results, such as medications taken, is included
- Specimen collection from the correct client is confirmed by checking the identification band
- Laboratory results are placed in the correct medical record

VENIPUNCTURE

Various members of the health care team can perform venipuncture. Although laboratories employ **phlebotomists** (individuals who perform venipuncture) to collect blood specimens, nurses must know how to perform venipuncture,

TABLE 28-3 Protocol: Care of the Client after Diagnostic Testing

Purpose	To restore the client's prediagnostic level of functioning by providing care and teaching relative to both those things the client can expect after a test and the outcomes or side effects of the test
Supportive Data	Decrease client anxiety by increasing the client's participation and knowledge of expected outcome measures after a diagnostic test Through proper postprocedure care and client teaching, alert the client to those signs and symptoms that must be reported to the practitioner
Assessment	Check the identification band and call the client by name Assess the client closely for signs of airway distress, adverse reactions to anesthetic or other medications, and other signs that may indicate accidental perforation of an organ Assess for bleeding in those areas where a biopsy was performed Assess the client's vital signs, including pain Assess vascular access lines or other invasive monitoring devices Assess the client's ability to expel air, if air was instilled during a gastrointestinal test Assess the client's knowledge of those things to expect during the recovery phase
Report to Practitioner	Notify the practitioner of any signs of respiratory distress, bleeding, or changes in vital signs; adverse reactions to anesthetic, sedative, or dye; and other signs of complications Notify the practitioner of client or family concerns or questions not answered in discussions with the nurse Notify the practitioner when any results are obtained from the diagnostic test Notify the practitioner when the client is fully alert and recovered (for an order to discharge)
Interventions	Implement the practitioner's orders regarding the postprocedure care of the client Institute Standard Precautions or surgical asepsis as appropriate to the client's care needs Position the client for comfort and accessibility so as to facilitate performance of nursing measures Monitor vital signs according to the frequency required for the specific test Observe the insertion site for hematoma or blood loss; replace pressure dressing, as needed Monitor the client's urinary output and drainage from other devices Enforce activity restrictions appropriate to the test Schedule client appointments as directed by the practitioner
Evaluation	Evaluate the client's respiratory status, especially if an anesthetic agent was used Evaluate the client's tolerance of oral liquids Evaluate the client's understanding of the procedural findings of when the practitioner expects to receive written results Evaluate the client's knowledge of those things to expect after discharge

TABLE 28-3 Protocol: Care of the Client after Diagnostic Testing (Continued)

Client Teaching	Based on client assessment and evaluation of knowledge, teach the client or family about the following: • Dietary or activity restrictions • Signs and symptoms that should be reported immediately to the practitioner • Medications
Documentation	Record in the client's medical record on the appropriate forms: • Assessment data, nursing interventions, and achievement of expected outcomes • Client or family teaching and demonstrated level of understanding • Written instructions given to the client or family members

because they routinely perform venipuncture in hospital critical care units, the home, and long-term care settings.

Venipuncture can be performed by using either a sterile needle and syringe or a vacuum tube holder with a sterile two-ended needle. Test tubes with different colored stoppers are used to collect blood specimens. The stoppers indicate the type of additive in the test tube. The tubes are universally color coded as follows:

- Red: no additive
- Lavender: ethylenediaminetetraacetic acid (EDTA)
- Light blue: sodium citrate
- Green: sodium heparin
- Gray: potassium oxalate
- Black: sodium oxalate

ARTERIAL PUNCTURE

Arterial blood gases reveal the lung's ability to exchange gases by measuring the partial pressures of oxygen (PaO_2) and carbon dioxide ($PaCO_2$) and evaluates the potential of hydrogen (pH) of arterial blood. Blood gases are ordered to evaluate:

- Oxygenation
- Ventilation and the effectiveness of respiratory therapy
- Acid–base balance in the blood

PROFESSIONALTIP

Arterial Blood Gases

To ensure an accurate determination of the client's actual blood gases, ABGs should not be drawn within 30 minutes after any respiratory treatment.

CLIENTTEACHING

Postarterial Puncture

The client should *immediately* notify the nurse if any pain or numbness occurs in the arm or leg after an arterial puncture. These symptoms indicate impaired circulation.

Arterial blood is drawn from a peripheral artery (e.g., radial or femoral) or from an arterial line. The blood is collected in a 5-mL heparinized syringe. The syringe is then rotated to mix the blood with the heparin to prevent clotting and then placed on ice.

In some agencies, it is within the scope of nursing practice to perform radial artery puncture, but femoral artery puncture is usually performed only by an advanced practitioner because of the associated increased risk of hemorrhage. It is not common practice for student nurses to draw ABG samples, but students often assist with the procedure and care for the client afterward.

The nurse is responsible for assessing the client for symptoms of postpuncture bleeding or occlusion. Apply direct pressure to the puncture site until all bleeding has stopped (a minimum of 5 minutes). Symptoms of impaired circulation include:

- Numbness and tingling
- Bluish color (cyanosis)
- Absence of a peripheral pulse

CAPILLARY PUNCTURE

When small quantities of capillary blood are needed for analysis or when the client has poor veins, a capillary puncture is performed. They are also used for blood glucose analysis. Figure 28-2 illustrates a capillary puncture of a fingertip.

CENTRAL LINES

A blood sample can also be collected from a **central line** (a venous catheter inserted into the superior vena cava through the subclavian or internal or external jugular vein). Central lines are used to treat fluid or electrolyte imbalances, such as severe dehydration caused by vomiting. Central lines are inserted when a peripheral route cannot be obtained, can be used for treatment, and to withdraw blood for analysis.

PROFESSIONALTIP

Common Sites for Capillary Puncture

- Inner aspect of a palmar fingertip is the most commonly used site.
- Earlobe is used when the client is in shock or the extremities are edematous.

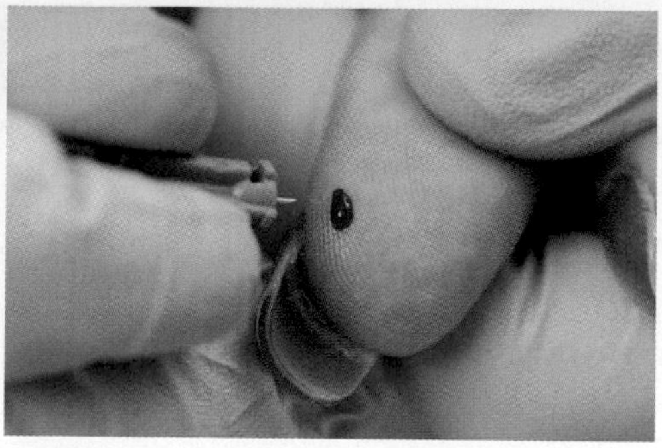

FIGURE 28-2 Capillary Puncture of Fingertip

The first blood sample drawn from a central line cannot be used for diagnostic testing. It must be discarded, with the volume of discard being the same as the dead space (catheter size). Agency protocol should specify the volume to discard relative to the type and size of catheter.

Central line care requires strict sterile technique. The practitioner must write an order for a blood sample to be obtained from a central line.

Peripherally inserted central catheters (PICC) are inserted into one of the major veins in the anticubital fossa or upper extremity and terminate in the superior vena cava. Blood samples can be collected from a PICC line. LPNs are required to successfully complete IV training to manage central lines and PICC lines. LPN nursing care of central lines varies from state to state. LPNs should know and follow the standards of practice for the state of clinical practice.

IMPLANTED PORT

Some clients have a **port-a-cath** (a port that has been implanted under the skin) over the third or fourth rib. The port's catheter is inserted into the superior vena cava or right atrium through the subclavian or internal jugular vein.

> **COMMUNITY/HOME HEALTH CARE**
>
> **Urine Collection in the Home**
>
> Clients in the home should place the urine container in a reclosable ("zipper") plastic bag and refrigerate until delivering to a laboratory. Doing so prevents bacteria growth and promotes accuracy of results.

> **COMMUNITY/HOME HEALTH CARE**
>
> **Central Line**
>
> Clients receiving prolonged therapy in the home environment usually have a central line in place. Because one of the primary complications of central venous catheter insertion is infection, the nurse must be alert for signs of infection (e.g., fever).

> **SAFETY**
>
> **Standard Precautions and Urine Collection**
>
> All urine collection requires the use of Standard Precautions to prevent transmission of microorganisms among nurses, clients, and other health care providers. All specimen containers should be sealed in a biohazard bag prior to transport to the laboratory.

This implanted port is used for the same purpose as a central line. Using strict sterile technique, blood can be withdrawn for analysis by accessing the port. This should be performed only by a nurse who has the education to properly do so.

URINE COLLECTION

Urine can be collected for various studies. The type of testing determines the method of collection. The different methods of urine collection are as follows:

- Random collection (routine analysis)
- Timed collection (24-hour urine)
- Collection from a closed urinary drainage system
- Sterile specimen (catheterized)
- Clean-voided specimen

The client's age and the method of collection determine client teaching. The collection method should be written on the laboratory requisition.

Random Collection The practitioner writes the order for a UA (routine urine analysis), also called a random collection. The specimen can be collected at any time using a clean, not sterile, cup. The specimen should be taken immediately to the laboratory to prevent bacterial growth and changes in the urine's analytes.

Timed Collection Timed collection is done over a 24-hour period. The urine is collected in a plastic gallon container that contains preservative(s), some of which are caustic.

For a timed collection, the client is told to **void** (eliminate urine) and discard the specimen at the beginning of the collection. Timing for a 24-hour urine collection begins after the first voiding has been discarded. For example, if the client voids at 1000 hours (24-hour [military] time), that urine should be discarded, but all urine is saved until 1000 hours the following day, when the last urine is saved. The client can void into a clean container and pour the urine into the collection bottle. Toilet tissue should not be dropped into the container used to catch the urine. The collection container should be refrigerated or kept on ice the entire 24 hours to stabilize the analytes and retard bacterial growth.

Collection from a Closed-Drainage System A sterile specimen can be collected from a client with an indwelling Foley catheter and closed-drainage system. A sterile specimen is used for urine culture. The urine specimen should *not* be obtained from the drainage bag because the analytes in the urine drainage bag change, leading to inaccurate results, and bacteria grows quickly in the drainage bag. The closed-drainage tubing has an aspiration port for sterile specimen collection.

Sterile Specimen When a sterile urine specimen is required and the client does not have an indwelling catheter and closed-drainage system, the client is catheterized. A small amount of urine is allowed to run out of the catheter into a basin, then the urine is allowed to flow into a sterile specimen bottle.

Clean-Voided Specimen Clean-voided (clean-catch, or midstream) specimen collection is done to have a specimen uncontaminated by skin flora. The collection technique is different for women and men. The female client is instructed to cleanse from the front to the back and then void into the specimen bottle; the male client is instructed to cleanse from the tip of the penis downward and then void into the specimen bottle.

Stool Collection

The reason for collecting a stool specimen should be explained to the client. The client is then instructed to defecate into a clean bedpan or container and discard used tissue in the toilet. Stools can be collected one time or over 24, 48, or 72 hours. Stools to be collected over a prolonged period must be placed into a container and refrigerated. Once all stools have been collected, the container should be labeled with the client's name, the date and time, and the test to be performed. All stool specimens are placed in a biohazard bag before being transported to the laboratory.

BLOOD TESTS

Many tests can be performed on the blood. Tests specific to the hematologic system are described in Table 28-4.

Type and Crossmatch

A **type and crossmatch** identifies the client's blood type and determines compatibility of blood between a potential donor and recipient (client). There are four basic blood types: A, B, AB, and O. The blood types are determined by the presence or absence of A or B antigens. **Antigens** are substances, usually proteins, that cause the formation of and react specifically with antibodies. **Antibodies** are immunoglobulins produced by the body in response to bacteria, viruses, or other antigenic substances. Type A and type B are antigens that are classified as **agglutinogens**, or substances that cause agglutination (clumping of RBCs). Agglutinins are specific kinds of antibodies whose interaction with antigens manifests as agglutination.

SAFETY

Collecting Stool from a Client with Hepatitis

Write on the requisition form that the client has hepatitis. Doing so alerts laboratory personnel to be especially careful when handling the specimen.

CRITICAL THINKING

Type and Rh

If a client's blood type is AB positive, what are the possible blood types of the client's parents? Can the client receive Rh-negative blood? Explain your answer.

Blood types are also identified as positive or negative, depending on the presence or absence of the Rh factor. The Rh factor is an antigen that may be found on the RBC. The designation *Rh positive* means the antigen is present; *Rh negative* means the antigen is absent. An individual's blood type and Rh are determined genetically.

Crossmatch identifies the compatibility of the donor's blood with that of the recipient. A sample of the recipient's blood is mixed with the blood of a possible donor in the laboratory. If the mixed sample does not agglutinate, it is compatible.

Blood Chemistry

Blood chemistry tests are often grouped together, requiring one requisition and one venous specimen. Tests performed include glucose, electrolytes, enzymes, lipids, creatinine, and protein values. Other tests that may be performed on a blood specimen are listed in Table 28-5.

Blood Glucose Blood for measuring glucose is obtained by either skin puncture or venipuncture and is either fasting (FBS) or nonfasting (usually 2 hours postprandial) blood sugar. If the results of this screening test for diabetes mellitus are abnormal, the practitioner may order a glucose tolerance test, the most accurate test for diagnosing hypoglycemia and hyperglycemia (diabetes mellitus).

Serum Electrolytes An **electrolyte** is a substance that, when in solution, separates into ions and conducts electricity. Some electrolytes act on the cell membrane to allow the transmission of electrochemical impulses in nerve and muscle fibers, whereas others determine the activity of cellular metabolism (Guyton & Hall, 2000).

Cations are ions that have a positive charge, such as sodium (Na^+), potassium (K^+), calcium (Ca^{++}), and magnesium (Mg^{++}). Anions are ions that have a negative charge, including chloride (Cl^-), bicarbonate (HCO_3^-), and phosphate (HPO_4^{--}).

Blood Enzymes Enzymes are globular proteins produced in the body that catalyze chemical reactions within the cells. Enzyme tests are key to diagnosing tissue damage, mainly to the myocardium and, to a lesser degree, to the brain.

Plasma levels of intracellular enzymes elevate in the presence of myocardial **necrosis** (tissue death as the result of disease or injury). Enzymes in the blood are directly proportional to the degree of cellular damage. The enzymes are not used alone in determining a diagnosis but, rather, are reviewed with other diagnostic studies.

Blood Lipids An elevated serum lipid level is one of the controllable contributing risk factors to congestive heart disease (CHD). **Lipoproteins** (blood lipids bound to protein) are measured along with cholesterol.

Text continues on page 626

TABLE 28-4 Tests Specific to the Hematologic System

TEST	EXPLANATION/NORMAL VALUES	NURSING RESPONSIBILITIES
Red blood cells (RBCs)	Number of RBCs per mm^3 of blood. May be low in clients with rheumatoid arthritis. Clients living in high altitudes may have an elevated RBC level. Normal: Male: 4.6–6.2 million/mm^3 Female: 4.2–5.5 million/mm^3	The client is not required to fast for the test.
White blood cells (WBCs)	Number of WBCs per mm^3 of blood. Elevation is associated with infectious processes. Normal: 4,100–10,800 mm^3	The client is not required to fast for the test. Exercise, stress, last month of pregnancy, labor, previous splenectomy, and eating may increase level and alter differential values. Note medications taken that may affect test; aspirin, heparin, and steroids may increase WBC level, whereas antibiotics and diuretics may decrease WBC level.
Differential count	Percentage of types of WBCs in 1 mm of blood.	The client is not required to fast for the test.
Neutrophilis	Increase in bacterial infections and trauma. Normal:	
Segs (mature neutrophils)	Segs: 50%–65%	
Bands (immature neutrophils)	Bands: 0%–5%	
Eosinophils	Increased in allergic reactions or parasitic infestation. Normal: 1%–3%	Corticosteroid therapy causes a decreased level.
Basophils	Increased in allergic reactions and during healing periods. Normal: 0.4%–1.0%	Steroids cause a decreased level.
Lymphocytes	Increased in viral infections and other diseases, such as pertussis and tuberculosis (TB). Decreased in acquired immunodeficiency syndrome (AIDS). Normal: 25%–35%	Steroids cause a decreased level.
Monocytes	Increased in chronic diseases, such as malaria, TB, Rocky Mountain spotted fever. May be low in clients with rheumatoid arthritis. Normal: 4%–6%	
Hemoglobin (Hgb)	Measures the oxygen-carrying compound in RBCs. Normal: Male: 14–18 g/dL Female: 12–16 g/dL Critical value: <5 g/dL	The client is not required to fast for the test. Sample may be drawn from a finger of a child or the heel of an infant.
Hemoglobin electrophoresis	Detects abnormal forms of hemoglobin. Performed after positive sickle cell test. If the hemoglobin electrophoresis is negative, the client has the sickle cell trait. If the hemoglobin electrophoresis is positive, the client has sickle cell anemia. Normal: Hgb S: 0% Hgb F: <2% Hgb Ca: 0%	If the client has had a blood transfusion within the last 12 weeks, the results of the test may be altered.

TABLE 28-4 Tests Specific to the Hematologic System (Continued)

TEST	EXPLANATION/NORMAL VALUES	NURSING RESPONSIBILITIES
Hematocrit (Hct)	Measures the percentage of blood cells in a volume of blood. Clients living in high altitudes may have an increased level. Normal: Male: 40%–54% Female: 38%–47% Critical value: <15% or >60%	The client is not required to fast for the test.
Platelet count	Measures the number of platelets per cubic milliliter of blood. Normal: 150,000–450,000/mm^3 Critical level: <50,000 and >1 million/mm^3	Instruct the client that strenuous exercise and oral contraceptives increase platelet level. Instruct the client that aspirin, acetaminophen, and sulfonamides decrease platelet level. If the client has a low platelet count, maintain digital pressure to the puncture site.
Bleeding time	Measures the length of time for a platelet plug to occlude a small puncture wound. Normal: 1–9 minutes (Ivy method) Critical value: >15 minutes	Notify the laboratory if the client is taking aspirin, anticoagulants, or other medications that may affect the clotting process.
Prothrombin time (PT, protime)	Measures the effectiveness of several blood-clotting factors. Normal: 10–13.4 seconds INR: 2.0–3.0 In the presence of anticoagulant therapy, the values should be 1½–2 times the normal value. Critical value: >20 seconds In the presence of anticoagulant therapy, the critical value should be >3 times the normal critical value.	Ensure that the blood specimen is drawn before the daily dose of warfarin (Coumadin) is administered. Instruct the client that alcohol intake may increase PT and that a diet high in fat may decrease PT. Note those medications taken that may affect results; salicylates, sulfonamides, and methyldopa (Aldomet), as these may increase PT, whereas digitalis and oral contraceptives decrease the level. Instruct the client not to take any medication without notifying the physician, as medications may affect the PT level.
International normalized ratio (INR)	Normal: 0.9–1.1 Clients on anticoagulant drugs should have an INR of 2–3 (2.5–3.5 for the client with a mechanical prosthetic heart valve). The INR is more accurate than PT in monitoring warfarin (Coumadin) therapy.	The daily warfarin (Coumadin) dose should be given after blood has been drawn for the INR.
Partial thromboplastin time (PTT), also called activated partial throboplastin time (APTT)	Normal: PTT: 60–70 sec APTT: 21–35 sec In the presence of anticoagulant therapy, the normal value is 1.5–2.5 times the control value. Critical value: APTT: >70 seconds PTT: >100 seconds	If the client is receiving intermittent heparin doses, schedule the APTT to be drawn 30–60 minutes before the next heparin dose. If heparin is given continuously, the blood specimen can be drawn at any time. If PTT is greater than 100 seconds, the client is at risk for bleeding, and the physician is notified. The antidote for heparin is protamine sulfate. Note whether the client is taking antihistamines, vitamin C, or salicylates, as these prolong PTT time.

(Continues)

Table 28-4 Tests Specific to the Hematologic System (Continued)

TEST	EXPLANATION/NORMAL VALUES	NURSING RESPONSIBILITIES
D dimer test (fragment D dimer, fibrin degradation fragment)	Measures a fibrin split product that is released when a clot breaks. Confirms the diagnosis of disseminated intravascular coagulation (DIC). Screens for deep vein thrombosis (DVT) and pulmonary emboli. Normal: <10 mg/mL	Note whether the client is on thrombolytic therapy, as the results of this test would be increased from negative to positive.

Table 28-5 Additional Tests Performed on Blood Specimen

TEST	EXPLANATION/NORMAL VALUES	NURSING RESPONSIBILITIES
Acid phosphatase	Acid phosphatase is an enzyme found in the prostate gland, seminal fluid, and RBCs. An elevated level is seen in clients with prostatic cancer and hemolytic anemias. If tumors are treated successfully, the level will decrease. A rising level may indicate a poor prognosis. Normal: 0–0.80 U/L	Tell the client that no food or drink restrictions are associated with this test. Apply pressure to the venipuncture site. Observe the site for bleeding. Used in rape investigations.
Adrenocorticotropic hormone (ACTH), corticotropin	Determines the function of the anterior pituitary. Because of diurnal variation, specimens should be drawn in both morning and evening. Normal: 4–22 pmol/L	Emotional or physical stress or recent radioisotope scans can interfere with test results. Drugs that may increase ACTH level include corticosteroids, estrogens, ethanol, and spironolactone. Explain the procedure to the client. This is especially important to decrease the client's stress level. Evaluate the client for increased stress level. Initiate NPO status 12 hours before test. The blood specimen must be drawn with a heparinized syringe, chilled by placing the specimen on ice, and immediately transported to the lab.
ACTH stimulation test, cortisol stimulation test, cosyntropin test	Monitors plasma cortisol level to indicate adrenal gland response to ACTH. Normal: 1 hour: ↑ 20 μg/dL at least above baseline	Note those medications taken that may affect results: cortisone, estrogens, hydrocortisone, and spironolactone may increase plasma cortisol level. Explain the procedure to the client. Initiate NPO status after midnight. For all tests, obtain baseline serum cortisol level. Administer injection of cosyntropin IM or IV. Draw blood specimen 30 to 60 minutes after injection.
Alanine aminotransferase (ALT, formerly serum glutamic pyruvic transaminase [SGPT])	ALT is an enzyme released in response to liver injury. Normal: varies with testing method	Note those medications taken that affect results: many medications may increase level, including antibiotics, narcotics, oral contraceptives, and many others.
Alkaline phosphatase (ALP)	Alkaline phosphatase is an enzyme found primarily in the liver, biliary tract, and bone. Detection is important for determining possible liver and bone disease. Normal: varies widely depending on method	Fasting may be required. Apply pressure to the venipuncture site. Observe the site for bleeding.

TABLE 28-5 Additional Tests Performed on Blood Specimen (Continued)

TEST	EXPLANATION/NORMAL VALUES	NURSING RESPONSIBILITIES
Alpha-fetoprotein (AFP)	Test for tumor marker; elevated in nonseminomatous testicular cancer. Performed between 16 and 18 weeks of pregnancy. A high level is suggestive of neural tube defects. Normal: 0.9 ng/mL 16–18 weeks gestation: 30–43 μg/mL	Apply pressure to site and watch for bleeding or hematoma. Sample must be drawn between 15–20 weeks of gestation.
Amylase (AMS)	Amylase is an enzyme secreted by the pancreas. Elevation indicates pancreatitis. Normal: 25–125 IU/L	Note those medications taken that affect test results; steroids, aspirin, alcohol, some narcotics, some diuretics, and other drugs may increase level, whereas citrate, glucose, and oxalates may decrease level.
Antidiuretic hormone (ADH), vasopressin	Determines the production of ADH by the posterior pituitary. Normal: <1.5 pg/L	Explain the procedure to the client. Note those medications taken that may interfere with test results. Drugs that elevate ADH level include acetaminophen, barbiturates, cholinergic agents, estrogen, nicotine, oral hypoglycemic agents, some diuretics such as thiazides, and tricyclic antidepressants. Drugs that decrease ADH level include alcohol, beta-adrenergic agents, morphine antagonists, and phenytoin (Dilantin). Client should fast for 12 hours before the test. Evaluate the client for high level of physical or emotional stress.
Antinuclear antibodies (ANAs)	ANAs attack cell nuclei. The result is positive in 95% of clients with systemic lupus erythematosus. Levels are low in clients with mononucleosis, rheumatic fever, and liver diseases. Normal: negative at 1:20 dilution	Fasting is not required. Hydralazine (Apresoline) and procainamide (Pronestyl) may increase level. A radioactive scan in the past week may alter results; inform the lab, if applicable.
Antistreptolysin O (ASO)	High titer indicates presence of *beta-hemolytic streptococcus*, which may cause rheumatic fever or acute glomerulonephritis. Upper limit of normal varies with age, season, and geographic area. Normal: Adult: <1:100 12–19 years: <1:200 2–5 years: <1:100	There are no food or fluid restrictions. Antibiotics decrease ASO level. Check urine output if ASO is elevated. Urine output of less than 600 mL/24 h is associated with acute glomerulonephritis.
Antithyroid microsomal antibody, antimicrosomal antibody, microsomal antibody, thyroid autoantibody, thyroid antimicrosomal antibody	Used to detect thyroid microsomal antibodies found in clients with Hashimoto's thyroiditis. Normal: titer <1:100	Explain the procedure to the client.

(Continues)

TABLE 28-5 Additional Tests Performed on Blood Specimen (Continued)

TEST	EXPLANATION/NORMAL VALUES	NURSING RESPONSIBILITIES
Aspartate aminotransferase (AST, formerly serum glutamic oxaloacetic transaminase [SGOT])	AST is an enzyme that indicates inflammation of heart, liver, skeletal muscle, pancreas, or kidneys. Normal: Male: 8–46 U/L Female: 7–31 U/L	Avoid intramuscular (IM) injections; record date and time of any injections. Avoid hemolysis. Withhold medications that affect results, for 12 hours if possible; several medications, such as antihypertensives, cholinergic agents, anticoagulants, digitalis, and others, may increase level, as may exercise.
Arterial blood gases (ABGs)	Direct measurement of the pH, PaO_2, and $PaCO_2$, and calculated measurement of HCO_3^- and SaO_2 from samples of arterial blood. pH = expresses the acidity or alkalinity of the blood. PaO_2 = partial pressure of oxygen in the blood. $PaCO_2$ = partial pressure of carbon dioxide in the blood. SaO_2 = arterial oxygen saturation. HCO_3^- = bicarbonate ion concentration in the blood. The oxygen content of the blood expressed as a percentage of the oxygen carrying capacity of the blood. Normal: / Critical level: pH: 7.35–7.45 / <7.2 or >7.6 PaO_2: 75–100 mm Hg / <40 mm Hg $PaCO_2$: 35–45 mm Hg / <20 or >70 HCO_3^-: 24–28 mEq / <10 or >40 SaO_2: >95% (at sea level) / <60%	Explain that an arterial sample of blood is required. Arterial punctures cause more discomfort than venous. Instruct the client not to move. Assess the adequacy of collateral circulation. The blood sample is drawn in a syringe containing heparin. After the specimen has been obtained, rotate the syringe to mix the blood and heparin. The blood sample is placed on ice and taken immediately to the lab. Apply pressure to the arterial site for 3 to 5 minutes or 15 minutes if client is on an anticoagulant. Assess site for bleeding.
Bilirubin	Measures bilirubin in the blood. Indicates how well the liver is functioning. Normal: Total: 0.1–1.3 mg/dL Direct: 0.0–0.3 mg/dL Indirect: 0.1–1.0 mg/dL	Note those medications taken that affect results; steroids, antibiotics, oral hypoglycemics, narcotics, as well as others may cause increased level, whereas barbiturates, caffeine, penicillins, and salicylates may cause decreased level. Fasting may be required. Do not shake the tube; protect the tube from light.
Blood glucose, fasting blood sugar (FBS)	Measures blood level of glucose (serum values). Results depend on method used by laboratory. Normal fasting glucose: 70–99 mg/dL (3.9–5.5 mmol/L) Impaired fasting glucose (prediabetes): 100–125 mg/dL (5.6–6.9 mmol/L) Diabetes: 126 mg/dL (7.0 mmol/L) and above on more than one testing occasion Critical values: >400 mg/dL <50 mg/dL	Client must fast (except for water) for 12 hours before test. Withhold insulin or oral antidiabetic medications until blood is drawn. Be certain client receives medications and meal after fasting specimen drawn. Cortisone, thiazide, and loop diuretics cause increase.

Table 28-5 Additional Tests Performed on Blood Specimen (Continued)

TEST	EXPLANATION/NORMAL VALUES	NURSING RESPONSIBILITIES
2 hour postprandial glucose (2h PPG) or 2 hour postprandial blood sugar (2h PPBS)	Measures blood glucose 2 hours after a meal. Normal: 70–140 mg/dL Diabetic: >140 mg/dL	Instruct the client to eat entire meal and then to not eat anything else until blood is drawn. Notify the laboratory of the time meal was completed.
Blood urea nitrogen (BUN)	Measures urea, end product of protein metabolism. Normal: 5–20 mg/dL	Initiate NPO status 8 hours prior to test, if possible. Note the client's hydration status. Note those medications taken that may affect results, including phenothiazines, nephrotoxic drugs, diuretics (hydrochlorothiazide [Hydro-Diuril], ethacrynic acid [Edecrin], furosemide [Lasix]); antibiotics (bacitracin, gentamicin, kanamycin, methicillin, neomycin); antihypertensives (methyldopa [Aldomet], guanethidine [Ismelin]), sulfonamides, propranolol, morphine, lithium, salicylates.
B-type natriuretic peptide (BNP)	Enables doctors to make the correct diagnosis of heart failure. Secreted from the ventricles of the heart in response to changes in pressure when heart failure develops and worsens. No heart failure: <100 pg/mL Suggests heart failure is present: 100–300 pg/mL Mild heart failure: >300 pg/mL Moderate heart failure: >600 pg/mL Severe heart failure: >900 pg/mL	Explain to client that a blood sample is needed. The test takes about 15 minutes.
CA-15-3	CA-15-3 (cancer antigen) is a tumor marker for monitoring breast cancer. Because benign breast or ovarian disease can also cause elevations, it has limited use in diagnosis. Normal: <22 U/mL	Fasting is not required. Apply pressure to the venipuncture site. Observe the site for bleeding.
CA-19-9	CA-19-9 (cancer antigen) is a tumor marker used primarily in the diagnosis of pancreatic carcinoma. Normal: <37 U/mL	Fasting is not required. Apply pressure to the venipuncture site. Observe the site for bleeding.
CA-125	CA-125 (cancer antigen) is a tumor marker especially helpful in making the diagnosis of ovarian cancer. Normal: 0–35 U/mL	Fasting is not required. Apply pressure to the venipuncture site. Observe the site for bleeding.
Calcitonin, HCT, thyrocalcitonin	Determines thyroid and parathyroid activity. Also used as a tumor marker to detect thyroid cancer and several other cancers. Normal: basal <151 pg/mL	Note those medications taken that may increase calcitonin level, including calcium, cholecystokinin, epinephrine, glucagon, pentagastrin, and oral contraceptives. Explain the procedure to the client. The client should fast 8 hours but may have water.

(Continues)

TABLE 28-5 Additional Tests Performed on Blood Specimen (Continued)

TEST	EXPLANATION/NORMAL VALUES	NURSING RESPONSIBILITIES
Carcinoembryonic antigen (CEA)	CEA is found in clients with cancer, especially colorectal cancer. It is especially useful in monitoring treatment response and is occasionally the first sign of tumor recurrence. Normal: <5 ng/mL Smoker <2.5 ng/mL Nonsmoker	Fasting is not required. Apply pressure to the venipuncture site. Observe the site for bleeding. Note whether the client smokes or has a disease that will alter results, such as hepatitis, cirrhosis, or colitis.
Cardiac enzymes Serum AST	Indicates possible tissue damage if elevated. Normal: Male: 7–21 U/L Female: 6–18 U/L	Neither fasting nor NPO status is necessary. Pattern of elevated levels of AST, CPK, and LDH is indicative of myocardial infarction (MI).
Creatine kinase CPK (CK)	Normal: Male: 55–170 U/L Female: 30–135 U/L	CPK is the first enzyme elevated after MI, and peaks within the first 24 hours.
CK isoenzymes	Present in skeletal muscle, brain, lungs, and heart muscle. Normal:	Elevation of an isoenzyme indicates damage to tissue in a specific organ; CK-MB is specific for myocardial cells. Level increases 3–6 hours following MI, peaks in 12–24 hours and returns to normal in 18–24 hours.
CK-MM (muscle)	100%	
CK-BB (brain)	0%	
CK-MB (heart)	0%	
Lactic dehydrogenase (LDH)	Normal: 45–90 U/L Critical level: 300–800 U/L following myocardial infarction	LDH_1 value greater than LDH_2 value is indicative of an acute MI. LDH_5 is elevated with congestive heart failure (CHF).
LDH isoenzymes		
LDH_1 (heart and erythrocytes)	*17.5%–28.3%	
LDH_2 (reticuloendothelial system)	*30.4%–36.4%	
LDH_3 (lungs and other tissues)	*18.8%–26.0%	
LDH_4 (kidney, placenta, pancreas)	*9.2%–16.5%	
LDH_5 (liver and striated muscles)	*5.3%–13.4%	
Cardiac troponin I and T	Proteins found in cardiac muscle. Protein is released when the muscle is injured or dead. Troponin I elevated level in 4–6 hours Normal: <1.5 ng/mL Troponin T elevated level in 4–6 hours Normal: <0.6 ng/mL	Explain to client that blood sample is needed. Test very expensive. Often used in the ED.

*% of total LDH

TABLE 28-5 Additional Tests Performed on Blood Specimen (Continued)

TEST	EXPLANATION/NORMAL VALUES	NURSING RESPONSIBILITIES
CD4 T-cell count	Predictor of HIV progression; baseline taken after positive HIV test. Normal: 500–1,000/mm^3 Critical value: <200/mm^3	Explain the meaning of the test. Provide follow-up explanation of test results.
Cholesterol (lipid profile)	Lipid necessary for steroid, bile, and cell membrane production. Normal: <200 mg/dL (total)	Have client fast 12–14 hours prior to test. No alcohol 24 hours prior to test. Diet intake 2 weeks prior to test will affect results. Note those medications taken that may affect results; steroids, phenytoin, diuretics, and others may elevate level, whereas MAO inhibitors, some antibiotics, lovastatin, and others may decrease level. If elevated, increased risk of coronary artery disease (CAD), hypertension, and MI.
High density lipoprotein (HDL)	Normal: 30–70 mg/dL	
Low density lipoprotein (LDL)	Normal: 60–160 mg/dL	
Very low density lipoprotein (VLDL)	Normal: 25%–50%	
Triglycerides	Normal: 40–150 mg/dL	Elevated level in CAD; level increases when LDL level increases.
Complement assay (total complement, C3 and C4)	Decreased levels in autoimmune diseases due to depletion of complement by antibody–antigen complexes. Normal: C3: Male: 80–180 mg/dL Female: 76–120 mg/dL C4: 15–45 mg/dL	Fasting is not required.
Coombs' test (direct antiglobulin test)	Detects whether immunoglobulins are attached to RBCs. Normal: negative	Note whether the client is taking ampicillin (Unasyn), captopril (Capoten), indomethacin (Indocin), or insulin, as these cause false-positive results.
Cortisol, hydrocortisone	Determines adrenal cortex function. There is normally a diurnal variation, with higher level around 6 to 8 A.M. and lowest levels around midnight. Normal: 8 A.M.: 6–28 µg/dL, or 170–625 nmol/L 4 P.M.: 2–12 µg/dL, or 80–413 nmol/L	Note whether the client has been under physical or emotional stress as either can artificially elevate plasma cortisol level. Likewise, recent use of radioisotopes can interfere with test results. Note those medications taken that may affect results. Drugs that may increase plasma cortisol level include estrogen, oral contraceptives, and spironolactone (Aldactone). Drugs that may decrease plasma cortisol level include androgens and phenytoin (Dilantin). Explain the procedure to the client. Two specimens are drawn—one at 8 A.M. and another at 4 P.M. Assess the client for physical or emotional stress and report to the physician. Indicate times of collection on laboratory requisitions.

(Continues)

Table 28-5 Additional Tests Performed on Blood Specimen (Continued)

TEST	EXPLANATION/NORMAL VALUES	NURSING RESPONSIBILITIES
C-reactive protein test (CRP)	An abnormal protein appears in the blood of clients with an acute inflammatory process. Used to monitor the progress of clients with autoimmune disorders such as rheumatoid arthritis. More sensitive than erythrocyte sedimentation rate (ESR). Normal: <6 mg/L	Fast, except for water, for 8 hours. Note those medications that may affect results: nonsteroidal antiinflammatory drugs (NSAIDs), steroids, and salicylates may decrease level; oral contraceptives and intrauterine devices (IUDs) may increase level. Inform laboratory, if applicable.
Culture	Identifies pathogens in blood. Normal: none	There are no food or fluid restrictions. Specimen should be taken immediately to the laboratory. All specimens should be collected prior to initiating antibiotic therapy.
Dexamethasone suppression test (DST), prolonged/rapid DST, cortisol suppression test (ACTH suppression test)	Monitors plasma cortisol level to measure adrenal gland function. Normal: <5 mg/dL	Stress can interfere with test results. Note those medications taken that may affect results, including barbiturates, estrogens, oral contraceptives, phenytoin (Dilantin), spironolactone, steroids, and tetracyclines. Explain the procedure to the client. Weigh the client for baseline weight. Rapid test: Administer dexamethasone 1 mg orally at 11 P.M. with milk or antacid. Administer sedative, if ordered. At 8 A.M., before client rises, draw plasma cortisol level. Overnight 8-mg dexamethasone suppression test: If no cortisol suppression occurs, repeat test using 8 mg dexamethasone. If there is still no cortisol suppression, a prolonged test over 6 days involving six 24-hour urine collections should be done.
Electrolytes	Determines blood electrolyte levels. First four are the most commonly measured.	Sodium and potassium are necessary for cardiac electrical conduction.
Sodium (Na^+)	Measures level of serum sodium. Function in the body: Major electrolyte in extracellular fluid, regulates fluid balance, stimulates conduction of nerve impulses, helps maintain neuromuscular activity. Normal: 135–145 mEq/L	There are no food or fluid restrictions.
Potassium (K^+)	Measures level of serum potassium. Function in the body: Major electrolyte in intracellular fluid, maintains normal nerve and muscle activity, assists in cellular metabolism of carbohydrates and proteins. Normal: 3.5–5.5 mEq/L	There are no food or fluid restrictions. If the client has hypokalemia or hyperkalemia, evaluate the client for cardiac dysrhythmias.

TABLE 28-5 Additional Tests Performed on Blood Specimen (Continued)

TEST	EXPLANATION/NORMAL VALUES	NURSING RESPONSIBILITIES
Electrolytes Continued		
Chloride (Cl^-)	Measures level of serum chloride Function in the body: Major electrolyte in extracellular fluid, functions in combination with sodium to maintain osmotic pressure, assists in maintaining acid–base balance Normal: 100–110 mEq/L	There are no food or fluid restrictions.
Calcium, total/ionized Ca^{++}	Indicates parathyroid gland function and calcium metabolism. Because ionized calcium is unaffected by serum albumin, it can give more accurate results; however, most laboratories do not have the equipment to perform the test. Normal: Total: 8.5–10.5 mg/dL, or 2.25–2.75 nmol/L Ionized: 4.5–5.6 ng/dL, or 1.05–1.30 nmol/L	Note those medications taken that may affect results. Drugs that may increase serum calcium level include calcium salts, hydralazine, lithium, thiazide diuretics, parathyroid hormone (PTH), thyroid hormone, and vitamin D. Drugs that may decrease serum calcium level include acetazolamide, anticonvulsants, asparaginase, aspirin, calcitonin, cisplatin, corticosteroids, heparin, laxatives, loop diuretics, magnesium salts, and oral contraceptives. Vitamin D and excessive milk ingestion can also interfere with test results. Explain the procedure to the client. Fasting is not required for serum calcium, but might be required if other blood chemistry tests are to be drawn.
Magnesium (Mg^{++})	Measures level of serum magnesium Function in the body: Combines with calcium and phosphorous in intracellular bone tissue, essential for neuromuscular contraction, synthesis of protein, and body temperature regulation Normal: 1.6–2.6 mEq/L	There are no food or fluid restrictions.
Phosphate (PO_4^{--})	Measures level of serum phosphate Function in the body: An essential intracellular electrolyte, exists in an inverse relationship with calcium Normal: 3–4.5 mg/dL	Initiate NPO status after midnight. Intravenous fluids containing glucose are sometimes discontinued several hours before the test.
Bicarbonate (HCO_3^-) (total carbon dioxide content or carbon dioxide capacity)	Always in a 20:1 ratio with carbonic acid. Normal: venous 22–29 mEq/L arterial 21–28 mEq/L	There are no food or fluid restrictions. Loss of gastric contents is the most common reason for increased level.
ELISA	Screening test used to indicate the presence of HIV Normal: negative	Inform the client that if the first ELISA test is positive, a second ELISA will be drawn before confirmation is done with Western blot. Provide pretest counseling. Obtain informed consent. Provide or arrange for posttest counseling.

(Continues)

Table 28-5 Additional Tests Performed on Blood Specimen (Continued)

TEST	EXPLANATION/NORMAL VALUES	NURSING RESPONSIBILITIES
Erythrocyte sedimentation rate (ESR or sed rate test)	Measures, in mm, RBC descent in a normal saline solution after 1 hour. Level is increased in inflammatory, infectious, necrotic, or cancerous conditions, due to increased protein content in plasma. Used to monitor the course of therapy for clients with autoimmune diseases, such as rheumatoid arthritis. Normal: Male: 0–13 mm/h Female: 0–20 mm/h	The test should be performed within 3 hours after the blood is drawn. Menstruation or pregnancy may increase level. Ethanbutal, quinine, aspirin, cortisone, and prednisone may alter results.
Folic acid (Folate level)	Measures folic acid level in the blood. Normal: 5–20 ug/mL, or 14–34 mmol/L	Fasting is not required. Instruct the client not to drink any alcoholic beverages before the test. The test is drawn before folic acid medications are administered. Note whether the client is taking phenytoin (Dilantin), primidone (Mysoline), methotrexate, antimalarial agents, or oral contraceptives, as these cause decreased level.
Follicle-stimulating hormone (FSH)	Determines anterior pituitary function. Usually measured with luteinizing hormone level. Normal: varies with phase of menstrual cycle Follicular: 5–20 mU/mL Midcycle peak: 15–30 mU/mL Luteal: 5–15 mU/mL Postmenopause: 50–100 mU/mL Male: 5–20 mU/mL	Note whether client is taking estrogen or progesterone, as these may decrease FSH level. Recent use of radioisotopes can also interfere with test results. Explain the procedure to the client. Indicate on the laboratory requisition the date of the last menstrual period (LMP) or that the client is postmenopausal. Indicate use of estrogen or progesterone on laboratory requisition. The client should be relaxed and recumbent for 30 minutes before the test.
Gamma-glutamyl transpeptidase (GGT or GGTP)	Enzyme that detects liver cell dysfunction. Normal: 5–38 IU/L	The client must fast for 8 hours prior to test. Note alcohol, Dilantin, and phenobarbital may elevate results, whereas oral contraceptives and clofibrate may decrease results.
Globulin	Key for antibody production. Indicates how well the liver is functioning. Normal: 2.3–3.5 g/dL	Note those medications taken that affect results (see albumin).
Glucose tolerance test (GTT)	Evaluates blood and urine glucose 30 minutes before, and 1, 2, and 3 hours after a standard glucose load. Normal: fasting 70–99 mg/dL 1 hr 160 mg/dL 2 hr 115 mg/dL 3 hr 70–110 mg/dL	The client must fast (except for water) for 6–8 hours prior to the test. Withhold drugs that interfere with results. After administration of glucose load, withhold all food. The client should drink water, however. Collect urine specimens at hourly periods. Administer meal and medications after test is completed.

TABLE 28-5 Additional Tests Performed on Blood Specimen (Continued)

TEST	EXPLANATION/NORMAL VALUES	NURSING RESPONSIBILITIES
Hemoglobin A1c (Hb_{A1c})	Measures the amount of glycated or glycosylated hemoglobin, evaluating average blood glucose level over the past 120 days. Range varies with lab: Normal: <6% Good control: <7% Poor Control: >8%	Fasting is not required. Blood can be drawn at any time.
Hepatitis B surface antigen (HB_sAG)	A positive result indicates presence of hepatitis or that the person is a carrier. Normal: negative	
Human chorionic gonadotropin (hCG)	Test for tumor marker; elevated in germ cell testicular cancer. Normal: negative Female, pregnant: positive, peaks at 8–12 weeks then falls Female, abnormal pregnancy or choriocarcinoma: remains high or increases	Apply pressure to the site and observe for bleeding or hematoma.
Human leukocyte antigen DW4 (HLA-DW4)	Positive (present in 50% of clients with rheumatoid arthritis). Normal: negative	Fasting is not required.
Lead (Pb)	Evaluation or screen for lead toxicity. Especially used in children.	Explain the procedure to the client. Inform client that a blood sample is needed.
Lupus erythematosus test (LE prep)	Positive in 70%–80% of clients with systemic lupus erythematosus. May be positive in clients with rheumatoid arthritis. Used to diagnose and monitor the course of treatment for clients with systemic lupus erythematosus. Normal: negative	Fasting is not required. May be ordered daily for 3 days. Note whether the client is taking Apresoline, Pronestyl, oral contraceptives, quinidine, penicillin, Aldomet, tetracycline, isoniazid, or reserpine, as these may cause false-positive results.
Luteinizing hormone (LH) assay	Determines anterior pituitary function. It can be used to determine whether ovulation has occurred. Can also determine whether gonadal insufficiency is primary or secondary. Normal: Males: 7–24 mU/mL Females: 6–30 mU/mL	Note whether the client is taking estrogen or progesterone, as these may decrease LH level. Recent use of radioisotopes can also interfere with test results. Explain the procedure to the client. Indicate on the laboratory requisition the date of the LMP or that the client is postmenopausal.
Parathyroid hormone (PTH), parathormone	Measures the quantity of PTH to determine hyperparathyroidism or whether hypercalcemia is caused by parathyroid glands. Normal: 10–60 pg/mL	Recent use of radioisotope can interfere with test results. Explain the procedure to the client. Initiate NPO status after midnight, except for water. Obtain morning blood specimen and indicate time of collection.

(*Continues*)

Table 28-5 Additional Tests Performed on Blood Specimen (Continued)

TEST	EXPLANATION/NORMAL VALUES	NURSING RESPONSIBILITIES
Phosphorus	Determines the level of phosphorus in the blood. Normal: 3.0–4.5 mg/dL, or 0.97–1.45 nmol/L	Laxatives or enemas containing sodium phosphate can increase serum phosphorus level. Note those medications taken that may affect results. Drugs that may increase serum phosphorus level include methicillin and excessive vitamin D. Recent carbohydrate ingestion including IV administration causes decreased serum phosphorus level, as do antacids and mannitol. Explain the procedure to the client. Initiate NPO status 12–14 hours before test. Discontinue IV fluids containing glucose for several hours before test, if possible.
Polymerase chain reaction (PCR)	Detects HIV-specific DNA (virus). Normal: negative	Explain the meaning of the test. Provide follow-up explanation of test results.
Progesterone assay	Determines ovulation and function of corpus luteum. Adrenal tumors can elevate level. Normal: Male: <100 ng/dL Female: midcycle: 300–2,400 ng/dL Pregnancy 7–13 weeks 1,500–5,000 ng/dL 14+ weeks 6,500–20,000 ng/dL	Recent use of radioisotopes or hemolysis resulting from rough handling of blood specimen can interfere with test results. Note those medications taken that may interfere with test results, including estrogen and progesterone. Explain the procedure to the client. Indicate the date of LMP on the laboratory requisition.
Prolactin level (PRL)	Determines anterior pituitary secretion. Among the problems indicated by an elevated level are pituitary tumors or primary hypothyroidism. Normal: Female, or male: 0–20 ng/mL Pregnant: 20–400 ng/mL	Note those medications taken that may affect results. Drugs that may increase prolactin level include phenothiazines, oral contraceptives, reserpine, opiates, verapamil, histamine antagonists, monoamine oxidase (MAO) inhibitors, and antihistamines. Drugs that may decrease prolactin level include ergot alkaloid derivatives, clonidine, levodopa, and dopamine. Explain the procedure to the client. The blood specimen should be obtained in the morning and placed on ice if not taken immediately to the laboratory.
Prostate-specific antigen (PSA)	PSA is an antigen detected in all males; level increases with prostatic cancer. It is more sensitive and specific than the acid phosphatase. Normal: <4 ng/mL	Fasting is not required. Apply pressure to the venipuncture site. Observe the site for bleeding.
Protein	Measures total protein in the blood. Normal: 6–8 g/dL	Note those medications taken that may affect results; steroids and hormones such as insulin, and growth hormones may increase level, whereas oral contraceptives and liver toxic drugs may decrease level.

Table 28-5 Additional Tests Performed on Blood Specimen (Continued)

TEST	EXPLANATION/NORMAL VALUES	NURSING RESPONSIBILITIES
Renin assay, plasma renin activity (PRA)	Measures the amount of renin and is used as a screening procedure to detect essential or renal hypertension. When combined with plasma aldosterone level, determines adrenal cortex activity. Normal: Upright position, sodium depleted or restricted diet: 20–39 years: 2.9–24 ng/mL/h >40 years: 2.9–10.8 ng/mL/h Upright position, sodium repleted or normal diet: 20–39 years: 0.1–4.3 ng/mL/h >40 years: 0.1–3.0 ng/mL/h	Pregnancy, salt intake, or licorice ingestion can interfere with test results. Time of day (early in the day), a low-salt diet, or an upright position increases renin value. Note those medications taken that may interfere with test results, including antihypertensives, diuretics, estrogens, oral contraceptives, and vasodilators. Explain the procedure to the client. The client should maintain a normal diet with sodium restricted to 3 grams per day for 3 days before the test. Drugs and licorice should be discontinued for 2 to 4 weeks before the test. The client should stand or sit upright for 2 hours before blood is drawn. Client position, dietary status, time of day, and drugs should be recorded on the laboratory requisition. Blood specimen should be placed in ice and taken immediately to the laboratory. After blood specimen is obtained, the client may resume a normal diet and restart medications.
Rheumatoid factor (RF)	Abnormal protein in serum of approximately 80% of clients with rheumatoid arthritis. Formed as a result of the reaction of IgM to an abnormal IgG. Also elevated in clients with other autoimmune diseases such as systemic lupus erythematosus. Normal: negative	Fasting is preferred.
Sensitivity	Used to identify a pathogen's susceptibility to commonly used antibiotics. Allows the selection of appropriate antibiotic therapy. Normal: none	Specimen should be taken immediately to the laboratory.
Serum acid phosphatase (prostatic) (ACP)	Serum measurement of prostatic acid phosphatase, elevated in malignancy; because it detects cancer in the later stages, no longer commonly used. Normal: 0.0–0.8 U/L	Apply pressure to the site. Observe the site for bleeding or hematoma.
Serum alkaline phosphatase (ALP)	Serum measurement of alkaline phosphates, elevated in malignancy. Normal: 30–120 U/L	Apply pressure to the site. Observe the site for bleeding or hematoma.
Serum creatinine	Specific indicator of renal disease. Normal: 0.4–1.5 mg/dL	Note those medications taken that may affect results, including amphotericin B, cephalosporins (cepfazolin [Ancef]; cephalothin [Keflin]); methicillin; ascorbic acid; barbiturates; lithium carbonate; methyldopa (Aldomet); triamterene (Dyrenium).

(Continues)

TABLE 28-5 Additional Tests Performed on Blood Specimen (Continued)

TEST	EXPLANATION/NORMAL VALUES	NURSING RESPONSIBILITIES
Sickledex (sickle-cell test)	Screening test to determine the presence of Hgb S. Normal: no Hgb S If results are positive, a hemoglobin electrophoresis test is done.	There are no food or fluid restrictions. Note on the laboratory requisition whether the client had a blood transfusion in the past 3 to 4 months.
Thyroid-stimulating hormone (TSH), thyrotropin	Determines thyroid function as well as monitors exogenous thyroid replacement. Normal: 2–10 μU/mL, or 2–10 mU/L	Recent use of radioisotopes may affect test results. Severe illness may decrease TSH level. Drugs that may increase TSH level include antithyroid drugs, lithium, potassium iodide, and TSH injection. Drugs that may decrease TSH level include aspirin, dopamine, heparin, steroids, and T_3. Explain the procedure to the client. The client should be relaxed and recumbent for 30 minutes before the test.
TSH stimulation test	Differentiates between primary and secondary hypothyroidism. Normal: none given	Explain the procedure to the client. Obtain baseline level of radioactive iodine intake or serum T_4. Administer 5–10 units of TSH intramuscularly for 3 days. Repeat radioactive iodine intake or T_4 as indicated for comparison studies.
Thyrotropin-releasing hormone (TRH) test, thyrotropin-releasing factor (TRF) test	Assesses the responsiveness of the anterior pituitary by its secretion of TSH in response to an IV injection of TRH. Also tests the function of the thyroid gland. Normal: undetectable to 15 μU/mL	Pregnancy may increase TSH response to TRH. Note those medications taken that may modify TSH response, including antithyroid drugs, aspirin, corticosteroids, estrogens, levodopa, and T_4. Explain the procedure to the client. Any thyroid preparations should be discontinued for 3–4 weeks before the test.
Thyroxine (T_4) screen	Directly measures the amount of T_4 present. Normal: radioimmunoassay: 5–12 μg/dL, or 65–155 nmol/L	X-ray iodinated contrast studies may increase T_4 levels. Pregnancy will increase T_4 level. Note those medications taken that may affect results. Drugs that may increase T_4 level include clofibrate, estrogens, heroin, methadone, and oral contraceptives. Drugs that may decrease T_4 level include anabolic steroids, androgens, antithyroid drugs, lithium, phenytoin (Dilantin), and propranolol (Inderal). Explain the procedure to the client. Evaluate the client's drug history. If needed, instruct the client to stop exogenous T_4 medications for 1 month prior to test.

TABLE 28-5 Additional Tests Performed on Blood Specimen (Continued)

TEST	EXPLANATION/NORMAL VALUES	NURSING RESPONSIBILITIES
Thyroxine free, FTI, FT_4	Measures the amount of free T_4 that actually enters the cells and is active in metabolism. A true indicator of thyroid activity. Can be used to diagnose thyroid status in pregnant females or clients on drugs that can interfere with results of other tests. Normal: 280–480 pg/dL	Recent radionuclear scans can interfere with test results. Explain the procedure to the client. Blood specimens for T_4 and T_3 uptake must be obtained to calculate T_4.
Total iron-binding capacity (TIBC)	Determines the ability of iron to bind to a protein called transferrin. Normal: 300–360 mg/dL	NPO 12 hours prior to the test. A recent blood transfusion or a diet high in iron may affect test results. Note whether the client is taking oral contraceptives, as these increase TIBC level.
Triglycerides	Form of fat produced in the liver. Normal: 30–150 mg/dL	Client to fast 12–14 hours prior to the test, and have no alcohol for 24 hours before. Diet of prior 2 weeks affects results.
Triiodothyronine (T_3) radioimmunoassay (T_3 by RIA)	Determines thyroid gland function Normal: 110–230 ng/dL, or 1.2–1.5 nmol/L	Radioisotope administration may interfere with test results. Pregnancy increases T_3 results. Note those medications taken that may affect results. Drugs that may increase T_3 level include: estrogen, methadone, and oral contraceptives. Drugs that may decrease T_4 level include anabolic steroids, androgens, phenytoin (Dilantin), propranolol (Inderal), reserpine, and salicylates (high dose). Explain the procedure to the client. Determine whether exogenous T_3 is being taken. With physician's approval, withhold those drugs that would interfere with test results.
Triiodothyronine (T_3) serum free	Measures the amount of free T_3 that actually enters the cells and is active in metabolism. A true indicator of thyroid activity. Can be used to diagnose thyroid status in pregnant females or clients on drugs that can interfere with results of other tests. Normal: 0.2–0.6 ng/dL	Explain the procedure to the client. Blood specimens for T_3 and T_4 uptake must be obtained to calculate T_3.
Troponin I and Troponin T Cardiac-specific (TnI, TnT, cTnI, cTnT)	Used to diagnose a myocardial infarction, to detect and evaluate mild to severe cardiac injury, and to distinguish angina that may be due to other causes. Normal: 0.6 ng/mL	Explain the procedure to the client. Apply pressure to venipuncture site.
Uric acid	Elevated in gout. Normal: Male: 2.1–8.5 mg/dL Female: 2.0–8.0 mg/dL	There are no food or drink restrictions. Note those medications and other substances taken that may affect results, including ascorbic acid, diuretics, levadopa, allopurinol, and Coumadin.

(Continues)

Table 28-5 Additional Tests Performed on Blood Specimen (Continued)

TEST	EXPLANATION/NORMAL VALUES	NURSING RESPONSIBILITIES
VDRL (Venereal Disease Research Laboratory), RPR (rapid plasma reagin), FTA-ABS (fluorescent treponemal antibody-absorption test), Reiter test, fluorescent antibody Treponema pallidum immobilization (TPI) test (performed only at Centers for Disease Control and Infection [CDC] in Atlanta, GA)	Blood tests for presence of syphilis. Normal: negative or nonreactive	Explain the test to the client, including amount of blood to be drawn.
Western blot	Confirmatory test for the presence of antibodies to HIV. Normal: negative	Provide pretest counseling. Obtain informed consent. Provide or arrange posttest counseling.

Urine Tests

Urinalysis assists in the diagnosis of various conditions. Substances not normally found in the urine include RBCs, white blood cells (WBCs), protein, glucose, ketones, and casts. Tests often performed on a urine specimen are found in Table 28-6.

Urine pH

The hydrogen ion concentration in the urine determines the pH. Diabetes mellitus, diarrhea, dehydration, emphysema, and starvation make the urine acidic. Urinary tract infections, chronic renal failure, renal tubular acidosis, and salicylate poisoning make the urine alkaline.

Specific Gravity

Specific gravity measures the number of solutes in a solution. Urea and uric acid, by-products of nitrogen metabolism, are the greatest influence on urine specific gravity.

Specific gravity increases with excess fluid loss from the body. Renal disease decreases specific gravity.

Urine Glucose

Glucose spills into the urine when the blood level of glucose exceeds the renal threshold (180 mg/dL). Measuring urine glucose is not as accurate as measuring the blood glucose level.

PROFESSIONALTIP

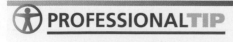

Drugs and Laboratory Tests

Note drugs the client is taking when those drugs may influence the results of laboratory tests.

Urine Ketones

Ketones, products of incomplete fat metabolism, are completely metabolized by the liver under normal conditions. The most common cause of ketonuria (excessive ketones in the urine) is diabetes.

Urine Cells and Casts

The urine is normally free of blood cells and casts. In cases of nephritis, renal damage or failure, and urinary stones or infections, the following can occur:

- Bleeding, resulting in RBCs in the urine
- Accumulation of epithelial cells accompanied by cast formation
- WBCs in the urine, indicating infection

Stool Tests

Stool specimens are examined for normal substances (such as urobilinogen) and blood, bacteria, and parasites (Table 28-7).

Urobilinogen

Urobilinogen, a colorless derivative of bilirubin, is formed by the normal action of intestinal flora on bilirubin. It increases in situations of severe hemolysis and decreases with most biliary obstructions.

PROFESSIONALTIP

Testing for Blood Lipid Level

To allow for the proper balance between the vascular and extravascular compartment and ensure valid test results, the blood should always be drawn after the client has been sitting quietly for 5 minutes.

TABLE 28-6 Tests Performed on Urine

TEST	EXPLANATION/NORMAL VALUES	NURSING RESPONSIBILITIES
Urinalysis Color Odor pH Specific gravity Glucose Acetone (ketone) Casts Albumin (protein) RBCs WBCs Bilirubin Bacteria Leukocyte esterase Nitrites	 Clear amber Pleasantly aromatic until left standing; offensive and unpleasant in kidney infection. 4.6–8.0 1.015–1.030 Negative Negative Rare Negative 2–3/HPF 4–5/HPF Negative Negative Negative Negative	Explain the procedure and purpose to the client and assist with specimen collection, if needed. Ensure that the specimen is taken to the laboratory in a timely manner.
Aldosterone assay	A blood test or 24-hour urine collection to evaluate the adrenal cortex, especially for tumors. The 24-hour urine is more reliable, but the blood specimen is more convenient. Normal, blood: Male: 6–22 ng/dL, or 0.17–0.61 nmol/L Female: 5–30 ng/dL, or 0.14–0.80 nmol/L Normal, urine: 2–80 µg/24 h, or 5.5–72.0 nmol/24 h	Strenuous exercise and stress can increase aldosterone level. Excessive licorice ingestion can decrease aldosterone level. Client should be upright (sitting or standing) for 4 hours before test. Explain the procedure to the client. The client should follow a normal diet with 3 grams of sodium/day and no licorice for at least 2 weeks before the test. Medications should be stopped for at least 2 weeks before the test, if possible. Initiate 24-hour urine collection. Send collection to laboratory immediately upon conclusion.
Bence Jones protein	Bence Jones proteins are immunoglobulins typically found in the urine of clients with multiple myeloma. They may also be associated with tumor metastases to the bone and chronic lymphocytic leukemia. Normal: negative	Instruct the client for a clean-catch or 24-hour urine specimen. Instruct the client not to contaminate specimen with toilet paper or stool.
Creatine clearance	Normal: Male: 95–135 mL/min Female: 85–125 mL/min Minimum: 10 mL/min to maintain life	Instruct the client about the 24-hour urine test. Encourage hourly water intake. Keep urine on ice or in special refrigerator. Cephalosporins and vigorous exercise affect results.
17-hydroxycortico-steriods (17-OHCS)	24-hour urine test that measures adrenal cortex function. Normal: Male: 3–10 mg/24 h Female: 2–6 mg/24 h	Emotional or physical stress or licorice ingestion may increase adrenal activity. Note those medications taken that may affect results. Drugs that may increase 17-OHCS level include acetazolamide, chloral hydrate, ascorbic acid, and erythromycin. Drugs that may decrease 17-OHCS level include estrogens, oral contraceptives, phenothiazines, and reserpine. Explain the procedure to the client. Initiate 24-hour urine collection. Send collection to laboratory immediately upon conclusion.

(*Continues*)

Table 28-6 Tests Performed on Urine (Continued)

TEST	EXPLANATION/NORMAL VALUES	NURSING RESPONSIBILITIES
17-ketosteroids (17-KS)	24-hour urine test that measures adrenal cortex function. Normal: Male: 5–23 mg/24 h, or 24–88 μmol/24 h Female: 2–15 mg/24 h, or 14–52 μmol/24 h	Stress may increase adrenal activity. Note medications taken that may affect results. Drugs that increase 17-KS level include antibiotics and dexamethasone. Drugs that may decrease 17-KS level include estrogen and oral contraceptives. Explain the procedure to the client. With physician's approval, withhold all drugs for several days before test. Monitor client for stress and report to physician. Initiate 24-hour urine collection. Send collection to laboratory immediately upon conclusion.
Schilling test	Determines vitamin B_{12} absorption by the intestine. Differentiates between pernicious anemia and gastrointestinal malabsorption problems. Normal: 8%–40% of the radioactive vitamin B_{12} is excreted in the urine within 24 hours.	Collect the urine for a 24- to 48-hour period. Laxatives are not given during the test, as they decrease the absorption of vitamin B_{12}.
Urine cortisol, hydrocortisone	24-hour urine test that measures adrenal cortex function. Normal: 22–69 μmol/24 h, or 8–25 mg/24 h	Pregnancy or stress increases cortisol level. Recent radioisotope scans can interfere with test result. Note medications taken that may interfere with test result, including oral contraceptives and spironolactone. Explain the procedure to the client. Assess for stress and report to physician. Initiate 24-hour urine collection. Send collection to laboratory immediately upon conclusion.
Vanillylmandelic acid (VMA) and catecholamines (epinephrine, norepinephrine, metaneprine, normetanephrine, dopamine)	24-hour urine test that diagnoses pheochromocytoma and other adrenal tumors. Normal: VMA: 2–7 mg/24 h, or 10–35 μmol/24 h Epinephrine: 0.5–20.0 μg/24 h, or <275 nmol/24 h Norepinephrine: 15–80 μg/24 h Metanephrine: 24–96 μg/24 h Normetanephrine: 75–375 μg/24 h Dopamine: 65–400 μg/24 h	Certain foods (e.g., tea, coffee, cocoa, vanilla, chocolate), vigorous exercise, stress, or starvation may increase VMA level. Uremia, alkaline urine, or iodinated contrast dyes may falsely decrease VMA level. Note those medications taken that may affect results. Drugs that may increase VMA level include caffeine, epinephrine, levodopa, lithium, and nitroglycerine. Drugs that may decrease VMA level include clonidine, disulfiram (Antabuse), guanethidine, imipramine, MAO inhibitors, phenothiazines, and reserpine. Drugs that may increase catecholamine level include ethyl alcohol, aminophylline, caffeine, chloral hydrate, clonidine (chronic therapy), contrast media (iodine containing), disulfiram (Antabuse), epinephrine, erythromycin, insulin, methenamine, methyldopa, nicotinic acid (large doses), nitroglycerin, quinidine, riboflavin, and tetracyclines. Drugs that may decrease catecholamine level include guanethidine, reserpine, and salicylates.

Table 28-6 Tests Performed on Urine (Continued)

TEST	EXPLANATION/NORMAL VALUES	NURSING RESPONSIBILITIES
Vanillylmandelic acid (VMA) and catecholamines (Continued)		Explain the procedure to the client. The client should be on a VMA-restricted diet for 2–3 days before the test. Items restricted include coffee, tea, bananas, chocolate, cocoa, licorice, citrus fruit, anything with vanilla, and aspirin. Client should not take antihypertensive drugs before the test. Initiate 24-hour urine collection.

Table 28-7 Tests Performed on Stool

Stool occult blood (guaiac) Fecal occult blood test (FOBT) Hemoccult	Fecal occult blood screening studies may be utilized as possible indicators of colorectal cancer. Normal: negative for blood	Place a smear of stool on a card. Medications such as anticoagulants, aspirin, iron preparations, NSAIDs, and steroids may cause a false-positive result, whereas vitamin C may cause a false negative. Red meat should not be ingested for 3 days prior to the test. For premenopausal women, wait at least 4 days after menstrual period. Wear gloves when obtaining and handling the specimen.
Clostridium difficile (*C. difficile* toxin)	Evaluation for the etiology of diarrhea, especially postantibiotic diarrhea. Normal: negative	Adhere to standard precautions. Client should be placed in contact isolation.
Fecal fat	Evaluation for malabsorption. Fat in stool is assessed by collecting the client's stool over a 72-hour period. Normal: negative	Instruct client to inform nurse as soon as possible after defecation to collect specimen. Ensure that the client is properly cleaned and dry.
WBC or leukocyte cell count	Evaluation of diarrhea for inflammation and/or infection of the bowel. Evaluates the presence of leukocytes in a single stool specimen. Normal: negative	Explain the procedure to the client. Give client privacy for defecation.
Stool O&P (ova & parasite)	A positive result indicates infection. Normal: negative	Place the stool specimen in a container and take warm to the laboratory. Usually done 3 times.

Occult Blood

Occult blood is invisible blood in the stool that can be detected only by chemical means or with a microscope. The digestive process in the GI tract acts on blood, making it occult. Random sampling for occult blood is done to diagnose gastrointestinal bleeding, ulcers, and malignant tumors (Figure 28-3).

To decrease the possibility of a false-positive result when occult blood is to be used to confirm suspicions of a gastrointestinal disorder, the client is placed on a 3-day diet free of meat, poultry, and fish. Drugs causing a false-positive test for occult blood are salicylate, steroids, and indomethacin.

Parasites

The gastrointestinal tract can harbor parasites and their eggs (ova). Whereas some of these parasites are harmless, others cause clinical symptoms. Most common parasites except pinworms (which can enter the body through both the oral and anal routes) enter the body through the mouth when contaminated water or food is ingested.

Culture and Sensitivity Tests

Culture is the growing of microorganisms to identify the pathogen. Culture and **sensitivity** (C&S) tests are performed

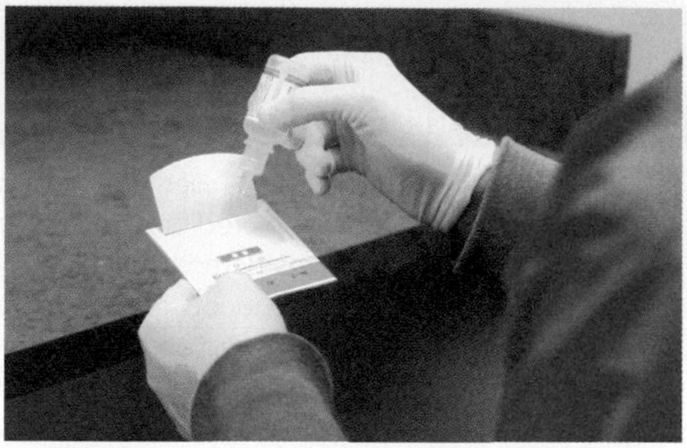

FIGURE 28-3 Applying the Developing Solution to a Stool Sample to Test for Occult Blood

to identify both the pathogen and its susceptibility to commonly used antibiotics. Sensitivity allows the selection of appropriate antibiotic therapy. All C&S specimens should be immediately taken to the laboratory.

Blood Culture

Bacteremia is bacteria in the blood. A blood culture should be procured while the client is having chills and fever. A series of three collections are performed using strict sterile technique. The needle should be changed after the specimen is collected and before injecting the blood sample into the test tube.

Throat (Swab) Culture

The throat normally hosts many organisms. Throat cultures identify such pathogens as beta-hemolytic streptococci, *Staphylococcus aureus*, meningococci, gonococci, *Bordetella pertussis*, and *Corynebacterium diphtheria*. A throat swab is commonly done to identify streptococcal infections, which can cause rheumatic fever or glomerulonephritis if left untreated.

To obtain a throat swab, use a wooden blade to depress the tongue and swab the white patches, exudate, or ulcerations of the throat with a sterile applicator (Figure 28-4). The applicator should not touch any other parts of the mouth. The applicator is then placed in a sterile container.

Sputum Culture

Sputum tests include culture, smear, and cytology. Sputum, created by the mucous glands and goblet cells of the tracheobronchial tree, is sterile until it reaches the throat and mouth, where it comes in contact with normal flora. For a more accurate identification of pulmonary organisms, sputum can be obtained by tracheobronchial suctioning and transtracheal aspiration.

In addition to the organism(s) found in a culture, a sputum smear identifies eosinophils, epithelial cells, and other substances. Smears help diagnose asthma (eosinophils) and fungal infections. The specimen must be refrigerated if it cannot be taken immediately to the laboratory.

Sputum **cytology** (the study of cells) is performed to diagnose cancer of the lungs. The specimen should be collected early in the morning and after a deep cough.

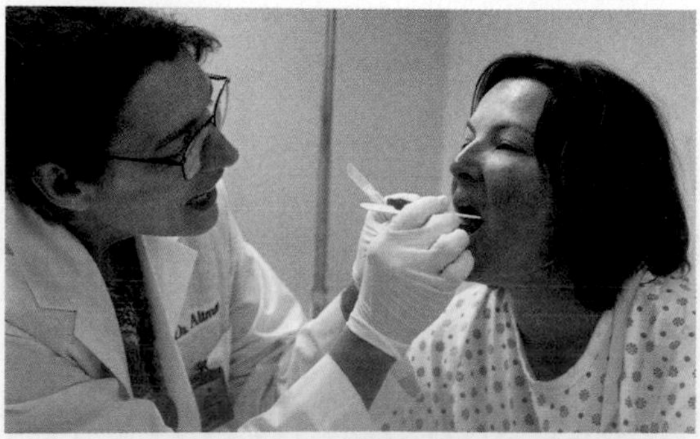

FIGURE 28-4 Swab the sample area using a quick, gentle motion.

PROFESSIONAL TIP

Cultures

All culture tests should be performed before initiating antibiotic therapy so as to identify the type of pathogen and its sensitivity to specific antibiotics.

CLIENT TEACHING

Pap Smear

Advise female clients to prepare for a Pap smear by:

- Avoiding intercourse, douches, and vaginal creams for 24 hours before the test.
- Informing the practitioners if they are menstruating, as the test will need to be delayed.

Cervical Pap smear testing is recommended every 2 to 3 years after the onset of sexual activity. Annual testing is indicated for those women who:

- Are over 40 years of age.
- Have a family history of cervical cancer.
- Previously had a positive Pap smear.

Urine Culture

Urinary C&S tests are performed whenever a urinary tract infection is suspected.

Stool Culture

Stool C&S is performed to identify bacterial infections. If the client has diarrhea, a rectal swab can be taken and used as a specimen, but fecal material must be visible on the swab for the laboratory to perform the test.

PAPANICOLAOU TEST

The **Papanicolaou test** (a smear method of examining stained exfoliative cells), commonly called a Pap smear, evaluates the metabolic activity, cellular maturity, and morphological variations of cervical tissue. Papanicolaou testing can also be done on specimens from other organs, such as gastric secretions and bronchial aspirations.

PROFESSIONALTIP

Contrast Media

Carefully monitor those clients scheduled for dye injection studies who have a history of allergies to any foods or drugs because such allergies may predispose them to allergic reactions to contrast media.

SAFETY

X-rays

- Question the client about the possibility of pregnancy, asthma, and allergic reactions to contrast media (iodine), as well as to other foods and drugs, before scheduling x-rays.
- If the client has not previously received iodine, note this on the requisition to indicate that allergic status is unknown.

RADIOLOGICAL STUDIES

Radiography (the study of film exposed to x-rays or gamma rays through the action of ionizing radiation) is used by the practitioner to study internal organ structure. When used in conjunction with a **contrast medium** (a radiopaque substance that facilitates roentgen imaging of the body's internal structures), **fluoroscopy** (immediate, serial images of the body's structure and function) reveals the motion of organs. X-rays are valuable in formulating a diagnosis and helping to determine if other studies (e.g., a lung lesion requiring biopsy to differentiate between a benign or malignant tumor) are necessary.

Some radiological tests require a contrast medium such as barium and iodine that often interferes with other diagnostic studies. Draw a blood sample for thyroid function before beginning an intravenous pyelogram (IVP), where radioactive iodine dye is administered. If a client needs both an IVP and a barium enema, perform the IVP first because the barium is likely to decrease kidney visualization. Commonly performed radiological studies are described in Table 28-8.

CHEST X-RAY

The chest x-ray is the most common radiological study. Chest x-rays are taken from various views (Figure 28-5, p. 636) because multiple views of the chest are needed to assess the entire lung field. To prepare for a chest x-ray, the client should remove all clothing from the waist up and don a gown. The client should also remove all metal objects (jewelry) because metal will appear on the x-ray film, thereby obscuring visualization of parts of the chest. Pregnant women are advised against x-rays; however, if x-ray is absolutely necessary, the woman should be draped with a lead apron to protect the fetus.

COMPUTED TOMOGRAPHY

Computed tomography (CT) is the radiological scanning of the body. X-ray beams and radiation detectors transmit data to a computer that transcribes the data into quantitative measurement and multidimensional images of the internal structures. Figure 28-6 (p. 637) illustrates the sagittal, transverse, and coronal planes used in CT scanning.

The procedure requires the client's informed consent. The client's cooperation is essential during CT scanning because the client will be positioned and asked to remain motionless. Prepare the client by providing an explanation and pictures of what to expect.

BARIUM STUDIES

Barium (a chalky white contrast medium) is a preparation that permits roentgenographic visualization of the internal structures of the digestive tract. Barium studies can reveal congenital abnormalities, reflux, spasm, stricture, obstruction, inflammation, ulceration, lesions, varices, and fistula.

ANGIOGRAPHY

Angiography allows visualization of vascular structures by using fluoroscopy and a contrast medium. It shows blood flow to the heart, lungs, brain, kidneys, lower extremities, and is useful in diagnosing an **aneurysm** (weakness in the wall of a blood vessel).

TABLE 28-8 Radiologic Studies

TEST	EXPLANATION/NORMAL VALUES	NURSING RESPONSIBILITIES
Radiograph (x-ray)	Most common diagnostic study. Identifies traumatic disorders, i.e., fractures, dislocations, tumors, bone disorders, joint deformities, bone density, and changes in bone relationships. Performed by a technician.	Explain the procedure to the client. Prepare the client as ordered. No specific postprocedure care is required. Administer an analgesic, especially for the arthritic client.
Abdominal x-rays	Determines diaphragm position and gas and fluid distribution in the abdomen.	No preparation is required.

(Continues)

Table 28-8 Radiologic Studies (Continued)

TEST	EXPLANATION/NORMAL VALUES	NURSING RESPONSIBILITIES
Adrenal angiography, Adrenal arteriogram	Study of adrenal glands and arterial system after injection of radiopaque dye to detect benign or malignant tumors or hyperplasia of the adrenal glands. Normal: no growth or enlargement	Assess for allergy to shellfish or iodine, arteriosclerosis, pregnancy, or blood disorders, as they preclude the test. Explain the procedure to the client. Assess for allergies. Informed and written consent must be obtained before the procedure. Note whether client has been taking anticoagulants. Initiate NPO status after midnight. Mark peripheral pulses with a pen before the procedure. Inform the client that a warm flush may be felt when the dye is injected. Observe the puncture site. Monitor vital signs. Monitor peripheral pulses, color, and temperature of extremities. Institute bed rest for 12–24 hours. Apply cold compresses to puncture site, if needed. Force fluids to prevent possible dehydration from the dye.
Adrenal venography	Involves insertion of a catheter through the femoral vein and into the adrenal vein to withdraw a blood specimen to detect the function of each adrenal gland. A contrast dye is injected to visualize size and position of the adrenal glands. Normal: no growth or enlargement	Explain the procedure to the client. Assess for allergies. Obtain informed and written consent. Inform the client that a burning sensation may be experienced when the dye is injected. Although this study involves the venous system, monitor vital signs and injection site as well as pulses, temperature, and color of extremities.
Angiography (cardiac angiogram)	Performed when vessels in a specific organ or vascular area (e.g., heart, kidney) need to be visualized to identify obstruction or abnormality. Involves the insertion of a catheter into a venipuncture site with the injection of a contrast medium, after which angiographic films are taken as the contrast medium enters into the area being studied. Normal: normal vessel	Explain the procedure to the client. Obtain baseline vital signs. Assess for potential allergies to contrast medium.
Arteriography (arteriogram)	Assesses for pathology such as narrowing from atherosclerosis. Normal: normal vessels	Explain the procedure to the client. Assess for potential allergies to contrast medium.
Arthrogram (-graphy)	Visualization of a joint. Radiopaque dye or air is injected into the joint cavity to outline soft tissue, usually on knee/shoulder joints. Local anesthetic and sterile technique are used. Performed by a physician; takes approximately 30 minutes. Normal: absence of lesions, fractures, or tears	Explain the procedure to the client. Obtain informed consent. Client wears an elastic bandage for several days; check for edema. Administer a mild analgesic for pain. Monitor for increased pain. Neither fasting nor sedation is required.
Barium enema	An enema of barium is given while x-rays are taken of the large intestine.	Initiate NPO status the night before. Administer the ordered medication to clean the bowel. Observe the results of the laxatives, and inform the x-ray department if there have been no results. After the test, force oral fluids and administer a cleansing enema, as ordered. Document status of abdomen and stools.

Table 28-8 Radiologic Studies (Continued)

TEST	EXPLANATION/NORMAL VALUES	NURSING RESPONSIBILITIES
Barium swallow	The client drinks a glass of barium while x-rays are taken of the esophagus and cardiac sphincter.	Initiate NPO status the evening before. Explain the procedure and the time frame for results. Encourage the client to drink fluids and eat fiber after the test. A laxative is sometimes given after the test. The client should be instructed that bowel movements will be white for 1–2 days. During the test, the client will be tilted on the x-ray table in various positions. There may be repeated pictures taken at half-hour intervals as the barium moves through the bowel. Document the client's tolerance of the procedure and passage of the barium. Because the procedure can be lengthy, encourage the client to take reading material.
Cardiac catheterization (cardiac angiogram, coronary arteriogram)	A catheter is passed into the right and/or left side of the heart to determine oxygen level, cardiac output, and pressure within the heart chambers.	Assess the client for allergy to iodine or shellfish. The client is to fast for 6 hours prior to the test, but medications can be taken with sips of water. Inform the client of the possibility of feeling warm or flushed during the test. After the procedure, assess the peripheral pulses every 15 minutes for 2–4 hours, or according to physician's orders. Assess color, temperature, and pulse in the extremity below the catheter insertion site. Instruct the client to keep the involved extremity straight for 6–8 hours.
Chest x-ray	Provides a two-dimensional image of the lungs without using contrast media. Used to detect the presence of fluid within the interstitial lung tissue or the alveoli; tumors or foreign bodies; and the presence and size of a pneumothorax. The size of the heart can also be determined by chest x-ray.	Explain the test to the client. If appropriate, inquire whether the client may be pregnant, to prevent exposure of the fetus to x-ray. The client is generally required to stand for various views; if the client is unable to stand, views may be obtained with the client in a sitting position, or a portable x-ray may be obtained. Instruct the client to inspire deeply and hold the breath. Instruct the client to remove all metal objects from the chest and neck area and to don a hospital gown that does not have snap closures.
Computed tomography (CT) scan	Provides a three-dimensional cross-sectional view of tissues. Computer-constructed picture interprets densities of various tissues. Most useful for viewing tumors in the chest, abdominal cavity, and brain. There are several different types of CT scans depending on what is being assessed (e.g., brain, cardiac, thoracic, bone, abdomen, pelvic). Angiography or myelography can also be performed via CT scanning.	Explain the procedure to the client. Obtain informed consent. Remove wigs and hairpins and clips for head CT. Initiate NPO status 8 hours prior to scan. Assess for iodine allergy. Observe for signs of anaphylaxis, if dye is used. Check for claustrophobia. Inform the client that the test will take approximately 45 minutes to 1 hour. The client must lie still on a hard, flat table and will be put through a large machine. Because barium will interfere with the test, schedule tests using barium either after or 4 or more days before the scan.

(Continues)

Table 28-8 Radiologic Studies (Continued)

TEST	EXPLANATION/NORMAL VALUES	NURSING RESPONSIBILITIES
Conduitogram	Radiopaque dye is injected through a catheter into either the conduit or a piece of ileum to assess by means of x-ray the length and emptying ability of the conduit as well as the presence of stricture or obstruction.	A conduit is a connection between the bladder or pouch and the outside of the body. Explain the procedure to the client. Assess the client for allergies to iodine-based dye.
Fistula gram	Radiopaque dye or barium is given to drink, and x-rays are taken as the dye or barium passes through the gastrointestinal tract. The dye shows the location of the fistula and how it is connected to the gastrointestinal tract.	Initiate NPO status as ordered. Explain the procedure and the time frame for the results and identify the person who will give the client the results.
Fluoresce in angiography	Following IV injection of sodium fluorescein, rapid-sequence photographs of the fundus are taken with a special camera. Visualization of microvascular structures of the retina and choroid are enhanced, allowing evaluation of the entire retinal vascular bed.	Instill eye drops to dilate the pupils. Start an IV so the sodium fluorescein can be injected. Remove the IV following completion of the test. Inform the client that skin and urine may be yellow for 24–48 hours.
Hysterosalpin-gogram	Radiopaque dye is instilled through the cervix. Used to diagnose uterine cavity and tubal abnormalities. Performed as a part of an infertility workup.	Explain the procedure and prepare the client in the lithotomy position. The test is done in the radiology department. Inquire about allergies to iodine or other dyes. Assist the physician.
Intravenous pyelogram (IVP)	Infusion of radiopaque dye into a vein, allowing visualization of the urinary system. The renal pelvis, ureters, and bladder can be seen. If BUN is over 40 mg/dL, the test may not be performed.	Explain the procedure to the client. Explain that the client will experience a warm feeling during dye injection. Ask the client about allergies. Serve a light supper, then initiate NPO status overnight. Administer a laxative or enema. Schedule test before barium studies. Posttest, observe for untoward reaction to dye. Encourage fluids for 24 hours to eliminate dye.
Kidney-ureter-bladder x-ray (KUB)	Shows abnormalities such as calculi, tumors, or changes in anatomic position.	Explain the procedure to the client. No preparation is required.
Long bone x-rays	Serial x-rays of the long bones to determine bone growth.	Explain the procedure to the client. Instruct the client to keep extremities still while the x-ray is being taken. Shield ovaries, testes, or pregnant uterus. Remove all metallic objects from area being x-rayed.
Lymphangiogram	A contrast dye is injected into the lymph vessels in the hands or feet to examine the lymph vessels and nodes. Used to stage lymphomas and evaluate the effectiveness of chemotherapy and radiation therapy. Normal: normal-sized lymph nodes with no malignant cells	The dye remains in the lymph nodes for 6 months to 1 year, so disease progress can be evaluated with an x-ray. Obtain informed consent. Inform the client that if a blue-colored dye is used, the skin and urine may have a bluish discoloration. Assess the client's breath sounds after the procedure, as lipoid pneumonia is a possible complication if the dye gets into the thoracic duct.

Table 28-8 Radiologic Studies (Continued)

TEST	EXPLANATION/NORMAL VALUES	NURSING RESPONSIBILITIES
Mammography	Used to diagnose benign and malignant disorders of the breast.	Explain the procedure to the client. The breast will be compressed, possibly causing discomfort for several seconds. Explain that it is important to have a baseline mammogram done between the ages of 35 and 40 and a breast examination done by a physician or nurse practitioner every 3–4 years. For women ages 40–49, a mammogram should be performed every 1–2 years; for those over 50, an annual mammogram is recommended along with an annual breast examination by physician or nurse practitioner.
Myelogram	X-ray of spinal subarachnoid space following injection of an opaque medium.	Follow nursing responsibilities for lumbar puncture in Table 28-14. Inform the client that the table may be tilted during the procedure. Obtain informed consent according to facility guidelines. Withhold the meal prior to procedure. Administer a light sedative, if ordered. Postprocedure care is determined by the type of medium used; follow physician's orders for activity and fluids.
Orbital CT scan	Allows visualization of abnormalities not readily seen on standard x-rays, delineating size, position, and relationship to adjoining structures. The orbital CT is a series of images reconstructed by a computer and displayed as anatomic slices on an oscilloscope. It identifies space-occupying lesions earlier and more accurately than do other x-ray techniques. It also provides three-dimensional images of orbital structures, especially the ocular muscles and optic nerve. Enhancement with a contrast agent may help define ocular tissue and circulation abnormalities.	Explain the test and the procedure to the client: that the client is positioned on an x-ray table; that the head of the table is moved into the scanner; that the scanner rotates during the test and may make loud, crackling sounds; that if an IV contrast agent is required, the client may feel flushed and warm or experience a transient headache; and that salty taste, nausea, and vomiting may occur following injection of the IV contrast dye. Reassure the client that the reaction is common and that she may signal the technician if she is unable to tolerate the test.
Positron emission tomography (PET) scan	Radioactive tracers are injected intravenously prior to the test. Nuclear imaging is used to confirm tissue that has adequate blood supply and tissue that has become impaired due to a lack of blood.	Instruct the client not to smoke or consume caffeine or alcohol for 24 hours prior to the test. Initiate NPO status from 10 P.M. the evening before the test, except for medications and water. Obtain informed written consent. Encourage the client to drink fluids after the procedure to facilitate faster excretion of the radioactive material.
Pouchogram	Installation of radiopaque dye into the Kock or Indiana pouch. Done with the continent ostomies to determine the state of healing and size of the pouch created.	Assess the client for allergy to iodine. Explain the procedure to the client.

(Continues)

TABLE 28-8 Radiologic Studies (Continued)

TEST	EXPLANATION/NORMAL VALUES	NURSING RESPONSIBILITIES
Pulmonary angiography	Assesses the arterial circulation of the lungs. Most often used to detect pulmonary emboli.	Explain the procedure to the client. Assess for allergy to iodine or shellfish. Inform the client that an arterial puncture is required, usually of the femoral artery, and that injection of the dye may cause a flushing or warm sensation due to vasodilation. After the study, assess the arterial puncture site frequently for evidence of bleeding. Assess vital signs and respiratory status. The client may be required to lie flat for up to 6 hours if the femoral artery is used for access. Obtain informed consent per facility policy.
Renal angiography	A catheter is inserted into the femoral artery and threaded into the renal artery. Dye is injected to show blood vessels in the kidney.	Initiate NPO status; administer enema. Assess client for allergy to iodine or shellfish. Check vital signs and peripheral pulses. Institute posttest bed rest, with leg straight. Monitor vital signs, peripheral pulses, urine output, and puncture site.
Voiding cystourethrography	The bladder is filled with dye, and x-rays are taken to observe bladder filling and emptying. Detects structural abnormalities of the bladder and urethra and reflux into the ureters.	Administer enema. Insert a Foley catheter and inject dye into bladder while x-rays are taken. Remove catheter and ask the client to void while more x-rays are taken. Allow the client to express feelings, as this test may be embarrassing.

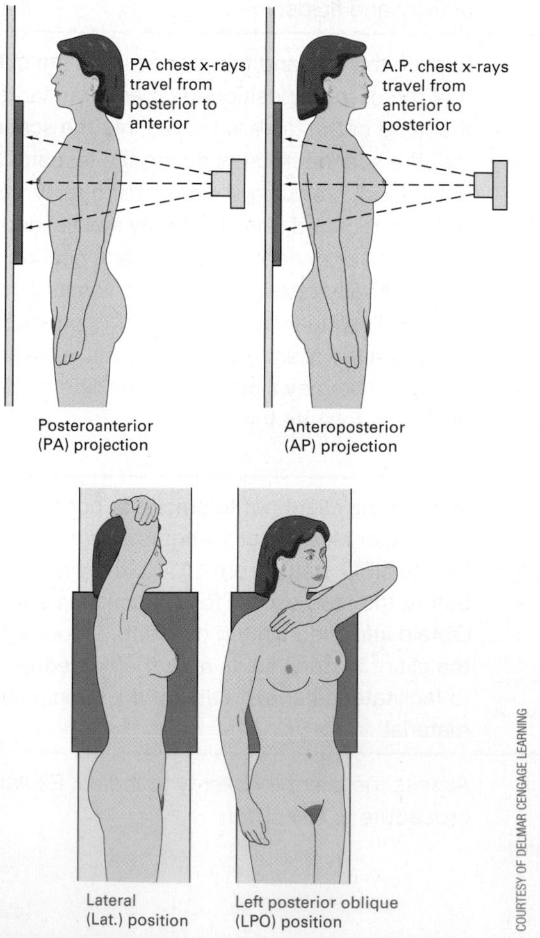

FIGURE 28-5 Radiographic Projection Positions

ARTERIOGRAPHY

Arteriography is the radiographic study of the vascular system after radiopaque dye is injected through a catheter. Using fluoroscopy, the catheter is threaded through a peripheral artery into the area to be studied, such as the aorta or the cerebral, coronary, pulmonary, renal, iliac, femoral, or popliteal artery. With the client on a cardiac monitor, dye is injected through the vascular catheter, and a rapid sequence of films is taken.

PROFESSIONALTIP

Computed Tomography

Assess the client's ability to relax, and review imagery relaxation. Sedation can be administered with an order from the practitioner.

SAFETY

Contrast Media

If a contrast medium is used, observe the client for indicators of allergic reaction to the dye, such as respiratory distress, urticaria, hives, nausea, vomiting, decreased production of urine (oliguria), and decreased blood pressure.

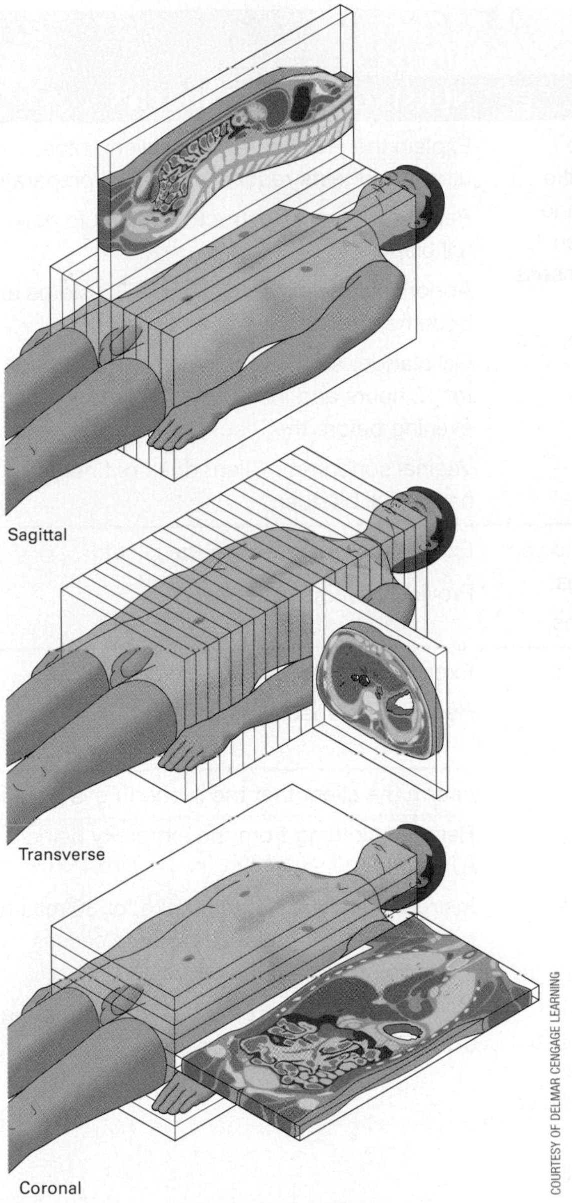

FIGURE 28-6 Computed Tomography

DYE INJECTION STUDIES

Iodine, a common dye used in radiographic studies, might cause the client to experience the following temporary symptoms: shortness of breath, nausea, and a warm to hot flushed sensation. Most dye injection studies are invasive and thus require written informed consent. Assess the client for allergies to iodine and/or the contrast agent prior to administration.

ULTRASONOGRAPHY

An **ultrasound**, also called an echogram or sonogram, is a noninvasive procedure using high-frequency sound waves to visualize deep body structures. To ensure accuracy, this procedure should be scheduled before studies using a contrast medium or air, because the contrast medium would reflect the sound waves differently than body structures do. The client must lie still during the procedure.

Ultrasound is used to evaluate the brain, thyroid gland, heart, abdominal aorta, vascular structures, liver, gallbladder, pancreas, spleen, and pelvis. During pregnancy, an ultrasound is commonly done to evaluate the size of the fetus and placenta. A full bladder is needed to ensure visualization.

To increase the contact between the skin and the **transducer** (instrument that converts electrical energy to sound waves), a coupling agent (lubricant) is placed on the surface of the body area to be studied. The transducer sends sound waves through the body tissue, which are reflected back and recorded. The varying density of body tissues deflects the waves into a differentiated pattern on an oscilloscope. Photographs are taken of the sound wave pattern on the oscilloscope. Table 28-9 describes some ultrasound tests.

MAGNETIC RESONANCE IMAGING

Magnetic resonance imaging (MRI) uses radio waves and a strong magnetic field to make continuous cross-sectional images of the body. During the study, a noniodine IV paramagnetic contrast agent may be used. The study reveals lesions and changes in the body's organs, tissues, and vascular and skeletal structures (Table 28-10).

NUCLEAR SCANS

Radionuclide imaging (nuclear scanning) uses radionuclides (or radiopharmaceuticals) to show morphological and functional changes in the body's structure. A scintigraphic scanner, placed over the area of study, detects emitted radiation and produces a visual image. The results reveal congenital abnormalities, skeletal changes, infections, lesions, and glandular and organ enlargement (Table 28-11). For all nuclear scans, written informed consent is required. The client must remove all jewelry and metal objects.

ELECTRODIAGNOSTIC STUDIES

Electrodiagnostic tests measure electrical activity of the brain, heart, and skeletal muscles. Electrical sensors (electrodes) are placed at certain points to measure the velocity, tone, and direction of the impulses. The impulses are then transmitted to an oscilloscope or printed on graphic paper. Table 28-12 describes the various electrodiagnostic studies.

ELECTROENCEPHALOGRAPHY

An **electroencephalogram (EEG)** is the graphic recording of the brain's electrical activity. During the procedure, electrodes are placed on the client's scalp. The electrodes transmit impulses from the brain to an EEG machine. The machine amplifies the brain's impulses and records the waves on strips of paper. An EEG can reveal not only the presence of a seizure disorder or intracranial lesion but also the type. The absence of the brain's electrical activity is used to confirm death.

ELECTROCARDIOGRAPHY

An **electrocardiogram (EKG or ECG)** is a graphic, noninvasive recording of the heart's electrical activity.

TABLE 28-9 Ultrasound Tests

TEST	EXPLANATION/NORMAL VALUES	NURSING RESPONSIBILITIES
Ultrasound	High-frequency ultrasound waves are sent into the body, and echoes are recorded as they strike tissues of different densities, producing an image or photograph. Useful in distinguishing between cystic and solid masses. Most often used to assess the pelvis, heart, and abdomen. Diagnostic for cysts, tumors, pregnancy, fetal gestational age, and multiple gestation.	Explain the procedure to the client. Most ultrasound tests require no special preparation: Pelvic sonogram: Instruct the client to have a full bladder. Abdominal sonogram: Initiate NPO status at bedtime; prepare bowel as directed. Gallbladder sonogram: Initiate NPO status for 12 hours and institute a fat-free diet the evening before the test. Vaginal sonogram: Client does not need to have a full bladder.
Breast ultrasound	Differentiates between solid and cystic lesions and can be used in conjunction with mammogram findings. Normal: no abnormalities or pathological lesions	Explain the procedure to the client. Provide privacy as needed.
Carotid Doppler	Evaluates carotid arteries in client at high risk or having symptoms of cerebrovascular disease. Normal: no occlusion or stenosis	Explain the procedure to the client. Requires no special preparation.
Doppler ultrasound	Determines patency of veins and arteries in conditions such as arterial occlusive disease, arteriosclerotic disease, or Raynaud's disease. Normal: audible "swishing" sound of the Doppler when placed over vessel A Doppler unit with blood pressure cuffs can measure the pulse volume of arteries and veins. An AB index is obtained by dividing the blood pressure reading in the ankle by the blood pressure reading in the arm (brachial artery). This is known as the ankle-to-brachial arterial blood pressure. There should be a less than 20 mm Hg difference between the pressure in the lower extremity as compared to the pressure in the upper extremity. Normal, AB index: 0.85 or greater	Inform the client that the procedure is painless. Remove clothing from the extremity being evaluated. Instruct the client not to smoke for 30 minutes prior to the test, because nicotine causes vasoconstriction of the vessels. Remove conductive or acoustic gel from the skin after the test is completed.
Echocardiogram	An ultrasound of the heart to determine hypertrophies, cardiomyopathies, or congenital defects. Very helpful in diagnosing valve abnormalities and pericardial effusion. The Doppler technique assesses coronary blood flow and evaluates cardiac valvular disease.	Explain the procedure to the client and assure the client that there is no discomfort during the procedure, although some pressure may be felt on the chest wall from the transducer.
Postvoid bladder ultrasound	Evaluation of urinary bladder for urine retention. Normal: normal size, shape, and position of the bladder; no masses or residual urine	Provide for privacy. Assist client in removing clothing from the waist down.
Thyroid ultrasound	Detects the size, shape, and position of the thyroid gland.	Explain the procedure to the client: that the client will lie supine, with the neck hyperextended; that breathing or swallowing will not be affected by the sound transducer; that a liberal amount of lubricating gel will be placed on the neck for the transducer; and that a series of photos will be taken over a 15-minute period. Assist the client in removing the lubricant.

TABLE 28-9 Ultrasound Tests (Continued)

TEST	EXPLANATION/NORMAL VALUES	NURSING RESPONSIBILITIES
Transrectal bladder ultrasound	Produces an image of the prostate or bladder and surrounding tissue.	Explain the procedure to the client.

TABLE 28-10 Magnetic Resonance Imaging

TEST	EXPLANATION/NORMAL VALUES	NURSING RESPONSIBILITIES
Magnetic resonance imaging (MRI)	Uses magnetic field and radio waves to detect edema, hemorrhage, blood flow, infarcts, tumors, infections, aneurysms, demyelinating disease, muscular disease, skeletal abnormalities, intervertebral disk problems, and causes of spinal cord compression. Can be used in conjunction with a magnetic resonance angiogram (MRA). Provides greater tissue discrimination than do chest x-ray or CT scans. Performed by qualified technologist. Takes approximately 1 hour.	Assess the client for the presence of metal objects within the body (i.e., shrapnel, cochlear implants, pacemakers). Explain the procedure to the client: the client will be required to lie still for up to 20 minutes at a time; the client will be placed within a scanning tunnel; sedation may be required if the client has claustrophobic tendencies; the magnet will make a loud thumping noise as images are obtained (provide earplugs as necessary). As the test may require up to 2 hours to perform, have the client void prior to entering the scanning tunnel. Obtain informed written consent, per facility policy.
Brain MRI	Scans for tumors, pathological lesions and masses, and abnormalities.	Explain the procedure to the client. Evaluate for claustrophobia.
Breast MRI	Delineates and/or differentiates breast disease.	Explain the procedure to the client. Provide privacy as needed. Evaluate for claustrophobia.
Joint MRI	Scans for ligament injuries and abnormalities.	Explain the procedure to the client. Position the client for comfort. Evaluate for claustrophobia.
Soft tissue MRI	Scans for abscesses, masses, tumors, and abnormalities.	Explain the procedure to the client. Evaluate for claustrophobia.
Vertebral MRI	Detects disk disease and used for clarifying x-ray findings.	Explain the procedure to the client and assure that there is no discomfort. Evaluate for claustrophobia.

TABLE 28-11 Nuclear Scans

TEST	EXPLANATION/NORMAL VALUES	NURSING RESPONSIBILITIES
Scan (radioisotope test)	A radioactive substance or isotope is taken up by the part of the body being examined. Sites most frequently studied are the bone, liver, spleen, lungs, heart, urinary tract, thyroid, and brain. The radioactive substance is given orally or intravenously by nuclear medicine personnel.	Explain the procedure to the client: that the client must lie still for 30–60 minutes and that the machine makes clicking noise at times. For liver, spleen, lung, thyroid, and brain scans, no special preparation is required. For a heart scan, initiate NPO status the evening before. For a kidney scan, hydrate as ordered.

(Continues)

Table 28-11 Nuclear Scans (Continued)

TEST	EXPLANATION/NORMAL VALUES	NURSING RESPONSIBILITIES
Radioactive iodine uptake (RAIU), iodine uptake,[131] I uptake	Uses oral radioactive iodine to determine thyroid function by the thyroid's ability to trap and retain iodine. Normal: 2 hours: 4% to 12% absorbed 6 hours: 6% to 15% absorbed 24 hours: 8% to 30% absorbed	The client who is allergic to iodine or shellfish or is pregnant should not have the test. Client should fast overnight. Drugs that decrease RAIU level include ACTH, antihistamines, saturated solution of potassium iodine, thyroid drugs, antithyroid drugs, and tolbutamide.
Radionuclide angiography (multiplegated radioisotope scan, multigated acquisition scanning, MUGA)	A radioisotope is injected to evaluate the function of the left ventricle. The ejection fraction (a comparison of the volume of blood pumped by the left ventricle to the total volume of blood left in the ventricle) is measured.	
Technetium pyrophosphate scanning	Important in diagnosing acute MIs, with the best accuracy obtained at 48 hours after the client experiences symptoms suggestive of an infarct. A tracer or radioisotope, which is injected intravenously, accumulates in the damaged or infarcted tissue areas, called "hot spots."	Instruct the client not to smoke or consume caffeine or alcohol for 3 hours before the test. Inform the client that the test will take 45–60 minutes.
Ventilation-perfusion scan (lung scan)	Assesses ventilation and perfusion of the lungs. Most often used to detect the presence of pulmonary emboli.	Assess for allergy to iodine and shellfish. Explain the procedure to the client: that a radioactive contrast media will be introduced via an IV access and inhalation of radioactive gas and that the client will be required to hold the breath for short periods as images are obtained.

Table 28-12 Electrodiagnostic Studies

TEST	EXPLANATION/NORMAL VALUES	NURSING RESPONSIBILITIES
Cardiac event monitor	Similar to a Holter monitor but worn for an extended period of time (weeks to months) with recording triggered by the client when symptoms occur.	Explain the procedure to the client. Instruct the client to engage in normal daily activities.
Electrocardiogram (EKG or ECG)	Electrodes are placed on the skin to record wave patterns of the electrical conduction of the heart. Detects myocardial damage, rhythmic disturbances, and hyperkalemia.	Explain the procedure to the client. Inform the client that the test is painless.
Electroencephalogram (EEG)	Record of electrical activity generated in the brain and obtained through electrodes applied to the scalp or microelectrodes placed in brain tissue during surgery.	Withhold caffeine due to stimulant effect. Serve meal so that blood sugar will not be altered. Shampoo hair night before test. Explain the procedure to the client: that the test takes approximately 45 minutes to 2 hours; the procedure is painless; the client may be asked to open and close the eyes during the test and that there may be flashing lights or small electrical stimulations.

TABLE 28-12 Electrodiagnostic Studies (Continued)

TEST	EXPLANATION/NORMAL VALUES	NURSING RESPONSIBILITIES
Electromyography (EMG)	Detects primary muscular disorders. A needle electrode is inserted into the muscle being examined. Measures electrical activity of skeletal muscle at rest and during voluntary muscle contraction.	Explain the procedure to the client. Obtain informed written consent. Instruct the client to refrain from consuming caffeine and smoking for 3 hours before the test. Assure client that the needle will not cause electrocution. Inform the client that there will be temporary discomfort when the needle electrode is inserted.
Electromyography (EMG) (Continued)		Observe the site for hematoma or inflammation after the test. The procedure takes approximately 1 hour.
Electroretinogram (ERG)	A record of the changes in the retina's electric potential following stimulation by light. Clinically useful in some clients with retinal disease. Performed by placing a contact lens electrode on the anesthetized cornea. The electrical potential recorded on the cornea is identical to the response that would be obtained if the electrodes were placed directly on the surface of the retina.	Explain the test and procedure to the client.
Esophageal motility studies (manometry)	Evaluates muscle contractions and coordination by using a tube with transducers. Used as a diagnostic tool for disorders of the esophagus and lower esophageal sphincter (LES).	Initiate NPO status 6–8 hours prior to the test.
Holter monitor	A portable EKG monitors and records the electrical conduction of the heart for a period of 24 hours. The heart rhythm is compared to client activities.	Instruct the client to engage in normal daily activities and to keep a journal of symptoms experienced in performing these activities.
Stress test	An EKG taken as the client exercises. Evaluates the effects of exercise on the heart. Often, the client is asked to walk on a treadmill, the incline of which is elevated at various times throughout the test. Used frequently on clients who have CAD.	Explain the procedure to the client. Encourage the client to wear good walking shoes during the test.
Thallium test (myocardial perfusion scan)	A radioactive tracer (Thallium^{201}) is injected and accumulates in myocardial tissue that is well perfused. Accumulation is lessened in areas of myocardial tissue that are not well perfused, areas called "cold spots." The client may be asked to perform exercise, such as riding a bike, during the test to evaluate the perfusion of myocardial tissue during exercise.	Instruct the client to refrain from eating and drinking for 3 hours prior to the test.

Lubricated electrodes are applied to the chest wall and extremities. The client is asked to lie still during the test. The pain-free test can reveal abnormal transmission of impulses and electrical position of the heart's axis.

A portable cardiac monitor (Holter monitor) records the heart's electrical activity, producing a continuous recording over a specified time (e.g., 24 hours) (Figure 28-7). It allows the client to ambulate and perform regular activities. Clients keep a log of activities resulting in the heart beating faster or irregularly. The EKG tracing is reviewed in relation to the client's log to determine if certain activities, such as walking, are associated with abnormal transmission of impulses.

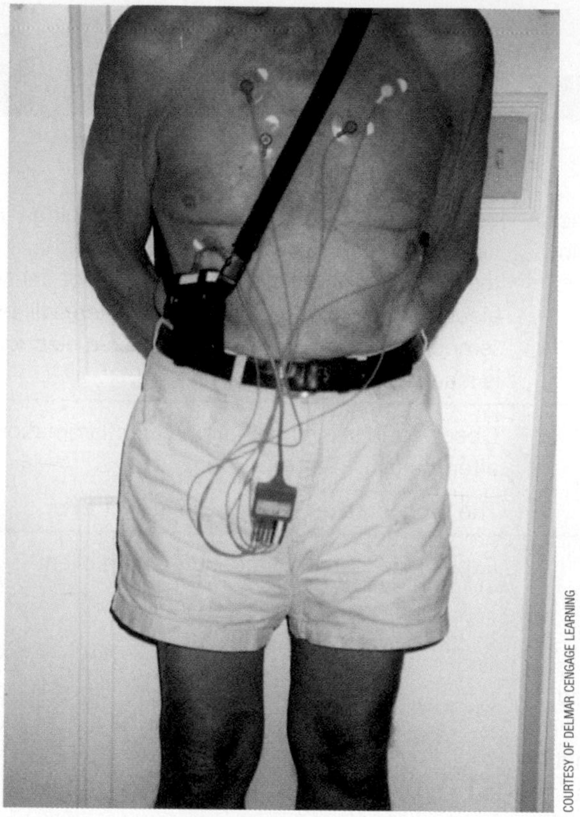

FIGURE 28-7 Holter Monitor

Stress Test

A **stress test** measures the client's cardiovascular fitness. It shows the myocardium's ability to respond to increased oxygen requirements (the result of exercise) by increasing the blood flow to the coronary arteries.

The client walks on a treadmill while connected to an EKG machine. Continuous EKG recordings are made during frequent changes in the treadmill's slope and speed. If the client experiences any symptoms of decreased cardiac output (chest pain, dyspnea, fatigue, or ischemic changes revealed by the EKG monitor), the test is stopped immediately.

Thallium Test

Thallium^{201} is a radioactive isotope that emits gamma rays and closely resembles potassium. Although a radioactive study, the thallium test is discussed here because it is often performed in conjunction with an EKG. Thallium is rapidly absorbed by normal myocardial tissue but is slowly absorbed by areas with poor blood flow and damaged cells. During the test, thallium is administered intravenously, and the scanner detects the radiation and makes a visual image. The light areas on the image represent heavy isotope uptake (normal myocardial tissue), whereas the dark areas represent poor isotope uptake (poor blood flow and damaged cells).

There are two types of thallium test: resting imaging and stress imaging. Resting imaging can detect a myocardial infarction within its first few hours. Stress imaging (thallium stress test) is performed while the client is on a treadmill and being monitored with an EKG. At peak stress, the IV thallium is injected. Scanning is performed in 3 to 5 minutes and again in 2 to 3 hours. The test is stopped immediately if the client becomes symptomatic for ischemia.

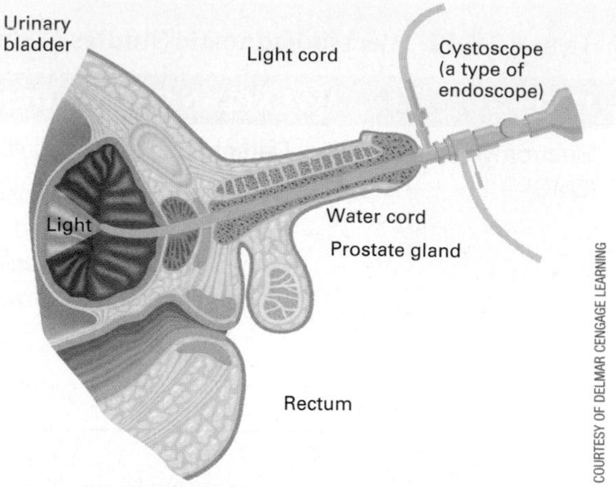

FIGURE 28-8 Cystoscope

ENDOSCOPY

Endoscopy is the visualization of a body organ or cavity through a scope. An endoscope (a metal or fiber-optic tube) is inserted directly into the body structure to be studied (Figure 28-8). A light and, in some studies, a camera at the end of the scope allow the practitioner to assess, via direct visualization or television picture, for lesions and structural problems. The endoscope has an opening at the distant tip that allows the practitioner to administer an anesthetic agent and to lavage, suction, and biopsy tissue. Common endoscopic procedures are listed in Table 28-13.

After the procedure, monitor vital signs, observe for bleeding, and assess for procedural risks (e.g., return of the gag and swallowing reflexes following a bronchoscopy performed under local anesthesia).

ASPIRATION/BIOPSY

Aspiration is performed to withdraw fluid that has abnormally collected or to obtain a specimen. To minimize client discomfort when the skin is pierced by the needle, a local anesthetic is administered in the area to be studied.

A hollow-bore needle with stylet is used to pierce the skin. The stylet is withdrawn once the needle is in place, leaving only the outer needle to aspirate the fluid. A **biopsy** (excision of a small amount of tissue) can be obtained during aspiration or in conjunction with other diagnostic tests (e.g., bronchoscopy). Table 28-14 outlines various aspiration/biopsy procedures.

BONE MARROW ASPIRATION/BIOPSY

The iliac crest and sternum are common sites for bone marrow puncture. A fluid specimen (aspiration) or a core of marrow cells (biopsy) can be obtained. Both tests are often done to obtain the best possible marrow specimen. The test identifies anemias; cancers such as multiple myeloma, leukemia, or Hodgkin's disease; or the client's response to chemotherapy.

Client positioning is determined by the site used: supine for the sternum and side lying for the iliac crest. The site is prepped to decrease the skin's normal flora. Explain to the client that pressure may be experienced as the specimen is withdrawn. The client should hold still because a sudden movement may dislodge the needle.

TABLE 28-13 Endoscopic Procedures

TEST	EXPLANATION/NORMAL VALUES	NURSING RESPONSIBILITIES
Endoscopy	Permits visual examination of internal structures of the body using specially designed instruments. The observation may be done through a natural body opening or through a small incision. A biopsy of suspicious areas may then be done for further study.	Explain the procedure to the client. Initiate NPO status 8–10 hours before test, except for sigmoidoscopy, before which a liquid diet should be followed for several days prior to the examination. Administer a laxative and then a cleansing enema.
Arthroscopy	Endoscopic procedure for direct visualization of a joint. Done in an operating room under sterile conditions and local or general anesthesia.	Perform frequent neurovascular checks. Elevate the client's leg. Apply compression dressing. Administer analgesic for discomfort.
Bronchoscopy	Direct visual examination of the bronchi through a fiber optic scope. Used to remove foreign bodies, for aggressive pulmonary cleansing, and to obtain sputum and tissue specimens.	Obtain written informed consent per facility policy. Explain the procedure to the client: that the client must be NPO for at least 6 hours prior to the test; that, if ordered, preprocedure sedation is administered; that an IV access will be obtained and sedation given during the procedure via this route. Following the procedure, frequently assess vital signs and respiratory status. Assess the client for unusual amounts of bleeding. Inform the client that sputum may be blood tinged initially following the procedure. Maintain the client in a side-lying position until the gag reflex returns. Withhold all food and fluids until the client is fully awake and has a gag reflex.
Colonoscopy	Examination of the rectum, colon, cecum, and ileocecal valve.	Initiate sedation. Cleanse the bowel. Offer only clear liquids after cleansing. Initiate NPO status for 6–8 hours prior to the test. Inform the client that flatulence and cramping will be experienced after the test.
Colposcopy	Direct visualization of the vagina and cervix through a high-powered microscope. Acetic acid is applied to the tissue to dehydrate the cells for improved visualization. Used to diagnose cervical dysplasia or carcinoma in situ of the cervix. Biopsies may be obtained as needed.	Explain the procedure and prepare the client in the dorsal lithotomy position. Assist with the procedure. Prepare biopsy specimens for pathological examination.
Cytoscopy	A cystoscope is passed through the urethra and into the bladder to examine the interior of the bladder for inflammation, stones, tumors, or congenital abnormalities. A biopsy may be performed, and small stones may be removed. Ureteral catheters may be inserted to obtain urine from each kidney. May require topical, spinal or general anaesthesia.	Explain the procedure to the client. Obtain informed written consent. Check vital signs. Instruct in deep breathing, if general anesthesia is to be used. Allow a full liquid diet if topical anesthetic is to be used. Monitor I&O.
Endoscopic retrograde cholangiopan-creatogram (ERCP)	Examination of the common bile duct (CBD) and biliary and pancreatic systems following injection of dye. Sphincterotomy, stone crushing, and stone removal can be done.	Initiate sedation. X-ray is used in conjunction. Initiate NPO status 6–8 hours prior to examination. Inform the client that the test can last up to 2 hours.

(Continues)

Table 28-13 Endoscopic Procedures (Continued)

TEST	EXPLANATION/NORMAL VALUES	NURSING RESPONSIBILITIES
Esophagogastro-duodenoscopy (EGD)	Examination of the esophagus, stomach, and duodenum. Biopsies can be taken, and dilations done.	Initiate sedation. Initiate NPO status 6–8 hours prior to the examination. Remove dentures and eye wear.
Flexible sigmoidoscopy	Examination of the sigmoid colon and rectum.	Sedation is optional. Administer enemas prior to examination. Inform the client to expect some flatulence and cramping after the examination.
Histeroscopy/ hysteroscopy	Provides a visual evaluation of the endometrium to diagnose or treat a uterine problem, and to perform a procedure such as endometrial ablation.	Explain the procedure to the client. Obtain written informed consent. Client may be asked not to eat or drink for a certain time before the procedure. Some routine lab tests may be done. Client will be asked to empty bladder. Explain to the client that the vaginal area will be cleansed with an antiseptic. The client may feel faint or sick or may have slight vaginal bleeding and cramps for a day or two.
Laparoscopy	Examination of the internal pelvic structures by direct visualization with a laparoscope. Usually performed under general anesthesia. Diagnostic for pelvic disorders and infertility problems.	Explain the procedure to the client. Prepare the client, conduct pre- and postoperative assessment, and institute interventions. Provide discharge instructions on activity and follow-up.
Peg tube placement	Transcutaneous placement of a gastric tube via endoscopy for nutritional (medical) support.	Obtain written informed consent per facility policy. Explain the procedure to the client. Prepare the client, conduct pre- and postoperative assessment, and implement interventions. Assess the site for bleeding after the procedure.

Table 28-14 Aspiration/Biopsy Procedures

TEST	EXPLANATION/NORMAL VALUES	NURSING RESPONSIBILITIES
Aspiration procedures		
Arthrocentesis	Procedure to obtain fluid from a joint using strict sterile technique. The knee is anesthetized, the sterile needle is inserted into joint space, and synovial fluid is aspirated. Used to diagnose infections, crystal-induced arthritis, and synovitis, and to inject anti-inflammatory medications. Normal: RBCs, 0; WBCs, 0–150/mm^3, neutrophils, >25%	Explain the procedure to the client. Obtain written informed consent. Assess site for edema, pain. The client should fast if possible. Apply pressure dressing and ice.
Bone marrow aspiration	Evaluates how well the bone marrow is producing RBCs, WBCs, and platelets. Normal: adequate numbers of RBCs, WBCs, and platelets.	Obtain written informed consent. Inform the client that pressure will be felt when the physician aspirates the bone marrow. Assess the site for bleeding after the procedure is completed. Bed rest for 30 minutes.
Gastric acid stimulation	Determines the amount of hydrochloric (HCl) acid in the stomach. If no HCl acid is present, that indicates parietal cells are malfunctioning. Parietal cells secrete the	If the client is having the tube test, initiate NPO status after midnight and instruct the client not to smoke prior to the test. Inform the client that a nasogastric tube is inserted prior to the test so

TABLE 28-14 Aspiration/Biopsy Procedures (Continued)

TEST	EXPLANATION/NORMAL VALUES	NURSING RESPONSIBILITIES
Gastric acid stimulation (Continued)	intrinsic factor that is essential for vitamin B_{12} absorption. Used to diagnose pernicious anemia. Normal tube test: Basal acid output: 2–6 mEq/h Maximal acid output: 16–26 mEq/h Normal, tubeless test: presence of dye in urine (usually blue or blue-green in color)	that gastric contents can be aspirated after the administration of pentagastrin. If the client is having the tubeless test, inform the client of the possibility of a blue or blue-green discoloration of urine. Note any medications taken that affect results; antacids, anticholinergics, and cimetidine (Tagamet) decrease HCl level, whereas adrenergic-blocking agents, cholinergics, steroids, and alcohol elevate HCl level.
Lumbar puncture (LP) (spinal tap)	A needle is inserted into the subarachnoid space to measure cerebrospinal fluid (CSF) pressure and/or to obtain a specimen. Normal pressure: 60–180 mm water pressure Normal specific gravity: 1.007 Normal glucose: 45–100 mg/100 mL Normal complete blood count (CBC): 0 Normal WBC: 0–5 cells/mm^3	Obtain informed written consent. Have the client empty the bowel and bladder prior to procedure. Assist in setting up a sterile field and pouring solutions, if not included in the tray. Assist the client to maintain the position. Postprocedure, deliver the specimen to the lab for testing, keep the client flat in bed for 3–24 hours or as ordered by physician; encourage fluid intake to replace fluids lost; and monitor vital and neurological signs.
Paracentesis	Fluid is withdrawn from the abdominal cavity by inserting a needle into the abdomen. The specimen is analyzed for infection or bleeding.	Have the client empty the bladder prior to the procedure. Prepare the abdomen by scrubbing it with a surgical prep solution and draping it with a sterile drape. Postprocedure, dress the site with a sterile dressing and monitor the site for further drainage. Assess vital signs one time postprocedure.
Pericardiocentesis	Fluid is removed from the pericardial sac for analysis or to relieve pressure.	Obtain written informed consent. Position the client in the semi-Fowler's position during the procedure and attach to an EKG monitor. Postprocedure, take vital signs every 15 minutes and monitor EKG rhythm.
Thoracentesis	Removal of fluid for diagnostic purposes. May also obtain biopsy, instill medications, and remove fluid for client comfort and safety.	Explain the procedure to the client. Obtain written informed consent. Position the client in an upright sitting position, leaning forward. Have client rest the arms on an over-bed table to facilitate this position. Explain to the client that the area will be anesthetized prior to the procedure. Instruct the client to hold as still as possible during the insertion of the thoracentesis needle. Assist the physician during the procedure. Deliver the specimen to the laboratory as soon as possible. Observe the thoracentesis site for bleeding following the procedure. Assess breath sounds before and after the procedure. Report absent breath sounds immediately.
Biopsy procedures	Removal of sample tissue for microscopic study. Tissue may be quickly frozen or placed in formalin before it is chemically stained	Explain the procedure to the client. Follow the physician's orders and/or agency protocol for client preparation.

(Continues)

TABLE 28-14 Aspiration/Biopsy Procedures (Continued)

TEST	EXPLANATION/NORMAL VALUES	NURSING RESPONSIBILITIES
Biopsy procedures (Continued)	and thinly sliced for analysis. Frozen section analysis takes only a few minutes and is often completed while a client is still in surgery. The full biopsy analysis takes 24–48 hours to complete but is the most accurate means of establishing a cancer diagnosis. Tissue biopsy is essential to confirming the type of cancer, the amount of lymph node involvement, and whether the cancer was successfully removed.	Obtain informed written consent.
Breast biopsy	Performed with or without local or general anesthesia and by aspiration, needle biopsy, excision, or incision. Tissue or fluid is obtained and sent to pathology for examination and identification of abnormal cells. Evaluates cystic breast lesions for malignancy. New method of obtaining breast biopsies may be done with the stereotactic mammography studies.	Explain the procedure to the client. Have the client undress down to the waist. Cleanse the biopsy region and shave the area, if needed. Drape the breast and adjacent skin. Provide emotional support prior to, during, and following the procedure. Monitor vital signs. Apply a sterile dressing or bandage. Instruct the client in postbiopsy wound care.
Cardiac biopsy	Done during a cardiac catheterization. The tissue sample is taken from the apex or septum to determine toxicity related to drugs; inflammation; or rejection of a transplanted heart.	Preparation is the same as for cardiac catheterization (see Table 28-8). After the procedure, observe the client for symptoms of a perforation, such as chest pain, decreased blood pressure, or dyspnea.
Endometrial biopsy	Obtained with special biopsy instruments and used to diagnose endometrial tissue abnormalities.	Explain the procedure to the client. Prepare the tissue preservation agent and label and send the sample to pathology. Assist the client in relaxing during the procedure, to offset the discomfort/cramping she may experience.
Liver biopsy	Obtained by inserting a needle into the liver. May be done with ultrasound or CT scan to guide needle placement. Evaluates cirrhosis, cancer, and hepatitis.	Schedule H&H, PT, PTT, and platelet tests prior to the procedure. Instruct the client to refrain from using NSAIDs including aspirin for 1 week prior to the procedure. Prepare the site by scrubbing it with a surgical prep solution and draping with a sterile towel. Monitor for signs of hemorrhage postprocedure by frequently monitoring vital signs and pain. Have the client lie on the right side. Support the biopsy site with a towel or bath blanket for 2 hours. Monitor the site for ecchymosis.
Prostatic biopsy	Removal of a small piece of tissue for microscopic examination.	Monitor for and educate the client about signs and symptoms of hemorrhage, infection, and postprocedure pain.
Testicular biopsy	Determines presence of sperm and rules out vas deferens obstruction.	Monitor for and educate the client about signs and symptoms of infection or hemorrhage.
Thyroid biopsy	Excision of thyroid tissue for histological examination after noninvasive tests prove abnormal or inconclusive. Can be obtained through needle biopsy or open surgical biopsy under general anesthesia.	Explain the procedure to the client. Obtain informed written consent. Assess for allergies. Have coagulation blood studies done. Assess for bleeding and respiratory and swallowing difficulties after the test. To prevent undue strain on the biopsy site, instruct the client to put both hands behind the neck when sitting up. Warn the client that a sore throat is possible after the biopsy.

After the procedure, the client should be kept on bed rest for 1 hour. Monitor vital signs to assess for bleeding (rapid pulse rate, low blood pressure). Instruct the client to report to the practitioner any bleeding or signs of inflammation.

PARACENTESIS

Paracentesis is the aspiration of fluid from the abdominal cavity. It can be diagnostic, therapeutic, or both. With end-stage liver or renal disease, for instance, **ascites** (an accumulation of fluid in the abdomen) occurs. Pressure from ascites can interfere with breathing and gastrointestinal functioning. In this instance, aspiration is therapeutic. If a specimen for culture is taken, it is also diagnostic.

The client should void and be weighed before the procedure. The client should be placed in a high-Fowler's position in a chair or sitting on the side of the bed. The skin is prepped, anesthetized, and punctured with a **trocar** (a sharply pointed surgical instrument contained in a cannula). The trocar is held perpendicular to the abdominal wall and advanced into the peritoneal cavity. The trocar is removed when fluid appears, leaving the inner catheter in place to drain the fluid. The client is observed for changes resulting from the rapid removal of fluid.

After the procedure, a sterile dressing is applied to the puncture site, and the client is monitored for changes in vital signs and electrolytes. Instruct the client to record the color, amount, and consistency of drainage on the dressing after discharge.

THORACENTESIS

Thoracentesis is the aspiration of fluids from the pleural cavity. The pleural cavity normally has a small amount of fluid to lubricate the lining between the lungs and pleura. Inflammation, infection, and trauma may cause increased fluid production, which can impair ventilation.

To facilitate access to the rib cage, position the client with the arms crossed and resting on a bedside table (Figure 28-9). The client should not cough during insertion of the trocar. The practitioner selects, preps, and anesthetizes the puncture site. The trocar is usually inserted into the intercostal space at the place of maximum dullness to percussion. This should be above the seventh rib laterally and above the ninth rib posteriorly.

During the procedure, the client must be carefully monitored for symptoms of a **pneumothorax** (collection of air or gas in the pleural space, causing the lungs to collapse), such as dyspnea, pallor, tachycardia, vertigo, and chest pain. After the procedure, assess for signs of cardiopulmonary changes and a mediastinum shift, as indicated by bloody sputum and changes in vital signs.

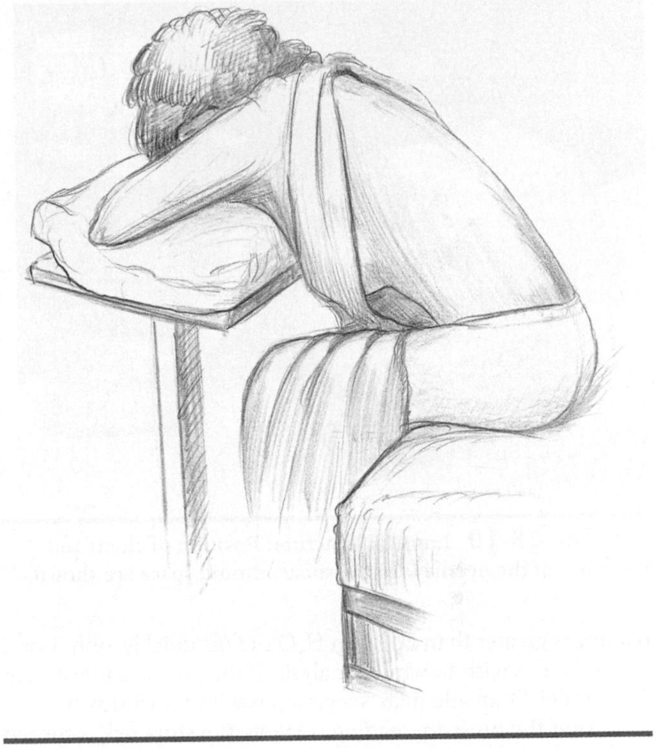

COURTESY OF DELMAR CENGAGE LEARNING

FIGURE 28-9 Client Position for Thoracentesis

CEREBROSPINAL FLUID ASPIRATION

Lumbar puncture (LP, "spinal tap") is the aspiration of cerebrospinal fluid (CSF) from the subarachnoid space. The specimen is examined for organisms, blood, and tumor cells. A spinal tap is also performed:

- To obtain a pressure measurement when blockage is suspected
- During a myelogram
- To instill medications (anesthetics, antibiotics, or chemotherapeutic agents)

The client assumes a lateral recumbent position, with the craniospinal axis parallel to the floor, the flat of the back perpendicular to the procedure table. The client should assume a flexed knee-chest position to bow the back, thereby separating the vertebrae. Most clients require assistance in maintaining this position throughout the procedure. Face the client and place one hand across the client's shoulder blades and the other hand over the client's buttocks.

The practitioner selects, preps, and anesthetizes the puncture site (usually interspace L3–L4, L4–L5, or L5–S1). The needle and stylet are inserted into the midsagittal space and advanced through the longitudinal subarachnoid space (Figure 28-10).

When positioned, the stylet is removed, leaving the needle in place. An initial CSF pressure reading is taken. If the pressure

CRITICAL THINKING

Thoracentesis

Thoracentesis is an invasive biopsy procedure to remove fluid for diagnostic purposes. What are potential complications associated with a thoracentesis? Why does a physician order a chest x-ray following the procedure?

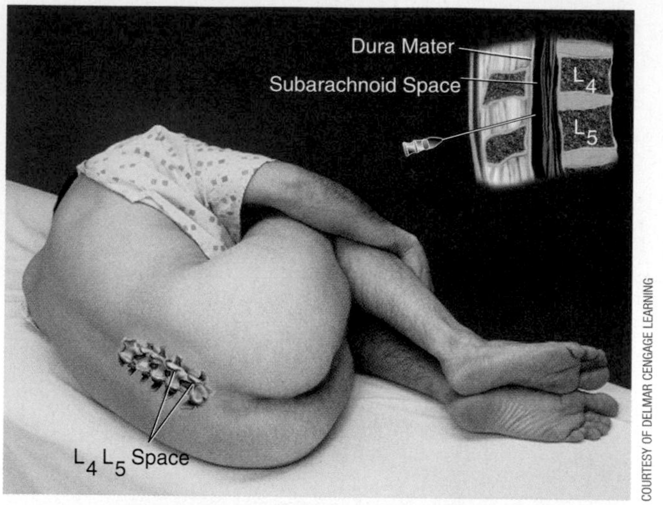

FIGURE 28-10 Lumbar Puncture: Position of client and insertion of the needle into the subarachnoid space are shown.

reading is greater than 200 mm H_2O or falls quickly, only 1 or 2 mL of CSF is withdrawn for analysis. If the pressure is less than 200 mm H_2O, an adequate specimen is withdrawn slowly.

After the pressure reading is taken, the stopcock is turned so the CSF slowly flows into a sterile test tube. A sterile cap is placed on the test tube, and the sample is taken to the laboratory. Rapid withdrawal of CSF can cause a transient postural headache. The client's cardiorespiratory status is monitored throughout the procedure.

> **PROFESSIONALTIP**
>
> **CSF Pressure**
>
> The client should be relaxed and quiet during the initial pressure reading because straining increases CSF pressure.
>
> After the procedure, pressure is applied to the puncture site, followed by a sterile bandage to prevent leakage of CSF. The client's neurological and cardiorespiratory statuses are then assessed. A postural headache is the most common complication of a lumbar puncture.

OTHER TESTS

Other diagnostic tests are described in Table 28-15.

TABLE 28-15 Other Tests

TEST	EXPLANATION/NORMAL VALUES	NURSING RESPONSIBILITIES
Arterial plethysmography (pulse volume recorder)	Determines arteriosclerotic disease in the upper extremities and occlusive disease in the lower extremities. Done by applying three blood pressure cuffs to an extremity. The cuffs are connected to a pulse volume recorder, which records the amplitude of each pulse wave. If there is a decrease in the amplitude of the pulse wave, an occlusion is in the artery proximal to the cuff. A decrease of 20 mm Hg of pressure indicates arterial occlusion. The test is not as reliable as arteriography but also does not have the risks associated with an arteriogram. Normal: normal arterial pulse waves	Explain to the client that the test is painless. Instruct the client to lie still during the test. Instruct the client not to smoke for 30 minutes prior to the test. Instruct the client to remove clothing from the extremity on which the test is to be done.
Audiometric testing	Evaluates both bone and air conduction and determines the degree of hearing loss. The client wears headphones, through which a series of tones is delivered at different frequencies. The client signals to the audiologist when the tones are audible. The results are recorded on an audiogram. The client is kept in a soundproof booth during the test.	Explain the procedure and its purpose to the client. Ensure that the client is not claustrophobic.

TABLE 28-15 Other Tests (Continued)

TEST	EXPLANATION/NORMAL VALUES	NURSING RESPONSIBILITIES
Brainstem auditory-evoked response (ErA and BAER)	Detects hearing dysfunctions of the central nervous system and cochlear nerve (cranial nerve VII). Valuable for testing comatose clients, clients with neurological damage, and children. An altered appearance of the brainstem waveforms or a delay or loss of a waveform indicates an abnormality including a possible cochlear lesion or acoustic neuroma.	Explain the procedure and its purpose to the client particularly that the client will be in a darkened room and will have both electrodes attached to the head and earphones in place.
Caloric test	Assesses alteration in vestibular function. The client is placed in a supine or Fowler's position and each ear is irrigated with cold and then warm water. Cold water causes rotary nystagmus away from injected ear and back to midline; warm water toward injected ear. Most commonly done on comatose clients. A punctured eardrum or Ménière's disease may contraindicate the test.	Explain the procedure and its purpose to the client. Tell the client that nystagmus, vertigo, nausea, vomiting, and an unsteady gait represent a normal response. Stay with the client and have an emesis basin and tissues available.
Color vision tests	Most common color vision tests use pseudoisochromatic (seemingly the same color) plates comprising patterns of dots of the primary colors superimposed on backgrounds of randomly mixed colors. A client with normal vision can identify the patterns; a client with a color deficiency cannot distinguish between pattern and background.	Explain the test and procedure to the client.
Culture and sensitivity (C&S)	Determines presence of microorganism and identifies the antibiotic that will kill or inhibit growth of microorganism. Drainage from infected lesions is obtained with a sterile swab and is incubated in order to identify the causative organism and to determine antibiotic sensitivity. Normal: negative for microorganism growth.	Ensure that the specimen has been obtained before initiating antibiotic therapy. Specimens should be taken to the laboratory within 30 minutes of being obtained.
Cytology	The study of cells and fluids obtained from various organs by scrapings, brushings, or needle aspiration. Cytologic smears, such as the Pap smear, are routinely done to study cells from the female genital tract. A cytological smear showing evidence of malignancy is followed by a biopsy to facilitate a more comprehensive diagnosis.	Explain the procedure to be used for obtaining cells and fluids for study. Follow agency protocol for client preparation.
Dark field examination of wart scrapings	Microscopic examination to differentiate genital warts from syphilis condylomata.	Take a careful client history. Examine the genital area carefully and provide scalpel and slide, if specimen is to be obtained. Explain the procedure thoroughly to the client.
Dilation and curettage (D&C)	Surgical scraping of the endometrial lining, performed under general, epidural, or paracervical anesthesia and on an outpatient basis. Diagnostic or therapeutic for uterine bleeding disorders.	Explain the procedure to the client. Perform pre- and postoperative assessment and provide care. Provide discharge instructions related to activities and follow-up appointments.

(Continues)

Table 28-15 Other Tests (Continued)

TEST	EXPLANATION/NORMAL VALUES	NURSING RESPONSIBILITIES
Dynamic infusion cavernosometry and cavernosography (DICC)	Group of diagnostic tests that measure neurovascular events of penile erection.	Perform baseline assessment, monitor during the procedure, and assess for postoperative complications; advise the client of possible discomfort related to the injection. Explain the procedure to the client. Assess for allergies. If preferred by the laboratory, initiate NPO status after midnight. Restrict iodine and thyroid preparations a week before test. Inform the client that radioactive iodine may be given orally or intravenously. Withhold food for 45–60 minutes after the iodine is given. Provide the client with a list of times to report to radiology. Tell the client that he will lie supine for test, which takes about 30 minutes, and that neither isolation nor specific urine precautions are necessary.
Huhner test (postcoital test)	Performed in the office. The couple has intercourse 2 hours before the appointment. A sample of secretions is removed from the vagina and placed on a microscopic slide. The sperm are observed for number and motility in the cervical mucous. Normal: a minimum of 20 sperm per field that demonstrate good motility	Explain the procedure to the client and schedule it near client's normal ovulation. Prepare the client in the lithotomy position. Assist the physician or nurse practitioner with the procedure. Perform microscopic observations as directed.
Nocturnal tumescence penile monitoring	Various devices are attached to the penis at night to monitor swelling (tumescence).	Explain to the client that the test will require application of a device to the penis and that the device is to be worn while sleeping. Show the client the device and explain how to apply it.
Papanicolaou (Pap) smear	Cells are obtained from the external and internal cervical canal. Screening tool for premalignant and malignant cervical changes.	Explain the procedure. Have client empty bladder and undress. Position client in dorsal lithotomy position. Help client relax during procedure. Prepare microscopic slides for pathology. Instruct the client on the importance of having an annual Pap smear.
Past-point testing	Measures the ability or inability to accurately place a finger on some part of the body, usually the client's or examiner's face and fingers. For example, the examiner will instruct the client to close her eyes and touch her nose, then, with eyes open, touch the examiner's nose or the examiner's index finger.	Explain the test and procedure to the client. Explain that it is painless and represents a helpful measure of vestibular function (coordination).
Patch testing	Allergens within occlusive patches are applied to normal skin (usually the upper back) for 48 hours. If the client is allergic to a specific allergen, an erythematous skin reaction will occur.	Clean and dry the skin where the patches are to be applied. Tell the client that the patches must be left in place for the full 48 hours.

Table 28-15 Other Tests (Continued)

TEST	EXPLANATION/NORMAL VALUES	NURSING RESPONSIBILITIES
Pelvic examination (Recommended about 3 years after the beginning of sexual intercourse but no later than age 21 and continue screening through menopause. Screening should be performed every year with the regular Pap test or every 2 years using the newer liquid-based Pap test.)	Performed by a physician or nurse practitioner. The external and internal pelvic structures are visualized, the pelvic organs are palpated via bimanual examination, and the cervix is examined via a speculum. A Pap smear and rectovaginal exam are also performed, and cultures and wet smears may be obtained.	Explain the procedures to the client, prepare the client by having her void and undress, position the client on the examination table in a dorsal lithotomy position, help the client to relax during the examination, prepare slides and culture medium, obtain other supplies, and assist with the procedure.
Postvoid residual (PVR)	Urinary bladder catheterization for the quantification of urine retention.	Explain the procedure to the client. Have the client void prior to the catheterization. Use strict sterile technique during the procedure. Measure and record urine output from the catheterization.
Prostatic smears	Microscopic examination of prostatic secretions obtained via rectal massage performed by a physician.	Explain to the client that to obtain the specimen, the prostate must be massaged via the rectum and that this will cause some discomfort.
Pulmonary function tests (PFTs)	A group of studies used to evaluate ventilatory function. Measurements are obtained directly via spirometer or calculated from the results of spirometer measurements. Bronchodilators may be used during the study. Measurements included are: Tidal volume: the amount of air inhaled and exhaled in one breath: 500 mL at rest. Inspiratory reserve volume: the amount of air inspired at the end of a normal inspiration. Expiratory reserve volume: the amount of air expired following a normal expiration. Residual volume: the amount of air left in lungs after maximal expiration. Vital capacity: the total volume of air that can be expired after maximal inspiration. Total lung capacity: the total volume of air in the lungs when maximally inflated. Inspiratory capacity: the maximum amount of air that can be inspired after normal expiration. Forced vital capacity: the capacity of air exhaled forcefully and rapidly following maximal inspiration. Minute volume: the amount of air breathed per minute.	Explain the procedure to the client. PFTs should not be done within 1–2 hours after a meal. After the test, monitor respiratory status. Advise the client to avoid activity and to rest following the test, as fatigue may result.

(Continues)

TABLE 28-15 Other Tests (Continued)

TEST	EXPLANATION/NORMAL VALUES	NURSING RESPONSIBILITIES
Pulse oximetry	A noninvasive procedure. A transdermal clip is placed on a finger or earlobe to detect the arterial oxygen saturation (SaO_2). Normal: >95% (at sea level)	Explain the procedure to the client. Assess peripheral circulation, as this may alter results. Place the sensor on the earlobe, fingertip, or pinna of the ear. Keep the sensor intact until a consistent reading is obtained. Observe and record readings. Report to the physician measurements below 95%.
Rinne test (tuning fork)	Detects loss of hearing in one or both ears. Tuning fork is struck and placed against the mastoid bone to measure the sound conduction through the bone. The tuning fork is then placed beside and parallel to the ear to test conduction through the air. If the sound is louder when the tines are placed beside the ear, hearing is normal or the hearing loss is sensorineural. If the sound is louder when conducted through the bone, the hearing loss is conductive.	Explain the procedure and its purpose to the client.
Romberg test	Assesses vestibular (balance) function. The client stands with the eyes closed, arms extended in front, and feet together. Normal: slight swaying.	Explain the procedure and its purpose to the client. Stand close and reassure the client that someone will catch him if he begins to fall.
Schiller test	Performed during colposcopy. An iodine solution is applied to the cells of the cervix. Abnormal cells turn white or yellow. Aids in visualization of abnormal tissue and indicates areas for biopsy. Normal: cells turn brown	Explain the reason for the application of the solution. Assist with the biopsy procedure as necessary. Label tissue specimens and send to histology.
Segmented bacteriologic localization cultures	The first 5–10 mL of urine is collected, the next 200 mL is discarded, then 5–10 mL is collected midstream. The prostate is then massaged until prostatic secretions can be collected. Finally, 5–10 mL urine is collected before the bladder is emptied. Four samples are needed in sterile culture tubes.	Ensure that the client is well hydrated and has a full bladder.
Semen analysis	Determines the presence, number, and motility of sperm.	Teach the client about proper collection of sperm.
Skin scrapings	A lesion is scraped with an oiled scalpel blade. The cells are then examined under a microscope. Used to diagnose fungal lesions.	Explain the procedure and its purpose to the client.
Slit-lamp examination	The cornea is examined with the aid of a slit lamp. Provides a visual evaluation and possible treatment of corneal lesions. The exam may reveal disorders such as iritis, corneal abrasions, conjunctivitis, and cataracts.	Explain the procedure and its purpose to the client.
Speech audiometry (Spondee threshold)	Evaluates ability to hear and understand the spoken word. A series of two-syllable words commonly recognized by their vowel sounds (like *toothbrush* and *baseball*) are delivered through earphones. When the client correctly repeats the word, the sound intensity is recorded in decibels. The test is normally conducted in a soundproof booth.	Explain the procedure and its purpose to the client. Ensure that the client is not claustrophobic.

TABLE 28-15 Other Tests (Continued)

TEST	EXPLANATION/NORMAL VALUES	NURSING RESPONSIBILITIES
Sputum analysis	Sputum samples are examined for the presence of bacteria, fungi, molds, yeasts, and malignant cells. Appropriate antibiotic therapy is determined via C&S studies.	Explain the procedure and its purpose to the client. Obtain specimens early in the morning to prevent contamination via ingested food or fluids. Instruct the client to breathe deeply and cough, so as to facilitate collection of a specimen originating from the lower respiratory tract. If necessary, pulmonary suctioning may be used to induce such a specimen. Instruct the client to expectorate sputum into the appropriate container. Deliver specimens to the laboratory as soon as possible.
Tonometry	Used to measure intraocular pressure and to aid in the diagnosis and follow-up evaluation of glaucoma. Two types of tonometric devices are used for assessment: applanation and indentation. An applanation tonometer is the most accurate and commonly used device and measures the force (delineated by the reading on the tension dial on the tonometer) required to flatten a small, standard area of the cornea. An indentation tonometer measures the deformation of the globe in response to a standard weight placed on the cornea. Before use of either apparatus, the eyes are anesthetized with a local ophthalmic solution, such as benoxinate with fluorescein or tetracaine, so that the pressure from the tonometer will not be felt. Normal: 20 mm Hg or lower	Explain the procedure and its purpose to the client. Explain to the client that this test measures the pressure within the eyes and that although the test requires the client's eyes to be anesthetized, the anesthesia will wear off shortly after the examination is complete. Reassure the client that the procedure is painless.
Tympanometry	Measures the movement of the eardrum in response to air pressure in the ear canal. Evaluates the presence of fluid in the middle ear and is commonly used to evaluate otitis media in children or adults.	Explain the procedure and its purpose to the client. Inform the client a small burst of air is introduced through the otoscope, which may produce an uncomfortable sensation.
Tzanck smear	Fluid from the base of a vesicle is applied to a glass slide, stained, and examined under a microscope. Used to diagnose herpes zoster, herpes simplex, varicella, or pemphigus. Normal: negative	Describe to the client how the laboratory technician will obtain the specimen and that although the procedure will likely not be painful, the client must remain still to prevent injury. Provide scalpel blade, glass slide, and stain for collection.
Urethra pressure profile (UPP)	Assesses functional urethral length and general competency of the urethra and sphincter, either at rest or during coughing, straining, or voiding. Functional profile length is the length from bladder outlet to the point in the urethra where urethral pressure equals intravesical pressure. Used to diagnose stress or overflow incontinence or urethral obstruction. Normal: Male: bladder outlet through membranous urethra Female: bladder outlet through mid-urethra	Explain the procedure and its purpose to the client: that it is often performed when the bladder is empty and the client is at rest; that it may be performed simultaneously with CMG; and that the client may be asked to cough or void. Provide privacy, as the test can be embarrassing.

(Continues)

Table 28-15 Other Tests (Continued)

TEST	EXPLANATION/NORMAL VALUES	NURSING RESPONSIBILITIES
Uroflowmetry	Noninvasive assessment of urination. An electronic device connected to a funneled commode calculates the rate of urine flow, volume voided, and time taken to void.	Explain the procedure and its purpose to the client. Instruct the client to void as usual, leaving client alone to do so, if possible.
Weber test (tuning fork)	Detects loss of hearing in one or both ears. Tuning fork is struck and the handle is placed in the middle of the forehead. Clients with normal hearing or bilateral deafness will hear or not hear the sound equally in both ears. Clients with unilateral hearing loss will hear the sound only in the unaffected ear.	Explain the procedure and its purpose to the client.
Wood's light examination	Skin and hair are examined under ultraviolet light (black light) in a darkened room. Used to diagnose fungal infections (tinea) of hair and skin.	Explain the procedure and its purpose to the client. Reassure the client that the rays are not harmful.

CASE STUDY

A 68-year-old male client is admitted to the hospital with a hemoglobin of 9 g/dL and hematocrit of 28%. He is pale, fatigued, complains of muscle weakness, and has a family history of colon cancer. The physician orders a colonoscopy to be performed.

Questions

1. What nursing measures are taken to ensure the client's safety for the colonoscopy?
2. What are the nurse's responsibilities when preparing the client for the colonoscopy?
3. What are the nursing responsibilities when caring for the client during the colonoscopy?
4. What postprocedure nursing care is provided?

SUMMARY

- Most invasive procedures require that the client give written informed consent.
- Prepare clients for diagnostic testing by ensuring client understanding and compliance with preprocedural requirements.
- Clients, families, and significant others must be involved in the testing process; advise them of the estimated procedure time.
- To help offset the discomfort and anxiety experienced during procedures, teach the client how to perform relaxation techniques such as imagery.
- After a diagnostic test, provide care and teach the client those things to expect, including the outcomes or side effects of the test.
- The nurse facilitates the scheduling of diagnostic tests, performs client teaching, performs or assists with procedures, and assesses clients for adverse responses.
- Schedule diagnostic procedures to promote client comfort and cost containment.
- Standard Precautions are used when obtaining a specimen or assisting with an invasive procedure.
- Before a procedure, obtain baseline vital signs and assess the client's preparation for testing.
- After a procedure, assess the client for secondary procedural complications and perform any necessary nursing interventions.

REVIEW QUESTIONS

1. After the client voided, he reports feeling lower abdominal pressure, fullness, and a need to void again. When the client tries to urinate, no urine is voided. Which diagnostic test will the physician order?
   1. Uric acid.
   2. 17-ketosteroids (17-KS).
   3. Postvoid residual.
   4. Urine cortisol.
2. When preparing a client for diagnostic testing, nursing measures to ensure client safety include: (Select all that apply.)
   1. establishing baseline vital signs.
   2. identifying known allergies.
   3. assessing teaching effectiveness.
   4. checking the identification band.
   5. evaluating the client's respiratory status.
   6. obtaining written informed consent for invasive procedures.
3. The nurse is preparing a client for a bronchoscopy. Which statement made by the client indicates the need for further teaching?
   1. "The procedure is invasive and requires a signed consent."
   2. "The nurse will start an IV in my hand or arm."
   3. "The nurse will check my vital signs frequently."
   4. "I will be able to drink water again as soon as the procedure is over."
4. When scheduling a series of tests, the nurse knows to schedule:
   1. a barium enema before an upper GI.
   2. an ultrasound after all other tests.
   3. an upper GI before a gallbladder x-ray.
   4. a gallbladder x-ray before any barium studies.
5. A test that combines a radioactive scan with an electrodiagnostic study is a:
   1. MUGA.
   2. brain scan.
   3. thallium stress test.
   4. radioactive iodine uptake test.
6. Place the nursing actions in the correct order when providing care for a client undergoing diagnostic testing:
   A. Correctly label specimen(s)
   B. Obtain baseline vital signs
   C. Provide written discharge instructions
   D. Ensure client is wearing identification band
   E. Monitor for signs of complications
   1. C, B, D, A, E
   2. D, B, A, E, C
   3. B, D, C, A, E
   4. B, D, E, C, A
7. A newly diagnosed diabetic client asks the nurse, "What is a hemoglobin A1C test?" The best response by the nurse is:
   1. "The procedure is ordered once a year and requires a 12-hour fasting prior to the blood draw."
   2. "The urine test evaluates the amount of glucose in the bloodstream."
   3. "The blood test evaluates the average blood glucose over 120 days."
   4. "The test requires a finger stick blood sample that evaluates the average blood glucose over 180 days."
8. Nursing responsibilities for common diagnostic testing procedures include: (Select all that apply.)
   1. remaining with the client during induction of anesthesia.
   2. placing the client in the correct position for the procedure.
   3. assessing the client's allergies to dye and contrast agents.
   4. referring the client's medical questions and concerns to family.
   5. creating an individualized care plan for the client's procedure.
   6. assessing the client's comfort level (pain).
9. The physician has ordered an occult blood stool test to confirm suspicions of a GI disorder. Which of the following does not cause a false-positive test result?
   1. Steroids.
   2. Grapefruit.
   3. Salicylate.
   4. Meat.
10. Nursing responsibilities when caring for a client that is scheduled for a chest x-ray include:
    1. instructing the client to inspire deeply and hold the breath.
    2. inquiring whether the client may be pregnant.
    3. instructing the client to remove all metal objects from the chest and neck area.
    4. all of the above.

REFERENCES/SUGGESTED READING

Ahmed, D. (2000). Hidden factors in occult blood testing. *American Journal of Nursing, 100*(12), 25.

Beattie, S. (2007). Bone marrow aspiration and biopsy. *RN, 70*(2), 41–43.

Bourg, M. (2007). Screening for microalbuminuria. *Nursing2007, 37*(2), 70.

Carr, M., & Grey, M. (2002). Magnetic resonance imaging. *American Journal of Nursing, 102*(12), 26–33.

Clinical Rounds. (2002). Quick blood test identifies heart failure. *Nursing2002, 32*(6), 34.

Connolly, M. (2001). Chest X-rays: Completing the picture. *RN, 64*(6), 56–62.

Daniels, R. (2010). Delmar's guide to laboratory and diagnostic tests 2nd edition. Clifton Park, NY: Delmar Cenage Learning.

Darty, S., Thomas, M., Neagle, C., Link, H., Wesley-Farrington, D., & Hundley, G. (2002). Cardiovascular magnetic resonance imaging. *American Journal of Nursing, 102*(12), 34–38.

Deatcher, J. (2008). Diabetes under control: Prediabetes. Are you or your patients at risk for type 2 diabetes? *American Journal of Nursing, 108*(7), 77–79.

Ernst, D. (1999). Collecting blood culture specimens. *Nursing99, 29*(7), 56–58.

Gallauresi, B. (1998). Pulse oximeters. *Nursing98, 28*(9), 31.

Guyton, A., & Hall, J., (2000). *Textbook of medical physiology* (10th ed.). Philadelphia: W. B. Saunders.

Hill, J., & Newton, J. (1998). Contrast echo: Your role at the bedside. *RN, 61*(10), 32–35.

Josephson, D. (2004). *Intravenous infusion therapy for nurses: Principles and practice.* Clifton Park, NY: Delmar Cengage Learning.

Kayyali, A., Singh Joy, S., & Cutugno, C. (2008). Informing practice: "Point-of-care" glucometers. *American Journal of Nursing, 108*(9), 72cc.

Kee, J. (2006). *Laboratory and diagnostic tests with nursing implications* (7th ed.). Upper Saddle River, NJ: Prentice Hall.

Lawrence, B., & Tasota, F. (2003). Detecting neuromuscular problems with electromyography. *Nursing2003, 33*(4), 82.

Lewis, K. (2000). *Sensible analysis of the 12-lead ECG.* Clifton Park, NY: Delmar Cengage Learning.

McEnroe-Ayers, D. (2002a). EBCT: Beaming in on coronary artery disease. *Nursing2002, 32*(4), 81.

McEnroe-Ayers, D. (2002b). Preparing a patient for cardiac catheterization. *Nursing2002, 32*(9), 82.

Montes, P. (1997). Managing outpatient cardiac catheterization. *American Journal of Nursing, 97*(8), 34–37.

Neighbors, M., & Tannehill-Jones, R. (2006). *Human disease* (2nd ed.). Clifton Park, NY: Delmar Cengage Learning.

Nursing2002. (2002). Teaching your patient about cardiovascular tests. *Nursing2002, 32*(1), 62–64.

Prue-Owens, K. (2006). Use of peripheral venous access devices for obtaining blood samples for measurement of activated partial thromboplastin time. *Critical Care Nurse, 26*(1), 30–38.

Rushing, J. (2007). Obtaining a throat culture. *Nursing2007, 37*(3), 20.

Ryan, D. (2000). Is it an MI? A lab primer. *RN, 63*(2), 26–30.

Tasota, F. (2002). Full-body scans: Screening for problems. *Nursing2002, 32*(7), 22.

Tasota, F., & Tate, J. (2001a). Assessing thyroid function with serum tests. *Nursing2001, 31*(1), 22.

Tasota, F., & Tate, J. (2001b). Diagnosing pulmonary embolism with spiral CT. *Nursing2001, 31*(5), 75.

Tasota, F., & Tate, J. (2001c). Digital mammography: Enhanced imaging in real time. *Nursing2001, 31*(4), 70.

Tasota, F., & Tate, J. (2001d). Interpreting the highs and lows of platelet counts. *Nursing2001, 31*(2), 25.

Tasota, F., & Tate, J. (2001e). Teaching patients about lipid levels. *Nursing2001, 31*(3), 68.

Tasota, F., & Tate, J. (2001f). Using PET to detect abnormalities. *Nursing2001, 31*(11), 24.

White, L., & Duncan, G. (2002). *Medical-surgical nursing: An integrated approach* (2nd ed.). Clifton Park, NY: Delmar Cengage Learning.

Wong, F. (1999). A new approach to ABG interpretation. *American Journal of Nursing, 99*(8), 34–36.

RESOURCES

Harvard Health Publications, Harvard Medical School, http://www.health.harvard.edu/diagnostic-tests

National Library of Medicine, http://www.nlm.nih.gov

The Cleveland Clinic, http://my.clevelandclinic.org

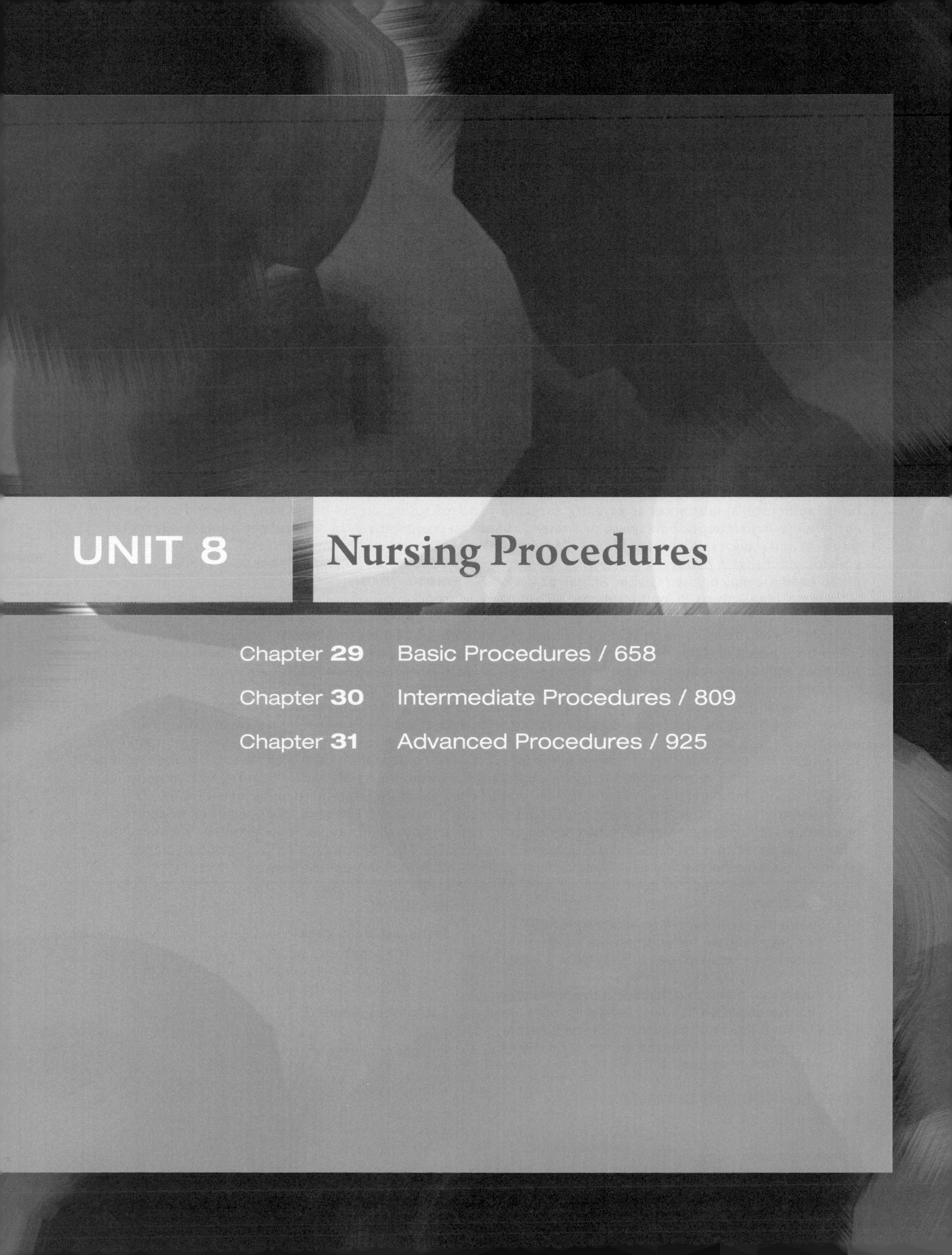

UNIT 8 Nursing Procedures

CHAPTER 29
Basic Procedures

PROCEDURE 29-1 Hand Hygiene

OVERVIEW

Hand hygiene is a general term that includes *hand washing* (using plain soap and water), *antiseptic hand wash* (using antimicrobial substances and water), *antiseptic hand rub* (using alcohol-based hand rub), and *surgical hand antisepsis* (using antiseptic hand wash or antiseptic hand rub preoperatively by surgical personnel to eliminate transient and reduce resident hand flora) (Centers for Disease Control and Prevention [CDC], 2007). *When hands are visibly dirty, wash hands with soap (plain or antimicrobial) and water. If hands are not visibly soiled, an alcohol-based hand rub may be used* (Siegel, Rhinehart, Jackson, & Chiarello, 2007).

Hand washing is the rubbing together of all surfaces and crevices of the hands using a soap or chemical and water. Hand washing is a component of all types of isolation precautions and is the most basic and effective infection-control measure to prevent and control the transmission of infectious agents.

The three essential elements of hand washing are soap or chemical, water, and friction. Soaps that contain antimicrobial agents are frequently used in high-risk areas such as emergency departments and nurseries. Friction is the most important element of the trio because it physically removes soil and transient flora.

Hand washing is performed after arriving at work, before leaving work, between client contacts, after removing gloves, when hands are visibly soiled, before eating, after excretion of body waste (urination and defecation), after contact with body fluids, before and after performing invasive procedures, and after handling contaminated equipment. The exact duration of time required for hand washing depends on the circumstances. A washing time of 10 to 15 seconds is recommended to remove transient flora from the hands. High-risk areas, such as nurseries, usually require about a minimum 2-minute hand wash. Soiled hands usually require more time (CDC, 2007). According to the CDC Standard Precautions (Siegel, Rhinehart, Jackson, & Chiarello, 2007), artificial fingernails or extenders are not recommended when having direct contact with clients at risk for infection or with potential adverse outcomes, that is, clients in intensive care or surgery. The CDC recommends following agency policy regarding wearing nonnatural nails when caring for clients other than those previously mentioned.

ASSESSMENT

1. Assess the environment **to establish if facilities are adequate for washing the hands.** Is the water clean? Is soap available? Is there a clean towel to dry hands?
2. Assess your hands **to determine if they have open cuts, hangnails, broken skin, or heavily soiled areas.**
3. Maintain short natural nails. **Short nails harbor fewer microorganisms and do not harm clients when providing care.**

POSSIBLE NURSING DIAGNOSIS

Risk for Infection

PLANNING

Expected Outcomes

1. The caregiver's hands are washed adequately to remove microorganisms, transient flora, and soiling from the skin.

Equipment Needed

- Soap
- Paper or cloth towels
- Sink
- Running water

delegation tips

All hospital personnel are expected to maintain proper hand hygiene technique and routinely practice Standard Precautions.

PROCEDURE 29-1 Hand Hygiene (Continued)

IMPLEMENTATION—ACTION/RATIONALE

ACTION	RATIONALE
Handwashing	
1. Remove jewelry. Wristwatch may be pushed up above the wrist (mid-forearm). Push sleeves of uniform or shirt up above the wrist at mid-forearm level.	1. Provides access to skin surfaces for cleaning. Facilitates cleaning of fingers, hands, and forearms.
2. Assess hands for hangnails, cuts, or breaks in the skin, and areas that are heavily soiled.	2. Intact skin acts as a barrier to microorganisms. Breaks in skin integrity facilitate development of infection and should receive extra attention during cleaning.
3. Turn on the water. Adjust the flow and temperature. Temperature of the water should be warm.	3. Running water removes microorganisms. Warm water removes less of the natural skin oils.
4. Wet hands and lower forearms thoroughly by holding under running water. Keep hands and forearms in the down position with elbows straight. Avoid splashing water and touching the sides of the sink or faucet.	4. Water should flow from the least contaminated to the most contaminated areas of the skin. Hands are considered more contaminated than arms. Splashing of water facilitates transfer of microorganisms. Touching of any surface during cleaning contaminates the skin.
5. Apply about 5 mL (1 teaspoon) of liquid soap. Lather thoroughly.	5. Lather facilitates removal of microorganisms. Liquid soap harbors less bacteria than bar soap.
6. Thoroughly rub hands together for about 10 to 15 seconds. Interlace fingers and thumbs and move back and forth to wash between digits. Wash palms, back of hands, and wrists with firm rubbing and circular motions (Figure 29-1-1). Special attention should be provided to areas such as the knuckles and fingernails, which are known to harbor organisms (Figure 29-1-2).	6. Friction mechanically removes microorganisms from the skin surface. Friction loosens dirt from soiled areas.
7. Rinse with hands in the down position, elbows straight. Rinse in the direction of forearm to wrist to fingers.	7. Flow of water rinses away dirt and microorganisms.
8. Blot hands and forearms to dry thoroughly. Dry in the direction of fingers to wrist and forearms. Discard the paper towels in the proper receptacle.	8. Blotting reduces chapping of skin. Drying from cleanest (hand) to least clean area (forearms) prevents transfer of microorganisms to cleanest area.
9. Turn off the water faucet with a clean, dry paper towel (Figure 29-1-3).	9. Prevents contamination of clean hands by a less clean faucet.

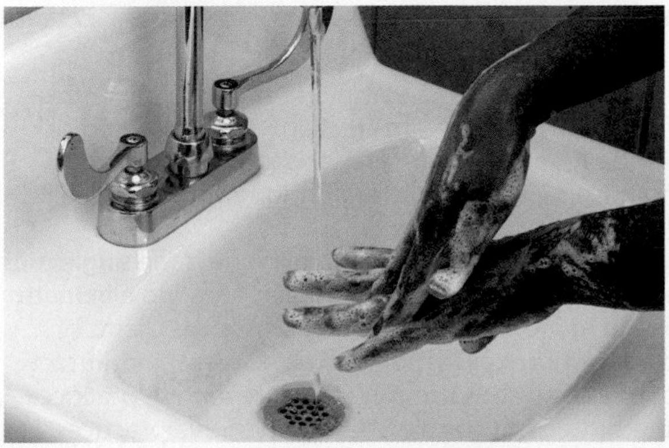

FIGURE 29-1-1 Lather thoroughly and rub hands together.

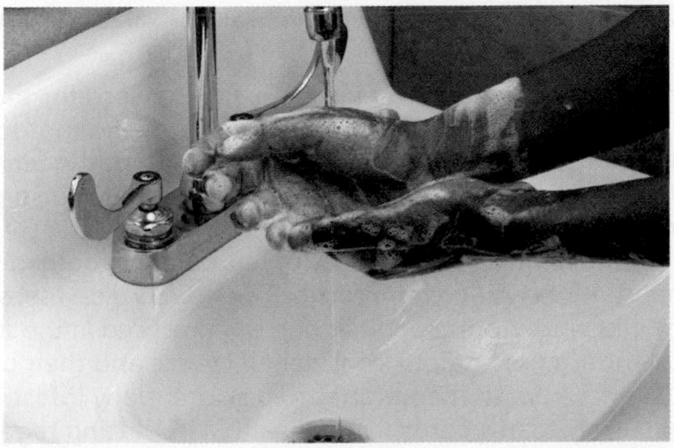

FIGURE 29-1-2 Give special attention to fingernails and knuckles.

(Continues)

PROCEDURE 29-1 Hand Hygiene (Continued)

ACTION	RATIONALE

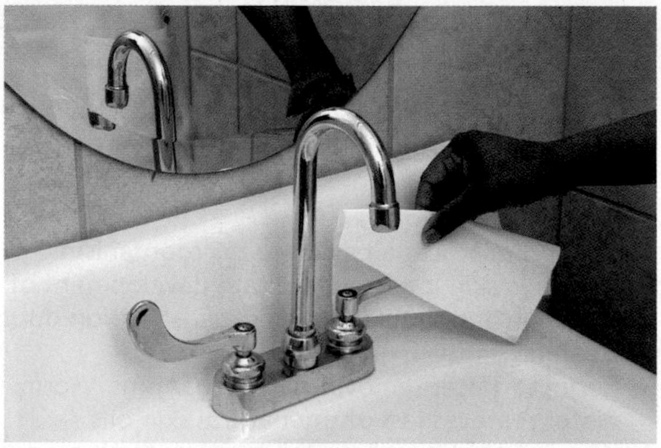

FIGURE 29-1-3 Turn off faucet with a clean, dry paper towel.

Alcohol-Based Hand Rub

ACTION	RATIONALE
10. Apply the manufacturer's recommended amount of product to one hand.	10. Amount of rub required varies by product.
11. Rub hands together, covering hands and fingers on all sides.	11. Spreads rub to cover all aspects of hands and fingers.
12. Continue rubbing until hands are dry.	12. Allows the alcohol-based hand rub to remove or destroy transient microorganisms and reduce resident flora.

EVALUATION

- The hand hygiene was adequate to control topical flora and infectious agents on the hands.
- The hands were not recontaminated during or shortly after the hand hygiene.

DOCUMENTATION

No documentation is needed for routine hand hygiene by the nurse.

PROCEDURE 29-2 Use of Protective Equipment

OVERVIEW

Infection control is an essential area of concern for the nurse in any setting. Effective implementation prevents or reduces the incidence of health care associated (nosocomial) infections. The hospitalized client is at increased risk for infection because of added exposure to pathogens, compromised immunologic state, and potential invasive procedures. Development of infection can delay healing, prolong hospital stay, or cause permanent disability or even loss of life.

Medical asepsis is the process of reducing microorganisms and preventing their spread. Hand hygiene is the single most important technique for infection control. Surgical asepsis takes this further with procedures implemented to eliminate any microorganisms. Medical asepsis is practiced in the surgical arena to reduce the risk of infection for the client.

Standard Precautions consider all clients and their bodily fluids, secretions, excretions (except sweat), nonintact skin, and mucous membranes to be potentially infectious. Standard Precautions are infection preventive practices that apply to all clients in any health care setting regardless of their infection status. These preventive practices include hand hygiene; wearing gloves, gown, masks, and eye protection or face shield; and injection safety.

(Continues)

PROCEDURE 29-2 Use of Protective Equipment (Continued)

Appropriate protective items are worn according to the interaction with the client (Siegel, Rhinehart, Jackson, & Chiarello, 2007):

- Gloves are required when hand contact with any body fluids is anticipated. This includes touching mucous membranes and nonintact skin. Latex-free and powder-free gloves are recommended. Hands are washed after the gloves are removed.
- Impervious gowns must be worn by health care workers to prevent soiling of clothing by splashes of blood or body fluids, and masks, along with eye protection, are mandated if splashes toward the face are anticipated.
- Masks are worn when caring for clients on airborne and/or droplet precautions and immunocompromised clients.
- Hair is covered by a cap when in the semirestricted and restricted areas of the surgical suite and in areas of the hospital where special procedures are done (i.e., bone marrow transplant).
- Eye protection (goggles) or face shields are worn during care activities that may be associated with splashes or sprays of blood or body fluids.
- Soiled protective items are removed promptly after use and disposed of as appropriate.

ASSESSMENT

1. Assess if Standard Precautions are followed or if specific isolation precautions are needed for the client's condition. **The type of microorganism and mode of transmission determine the degree of precautions.**
2. Assess the client's laboratory results **to learn which organism the client is infected with and the client's immune responses.**
3. Assess what nursing measures are required before entering the room **to have all the necessary equipment ready.**
4. Assess the client's knowledge for the need to wear a cap, gown, and mask during care **to direct client teaching.**
5. Assess whether the isolation is airborne, droplet, or contact and which isolation attire is necessary.

POSSIBLE NURSING DIAGNOSIS

Ineffective Protection
Social Isolation
Situational Low Self-Esteem

PLANNING

Expected Outcomes

1. The client and staff will remain free of health care associated infection.
2. The health care provider will be protected from infection when caring for the client.
3. The staff will avoid transmitting microorganisms to others.
4. The client will interact on a social level with nurse, family members, and other visitors.

Equipment Needed

- Gloves, clean—sterile if necessary
- Gown, sterile or clean
- Cap
- Mask
- Goggles
- Face mask

delegation tips

Donning and removing gloves, caps, and masks is a skill that is required of all personnel, including ancillary personnel. Proper technique should be monitored by the nursing staff.

IMPLEMENTATION—ACTION/RATIONALE

* Check client's identification band * Explain procedure before beginning *

ACTION	RATIONALE
1. Wash hands.	1. Reduces the transmission of microorganisms.
2. First put on the cap or surgical hat/hood. Hair should be tucked in a manner so that all hair is covered (Figure 29-2-1).	2. Because hair acts as a filter when left uncovered, it collects bacteria in proportion to its length, curliness, and oiliness. Loose hair may fall in the surgical area. Shedding hair may lead to surgical wound infection.

(Continues)

PROCEDURE 29-2 Use of Protective Equipment (Continued)

ACTION | **RATIONALE**

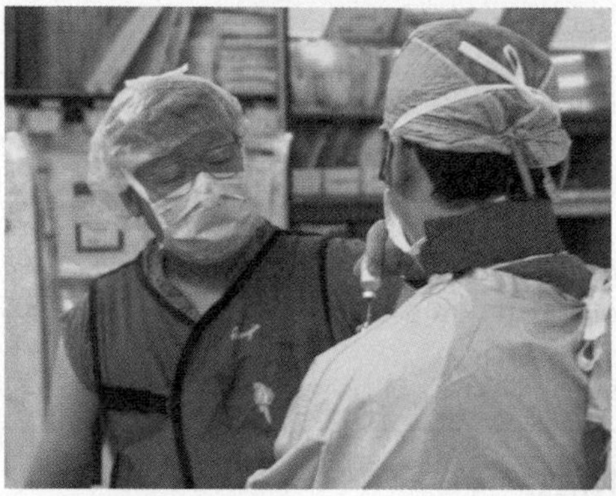

FIGURE 29-2-1 Caps and surgical caps cover the head, and hair is tucked in.

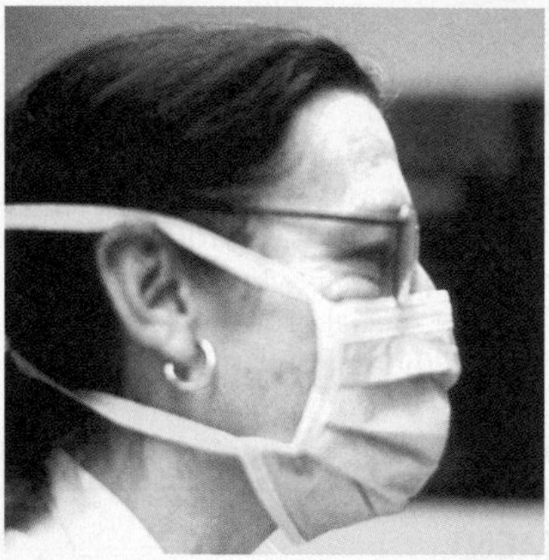

FIGURE 29-2-2 Bottom of the mask fits snugly under the chin.

3. Apply a mask around mouth and nose and secure in a manner that prevents venting. For masks with strings:
   a. Hold mask by top and pinch center (metal strip) over bridge of nose.
   b. Pull top two strings over ears and secure at top, back of head.
   c. Tie two lower ties around back or nape of neck so bottom of mask fits snugly under chin (Figure 29-2-2).

3. Masks are worn to contain and filter droplets of microorganisms that are expelled when talking, sneezing, or coughing. Masks prevent the transmission of oral and nasopharyngeal organisms between the nurse and client.

4. Open gown, slip arms into sleeves, and secure at neck and waist (Figure 29-2-3 A and B).

4. Gowns act as a protective barrier and should be worn to reduce exposure to blood, body fluid, or other potentially infectious liquids

5. Protective eyewear is worn whenever health care provider or client are at risk for splash and contamination. These are applied as goggles/glasses or face shields that have elastic ties for around the ears.

5. Protective eyewear reduces the incidence of contamination to the eyes. If eyewear or face shields become contaminated, they should be discarded immediately and replaced with a clean barrier.

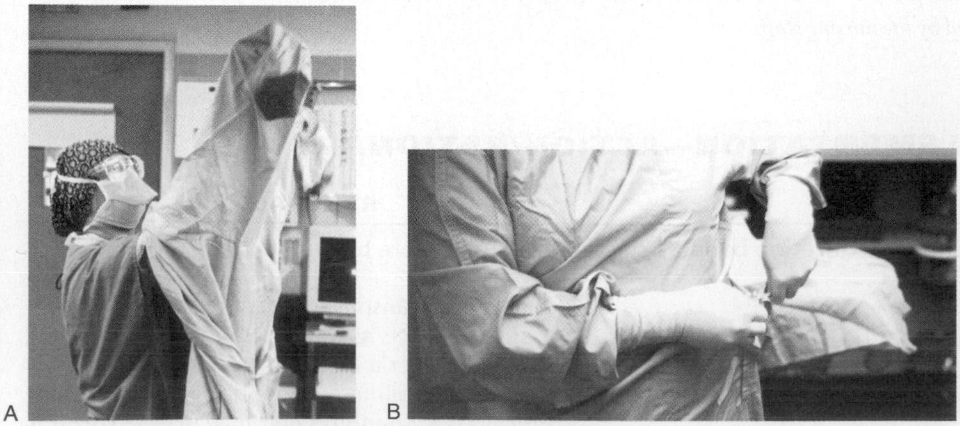

FIGURE 29-2-3 ***A,*** **The gown is put on before the gloves.** ***B,*** **Tie the gown at the neck and waist.**

(Continues)

PROCEDURE 29-2 Use of Protective Equipment (Continued)

ACTION	RATIONALE
6. Don clean gloves. If sterile gloves are required for a procedure, use open or closed method.	6. Gloves are worn to prevent gross contamination of the hands. They should be changed between clients and hands washed. The open method is used when performing procedures that require sterile technique but do not require donning a sterile gown or when both gloves need to be changed without assistance during a surgical procedure (Procedure 30-2). The closed method is used by scrubbed personnel in the operating room.
7. The open glove technique: a. Slide the hands into the gown all the way through the cuffs on the gown. b. Pick up the cuff of the left glove using the thumb and index finger of the right hand. c. Pull the glove onto the left hand, leaving the cuff of the glove turned down. d. Take the gloved left hand and slide the fingers under the cuff of the right glove, keeping the gloved fingers under the folded cuff. e. Pull the glove onto the right hand. f. Rotate the arm as the cuff of the glove is pulled over the gown.	7. The open glove method is commonly used for sterile procedures or when both gloves need to be changed without assistance during a surgical procedure.
8. The closed glove technique: a. Slide the hands into the gown all the way through the cuffs on the gown. b. Use right hand to pick up left glove. c. Place the glove on the upward-turned left hand—palm side down thumb to thumb with the fingers extending along the forearm pointing toward the elbow. d. Hold the glove cuff and sleeve cuff together with the thumb of the left hand. e. The right hand stretches the cuff of the left glove over the opened end of the sleeve. f. Work the fingers into the glove as the cuff is pulled onto the wrist. g. The right glove is done in the same manner.	8. The closed glove technique is used by the scrubbed personnel in the operating room. This is preferred because the possibility of the glove touching the skin is eliminated.
9. Enter the client's room and explain the rationale for wearing the attire.	9. Minimizes anxiety and feelings of isolation.
10. After performing necessary tasks, remove gown, gloves, mask, and cap before leaving the room.	10. Reduces transmission of organisms.
11. Removal of gown: Untie gown and remove from shoulders. Fold and roll gown down in front into a ball, so contaminated area is rolled onto center of gown. Dispose in approved receptacle.	11. Reduces transmission of organisms.
12. Removal of gloves:	12.
a. Grasp outside cuff of one glove and pull off, turning inside out. Hold it with the remaining gloved hand (Figures 29-2-4 and 29-2-5).	a. Reduces risk of contamination.
b. Pull the second glove off without touching the outside of the second glove (Figure 29-2-6). Turn the second glove over the first glove as it is removed (Figure 29-2-7). Dispose into receptacle with first glove (Figure 29-2-8).	b. Reduces risk of contamination.
13. Removal of mask: Untie bottom strings of mask first, then top strings, and lift off face. Hold mask by strings and discard.	13. Prevents contaminated surface of mask from contacting uniform.

(Continues)

PROCEDURE 29-2 Use of Protective Equipment (Continued)

ACTION	RATIONALE

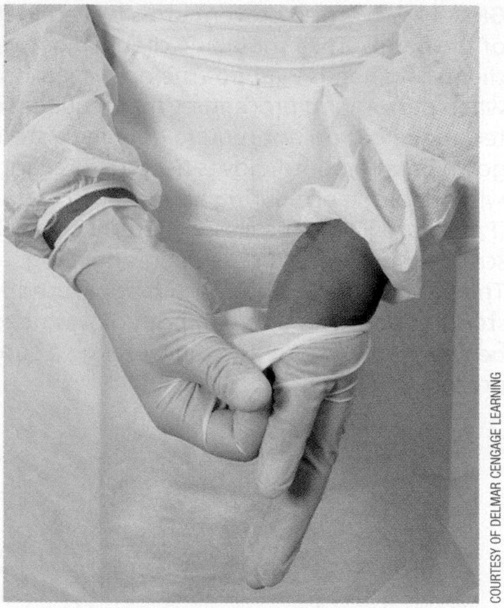

FIGURE 29-2-4 Grasp the outside cuff to remove the gown.

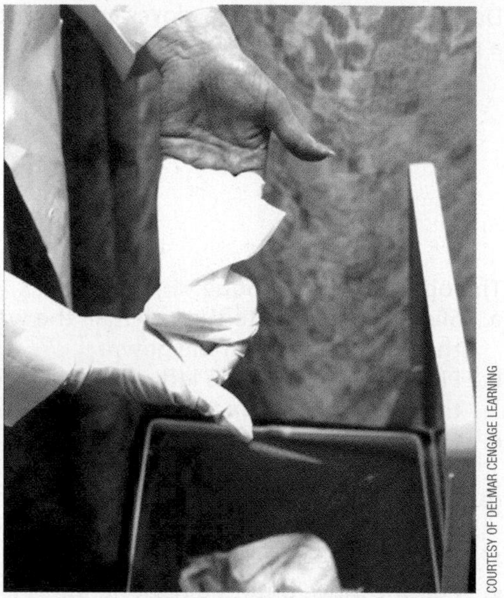

FIGURE 29-2-5 As the glove is removed, turn the glove inside out.

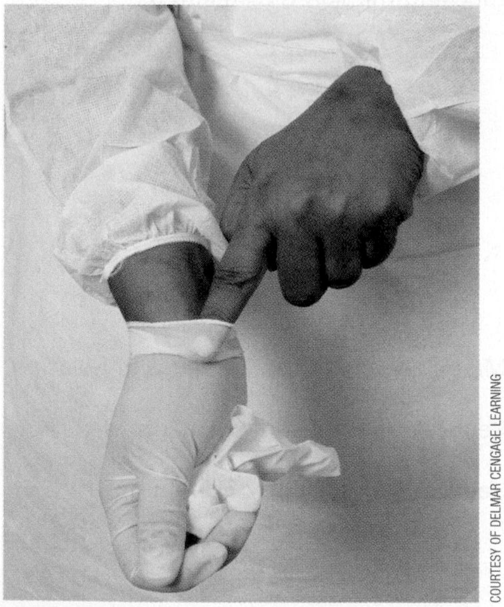

FIGURE 29-2-6 As the first glove is removed, place it inside the palm of the second glove. To remove the second glove, place a finger inside the glove and slide the glove down the hand.

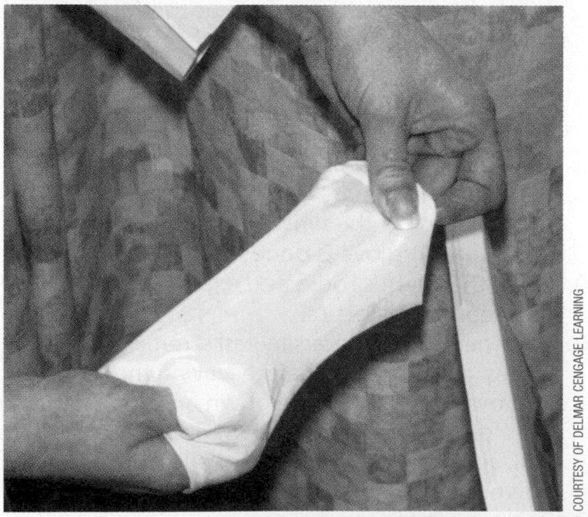

FIGURE 29-2-7 The second glove covers the first glove so that only the clean side of the glove is exposed.

ACTION	RATIONALE
14. Removal of cap: Grasp top surface of cap and lift from head.	14. Minimizes contact of hands to hair.
15. Wash hands.	15 Reduces transmission of microorganisms.

(Continues)

PROCEDURE 29-2 Use of Protective Equipment (Continued)

ACTION	RATIONALE

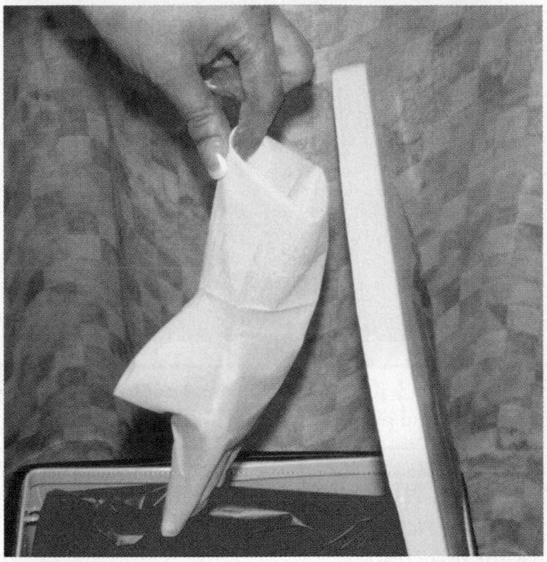

FIGURE 29-2-8 Place the contaminated gloves in the trash.

EVALUATION

- The client remains free of any health care associated infection.
- The health care provider and staff are protected from infection and microorganisms are contained without cross contamination.
- The client interacts on a social level with nurse, family members, and other visitors.

DOCUMENTATION

Nurses' Notes

- Type of protective barriers used and any breaks in isolation technique
- Client's compliance with and verbalization of understanding and adjustment to isolation
- Family members' compliance of isolation procedures

PROCEDURE 29-3 Taking a Temperature

OVERVIEW

Vital signs are generally taken with automatic measurement devices or a Dinamap with the results displayed on an electronic panel (Figure 29-3-1). The same basic procedural steps are used when obtaining the vital signs manually, such as with a BP cuff and stethoscope or thermometer. With the Dinamap, the temperature (T), pulse (P), blood pressure (BP), and pulse oximetry are automatically taken by applying a BP cuff and pulse oximetry sensor and correctly placing a thermometer probe. The electronic device promptly provides vital information to the nurse. Automated measurement devices simplify taking vital signs, but the nurse learns to manually take vital signs correctly and accurately in case of a malfunction of the electronic device or if one is not available. Therefore, the manual methods of obtaining vital signs are explained in Procedures 29-3 to 29-7. Specific vital signs are defined in the separate procedures. Refer to Chapter 26, Assessment"; Chapter 35, "Respiratory System"; and Chapter 36, "Cardiovascular System" for more detailed information on vital sign assessment.

Monitoring body temperature is a basic skill necessary in nursing and medical decision making. When heat production exceeds heat loss and body temperature rises above the normal range, pyrexia (fever) occurs. Pyrexia can accompany any inflammatory response, loss of body fluid, or prolonged exposure to high temperatures. When

(Continues)

PROCEDURE 29-3 Taking a Temperature (Continued)

the body is exposed to temperatures lower than normal for a prolonged length of time, hypothermia occurs. Hospitalized clients are at particular risk for infection and accompanying fever. Clients are stressed by their presenting conditions, and their bodies are further stressed by the hospital environment; thus, they are more susceptible to the infectious agents found there. Hypothermia generally occurs in response to prolonged exposure to cold weather or as a result of being immersed in cold water. Accurate monitoring and recording of a client's temperature is essential for diagnosis, treatment, and monitoring of the client.

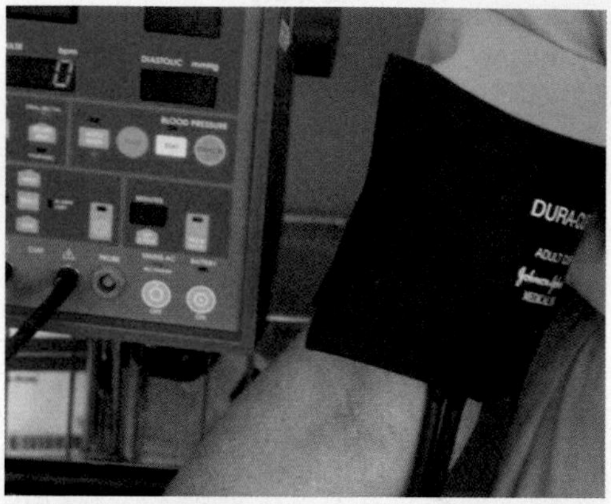

COURTESY OF DELMAR CENGAGE LEARNING

FIGURE 29-3-1 Health care personnel automatically take the T, P, BP, and pulse oximetry with the Dinamap.

ASSESSMENT

1. Assess body temperature for changes when exposed to pyrogens (endogenous or exogenous substances that cause fever) or to extreme hot or cold external environments **because such environments may indicate the cause of an infection.**
2. Assess the client for the most appropriate site to check temperature **to obtain an accurate reading.**
3. Confirm that the client has not consumed hot or cold food or beverage nor smoked for 15 to 30 minutes before the measurement **because these activities may alter the oral reading.**
4. Assess for mouth breathing and tachypnea **because both can cause an inaccurate oral reading.**
5. Assess for oral lesion, especially herpetic lesions, **because herpes viruses are extremely contagious and require implementation of Standard Precautions of the Centers for Disease Control and Prevention. Clients with herpetic lesions should have their own glass thermometer or disposable thermometer to prevent transmission to others.**

POSSIBLE NURSING DIAGNOSES

Ineffective Health Maintenance
Risk for Infection
Hypothermia
Hyperthermia
Ineffective Thermoregulation
Deficient Fluid Volume
Risk for Imbalanced Body Temperature

PLANNING

Expected Outcomes

1. An accurate temperature reading will be obtained.
2. The client will verbalize understanding of the reason for the procedure.

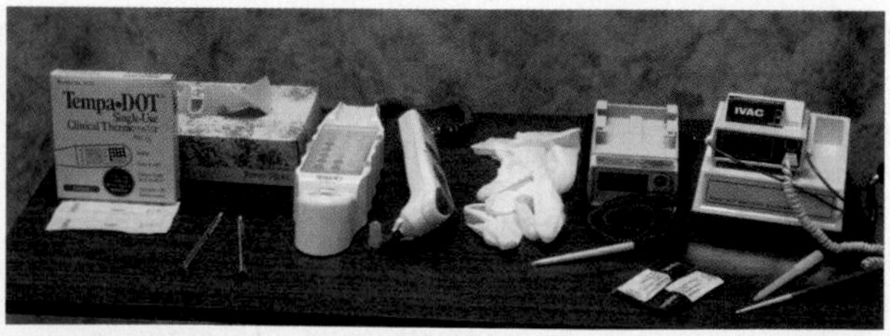

COURTESY OF DELMAR CENGAGE LEARNING

FIGURE 29-3-2 Various types of thermometers are used to take a client's temperature.

Equipment Needed (Figure 29-3-2)

- Vital signs automatic measurement device (Dinamap) or manual thermometer (one of the following)
  - — Electronic thermometer with disposable protective sheath
  - — Tympanic membrane thermometer with probe cover
  - — Disposable, single-use chemical strip thermometer
  - — Glass (mercury free): oral or rectal at client's bedside, usually color coded to avoid cross use
- Lubricant for rectal and glass thermometer
- Two pairs of nonsterile gloves
- Tissues

(Continues)

PROCEDURE 29-3 Taking a Temperature (Continued)

delegation tips

The skill of temperature measurement is often delegated to ancillary personnel; however, the nurse retains responsibility for knowledge of the client's temperature and appropriate actions. The expectation is that ancillary personnel will have documented instruction and competency validation of their ability to:

- *Select the correct route for measurement of the temperature.*
- *Correctly position the client for measurement.*
- *Correctly perform the measurement according to established guidelines and record on the appropriate flow sheet (clinical record).*
- *Recognize and report abnormal findings to the nurse.*

IMPLEMENTATION—ACTION/RATIONALE

ACTION	RATIONALE
* Check client's identification band * Explain procedure before beginning *	
1. Review medical record for baseline data and factors that influence vital signs.	1. Establishes baseline, provides direction in device selection, and helps determine site to use for measurement. Vital signs are measured in the order of temperature, pulse, and respiration (TPR); blood pressure (BP); and pulse oximetry, usually without interruptions, to provide the nurse with an objective clinical database to direct decision making.
2. Explain to the client that vital signs will be assessed. Encourage the client to remain still and refrain from drinking, eating, and smoking, and to avoid mouth breathing, if possible. Do not take vital signs within 30 minutes of the client drinking, eating, or smoking, as these activities give false readings.	2. Encourages participation, allays anxiety, and ensures accurate measurements. Cold or hot liquids and smoking alter circulation and body temperature. Mouth breathing can alter temperature.
3. Assess client's toileting needs and proceed as appropriate.	3. Prevents interruptions during measurements, communicates caring, and promotes client comfort.
4. Gather equipment.	4. Facilitates organization and establishes client trust when the health care worker is prepared and does not have to leave the room for supplies multiple times.
5. Provide for privacy.	5. Decreases embarrassment.
6. Wash hands and apply gloves when appropriate.	6. Hands are washed before and after every contact with a client to reduce the transmission of microorganisms. Gloves are worn to avoid contact with bodily secretions and to reduce transmission of microorganisms.
Oral Temperature—Electronic Thermometer	
7. Repeat Actions 1 to 6.	7. See Rationales 1 to 6.
8. Place disposable protective sheath over probe.	8. Reduces transmission of microorganisms.
9. Grasp top of the probe's stem. Avoid placing pressure on the ejection button (Figure 29-3-3).	9. Pressure on the ejection button releases the sheath from the probe.
10. Place tip of thermometer under the client's tongue and along the gumline to the posterior sublingual pocket lateral to center of lower jaw (Figure 29-3-4).	10. Sublingual pocket contains superficial blood vessels.
11. Instruct client to keep mouth closed around thermometer.	11. Maintains thermometer in proper place and decreases amount of time required for an accurate reading.
12. Thermometer will signal (beep) when a constant temperature registers (Figure 29-3-5).	12. Signal indicates final temperature reading.

(Continues)

PROCEDURE 29-3 Taking a Temperature (Continued)

ACTION | **RATIONALE**

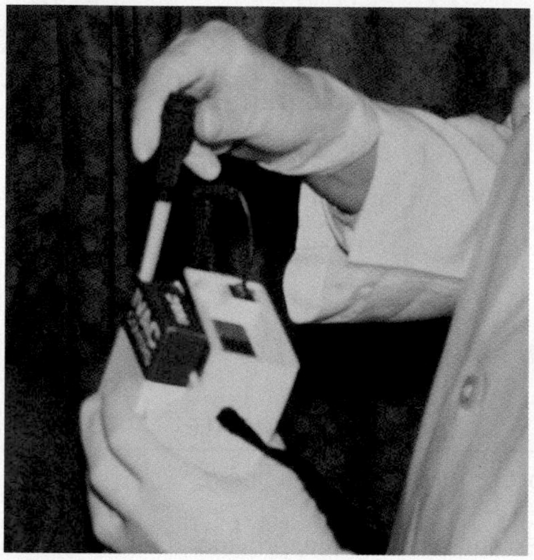

COURTESY OF DELMAR CENGAGE LEARNING

FIGURE 29-3-3 Place disposable protective sheath over probe.

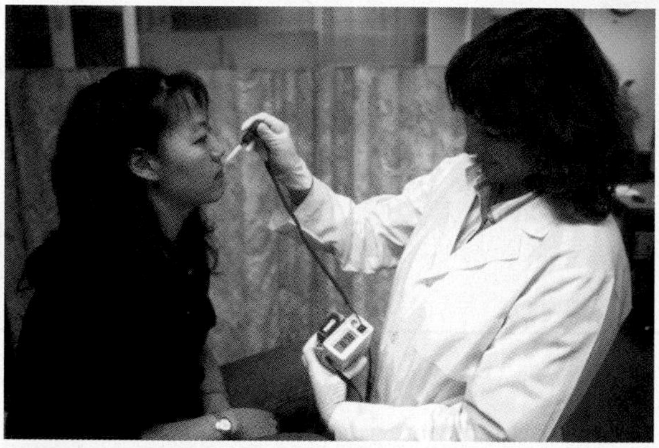

COURTESY OF DELMAR CENGAGE LEARNING

FIGURE 29-3-4 Place probe tip in the posterior sublingual pocket.

13. Read measurement on digital display of electronic thermometer. Push ejection button to discard disposable sheath into receptacle and return probe to storage well.
    - Rationale: Reduces transmission of microorganisms. Ensures that the electronic system is ready for next use.
14. Inform client of temperature reading.
    - Rationale: Promotes client's participation in care.
15. Remove gloves and wash hands.
    - Rationale: Reduces transmission of microorganisms.
16. Record reading according to institution policies.
    - Rationale: Accurate documentation by site allows for comparison of data.
17. Return electronic thermometer unit to charging base, checking that it is plugged in.
    - Rationale: Ensures charging base is plugged into electrical outlet and thermometer is ready for next use.
18. Wash hands.
    - Rationale: Reduces transmission of microorganisms.

Tympanic Temperature: Infrared Thermometer

19. Repeat Actions 1 to 6.
    - Rationale: See Rationales 1 to 6.
20. Position client in Sims' or sitting position.
    - Rationale: Promotes access to ear.
21. Remove probe from container and attach probe cover to tympanic thermometer unit (Figure 29-3-6).
    - Rationale: Prevents contamination.

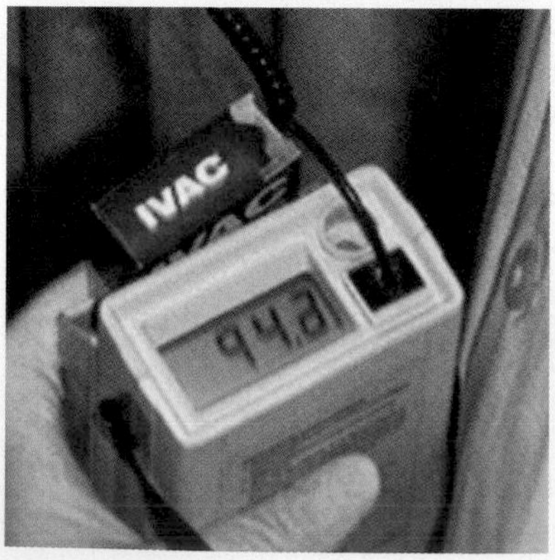

COURTESY OF DELMAR CENGAGE LEARNING

FIGURE 29-3-5 Listen for audible beep signal when temperature registers.

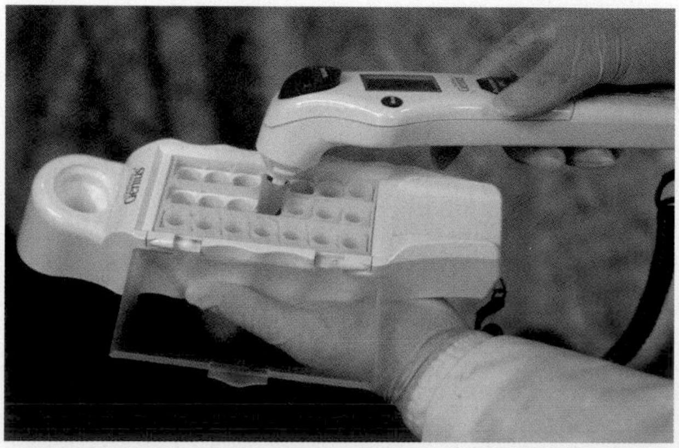

COURTESY OF DELMAR CENGAGE LEARNING

FIGURE 29-3-6 Attach disposable probe cover to unit.

(Continues)

PROCEDURE 29-3 Taking a Temperature (Continued)

ACTION	RATIONALE
22. Turn client's head to one side. For an adult, pull pinna upward and back; for a child, pull down and back. Gently insert probe with firm pressure into ear canal (Figure 29-3-7).	22. Provides access to ear canal. Gentle insertion prevents trauma to external canal. Firm pressure is needed to ensure probe will record an accurate temperature.
23. Remove probe after the reading is displayed on digital unit (usually 2 seconds).	23. Reading is displayed within seconds.
24. Discard probe cover into receptacle and replace probe in storage container.	24. Reduces transmission of microorganisms. Protects reusable probe from damage.
25. Return tympanic thermometer to storage unit.	25. Recharges batteries of unit for future use.
26. Record reading according to institution policy.	26. Promotes accurate documentation for data comparison.
27. Wash hands.	27. Reduces transmission of microorganisms.
Using a "Tempa-Dot"	
28. Repeat Actions 1 to 6.	28. See Rationales 1 to 6.
29. Position the client in a sitting or lying position.	29. Promotes client's comfort, and promotes site access for temperature measurement.
30. Prepare Tempa-Dot according to directions (Figure 29-3-8). • Oral measurement: Place Tempa-Dot under tongue as far back as possible. Have client press tongue down on thermometer and keep mouth closed for 60 seconds. Remove thermometer; read the last blue dot; ignore any skipped dot. • Axillary measurement: Place thermometer high in the armpit, vertical to the body, with dots against the torso. Lower client's arm to hold thermometer in place. Remove thermometer after 3 minutes.	30. Promotes accurate measurement and client safety.
31. Record temperature, indicate the method, and discard the thermometer.	31. Nursing documentation, practice clean technique.
32. Wash hands.	32. Reduces transmission of microorganisms.

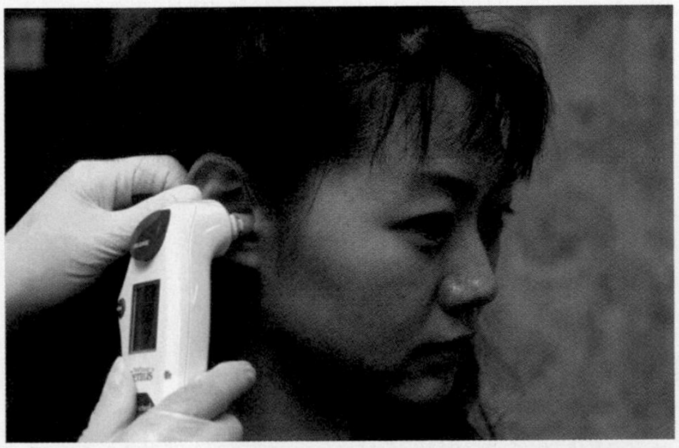
COURTESY OF DELMAR CENGAGE LEARNING

FIGURE 29-3-7 Insert temperature probe into ear canal.

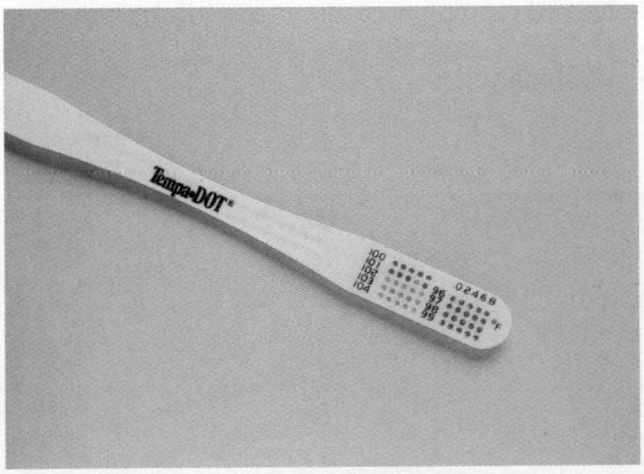

COURTESY OF DELMAR CENGAGE LEARNING

FIGURE 29-3-8 "Tempa-Dot" Single-Use Disposable Thermometer

(Continues)

PROCEDURE 29-3 Taking a Temperature (Continued)

ACTION	RATIONALE
Oral Temperature: Plastic Thermometer	
A glass thermometer is not generally used. Mercury glass thermometers are no longer recommended for use (National Institutes of Health, 2008).	
33. Repeat Actions 1 to 6.	33. See Rationales 1 to 6.
34. Select correct color tip of thermometer from client's bedside container (Figure 29-3-9).	34. Identifies correct device; a blue tip usually denotes an oral thermometer.
35. Remove thermometer from storage container, hold at end away from bulb and rinse under cool water.	35. Cleansing removes disinfectant, which can irritate oral mucosa. Cool water prevents expansion of the colored solution. Touching the bulb will heat the solution and cause an inaccurate reading.
36. Use a tissue to dry thermometer from bulb's end toward fingertips.	36. Wipe from area of least contamination to most contaminated area.
37. Read thermometer by locating colored solution level. It should read 35.5°C (96°F).	37. Thermometer must be below normal body temperature to ensure an accurate reading.
38. If thermometer is not below normal body temperature reading, grasp thermometer with thumb and forefinger and shake vigorously by snapping the wrist in a downward motion to move colored solution to a level below normal.	38. Shaking briskly lowers level of colored solution in column. Because glass thermometers break easily, make sure that nothing in the environment comes in contact with the thermometer when shaking it.
39. Place thermometer in client's mouth under the tongue and along the gumline to the posterior sublingual pocket. Instruct client to hold lips closed (Figure 29-3-10).	39. Ensures contact with large blood vessels under the tongue. Prevents environmental air from coming in contact with the bulb.
40. Leave in place as specified by institution policy, usually 3 to 5 minutes.	40. Thermometer must stay in place long enough to ensure an accurate reading.
41. Remove thermometer and wipe with a tissue away from fingers toward the bulb's end (Figure 29-3-11).	41. Mucus on thermometer may interfere with the effectiveness of the disinfectant solution. Wipe from area of least contamination to most contaminated area.
42. Read at eye level and rotate slowly until colored solution level is visualized.	42. Ensures an accurate reading.
43. Shake thermometer down, cleanse glass thermometer with soapy water, rinse under cold water, and return to storage container.	43. Mechanical cleansing removes secretions that promote growth of microorganisms. Hot water may cause coagulation of secretions and cause expansion of colored solution in the thermometer.
44. Remove and dispose of gloves in receptacle. Wash hands.	44. Reduces transmission of microorganisms.
45. Record reading according to institution policy.	45. Accurate documentation by site allows for comparison of data.
46. Wash hands.	46. Reduces transmission of microorganisms.

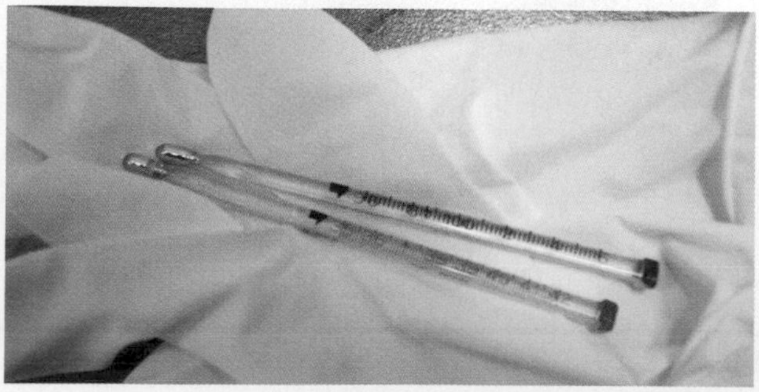
COURTESY OF DELMAR CENGAGE LEARNING

FIGURE 29-3-9 Oral (blue tip) and rectal (red tip) glass thermometer

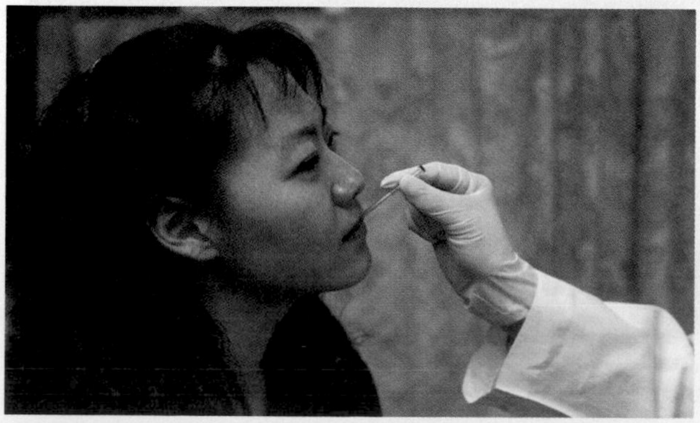
COURTESY OF DELMAR CENGAGE LEARNING

FIGURE 29-3-10 Place bulb of thermometer in the posterior sublingual pocket. Have client close lips around thermometer.

(Continues)

PROCEDURE 29-3 Taking a Temperature (Continued)

ACTION	RATIONALE
Rectal Temperature	
47. Repeat Actions 1 to 6.	47. See Rationales 1 to 6.
48. Place client in the Sims' position with upper knee flexed. Adjust sheet to expose only anal area.	48. Proper positioning ensures visualization of anus. Flexing knee relaxes muscles for ease of insertion.
49. Place tissues in easy reach. Apply gloves.	49. Tissue is needed to wipe anus after device is removed.
50. Prepare the thermometer.	50. Ensures a smooth procedure and an accurate reading.
51. Lubricate sheath or probe covering tip of rectal thermometer. (A rectal thermometer usually has a red tip or cap.)	51. Promotes ease of insertion of thermometer or probe.
52. With dominant hand, grasp thermometer. With other hand, separate buttocks to expose anus (Figure 29-3-12).	52. Aids in visualization of anus.
53. Instruct the client to take a deep breath. Insert the thermometer or probe gently into anus: infant, 1.2 cm (0.5 inches); adult, 3.5 cm (1.5 inches). If resistance is felt, do not force insertion.	53. Relaxes anal sphincter. Gentle insertion decreases discomfort to client and prevents trauma to mucous membranes.
54. Hold plastic thermometer in place for 3 to 5 minutes. If taking the rectal temperature with an electronic probe, remove it after the reading is displayed on digital unit (usually 2 seconds).	54. Prevents trauma to mucosa and breakage of glass thermometer.
55. Wipe off secretions on the glass thermometer with a tissue. Dispose of tissue in a receptacle.	55. Removes secretions and fecal material for visualization of mercury level. Prevents transmission of microorganisms.
56. Read measurement and inform the client of the temperature reading.	56. Promotes client's participation in care.
57. While holding glass thermometer in one hand, use other hand to wipe anal area with tissue to remove lubricant or feces. Dispose of soiled tissue. Cover client.	57. Prevents contamination of clean objects with soiled thermometer, decreases skin irritation, and promotes client comfort. Prevents embarrassment.
58. Wash thermometer.	58. Reduces transmission of microorganisms.
59. Remove and dispose of gloves in receptacle. Wash hands.	59. Reduces transmission of microorganisms.
60. Record reading according to institution policy.	60. Accurate documentation by site allows for comparison of data.

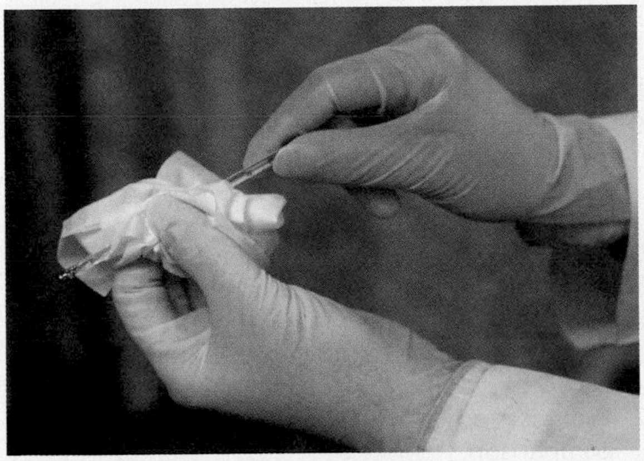

COURTESY OF DELMAR CENGAGE LEARNING

FIGURE 29-3-11 Wipe the thermometer with a tissue from fingertips to bulb end.

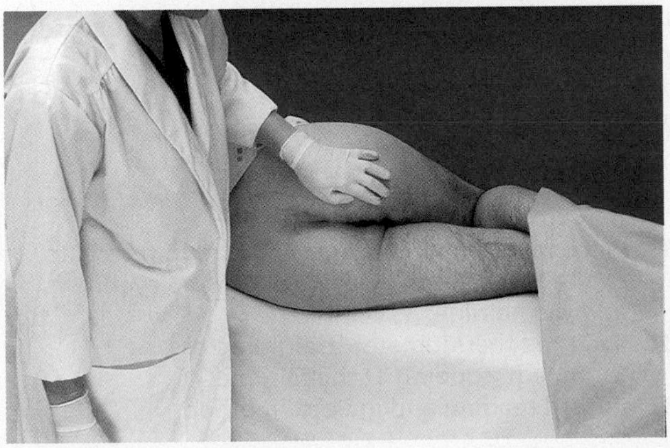

COURTESY OF DELMAR CENGAGE LEARNING

FIGURE 29-3-12 Preparation for the insertion of a rectal thermometer.

(Continues)

PROCEDURE 29-3 Taking a Temperature (Continued)

ACTION	RATIONALE
Axillary Temperature	
61. Repeat Actions 1 to 6.	61. See Rationales 1 to 6.
62. Remove client's arm and shoulder from one sleeve of gown. Avoid exposing chest.	62. Exposes axillary area.
63. Make sure axillary skin is dry; if necessary, pat dry.	63. Removes moisture and prevents a false low reading.
64. Prepare thermometer.	64. Ensures accurate use of thermometer.
65. Place thermometer or probe into center of axilla. Fold the client's upper arm straight down, and place arm across the client's chest. On a thin client, make sure flesh rather than a hollow armpit surrounds the thermometer or probe.	65. Puts device in contact with axillary blood supply. Maintains the device in proper position.
66. Leave glass thermometer in place as specified by institution policy (usually 6 to 8 minutes). Leave an electronic thermometer in place until signal is heard.	66. Device must stay in place long enough to ensure an accurate reading. Signal indicates final temperature reading.
67. Remove and read thermometer.	67. Allows accurate reading of temperature.
68. Inform client of temperature reading.	68. Promotes client's participation in care.
69. If using a thermometer, shake down the solution. Wash glass thermometer with soapy water, rinse under cold water, and return to storage container. If using an electronic thermometer, push ejection button to discard disposable sheath into receptacle and return probe to storage well.	69. Prevents breakage of glass thermometer and transmission of microorganisms. Removing the disposable sheath reduces transmission of microorganisms and ensures that the electronic system is ready for next use.
70. Assist the client with replacing the gown.	70. Promotes comfort.
71. Record reading according to institution policy.	71. Promotes accurate documentation for data comparison.
72. Wash hands.	72. Reduces transmission of microorganisms.
Disposable (Chemical Strip) Thermometer	
73. Repeat Actions 1 to 6.	73. See Rationales 1 to 6.
74. Apply tape to appropriate skin area, usually forehead.	74. Tape must be in direct contact with the client's skin.
75. Observe tape for color changes.	75. Color indicates temperature reading (refer to the manufacturer's instructions).
76. Record reading and indicate method.	76. Promotes accurate documentation for data comparison.
77. Wash hands.	77. Reduces transmission of microorganisms.
Noninvasive Temporal Artery Scan Thermometer (Temporal Scanner)	
78. Repeat Actions 1 to 6.	78. See Rationales 1 to 6.
79. Locate the client's exposed temporal artery.	79. The temporal artery has an accurate arterial temperature because the vessel has little vasomotor control and a reliable rate of perfusion (Exergen Corporation, 2009).
80. Place the thermometer sensor head in the center of the forehead halfway between the eyebrows and the hairline.	80. The scanner crosses the temporal artery by scanning across half of the forehead.
81. Slide the thermometer straight across the forehead, stopping at the hairline.	81. Maintain direct contact with the skin for an accurate reading.
82. Record reading and indicate method.	82. Promotes accurate documentation for data comparison.
83. Wash hands.	83. Reduces transmission of microorganisms.

(Continues)

PROCEDURE 29-3 Taking a Temperature (Continued)

ACTION	RATIONALE

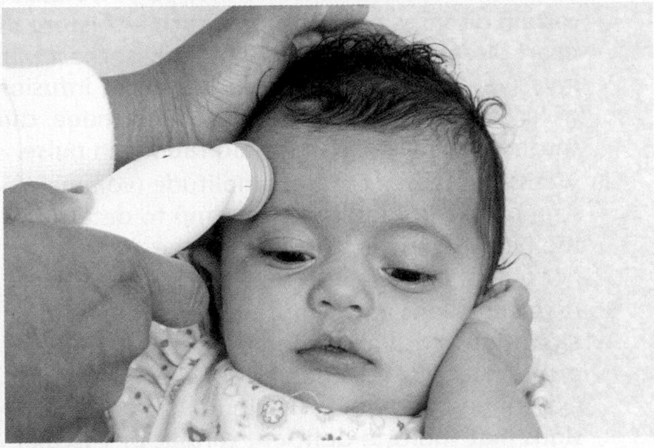

COURTESY OF DELMAR CENGAGE LEARNING

FIGURE 29-3-13 The child's temperature is taken with a temporal artery thermometer.

EVALUATION

- Establish client's baseline temperature.
- Compare temperature with the client's baseline temperature.
- Evaluate the client's condition for trauma caused by the instrument.

DOCUMENTATION

Vital Signs Flow Sheet or Electronic Medical Record

- Temperature measurement and site
- If using a paper flow sheet, plot the temperature on a graph to identify patterns, or sudden elevations and drops (a condition known as spiking). If the facility uses electronic medical records, enter the vital signs in the computer.

Medication Administration Record

- Antipyretic (fever-reducing) medications and temperature reading

Nurses' Notes

- Response to antipyretic medications

PROCEDURE 29-4 Taking a Pulse

OVERVIEW

A pulse is the number of heart beats in 1 minute. Pulse assessment is the measurement of a pressure pulsation created when the heart contracts and ejects blood into the aorta. Assessment of pulse characteristics provides clinical data regarding the heart's pumping action and the adequacy of peripheral artery blood flow. The radial pulse is most often used for basic assessment; however, other site areas are used in total assessment and when determining circulation to specific areas. Pulse rate is an indirect measurement of cardiac output obtained by counting the number of peripheral pulse waves over a pulse point. A normal pulse rate for adults is between 60 and 100 beats per minute. Pulse rhythm is the regularity of the heartbeat. It indicates how evenly the heart is beating. Pulse amplitude (also called pulse strength or volume) is a measurement of the strength or force exerted by the blood against the arterial wall with each heart contraction. It is described as normal (full, easily palpable), weak (thready and usually rapid), or strong (bounding).

PULSE-TAKING TECHNIQUES

Palpation

- Palpation of a pulse involves the index and middle fingers of one hand. Start with gentle pressure to locate the strongest pulsation and then use firmer palpation for the counting. When counting, also assess the rhythm and quality of the pulse. Measure the pulse for 30 and 60 seconds and then multiply the counts if need be to obtain the 1-minute reading.

(Continues)

PROCEDURE 29-4 Taking a Pulse (Continued)

Auscultation

- Auscultation is usually used to assess the apical pulse. The apical pulse is the most accurate pulse, especially when the peripheral pulse is difficult to locate. Auscultation requires the stethoscope. The stethoscope is equipped with a bell and a diaphragm. The diaphragm side is normally used for low-pitch sound, such as normal heart sound, bowel sound, or breath sound; the bell side is used for high-pitch sound, such as murmur and abnormal heart sound.

Doppler

- An ultrasonic Doppler device is used when the pulse cannot be detected by palpation. The Doppler detects the peripheral pulses in situations such as cardiopulmonary collapse in obese clients, infants with small arms, or clients with edema or peripheral vascular disease in which palpation of the pulse is difficult.
- A vendor-recommended conductive gel be applied to the skin as a coupling medium for ultrasound transmission. The transmitting device (probe) is then placed over the artery assessed. The Doppler usually is equipped with both high- and low-frequency probes. A high-frequency (8 to 10 Hz) probe is usually used on the surface vessel sites. A low-frequency (2 to 3 Hz) probe often is used for deeper sites, such as obstetric assessment.
- The sounds are amplified and heard through an earpiece or speaker attached to the device, assessing with low volume initially. Tilt the back of the probe toward the hand at an angle of about 45 degrees. Search the area of the assessed artery and tilt the probe for best Doppler sounds. Adjust the sound volume control to a comfort level for counting.

ASSESSMENT

1. Assess client for need to monitor pulse **because certain diseases or conditions, such as history of heart disease or cardiac dysrhythmias, chest pain, invasive cardiovascular diagnostic tests, infusion of large volume of IV fluids, or hemorrhage, can cause an increased risk for alterations in pulse.**
2. Assess the pulse for rate, amplitude (volume, strength), and regularity (rhythm) to determine the heart's pumping action and the adequacy of peripheral artery blood flow.
3. Assess for signs and symptoms of cardiovascular alterations, such as dyspnea, chest pain, orthopnea, syncope, palpitations, edema of extremities, cyanosis, or fatigue, **because these signs may indicate deficient cardiac or vascular function.**
4. Assess client for factors that may affect the character of the pulse, such as age, medications, exercise, change in position, or fever. **This enables the nurse to accurately assess for the significance of an alteration in pulse.**
5. Assess for the appropriate site for measuring pulse **so the pulse will be accurate.**
6. Assess the baseline heart rate and rhythm in the client's chart **to compare it with the current measurement.**
7. Assess circulatory status by using appropriate site (Table 29-4-1) **because pulses may be affected by surgery, medical condition, arterial blood draws, or poor circulation.**

POSSIBLE NURSING DIAGNOSES

Decreased Cardiac Output
Ineffective Peripheral Tissue Perfusion

TABLE 29-4-1 Pulse Point Assessment

PULSE POINT	LOCATION	ASSESSMENT CRITERIA
1. Temporal	Over the temporal bone, lateral to the eye, upper to the ear	Accessible; used routinely for infants and when radial is inaccessible
2. Carotid	Bilateral, under the lower jaw, beneath the sternomastoid muscles. Carotid pulse best represents the aortic pulse for its close location to the central circulation. Palpation of the carotid artery on the neck may cause stimulation of the carotid sinus and result in decrease of the pulse rate	Accessible; used routinely for infants and during shock or cardiac arrest when other peripheral pulses are too weak to palpate; also used to assess cranial circulation. Take a carotid pulse on only one side of the neck at a time (Figure 29-4-1)
3 Apical	Left ventricle, fourth to fifth intercostal space, on the midclavicular line	Used to auscultate heart sounds and assess apical-radial deficit

(Continues)

PROCEDURE 29-4 Taking a Pulse (Continued)

TABLE 29-4-1 Pulse Point Assessment (Continued)

PULSE POINT	LOCATION	ASSESSMENT CRITERIA
4. Brachial	Inner side between the groove of bicep and tricep muscles at the antecubital fossa	Used in cardiac arrest for infants, to assess lower arm circulation, and to auscultate blood pressure
5. Radial	On the thumb side, inner aspect of the wrist	Accessible; used routinely in adults to assess character of peripheral pulse
6. Ulnar	On the little finger side, outer aspect of the wrist	Used to assess circulation to ulnar side of hand and to perform the Allen test
7. Femoral	Below the inguinal ligament, in the anterior medial aspect of the thigh, midway to the anterior-superior iliac spine and symphysis pubis	Used to assess circulation to legs and during cardiac arrest
8. Popliteal	Behind the knee. Medial or lateral to the popliteal fossa	Used to assess circulation to legs and to auscultate leg blood pressure
9. Posterior Tibial	Inner side of the ankle, between the Achilles tendon and tibia	Used to assess circulation to feet
10. Pedal/Dorsal Pedal	Lateral to the extension tendon, from the great toe toward the ankle or between the first and second metatarsal bones on the dorsum (upper) part of the foot (General Practice Notebook, 2009)	Used to assess circulation to feet

PLANNING

Expected Outcomes

1. Pulse rate, quality, rhythm, and volume will be within normal range for the client's age group.
2. The client will be comfortable with the procedure and demonstrate an understanding regarding its importance.

Equipment Needed

- Vital signs automatic measurement device (Dinamap) or watch with a second hand or digital display
- Stethoscope
- Alcohol swab
- Gloves

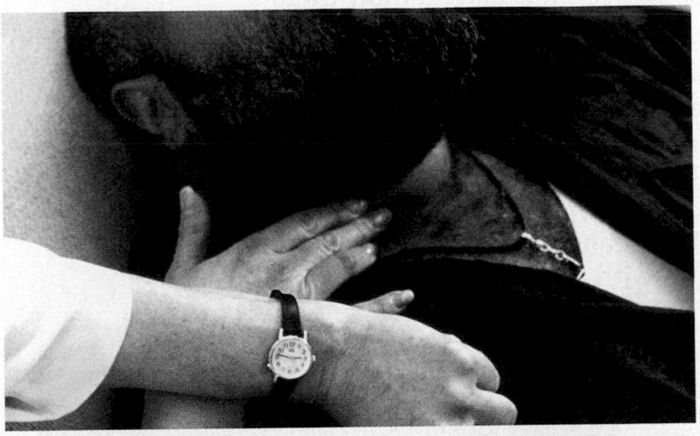

FIGURE 29-4-1 Take a carotid pulse on only one side of the neck at a time.

delegation tips

The radial pulse assessment is often delegated to trained ancillary personnel; however, the nurse is responsible for knowing the results. Assessment of the apical pulse may be delegated to specially prepared staff. The assessment of peripheral circulation is delegated after proper training in the monitoring of peripheral sites for the presence of abnormal color, motion, or sensation in the extremity. The absence of pulses is immediately reported for further assessment by the nurse, and the nurse is responsible for reviewing the data collected in a timely manner and revalidating the results, if indicated. The institution's policy should clearly indicate the training and validation requirements before the nurse delegates the monitoring of apical pulses and peripheral vascular assessments on stable clients. These tasks should not be delegated if the client is unstable.

(Continues)

PROCEDURE 29-4 Taking a Pulse (Continued)

IMPLEMENTATION—ACTION/RATIONALE

ACTION	RATIONALE
* Check client's identification band * Explain procedure before beginning *	
Taking a Radial (Wrist) Pulse	
1. Wash hands.	1. Reduces transmission of microorganisms.
2. Inform client of the site(s) at which you will measure pulse.	2. Encourages participation and allays anxiety.
3. Flex client's elbow and place lower part of arm across chest.	3. Maintains wrist in full extension and exposes artery for palpation. Placing client's hand over chest will facilitate later respiratory assessment without undue attention to your action. (It is difficult for any person to maintain a normal breathing pattern when someone is observing and measuring.)
4. Support client's wrist by grasping outer aspect with thumb.	4. Stabilizes wrist and allows for pressure to be exerted.
5. Place your index and middle fingers on inner aspect of client's wrist over the radial artery and apply light but firm pressure until pulse is palpated (Figure 29-4-2).	5. Fingertips are sensitive, facilitating palpation of pulsating pulse. The nurse may feel his or her own pulse if palpating with thumb. Applying light pressure prevents occlusion of blood flow and pulsation.
6. Identify pulse rhythm or regularity.	6. Palpate pulse until rhythm is determined. Describe as regular or irregular.
7. Determine pulse volume or amplitude.	7. Quality of pulse strength is an indication of stroke volume. Describe as normal, weak, strong, or bounding.
8. Count pulse rate by using second hand on watch. For a regular rhythm, count number of beats for 30 seconds and multiply by 2. For an irregular rhythm, count number of beats for a full minute, noting number of irregular beats.	8. An irregular rhythm requires a full minute of assessment to identify the number of inefficient cardiac contractions that fail to transmit a pulsation, referred to as a "skipped" or irregular beat.
Taking an Apical Pulse	
9. Wash hands.	9. Reduces transmission of microorganisms.
10. Raise client's gown to expose sternum and left side of chest.	10. Allows access to client's chest for proper placement of stethoscope.
11. Cleanse earpiece and diaphragm of stethoscope with an alcohol swab.	11. Decreases transmission of microorganisms from one health care practitioner to another (earpiece) and from one client to another (diaphragm).

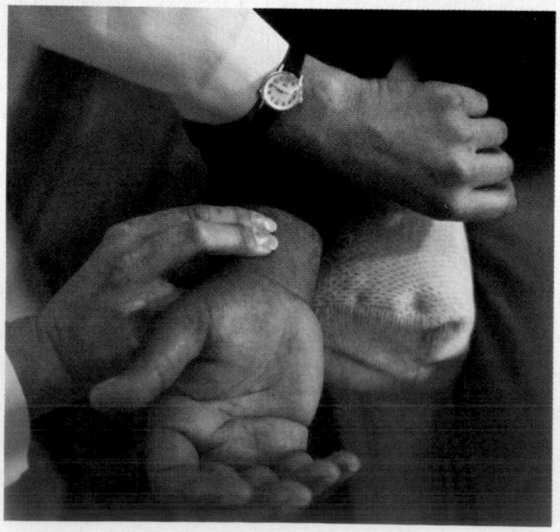

FIGURE 29-4-2 Place index and middle finger over radial artery and apply light but firm pressure until pulse is palpated.

(Continues)

PROCEDURE 29-4 Taking a Pulse (Continued)

ACTION | **RATIONALE**

TABLE 29-4-2 3-Point And 4-Point Scales for Measuring Pulse Volume

3-POINT SCALE		4-POINT SCALE	
SCALE	DESCRIPTION OF PULSE	SCALE	DESCRIPTION OF PULSE
0	Absent	0	Absent
1+	Thready/weak	1+	Thready/weak
2+	Normal	2+	Normal
3+	Bounding	3+	Increased
		4+	Bounding

12. Put stethoscope around your neck.
    - *Rationale:* 12. Ensures stethoscope is nearby for frequent use.
13. Locate apex of heart:
    - With client lying on left side, palpate and locate suprasternal notch.
    - Then, move to the left of the sternum and palpate for the second intercostal space. Palpate second intercostal space to left of sternum.
    - Place index finger in intercostal space, counting downward until fifth intercostal space is located.
    - Move index finger along fourth intercostal space left of the sternal border and to the fifth intercostal space, on the midclavicular line to palpate the apical impulse, called the point of maximal impulse (PMI) by some practitioners (Figure 29-4-3).
    - Keep index finger of nondominant hand on the apical impulse.
    - *Rationale:* 13. Identification of landmarks facilitates correct placement of the stethoscope at the fifth intercostal space in order to hear apical impulse.
      - Ensures correct placement of stethoscope.
14. Inform client that you are going to listen to his or her heart. Instruct client to remain silent.
    - *Rationale:* 14. Elicits client support. Stethoscope amplifies noise.
15. With dominant hand, put earpiece of the stethoscope in your ears and grasp diaphragm of the stethoscope in palm of your hand for 5 to 10 seconds.
    - *Rationale:* 15. Dominant hand facilitates psychomotor dexterity for placement of earpiece with one hand. Heat warms metal or plastic diaphragm and prevents startling client.
16. Place diaphragm of stethoscope over the apical impulse and auscultate for sounds S1 and S2 to hear lub-dub sound (Figure 29-4-4).
    - *Rationale:* 16. Movement of blood through the heart valves creates S1 and S2 sounds. Listen for a regular rhythm (heartbeats are evenly spaced) before counting.
17. Note regularity of rhythm.
    - *Rationale:* 17. Establishment of a rhythmic pattern determines length of time to count the heartbeats to ensure accurate measurement.
18. Start to count while looking at second hand or digital display of watch. Count lub-dub sound as one beat:
    - For a regular rhythm, count rate for 30 seconds and multiply by 2.
    - For an irregular rhythm, count rate for a full minute, noting number of irregular beats.
    - *Rationale:* 18. Ensures sufficient time to count irregular beats.
19. Share your findings with client.
    - *Rationale:* 19. Promotes client participation in care.

(Continues)

PROCEDURE 29-4 Taking a Pulse (Continued)

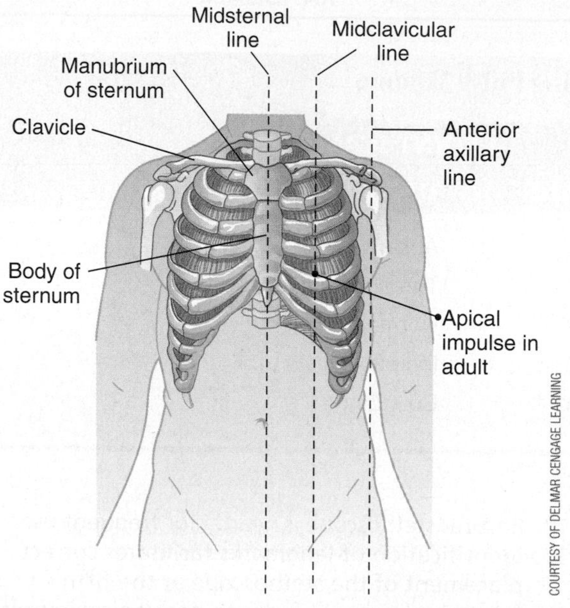

FIGURE 29-4-3 The apical impulse (still called PMI by some practitioners) is located along the fourth intercostal space left of the sternal border and to the fifth intercostal space on the midclavicular line.

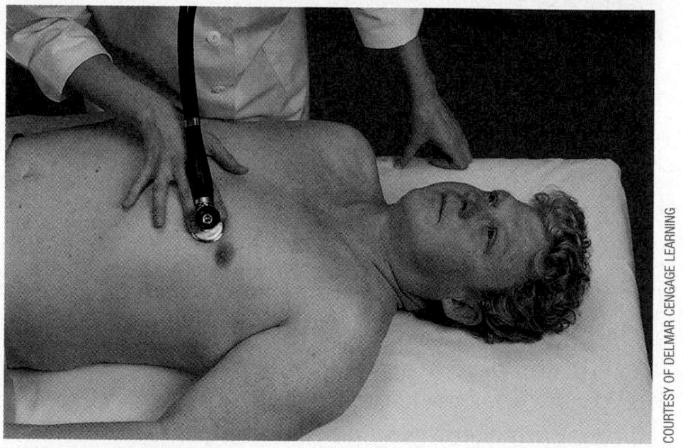

FIGURE 29-4-4 Place diaphragm of stethoscope over the apical impulse to hear the heart rate.

20. Record by site the rate, rhythm, and, if applicable, number of irregular beats.
21. Wash hands.

20. Record rate and characteristics at bedside to ensure accurate documentation.
21. Reduces transmission of microorganisms

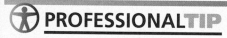

PROFESSIONALTIP

PMI versus Apical Impulse

The term *point of maximal impulse* (PMI) is not used as frequently because a cardiac abnormality can cause a stronger impulse in a different area. Therefore, the mitral landmark is now called the apical impulse (Estes, 2010).

EVALUATION

- Compare client's pulse with baseline rate, amplitude (volume, strength), and rhythm (regularity) to detect any changes.
- If pulse is irregular or abnormal, ask another nurse to check the pulse and then report to health care provider.
- Evaluate pulse site as required by client's condition and compare bilateral pulses. Example: For clients with poor peripheral circulation in the lower extremities, compare both pedal/dorsal or both posterior tibial pulses.

DOCUMENTATION

Nurses' Notes and/or Flow Sheet or Electronic Medical Record

- Pulse rate
- Observations regarding regularity, volume, or rate
- New irregularities in pulse reported to the client's health care provider

PROCEDURE 29-5 Counting Respirations

OVERVIEW

Respiratory assessment is the measurement of the breathing pattern. Assessment of respirations provides clinical data regarding the pH of arterial blood.

Normal breathing is slightly observable, effortless, quiet, automatic, and regular. It can be assessed by observing chest wall expansion and bilateral symmetric movement of the thorax or by placing the back of the hand next to the client's nose and mouth to feel the expired air.

When assessing respiration, ascertain the rate, depth, and rhythm of ventilatory movement. Assess the rate by counting the number of breaths taken per minute. Note the depth and rhythm of ventilatory movements by observing for the normal thoracic and abdominal movements and symmetry in chest wall movement. Normal respirations are characterized by a rate ranging from 12 to 20 breaths per minute.

One inspiration and expiration cycle is counted as one breath. The nurse can observe the rise and fall of the chest wall and count the rate by placing the hand lightly on the chest to feel it rise and fall (Figure 29-5-1). Count the number of respirations for a 30-second interval and multiply by 2 if respirations are regular and even. If the client is experiencing any respiratory difficulty, count the rate for a full minute.

Also observe alterations in the movement of the chest wall: Costal (thoracic) breathing occurs when the external intercostal muscles and the other accessory muscles are used to move the chest upward and outward; diaphragmatic (abdominal) breathing occurs when the diaphragm contracts and relaxes as observed by movement of the abdomen. Dyspnea refers to difficulty in breathing as observed by labored or forced respirations through the use of accessory muscles in the chest and neck to breathe. Dyspneic clients are acutely aware of their respirations and complain of shortness of breath.

Respiratory alterations may cause changes in skin color as observed by a bluish appearance of the nail beds, lips, and skin. The bluish color (cyanosis) results from reduced oxygen level in the arterial blood. Changes in the level of consciousness (restlessness, anxiety, and dyspnea) may also occur with decreased oxygen level. Clients assume a forward-leaning position or may have to stand to increase the expansion capacity of the lungs.

Metabolic alterations such as diabetic ketoacidosis can cause Kussmaul's respirations, which are abnormally deep but regular.

Apnea is the cessation of breathing for several seconds. Persistent apnea is called respiratory arrest. Irregular rhythm with alternating periods of apnea and hyperventilation is called Cheyne-Stokes respirations. The cycle begins with slow, shallow breaths that gradually increase to abnormally deep and rapid respirations, which then gradually slow and return to shallow breathing followed by apnea. This is common in clients who are dying.

ASSESSMENT

1. Assess the movement of client's chest wall **to see if it is equal bilaterally, if the movement is labored, or if the client is using accessory muscles to breathe.**
2. Assess the rate of respirations **to identify slow, rapid, or irregular respirations or even periods of apnea.**
3. Assess the depth of the client's breaths **to monitor shallow, deep, or uneven respirations. Think if there might be something influencing the client's respirations. Is the client in pain, frightened, talking, or smoking?**
4. Assess for risk factors such as fever, pain, anxiety, diseases, or trauma to the chest wall **that may alter the respirations because certain conditions may cause increased risk of alterations in respirations.**
5. Assess for factors that normally influence respirations such as age, exercise, anxiety, pain, smoking, medications, or postural changes **so that an accurate assessment can be made.**

POSSIBLE NURSING DIAGNOSES

Impaired Gas Exchange
Impaired Spontaneous Ventilation
Ineffective Airway Clearance
Ineffective Breathing Pattern

PLANNING

Expected Outcomes

1. An accurate evaluation of a client's respiratory rate and character is obtained.
2. The respiratory rate and character is normal.

Equipment Needed

- Watch with a second hand or digital display
- Stethoscope if needed

delegation tips

The skill of respiratory rate measurement is often delegated to properly trained ancillary personnel; however, the nurse is responsible for this information and appropriate action. Respiration counts over 30 (adult) or 60 (child) should be immediately reported to the nurse for further assessment.

(Continues)

PROCEDURE 29-5 Counting Respirations (Continued)

IMPLEMENTATION—ACTION/RATIONALE

ACTION	RATIONALE
* Check client's identification band * Explain procedure before beginning *	
1. Wash hands.	1. Reduces transmission of microorganisms.
2. Be sure chest movement is visible. Client may need to remove heavy clothing.	2. Facilitates observation of chest wall and abdominal movements.
3. Observe one complete respiratory cycle. If it is easier, place the client's hand across the abdomen and your hand over the client's wrist.	3. Helps determine what constitutes a breath. Helps to determine what to count. Hand rises and falls with inspiration and expiration.
4. Start counting with first inspiration while looking at the second hand of a watch (Figure 29-5-1). • Infants and children: Count a full minute. • Adults: Count for 30 seconds and multiply by 2. If an irregular rate or rhythm is present, count for 1 full minute.	4. Respiratory rate is one complete cycle (inspiration and expiration). • Infants and children usually have an irregular rate.
5. Observe character of respirations: • Depth of respirations by degree of chest wall movement (shallow, normal, or deep) • Rhythm of cycle (regular or interrupted)	5. Reveals volume of air movement into and out of the lungs.
6. Observe skin color and level of consciousness	6. Reveals reduced oxygen level in arterial blood.
7. Replace client's gown if needed.	7. Prevents embarrassment and chilling.
8. Record rate and character of respirations.	8. Record rate and characteristics at bedside to ensure accurate documentation.
9. Wash hands.	9. Reduces transmission of microorganisms.

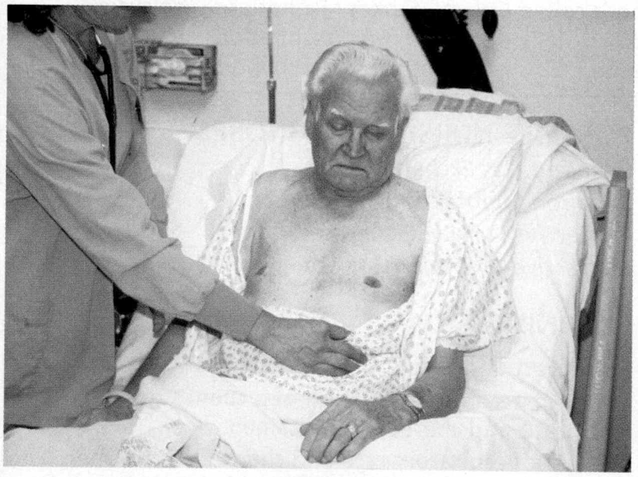

FIGURE 29-5-1 **Observe the depth of respirations and rhythm of cycle. Placing the client's hand across the abdomen and your hand over the client's wrist may make counting respirations easier.**

EVALUATION

- Evaluate client's respirations as a baseline value.
- Compare respirations with baseline to detect any alterations.

DOCUMENTATION

Vital Signs Flow Sheet or Electronic Medical Record

- Respiratory rate

Nurses' Notes

- Depth, rhythm, and character of respirations
- Respiratory rate outside the normal age range, an irregular rhythm, inadequate depth, or any abnormal characteristics such as dyspnea

PROCEDURE 29-6

Taking Blood Pressure

OVERVIEW

Blood pressure is the pressure exerted on the walls of blood vessels because of cardiac output and volume of circulating blood. Blood pressure measurement is performed during a physical examination, at initial assessment, and as part of routine vital signs assessment. Depending on the client's condition, the blood pressure is measured by either a direct or indirect technique.

The indirect method requires use of the sphygmomanometer and stethoscope for auscultation and palpation as needed. The most common site for indirect blood pressure measurement is the client's arm over the brachial artery. When the client's condition prevents auscultation of the brachial artery, assess the blood pressure in the forearm or leg sites. When pressure measurements in the upper extremities are not accessible, the popliteal artery, located behind the knee, is the site of choice. See Figure 29-6-1 for the location of the artery sites. Blood pressure can also be assessed in other sites, such as the radial artery in the forearm and the posterior tibial or dorsalis pedis artery in the lower leg. Because it is difficult to auscultate sounds over the radial, tibial, and dorsalis pedis arteries, these sites are usually palpated to obtain a systolic reading.

The direct method requires an invasive procedure in which an intravenous catheter with an electronic sensor is inserted into an artery and the artery-transmitted pressure on an electronic display unit is read.

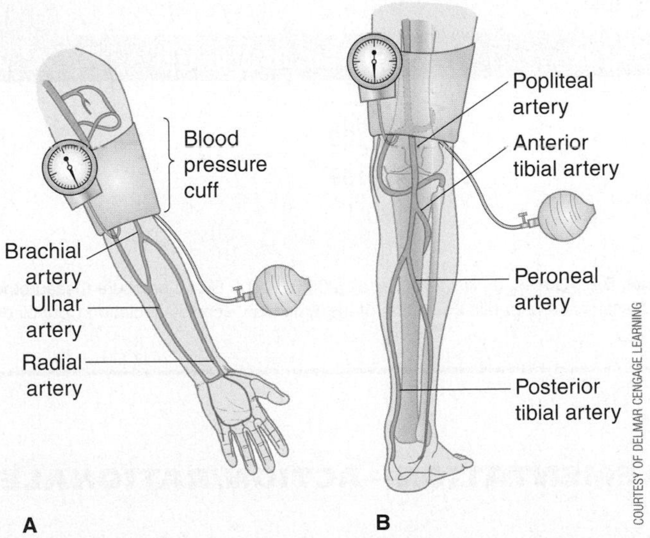

FIGURE 29-6-1A & B: Alternative blood pressure artery sites.

ASSESSMENT

1. Assess the condition of the potential blood pressure (BP) site **so that a site with an injury or surgery proximal to the site can be avoided.**
2. Assess the artery for any compromise to it **so that compressing the artery briefly will not cause decrease in circulation.**
3. Assess the distal pulse **to check if it is intact and palpable.**
4. Assess the circumference of the extremity for the right size cuff **so an accurate reading can be obtained.**
5. Assess for factors that affect blood pressure, such as age, anxiety, fear, medications, smoking, eating, or exercising within 30 minutes before BP assessment, and postural changes **so an accurate reading can be obtained.**
6. Determine client's baseline blood pressure by reading the medical record **so a comparison can be made with each BP reading.**

(Continues)

PROCEDURE 29-6 Taking Blood Pressure (Continued)

POSSIBLE NURSING DIAGNOSES

Ineffective Peripheral Tissue Perfusion
Decreased Cardiac Output
Deficient Knowledge (blood pressure control)

PLANNING

Expected Outcomes

1. An accurate estimate of the arterial pressure at diastole and systole is obtained.
2. Blood pressure is within the expected range for the client.
3. Client understands why the blood pressure is taken and what it means.

Equipment Needed

- Vital signs automatic measurement device (Dinamap) or stethoscope and sphygmomanometer/bladder with aneroid dial
- Gloves, if required
- Alcohol swabs

delegation tips

The measurement of blood pressure is often delegated to ancillary personnel who have been properly educated to use both manual and electronic equipment; however, the nurse is responsible for carefully monitoring this information for significant changes and taking appropriate action. The delegation of blood pressure measurement would be reserved for a client in stable physical condition and measured at sites without intravenous solutions infusing, dialysis shunt or fistula, painful extremity, or recent mastectomy.

TABLE 29-6-1 Classification of Hypertension and Prehypertension from the Joint National Committee on Prevention, Detection, Evaluation, and Treatment of High Blood Pressure

CLASSIFICATION BY BP CATEGORY	SYSTOLIC BP (mm Hg)	DIASTOLIC BP (mm Hg)
Normal	<120	<80
Prehypertension	120–139	80–89
Stage 1 hypertension	140–159	90–99
Stage 2 hypertension	≥160	≥100

BP, Blood Pressure

Pickering, T.G., Hall, J.E., Appel, L.J., Falkner, B.E., Grares, J., Hill, M.N., et al. (2005). Part I: Blood pressure measurement in humans: A statement for professionals from the subcommittee of professional and public education of the American Heart Association Council on high blood pressure research. Hypertension, 45, 142–161.

IMPLEMENTATION—ACTION/RATIONALE

ACTION	RATIONALE
* Check client's identification band * Explain procedure before beginning *	
Asculation Method Using Brachal Artery	
1. Wash hands.	1. Reduces transmission of microorganisms.
2. Determine which extremity is most appropriate for reading. Do not take a pressure reading on an injured or painful extremity or one in which an intravenous line is running.	2. Cuff inflation can temporarily interrupt blood flow and compromise circulation in an extremity already impaired or a vein receiving intravenous fluid.
3. Select a cuff size appropriate for the client. Estimate by inspection, or measure with a tape, the circumference of the bare upper arm at the midpoint between the shoulder (acromion) and the elbow (olecranon process) (Figure 29-6-2).	3. The bladder inside the cuff should encircle 80% of the arm in adults and 100% of the arm of children less than 13 years old. If in doubt, use a larger cuff to ensure equalization of pressure on the artery and accurate measurement.

(Continues)

PROCEDURE 29-6 Taking Blood Pressure (Continued)

ACTION	RATIONALE

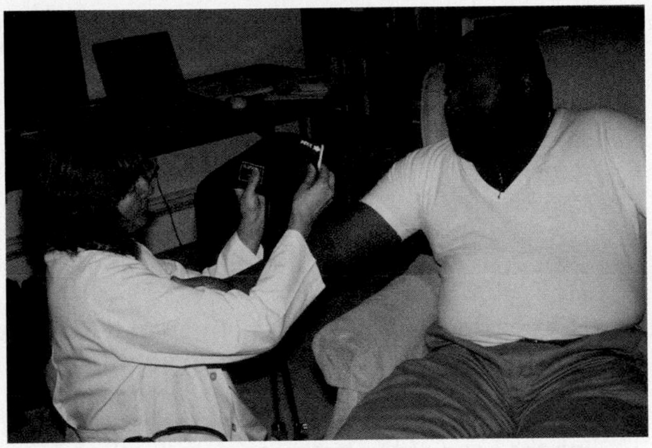

COURTESY OF DELMAR CENGAGE LEARNING

FIGURE 29-6-2 Select a cuff size appropriate for the client.

ACTION	RATIONALE
4. Have the client's bared arm resting on a support so the midpoint of the upper arm is at the level of the heart. Extend the elbow with palm turned upward.	4. Blood pressure increases when the arm is below the level of the heart and decreases when the arm is above the level of the heart.
5. Make sure the bladder cuff is fully deflated and the pump valve moves freely. Place the manometer so the center of the aneroid dial is at eye level and easily visible to the observer.	5. Equipment must be visible and function properly to obtain an accurate reading.
6. Palpate the brachial artery, in the antecubital space, and place the cuff so that the midline of the bladder is over the arterial pulsation. Next, wrap and secure the cuff snugly around the client's bare upper arm. The lower edge of the cuff should be 1 inch (2 cm) above the antecubital fossa (bend of the elbow) (Figures 29-6-3 and 29-6-4).	6. Ensures even pressure distribution over the brachial artery. Rolling up the sleeve may form a tourniquet around the upper arm. Always use a bare arm.

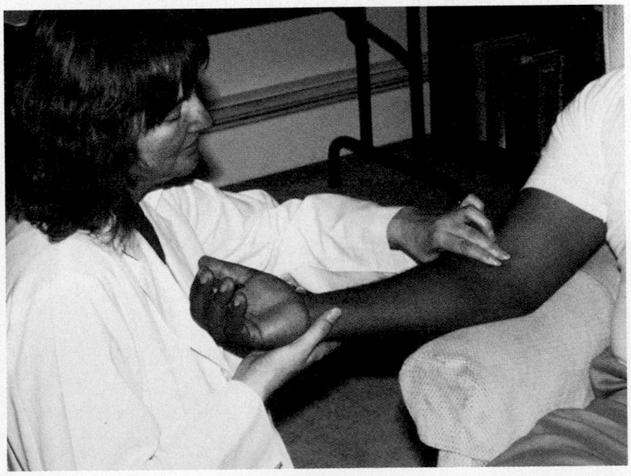

COURTESY OF DELMAR CENGAGE LEARNING

FIGURE 29-6-3 Palpate the brachial artery to determine placement of the stethoscope.

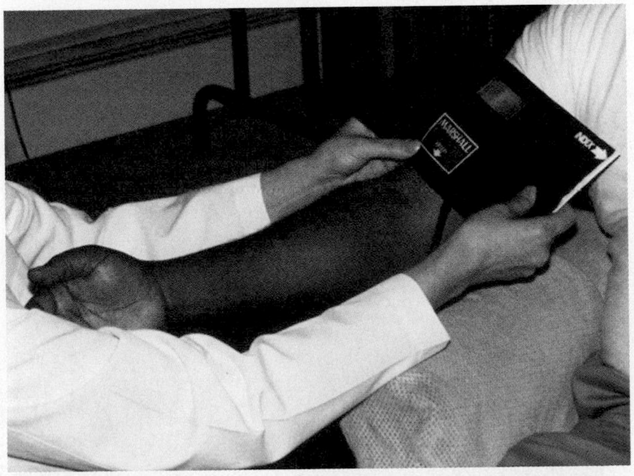

COURTESY OF DELMAR CENGAGE LEARNING

FIGURE 29-6-4 Center the blood pressure cuff over the brachial artery.

(Continues)

PROCEDURE 29-6 Taking Blood Pressure (Continued)

ACTION	RATIONALE
7. Inflate the cuff rapidly to 70 mm Hg and increase by 10-mm increments while palpating the radial pulse. Note the level of pressure at which the pulse disappears and subsequently reappears during deflation. Let all the air out of the cuff in preparation for reinflating the cuff to take the BP reading. Let the arm rest 1 minute before reinflating the cuff. This is called the two-step method of obtaining a BP by obtaining a baseline prior to obtaining the BP reading.	7. The palpatory method provides the necessary preliminary approximation of systolic blood pressure to ensure an accurate reading. When frequent measurements are required, such as every 15 minutes, the palpatory method is generally not incorporated with each pressure check.
8. Insert the earpieces of the stethoscope into the ear canals with a forward tilt to fit snugly.	8. The bell, the low-frequency position of the stethoscope, enhances sound transmission from chest piece to ears.
9. Relocate the brachial artery with your nondominant hand, and place the bell of the stethoscope over the brachial artery pulsation. The bell is held firmly in place, ensuring that the head is in direct contact with the skin and not touching the cuff (Figure 29-6-5).	9. Sound is heard best directly over the artery. Wedging the head of the stethoscope under the edge of the cuff results in considerable extraneous noise and may cause an inaccurate reading.
10. With the dominant hand, turn the valve clockwise to close. Compress the pump to inflate the cuff rapidly and steadily until the manometer registers 20 to 30 mm Hg above the level previously determined by the palpation.	10. Prevents air leaks during inflation. Ensures the cuff is inflated to a pressure greater than the client's systolic pressure.
11. Partially unscrew (open) the valve counterclockwise to deflate the bladder at 2 mm/sec while listening for the appearance of the five phases of the Korotkoff sounds. Note the manometer reading for these sounds. 1. A faint, clear tapping sound that increases in intensity 2. Swishing sound 3. Intense sound 4. Abrupt, distinctive muffled sound 5. No sound	11. Maintains constant release of pressure to ensure hearing first systolic sound. Identify manometer readings for each of the five phases. • Identify two consecutive tapping sounds to confirm systolic reading. • The American Heart Association (2002) recommends using Phase 4 as the diastolic level in children less than 13 years old. Even though 5 phases of Korotkoff sounds have been identified, most clients have only 2 clearly distinct sounds (Phases 1 and 5), identified as the systolic and diastolic sounds.

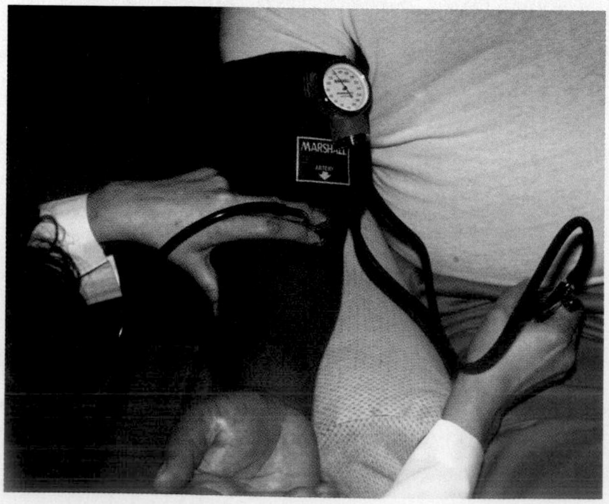

COURTESY OF DELMAR CENGAGE LEARNING

FIGURE 29-6-5 The stethoscope diaphragm should not touch the blood pressure cuff.

(Continues)

PROCEDURE 29-6 Taking Blood Pressure (Continued)

ACTION	RATIONALE
12. After the last Korotkoff sound is heard, deflate the cuff slowly for at least another 10 mm Hg to ensure that no other sounds are audible; then, deflate rapidly and completely.	12. Prevents arterial occlusion and client discomfort from numbness or tingling.
13. Allow the client to rest for at least 30 seconds and remove cuff. (A measurement should be repeated after 30 seconds and the two readings averaged. It may be done in the same or opposite arm) (American Heart Association, 2005).	13. Releases trapped blood in the vessels. Ensures accurate measurement.
14. Inform the client of the reading.	14. Promotes client's participation in health care.
15. The systolic (Phase 1) and diastolic (Phase 5) pressure should be immediately recorded, rounded off (upward) to the nearest 2 mm Hg. (In children and when sounds are heard nearly to the level of 0 mm Hg, the Phase 4 pressure should also be recorded, e.g., 136/104/96).	15. Ensures accuracy.
16. If appropriate, lower bed and place call light in easy reach.	16. Promotes client's safety.
17. Put all equipment in proper place.	17. Fosters maintenance of equipment.
18. Wash hands.	18. Reduces transmission of microorganisms.

EVALUATION

- Evaluate the blood pressure reading for accuracy by comparing with the medical record.
- Evaluate the client's blood pressure for being within the normal range.
- Identify variations in the client's blood pressure of more than 5 to 10 mm Hg from one arm to the other.
- Evaluate if the client's blood pressure changes significantly when he or she stands up.
- Report abnormal measurements to charge nurse or health care provider.

DOCUMENTATION

Vital Signs Flow Sheet or Electronic Medical Record

- Blood pressure measurement
- Site where recording was done
- Method of obtaining the pressure—auscultation or palpation

PROCEDURE 29-7 Performing Pulse Oximetry

OVERVIEW

Pulse oximetry is a quick, easy, noninvasive method to assess the arterial blood oxygen saturation of a client by using an external sensor. There are several types of sensors; however, the most common for adult use is a finger sensor. The finger is placed between a clip mechanism. On one side of the clip are light-emitting diodes (a red and an infrared); a photon detector is on the other side. The beam of light goes through the tissue and blood vessels, and the photon detector receives the light and measures the amount of light absorbed by oxygenated and unoxygenated hemoglobin. Unoxygenated hemoglobin absorbs more red light and oxygenated hemoglobin absorbs more infrared light. The amount of each light and, hence, the arterial blood oxygen saturation (SaO_2) is determined by the spectrum of light. Other types of sensors, using the same principle of spectrometry, are used on the toes, nose, ear, forehead, or around the hand or foot. Special sensors are available for the neonatal hand and pediatric toe.

(Continues)

PROCEDURE 29-7 Performing Pulse Oximetry (Continued)

ASSESSMENT

1. Assess the client's hemoglobin level. **Because pulse oximetry measures the percent of SaO_2, the results of the oxygenation status are affected. The results appear normal if the hemoglobin level is low because all hemoglobin available to carry O_2 is completely saturated; therefore, it is important to know the hemoglobin level.**
2. Assess the client's color. **If the client has vasoconstriction of the extremities, an inaccurate recording may be obtained.**
3. Assess the client's mental status **as this assists in general evaluation of oxygen delivery to the brain and indicates a high level of CO_2.**
4. Assess the client's pulse rate. The pulse oximeter measures pulse rate. **Manually assessing the pulse is a cross-reference to indicate functioning of the oximeter.**
5. Assess the area where the sensors are placed **to determine whether it is an area with adequate circulation (no scars or thickened nails).**
6. Remove nail polish and/or acrylic nails, **which interfere with sensor measurements.**

POSSIBLE NURSING DIAGNOSES

Impaired Gas Exchange
Ineffective Tissue Perfusion
Risk for Impaired Skin Integrity

PLANNING

Expected Outcomes

1. The SaO_2 will be in a normal range for the client (95%– 100% in the absence of chronic respiratory disease).
2. The client will be alert and oriented.
3. The client's color will remain normal.
4. The client will tolerate the placement of sensors.
5. There will not be any skin irritation or pressure from sensors.

Equipment Needed

- Vital signs automatic measurement device (Dinamap) with pulse oximetry or hand-held pulse oximeter
- Proper sensor
- Alcohol wipe or soap and water
- Nail polish remover if necessary

delegation tips

Ancillary personnel routinely perform pulse oximetry. They should be instructed on acceptable parameters and to report any abnormal findings to the nurse.

IMPLEMENTATION—ACTION/RATIONALE

ACTION	RATIONALE
* Check client's identification band * Explain procedure before beginning *	
1. Wash hands.	1. Reduces transmission of microorganisms.
2. Select an appropriate sensor. Sensors are commonly used for the fingertips. (See Figure 29-7-1.)	2. The sensor is selected based on the size of the person and the site to be used.
3. Select an appropriate site for the sensor. Fingers are most commonly used; however, toes (Figure 29-7-2), earlobes, nose, forehead (Figure 29-7-3), hands, and feet are used. Assess for capillary refill and proximal pulse. If the client has poor circulation, use an earlobe, forehead, or nasal sensor instead. In children, sensors are used on the hand, foot, or trunk. If elderly clients have thickened nails, pick another site.	3. Decreased circulation alters the O_2 saturation measurement.
4. Clean the site with an alcohol wipe. Remove artificial nails or nail polish if present or select another site. Clean any tape adhesive. Use soap and water if necessary to clean the site.	4. Polish and artificial fingernails alter the results.

(Continues)

PROCEDURE 29-7 Performing Pulse Oximetry (Continued)

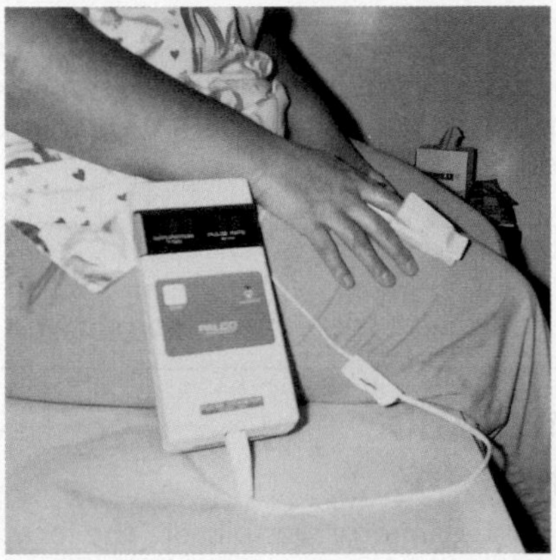

COURTESY OF DELMAR CENGAGE LEARNING

FIGURE 29-7-1 A pulse oximeter determines a client's O_2 saturation.

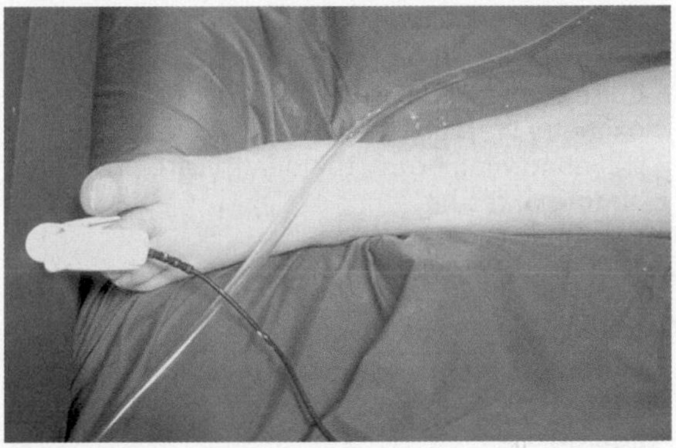

COURTESY OF DELMAR CENGAGE LEARNING

FIGURE 29-7-2 A pulse oximeter sensor may be place on a toe.

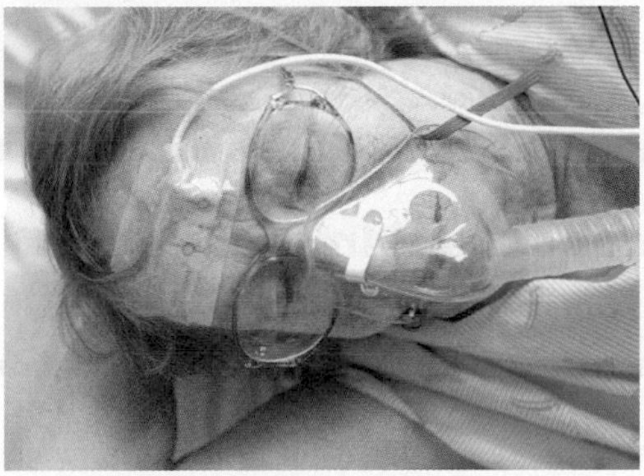

COURTESY OF DELMAR CENGAGE LEARNING

FIGURE 29-7-3 A pulse oximeter sensor may also be placed on the forehead.

ACTION	RATIONALE
5. Apply the sensor. Make sure the photon detectors are aligned on opposite sides of the selected site.	5. Proper application is necessary for accurate results.
6. Connect the sensor to the oximeter with a sensor cable. Turn on the machine. Initially a tone is heard, followed by an arterial wave-form fluctuation with each arterial pulse. In most oximeters if the battery is low, a low-battery light illuminates when 15 minutes of battery life are remaining. Plug in oximeters even when not in use.	6. The tone and wave-form fluctuation indicate the machine is detecting blood flow with each arterial pulsation.
7. Adjust the alarm limits for high and low O_2 saturation levels according to the manufacturer's directions. Pulse rate limits usually are also set. Adjust volume.	7. The alarms indicate that the saturation levels or pulse rates are outside the designated levels and alert the nurse of abnormal O_2 saturation levels and pulse rates.
8. If taking a reading, note the results. If the oximeter is being used for constant monitoring, move the site of spring sensors every 2 hours and adhesive sensors every 4 hours.	8. Prevents skin breakdown from pressure and skin irritation from the adhesive.
9. Cover the sensor with a sheet or towel to protect it from exposure to bright light.	9. Ambient light sources such as sunlight or warming lights may interfere with the sensor and alter the SaO_2 results.

(Continues)

PROCEDURE 29-7 Performing Pulse Oximetry (Continued)

ACTION	RATIONALE
10. If abnormal results are obtained, first assess the client. Are the client's hands cold? Is the sensor correctly placed on the client's finger? Is the pulse oximetry device broken? Obtain the pulse oximetry with another device. If the results are still abnormal, notify the health care provider of abnormal results.	10. A low SaO_2 level requires medical attention because permanent tissue damage may result from low oxygen saturation.
11. Wash hands.	11. Reduces transmission of microorganisms.

EVALUATION

- The SaO_2 is in the normal range for the client (95%– 100% in the absence of chronic respiratory disease).
- The client is alert and oriented.
- The client's color is normal.
- The client tolerates the placement of sensors.
- There is no skin irritation or pressure from sensors.

DOCUMENTATION

Nurses' Notes

- Time pulse oximetry was placed, the location of the sensor, baseline readings, and hemoglobin level

Flow Sheet

- Pulse, oxygen, flow rate, and saturation readings

PROCEDURE 29-8 Weighing a Client, Mobile and Immobile

OVERVIEW

A client's weight is essential data used in monitoring his or her response to a variety of therapies. Changes in a client's weight could necessitate an alteration in the assessment and intervention plans. Weigh a client on the same scale, the same time of day, and wearing the same amount of clothing. An accurate weight is important to ensure appropriate care.

ASSESSMENT

1. Assess the client's ability to stand independently and safely on a scale. **Consider factors requiring the use of a sling scale: The client is somnolent or comatose; paralyzed; too weak to stand; or unsteady when standing.**
2. Determine if clothing is similar to that worn during previous weight measurement **to help determine accuracy of the new weight.**

POSSIBLE NURSING DIAGNOSES

Imbalanced Nutrition: More Than Body Requirements
Imbalanced Nutrition: Less Than Body Requirements
Excess Fluid Volume
Deficient Fluid Volume

PLANNING

Expected Outcomes

1. Health care provider obtains accurate weight.
2. Client incurs no injuries.
3. Client maintains privacy.

Equipment Needed

- Scale: standing electronic or balance scale (see Figure 29-8-1), wheelchair scale, sling scale (Figure 29-8-2), or bed scale.
- Recommended disinfectant
- 1 to 3 other staff members to assist when using sling scale
- Plastic cover for sling scale
- Gloves (when applicable)

(Continues)

PROCEDURE 29-8 Weighing a Client, Mobile and Immobile (Continued)

delegation tips

The skill of weighing the mobile and immobile client is routinely delegated to trained ancillary personnel. The personnel should be instructed to do the following:

- *Select the correct scale for measurement.*
- *Properly and safely position the client for measurement.*
- *Correctly and safely perform the measurement according to established guidelines and record on the appropriate flow sheet (clinical record).*
- *Recognize and report abnormal findings promptly to the nurse.*

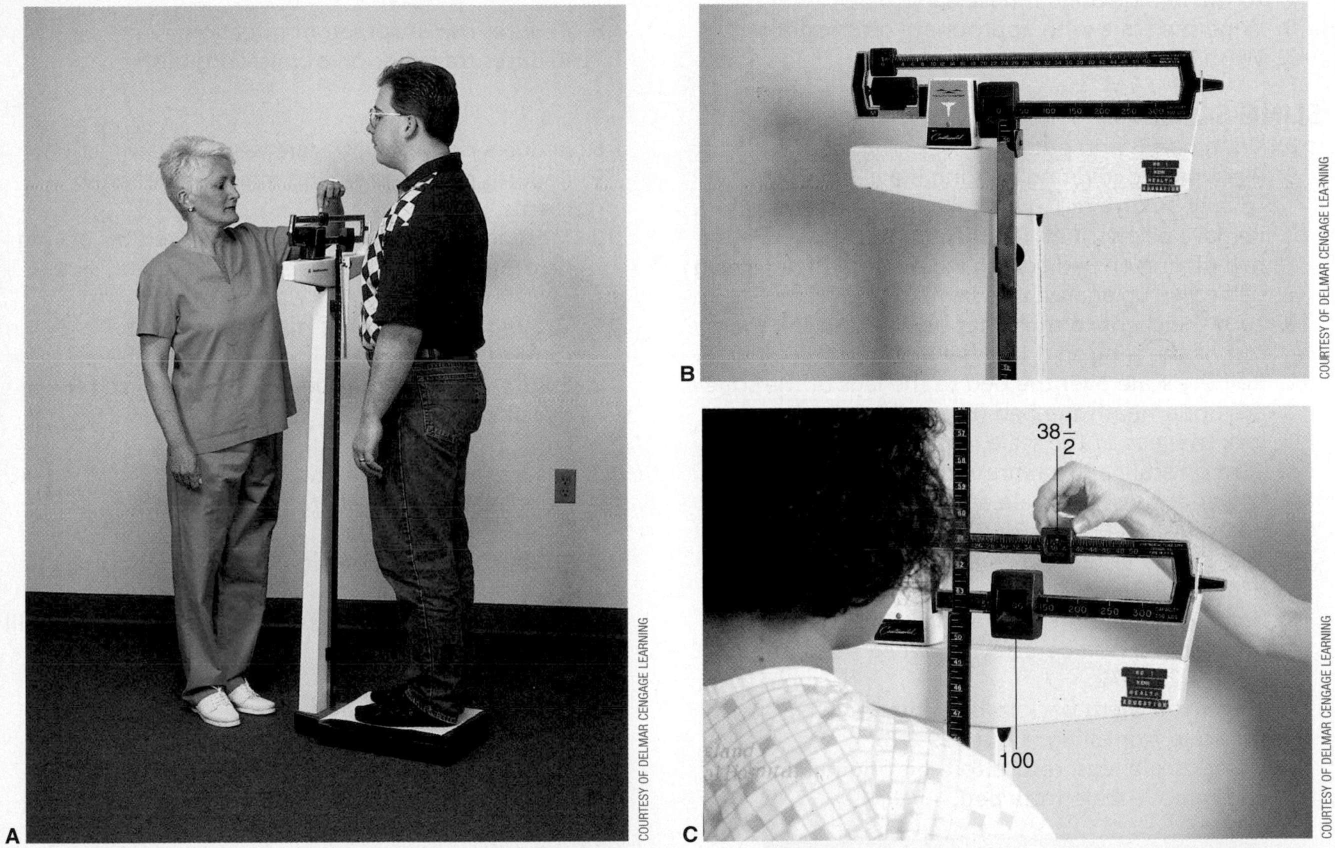

FIGURE 29-8-1 ***A,*** **The standing balance or digital scale weighs ambulatory clients.** ***B,*** **Prior to weighing the client, set both weight indicators to zero and make sure the tip of the balance beam is balanced in the middle of the mark.** ***C,*** **Move the both weight indicators on the balance beam until the tip of the beam is balanced in the middle of the mark. In the photo, the lower weight indicator is on 100, and the top one is on 38½, indicating the client weighs 138½ pounds.**

IMPLEMENTATION—ACTION/RATIONALE

ACTION	RATIONALE
* Check client's identification band * Explain procedure before beginning *	
STANDING SCALE	
1. Wash hands.	1. Reduces transmission of microorganisms.
2. Place the scale near the client.	2. Reduces risk of fall or injury.
3. Turn on the electronic scale and calibrate it to zero.	3. Ensures accurate reading.

(Continues)

PROCEDURE 29-8 Weighing a Client, Mobile and Immobile (Continued)

ACTION	RATIONALE
4. Ask client to remove shoes if necessary, step up on the scale, and stand still.	4. Obtains weight.
Electronic scale: Read weight after digital numbers have stopped fluctuating.	Reading is not accurate when the numbers are still fluctuating.
Balance scale: Slide the larger weight into the notch most closely approximating the client's weight. Slide the smaller weight into the notch so the balance rests in the middle. Add the two numbers for the client's weight.	Weights on scale must be balanced to obtain accurate reading.
5. Ask the client to step down. Assist the client back to the bed or chair, if necessary.	5. Reduces risk of injury if client needs assistance.
6. Wipe the scale with appropriate disinfectant.	6. Reduces risk of spread of infection.
7. Wash hands.	7. Reduces transmission of microorganisms.
SLING SCALE	
8. Wash hands and put on gloves if needed.	8. Reduces risk of health care associated infection.
9. Place plastic covering on sling if available (can usually be ordered in bulk from the manufacturer).	9. Reduces risk of spreading infection between clients.
10. Remove pillows. Turn the client to one side and place half of sling on bed next to the client, with remaining half rolled up against the client's back (Figure 29-8-3).	10. Most accurate weight will be obtained by leaving no other bedding between the client and sling.
11. Turn the client to the other side, and unroll the rest of the sling so it lays flat beneath the client.	11. Turning in this manner maximizes client comfort.
12. Roll the scale over the bed so the legs of the scale are underneath the bed (Figure 29-8-4). Open and lock the legs of the scale.	12. Ensures equipment is being used safely to reduce risk of injury.
13. Turn on scale and calibrate to zero.	13. Ensures accurate reading.
14. Lower arms of the scale and slip hooks through holes in sling (Figure 29-8-5).	14. Attaches sling to scale to obtain weight.
15. Pump scale until sling rests completely off the bed (Figure 29-8-6).	15. Ensures accurate weight.
16. Remind the client to remain still. Read weight after digital numbers have stopped fluctuating (Figure 29-8-7).	16. Reading is not accurate when the numbers are still fluctuating.
17. Lower the client back to bed and remove arms of the scale from sling (Figure 29-8-8).	17. Prepares for removal of sling.
18. Unlock scale legs, return to their original position, and remove scale from bed.	18. Allows for removal of equipment that obstructs proximity to the client, thereby facilitating removal of the sling.

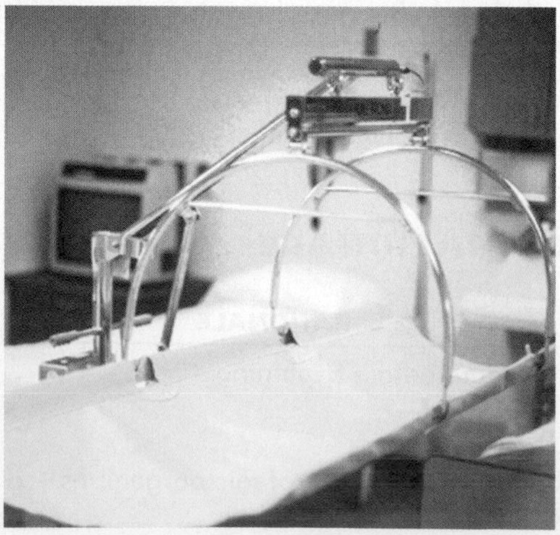

FIGURE 29-8-2 The sling scale weighs clients in bed.

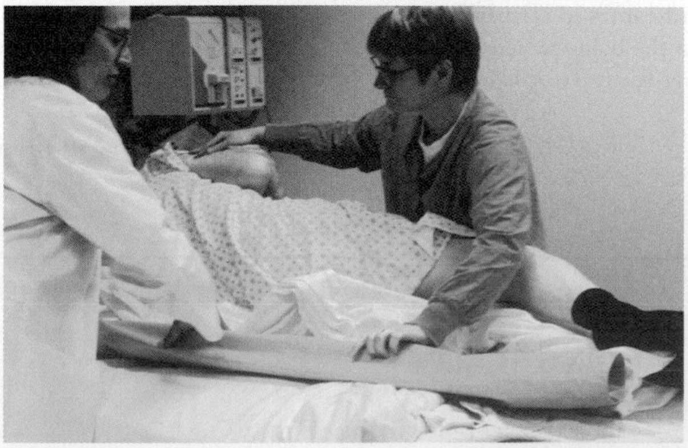

FIGURE 29-8-3 Turn client on one side and place sling on the bed.

(Continues)

PROCEDURE 29-8 Weighing a Client, Mobile and Immobile (Continued)

ACTION | **RATIONALE**

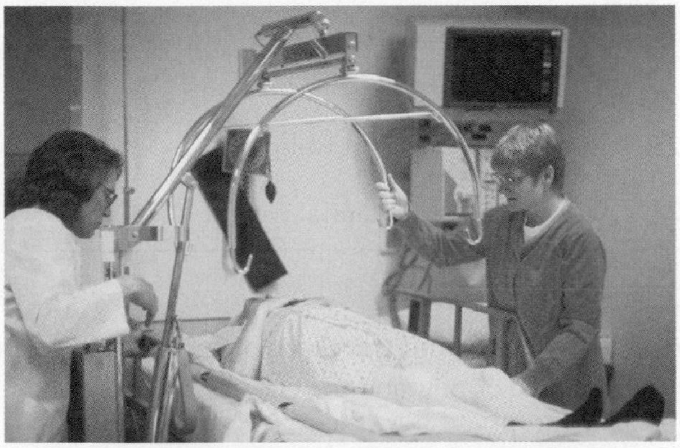

FIGURE 29-8-4 After unrolling the rest of the sling under the client, move the scale into position over the bed.

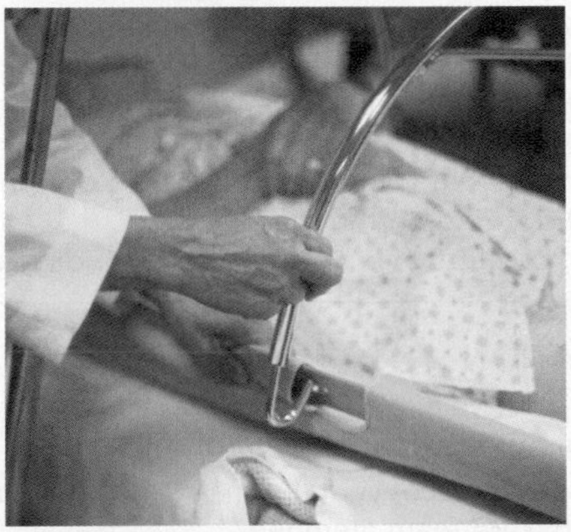

FIGURE 29-8-5 Attach the hooks through the holes in the sling.

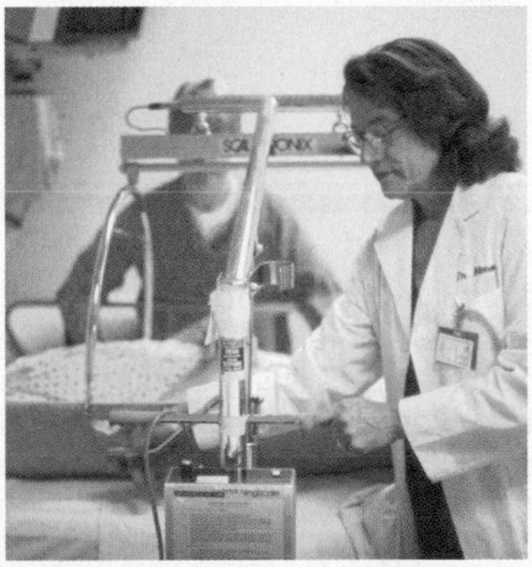

FIGURE 29-8-6 Pump the scale until the sling lifts completely off the bed.

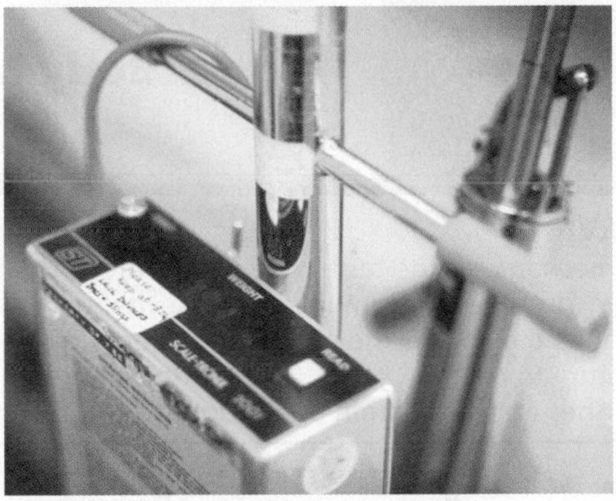

FIGURE 29-8-7 Read the weight after the numbers have stopped fluctuating.

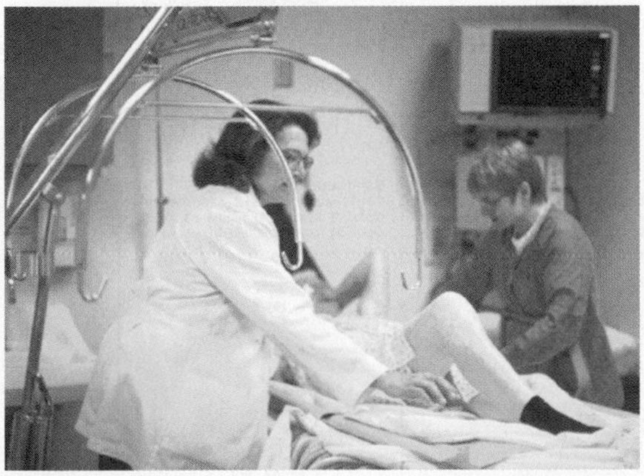

FIGURE 29-8-8 Lower the client back to the bed and remove the sling.

ACTION	RATIONALE
19. Turn the client on his or her side, roll up sling, turn client to the other side.	19. Facilitates removal of the sling.
20. Realign the client with pillows and covers.	20. Ensures comfort and privacy.
21. Remove plastic covering from the sling and discard as per hospital policy.	21. Reduces risk of spread of infection and health care associated infection.
22. Remove gloves and wash hands.	22 Reduces transmission of microorganisms.

(Continues)

PROCEDURE 29-8 Weighing a Client, Mobile and Immobile (Continued)

ACTION	RATIONALE
Bed Scale or Under-Bed Pod Scale Some beds have scales built into the bed that electronically weigh the client. Other beds weigh clients after rolling the bed onto four pods that are connected to a digital monitor.	
23. Place the same amount of bedding on the bed and clothing on the client.	23. Ensures accurate client weight.
24. Turn on electronic weight monitor and weigh client.	24. Obtain an accurate digital weight.

EVALUATION

- Compare weight obtained to previously recorded weight. Repeat weight if large discrepancy is noted.
- If large discrepancy still remains, notify appropriate health care team members.

DOCUMENTATION

Vital Signs Flow Sheet or Electronic Medical Record

- Date, time of day, and the weight of the client on the appropriate flow sheet

PROCEDURE 29-9 Proper Body Mechanics

OVERVIEW

Body mechanics is the term used when referring to lifting techniques and involves proper body alignment, balance, and synchronized movements that are vital when lifting and ambulating clients (Daniels, 2010). Proper use of body mechanics maximizes the power and energy of the musculoskeletal and neurological systems and prevents strains and injury to muscles, joints, and tendons. Correct body mechanics decreases work-related musculoskeletal injuries, diminishes excessive strain and fatigue, and minimizes the potential for injury (Figure 29-9-1). It is imperative that

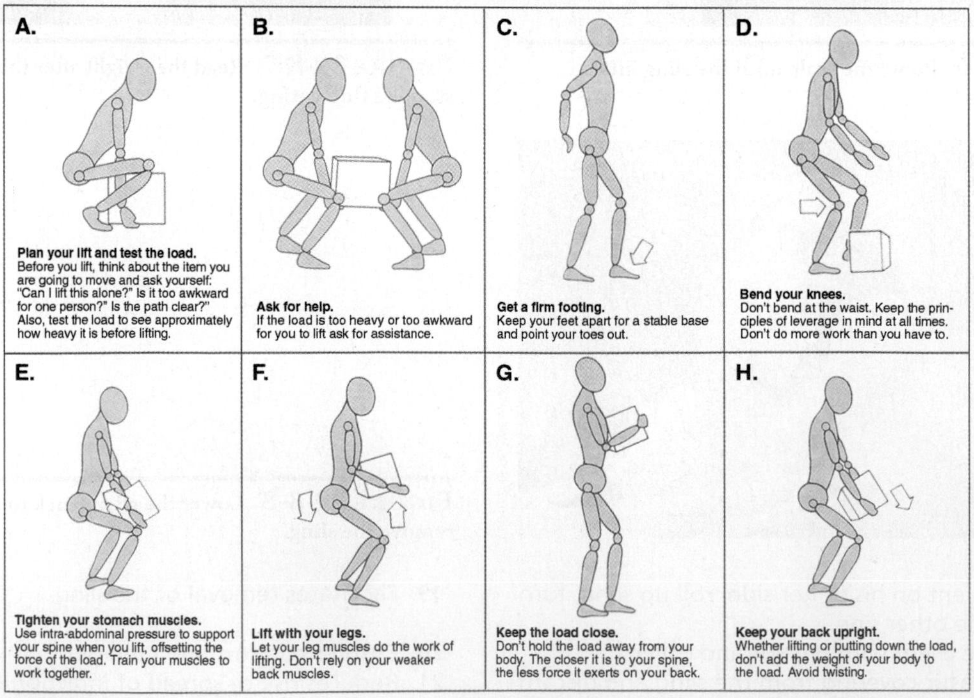
A.
Plan your lift and test the load.
Before you lift, think about the item you are going to move and ask yourself: "Can I lift this alone?" Is it too awkward for one person?" Is the path clear?" Also, test the load to see approximately how heavy it is before lifting.
B.
Ask for help.
If the load is too heavy or too awkward for you to lift ask for assistance.
C.
Get a firm footing.
Keep your feet apart for a stable base and point your toes out.
D.
Bend your knees.
Don't bend at the waist. Keep the principles of leverage in mind at all times. Don't do more work than you have to.
E.
Tighten your stomach muscles.
Use intra-abdominal pressure to support your spine when you lift, offsetting the force of the load. Train your muscles to work together.
F.
Lift with your legs.
Let your leg muscles do the work of lifting. Don't rely on your weaker back muscles.
G.
Keep the load close.
Don't hold the load away from your body. The closer it is to your spine, the less force it exerts on your back.
H.
Keep your back upright.
Whether lifting or putting down the load, don't add the weight of your body to the load. Avoid twisting.

FIGURE 29-9-1 Always follow these eight rules for lifting. *(Reprinted with permission from Ergodyne Corporation, St. Paul, MN.)*

(Continues)

PROCEDURE 29-9 Proper Body Mechanics (Continued)

nurses know and use proper lifting techniques and seek assistance as needed to avoid injury to self and clients. Knowledge of various client transfer techniques, specialized lifting skills of transfer from bed to stretcher and from bed to chair or wheelchair, and the use of the bed transfer board and a hydraulic lift are reviewed in the following procedure. Specific tips for client and staff safety are highlighted.

ASSESSMENT

1. Assess the need and degree to which the client requires assistance to achieve physical movement. **Identifies client's ability to attain maximum level of self-help before initiating intervention.**
2. Identify the type of physical movement required **to ensure the use of proper body mechanics such as pushing, pulling, or lifting.**
3. Identify the potential need for assistive equipment to accomplish the goal of safe lifting **to minimize the risk of client/nurse injury.**
4. Identify any unusual risks to safe lifting, such as an extra-heavy client or a home care setting. **Allows nurse to plan modifications to ensure good body mechanics and reduce the risk of injury.**
5. Assess the situation for obstacles, heavy clients, poor handholds, or equipment or objects in the way. Reduce or remove safety hazards prior to lifting the client or object.
6. Assess the situation for slippery surfaces, including wet floors; slippery shoes on client, helper, or nurse; and towels, linen, or paper on the floor. Resolve the slippery surface before lifting the client or object.
7. Assess the situation for hidden risks, including client confusion, combativeness, orthostatic hypotension, drug effects, pain, or fear.
8. Assess the client's vital signs, pain status, and need for pain medications before ambulating. Assess incisional areas and/or areas of injury.
9. Check equipment to ensure that it is in working order to facilitate a safe and uninterrupted transfer. Especially check locks on wheelchair.
10. Identify all equipment and tubes connected to the client and take appropriate preventive measures. Frequently, clients that require lifting or transfer have intravenous tubing, other tubing, and/or orthopedic equipment.
11. Assess the client's understanding of the steps required to achieve the goal of a safe transfer and the ability to assist. **Explanation of the steps in a clear, concise fashion will decrease anxiety, secure cooperation, and ease physical requirements for both the client and the nurse/caregiver.**

POSSIBLE NURSING DIAGNOSES

Risk for Injury
Impaired Physical Mobility

PLANNING

Expected Outcomes

1. Clients will be safely lifted/transferred by staff utilizing appropriate equipment and correct body mechanics.
2. Accidents during lifting of clients will be avoided by using proper body alignment and mechanics.
3. Heavy lifting will be facilitated by mechanical devices and a team effort.
4. Clients and families will be taught safe lifting/transfer techniques to facilitate this process in home and extended-care environments.
5. The nurse will practice safe lifting and proper body mechanics when performing nursing care that requires bending or lifting.
6. Staff and clients are not injured by using correct body mechanics and utilizing appropriate equipment.

Equipment Needed

- Transfer or gait belts
- Wheelchair equipped with working locks
- Transfer board
- Draw or lift sheet
- Nonslip shoes or slippers
- Safety or gait belt
- Stretcher equipped with working locks
- Hydraulic lift

delegation tips

Delegation to ancillary personnel of the moving, transferring, and lifting of clients is an expectation of their role after proper instruction and/or certification. Ancillary personnel are routinely expected to place the bed at proper height, use a wide base of support, properly position the client, and safely use assistive devices. After repositioning the client, ancillary personnel are expected to evaluate the client's level of comfort. The client who requires complex turning or lifting devices needs the supervision of the professional nurse.

(Continues)

PROCEDURE 29-9 Proper Body Mechanics (Continued)

IMPLEMENTATION—ACTION/RATIONALE

ACTION	RATIONALE
* Check client's identification band * Explain procedure before beginning *	
1. Wash hands.	1. Reduces the transmission of microorganisms.
2. Assess the client situation as stated in previous **Assessment** section.	2. Allows the nurse to anticipate and plan for unexpected events.
3. Maintain low center of gravity by bending at the hips and knees, not the waist. Squat down rather than bend over to lift and lower (Figure 29-9-2).	3. Provides for the equal distribution of body weight and assists in maintaining safe balance.
4. Establish a wide support base with feet spread apart (Figure 29-9-3).	4. Provides stability and lowers the center of gravity.
5. Use feet to move, not a twisting or bending motion from the waist.	5. Assists in maintaining correct body alignment, which increases strength to lift, push, pull, and carry.
6. When pushing or pulling, stand near the object and stagger one foot partially ahead of the other.	6. Provides a safety net for avoiding potential back injuries.
7. When pushing a client or an object, lean into the client or object and apply continuous light pressure. When pulling a client or an object, lean away and grasp with light pressure. Never jerk or twist your body to force a weight to move.	7. Firm pressure will provide continuous movement of the object and will avoid abrupt movements that require the expenditure of increased energy.
8. When stooping to move an object, maintain a wide base of support with feet, flex knees to lower body, and maintain straight upper body.	8. Provides the appropriate mechanics for the strength and endurance to achieve the task and to stand up straight upon completion.
9. When lifting or carrying an object, squat in front of the object, take a firm hold, and assume a standing position by using the leg muscles and keeping the back straight.	9. This stance will avoid the use of the back, diminish the potential for spinal twisting, and provide the lifter with a firm center of gravity and strength to lift the required weight.
10. When rising up from a squatting position, arch your back slightly. Keep the buttocks and abdomen tucked in and rise up with your head first.	10. Keeps the back from bowing and increasing the strain on the back muscles.
11. When lifting or carrying heavy objects, keep the weight as close to your center of gravity as possible.	11. Reduces the strain on arm, leg, and back muscles.
12. When reaching for a client or an object, keep the back straight. If the client or object is heavy, do not try to lift the client or object without repositioning yourself closer to the weight (Figure 29-9-4).	12. Avoids straining the back and arm muscles.

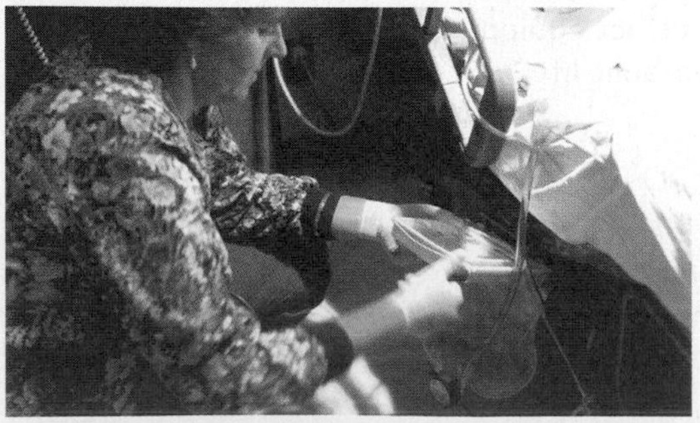

COURTESY OF DELMAR CENGAGE LEARNING

FIGURE 29-9-2 Squat rather than bend to maintain good posture.

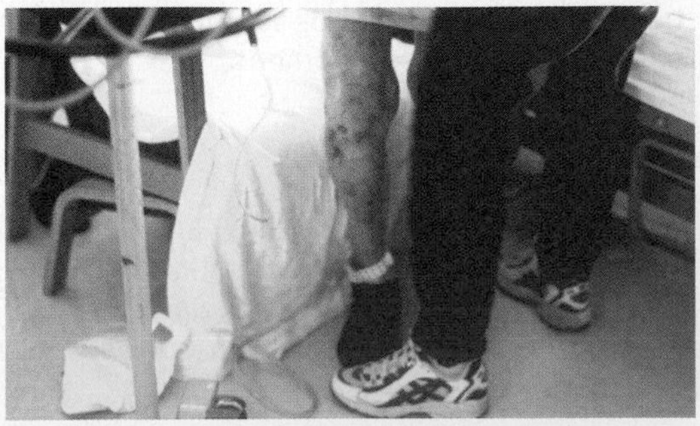

COURTESY OF DELMAR CENGAGE LEARNING

FIGURE 29-9-3 Spread feet apart to establish a wide base of support.

(Continues)

PROCEDURE 29-9 Proper Body Mechanics (Continued)

ACTION	RATIONALE
13. Use safety aids and equipment. Use gait belts (Figure 29-9-5), lifts (Figure 29-9-6), draw sheets, and other transfer assistance devices (Figure 29-9-7). Encourage clients to use handrails and grab bars (Figure 29-9-8). Wheelchair, cart, and stretcher wheels are locked when they are not actually being moved.	13. Reduces the strain on the nurse and improves the safety for the client.

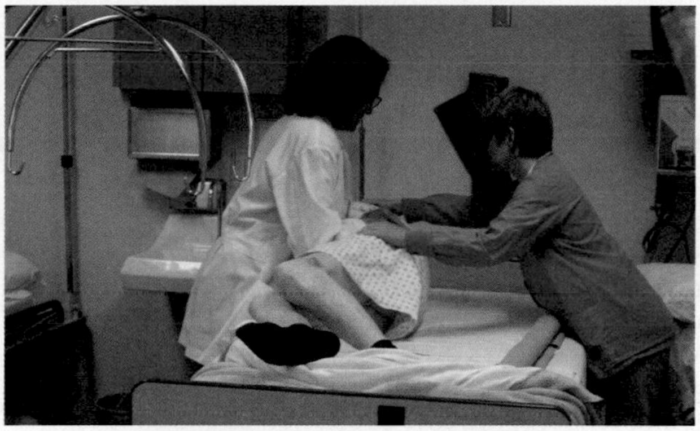

FIGURE 29-9-4 Keep your back straight when reaching.

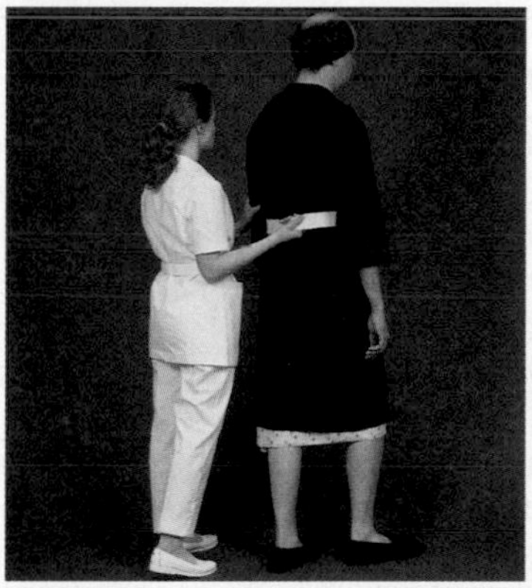

FIGURE 29-9-5 Use gait belts for better grip and control.

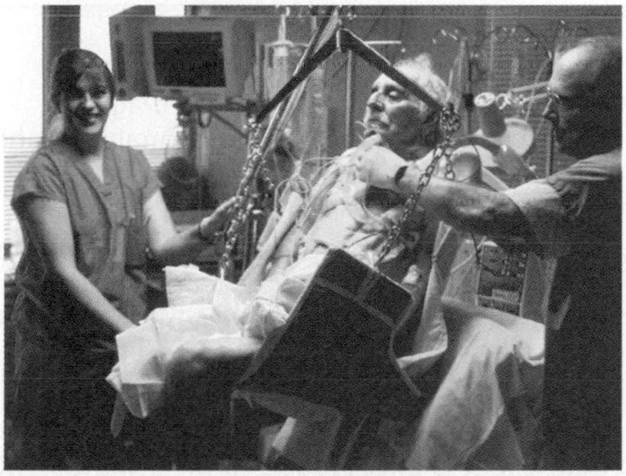

FIGURE 29-9-6 Use lifts to carry the weight of the client. Monitor equipment, lines, tubes, and drains and adjust as needed to prevent them from being dislodged.

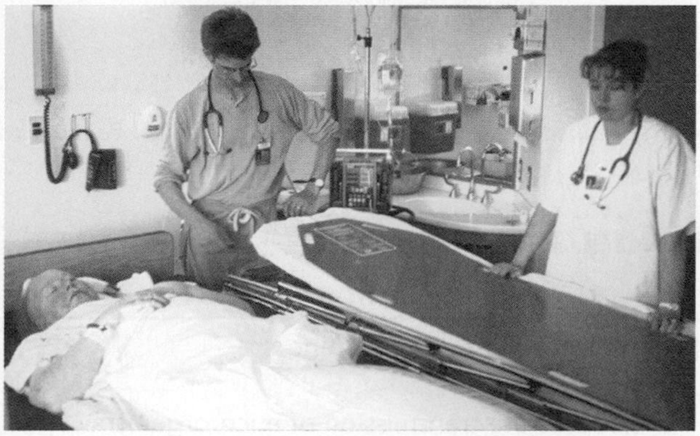

FIGURE 29-9-7 Use a transfer board to reduce shearing forces and to reduce effort needed to slide the client.

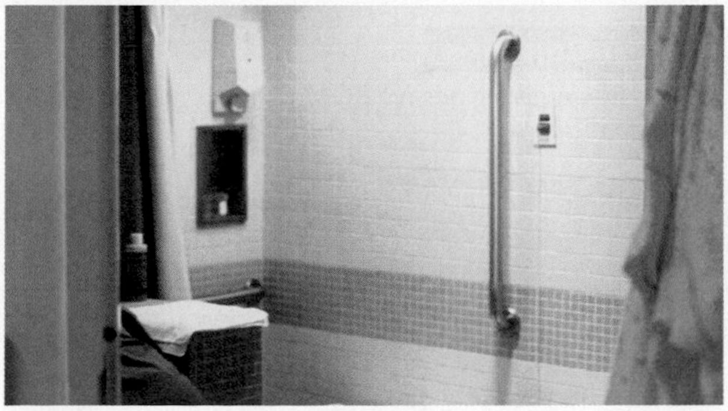

FIGURE 29-9-8 Encourage clients to use handrails and grab bars.

(Continues)

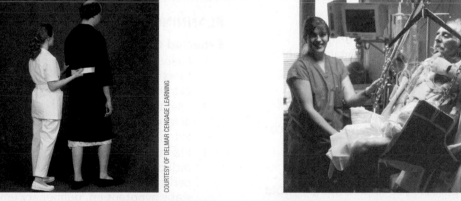

PROCEDURE 29-9 Proper Body Mechanics (Continued)

EVALUATION

- The client or object is lifted and/or moved without sustaining injury or damage.
- The nurse who is lifting and moving clients or objects is not injured.

DOCUMENTATION

Nurses' Notes

- Type of lift or transfer in the progress notes
- Client's tolerance of the lift or move

PROCEDURE 29-10 Performing Range-of-Motion (ROM) Exercises

OVERVIEW

Range of motion (ROM) is the natural range of movement of muscles and joints. When an individual is capable of moving the muscles and joints through their full range of movements in daily activities, he is performing active ROM exercises.

Clients recovering from a stroke or any client with limited movement may need health care personnel to do passive ROM and move the muscles and joints through the natural ROM for the joint. Passive ROM (PROM) exercises seek to maintain or improve the current level of functional mobility of a client's extremities. The nurse provides, assists with, and teaches the client functional movements in all available planes and directions of involved joints. ROM exercises prevent contractures and shortening of muscles and tendons, increase circulation to extremities, decrease vascular complications of immobility, and facilitate comfort for the client.

ASSESSMENT

1. Be aware of the client's medical diagnosis. **Understand the expected functional limits of a client with this diagnosis.**
2. Familiarize yourself with the client's current range of motion. Note any joint pain, stiffness, or inflammation that might limit the client's motion. **Understanding the client's current ROM will help you assess the functional limits of movement of each joint.**
3. Assess client consciousness and cognitive function. **Client is encouraged to participate in ROM as actively as possible.**

POSSIBLE NURSING DIAGNOSES

Impaired Physical Mobility
Risk for Activity Intolerance

PLANNING

Expected Outcomes

1. Client will maintain or improve current functional mobility in all involved joints and extremities.
2. Client will regain or improve strength and/or voluntary movement in involved joints and extremities.
3. Client will avoid complications of immobility, including pressure ulcers, contractures, decreased peristalsis, constipation, fecal impaction, orthostatic hypotension, pulmonary embolism, and thrombophlebitis.

Equipment Needed

- No special equipment is needed, except gloves when contact with body fluids is possible.

delegation tips

Administering passive ROM exercises may be delegated to properly trained ancillary personnel. Outcomes must be reported to the nurse.

IMPLEMENTATION—ACTION/RATIONALE

* Check client's identification band * Explain procedure before beginning *

ACTION	RATIONALE
1. Wash hands, wear gloves if contact with body fluids is possible.	1. Reduces the transmission of microorganisms.
2. Provide for privacy, including exposing only the extremity to be exercised.	2. Decreases physical exposure and embarrassment.

(Continues)

PROCEDURE 29-10 Performing Range-of-Motion (ROM) Exercises (Continued)

ACTION	RATIONALE
3. Adjust bed to comfortable height for performing ROM.	3. Prevents muscle strain and discomfort for nurse.
4. Lower bed rail only on the side you are working.	4. Prevents falls.
5. Describe the passive ROM exercises you are performing, or verbally cue client to perform ROM exercises with your assistance.	5. Exercises all joint areas.
6. Start at the client's head and perform ROM exercises down each side of the body.	6. Provides a systematic method to ensure that all body parts are exercised.
7. Repeat each ROM exercise three to five times as the client tolerates, with five times as maximum. Perform each motion in a slow, firm manner. Encourage full joint movement, but do not go beyond the point of pain, resistance, or fatigue.	7. Provides exercise to the client's tolerance or to a level that will maintain the joint function.
8. Perform the movements listed in Table 29-10-1. Figures 29-1 through 29-4 give examples to follow.	8. The ROM exercises optimize the performance of the movements, to preserve muscle tone and joint flexibility.

TABLE 29-10-1 Defining Joint Range of Motion

JOINT MOVEMENT	RANGE	MUSCLE GROUP(S)	
1. Temporomandibular Joint (TMJ) (Synovial Joint)			
a. Open mouth.	1–2.5 in.	Masseter, temporalis	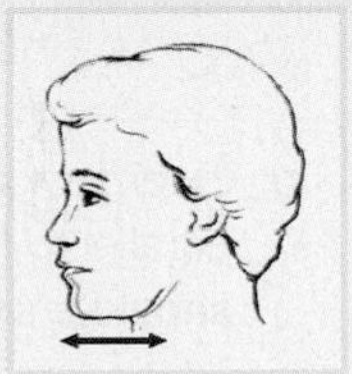
b. Close mouth.	Complete closure		
c. *Protrusion:* Push out lower jaw.	0.5 in.	Pterygoideus lateralis	
d. *Retrusion*: Tuck in lower jaw.	0.5 in.		
e. *Lateral motion*: Slide jaw from side to side.	0.5 in.	Pterygoideus lateralis, pterygoideus medialis	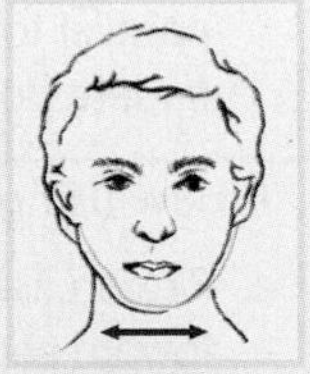
2. Cervical Spine (Pivot Joint)			
a. *Flexion*: Rest chin on chest.	45° each side	Sternocleisdomastoid	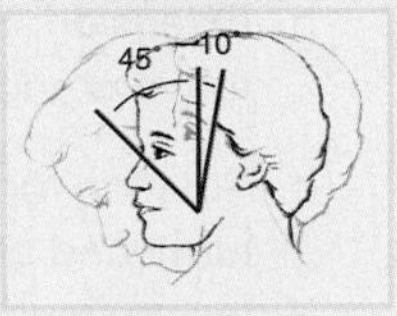
b. *Extension*: Return head to midline.	45°	Trapezius	
c. *Hyperextension*: Tilt head back.	10°	Trapezius	
d. *Lateral flexion*: Move head to touch ear to shoulder.	40° each side	Sternocleidomastoid	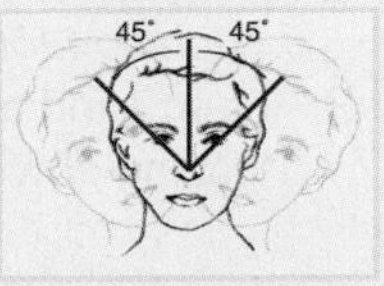
e. *Rotation*: Turn head to look to side.	90° each side	Sternocleidomastoid, trapezius	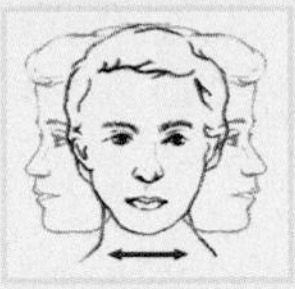

(Continues)

PROCEDURE 29-10 Performing Range-of-Motion (ROM) Exercises (Continued)

TABLE 29-10-1 Defining Joint Range of Motion (Continued)

JOINT MOVEMENT	RANGE	MUSCLE GROUP(S)
3. Shoulder (Ball-and-Socket Joint)		
a. *Flexion*: Raise straight arm forward to a position above the head.	180°	Pectoralis major, coracobrachialis, deltoid, biceps brachii
b. *Extension*: Return straight arm forward and down to side of body.	180°	Latissimus dorsi, deltoid, triceps brachii, teres major
c. *Hypertension*: Move straight arm behind body.	50°	Latissimus dorsi, deltoid, teres major
d. *Abduction*: Move straight arm laterally from side to a position above the head, palm facing away from head.	180°	Deltoid, supraspinatus
e. *Adduction*: Move straight arm download laterally and across front of body as far as possible.	230°	Pectoralis major, teres major
f. *Circumduction*: Move straight arm in a full circle.	360°	Deltoid, coracobrachialis, latissimus dorsi, teres major
g. *External rotation*: Bent arm lateral, parallel to floor, palm down, rotate shoulder so fingers point up.	90°	Infraspinatus, teres minor, deltoid
h. *Internal rotation*: Bent arm lateral, parallel to floor, rotate shoulder so fingers point down.	90°	Subscapularis, pectoralis major, latismus dorsi, teres major
4. Elbow (Hinge Joint)		
a. *Flexion*: Bend elbow, move lower arm toward shoulder, palm facing shoulder.	150°	Biceps brachii, brachialis, brachioradialis
b. *Extension*: Straighten lower arm forward and downward.	150°	Triceps brachii
c. *Rotation for supination*: Elbow bent, turn hand and forearm so palm is facing upward.	70°–90°	Biceps brachii, supinator
c. *Rotation for pronation*: Elbow bent, turn hand and forearm so palm is facing downward.	70°–90°	Pronator teres, pronator quadratus

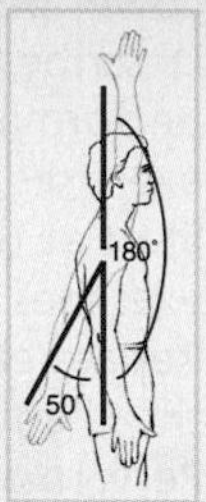

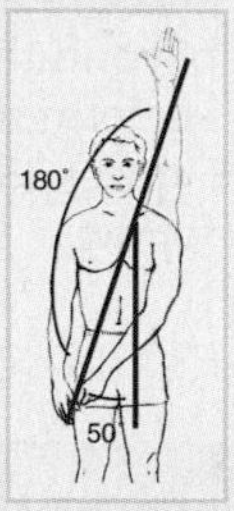

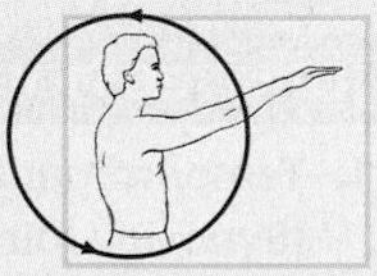

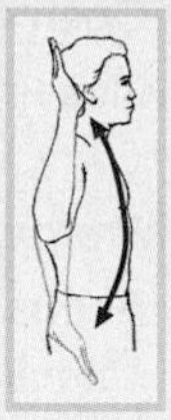

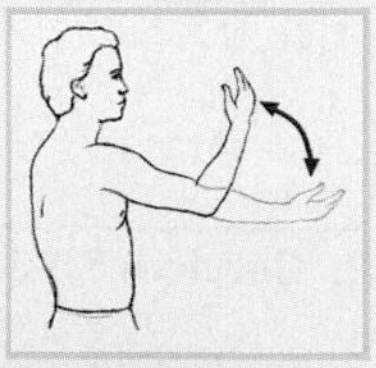

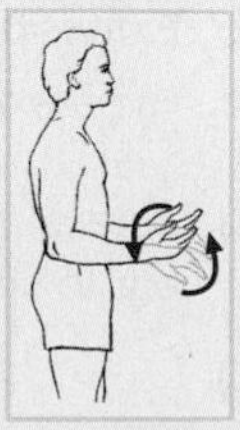

PROCEDURE 29-10 Performing Range-of-Motion (ROM) Exercises (Continued)

TABLE 29-10-1 Defining Joint Range of Motion (Continued)

JOINT MOVEMENT	RANGE	MUSCLE GROUP(S)
5. Wrist (Condyloid Joint)		
a. *Flexion*: Bend wrist so fingers move toward inner aspect of forearm.	80°–90°	Flexor carpi radialis, flexor carpi ulnaris
b. *Extension*: Straighten hand to same plane as arm.	80°–90°	Extensor carpi radialis longus, extensor carpi radialis brevis, extensor carpi ulnaris
c. *Hypertension*: Bend wrist so fingers move back as far as possible.	80°–90°	Extensor carpi radialis longus, extensor carpi radialis brevis, extensor carpi ulnaris
d. *Radial flexion*: abduction—Bend wrist laterally toward thumb.	Up to 20°	Extensor carpi radialis longus, extensor carpi radialis brevis, flexor carpi radialis
e. *Ulnar flexion*: adduction—Bend wrist laterally away from thumb.	30°–50°	Extensor carpi ulnaris, flexor-carpi ulnaris

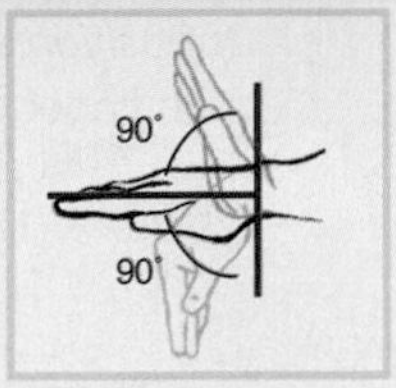

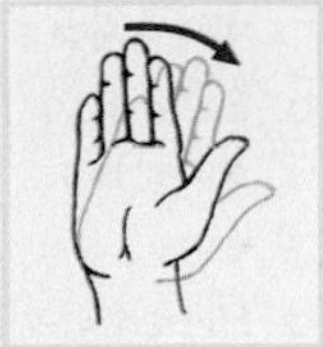

JOINT MOVEMENT	RANGE	MUSCLE GROUP(S)
6. Hand and Fingers (Condyloid and Hinge Joints)		
a. *Flexion*: Make a fist.	90°	Interosseus dorsales manus, flexor digitorum superficialis
b. *Extension*: Straighten fingers.	90°	Extensor indicis, extensor digiti minimi
c. *Hyperextension*: Bend fingers back as far as possible.	30°–50°	Extensor indicis, extensor digiti minimi
d. *Abduction*: Spread fingers apart.	25°	Interosseus dorsales manus
e. *Adduction*: Bring fingers together.	25°	Interosseus palmares

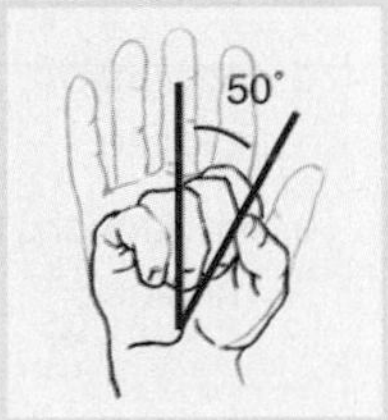

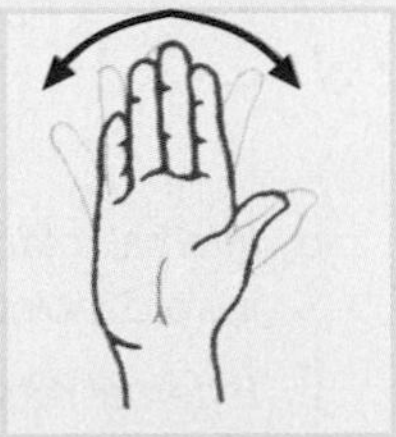

JOINT MOVEMENT	RANGE	MUSCLE GROUP(S)
7. Thumb (Saddle Joint)		
a. *Flexion*: Move thumb across palmar surface of hand.	90°	Felxor pollicis brevis, opponens pollicis
b. *Extension*: Move thumb away from hand.	90°	Extensor Pollicis brevis, extensor pollicis longus
c. *Abduction*: Move thumb laterally.	30°	Abductor pollicis brevis, abductor pollicis longus
d. *Adduction*: Move thumb back to hand.	30°	Adductor pollicis transversus, adductor pollicis obliquus

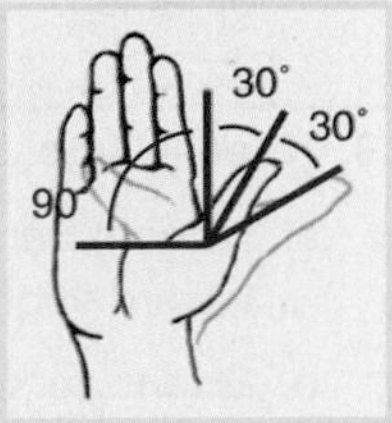

(Continues)

PROCEDURE 29-10 Performing Range-of-Motion (ROM) Exercises (Continued)

TABLE 29-10-1 Defining Joint Range of Motion (Continued)

JOINT MOVEMENT	RANGE	MUSCLE GROUP(S)
e. *Opposition*: Touch thumb to tip of each finger of same hand.	Touching	Opponens pollicis, flexor pollicis brevis

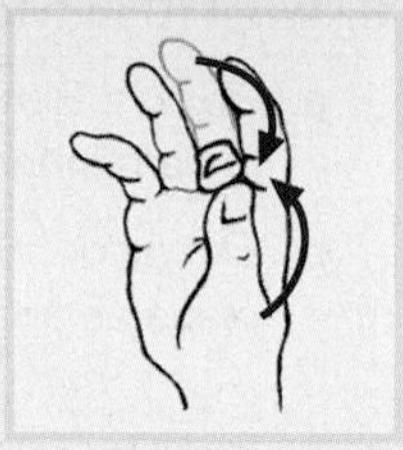

JOINT MOVEMENT	RANGE	MUSCLE GROUP(S)
8. Hip (Ball-and-Socket Joint)		
a. *Flexion*: Move straight leg forward and upward.	90°–120°	Psoas major, iliacus, iliopsoas
b. *Extension*: Move leg back beside the other leg.	90°–120°	Gluteus maximus, adductor magnus, semitendinosus, semimembranosus
c. *Hyperextension*: Move leg behind body.	30°–50°	Gluteus maximus, semitendinosus, semimembranosus
d. *Abduction*: Move leg laterally from midline.	40°–50°	Gluteus medius, gluteus minimus
e. *Adduction*: Move leg toward and past midline.	20°–30° past midline	Adductor magnus, adductor brevis, adductor longus
f. *Circumduction*: Move leg backward in a circle.	360°	Psoas major, gluteus maximus, gluteus medius, adductor magnus
g. *Internal rotation*: Turn foot and leg inward, pointing toes toward other leg.	90°	Gluteus minimus, gluteus medius, tensor fasciae latae
h. *External rotation*: Turn foot and leg outward, pointing toes away from other leg.	90°	Obturator externus, obturator internus, quadratus femoris

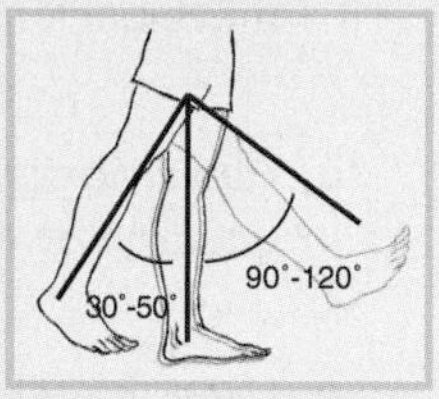

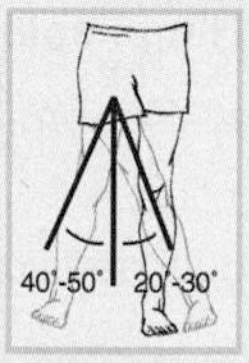

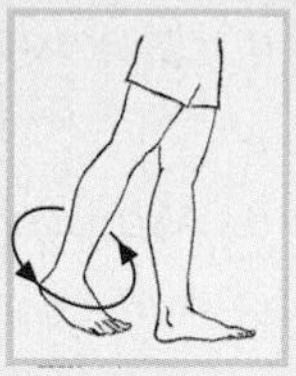

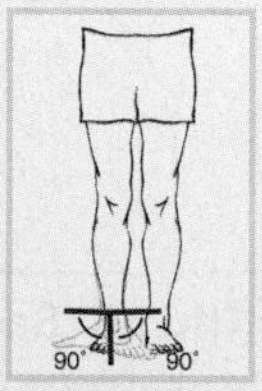

JOINT MOVEMENT	RANGE	MUSCLE GROUP(S)
9. Knee (Hinge Joint)		
a. *Flexion*: Bend knee to bring heel back toward thigh.	120°–130°	Biceps femoris, semitendinosus, semimembranosus
b. *Extension*: Straighten each leg, place foot beside other foot.	120°–130°	Rectus femoris, vastus lateralis, vastus medialis, vastus intermedius

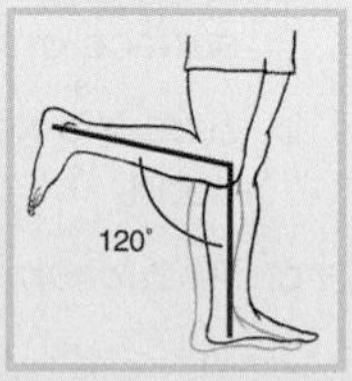

JOINT MOVEMENT	RANGE	MUSCLE GROUP(S)
10. Ankle (Hinge Joint)		
a. *Plantar flexion*: Point toes downward.	45°–50°	Gastrocnemius, soleus
b. *Dorsiflexion*: Point toes upward.	20°	Peroneus, tertius, tibialis anterior

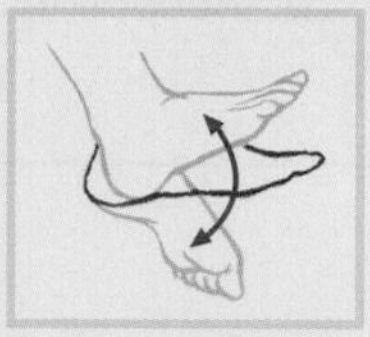

PROCEDURE 29-10 Performing Range-of-Motion (ROM) Exercises (Continued)

TABLE 29-10-1 Defining Joint Range of Motion (Continued)

JOINT MOVEMENT	RANGE	MUSCLE GROUP(S)
11. Foot (Gliding Joint) 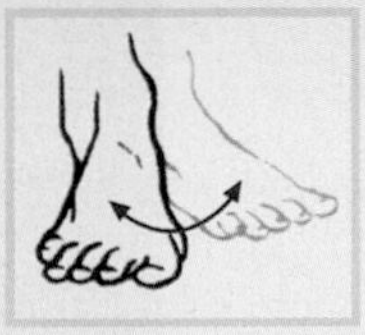		
a. *Eversion*: Turn sole of foot laterally.	5°	Perouеus longus, peroneus brevis
b. *Inversion*: Turn sole of foot medially.	5°	Tibialis posterior, tibialis anterior
12. Toes (Condyloid) 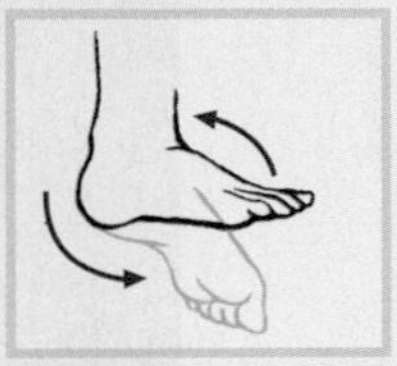		
a. *Flexion*: Curve toes downward.	35°–60°	Flexor hallucis brevis, lumbricales pedis, flexor digitorum brevis
b. *Extension*: Straighten toes.	35°–60°	Extensor digitorum longus, extensor digitorum brevis, extensor hallucis longus
c. *Abduction*: Spread toes apart.	Up to 15°	Interosseus dorsales pedis, abductor hallucis
d. *Adduction*: Bring toes together.	Up to 15°	Adductor hallucis, interosseus plantares

ACTION	RATIONALE

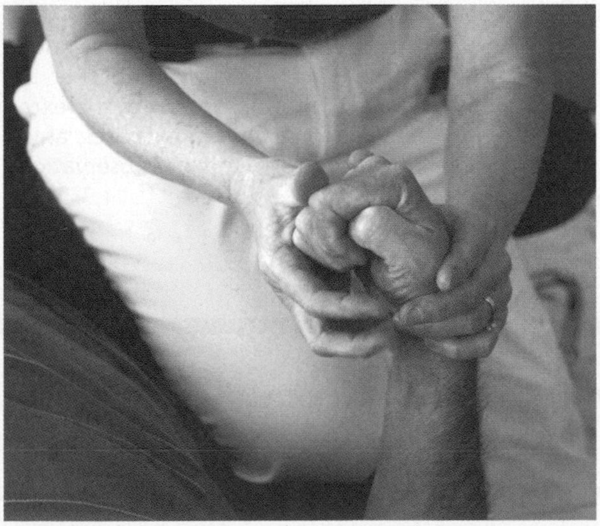

COURTESY OF DELMAR CENGAGE LEARNING

FIGURE 29-10-1 Flex and extend the wrist.

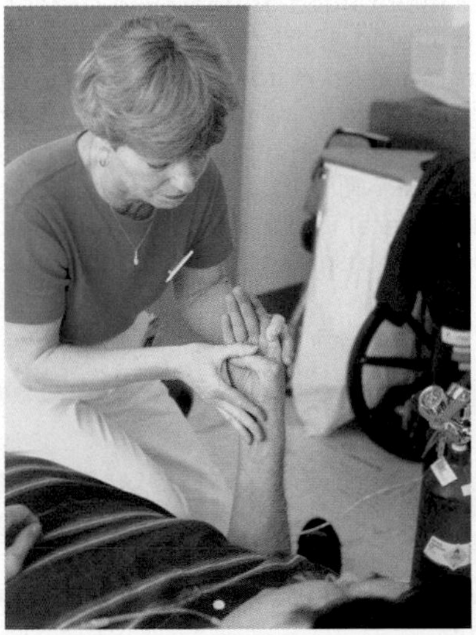

COURTESY OF DELMAR CENGAGE LEARNING

FIGURE 29-10-2 Flex and extend the fingers.

ACTION	RATIONALE
9. Observe client's joints and face for signs of exertion, pain, or fatigue during movement.	9. Alerts nurse to discontinue exercise.
10. Replace covers and position client in proper body alignment.	10. Promotes comfort.
11. Place side rails in original position.	11. Prevents falls.
12. Place call light within reach.	12. Facilitates communication.
13. Wash hands.	13. Reduces the transmission of microorganisms.

(Continues)

PROCEDURE 29-10 Performing Range-of-Motion (ROM) Exercises (Continued)

ACTION	RATIONALE

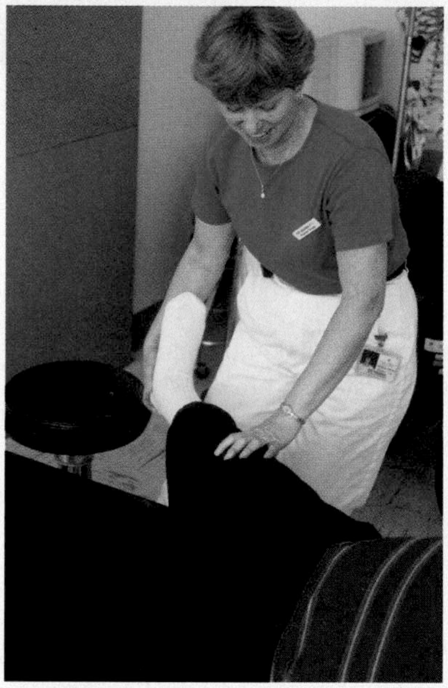

FIGURE 29-10-3 Slide the leg away from the client's midline, then return.

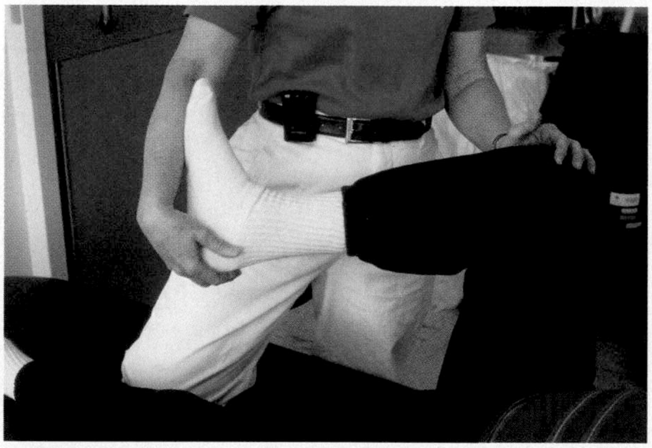

FIGURE 29-10-4 Flex and extend the knee.

EVALUATION

- Client has maintained or improved current functional mobility in all involved joints and extremities.
- Client has regained or improved strength and/or voluntary movement in involved joints and extremities.
- Client has avoided complications of immobility, including pressure ulcers, contractures, decreased peristalsis, constipation, fecal impaction, orthostatic hypotension, pulmonary embolism, and thrombophlebitis.

DOCUMENTATION

Nurses' Notes

- Performance of ROM exercises. Include joints and extremities on which ROM was performed, the types and degrees of limitation observed, the extent of the client's active involvement in exercises, any reports of pain or discomfort, and any observations of intolerance to exercise.
- Unusual findings

PROCEDURE 29-11 Ambulation Safety and Assisting from Bed to Walking

OVERVIEW

Client ambulation (assisted or unassisted walking) is encouraged soon after the onset of illness or surgery to prevent the complications of immobility. First, assess the strength, endurance, mobility, and orientation of the client. Assist with client ambulation, especially if equipment (IV infusions, urinary catheters, closed chest drainage systems, drainage tubes) is present. Evaluate client ambulation to plan the progression of activity.

Clients at high risk for falls include those with prolonged hospitalization, those taking sedatives or tranquilizers, confused clients, or those with a history of physical restraint use. A great majority of falls:

- Occur in the evening
- Occur in the client's room
- Involve wheelchairs
- Involve confused clients
- Involve unattended clients
- Involve clients with poor footwear

(Continues)

PROCEDURE 29-11 Ambulation Safety and Assisting from Bed to Walking (Continued)

- Occur with poor lighting
- Involve clients with poor vision
- Occur with clients experiencing neuromuscular impairment

Awareness of risk factors for falls allows many client injuries to be prevented. When the client is comfortably able to tolerate sitting on the side of the bed and then standing at the side of the bed, progressive ambulation activities are initiated. Disturbances in balance, coordination, proprioception (spatial position), as well as weakness, low endurance, and deconditioning often occur as consequences of medical/surgical procedures. These clients need assistance with ambulation. Gait belts provide client safety when ambulating.

Continually evaluate the client's strength and endurance during the entire ambulation process.

ASSESSMENT

1. Determine the client's most recent activity level and tolerance **to evaluate the client's current ambulatory ability.**
2. Assess the client's current status, including vital signs, fatigue, pain, and medications **to identify conditions that might adversely affect ambulation.**
3. **To evaluate the client's environment for safety:** Check for handrails to help the client stand and to hold onto while walking. Check that the floor is level, clean, and not slippery or wet. Make sure there is adequate lighting so the client can see where he or she is going.
4. Assess the client's ambulation equipment, including the use of a walker, cane, or other assistive device **to determine whether the equipment is in safe condition.**
5. Check the client's clothing **to determine that the client's shoes or slippers are safe to walk in and that he or she has adequate covering for warmth and privacy.**
6. While the client is ambulating, assess his or her gait and bearing. **Determines how well he or she is tolerating the activity and allows detection of hypotension, diaphoresis, breathlessness, or weakness.**
7. After ambulation, assess the client's ability to recover from the activity, including exhaustion, energy, and recovery times. **Determine if modifications need to be made in the distance, type of assistance, or length of time the client is ambulating.**

POSSIBLE NURSING DIAGNOSES

*Risk for **I**njury*
*Impaired **P**hysical Mobility*
***A**ctivity Intolerance*

PLANNING

Expected Outcomes

1. The client will be able to walk a predetermined distance, with assistance as needed, and return to the starting point.
2. While walking, the client will not suffer any injury.
3. The client will be able to increase the distance he or she can walk and/or will require less assistance to accomplish the distance on a regular basis.

Equipment Needed

- Gait belt (transfer) as needed (PRN)
- Assistive devices
- Shoes or nonslip footwear

delegation tips

The ambulation and safe movement of clients is routinely delegated after proper instruction regarding planning the move, arranging for adequate help, if necessary, and positioning oneself close to the client to prevent injury.

IMPLEMENTATION—ACTION/RATIONALE

ACTION	RATIONALE
* Wash hands * Check client's identification band * Explain procedure before beginning *	
Ambulation Safety	
1. When assisting a client with an intravenous (IV) infusion, place the IV pole with wheels at the head of the bed before having the client dangle the legs, so there is room to swing the legs from the bed to the floor. If orders allow, place a saline lock on the IV.	1. Prevents the client's legs from becoming tangled in the IV pole or tubing, causing a fall or causing the tubing to become dislodged. Provides more freedom of movement.
2. If the facility does not maintain IVs on IV poles, transfer the IV infusion from the bed IV pole to the portable IV pole. The client or the nurse can guide the portable IV pole ahead during ambulation (Figure 29-11-1).	2. Supports the IV while the client ambulates.

(Continues)

PROCEDURE 29-11 Ambulation Safety and Assisting from Bed to Walking (Continued)

ACTION	RATIONALE

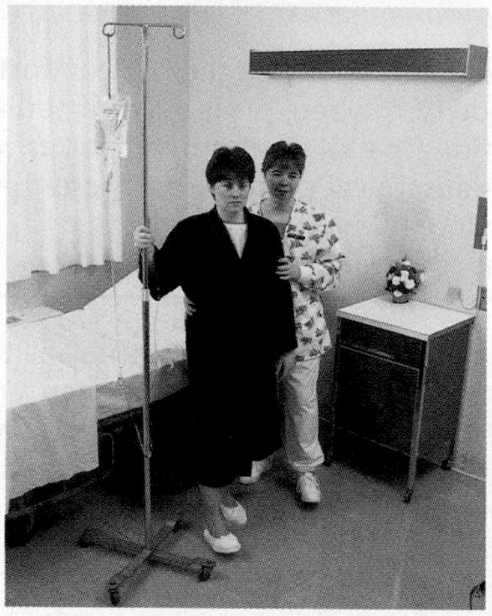

FIGURE 29-11-1 Ambulating client with an IV.

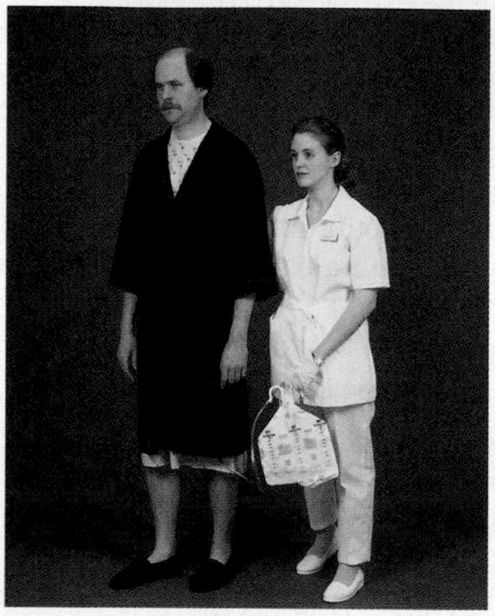

FIGURE 29-11-2 Ambulating client with a urinary drainage bag.

3. When assisting the client with a urinary drainage bag, empty the drainage bag before ambulation. Have the client sit on the side of the bed with legs dangling. Remove the urinary drainage bag from the bed. The nurse or client can hold the urinary drainage bag during ambulation. Make sure the drainage bag remains below the level of the bladder (Figure 29-11-2).

   Rationale: Emptying the bag reduces the weight of the bag. An empty bag kept below the level of the bladder reduces the risk of urine flowing back into the bladder, and, hence, reduces risk of contamination. Having the nurse hold the drainage bag allows the client to concentrate on safe ambulation.

4. When the client has a drainage tube such as a T-tube, Hemo Vac, or Jackson–Pratt drainage system, be sure to secure the drainage tube and bag before ambulation. Place a rubber band around the drainage tube near the drainage bag. Secure the drainage tube and bag with a safety pin through the rubber band. Allow slack. The safety pin is secured to the client's gown or robe (Figure 29-11-3). Make sure the safety pin is unfastened after the walk so that the tubing is not accidentally pulled when removing the gown.

   Rationale: Prevents the tubing from becoming dislodged or tangled in clothing or other tubes.

5. Ambulating the client with a closed chest tube drainage system often requires two nurses, one assisting the client and one nurse managing the closed chest tube drainage system. While the client is sitting on the edge of the bed with feet

   Rationale: Two nurses allow one to focus on the client's safety and ambulation while the other focuses on maintaining the chest drainage system and keeping tubes from becoming dislodged.

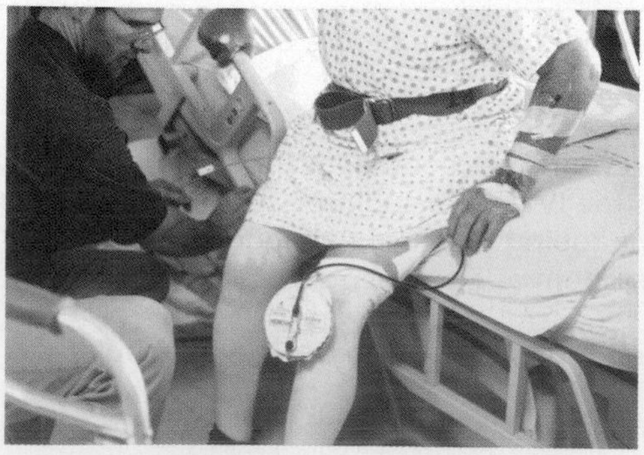

FIGURE 29-11-3 Secure tubes and drainage bags prior to ambulation so that they do not become dislodged.

(Continues)

PROCEDURE 29-11 Ambulation Safety and Assisting from Bed to Walking (Continued)

ACTION	RATIONALE
dangling, remove the hangers from the drainage system. Hold the closed chest tube drainage system upright at all times. Handle all IVs, tubes and chest tubes gently so as not to dislodge any drains.	
6. Use a transfer belt or gait belt when ambulating a client who is weak. For additional safety, a wheelchair can be pushed along behind the client for ready access if the client feels weak, tired, or faint.	6. The transfer belt is a 2-inch-wide webbed belt worn by the client for stabilization during transfers and ambulation. It provides more support for the client by having the nurse hold the back of the belt.
7. If a client feels faint or dizzy during dangling, return the client to a supine position in bed and lower the head of the bed. Monitor the client's blood pressure and pulse.	7. Keeps the client from falling from the bed. Lowering the head of the bed allows gravity to support blood flow to the brain in the hypotensive client.
8. If the client feels faint or dizzy during ambulation, allow the client to sit in a chair. Stay with the client for safety. Request another nurse to secure a wheelchair if not already available to return the client to bed.	8. May stop the client from progressing to full syncope.
9. If the client feels faint or dizzy during ambulation and starts to fall, ease the client to the floor while supporting and protecting the client's head. Position yourself next to and slightly behind the ambulating client, thus being able to step behind the client and safely ease the client to the floor. Ask other personnel to assist you in returning the client to bed. Assess orthostatic blood pressures.	9. Easing the client to the floor prevents injury to the client.
10. Encourage the client to void before ambulating, especially with elderly clients.	10. Prevents need to interrupt ambulation. Restroom may not be readily available.
Bed to Walking	
11. Inform client of the purposes and distance of the walking exercise.	11. Reduces client anxiety and increases cooperation.
12. Elevate the head of the bed and wait several minutes.	12. Prevents orthostatic hypotension.
13. Lower the bed height.	13. Reduces distance client has to step down, thus decreasing risk of injury.
14. Encourage client to actively move legs, or this may be done passively.	14. Stimulates flow of blood, especially elevation of systolic blood pressure to prevent possible orthostatic hypotension.
15. With one arm on the client's back and one arm under the client's upper legs, move the client into the dangling position.	15. Provides client support and reduces risk of falling.
16. Encourage client to dangle at side of bed for several minutes.	16. Prevents orthostatic hypotension. Allows for assessing tolerance for the sitting position.
17. Place gait belt around client's waist; secure the buckle in front. Place ambulation device such as a walker within reach of the client, if necessary. Assist client into standing position (Figure 29-11-4). Make sure bed is locked and floor is not slippery. Client shoes should have nonslip soles.	17. Provides handholds for the caregiver to support the client. Provides for client and caregiver safety.
18. Stand in front of client with your knees touching client's knees.	18. Prevents client from sliding forward if dizziness or faintness occurs.
19. Place arms under client's axilla.	19. Supports client's trunk.
20. Assist client to a standing position, allowing client time to balance.	20. Reduces risk of fall.
21. If client is able to proceed with ambulating, assume a position beside the client and assist the client as necessary using the gait belt. Place yourself in a guarding position so as to assist client quickly and safely, if necessary. Use additional assistance, as necessary.	21. Provides for client and caregiver safety.

(Continues)

PROCEDURE 29-11 Ambulation Safety and Assisting from Bed to Walking (Continued)

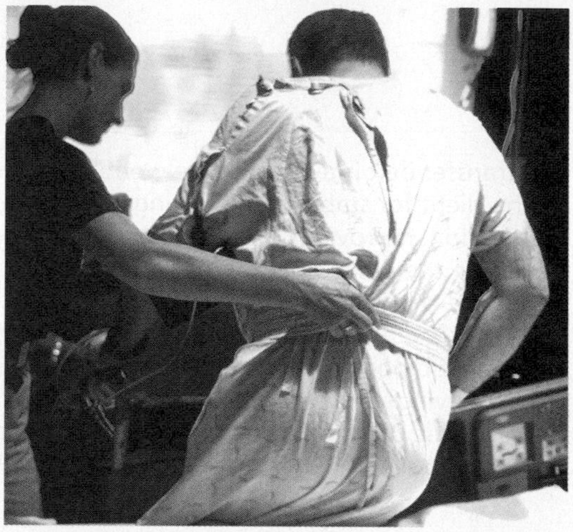

FIGURE 29-11-4 Assist the client to stand.

ACTION	RATIONALE
22. Following ambulation, return client to bed, remove gait belt, and monitor vital signs, as necessary. Make the client comfortable, and make sure all lines and tubes are secure.	22. Promotes safety and comfort.
23. Place the call light within reach of the client.	23. Provides for client safety.
24. Move the bedside table close to the bed and place items of frequent use within reach of the client.	24. Provides for client safety.
25. Wash hands.	25. Reduces the transmission of microorganisms.

EVALUATION

- The client was able to walk a predetermined distance, with assistance as needed, and return to the starting point.
- While walking, the client did not suffer any injury.
- The client was able to increase the distance walked and/or required less assistance to accomplish the distance on a regular basis.

DOCUMENTATION

Nurses' Notes

- Distance the client was able to ambulate and how the client tolerated the ambulation
- Assistive devices the client required and teaching done regarding using the device
- Special concerns or unusual findings observed while ambulating the client

PROCEDURE 29-12 Assisting with Crutches, Cane, or Walker

OVERVIEW

Mobility is an important part of everyone's life. Being able to move about in the environment can mean the difference between living at home and living in a health care facility. Being able to move independently improves a client's emotional, mental, and physical well-being.

Clients who cannot safely walk unassisted can use devices designed to aid them in walking independently. The three most common devices used are crutches, canes, and walkers.

The appropriate device for each client is determined by the client's health care provider, physical therapist, or nurse. These caregivers often work together to determine which device is best for the client. This decision is based on the client's ability to bear weight on the legs, upper arm strength, stamina, and the presence or absence of unilateral weakness.

(Continues)

PROCEDURE 29-12 Assisting with Crutches, Cane, or Walker (Continued)

Crutches are used by clients who cannot bear any weight on one leg, who can only bear partial weight on one leg, and who have full weight-bearing ability on both legs. Several types of crutches are available, depending on the length of time the client requires the assistance and the client's upper-body strength.

A cane is used by clients who can bear weight on both legs but one leg or hip is weaker or impaired. There are several types of canes as well. The standard, straight cane is used most often. There are also canes with three or four legs on the end, called quad canes, to increase a client's stability when walking.

Walkers are used by clients who require more support than a cane provides. Walkers are available with or without wheels. Walkers without wheels provide the most stability, but they must be lifted with each step. Walkers with wheels are somewhat less stable, but a client who does not have the upper-body strength to lift the walker repeatedly can push it along while walking.

ASSESSMENT

1. Assess the reason the client requires an assistive device. Is it a long-term need or a short-term need? **Helps determine which device to use.**
2. Assess the client's physical limitations. How much weight is the client able to bear? Can the client bear weight on both legs or just one? Is the upper body strength good? Does the client tire easily? **Assesses safety and comfort.**
3. Assess the client's physical environment. Is the client at home or in a medical facility? Is the environment suited to assistive needs and the assistive device the client will be using? Are the hallways wide enough? Well lit? Are the doorways wide enough? Are there stairs used frequently, and if so, how many? Do the doors swing open far enough? **Assesses safety and comfort.**
4. Assess the client's ability to understand and follow directions regarding use of an assistive device. Can the client understand the instructions? Can he or she remember them? Has the client used this device in the past? Is there a language barrier that might limit understanding? **Assesses safety, educational, comfort, and effectiveness.**

POSSIBLE NURSING DIAGNOSES

Impaired Physical Mobility
Risk for Trauma
Deficient Knowledge (assistive devices for mobility)

PLANNING

Expected Outcomes

1. The client will be able to demonstrate safe and independent ambulation with the assistance of crutches, a cane, or a walker.
2. The client will feel confident and safe while using the assistive device.

Equipment Needed

- Gait belt
- Assistive device: crutches, cane, or walker
- Tape measure
- Nonslip footwear

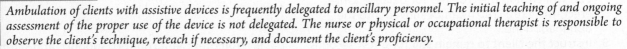

delegation tips

Ambulation of clients with assistive devices is frequently delegated to ancillary personnel. The initial teaching of and ongoing assessment of the proper use of the device is not delegated. The nurse or physical or occupational therapist is responsible to observe the client's technique, reteach if necessary, and document the client's proficiency.

IMPLEMENTATION—ACTION/RATIONALE

ACTION	RATIONALE
* Check client's identification band * Explain procedure before beginning *	
1. Assess client for strength, mobility, range of motion, visual acuity, perceptual difficulties, and balance. *Note:* The nurse and physical therapist often work together on assessment and choosing the correct assistive equipment of ambulation.	1. Helps determine the client's capabilities and amount of assistance required.
2. Measure client for size of crutches and adjust crutches to fit. While client is supine, measure client from heel to axilla. When client is standing, the crutch pad should fit 1.5 to 2 inches below axilla (Figure 29-12-1). Adjust hand grip so elbow is at 30-degree flexion.	2. Increases client safety and comfort. Space between crutch pad and axilla prevents pressure on radial nerves. Elbow flexion allows for space between crutch pad and axilla.

(Continues)

PROCEDURE 29-12 Assisting with Crutches, Cane, or Walker (Continued)

ACTION	RATIONALE

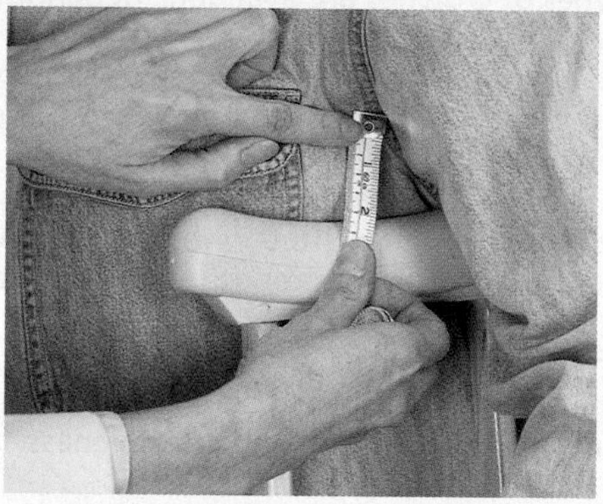

FIGURE 29-12-1 Adjusting the crutches to fit the client will increase comfort and stability.

Action	Rationale
3. Provide a robe or other covering as well as nonslip foot coverings or shoes.	3. Provides for privacy and safety.
4. Lower the height of the bed.	4. Allows client to sit with feet on the floor and increases safety.
5. Dangle the client at the side of the bed for several minutes. Assess for vertigo or nausea.	5. Allows for stabilization of blood pressure, thus preventing orthostatic hypotension.
6. Apply gait belt around the client's waist if balance and stability are unknown or unreliable. It is good practice to use a gait belt the first time the client is out of bed.	6. Provides support and promotes safety.
7. Demonstrate to client the method of holding crutches while he or she remains seated. This should be with elbows bent 30 degrees while hands are on the hand grips and pads 1.5 to 2 inches below the axilla. Instruct client to position crutches 4 to 5 inches laterally and 4 to 6 inches in front of feet. With weight on hands, not axilla.	7. Increases comprehension and cooperation, decreases anxiety.
8. Assist the client to a standing position by having client place both crutches in nondominant hand. Then, using the dominant hand, push off from the bed while using the crutches for balance. Once erect, the extra crutch can be moved into the dominant hand.	8. Allows for stability while promoting independence.
9. Instruct the client to remain still for a few seconds while assessing for vertigo or nausea. Stand close to the client to support as needed. While client remains standing, check for correct fit of the crutches.	9. Promotes client comfort, support, and safety. If the client becomes dizzy, sit client back down and wait before trying again.
Two-Point Gait (Figure 29-12-2A)	
10. Move the left crutch and right leg forward 4 to 6 inches. Move the right crutch and left leg forward 4 to 6 inches. Repeat the two-point gait.	10. The two-point gait (used for partial weight-bearing) provides a strong base of support. The client must be able to bear weight on both legs. This gait is faster than the four-point gait.
Three-Point Gait (Figure 29-12-2B)	
11. Advance both crutches and the weaker leg forward together 4 to 6 inches. Move the stronger leg forward, even with the crutches. Repeat the three-point gait.	11. The three-point gait (used for partial or non-weight-bearing) provides a strong base of support. This gait can be used if the client has a weak or non-weight-bearing leg.

(Continues)

PROCEDURE 29-12 Assisting with Crutches, Cane, or Walker (Continued)

ACTION	RATIONALE
Four-Point Gait (Figure 29-12-2C)	
12. Position the crutches 4.5 to 6 inches to the side and in front of each foot. Move the right crutch forward 4 to 6 inches and move the left foot forward, even with the left crutch. Move the left crutch forward 4 to 6 inches and move the right foot forward, even with the right crutch. Repeat the four-point gait.	12. The four-point gait (used for partial or full weight-bearing) provides greater stability. Weight bearing is on three points (two crutches and one foot or two feet and one crutch) at all times. The client must be able to bear weight with both legs.
Swing-Through Gait (Figure 29-12-2D)	
13. Move both crutches forward 4 to 6 inches. Move both legs forward in a swinging motion past the crutches. Repeat the swing-through gait.	13. The swing-through gait permits a faster pace. This gait requires greater balance, strength, and more practice.

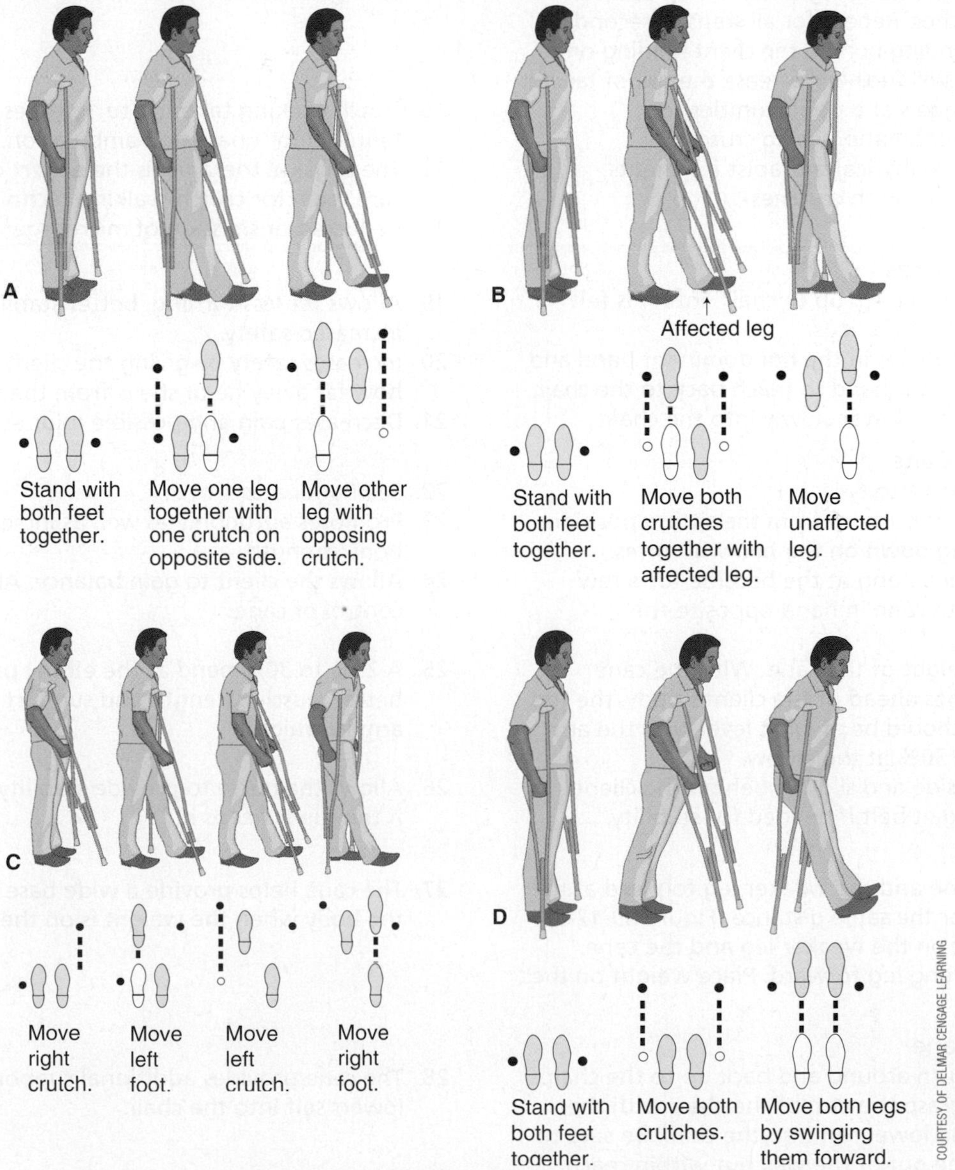
A
Stand with both feet together.
Move one leg together with one crutch on opposite side.
Move other leg with opposing crutch.
B
Affected leg
Stand with both feet together.
Move both crutches together with affected leg.
Move unaffected leg.
C
Move right crutch.
Move left foot.
Move left crutch.
Move right foot.
D
Stand with both feet together.
Move both crutches.
Move both legs by swinging them forward.
COURTESY OF DELMAR CENGAGE LEARNING

FIGURE 29-12-2 **Various crutch gaits; *A*, Two-point gait (partial weight bearing); *B*, Three-point gait (partial or non–weight bearing); *C*, Four-point gait (partial or full weight bearing); *D*, Swing through gait (non-weight-bearing)**

(Continues)

PROCEDURE 29-12 Assisting with Crutches, Cane, or Walker (Continued)

ACTION	RATIONALE
Walking Upstairs	
14. Stand beside and slightly behind client. Instruct client to position the crutches as if walking. Place body weight on hands. Place the strong leg on the first step. Pull the weak leg up and move the crutches up to the first step. Repeat for all steps.	14. Prevents weight bearing on the weaker leg. When ascending stairs, crutches should follow the legs, thereby allowing stability if the client's weight shifts down the stairs while moving. This allows the client to catch him or herself instead of falling backward.
Walking Downstairs	
15. Position the crutches as if walking. Place weight on the strong leg. Move the crutches down to the next lower step. Place partial weight on hands and crutches. Move the weak leg down to the step with the crutches. Put total weight on arms and crutches. Move strong leg to same step as weak leg and crutches. Repeat for all steps. A second caregiver standing behind the client holding on to the gait belt will further decrease the risk of falling.	15. Prevents weight bearing on the weaker leg. Crutches in front of the legs while descending stairs allow the client more forward stability if his or her weight shifts down the stairs while client is moving. This allows client to catch self before falling forward.
16. Set realistic goals and opportunities for progressive ambulation using crutches.	16. Crutch walking takes up to 10 times the energy required for unassisted ambulation.
17. Consult with a physical therapist for clients learning to walk with crutches.	17. The physical therapist is the expert on the health care team for crutch-walking techniques.
18. Wash hands.	18. Reduces transmission of microorganisms.
Sitting with Crutches	
19. Instruct client to back up to chair until it is felt with the back of the legs.	19. Allows for less turning, better stability, and increased safety.
20. Place both crutches in the nondominant hand and use the dominant hand to reach back to the chair.	20. Increases safety by giving the client an idea of how far away he or she is from the seat.
21. Instruct client to lower slowly into the chair.	21. Decreases pain and possible injuries.
Walking with a Cane	
22. Repeat Actions 1 to 6.	22. See Rationales 1 to 6.
23. Have the client push up from the sitting position while pushing down on the bed with arms.	23. Promotes autonomy as well as increases upper body strength.
24. Have the client stand at the bedside for a few moments with cane in hand opposite the affected leg.	24. Allows the client to gain balance. Allows more control of cane.
25. Assess the height of the cane. With the cane placed 6 inches ahead of the client's body, the top of the cane should be at wrist level with the arm bent 25% to 30% at the elbow.	25. A 25% to 30% bend at the elbow provides for better muscle strength and support than if the arm is straight.
26. Walk to the side and slightly behind the client, holding the gait belt if needed for stability.	26. Allows the nurse to provide stability or assistance if the client needs it.
Cane Gait	
27. Move the cane and the weaker leg forward at the same time for the same distance (Figure 29-12-3). Place weight on the weaker leg and the cane. Move the strong leg forward. Place weight on the strong leg.	27. The cane helps provide a wide base of support for the body when the weight is on the weaker leg.
Sitting with a Cane	
28. Have client turn around and back up to the chair. Have client grasp the arm of the chair with the free hand and lower self into the chair. Be sure to place the cane out of the way but within reach.	28. The cane provides additional support as client lowers self into the chair.
29. Consult with a physical therapist for clients learning to walk with a cane.	29. The physical therapist is the expert on the health care team for cane-walking techniques.
30. Wash hands.	30. Reduces transmission of microorganisms.

(Continues)

PROCEDURE 29-12 Assisting with Crutches, Cane, or Walker (Continued)

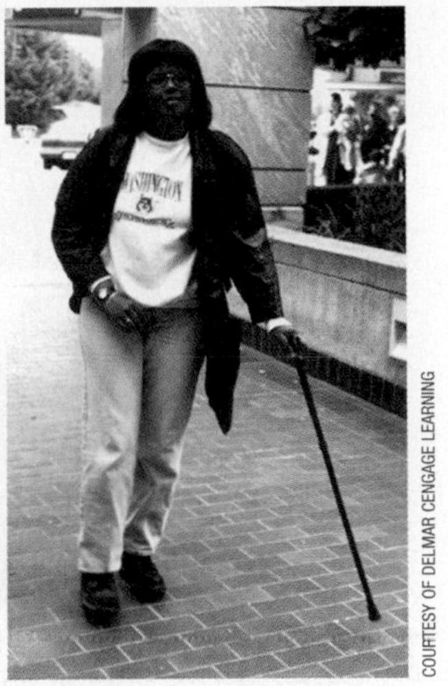

FIGURE 29-12-3 **Move the cane and the weaker leg forward. Cane should be in alignment with client.**

ACTION	RATIONALE
Walking with a Walker	
31. Repeat Actions 1 to 6.	31. See Rationales 1 to 6.
32. Place the walker in front of the client.	32. Positions the walker for use and provides stability when the client is standing.
33. Have the client put the nondominant hand on the front bar of the walker or on the hand grip for that hand, whichever is more comfortable. Then, using the dominant hand to push off from the bed and the nondominant hand for stabilization, help the client to an erect position.	33. Uses upper body strength and encourages independence.
34. Have the client transfer hand to the walker handgrips.	34. Allows the client to maintain balance while transferring weight.
35. Be sure the walker is adjusted so the handgrips are just below waist level and the client's arms are slightly bent at the elbow.	35. Provides maximum support from the arms while ambulating.
36. Walk to the side and slightly behind the client, holding the gait belt if needed for stability.	36. Provides stability or assistance if the client needs it.
Walker Gait	
37. Move the walker and the weaker leg forward at the same time (Figure 29-12-4). Place as much weight as possible or as allowed on the weaker leg, using the arms for supporting the rest of the weight. Move the strong leg forward and shift the weight to the strong leg (Figure 29-12-5).	37. Provides support for a weak or non–weight-bearing leg by using arm and upper body strength.
Sitting with a Walker	
38. Have the client turn around in front of the chair and back up until the back of the legs touch the chair. Have client place hands on the chair armrests, one hand at a time, then lower self into the chair using the armrests for support.	38. Using the armrests of the chair is a more stable support than using the walker.
39. Consult with a physical therapist for clients learning to walk with a walker.	39. The physical therapist is the expert on the health care team for walker techniques.
40. Wash hands.	40. Reduces transmission of microorganisms.

(Continues)

PROCEDURE 29-12 Assisting with Crutches, Cane, or Walker (Continued)

ACTION	RATIONALE

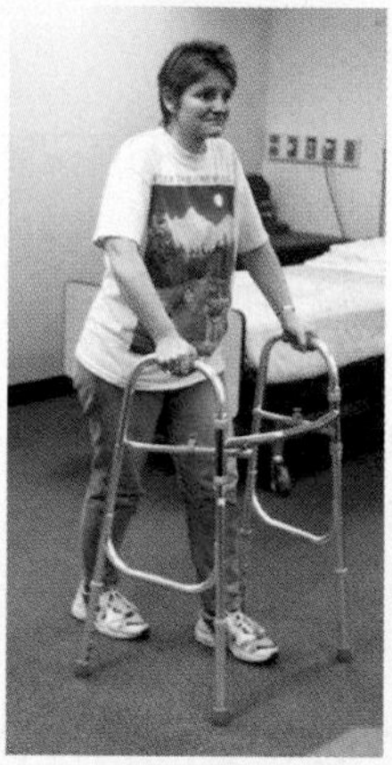

FIGURE 29-12-4 **Move the walker and the weaker leg forward.**

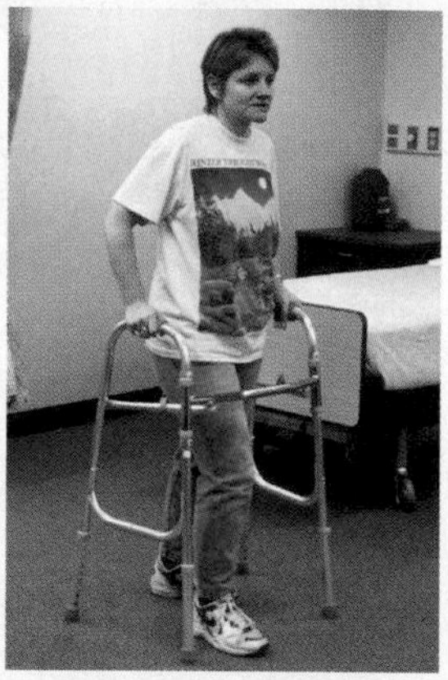

FIGURE 29-12-5 **Use the arms to support the rest of the weight and move strong leg forward.**

EVALUATION

- The client is able to demonstrate safe and independent ambulation with the assistance of crutches, a cane, or a walker.
- The client feels confident and safe while using the assistive device.

DOCUMENTATION

Nurses' Notes

- Type of device the client is using, the level of understanding regarding the use of the device, how far the client is able to walk using the device, and the client's response to the activity

Kardex

- Information that is pertinent to nurses or therapists regarding type of device or a particular client's needs

PROCEDURE 29-13 Turning and Positioning a Client

OVERVIEW

Clients are not always able to independently move and position themselves in bed. Proper turning and positioning allows the health care provider to make clients as comfortable as possible, prevent contractures and pressure sores, make portions of the client's body available for treatment or procedures, and allows clients greater access to their environment. There are three key concepts to remember when positioning a client: pressure, friction, and skin shear.

Any area that contacts the surface the client is lying on is a pressure site. Because of circulatory compromise, the pressure sites over bony prominences are at the highest risk of skin breakdown and ulceration. Always assess the blood flow to skin and tissue areas put under increased pressure when placing a client in a given position. When repositioning a client, be sure the sheets under the client are smooth. This helps prevent areas of increased pressure that could contribute to pressure sores.

Skin shear is caused when the skin is dragged across a hard surface. The deep layers of skin are torn by the resistance of being dragged. This damage to the skin can lead to skin breakdown and ulceration. To prevent skin shear, or friction burn from the sheets, do not drag a client across the bed. Lift the client into proper position or use a turning sheet.

(Continues)

PROCEDURE 29-13 Turning and Positioning a Client (Continued)

Friction is caused when the skin is dragged across a rough surface, thereby causing heat and damaging the skin's surface. Any damage to the skin's integrity can lead to infection and skin breakdown.

Clients who cannot reposition themselves must be repositioned at least every two hours and more frequently if they are uncomfortable, incontinent, or have poor circulation, fragile skin, decreased cognition, decreased sensation, or poor nutritional status. When repositioning a client, assess the skin for redness and integrity. Areas of redness should be resolved before the client is repositioned on that area. Areas of redness that do not resolve within 30 minutes after pressure relief should be documented. A plan to reposition the client more frequently may need to be instituted. Areas of prolonged redness are more likely to sustain tissue damage, as are tissue areas covering bony prominences. Hip, back, neck, or head conditions may require that a client be turned keeping the body in alignment, turning as one unit, as a log. This is called log rolling. Remember that proper body mechanics are essential to protect the caregiver's back and to ensure client safety.

ASSESSMENT

1. Assess the client's ability to move independently. **Determine if the client can assist with turning and repositioning.**
2. Assess the client's flexibility. **If clients have contractures or other flexibility limitations, their positions may need to be modified to allow for the restrictions.**
3. Assess the client's age, medical diagnosis, cognitive status, skin integrity, nutritional status, continence, altered sensation, as well as the overall condition of the musculoskeletal system. **Helps determine the client's potential for pressure sore development.**
4. Assess the physician's or qualified practitioner's orders for specific restrictions regarding client positioning **to ensure the correct positioning is implemented.**

POSSIBLE NURSING DIAGNOSES

Risk for Impaired Skin Integrity
Impaired Physical Mobility
Activity Intolerance
Acute Pain

PLANNING

Expected Outcomes

1. The client will maintain skin integrity without skin burns, pressure areas, or pressure ulcers.
2. The client will be comfortable as evident by verbal and nonverbal cues.

Equipment Needed

- Pillows
- Rolled blankets or towels
- Footboard
- Heel protectors
- Hand rolls
- Gloves (if chance of exposure to body fluids)

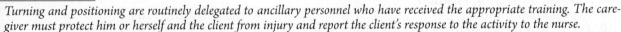

delegation tips

Turning and positioning are routinely delegated to ancillary personnel who have received the appropriate training. The caregiver must protect him or herself and the client from injury and report the client's response to the activity to the nurse.

IMPLEMENTATION—ACTION/RATIONALE

ACTION	RATIONALE
* Check client's identification band * Explain procedure before beginning *	
1. Wash hands.	1. Reduces the transmission of microorganisms.
2. Gather all necessary equipment. Provide for client privacy.	2. Ensures client dignity and allows for a smooth procedure.
3. Secure adequate assistance to safely complete task.	3. Prevents caregiver back and muscle strain as well as provides for client safety.
4. Adjust bed to comfortable working height. Lower side rail on side of bed from which you are assisting client.	4. Prevents caregiver back and muscle strain.
5. Follow proper body mechanics guidelines: When moving a client in bed, position the bed so that your legs are slightly bent at the knees and hips. Maintain the natural curves in your back while lifting. Position one foot slightly in front of	5. Prevents caregiver back injury and muscle strain and promotes client safety. Spreading feet to create a wide base helps prevent loss of balance.

(Continues)

PROCEDURE 29-13 Turning and Positioning a Client (Continued)

ACTION	RATIONALE
the other and spread feet apart to create a wide base for balance. When your arms are placed under the client, slowly lean backward onto your back leg using your body weight to help you lift the client to one side of the bed. Do not extend or rotate your back to move a client in bed. If you cannot move the client easily, always ask for and obtain assistance for both your and the client's safety (Figure 29-13-1). Be sure the floor is not slippery and that the bed is locked. Always use a turning sheet when rolling a client because this gives you better support and control of the client (Figure 29-13-2).	
6. Position drains, tubes, and IVs to accommodate for new client position.	6. Prevents accidental dislodgment and/or discomfort from movement by reduced mechanical tension.
7. Place or assist client into appropriate starting position. Monitor client status, and provide adequate rest breaks or support as necessary.	7. Prevents client injury.
Moving from Supine to Side-Lying Position	
8. Slide your hands underneath the client. Move the client to one side of the bed by lifting the client's body toward you in stages—first the upper trunk, then the lower trunk, and finally the legs. Lift the client's body; do not drag the client across the sheets. Move to other side of bed. Roll the client to side-lying position by placing the client's inside arm next to the client's body with the palm of the hand against the hip. Cross the client's outside arm and leg toward midline and log roll the client toward you using the client's outside shoulder and hip for leverage while maintaining stability and control of top arm and leg.	8. Prevents shearing of skin tissue. Maintains client body alignment. Protects caregiver's back and prevents muscle strain. Prevents client injury and shearing of skin tissue.
Maintaining Side-Lying Position	
9. Repeat Actions 1 to 8.	9. See Rationales 1 to 8.
10. Pillows may be placed to support the client's head and arms (Figure 29-13-3). An additional pillow	10. Provides support and comfort.

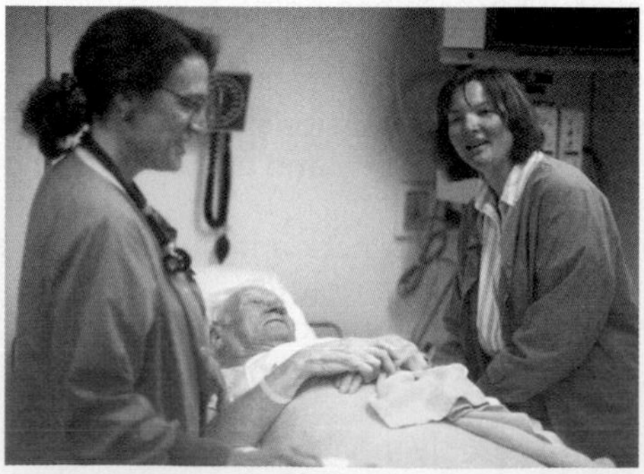

FIGURE 29-13-1 If the client is heavy or hard to move, always obtain assistance for both the client's and your safety.

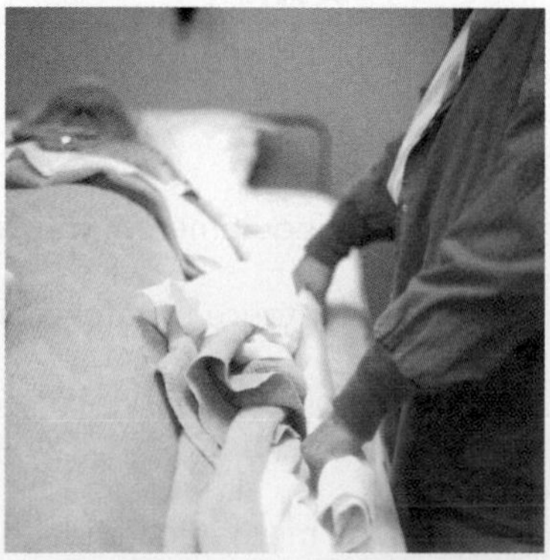

FIGURE 29-13-2 When rolling a client, use a turning sheet for better support and control.

(Continues)

PROCEDURE 29-13 Turning and Positioning a Client (Continued)

ACTION	RATIONALE

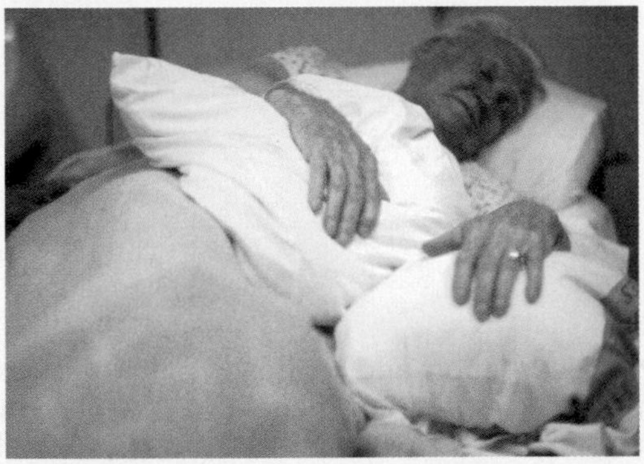

FIGURE 29-13-3 **Place pillows to support the head and arms.**

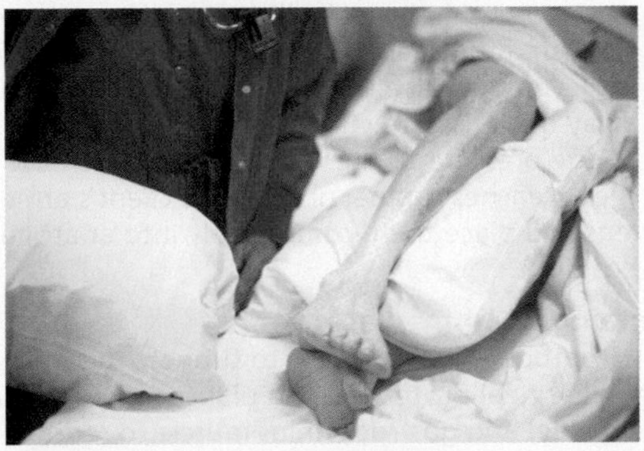

FIGURE 29-13-4 **Place pillows to support the leg, ankle, and foot.**

may be used to support the topside leg, and fully and equally support the thigh, knee, ankle, and foot (Figure 29-13-4). Move the lower arm forward slightly at the shoulder and bend the elbow for comfort. If the client is unstable, a pillow placed against the back will provide additional support and keep the client from rolling supine.

Moving from Side-Lying to Prone Position

ACTION	RATIONALE
11. Repeat Actions 1 to 8.	11. See Rationales 1 to 8.
12. Remove positioning towels, pillows, or other support devices. Assess whether the client's position in bed needs to be adjusted to accommodate the continued movement into prone. Move the client's inside arm next to the client's body with palm against hip. Roll the client onto the stomach using the shoulder and hip as key points of control. The head must be placed in a comfortable position to one side without excessive pressure to sensitive areas. Pillows under the trunk are placed as needed to relieve pressure and increase comfort. The client's arms are placed comfortably at the client's side and the legs are uncrossed with the feet approximately a foot apart.	12. Ensures comfort and safety in movement.

Maintaining Prone Position

ACTION	RATIONALE
13. A shallow pillow or a folded towel may be used to support the client's head comfortably as well as a pillow placed under the abdomen to support the back. An additional pillow may be placed under the lower leg to reduce the pressure of the toes and forefoot against the bed.	13. Provides support and comfort.

Moving from Prone to Supine Position

ACTION	RATIONALE
14. Repeat Actions 1 to 8.	14. See Rationales 1 to 8.
15. Remove positioning towels, pillows, or other supporting devices. Slide your hands underneath the client. Move the client segmentally to one side of the bed to accommodate the new position. Position the inside arm next to the client's body with the client's palm next to the hip. Roll the	15. Provides support and comfort.

(Continues)

PROCEDURE 29-13 Turning and Positioning a Client (Continued)

ACTION	RATIONALE
client to supine by log rolling the client toward you using the client's outside shoulder and hip for leverage. Have the client's face positioned away from the direction of the roll to prevent undue pressure to the face or neck. When the client reaches supine, uncross the client's arms and legs and place them comfortably into anatomic positions.	
Maintaining Supine Position	
16. A footboard may be used to support the foot as well as heel protectors or a pillow placed between the heel and gastrocnemius muscle to reduce the pressure on the heels. Assess and compare warmth, sensation, color, and movement of feet. To prevent excessive external rotation of the lower extremity, a trochanter roll is used. For comfort, additional pillows are used to support the client's head, arms, or lower back.	16. Provides support and comfort. Heel protectors and routine assessment of the feet help to prevent pressure sores. Trochanter rolls and pillows help to prevent displacement of the acetabulum (hip joint).
Log Rolling	
17. Repeat Actions 1 to 8.	17. See Rationales 1 to 8.
18. Use three nurses. Place a turning/draw sheet under client's head, back, and buttocks (if not already present).	18. Provides for client safety. Reduces shearing force.
19. Place pillow between client's legs.	19. Keeps legs in alignment with body.
20. Have client fold arms across chest.	20. Prevents getting the client's arms trapped or injured.
21. Roll up draw sheet on the far side until it is next to the client.	21. Provides support under the heavy parts of the client and places the nurses' hands close to the weight to be turned.
22. One nurse places hands under the client's far leg, another holds rolled draw sheet at client's buttocks, and third nurse holds rolled draw sheet at chest and shoulder level.	22. Ensures client is turned like a log, as a unit.
23. Nurse nearest the client's head gives the signal to turn: 1-2-3 turn.	23. Ensures a smooth, coordinated turn.
24. Tuck pillows at client's back and abdomen.	24. Helps maintain side-lying position.
25. Assess the client for comfort and proper alignment.	25. Comfort is subjective. Ensures alignment.
26. Procedure can be reversed to reposition client on back or opposite side.	26. Reduces pressure ulcer development.
27. Be sure to replace side rails to upright position as well as to lower bed to beginning position.	27. Provides for client safety.
28. Place call light within reach of the client.	28. Provides for client safety.
29. Move bedside table close to bed and place items of frequent use within reach of the client.	29. Provides for client safety.
30. Wash hands.	30. Reduces the transmission of microorganisms.

EVALUATION

- Safe and proper body alignment and movement were achieved for both client and caregiver.
- The client is comfortable in the new position as evident by verbal and nonverbal cues.
- The client's skin and underlying organs and tissues were protected from pressure, friction, and shear.

DOCUMENTATION

Nurses' Notes

- Client's new position and time of the position change
- Report or observation of pain, discomfort, or dyspnea
- Integumentary assessment, including color and integrity of skin and length of time redness persists over bony prominences

PROCEDURE 29-14 Moving a Client in Bed

OVERVIEW

Prolonged immobility is uncomfortable and presents an increased risk of many complications. Muscle wasting, clot formation, and skin breakdown are the most common risks associated with immobility. Clients who are unable to move themselves in bed or are only able to assist with moving in bed are at risk for discomfort and complications related to immobility. Often, clients' restlessness in bed will cause them to slide down toward the foot of the bed. This is especially true in beds where the head raises up to a Fowler's or semi-Fowler's position. If the client slides down toward the foot of the bed while the head is elevated, it leads to reduced respiratory effort, reduced lung capacity, and skin breakdown, thus impairing the client's recovery.

The nurse often moves a client to a more comfortable position. Repositioning a client is sometimes done by a single staff member, but often it requires two or more people to do this procedure safely.

ASSESSMENT

1. Assess the client's ability to assist with repositioning. Determine if the client can move with the aid of an overhead trapeze or the side rail. Judge how much assistance will be needed. **Determines safety for the client and the nurse and good body mechanics for the nurse.**
2. Assess the client's ability to understand and follow directions and assist and cooperate with the move. **Affects how the procedure is completed and client teaching.**
3. Assess the client's environment and bed for cleanliness. Has the client been restless, sweaty, or incontinent? Check to see if the sheets are turned or twisted. Tubes, lines, wires, traction, casts, or splints are moved carefully. **Affects how the procedure is completed. Affects what additional procedures are performed. Prepares the caregivers to keep tubes and equipment from becoming dislodged, tipped, or pulled.**

POSSIBLE NURSING DIAGNOSES

Impaired Physical Mobility
Activity Intolerance
Risk for Impaired Skin Integrity

PLANNING

Expected Outcomes

1. The client will be moved in bed without injury to self.
2. The client will be moved in bed without injury to the staff.
3. The client will report an increase in comfort following the move.
4. All tubes, lines, and drains will remain patent and intact.

Equipment Needed

- Hospital bed with side rails
- Trapeze if required
- Turn sheet or draw sheet

delegation tips

Turning and positioning is routinely delegated to ancillary personnel who have received appropriate training. The caregiver protects himself and the client from injury and reports the client's activity response to the nurse.

IMPLEMENTATION—ACTION/RATIONALE

ACTION	RATIONALE
* Check client's identification band * Explain procedure before beginning *	
Moving a Client Up in Bed with One Nurse	
1. Wash hands.	1. Reduces the transmission of microorganisms.
2. Elevate bed to just below waist height. Lower head of bed if tolerated by client. Lower side rails on the side where you are standing.	2. Lessens strain on nurse's back muscles.
3. Remove the pillow and place it against the headboard.	3. Prevents having to move against the pillow. Provides padding of the headboard if the client should be moved too high in the bed.
4. Have client hold on to the overhead trapeze, if available (Figure 29-14-1).	4. Promotes client autonomy by allowing the client to assist with the move.

(Continues)

PROCEDURE 29-14 Moving a Client in Bed (Continued)

ACTION	RATIONALE

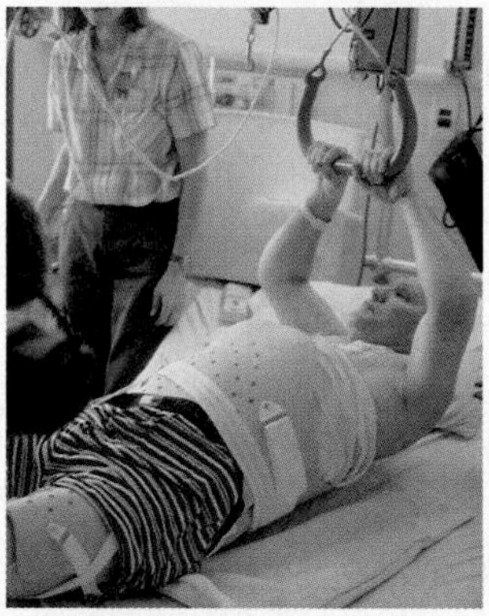

FIGURE 29-14-1 Have client hold onto the overhead trapeze, if one is available, to assist in the move.

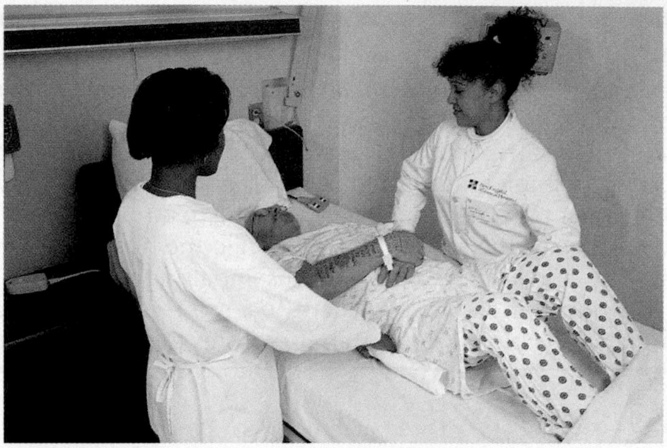

FIGURE 29-14-2 Have the client bend the knees and place feet on the bed.

ACTION	RATIONALE
5. Have the client bend the knees and place the feet flat on the bed if able (Figure 29-14-2).	5. Allows the client to assist in the move; promotes client autonomy.
6. Stand at an angle to the head of the bed, feet apart, knees bent, feet toward the head of the bed.	6. Promotes good body mechanics.
7. Slide one hand and arm under the client's shoulder, the other under the client's thigh.	7. Distributes the client's weight more evenly. Promotes good lifting technique.
8. Rock forward toward the head of the bed, lifting the client with you. Simultaneously have the client push with the legs.	8. Allows a smooth motion to lift the client. Client assistance lessens strain on nurse's back muscles; promotes client autonomy.
9. If the client has a trapeze, have the client pull up holding onto the trapeze as you move the client upward in bed.	9. Client assistance lessens strain on nurse's back muscles; promotes client autonomy.
10. Repeat these steps until the client is moved up high enough in bed.	10. Large or very immobile clients are often not moved far enough in one step.
11. Return the client's pillow under the head.	11. Promotes client comfort.
12. Elevate head of bed, if tolerated by client.	12. Promotes comfort; facilitates eating and drinking; facilitates communication.
13. Assess client for comfort.	13. Comfort is subjective.
14. Adjust the client's bedclothes as needed for comfort.	14. Promotes comfort.
15. Lower bed and elevate side rails.	15. Promotes client safety.
16. Wash hands.	16. Reduces the transmission of microorganisms.
Moving a Client Up in Bed with Two or More Nurses	
17. Wash hands and apply gloves if needed.	17. Reduces the transmission of microorganisms.
18. Elevate bed to just below waist height. Lower head of bed if tolerated by client. Lower side rails.	18. Lessens strain on nurses' back muscles.
19. With two nurses, place turn/draw sheet under client's back and head.	19. Reduces shearing force, which can precipitate skin breakdown.
20. Roll up the draw sheet on each side until it is next to the client (refer to Figure 29-14-3).	20. Provides support under the heavy parts of the body and places the nurse's hands close to the weight to be moved.
21. Follow previous Actions 3 to 5.	21. See Rationales 3 to 5.
22. The nurses stand on either side of the bed, at an angle to the head of the bed, with knees flexed, feet apart in a wide stance.	22. Promotes good body mechanics.

(Continues)

PROCEDURE 29-14 Moving a Client in Bed (Continued)

ACTION	RATIONALE

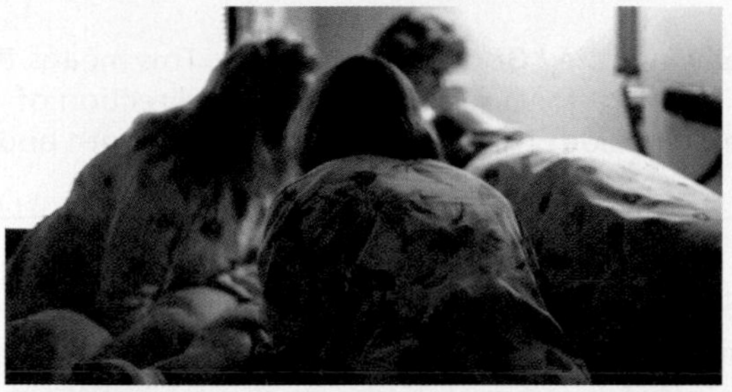

FIGURE 29-14-3 At the signal from the lead nurse, lift and pull in one smooth motion. A gentle, smooth, coordinated motion does not jar or injure the client.

ACTION	RATIONALE
23. The nurses hold their elbows as close as possible to their bodies.	23. Allows the muscles of the torso to assist the arm muscles in bearing and moving the weight of the client.
24. The lead nurse gives the signal to move: 1-2-3 go. The nurses lift the turn/draw sheet off the bed and toward the head of the bed in one smooth motion. Simultaneously, the client pushes with the legs or pulls using the trapeze. Nurses take care to move the client with a gentle, smooth, coordinated motion so as not to jar or injure the client.	24. Allows a smooth motion to lift the client. Client assistance lessens strain on the nurses' back muscles; promotes client autonomy.
25. Repeat previous Actions 10 to 16.	25. See previous Rationales 10 to 16.

EVALUATION

- The client was moved without injury to self or staff.
- The client reported an increase in comfort following the move.
- All tubes, lines, and drains remained intact.

DOCUMENTATION

Nurses' Notes

- Time and position the client was moved
- Unusual findings

PROCEDURE 29-15 Transferring from Bed to Wheelchair, Commode, or Chair

OVERVIEW

Client activity is an important part of the healing process. Activity improves muscle tone, increases venous return to the heart, and stimulates peristalsis. Moving a client from the bed to a chair is an important part of client activity.

Moving a client from the bed to a chair, wheelchair, commode, or stretcher is called a transfer. Transferring a client requires good planning to avoid injury to the client and the nurse. When transferring a client, consider the client's ability to assist with the transfer. If the client is unable to provide any assistance or is large, one or more staff members are needed to help perform the transfer safely.

The most frequent complication in transferring a client is falling during the transfer. Gait belts provide client safety during a transfer. If a client starts to fall during the transfer, lower him or her gently to the floor, making sure the head does not strike anything. If a client does fall, obtain assistance and perform a thorough assessment of the client before moving him or her.

Another possible hazard in client transfers is pulling on or dislodging indwelling tubes or catheters. Think ahead about ways tubes will move with the transfer and try to avoid snagging them. Take care to appropriately anchor all tubes and catheters before transferring a client.

Clients are also at risk of damage to their skin during a transfer. Sliding across the sheets, side rails, and wheelchair armrest can bruise or injure the client. Use a transfer board or pad any sharp exposed areas to help prevent injury to the client.

(Continues)

PROCEDURE 29-15 Transferring from Bed to Wheelchair, Commode, or Chair (Continued)

Be sure the client is wearing shoes or slippers with firm, nonslip soles when transferring a client. Even if the client is standing only briefly, the feet need protecting from potential injury and contamination from the floor and the client from slipping.

When transferring a client with weakness on one side of the body, use the "Good to go" maxim. This means that the client needs to lead off with the "good" or strong side of the body. Perform the transfer in the direction of the good side, so the client pivots and supports the weight on the good side. This allows maximum strength and stability on the client's part.

ASSESSMENT

1. Assess the client's current level of mobility. Determine how much the client is able to assist with the transfer. Assess for pain or confusion, which might impair ability to assist. Check for a "weak" side. **Affects how the procedure is completed.**
2. Assess for any impediments to mobility, including casts, drainage tubes, catheters, IVs, or intubation. **Affects how the procedure will be carried out. Prepares caregivers to keep tubes and equipment from becoming dislodged, tipping, or pulling.**
3. Assess the client's level of understanding and anxiety regarding the procedure. **Affects how the procedure is completed and client teaching.**
4. Assess the client's environment. Assess the available space for maneuvering the wheelchair to the bed. **Affects how the procedure is completed and safety and good body mechanics for caregivers.**
5. Assess the equipment. Check the bed and chair height. See whether they are adjustable. Check for chair footings and wheelchair brakes. **Affects safety for client and caregivers.**

POSSIBLE NURSING DIAGNOSES

Impaired Physical Mobility
Activity Intolerance
Risk for Injury

PLANNING

Expected Outcomes

1. The client will be transferred from the bed to the wheelchair, commode, or chair without pain or injury.
2. Drainage tubes, IVs, or other devices will be intact.
3. The client's skin will be intact and undamaged.

Equipment Needed

- Bed
- Wheelchair, chair, or commode
- Any splints, braces, or supportive equipment specific to the client
- Shoes or slippers with nonskid soles
- Gait belt
- Transfer board (if necessary)

delegation tips

Assisting a client from a bed to a wheelchair, commode, or chair is a skill routinely delegated to properly trained ancillary personnel.

IMPLEMENTATION—ACTION/RATIONALE

* Check client's identification band * Explain procedure before beginning *

ACTION	RATIONALE
1. Wash hands.	1. Reduces transmission of microorganisms.
2. Assess client for ability to assist with the transfer and for presence of cognitive or sensory deficits.	2. Allows planning regarding the amount of assistance and cooperation to expect from the client.
3. Lock the bed in position.	3. Prevents the bed from rolling during the procedure.
4. Place any splints, braces, or other devices on the client.	4. Provides support and prevents injury to the client.
5. Place the client's shoes or slippers on the client's feet.	5. Provides a nonslip surface for stability.
6. Lower the height of the bed to lowest possible position.	6. Reduces distance client has to step down, thus decreasing risk of injury.

(Continues)

PROCEDURE 29-15 Transferring from Bed to Wheelchair, Commode, or Chair (Continued)

ACTION	RATIONALE
7. Slowly raise the head of the bed if this is not contraindicated by the client's condition.	7. Minimizes lifting.
8. Place one arm under the client's legs and one arm behind the client's back. Slowly pivot the client so the client's legs are dangling over the edge of the bed and the client is in a sitting position on the edge of the bed (Figure 29-15-1).	8. Supports the client while sitting him or her upright.
9. Allow client to dangle for 2 to 5 minutes. Help support client if necessary (Figure 29-15-2).	9. Allows time for assessing client's response to sitting; reduces possibility of orthostatic hypotension.
10. Bring the chair or wheelchair close to the side of the bed. Place it at a 45-degree angle to the bed. If the client has a weaker side, place the chair or wheelchair on the client's strong side.	10. Minimizes transfer distance. Allows the client to pivot on the stronger leg.
11. Lock wheelchair brakes and elevate the foot pedals. For chairs, lock brakes if available.	11. Provides stability.
12. If using a gait belt to assist the client, place it around the client's waist.	12. Provides a secure handhold for the nurse during the transfer.
13. Assist client to side of bed until feet are firmly on the floor and slightly apart.	13. Moves client into proper position for transfer. Provides stable footing for client.
14. Grasp the sides of the gait belt or place your hands just below the client's axilla. Using a wide stance, bend your knees and assist the client to a standing position.	14. Wide stance increases nurse stability and minimizes strain on the back. Avoids putting pressure directly on the axilla, and risking nerve damage or shoulder subluxation.
15. Standing close to the client, pivot until the client's back is toward the chair.	15. Moves client into proper position to be seated.
16. Instruct the client to place hands on the arm supports, or place the client's hands on the arm supports of the chair.	16. Allows client to gain balance and judge distance to seat.
17. Bend at the knees and ease the client into a sitting position.	17. Increases stability and minimizes strain on back.
18. Assist client to maintain proper posture. Support weak side with pillow if needed.	18. Increases client comfort.
19. Secure the safety belt, place client's feet on feet pedals, and release brakes if you will be moving the client immediately. Make sure tubes and lines, arms, and hands are not pinched or caught between the client and the chair (Figure 29-15-3).	19. Ensures client safety; prepares client for movement.

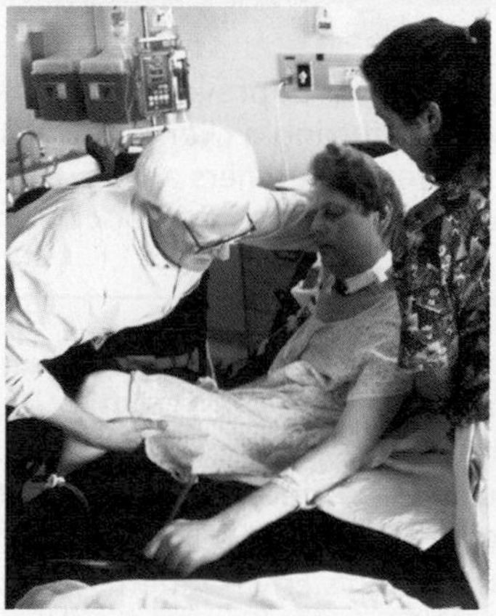

COURTESY OF DELMAR CENGAGE LEARNING

FIGURE 29-15-1 Pivot the client to a sitting position on the edge of the bed.

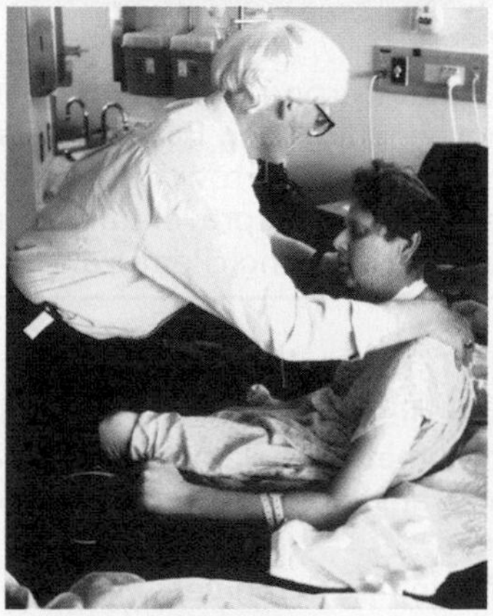

COURTESY OF DELMAR CENGAGE LEARNING

FIGURE 29-15-2 Support the client, if needed, while the client adjusts to the sitting position.

(Continues)

PROCEDURE 29-15 Transferring from Bed to Wheelchair, Commode, or Chair (Continued)

ACTION	RATIONALE
If a client is sitting in a wheelchair, position the footrests in a position of client comfort (Figure 26-15-4); if in a chair, offer a footstool if available.	
20. Wash hands.	20. Reduces the transmission of microorganisms.

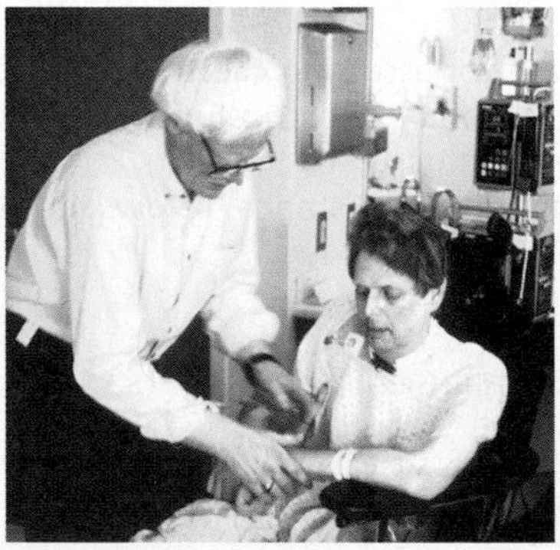

FIGURE 29-15-3 **Once the client is moved, make sure skin, tubing, or equipment is not pinched between the client and the chair.**

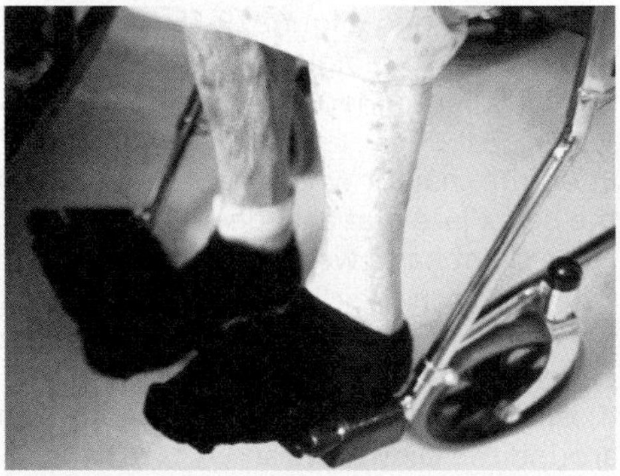

FIGURE 29-15-4 **Position the wheelchair footrests or use a footstool if the client is sitting in a chair.**

EVALUATION
- Client was transferred from the bed to the wheelchair without pain or injury.
- Drainage tubes, IVs, or other devices remain intact.
- Client's skin is intact and undamaged.

DOCUMENTATION
Nurses' Notes
- Client's tolerance of the activity, any aids that were required, how much assistance was required, and the client's ability to assist
- Unusual events during the transfer

PROCEDURE 29-16 Transferring from Bed to Stretcher

OVERVIEW
Some clients are not strong enough to sit erect in a wheelchair or have some injury that prevents them from sitting, so they are moved while lying flat. The most commonly used equipment for transferring a client is a stretcher (gurney). A stretcher is a narrow, cartlike bed that rolls on wheels. For client safety, stretchers are equipped with side rails or safety straps to prevent accidental falls during transport. The wheels on a stretcher lock to prevent accidental movement during client transfers.

ASSESSMENT
1. Assess the client's current level of mobility. **Knowing whether a client is able to assist with the transfer affects how the transfer is performed.**
2. Assess for injury. **Caregivers keep the client in the same alignment as much as possible.**
3. Assess for any impediments to mobility such as a cast, drainage tubes, IVs, or intubation. **This affects how the transfer is performed.**
4. Assess the client's level of understanding of the procedure. **This affects client comfort, anxiety, and cooperation.**
5. Assess the client's environment. Assess how close the stretcher will move to the bed and the height of the bed. **This allows for a safe transfer. Plan for good body mechanics.**

(Continues)

PROCEDURE 29-16 Transferring from Bed to Stretcher (Continued)

6. Make sure the stretcher is safe to use. Check for working brakes, side rails, safety straps that are intact and usable, and an IV pole attachment if needed. **This allows for a safe transfer. Plan for good body mechanics.**

POSSIBLE NURSING DIAGNOSES

Impaired Physical Mobility
Activity Intolerance

PLANNING

Expected Outcomes

1. The client will be transferred from the bed to the stretcher without pain or injury.
2. Drainage tubes, IVs, or other devices will remain intact.
3. The client's skin will be intact and undamaged.

Equipment Needed

Transferring a Client with Minimum Assistance

- Bed
- Stretcher

Transferring a Client with Maximum Assistance

- Bed
- Stretcher
- Pillows
- Transfer/slider boards
- Lift sheet
- Other qualified personnel to assist

delegation tips

Assisting a client from a bed to a stretcher is a skill routinely delegated to properly trained ancillary personnel.

IMPLEMENTATION—ACTION/RATIONALE

ACTION	RATIONALE
* Check client's identification band * Explain procedure before beginning *	
Minimum Assistance	
1. Wash hands.	1. Reduces the transmission of microorganisms.
2. Raise the height of bed to 1 inch higher than the stretcher and lock brakes of bed.	2. Reduces distance nurse must bend, thus preventing back strain; prevents bed from moving.
3. Instruct client to move to side of bed close to stretcher. Lower side rails of bed and stretcher. Leave side rails on opposite side up.	3. Decreases risk of client falling.
4. Stand at outer side of stretcher and push it toward bed.	4. Diminishes the gap between bed and stretcher; secures the stretcher position.
5. Instruct client to move onto stretcher with assistance as needed.	5. Promotes client independence.
6. Cover client with sheet or bath blanket.	6. Promotes comfort; protects privacy.
7. Elevate side rails on stretcher and secure safety belts about client. Release brakes of stretcher.	7. Prevents falls.
8. Stand at head of stretcher to guide it when pushing.	8. Pushing, not pulling, ensures proper body mechanics.
9. Wash hands.	9. Reduces the transmission of microorganisms.
Maximum Assistance	
10. Repeat Actions 1 and 2.	10. See Rationales 1 and 2.
11. Assess amount of assistance required for transfer. Usually 2 to 4 staff members are required for the maximum-assisted transfer.	11. Promotes client independence; ensures that enough staff are present before beginning transfer.
12. Lock wheels of bed and stretcher.	12. Prevents falls.
13. Have one nurse stand close to client's head.	13. Supports client's head during the move.
14. Log roll the client (keep in straight alignment) and place a lift sheet under the client's back, trunk, and upper legs. The lift sheet can extend under the head if client lacks head control abilities.	14. Prevents flexion and rotation of client's hips and spine; maintains correct body alignment.

(Continues)

29-16 Transferring from Bed to Stretcher (Continued)

ACTION	RATIONALE
15. Empty all drainage bags (e.g., T-tube, Hemovac, Jackson–Pratt). Record amounts. Secure drainage system to client's gown before transfer.	15. Decreases possibility of spills; prevents dislodging of tubes.
16. Move client to edge of bed near stretcher. Lift up and over to avoid dragging.	16. Prevents dragging, which causes shearing force.
17. Because the client is now on the side of the bed, without the side rail up, the nurse on nonstretcher side of bed holds the stretcher side of the lift sheet up (by reaching across the client's chest) to prevent the client from falling onto the stretcher or off the bed.	17. Protects the client from falling.
18. Place pillow and slider board overlapping the bed and stretcher (Figure 29-16-1).	18. Protects head from injury. Slider board eases movement of the client.
19. Have staff members grasp edges of lift sheet. Be sure to use good body mechanics (Figure 29-16-2).	19. Provides surface for client to slide on. Prevents dragging and shearing.
20. On the count of three, have staff members pull lift sheet and the client onto the stretcher.	20. Working in unison makes the overall job easier and prevents staff injury.
21. Position client on stretcher, place pillow under head, and cover with a sheet or bath blanket.	21. Promotes comfort and provides for privacy.
22. Secure safety belts and elevate side rails of stretcher.	22. Prevents falls.
23. If IV is present, move it from bed IV pole to stretcher IV pole after client transfer.	23. Prevents tubing from being pulled and IV from being dislodged.
24. Wash hands.	24. Reduces the transmission of microorganisms.

EVALUATION

- The client was transferred from the bed to the stretcher without pain or injury.
- All drainage tubes, IVs, or other devices remain intact.
- Assess whether the client's skin is intact and undamaged.

DOCUMENTATION

Kardex

- Amount of assistance the transfer required and amount the client was able to assist

Nurses' Notes

- Time, date, reason for transfer, type of transfer, and how the client tolerated the activity

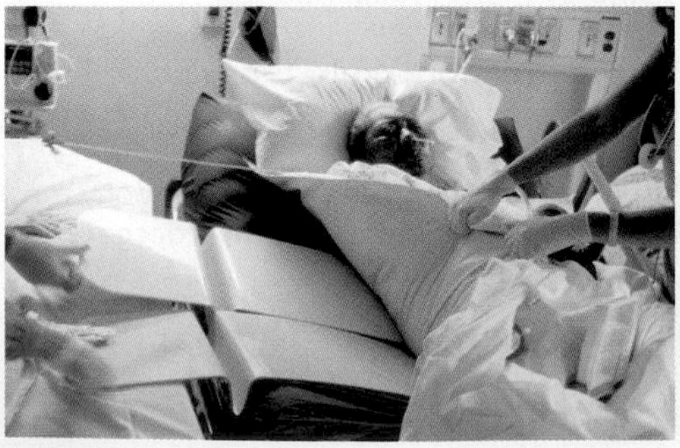

FIGURE 29-16-1 Place pillow and slider board overlapping the bed and stretcher.

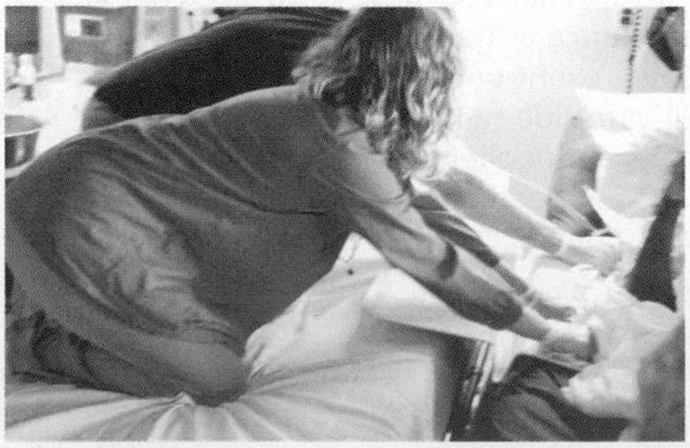

FIGURE 29-16-2 Firmly grasp edges of lift sheet.

PROCEDURE 29-17 Bed Making: Unoccupied Bed

OVERVIEW

After the client takes a bath, clean linens are placed on the bed to promote comfort and decrease transmission of microorganisms. If the client is able to get out of bed, assist the client to a chair and proceed with making the bed. After surgery, the client is returned to a clean bed with the linens folded to the foot of the bed to promote easy client transfer.

ASSESSMENT

1. Assess your equipment. Check for all linens necessary to change the bed. Check for a dirty linen hamper. **Facilitates a smooth procedure.**
2. Assess whether the bed needs cleaning before placing clean sheets on it. **Reduces the transmission of microorganisms.**
3. Assess the client's needs in the bed. Check for profuse drainage, incontinence, or special needs for comfort or skin integrity. **Determines how the procedure is performed.**
4. Assess the client's ability to be out of bed in a safe place while changing linens. **Assures client safety.**

POSSIBLE NURSING DIAGNOSIS

Risk for Impaired Skin Integrity

PLANNING

Expected Outcomes

1. The client will have clean linens on the bed.
2. The clean linens will be appropriate to the client's needs and condition.

Equipment Needed

- Bottom sheet (fitted, if available)
- Top sheet
- Protective disposable pad
- Draw sheet (regular top sheet may be used)
- Blanket
- Spread
- Pillowcase (each pillow on the bed)
- Mattress pad (optional)
- Antiseptic solution, washcloth, and towel
- Laundry bag
- Nonsterile gloves

delegation tips

Bed making is usually delegated to ancillary personnel. Their instruction should include safety precautions for themselves and the client, and understanding the appropriate use of Standard Precautions.

IMPLEMENTATION—ACTION/RATIONALE

* Wash hands * Check client's identification band * Explain procedure before beginning *

ACTION	RATIONALE
1. Place hamper by client's door if linen bags are not available. Assess condition of blanket and/or bedspread.	1. Provides for proper disposal of soiled linens. Allows for organization of supplies.
2. Gather linens and gloves. Place linens on a clean, dry surface in reverse order of usage at the client's bedside (pillowcases, top sheet, draw sheet, bottom sheet).	2. Provides easy access to items.
3. Inquire about the client's toileting needs and attend as necessary.	3. Provides for client comfort and prevents interruptions during bed making.
4. Assist client to a safe, comfortable chair.	4. Increases client's comfort and decreases risk of falls.
5. Apply gloves.	5. Reduces risk of infection from soiled, contaminated linens.
6. Position bed: flat, side rails down, adjust height to waist level.	6. Promotes good body mechanics and decreases back strain.
7. Remove and fold blanket and/or bedspread. If clean and reusable, place on clean work area.	7. Keeps reusable bed linens clean.

(Continues)

PROCEDURE 29-17 Bed Making: Unoccupied Bed (Continued)

ACTION	RATIONALE
8. Remove soiled pillowcases by grasping the closed end with one hand and slipping the pillow out with the other. Place the soiled cases on top of the soiled sheet, and place the pillows on clean work area.	8. Allows easy removal of the pillowcases without contamination of uniform by soiled linens and keeps pillows clean.
9. Remove soiled linens: Start on the side of the bed closest to you; free the bottom sheet and mattress pad (if used) by lifting the mattress and rolling soiled linens to the middle of the bed. Go to the other side of the bed, repeat action.	9. Prevents tearing and fanning of linens. Linens are folded from cleanest area to most soiled to prevent contamination.
10. Fold (do not fan or flap) soiled linens: head of bed to middle, foot of bed to middle. Place in linen bag, keeping soiled linens away from uniform.	10. Fanning or flapping linens increases the number of microorganisms in the air. Folding linens reduces the risk of transmission of infection to others.
11. Check mattress. If the mattress is soiled, clean it with an antiseptic solution and dry it thoroughly.	11. Reduces the transmission of microorganisms.
12. Remove gloves, wash hands, and apply a second pair of clean gloves (when appropriate).	12. Reduces the transmission of microorganisms to clean linens.
13. Open the clean mattress pad lengthwise onto the bed. Unfold half the pad's width to the center crease and smooth the pad flat. If there are elastic bands to hold the pad in place, slide them under the corners of the mattress.	13. Facilitates making bed in an organized, time-saving manner by not having to go from one side of the bed to the other.
14. Proceed with placing the bottom sheet onto the mattress. Linens differ from facility to facility. Bottom sheets may be fitted or they may be flat. Proceed to the appropriate action for the linen available.	14. Use linen available at the facility.
Fitted Bottom Sheet	
15. Position yourself diagonally toward the head of the bed.	15. Ensures good body mechanics and efficient procedure.
16. Start at the head with seamed side of the fitted sheet toward the mattress.	16. Placement of seamed side toward mattress prevents irritation to the client's skin.
17. Lift the mattress corner with your hand closest to the bed; with your other hand, pull and tuck the fitted sheet over the mattress corner; secure at the head of the bed.	17. Prevents straining of back muscles; decreases the chance that the sheet will pull out from under the mattress.
18. Pull and tuck the fitted sheet over the mattress corners at the foot of the bed.	18. Prevents straining of back muscles; decreases the chance that the sheet will pull out from under the mattress.
Flat Regular Sheet	
19. Unfold the bottom sheet with the seamed side toward the mattress. Align the bottom edge of the sheet with the edge of the mattress at the foot of the bed.	19. Placement of the seamed side toward the mattress prevents irritation to the client's skin. Ensure proper placement of the sheet so that it can be tightly secured at the top and on both sides of the bed.
20. Allow the sheet to hang 10 inches (25 cm) over the mattress on the side and at the top of the bed.	20. Proper placement of linens ensures adequate sheeting for all sides of the bed.
21. Position yourself diagonally toward the head of the bed. Lift the top of the mattress corner with the hand closest to the bed and smoothly tuck the sheet under the mattress.	21. Prevents straining of back muscles; decreases the chance that the sheet will pull out from under the mattress.
22. Miter the corner at the head of the bed using the following technique (Figure 29-17-1).	22. Secures sheet tightly to the mattress, with the triangular fold providing a smooth tuck to keep the linen in place.
23. Face the side of bed and lift and lay the edge of the sheet onto the bed to form a triangular fold.	23. Forms the base for the tuck.

(Continues)

PROCEDURE 29-17 Bed Making: Unoccupied Bed (Continued)

ACTION	RATIONALE

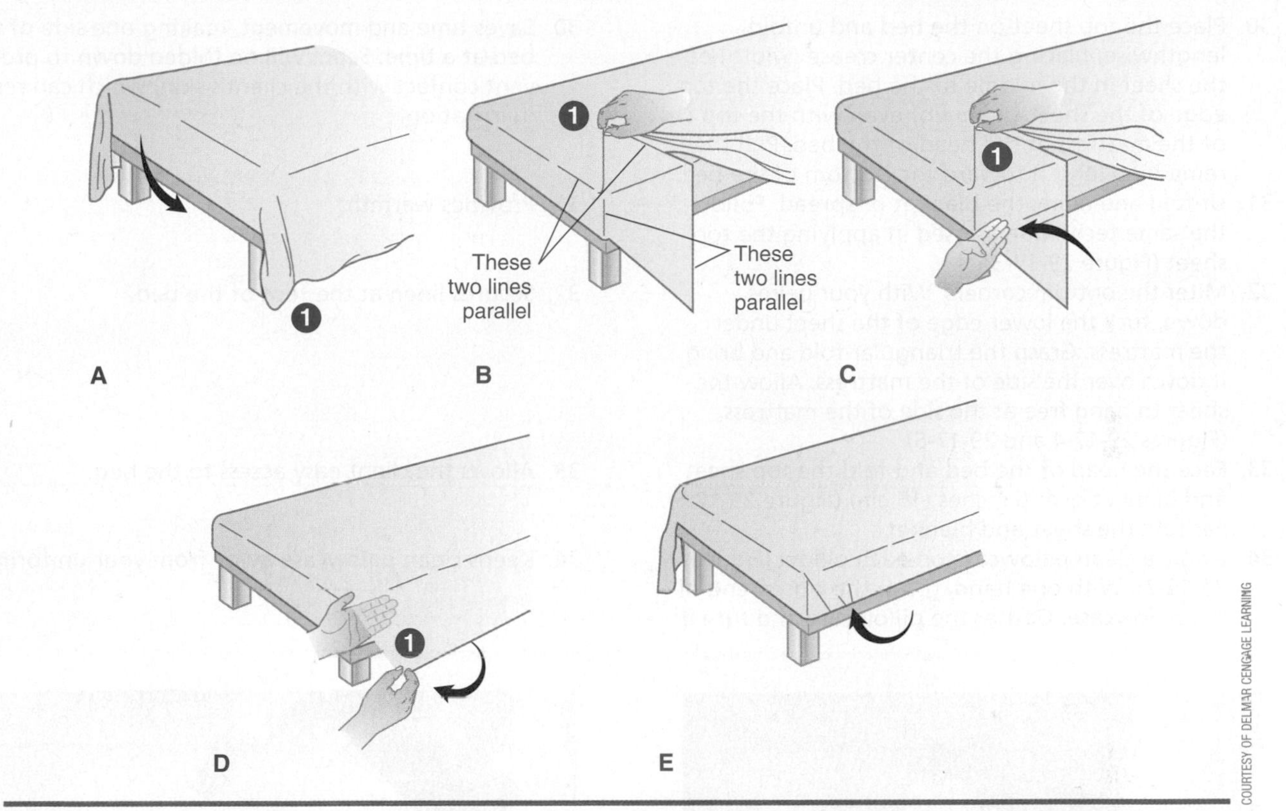

FIGURE 29-17-1 Steps in making a mitered corner; *A,* Tuck the lower edge of the sheet under the mattress; *B,* Grasp the triangular point of the sheet and raise it parallel to the edge of the mattress; *C,* Tuck the sheet that hangs below the mattress under the mattress; *D,* Bring the triangular point down alongside the bed; E, Tuck the sheet under the mattress with palms down.

ACTION	RATIONALE
24. With your palms down, tuck the lower edge of sheet (hanging free at the side of the mattress) under the mattress.	24. Forms the first half of the tuck.
25. Grasp the triangular fold; bring it down over the side of the mattress. Allow the sheet to hang free at the side of the mattress.	25. Will form the final portion of the mitered corner when tucked in.
26. Place the draw sheet on the bottom sheet and unfold it to the middle crease (Figure 29-17-2).	26. Provides a sheet to lift and move the client in bed without having to use the bottom sheet and remake the bed. Helps to keep the bottom sheet clean.
27. Face the side of the bed, palms of hands down. Tuck both the bottom and draw sheets under the mattress. Ensure that the bottom sheet is tucked smoothly under the mattress all the way to the foot of the bed.	27. Keeps sheet taut, in place, and wrinkle-free, thereby decreasing the risk of skin irritation.
28. Go to the other side of the bed, unfold the bottom sheet, and repeat the actions used to apply the mattress pad and bottom sheet.	28. Unfolding decreases air current; air currents can spread microorganisms.
29. Unfold the draw sheet, if used, and grasp the free-hanging sides of both the bottom and draw sheets. Pull toward you, keeping your back straight, and with a firm grasp (sheets taut) tuck both sheets under the mattress. Use your arms and open palms to extend the linen under the mattress. Place the protective pad on the bottom sheet.	29. Uses your body's weight in pulling the sheet taut and prevents strain on your back muscles.

(Continues)

PROCEDURE 29-17 Bed Making: Unoccupied Bed (Continued)

ACTION	RATIONALE
30. Place the top sheet on the bed and unfold lengthwise, placing the center crease (width) of the sheet in the middle of the bed. Place the top edge of the sheet (seam up) even with the top of the mattress at the head of the bed. Pull the remaining length toward the bottom of the bed.	30. Saves time and movement, making one side of the bed at a time. Seam will be folded down to prevent contact with the client's skin, which can result in irritation.
31. Unfold and apply the blanket or spread. Follow the same technique as used in applying the top sheet (Figure 29-17-3).	31. Provides warmth.
32. Miter the bottom corners. With your palms down, tuck the lower edge of the sheet under the mattress. Grasp the triangular fold and bring it down over the side of the mattress. Allow the sheet to hang free at the side of the mattress (Figures 29-17-4 and 29-17-5).	32. Secures linen at the foot of the bed.
33. Face the head of the bed and fold the top sheet and blanket over 6 inches (15 cm) (Figure 29-17-6). Fanfold the sheet and blanket	33. Allows the client easy access to the bed.
34. Apply a clean pillowcase on each pillow (Figure 29-15-7). With one hand, grasp the closed end of the pillowcase. Gather the pillowcase and turn it	34. Keeps clean pillowcase away from your uniform.

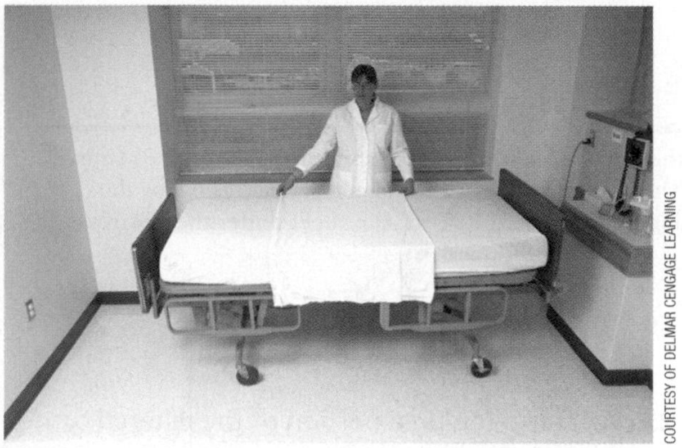

FIGURE 29-17-2 The draw sheet is placed on top of the bottom sheet and may be used as a turning sheet.

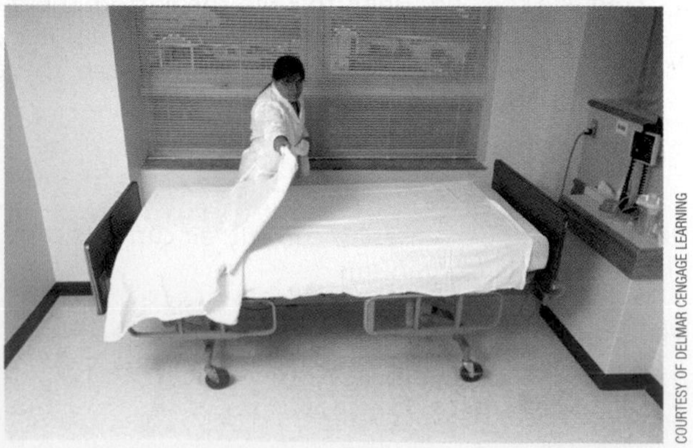

FIGURE 29-17-3 Place the blanket or spread over the top sheet.

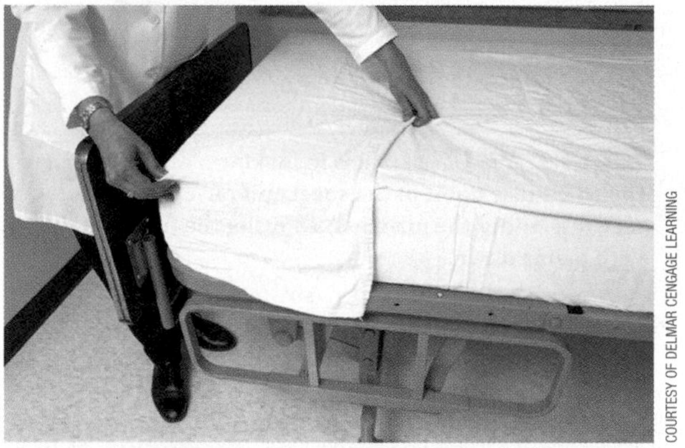

FIGURE 29-17-4 Lift and lay the edge of the sheet and blanket on the bed to form a triangular fold.

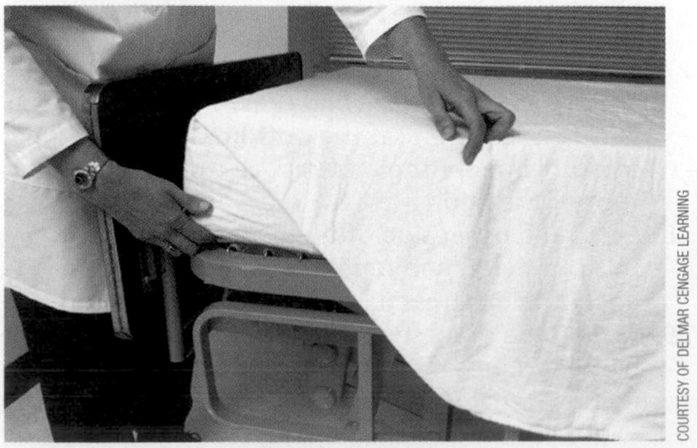

FIGURE 29-17-5 Bring the triangular fold down and let it hang freely at the side of the mattress.

(Continues)

PROCEDURE 29-17 Bed Making: Unoccupied Bed (Continued)

ACTION | **RATIONALE**

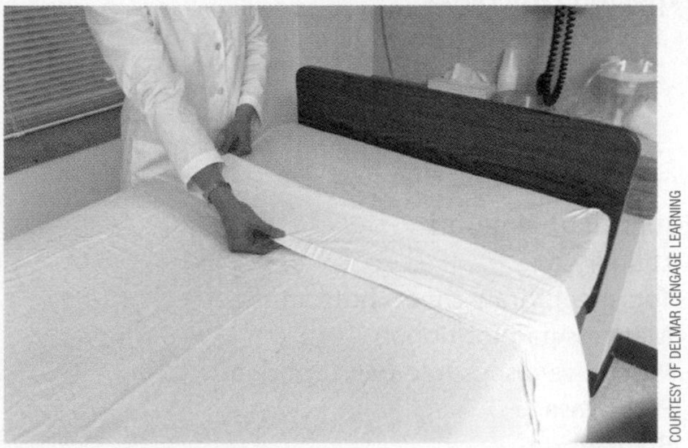

FIGURE 29-17-6 **Fold a cuff with the top sheet and blanket.**

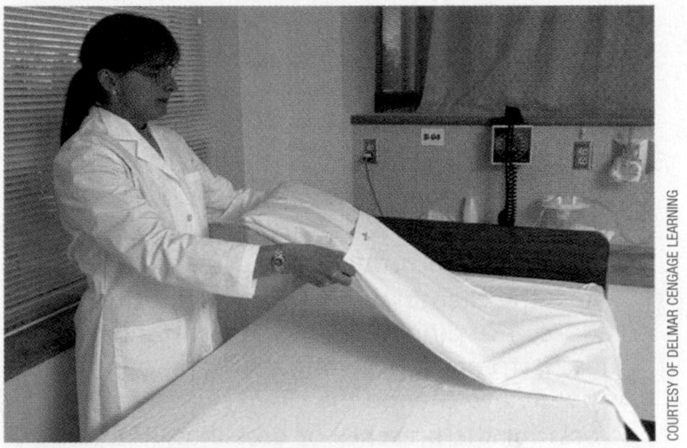

FIGURE 29-17-7 **A quick method of applying a clean pillowcase on a pillow.**

ACTION	RATIONALE
inside out over hand. With same hand, grasp the middle of one end of the pillow. With the other hand, pull the case over the length of the pillow. The corners of the pillow should fit snugly into the corners of the case.	
35. Return the bed to the lowest position and elevate the head of the bed 30 to 45 degrees. Put side rails up on side, farthest from client.	35. Provides for client safety.
36. Inquire about toileting needs of the client; assist as necessary.	36. Saves client energy and provides time to care for the client's needs.
37. Assist the client back into the bed and pull up the side rails; place call light in reach; take vital signs.	37. Promotes client safety and a means to call for assistance. Sitting up in a chair and movement may cause changes in the client's vital signs.
38. Remove gloves and wash hands.	38. Reduces the transmission of microorganisms.

EVALUATION
- Confirm that fresh linens were placed on the bed in a manner appropriate to the client's needs.

DOCUMENTATION
Nurses' Notes
- Client's tolerance to being out of bed. (Linen changes are not generally documented.)

PROCEDURE 29-18 Bed Making: Occupied Bed

OVERVIEW
After the client takes a bath, clean linens are placed on the bed to promote comfort and decrease the transmission of microorganisms. If the client is unable to get out of bed, change the linens around the client. Assistance is needed if the client is in traction or cannot be turned. Care is taken to avoid disturbing the traction weights. If the client cannot be turned, change the linens from head to toe. Place a waterproof draw sheet on the beds of clients who are incontinent or have profuse drainage. The type and amount of linens placed on the bed will vary based on the type of bed the client is using. Air beds and Clinitron beds, for example, use only minimal linens under the client.

(Continues)

PROCEDURE 29-18 Bed Making: Occupied Bed (Continued)

ASSESSMENT

1. Assess your equipment. **Facilitates a smooth procedure.**
2. Assess whether the bed needs cleaning before placing clean sheets on it. **Reduces the transmission of microorganisms.**
3. Assess the client's needs in the bed. Check for profuse drainage, incontinence, or special needs for comfort or skin integrity. **Determines how the procedure is performed.**
4. Assess the client's ability to assist with the procedure, including mobility, mental status, and muscle strength. **Determines whether assistance is needed to change the client's linens.**
5. Assess for the presence of dressings, IV lines, tubes, or any equipment that may be attached to the client. **Provides for client safety.**

POSSIBLE NURSING DIAGNOSIS

Risk for Impaired Skin Integrity

PLANNING

Expected Outcomes

1. The client will have clean linens on the bed.
2. The clean linens will be appropriate to the client's needs and condition.
3. The linens will be changed with a minimum of trauma to the client.

Equipment Needed

- Laundry bag
- Top sheet, draw sheet, bottom sheet
- Mattress pad (optional)
- Protective disposable pad (optional)
- Pillowcase
- Blanket
- Bath blanket
- Antiseptic solution, washcloth, and towel
- Nonsterile gloves (if needed)

delegation tips

Bed making is usually delegated to ancillary personnel. Their instruction should include the appropriate use of Standard Precautions and safety precautions for themselves and the client, such as the proper movement of the client in bed, how to manage drains and dressings, and the use of proper body mechanics. In certain situations where the client is in critical condition and multiple tubes, especially chest tubes, are present, the nurse assists.

IMPLEMENTATION—ACTION/RATIONALE

* Wash hands * Check client's identification band *

ACTION	RATIONALE
1. Explain procedure to client.	1. Promotes client cooperation.
2. Bring equipment to the bedside.	2. Facilitates procedure organization.
3. Cover client with a bath blanket (Figure 29-18-1). Remove top sheet and blanket. Loosen bottom sheet at foot and sides of bed. Lower side rail nearest the nurse, if necessary for access.	3. Bath blanket prevents exposure and chills. Facilitates easy removal of linens. Lowering only side rail close to nurse reduces client's risk of falls.
4. Position client on side, facing away from you. Reposition pillow under head.	4. Provides space to place clean linens.
5. Fanfold or roll bottom linens close to client toward the center of the bed (Figure 29-18-2).	5. Keeps soiled linen together. Promotes comfort when client later rolls to other side.
6. Place clean bottom linens with the center fold nearest the client. Fanfold or roll clean bottom linens nearest client and tuck under soiled linen (Figure 29-18-3). If fitted sheets are not available, maintain an adequate amount of sheet at head of bed for tucking. Have sheet even with bottom of mattress.	6. Provides for maximum fit of sheets and decreases chance of wrinkles.
7. If fitted sheets are not available, miter bottom sheet at head of bed. To miter, lift the mattress and tuck the sheet over the edge of the mattress, lift edge of sheet that is hanging to form a triangle, and lay upper part of sheet back onto bed; tuck the lower hanging section under the mattress. Repeat for each corner. Tuck the sides of the sheet under the mattress.	7. Holds linens firmly in place.

(Continues)

PROCEDURE 29-18 Bed Making: Occupied Bed (Continued)

ACTION | **RATIONALE**

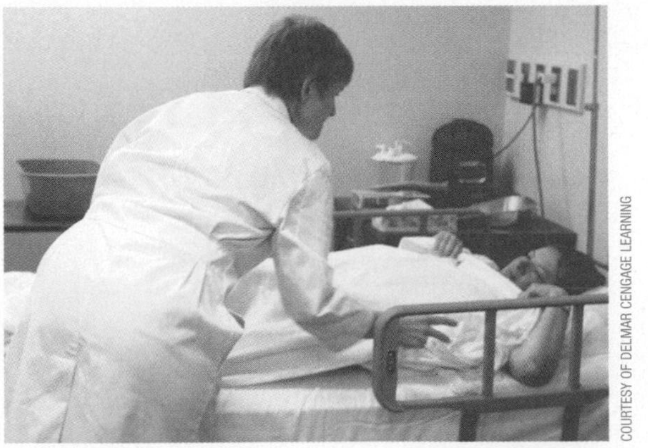

FIGURE 29-18-1 Cover the client with a bath blanket for warmth and modesty while top sheet and blanket are removed.

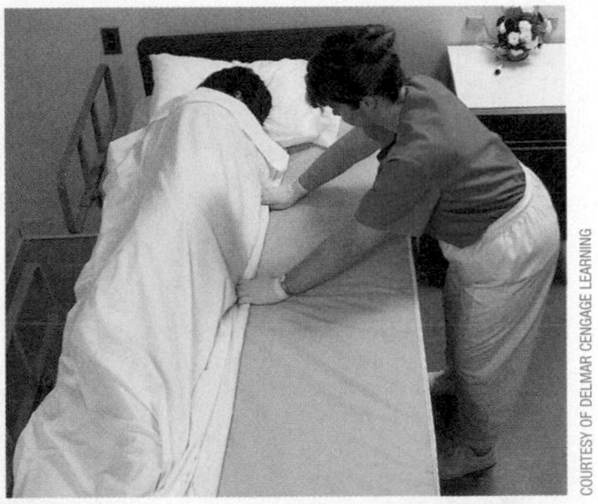

FIGURE 29-18-2 When changing an occupied bed, fanfold the bottom linens toward the center of the bed close to the client. Change gloves, if soiled, before handling clean linen.

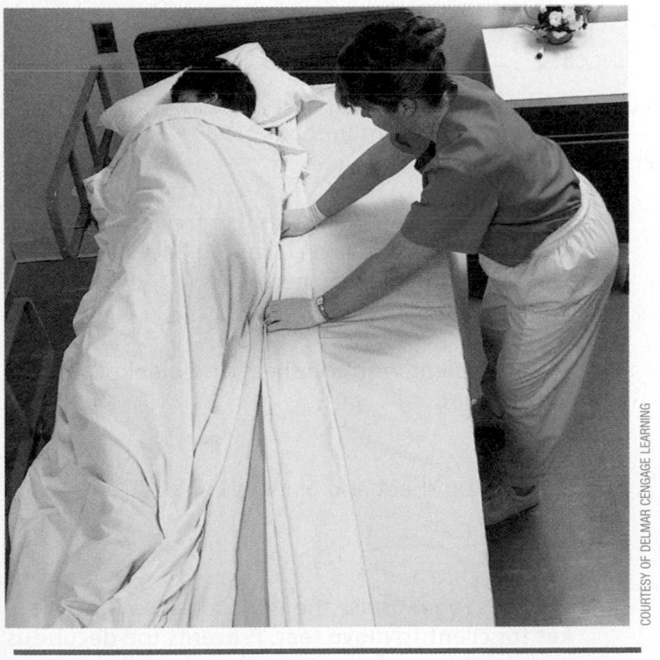

FIGURE 29-18-3 Fanfold or roll clean bottom sheet on the bed and tuck under soiled linen.

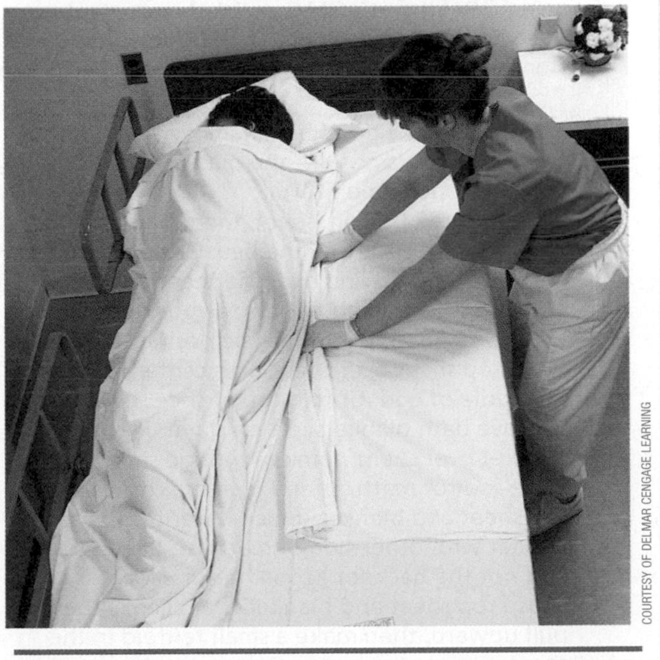

FIGURE 29-18-4 Fanfold or roll draw sheet on the bed and tuck under soiled linen.

8. Fold the draw sheet in half. Identify the center of the draw sheet and place it close to the client. Fanfold or roll draw sheet closest to client and tuck under soiled linen. Smooth linen (Figure 29-18-4). Add protective padding if needed. Tuck draw sheet under mattress, working from the center to the edges. Draw sheet should be positioned under the lower back and buttocks.

   Rationale: 8. Draw sheet facilitates moving and lifting clients while in bed.

9. Roll client over onto side facing you. Raise side rail.

   Rationale: 9. Positions client off soiled linen. Protects client from falling.

(Continues)

PROCEDURE 29-18 Bed Making: Occupied Bed (Continued)

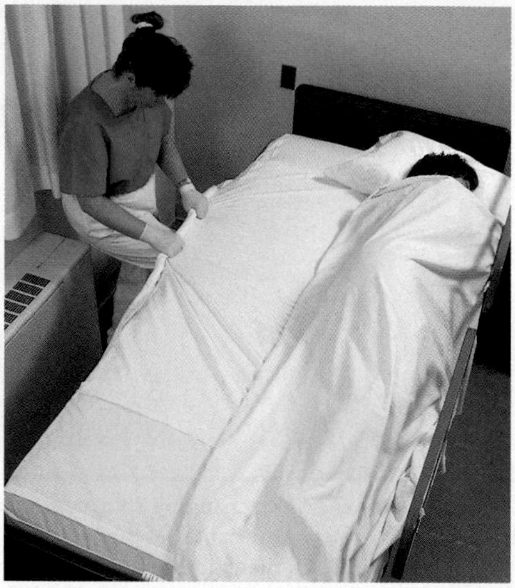

FIGURE 29-18-5 Unfold/unroll the bottom sheet and draw sheet. Grasp each sheet with knuckles up and over the sheet and pull tightly while leaning back with your body weight.

ACTION	RATIONALE
10. Move to other side of bed. Remove soiled linens by rolling into a bundle and place in linen bag without touching uniform.	10. Prevents cross contamination.
11. Unfold/unroll bottom sheet, then draw sheet. Look for objects left in the bed. Grasp each sheet with knuckles up and over the sheet and pull tightly while leaning back with your body weight (Figure 29-18-5). Client may be positioned supine.	11. Tight sheets keep linens wrinkle free and decrease the risk of skin irritation. Leaning back uses body weight for good body mechanics.
12. Place top sheet over client with center of sheet in middle of bed. Unfold top of sheet over client. Remove bath blankets left on client. Place top blanket over client, same as the top sheet.	12. Provides client with top sheet and blanket to prevent chilling.
13. Raise foot of mattress and tuck the corner of the top sheet and blanket under. Miter the corner. Repeat with other side of mattress. Bend knees and not the back for proper mechanics.	13. Secures top sheet and blanket in place.
14. Grasp top sheet and blanket over client's toes and pull upward, then make a small fanfold in the sheet.	14. Provides room under the tight top sheet and blanket for client to move feet. Prevents toe decubitus and sheet burns from pressure.
15. Remove soiled pillowcase. Grasp center of clean pillowcase and invert pillowcase over hand/arm. Maintain grasp of pillowcase while grasping center of pillow. Use other hand to pull pillowcase down over pillow. Place pillow under client's head.	15. Provides clean pillowcase without shaking pillow or pillowcase. Promotes comfort.
16. Wash hands.	16. Reduces the transmission of microorganisms.

EVALUATION

- The client has clean, unwrinkled linen.
- The linen placed on the bed is suitable for the client's special needs.
- The linen was changed with a minimum of pain and trauma to the client.

DOCUMENTATION

Nurses' Notes

- How the client tolerated the bed change, and any unusual findings. (Bed change is not generally documented.)

(Continues)

PROCEDURE 29-19 Bathing a Client in Bed

OVERVIEW

Bathing clients is an essential component of nursing care and a critical time to assess the client. Whether the nurse performs the bath or delegates the activity to another health care provider, the nurse is responsible for ensuring that the hygienic needs of the client are met. Cleansing baths are provided as routine client care for personal hygiene. Following are the five types of cleansing baths:

1. Shower
2. Tub
3. Self-help, or assisted bed bath
4. Complete bed bath
5. Partial bath

There are several variations of bed bath depending on the client's ability to assist with care. The complete bed bath is provided to dependent clients confined to bed. The nurse washes the client's entire body during a complete bed bath. A partial bed bath and a self-help bed bath are variations of the complete bed bath.

After washing a client's hair, cover the head with a towel even if still washing the rest of the body. Most heat is lost from the head, and older clients chill very quickly and have difficulty regulating their temperature.

ASSESSMENT

1. Assess the client's level of ability to assist with the bath. **Determine if the client is able to follow directions. Check the client's ability to assist with cleaning any portion of the body.**
2. Assess the client's level of comfort with the procedure. Check into potential cultural, sexual, or generational issues. **Determine whether the client is uncomfortable, tense, or nervous about being bathed by someone else.**
3. Assess the environment. Verify that the equipment needed is available. Assess if the client has skin intact or dressings, IV lines, or drainage tubes in place. Check whether clean, warm water is available. **Determine whether the need for modesty and privacy can be met. The environment should be conducive to a clean, safe, and comfortable procedure.**

POSSIBLE NURSING DIAGNOSES

Risk for Impaired Skin Integrity
Bathing/Hygiene Self-Care Deficit

PLANNING

Expected Outcomes

1. Clients will be cleaned without damage to their skin.
2. Clients' privacy will be maintained throughout the procedure.
3. Clients will participate in their own hygiene as much as possible.
4. Clients will not become overly tired or experience increased pain, cold, or discomfort as a result of the bath.

Equipment Needed

Some facilities provide packs of microwaveable pre-moistened cloths for baths. For the traditional bed bath, these items are needed:

- Bath towels
- Washcloths
- Bath blanket
- Washbasin
- Soap
- Soap dish
- Lotion
- Deodorant
- Clean gown
- Clean linen
- Disposable, latex-free gloves

delegation tips

This skill is routinely delegated to ancillary personnel who should allow the client to perform as much of the bath as possible or permitted. The caregiver employs Standard Precautions, properly positions the client, and observes and reports the client's skin condition and color to the nurse. The nurse retains the responsibility to assess the client.

(Continues)

PROCEDURE 29-19 Bathing a Client in Bed (Continued)

IMPLEMENTATION—ACTION/RATIONALE

* Check client's identification band * Explain procedure before beginning *

ACTION	RATIONALE
1. Assess the client's preferences about bathing.	1. Provides client opportunity to participate in care.
2. Prepare environment. Close doors and windows, adjust temperature, provide time for elimination needs, and provide privacy.	2. Protects from chills during bath and increases sense of privacy.
3. Wash hands. Apply gloves. Gloves should be changed when emptying water basin.	3. Reduces the transmission of microorganisms.
4. Lower side rail on the side close to you. Position client in a comfortable position close to the side near you.	4. Prevents unnecessary reaching. Facilitates use of good body mechanics.
5. If bath blankets are available, place bath blanket over top sheet. Remove top sheet from under bath blanket. Remove client's gown. Bath blanket should be folded to expose only the area being cleaned at that time. Towels may also be used for bath blankets. Top sheets are not used as bath blankets because they are not absorbent and do not prevent chilling.	5. Prevents exposure of client. Promotes privacy. Protects from chills.
6. Fill washbasin two-thirds full. Permit client to test temperature of water with hand. Water should be changed when a soap film develops or water becomes soiled.	6. Prevents accidental burns or chills.
7. Wet the washcloth and wring it out.	7. Prevents unnecessarily wetting of client.
8. Make a bath mitten with the washcloth. To make a mitten, grasp the edge of the washcloth with the thumb; fold a third over the palm of the hand; wrap remainder of cloth around hand and across palm, and grasp the second edge under the thumb; fold the extended end of the washcloth onto the palm and tuck under the palmar surface of the cloth.	8. Prevents ends of washcloth from dragging across skin. Promotes friction during bath.
9. Wash the face (Figure 29-19-1). Ask the client about preference for using soap on the face. Use a separate corner of the washcloth for each eye, wiping from inner to outer canthus. Wash neck and ears. Rinse and dry well. Male clients may want to shave at this time. Provide assistance with shaving as needed.	9. Some clients may not use soap on the face. Using separate corners of washcloth reduces risk of transmitting microorganisms from one eye to the other eye. Patting dry reduces skin irritation and drying.
10. Wash arms, forearms, and hands. Wash forearms and arms using long, firm strokes in the direction of distal to proximal. Arm may need to be supported while being washed. Wash axilla. Rinse and dry well. Apply deodorant or powder if desired. Immerse client's hand into basin of water. Allow hand to soak about 3 to 5 minutes. Wash hands, interdigit area, fingers, and fingernails. Rinse and dry well.	10. Long strokes promote circulation. Soaking hands softens nails and loosens soil from skin and nails. Strokes directed distal to proximal promote venous return.
11. Wash chest and abdomen. Place bath towel lengthwise over chest and abdomen, then fold bath blanket to waist. Lift bath towel and wash	11. Promotes privacy and prevents chills. Long strokes promote circulation. Perspiration and soil collect within skin folds.

(Continues)

PROCEDURE 29-19 Bathing a Client in Bed (Continued)

ACTION | **RATIONALE**

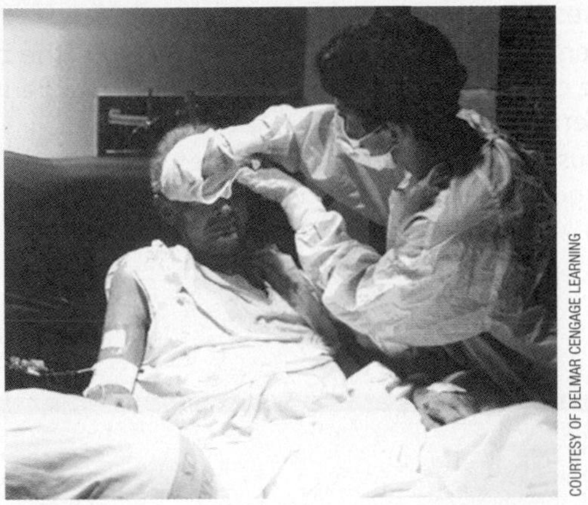

FIGURE 29-19-1 **Wash the client's face first.**

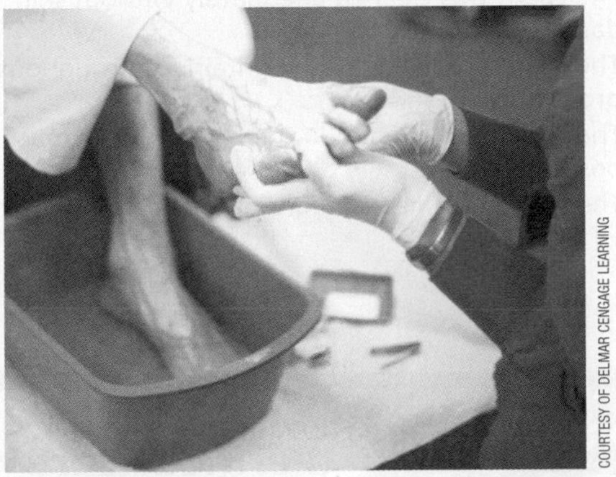

FIGURE 29-19-2 **Place feet in basin. Clean interdigits and soles of feet.**

chest in circular motions. Wash skin fold under the female client's breast by lifting each breast. Leave chest covered with dry towel and fold bath blanket down to suprapubic area. Wash abdomen including the umbilicus and other skin folds carefully. Rinse and dry all skin areas well. Replace bath blanket over chest and abdomen.

12. Wash legs and feet. Expose leg farthest from you by folding bath blanket to midline. Bend the leg at the knee. Grasp the heel, elevate the leg from the bed, and cover bed with bath towel. Place washbasin on towel. Place client's foot into washbasin (Figure 29-19-2). Allow foot to soak while washing the leg with long, firm strokes in the direction of distal to proximal Gently wash the legs of clients with deep vein thrombosis (DVT) or other coagulation issues; do not use firm strokes. Rinse leg and dry well. Clean soles, interdigits, and toes. Carefully examine the foot and between the digits of a diabetic for pressure sores or ulcerations. Rinse foot and dry well. Apply lotion to legs and feet if they are dry but do not massage legs, as an embolus may occur. Perform the same procedure with the other leg and foot.
    - *Rationale:* 12. Supports joints to prevent strain and fatigue. Soaking foot loosens dirt, softens nails, and promotes comfort.
13. Wash back. Assist client into prone or side-lying position facing away from you. Wash the back and buttocks using long, firm strokes. Rinse and dry well. Give back rub and apply lotion.
    - *Rationale:* 13. Exposes back and buttocks for washing. Back rub promotes relaxation and circulation.
14. Perineal care: Assist client to supine position. Perform perineal care (see Procedure 29-20).
    - *Rationale:* 14. Removes genital secretions and soil.
15. Apply lotion as desired or needed. Apply clean gown.
    - *Rationale:* 15. Lotion lubricates skin.
16. Wash hands.
    - *Rationale:* 16. Reduces the transmission of microorganisms.

(Continues)

PROCEDURE 29-19 Bathing a Client in Bed (Continued)

EVALUATION
- The client was cleaned adequately without skin damage.
- The client's modesty was maintained throughout the procedure.
- The client participated in the procedure as much as possible.
- The client remained comfortable during the procedure.

DOCUMENTATION
Nurses' Notes
- Client was bathed. Indicate how much of the bath the client assisted with and how well the client tolerated the activity.
- Unusual findings including rashes, open sores, poor turgor, and so on.

PROCEDURE 29-20 Perineal Care

OVERVIEW
The perineum is the external structure of the pelvic floor. It is composed of the skin and muscle surrounding the genitalia; it is the area between the scrotum and anus in the male and between the vulva and anus in the female. Care of the perineum and genitalia is directed toward maintaining a hygienic perineal environment. Perineal and genital care is usually self-care; however, alterations in the client's ability to perform self-care or alterations in the perineum and genitalia are reasons for nurses or other care providers to perform this skill. Perineal and genital care is an emotionally and culturally difficult subject. Many cultures have specific beliefs and taboos regarding the perineal/genital area. Many people are embarrassed by the idea of anyone else seeing or touching their genitals, particularly a stranger. Be aware of these possibilities when approaching genital/perineal care. In general, a professional, nonjudgmental approach will put the client more at ease with the procedure. Ask the client or the client's caregiver, if possible, about any preferences the client may have in this area.

ASSESSMENT
1. Evaluate client status: level of consciousness, ability to ambulate, ability to perform self-care, frequency of urination and defecation, skin condition. **This allows the nurse to decide who, where, how, and when to perform perineal care.**
2. Identify cultural preferences for perineal care. **Perineal care is strongly associated with cultural practices, for example, who may touch the perineal area and how, and the proper way to "wipe." To the extent possible, these preferences are identified and incorporated into the client's care.**
3. Assess the client's perineal health. Ask the male client if he has any perineal/genital itching or discomfort. Ask the female client if she has any urethral, vaginal, or anal discharge. **Determines the presence of signs and symptoms that may need additional assessment and intervention.**
4. Determine if the client is incontinent of urine or stool. **Affects how the procedure is done and what additional procedures may be necessary.**
5. Assess whether the client has recently had perineal/genital surgery. **Affects how the procedure is done and what additional procedures may be necessary.**

POSSIBLE NURSING DIAGNOSES
Risk for Impaired Skin Integrity
Bathing/Hygiene Self-Care Deficit

PLANNING
Expected Outcomes
1. Perineum and genitalia will be dry, clean, and free of secretions and unpleasant odors.
2. The client will report feeling comfortable and clean in the perineal area.
3. The client will not experience discomfort or undue embarrassment during the procedure.
4. The perineum will be free of skin breakdown or irritation.

Equipment Needed
- Personal protective equipment (gloves, gown)
- Toilet paper/washcloths
- Waterproof pads

(Continues)

PROCEDURE 29-20 Perineal Care (Continued)

- Cleansing solution, if needed
- Perineal wash bottle (fill with plain, warm water).
- Water receptacle (bedpan or toilet if client is ambulatory)
- Dry towels
- Perineal treatment (i.e., ointment or lotions) if necessary
- Linen receptacle
- Room deodorizer

delegation tips

This skill is routinely delegated to ancillary personnel who should be trained in Standard Precautions and proper client positioning, and to report color, odor, and amount of any discharge, if present, to the nurse.

IMPLEMENTATION—ACTION/RATIONALE

ACTION	RATIONALE
* Check client's identification band * Explain procedure before beginning *	
1. Wash hands and wear gloves. If appropriate and splashing is likely, wear gown, mask, and goggles.	1. Reduces the transmission of microorganisms.
2. Close privacy curtain or door.	2. Provides privacy.
3. Position client.	3. If client is ambulatory, perineal care may be done either with client on or standing at the toilet. If perineal care is to be performed in the bed, place the client on the side or over a deep bedpan.
4. Place waterproof pads under the client in the bed or under bedpan if used.	4. Protects bed linen.
5. Remove fecal debris with toilet paper and dispose in toilet.	5. May require several attempts. If performing at the bedside, may collect paper in disposable pad or linens until end of procedure.
6. Spray perineum with washing solution if indicated. Alternatively, plain water may be used.	6. Several perineal solutions are available, which may or may not require rinsing. Carefully evaluate this requirement. Solutions that require rinsing may cause skin breakdown if left on the skin.
7. Wash perineum with wet washcloths (front to back on females), changing to clean area on washcloth with each wipe (Figure 29-20-1). Wash the penis on the male (Figure 29-20-2).	7. Maximizes cleaning; prevents spread of rectal flora to vagina and meatus.
8. Carefully examine gluteal folds and scrotal folds for debris. Gently visualize vulva for debris.	8. Fecal material causes irritation and skin breakdown rapidly when left in contact with skin.
9. If soap is used, spray area with clean water from the peri-bottle.	9. Rinses soap, which can irritate the skin, from the area.
10. Change gloves.	10. Reduces the transmission of microorganisms.
11. Dry perineum carefully with towel.	11. Residual moisture provides an ideal environment for the growth of microorganisms.
12. If indicated, apply barrier lotion or ointment.	12. Barrier ointments may be used if client is incontinent or skin folds tend to harbor moisture.
13. Reposition or dress client as appropriate.	13. Promotes client comfort.
14. Dispose of linens and garbage according to hospital policy.	14. Prevents spread of disease or bacteria.
15. Wash hands.	15. Reduces the transmission of microorganisms.
16. Deodorize room if appropriate.	16. Promotes client comfort. This may also be done at the beginning of the procedure.

(Continues)

PROCEDURE 29-20 Perineal Care (Continued)

ACTION	RATIONALE

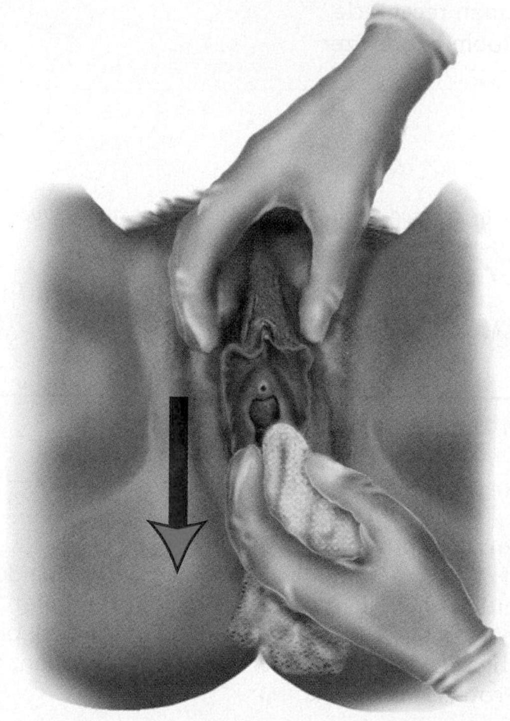

FIGURE 29-20-1 Wash the female perineum from front to back.

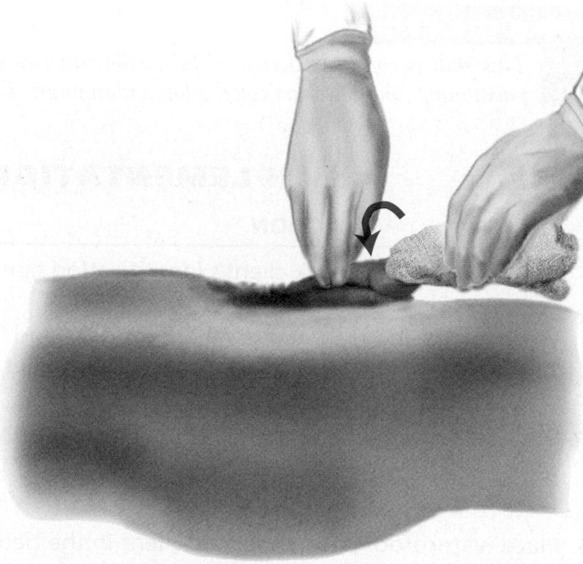

FIGURE 29-20-2 Wash the penis with a warm, wet washcloth in circular motions.

EVALUATION

- The perineum and genitalia are dry, clean, and free of secretions and unpleasant odors.
- The client reports feeling comfortable and clean in the perineal area.
- The client did not experience discomfort or undue embarrassment during the procedure.

DOCUMENTATION

Nurses' Notes

- Time and type of perineal care provided
- Unusual findings such as skin breakdown, infection, or unusual drainage
- Client special preferences or cultural considerations

Kardex

- Special preferences or cultural considerations

PROCEDURE 29-21 Routine Catheter Care

OVERVIEW

An indwelling catheter is used to provide continuous drainage of urine from the bladder. The catheter, which is attached to a drainage bag, may be used for episodic or long-term urinary drainage. Because the catheter is in the bladder through the urethra, bacteria may enter the urinary system; therefore, care must be taken to ensure that the surrounding area is clean to decrease contamination of the catheter by bacterial flora. Clients may be embarrassed or frightened by the catheter and related care and, therefore, require emotional support.

(Continues)

PROCEDURE 29-21 Routine Catheter Care (Continued)

ASSESSMENT

1. Assess catheter patency and urine color, consistency, and amount while performing the care **to determine if catheter and drainage system are functioning correctly.**
2. Determine the condition of the urinary meatus and perineal area **to monitor for redness, swelling, or drainage, stool, or vaginal discharge, as indicators of infection. External infections may migrate up the catheter and lead to urinary tract infection.**
3. Determine the client's emotional reaction and feelings related to the catheter. **This may prevent untoward reactions to the care and allow the nurse to help the client deal with some deeper emotional issues.**

POSSIBLE NURSING DIAGNOSES

Risk for Infection
Risk for Impaired Skin Integrity

PLANNING

Expected Outcomes

1. The client will be free of signs and symptoms of urinary tract infection.
2. The client will understand the reason for the catheter and related cares.
3. The meatus and surrounding area will be clean and free of drainage.

Equipment Needed

- Clean latex-free gloves
- Washcloth, soap, and water
- Waterproof pad
- Antiseptic solution
- Sterile swabs

delegation tips

Routine catheter care is a procedure ancillary personnel are able to perform after proper instruction and supervision. Instruction should include notifying the nurse regarding the appearance of catheter drainage and any problems with catheter tubing, such as leaks.

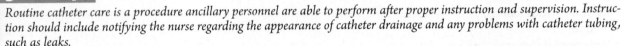

IMPLEMENTATION—ACTION/RATIONALE

* Check client's identification band * Explain procedure before beginning *

ACTION	RATIONALE
1. Wash hands.	1. Reduces the transmission of microorganisms.
2. Check institutional protocol or care plan.	2. Ensures proper procedure.
3. Provide privacy.	3. Protects client dignity.
4. Place client in supine position and expose perineal area and catheter.	4. Allows for visualization of field. If unable to visualize the perineal area with the client supine, try placing the client in a side-lying position.
5. Place waterproof pad under client.	5. Protects bed linens.
6. Put on clean gloves.	6. Reduces transmission of microorganisms.
7. After performing perineal care (Procedure 29-20), cleanse meatus if there is excessive purulent drainage with nonirritating antiseptic solutions on cotton balls.	7. Moving from the most clean area out decreases risk of recontamination.
8. Wash catheter from meatus out to end of catheter, taking care not to pull on catheter.	8. Moving from most clean area out does not transmit bacteria to meatal area predisposing the client to a urethral or bladder infection.
9. Be sure to repeat catheter care any time it becomes soiled with stool or other drainage.	9. Reduces chance of infection.
10. Place linen or cotton balls in proper receptacle for laundry or disposal.	10. Reduces transmission of infection to other clients.
11. Wash hands.	11. Reduces transmission of microorganisms.

(Continues)

PROCEDURE 29-21 Routine Catheter Care (Continued)

EVALUATION

- The client is free of signs and symptoms of urinary tract infection.
- The client understands the reason for the catheter and related care.
- The meatus and surrounding area are clean, intact, and free of drainage.

DOCUMENTATION

Nurses' Notes

- Time the procedure was performed and condition of area surrounding the catheter

PROCEDURE 29-22 Oral Care

OVERVIEW

The oral cavity functions in mastication, secretion of mucus to moisten and lubricate the digestive system, secretion of digestive enzymes, and absorption of essential nutrients. Common problems occurring in the oral cavity include the following:

- Bad breath (halitosis)
- Dental cavities (caries)
- Plaque
- Periodontal disease
- Inflammation of the gums (gingivitis)
- Inflammation of the oral mucosa (stomatitis)

Poor oral hygiene and loss of teeth may affect a client's social interaction and body image as well as nutritional intake. Daily oral care is essential to maintain the integrity of the mucous membranes, teeth, gums, and lips. Through preventive measures, the oral cavity and teeth can be preserved. Preventive oral care consists of fluoride rinsing, flossing, and brushing.

Fluoride

Researchers determined that fluoride can prevent dental caries. Fluoride is a common component of many mouthwashes and toothpastes; however, people with excessive dryness or irritated mucous membranes should avoid commercial mouthwashes because of the alcohol content, which causes drying of mucous membranes. Educate clients about fluoride being an excellent preventive measure against dental caries, but excessive fluoride exposure can affect the color of tooth enamel.

Flossing

Floss daily in conjunction with brushing of teeth. Flossing prevents the formation of plaque, removes plaque between the teeth, and removes food debris. Cavities and periodontal disease are prevented by regular flossing. Many floss holders are available to facilitate flossing.

Brushing

Teeth should be brushed after each meal. Brushing is performed using a dentifrice (toothpaste) that contains fluoride to aid in preventing dental caries. An effective homemade dentifrice is the combination of two parts salt with one part baking soda. Brushing removes plaque and food debris and promotes blood circulation of the gums. Dentures are brushed using the same brushing motion as that used for brushing teeth.

ASSESSMENT

1. Assess whether the client is able to assist with oral care and to what extent. **Promotes independence where possible.**
2. Evaluate whether the client has an understanding of proper oral hygiene. **Promotes self-care and teaching.**
3. Check whether the client has dentures. **Determines how oral care is performed.**

(Continues)

PROCEDURE 29-22 Oral Care (Continued)

4. Assess the condition of the client's mouth. **Determines how oral care is performed.**
5. Assess whether inflammation, bleeding, infection, or ulceration is present. **Determines how oral care is performed. Determines the need for additional assessment and intervention.**
6. Assess what cultural practices to consider. **Determines how oral care is performed.**
7. Assess whether there are any appliances or devices present in the client's mouth such as braces, endotracheal tube, or bridgework. **Determines how oral care is performed.**
8. Check that the proper equipment is available to perform oral care. **Ensures a smooth procedure.**

POSSIBLE NURSING DIAGNOSES

Risk for Infection
Impaired Oral Mucous Membrane
Bathing/Hygiene Self-Care Deficit
Deficient Knowledge-Oral Hygiene

PLANNING

Expected Outcomes

1. Client's mouth, teeth, gums, and lips will be clean and free of food particles.
2. Any inflammation, bleeding, infection, or ulceration present will be noted and treated.
3. The oral mucosa will be clean, intact, and well hydrated.

Equipment Needed

Brushing and Flossing

- Toothbrush
- Toothpaste with fluoride
- Emesis basin
- Towel
- Cup of water
- Nonsterile gloves
- Dental floss, floss holder
- Mirror
- Lip moisturizer

Denture Care

- Denture brush
- Denture cleaner
- Emesis basin
- Towel
- Cup of water
- Nonsterile gloves
- Tissue
- Denture cup

Special Care Items for Clients with Impaired Physical Mobility or Who Are Unconscious (comatose)

- Soft toothbrush or toothette
- Tongue blade
- 3 × 3 gauze sponges
- Cotton-tip applicators
- Prescribed solution
- Plastic Asepto syringe
- Suction machine and catheter

delegation tips

Oral care is routinely delegated to ancillary personnel, who allow the client to perform as much of the oral care as possible or permitted. The caregiver is educated to employ Standard Precautions, to properly position the client, and to observe and report the client's mucous membrane condition and color to the nurse.

IMPLEMENTATION—ACTION/RATIONALE

ACTION	RATIONALE
* Check client's identification band * Explain procedure before beginning *	
Self-Care Client: Flossing and Brushing	
1. Assemble articles for flossing and brushing.	1. Promotes efficiency.
2. Provide privacy.	2. Relaxes the client.
3. Place client in a high Fowler's position.	3. Decreases risk of aspiration.
4. Wash hands and apply gloves.	4. Reduces the transmission of microorganisms.
5. Arrange articles within client's reach.	5. Facilitates self-care.

(Continues)

PROCEDURE 29-22 Oral Care (Continued)

ACTION	RATIONALE
6. Assist client with flossing and brushing as necessary. Position mirror, emesis basin, water with straw near the client, and a towel across the chest (Figure 29-22-1).	6. Flossing and brushing decrease microorganism growth in the mouth. Use of mirror permits cleaning back and sides of teeth.
7. Assist client with rinsing mouth.	7. Removes toothpaste and oral secretions.
8. Reposition client, raise side rails, and place call button within reach.	8. Promotes comfort, safety, and communication.
9. Rinse, dry, and return articles to proper place.	9. Promotes a clean environment.
10. Remove gloves, wash hands, and document care.	10. Reduces the transmission of microorganisms and documents nursing care.
Self-Care Client: Denture Care	
11. Assemble articles for denture cleaning (Figure 29-22-2).	11. Promotes efficiency.
12. Provide privacy.	12. Relaxes the client.
13. Assist client to a high Fowler's position.	13. Facilitates removal of dentures.
14. Wash hands and apply gloves.	14. Reduces the transmission of microorganisms and exposure to body fluids.
15. Assist client with denture removal: a. Top denture: • With gauze, grasp the denture with thumb and forefinger and pull downward. • Place in denture cup. b. Bottom denture: • Place thumbs on the gums and release the denture. Grasp denture with thumb and forefinger and pull upward. • Place in denture cup.	15. Breaks seal created with dentures without causing pressure and injury to oral membranes. Prevents breaking of dentures.
16. Apply toothpaste to brush, and brush dentures either with cool water in the emesis basin or under running water in the sink. Pad sink with towel to protect dentures in case they are dropped. Some clients prefer to clean dentures by soaking them in a cup with water and an effervescent denture cleaning tablet.	16. Facilitates removal of microorganisms.
17. Rinse thoroughly.	17. Removes toothpaste.
18. Assist client with rinsing mouth and replacing dentures.	18. Freshens mouth and facilitates intake of solid food.

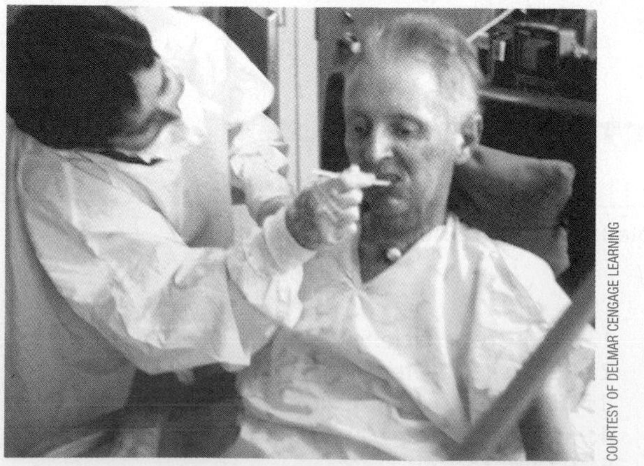

COURTESY OF DELMAR CENGAGE LEARNING

FIGURE 29-22-1 Promote independence but assist with flossing or brushing as necessary.

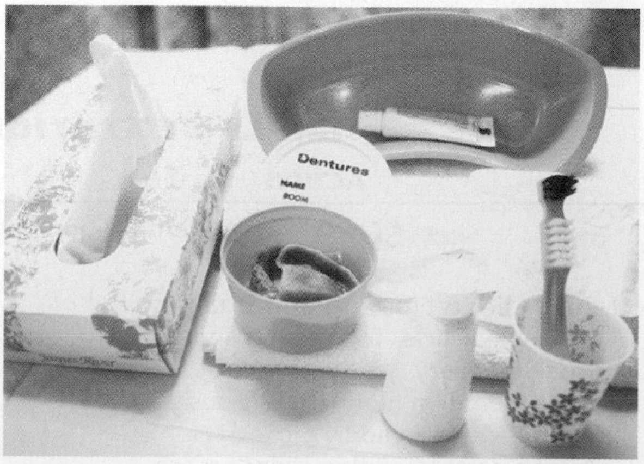

COURTESY OF DELMAR CENGAGE LEARNING

FIGURE 29-22-2 Assemble articles for denture care.

(Continues)

PROCEDURE 29-22 Oral Care (Continued)

ACTION	RATIONALE
19. Reposition client, with side rails up and call button within reach.	19. Promotes comfort, safety, and communication.
20. Rinse, dry, and return articles to proper place.	20. Maintains a clean environment.
21. Remove gloves and wash hands.	21. Reduces the transmission of microorganisms.
Full-Care Client: Brushing and Flossing	
22. Assemble articles for flossing and brushing.	22. Promotes efficiency.
23. Provide privacy.	23. Relaxes client.
24. Wash hands and apply gloves.	24. Reduces the transmission of microorganisms and exposure to body fluids.
25. Position client as condition allows: high Fowler's, semi-Fowler's, or lateral position, head turned toward side (Figure 29-22-3).	25. Decreases risk of aspiration.
26. Place towel across client's chest or under face and mouth if head is turned to one side.	26. Catches secretions.
27. Moisten toothbrush or toothette, apply small amount of toothpaste, and brush teeth and gums.	27. Moistens mouth and facilitates plaque removal.
28. Grasp the dental floss in both hands or use a floss holder and floss between all teeth; hold floss against tooth while moving floss up and down sides of teeth.	28. Removes plaque and prevents gum disease.
29. Assist the client in rinsing mouth.	29. Removes toothpaste and oral secretions.
30. Reapply toothpaste and brush the teeth and gums using friction in a circular motion. On inner and outer surfaces of teeth, hold brush at 45-degree angle against teeth and brush from sulcus to crowns of teeth. On biting surfaces, move brush back and forth in short strokes. All surfaces of teeth should be brushed from every angle.	30. Permits cleaning of back and sides of teeth and decreases microorganism growth in mouth.
31. Assist the client in rinsing and drying mouth.	31. Removes toothpaste and oral secretions.
32. Apply lip moisturizer, if appropriate.	32. Maintains skin integrity of lips.
33. Reposition client, raise side rails, and place call button within reach.	33. Promotes comfort, safety, and communication.
34. Rinse, dry, and return articles to proper place.	34. Provides an orderly environment.
35. Remove gloves and wash hands.	35. Reduces the transmission of microorganisms.

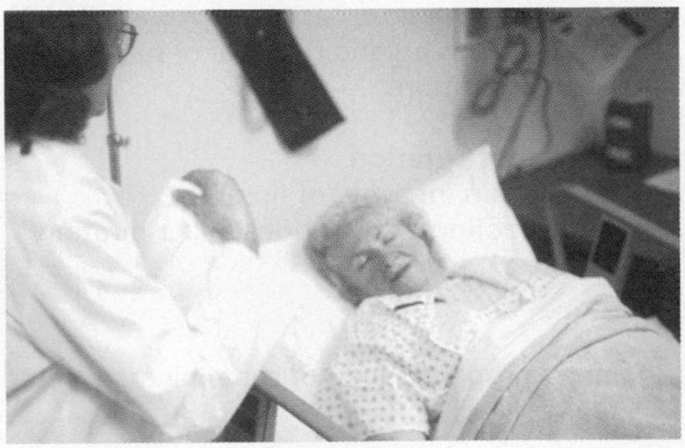

FIGURE 29-22-3 If client is unable to sit up, turn head to the side.

(Continues)

PROCEDURE 29-22 Oral Care (Continued)

ACTION	RATIONALE
Clients at Risk for or with an Alteration of the Oral Cavity	
36. Follow Actions 22 to 24.	36. See Rationales 22 to 24.
37. Bleeding:	37.
a. Assess oral cavity with a padded tongue blade and flashlight for signs of bleeding.	a. Determines whether bleeding is present, amount, and specific areas.
b. Proceed with the actions for oral care for a full-care client except:	b.
• Do not floss.	• Decreases risk of bleeding and trauma to gums.
• Use a soft toothbrush, toothette, or a tongue blade padded with 3 × 3 gauze sponges to gently swab teeth and gums.	• Decreases risk of bleeding and trauma to gums.
• Dispose of padded tongue blade into a biohazard bag according to institutional policy.	• Promotes proper disposal of contaminated waste.
• Rinse with tepid water.	• Cleanses mouth.
38. Infection or ulceration:	38.
a. Assess oral cavity with a tongue blade and flashlight for signs of infection.	a. Determines appearance, integrity, and general condition.
b. Culture lesions as ordered.	b. Identifies growth of specific microorganisms.
c. Proceed with the actions for oral care for a full-care client except:	c.
• Do not floss.	• Prevents irritation, pain, and bleeding.
• Use prescribed antiseptic solution.	• Antiseptic solutions decrease growth of microorganisms.
• Use a tongue blade padded with 3 × 3 gauze sponges to gently swab the teeth and gums.	
• Dispose of padded tongue blade into a biohazard bag according to institutional policy.	• Promotes proper disposal of contaminated materials.
• Rinse mouth with tepid water.	• Cleanses mouth.
• Apply additional solution as prescribed.	• Provides a coating that promotes healing of the tissue.
Unconscious (Comatose) Client	
39. Follow Actions 22–24.	39. See Rationales 22 to 24.
40. Place the client in a lateral position, with the head turned toward the side.	40. Prevents aspiration.
41. Use a floss holder and floss between all teeth.	41. Prevents transfer of microorganisms from a client bite.
42. Moisten toothbrush or toothette, and brush the teeth and gums using friction in a circular motion. Do not use toothpaste. Brush teeth as described in Action 30.	42. Permits cleaning of back and sides of teeth and decreases microorganism growth in mouth. Toothpaste may foam and cause aspiration.
43. After flossing and brushing, rinse mouth with an Asepto syringe (do not force water into the mouth) and perform oral suction.	43. Promotes cleansing and removal of secretions and prevents aspiration.
44. Dry the client's mouth.	44. Prevents skin irritation.
45. Apply lip moisturizer.	45. Maintains skin integrity of lips.
46. Leave the client in a lateral position with head turned toward side for 30 to 60 minutes after oral hygiene care. Suction one more time. Remove the towel from under the client's mouth and face.	46. Prevents pooling of secretions and aspiration.
47. Dispose of any contaminated items in a biohazard bag and clean, dry, and return all articles to the appropriate place.	47. Promotes proper disposal of contaminated materials.
48. Remove gloves and wash hands.	48. Reduces the transmission of microorganisms.

(Continues)

PROCEDURE 29-22 Oral Care (Continued)

EVALUATION

- The client's mouth, teeth, gums, and lips are clean and free of food particles.
- Inflammation, bleeding, infection, or ulceration are noted and cared for.
- The oral mucosa is clean, intact, and well hydrated.
- The oral care was performed with a minimum of trauma to the client.

DOCUMENTATION

Nurses' Notes

- Unusual findings

PROCEDURE 29-23 Eye Care

OVERVIEW

Eyes need little daily care and are continually cleansed by the production of tears and movement of eyelids over the eyes. Some clients, however, do have special eye care needs.

Contact Lenses

Self-care is the best method of care for a client with contact lenses; however, accidents or illness may render a client unable to remove or care for the lenses. Some lenses may be left on the cornea for up to a week without damage. Most must be removed daily for cleaning and to prevent hypoxia of the cornea. It is a nursing responsibility to determine whether the client is wearing contact lenses and to properly care for the lenses and the client's eyes. In acute care situations, encourage the client to wear glasses if possible and send the contact lenses home with a family member.

Prosthetic Eyes

Some clients have an artificial eye (ocular prosthesis) in place. Artificial eyes are created to look identical to the client's biologic eye. They are generally made from glass or plastic. Some artificial eyes are permanently implanted in the eye socket, but others must be removed daily for cleaning. The eye socket should also be gently cleansed to remove crusts and mucus, and the prosthesis replaced in the eye socket.

ASSESSMENT

1. Determine if the client is wearing contact lenses or has an ocular prosthesis. If the client is unable to answer questions, you will need to find out another way. Does it indicate in the client's chart if the client wears contact lenses or has a prosthesis? Are there family members present to ask? **This affects the eye care given.**
2. Are the eye care supplies needed available? If the client can tell you what kind of eye care products he or she normally uses, ask or have a family member bring these products from home. **This affects eye care given.**
3. Assess whether the client can do his or her own eye care. If not, evaluate what kind of assistance the client needs. **This promotes maximum independence in the client.**

POSSIBLE NURSING DIAGNOSES

*Ineffective **H**ealth Maintenance*
*Bathing/Hygiene **S**elf-Care Deficit*
*Disturbed Sensory **P**erception (Visual)*

PLANNING

Expected Outcomes

1. The client's contact lenses will be safely removed and stored.
2. The client's ocular prosthesis will be safely removed, cleaned, and either stored or returned to the client's eye socket.
3. The client's contacts or prosthesis will be cared for with a minimum of trauma to the client's eyes.
4. The client's eyes will be free of crusts and exudate.

Equipment Needed

Artificial Eye

- Storage container
- Mild soap
- 3 × 3 gauze sponges
- Cotton balls
- Towel
- Emesis basins

(Continues)

PROCEDURE 29-23 Eye Care (Continued)

- Eye irrigation syringe (optional)
- Running water
- Sterile gloves
- Biohazard bag
- Saline solution
- Protector pad

Contact Lenses

- Lens container
- Soaking solution—type used by client
- Towel
- Suction cup (optional)
- Scotch tape (optional)
- Nonsterile gloves

delegation tips

Eye care requires the assessment and intervention of the nurse and delegation to ancillary personnel is inappropriate.

IMPLEMENTATION—ACTION/RATIONALE

* Check client's identification band * Explain procedure before beginning *

Artificial Eye Removal

ACTION	RATIONALE
1. Inquire about client's care regimen and gather equipment accordingly.	1. Promotes continuity of care.
2. Provide privacy.	2. Relaxes the client.
3. Wash hands; apply gloves.	3. Reduces the transmission of microorganisms.
4. Place client in a semi-Fowler's position.	4. Facilitates procedure and client participation.
5. Place the cotton balls in an emesis basin filled halfway with warm tap water.	5. Dry cotton balls could cause irritation.
6. Place 3 × 3 gauze sponges in bottom of second emesis basin and fill halfway with mild soap and tepid water.	6. Gauze serves as padding to prevent breakage of the prosthesis.
7. Grasp and squeeze excess water from a cotton ball. Wash the eyelid with the moistened cotton ball, starting at the inner canthus and moving outward toward the outer canthus. After each use, dispose of cotton ball in biohazard bag. Repeat procedure until eyelid is clean (without dried secretions).	7. Eliminating the excess water prevents water from running down the client's face. Cleansing the eyelid prevents contamination of the lacrimal system (inner canthus area). Disposal of cotton balls reduces transmission of microorganisms to other health care workers.
8. Remove the artificial eye:	8. Cleanses the artificial eye.
a. Using dominant hand, raise the client's upper eyelid with index finger and depress the lower eyelid with thumb.	a. Promotes removal of artificial eye.
b. Cup nondominant hand under the client's lower eyelid.	b. Cupping reduces dropping and possible breaking of the eye.
c. Apply slight pressure with index finger between the brow and the artificial eye and remove it. Place it in an emesis basin filled with warm, soapy water.	c. Applying pressure will help the prosthesis to slip out.
9. Grasp a moistened cotton ball and cleanse around the edge of the eye socket. Dispose of the soiled cotton ball into biohazard bag.	9. Cleanses the eye socket. Disposal of cotton ball reduces transmission of microorganisms to other health care workers.
10. Inspect the eye socket for any signs of irritation, drainage, or crusting. Note: If the client's usual care regimen or physician order requires irrigation of the socket, proceed with Action 11; otherwise, go to Action 12.	10. Indicates an infection.

(Continues)

PROCEDURE 29-23 Eye Care (Continued)

ACTION	RATIONALE
11. Eye socket irrigation:	11. Cleanses the eye socket and removes secretions.
a. Lower the head of the bed and place the client in a supine position. Place protector pad on bed; turn head toward socket side and slightly extend neck.	a. Positioning of client facilitates ease in performing the procedure and client comfort.
b. Fill the irrigation syringe with the prescribed amount and type of irrigating solution (warm tap water or normal saline).	b. Ensures compliance with client's regimen or prescribed orders.
c. With nondominant hand, separate the eyelids with your forefinger and thumb while resting fingers on the brow and cheekbone.	c. Keeps the eyelid open and the socket visible.
d. Hold the irrigating syringe in dominant hand several inches above the inner canthus; with thumb, gently apply pressure on the plunger, directing the flow of solution from the inner canthus along the conjunctival sac.	d. Prevents injury to the client.
e. Irrigate until the prescribed amount of solution has been used.	e. Ensures compliance with client's regimen of prescribed orders.
f. Wipe the eyelids with a moistened cotton ball after irrigating. Dispose of soiled cotton ball in biohazard bag.	f. Reduces the transmission of microorganisms to prosthesis.
g. Pat the skin dry with the towel.	g. Prevents maceration of the skin.
h. Return the client to a semi-Fowler's position.	h. Promotes client comfort.
i. Remove gloves, wash hands, and apply clean gloves.	i. Reduces the transmission of microorganisms.
12. Rub the artificial eye between index finger and thumb in the basin of warm, soapy water.	12. Creates cleaning with friction and prevents breakage of the prosthesis.
13. Rinse the prosthesis under running water or place in the clean basin of tepid water. Do not dry the prosthesis. *Note:* Either reinsert the prosthesis (Action 14) or store in a container (Action 15).	13. Removes soap and secretions. Keeping the artificial eye wet prevents irritation from lint or other particles that might adhere to it and facilitates reinsertion.
14. Reinsert the prosthesis:	14. Allows for client comfort.
a. With the thumb of the nondominant hand, raise and hold the upper eyelid open.	a. Facilitates reinsertion of the prosthesis without discomfort to the client.
b. With the dominant hand, grasp the artificial eye so that the indented part is facing toward the client's nose and slide it under the upper eyelid as far as possible.	b. Positions the prosthesis for insertion.
c. Depress the lower lid.	c. Allows the prosthesis to slide into place.
d. Pull the lower lid forward to cover the edge of the prosthesis.	d. Holds the prosthesis in place.
15. Place the cleaned artificial eye in a labeled container with saline or tap water solution.	15. Protects the prosthesis from scratches and keeps it clean.
16. Grasp a moistened cotton ball and squeeze out excessive moisture. Wipe the eyelid from the inner to the outer canthus. Dispose of the soiled cotton ball in a biohazard bag.	16. Squeezing the cotton ball removes moisture. Cleansing the eyelid prevents contamination of lacrimal system. Disposal of cotton ball reduces the transmission of microorganisms to other health care workers.
17. Clean, dry, and replace equipment.	17. Promotes a clean environment.
18. Reposition the client, raise side rails, and place call light in reach.	18. Promotes client's comfort, safety, and communication.
19. Dispose of biohazard bag according to institutional policy.	19. Reduces the transmission of microorganisms to other health care workers.
20. Remove gloves and wash hands.	20. Same as Rationale 19.

(Continues)

PROCEDURE 29-23 Eye Care (Continued)

ACTION	RATIONALE
Contact Lens Removal	
21. Assess level of assistance needed and provide privacy.	21. Level of assistance determines level of intervention. Privacy reduces anxiety.
22. Wash hands.	22. Reduces the transmission of microorganisms.
23. Assist the client to a semi-Fowler's position if needed.	23. Facilitates removal of lens.
24. Drape a clean towel over the client's chest.	24. Provides a clean surface and facilitates the location of a lens if it falls during removal.
25. Prepare the lens storage case with the prescribed solution.	25. Hard lenses can be stored dry or in a special soaking solution. Soft lenses are stored in sterile normal saline without a preservative.
26. Instruct the client to look straight ahead. Assess the location of the lens. If it is not on the cornea, either you or the client should gently move the lens toward the cornea with pad of index finger (Figure 29-23-1).	26. Client's position promotes easy removal of lens. Positioning lens on the cornea aids removal. Use of the finger pad of the index finger prevents damage to cornea and lens.
27. Remove the lens.	27. Provides for cleaning and storage of the lens.
a. Hard lens:	a.
• Cup nondominant hand under the eye.	• Cupping the hand under eye helps catch the lens and prevent breakage.
• Gently place index finger on the outside corner of the eye and pull toward the temple and ask client to blink. Catch the lens in your nondominant hand.	• Pulling the corner of the eye tightens the eyelid against the eyeball. Pressure on the upper edge of lens causes the lens to tip forward.
b. Soft lens:	b.
• With nondominant hand, separate the eyelid with your thumb and middle finger.	• Separating the eyelid exposes the lower edge of lens.
• With the index finger of the dominant hand gently placed on the lower edge of the lens, slide the lens downward onto the sclera and gently squeeze the lens.	• Positions lens for easy grasping with the pad of the index finger, which prevents injury to the cornea and lens. Squeezing the lens allows air to enter and release the suction.
• Release the top eyelid (continue holding the lower lid down) and remove the lens with your index finger and thumb.	• Ensures control of the lens.
Note: If Action 27 is unsuccessful, secure a suction cup to remove the contact lens. If you are unable to remove the lens, notify the physician or qualified practitioner.	• Suction cup is used to remove a lens from an unconscious or dependent client.

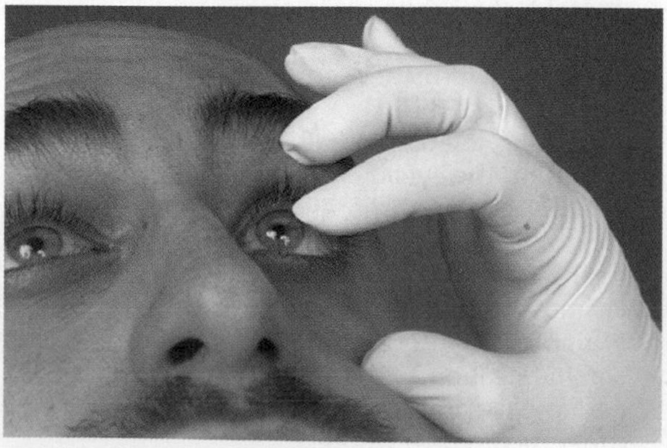

FIGURE 29-23-1 If the lens is not on the cornea, gently move it toward the cornea with the pad of the index finger.

(Continues)

PROCEDURE 29-23 Eye Care (Continued)

ACTION	RATIONALE
28. Store the lens in the correct compartment of the case ("right" or "left"). Label with the client's name. Note: Some soft lenses are thrown away after a timed usage. Check with client before disposing of contact lens.	28. Storage prevents damage to the lenses and ensures that each lens will be reinserted into the correct eye.
29. Remove and store the other lens by repeating Actions 27 and 28.	29. Refer to Rationales 27 and 28.
30. Assess eyes for irritation or redness.	30. Signs of corneal irritation.
31. Store the lens case in a safe place.	31. Prevents damage or loss.
32. Dispose of soiled articles and clean and return reusable articles to proper location.	32. Reduces the transmission of infection.
33. Reposition the client, raise side rails, and place call light in reach.	33. Promotes client comfort, safety, and communication.
34. Remove gloves and wash hands.	34. Reduces the transmission of infection.

EVALUATION

- The client's contact lenses were safely removed and stored.
- The client's ocular prosthesis was safely removed, cleaned, and either stored or returned to the client's eye socket.
- The client's contacts or prosthesis were cared for with a minimum of trauma to the client's eyes.
- The client's eyes are free of crusts and exudate.
- The client is comfortable.

DOCUMENTATION

Nurses' Notes

- Whether the client wears contact lenses
- Location and condition of the lenses
- Whether the client requires assistance to place and remove the contact lenses
- Whether the client has an ocular prosthesis and which eye
- Condition of the prosthesis and the condition of the eye socket
- Care performed on the prosthesis and the socket and how the client tolerated the activity
- Client teaching

Kardex

- Whether the client wears contact lenses or glasses or has an ocular prosthesis
- Special care requirements

PROCEDURE 29-24 Giving a Back Rub

OVERVIEW

Giving a back rub is a basic nursing skill. Back massage is an effective means of building a sense of trust and increased rapport between the nurse and client. Clients are often touch-deprived in the busy health care industry of today. The small amount of time that it takes to do a simple back massage can often soothe and relax a "difficult" client and increase the effectiveness of the nurse–client relationship.

Massage is performed in many different ways, from light strokes to heavy kneading. Various forms include effleurage, deep or gentle stroking, and petrissage, a kneading performed with the tips of the fingers and thumbs or palm of the hand. Massage stimulates circulation and promotes lymphatic drainage, thereby helping to rid the body of metabolic wastes, speed healing, and provide gentle relaxation. However, do not massage over areas of skin that are red or white and remain that color for over a minute. Massaging over these areas may damage the tissue. Do not massage over open skin areas or boney prominences that do not have fatty tissue. Massage can open lines of communication and improve the therapeutic relationship between a nurse and client.

(Continues)

PROCEDURE 29-24 Giving a Back Rub (Continued)

ASSESSMENT

1. Assess the client's willingness to have a massage. **The client may not want a massage or may not enjoy the tactile experience of a massage.**
2. Assess the client for contraindications of a back rub. Conditions include open sores or lesions, vertebral fractures, burns, and signs of pressure ulcers. **To prevent injuring the client.**
3. Assess any limitations the client has in positioning **to determine if the client has any conditions that prohibit a side-lying or prone position.**
4. Assess the client for fatigue, stiffness, or soreness in the back and shoulders. **Knowing areas of particular concern allows you to focus your energies toward "trouble areas."**
5. Assess the client for anxiety or emotional disturbances. **Massage can help reduce anxiety and calm people in distress.**
6. If possible, have the client quantify the degree of discomfort using a 1 to 10 rating scale. **Quantifying the results can provide more validity to the intervention.**

POSSIBLE NURSING DIAGNOSES

Anxiety (mild)
Impaired Physical Mobility

PLANNING

Expected Outcomes

1. The client will experience a reduction in tension, anxiety, pain, and fatigue.
2. The client's circulation to the back is improved.
3. The nurse will establish a better rapport with the client.

Equipment Needed

- Quiet environment, free of interruptions, with a comfortable room temperature
- Comfortable bed or massage table that allows a client to lie in a side-lying or prone position
- Bath blanket
- Bath towel, to absorb excess moisture, oils
- Lotion, baby powder, or massage oil
- Gloves if necessary

delegation tips

Giving a back rub to a client is routinely delegated to properly trained ancillary personnel, who communicate the client's response to a back rub to the nurse.

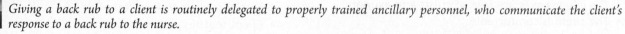

IMPLEMENTATION—ACTION/RATIONALE

* Check client's identification band * Explain procedure before beginning *

ACTION	RATIONALE
1. Wash your hands and apply gloves if necessary.	1. Reduces the transmission of microorganisms.
2. Help client to a prone or side-lying position.	2. Allows exposure of back and shoulder area.
3. Drape the bath blanket and undo the client's gown, exposing the back, shoulder, and sacral area but keeping the remainder of the body covered.	3. Prevents chilling and excess exposure.
4. Pour a small amount of lotion in your hand and warm between your palms for a few moments. The lotion bottle can also be submerged in a bowl of warm water for a few minutes to warm the lotion. Baby powder may be substituted for oils or lotions.	4. Prevents the shock of cold lotion being applied to the body. Some clients may be sensitive to oils or lotions.
5. Begin in the sacral area with smooth, circular strokes, moving upward toward the shoulders. Gradually lengthen the strokes to the upper back, scapulae, and upper arms. Apply firm, continuous pressure without breaking contact with the client (Figures 29-24-1).	5. Applying firm, continuous pressure increases circulation and relaxation.
6. Assess client's back as you are massaging for areas of redness and signs of decreased circulation.	6. Monitors for signs of early skin breakdown.
7. Provide a firm, kneading massage to areas of increased tension if desired, in areas such as the shoulders and gluteal muscles.	7. Firm, kneading strokes can decrease muscle tension, reducing pain and increasing relaxation.

(Continues)

PROCEDURE 29-24 Giving a Back Rub (Continued)

ACTION	RATIONALE

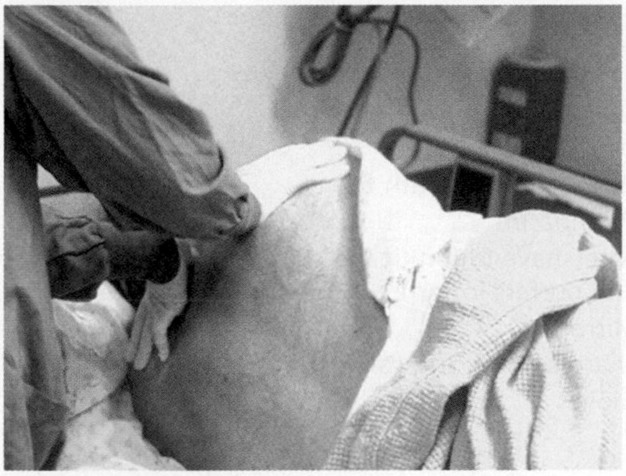

FIGURE 29-24-1 Apply firm, continuous pressure without breaking contact between your hands and the client's skin.

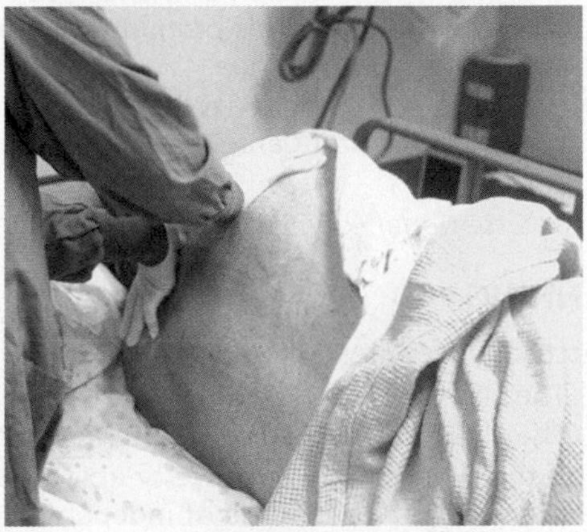

FIGURE 29-24-2 Finish the massage with light brushstrokes, using the fingertips.

ACTION	RATIONALE
8. Complete the massage with long, very light brushstrokes, using the tips of the fingers (Figure 29-24-2).	8. This is a very relaxing stroke and signals an end to the massage.
9. Gently pat or wipe excess lubricant off the client and cover the client.	9. Prevents soiling of the bed with excess lotions and keeps the client warm.
10. Wash hands.	10. Reduces the transmission of microorganisms.

EVALUATION
- The client experienced a reduction in tension, anxiety, pain, and fatigue.
- The nurse established better rapport with the client.

DOCUMENTATION
Nurses' Notes
- Time and date the back rub was performed
- Client's response to the back rub
- Complaints of pain or tension the client reported
- Unusual findings

PROCEDURE 29-25 Shaving a Client

OVERVIEW
Shaving is usually done after a bath or shower and as often as required to remove unwanted facial hair. Most men shave every day, although the facial hair of older clients does not grow as rapidly. If a beard or mustache is present, it is groomed daily and trimmed as appropriate. Do not shave off beards or mustaches without the client's permission. Some clients on anticoagulants may prefer to shave with an electric shaver instead of a safety razor.

ASSESSMENT
1. Assess whether the client is able to perform self-care. **Promote independence when possible.**
2. Assess the client's skin for areas of redness, skin breakdown, moles, or skin lesions. **Shaving could irritate the skin further.**
3. Assess whether the client has a bleeding tendency or is on anticoagulants. **If there is an increased risk of bleeding, an electric razor is used.**
4. If the client prefers to shave himself, assess the client's ability to manipulate the razor. **The client must be able to shave safely.**

(Continues)

PROCEDURE 29-25 Shaving a Client (Continued)

5. Assess the client's preference for the type of shaving, type of equipment, and type of lotion (if there are options). **This promotes independence.**

POSSIBLE NURSING DIAGNOSES

*Dressing/Grooming **S**elf-Care Deficit*
*Risk for **I**njury*
*Risk for Situational Low **S**elf-Esteem*

PLANNING

Expected Outcomes

1. The client will be neat and well groomed.
2. The client's skin integrity will remain intact.
3. If the client is able to shave or able to assist, the client will attain a sense of independence.
4. The client will be comfortable following the procedure.

Equipment Needed

- Electric razor or disposable razor
- Shaving cream or soap
- Warm water
- Washcloth and bath towel
- Washbasin
- Aftershave lotion (if the client has no skin irritation and prefers lotion)
- Mirror
- Sharp scissors and comb if mustache care required
- Gloves

delegation tips

Shaving the adult male client is routinely delegated. Exercise caution with intubated clients to maintain the integrity of their tubes.

IMPLEMENTATION—ACTION/RATIONALE

* Check client's identification band * Explain procedure before beginning *

ACTION	RATIONALE
1. Wash hands and apply gloves.	1. Reduces transmission of microorganisms.
2. Assist the client to a comfortable position. If the client can shave himself, set up the equipment and supplies, including warm water, and watch the client for safety. Adjust lighting as needed.	2. Facilitates comfort and ease of shaving. Encourages sense of self-control and independence.
3. Place a towel over the client's chest and shoulder.	3. Protects the client and gown from soil.
4. Raise the bed to a comfortable height.	4. Facilitates comfort of staff.
5. Fill a washbasin with water at approximately 44°C (110°F). Check temperature for comfort.	5. Warm water helps soften the skin and beard.
6. Place the washcloth in the basin and wring out thoroughly. Apply the cloth over the client's entire face.	6. Warm water helps soften the skin and beard. Warmth can be relaxing.
7. Apply shaving cream.	7. Helps soften the whiskers.
8. Take the razor in the dominant hand and hold it at a 45-degree angle to the client's skin. Start shaving across one side of the client's face. Use the nondominant hand to gently pull the skin taut while shaving. Use short, firm strokes in the direction hair grows (Figure 29-25-1). Use short, downward strokes over the upper lip area.	8. Holding the skin taut prevents razor cuts and discomfort during shaving.
9. Rinse the razor in water as cream accumulates.	9. Keeps the cutting edge of the razor clean.
10. Check the face to see if all the facial hair is removed.	10. Ensures a neat appearance.
11. After all the facial hair is removed, rinse the face thoroughly with a moistened washcloth.	11. Promotes comfort and cleanliness.
12. Dry the face thoroughly and apply aftershave lotion if desired.	12. Stimulates and lubricates the skin.
13. Assist the client to a comfortable position and allow him to inspect the results of the shave.	13. Facilitates comfort and a sense of control.

(Continues)

PROCEDURE 29-25 Shaving a Client (Continued)

ACTION	RATIONALE

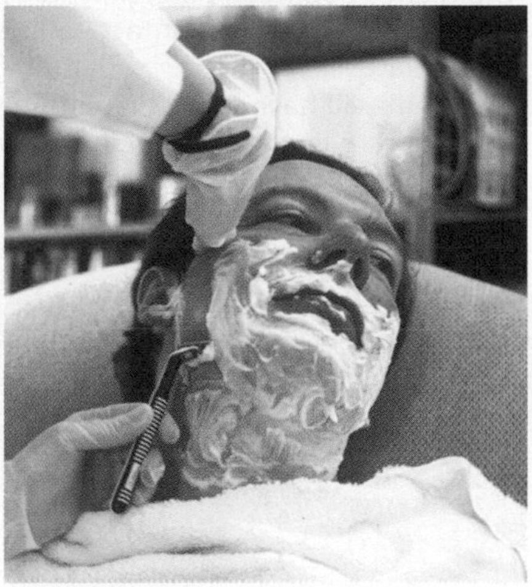

FIGURE 29-25-1 Shave with short, firm strokes in the direction the hair grows.

ACTION	RATIONALE
14. Dispose of equipment in proper receptacle.	14. Equipment should not be shared between clients in accordance with Standard Precautions because disruption of skin and bleeding may occur. The client may, however, keep his own razor. Clean and store it at the bedside.
15. Wash hands.	15. Reduces the transmission of microorganisms.

EVALUATION

- The client is neat and well groomed.
- The client's skin integrity remained intact.
- If the client was able to shave or able to assist, the client attained a sense of independence.
- The client is comfortable following the procedure.

DOCUMENTATION

Nurses' Notes

- Procedure, if the client was able to assist, and how the client tolerated the activity
- Unusual findings or injury that may have occurred

PROCEDURE 29-26 Applying Antiembolic Stockings

OVERVIEW

Antiembolic stockings also called TED® hose or elastic stockings, are used to promote circulation by compression and are useful to prevent thrombophlebitis. They are used on the legs of a client after surgery, on clients who are immobile, and on clients who have vascular disorders such as thrombophlebitis, varicose veins, and other conditions of impaired circulation of the lower extremities.

ASSESSMENT

1. Assess the condition of the client's lower extremities, noting edema, color, temperature, intact skin, ulcers, or infections. **Establishes a baseline for comparison.**
2. Assess the quality and equality of peripheral pulses in the legs (either dorsalis pedis or posterior tibial pulses) **to determine circulatory status.**
3. Assess the client's understanding of the reasons for, and the use of, the antiembolic stockings **to determine the amount of client teaching required.**

(Continues)

PROCEDURE 29-26 Applying Antiembolic Stockings (Continued)

4. Assess the client for signs and symptoms of deep vein thrombosis, such as increased calf size or color change, **to determine the appropriateness of the TED® hose placement.**

POSSIBLE NURSING DIAGNOSES

Risk for Impaired Skin Integrity
Decreased Cardiac Output
Ineffective Tissue Perfusion

PLANNING

Expected Outcomes

1. The client will experience no signs or symptoms of deep venous thrombosis or thrombophlebitis.
2. The client's venous return will be improved.
3. The client's popliteal, posterior tibial, and dorsalis pedis pulses will remain intact while stockings are in place.
4. The client will have good circulation while stockings are in place, as evident by warm skin temperature, capillary return within normal limits, sensation present, and no edema present in both extremities.

Equipment Needed

- Antiembolic stockings and package directions (latex-free, if necessary)
- Tape measure

delegation tips

Ancillary personnel routinely remove and reapply antiembolic stockings. Instruction is given to staff to apply stockings while client is supine in bed and to inspect and report any skin breakdown, impaired circulation, or excessive edema to the nurse.

IMPLEMENTATION—ACTION/RATIONALE

ACTION	RATIONALE
* Check client's identification band * Explain procedure before beginning *	
1. Wash hands.	1. Reduces transmission of microorganisms.
2. Review the orders with the client, including the reason for the stockings and the type of stockings ordered (e.g., knee or thigh high).	2. Facilitates compliance.
3. With the client in a supine position in bed, measure the client's leg for the correct size: • Thigh-high stockings: from Achilles tendon to the gluteal fold, circumference of the midthigh • Below-the-knee stockings: from the Achilles tendon to the popliteal fold, circumference of the midcalf	3. Supine position encourages venous return and decreases swelling, thereby allowing accurate measurement for size of stockings.
4. Compare the obtained measurements with the package insert to ascertain proper size.	4. Correct size is essential for stockings to apply the appropriate pressure for adequate venous return without compromise to circulation.
5. Apply stockings. The best time to apply stockings is early in the morning, before the client gets out of bed or immediately after surgery. Keep client in supine position until stockings are applied.	5. Feet are less swollen in the morning because the feet have been in a nondependent position during the night and most venous return has occurred. This, of course, is not the case in a client who has been up frequently during the night.
6. Open the package and turn stockings inside out over hand and arm. Place hand deep enough inside a stocking to grasp the stocking toe.	6. Because stockings contain strong elastic, application can be difficult if not initiated from the bottom up and if stockings are not turned inside out. Wrinkles in stockings can also occur if a systematic approach is not used for application.
7. Using the hand inside the stocking, hold onto the client's toes. Invert the stocking with the other hand and pull it over the hand and the client's toes. Release toes.	7. See Rationale 6.

(Continues)

PROCEDURE 29-26 Applying Antiembolic Stockings (Continued)

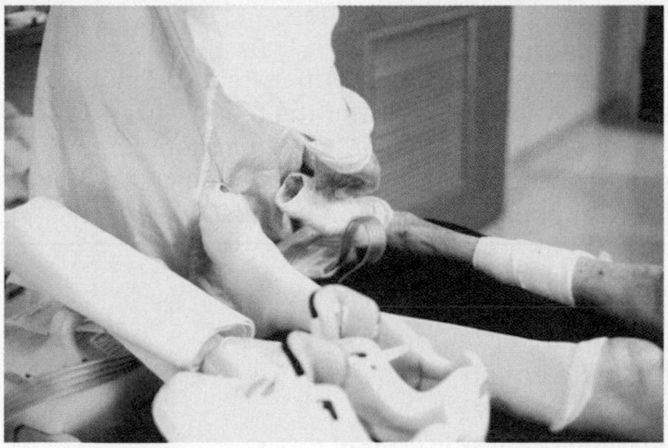

FIGURE 29-26-1 Place the stocking over the client's toes and foot.

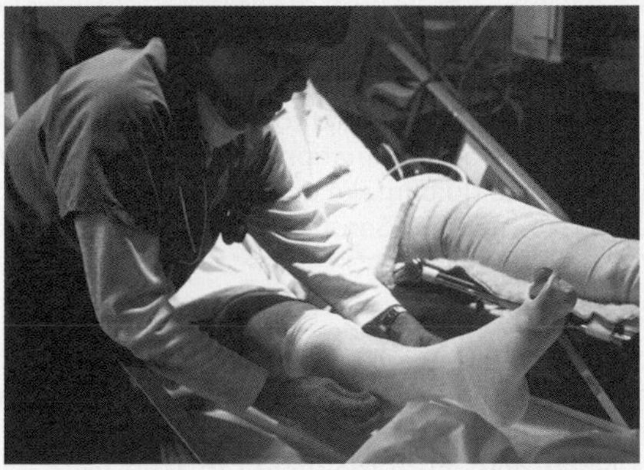

FIGURE 29-26-2 Pull the stocking smoothly and evenly up the client's leg.

ACTION	RATIONALE
8. Hold each side of the stocking and pull it from the client's toes to the heel in one motion (Figure 29-26-1).	8. See Rationale 6.
9. Continuing to hold each side of the stockings, firmly pull the stocking up by using the thumbs to guide the stockings upward over the ankles and up the client's leg (Figure 29-26-2).	9. See Rationale 6.
10. Repeat with the other leg, if necessary.	10. See Rationale 6.
11. Smooth and remove any wrinkles in the stockings.	11. Wrinkles can create skin breakdown and can cause a tourniquet effect on the leg.
12. Assess circulatory and neurostatus of feet. (CMS: circulatory, movement, sensation)	12. Establishes baseline assessment.
13. Wash hands.	13. Reduces transmission of microorganisms.

EVALUATION

- The client has not experienced any signs or symptoms of deep venous thrombosis or thrombophlebitis.
- The client's venous return is improved.
- The client's popliteal, posterior tibial, and dorsalis pedis pulses remain intact while stockings are in place.
- The client has good circulation while stockings are in place, as evident by warm skin temperature, capillary return within normal limits, sensation within normal limits, and no edema in either extremities.

DOCUMENTATION

Nurses' Notes

- Use of stockings
- Skin integrity, any presence of venous problems, and circulatory status of extremities
- Equality of pedal pulses
- Size and length of stockings

PROCEDURE 29-27

Assisting with a Bedpan or Urinal

OVERVIEW

Voiding and bowel elimination for the client confined to bed require a bedpan and/or a urinal. Reduced mobility, pain, privacy issues, the need for assistance, delays in getting assistance when needed, and the fear of interruption can all alter normal elimination patterns. Fear of creating embarrassing noises, sights, or odors may compel the client to reduce fluid intake or avoid the urge to eliminate while in the hospital. This can lead to an increased risk of urinary tract infection. Sensitivity and proper technique by caregivers support the client on bed rest.

ASSESSMENT

1. Assess your equipment. Do you have the necessary items within reach? **Prevents having to stop the procedure and leave the client's bedside.**
2. Assess how much the client can assist in positioning and removing the bedpan. **Determines how the procedure is done and whether assistance is required.**
3. Check whether the client is confused, combative, in traction, or immobile. **Determines how the procedure is done and whether assistance is required.**
4. Check for casts, braces, or dressings that need protecting from accidental contamination with waste products. **Determines how much preparation is needed before toileting.**
5. Check for privacy and unexpected interruptions. **Determines if extra steps are needed to ensure privacy before toileting.**
6. Assess if client has orders to record intake and output. **Determines need to take steps for measurement and may require containers with measurement markings.**

POSSIBLE NURSING DIAGNOSES

Constipation
Bowel Incontinence
Stress Urinary Incontinence
Urge Urinary Incontinence
Urinary Retention
Toileting Self-Care Deficit
Situational Low Self-Esteem
Powerlessness

PLANNING

Expected Outcomes

1. Clients will be able to void and defecate when necessary.
2. Clients will have as much privacy and comfort as allowable, given their physical condition.
3. Intake and output will be accurately measured as needed.
4. The urinal or bedpan will be placed without skin damage.
5. The bedpan will be removed and emptied without spillage.

Equipment Needed

- Bedpan (regular or fracture) or urinal
- Disposable gloves
- Bedpan cover
- Toilet paper
- Washcloth and towel

delegation tips

This skill is routinely delegated to ancillary personnel educated in Standard Precautions and proper body positioning, and to report color, odor, and amount of output to the nurse.

IMPLEMENTATION—ACTION/RATIONALE

ACTION	RATIONALE
* Check client's identification band * Explain procedure before beginning *	
Positioning a Bedpan	
1. Close curtain or door.	1. Provides for privacy.
2. Wash hands; apply gloves.	2. Reduces transmission of microorganisms.
3. Lower head of bed so client is in supine position.	3. The supine position will increase ability of client to move to side-lying position.
4. Elevate bed.	4. Ensures proper body mechanics.
5. Assist client to side-lying position using side rail for support.	5. Provides for best position for proper placement of bedpan.

(Continues)

PROCEDURE 29-27 Assisting with a Bedpan or Urinal (Continued)

ACTION	RATIONALE
6. Powder edge of bedpan if necessary.	6. For comfort; prevents bedpan from sticking to the skin.
7. While holding the bedpan with one hand, help the client roll onto his or her back, while pushing against the bedpan (toward the center of the bed) to hold it in place (Figure 29-27-1A).	7. Prevents dislocation or alignment of bedpan.
8. Alternate: Help the client raise the hips using the over-bed trapeze, and slide the pan in place (Figure 29-27-1B). Alternate: If the client is unable to turn or raise hips, use a fracture pan instead of a bedpan (Figure 29-27-2A&B). With a fracture pan, the flat side is placed toward the client's head.	8. Provides an alternate way to position the pan. Fracture pan reduces the amount of movement and lift required to place the pan.
9. Check placement of bedpan by looking between client's legs.	9. May prevent spillage from misalignment of bedpan.
10. If indicated, elevate head of bed to 45-degree angle or higher for comfort.	10. Check order of physician or qualified practitioner; bed remains flat if client has a spinal cord injury or spinal surgery. Elevating the head of bed creates a more normal elimination position.
11. Place call light within reach of client; place side rails in upright position, lower bed, and provide privacy.	11. Privacy allows for a more comfortable elimination environment; elevated side rails provide for safety.
12. Remove gloves; wash hands.	12. Reduces transmission of microorganisms.
Positioning a Urinal	
13. Repeat Actions 1 and 2.	13. See Rationales 1 and 2.
14. Lift the covers and place the urinal (Figure 29-27-2C) so the client may grasp the handle and position it. If the client cannot do this, you must position the urinal and place the penis into the opening (Figure 29-27-3).	14. Ensures proper placement of the urinal and reduces the risk of spillage.
15. Remove gloves; wash hands.	15. Reduces transmission of microorganisms.

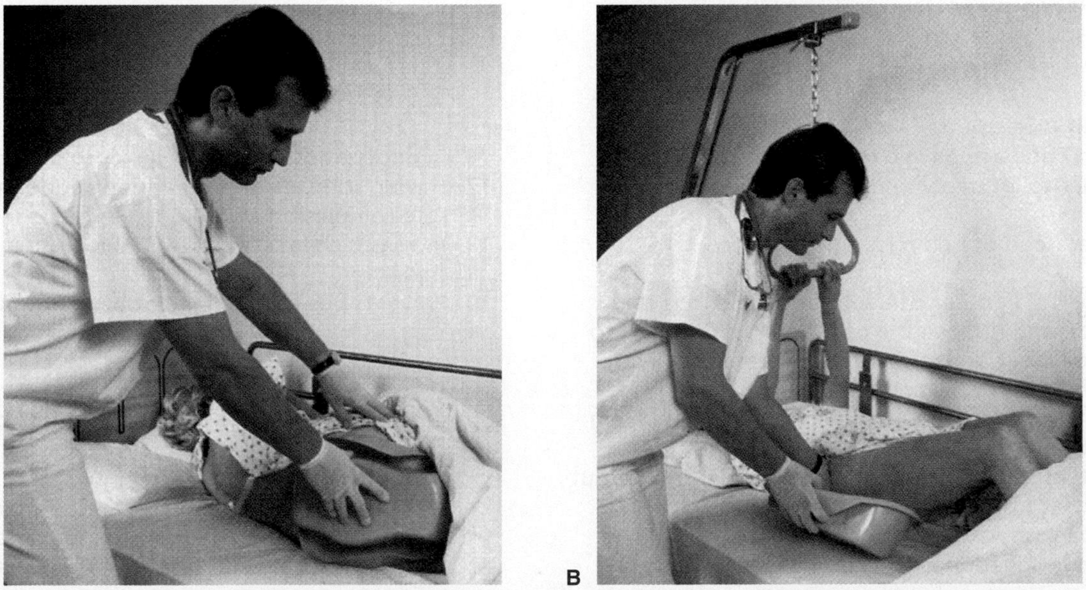

A B

COURTESY OF DELMAR CENGAGE LEARNING

FIGURE 29-27-1 Positioning a bedpan: *A*, Hold the bedpan in place with one hand and have the client roll onto the pan. *B*, A client uses the trapeze bar to raise hips when given a bed pan.

(Continues)

PROCEDURE 29-27 Assisting with a Bedpan or Urinal (Continued)

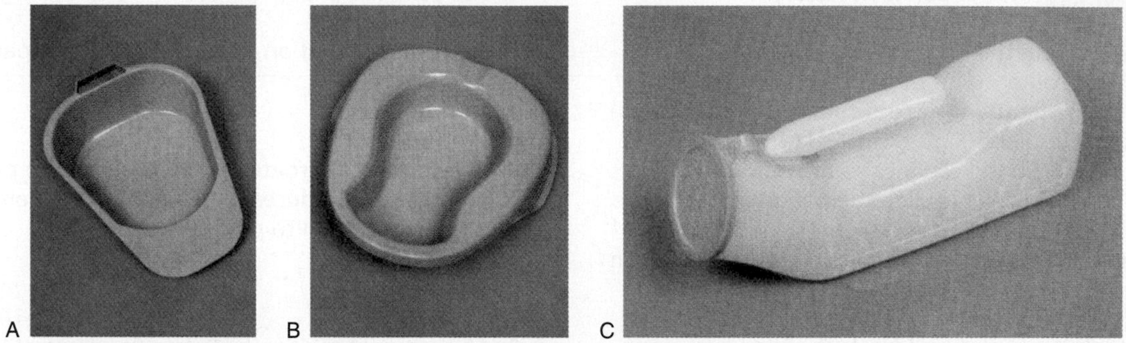

COURTESY OF DELMAR CENGAGE LEARNING

FIGURE 29-27-2 **Bedpans and urinals are used when clients are on bed rest; *A*, A fracture pan is used when the client is unable to turn or raise hips; *B*, A bedpan is offered to clients who do not have mobility problems; *C*, A urinal is used by a male when on bed rest.**

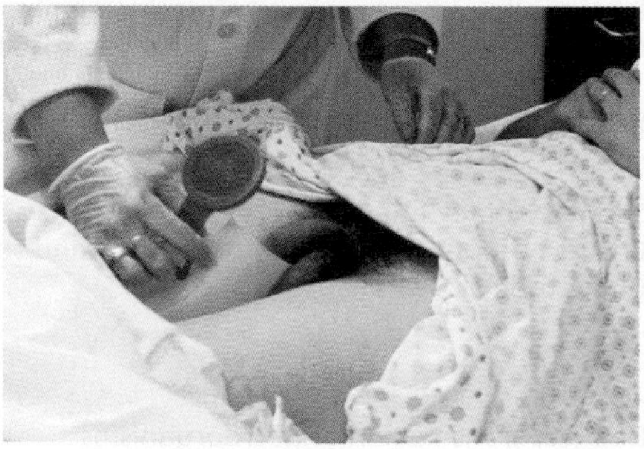

COURTESY OF DELMAR CENGAGE LEARNING

FIGURE 29-27-3 **If the client is unable to assist, place the penis into the opening of the urinal.**

Removing a Bedpan

ACTION	RATIONALE
16. Wash hands; apply gloves.	16. Reduces transmission of microorganisms.
17. Gather toilet paper and washing supplies.	17. Having supplies at the bedside allows smooth and safe completion of the procedure.
18. Lower head of bed to supine position.	18. Increases client's ability to move to side-lying position.
19. While holding bedpan with one hand, roll client to side and remove the pan, being careful not to pull or shear skin sticking to the pan and being careful not to spill contents.	19. Prevents possible spillage of bedpan contents.
20. Assist with cleaning or wiping; always wipe from front to back.	20. Client may not be able to clean self; wiping from front to back decreases chances of cross contamination from anus to urethra.
21. Empty bedpan (observe and measure urine output and check for occult blood if ordered), clean bedpan, and store it in proper place.	21. Promotes privacy and decreases the chance of spilling contents. Assess for constipation and diarrhea.
22. Remove soiled gloves. Wash hands.	22. Reduces transmission of microorganisms.

(Continues)

PROCEDURE 29-27 Assisting with a Bedpan or Urinal (Continued)

ACTION	RATIONALE
23. Allow client to wash hands.	23. Provides for physical hygiene and comfort.
24. Place call light within reach; recheck that side rails are in the upright position.	24. Ensures client safety and comfort.
25. Wash hands.	25. Reduces transmission of microorganisms.
Removing a Urinal	
26. Wash hands and apply gloves.	26. Reduces transmission of microorganisms.
27. Empty the urinal, measuring urine output if ordered; rinse the urinal; and replace it within the client's reach. Observe odor and color of urine before discarding.	27. Provides a way to measure the client's output. Keeping the urinal within reach promotes client autonomy. Helps evaluate for concentrated urine, infection, and renal problems.
28. Remove soiled gloves. Wash hands.	28. Reduces transmission of microorganisms.
29. Allow client to wash hands.	29. Provides for physical hygiene and comfort.
30. Place call light within reach; recheck that side rails are in the upright position.	30. Ensures client safety and comfort.
31. Wash hands.	31. Reduces transmission of microorganisms.

EVALUATION
- The client was able to void or defecate as needed.
- The client's request for assistance was answered promptly.
- The bedpan or urinal was removed and emptied without spillage.
- Ordered tests were performed and samples were collected.
- The client's skin integrity was maintained without skin shear or tearing.
- The client was provided with as much privacy and comfort as possible.

DOCUMENTATION
Nurses' Notes
- Elimination and voiding; include color, odor, consistency, and any unusual findings such as blood or mucus
- Client complaints such as constipation or burning with urination
- Condition of the client's skin

Intake and Output Record
- Time the client voided and the amount of urine voided

PROCEDURE 29-28 Applying a Condom Catheter

OVERVIEW
The condom catheter is an external drainage system that collects urine from male clients with incontinence. It is less invasive than a retention catheter and allows less contact of the skin with urine than a disposable brief or protective disposable underpad. Condom catheters require an order from an appropriate health care provider.

ASSESSMENT
1. Assess skin integrity around the penis and perineal area **to look for signs of irritation and skin breakdown.**
2. Assess the client for ability to cooperate with the application and retention of the condom catheter **to determine what type of teaching is necessary.**

(Continues)

PROCEDURE 29-28 Applying a Condom Catheter (Continued)

3. Assess the amount and pattern of urinary incontinence **to determine if the condom catheter is the best continence method for the client.**
4. Assess for latex allergy.

POSSIBLE NURSING DIAGNOSES

Impaired Urinary Elimination
Risk for Impaired Skin Integrity
Toileting Self-Care Deficit

PLANNING

Expected Outcomes

1. The client will have a condom catheter in place without leakage or discomfort.
2. The client will have no skin irritation from the condom catheter.
3. The client will understand the reason for, and cooperate with, the placement and retention of the condom catheter.

Equipment Needed

- Condom catheter kit with adhesive strip
- Urinary drainage bag
- Clean gloves
- Basin with warm water and soap
- Towel and washcloth

delegation tips

Application of a condom catheter may be delegated to properly trained ancillary personnel. The need for condom drainage and the ongoing assessment of the client's skin condition is followed up by the nurse.

IMPLEMENTATION—ACTION/RATIONALE

* Check client's identification band * Explain procedure before beginning *

ACTION	RATIONALE
1. Wash hands.	1. Reduces transmission of microorganisms.
2. Protect the client's privacy by closing the door and pulling curtains around the bed.	2. Allows privacy for the client.
3. Position the client in a comfortable position, preferably a supine position, if tolerated by the client. Raise the bed to a comfortable height for the nurse.	3. Facilitates the cleaning and application of the catheter. Raising the bed to a comfortable height promotes good body mechanics.
4. Apply nonsterile latex-free gloves.	4. Prevents possible transmission of microorganisms.
5. Fold the client's gown across the abdomen and the sheet just below pubic area.	5. Provides minimal exposure of the client, thereby reducing the client's embarrassment.
6. Assess the client's penis for any signs of redness, irritation, or skin breakdown.	6. A significant amount of skin breakdown may require an indwelling catheter. Provides baseline data for comparison with future assessments.
7. Clean the client's penis with warm soapy water. Retract the foreskin on the uncircumcised male and clean thoroughly in folds.	7. Removes microorganisms that could enter the urinary meatus and cause a urinary tract infection. Avoids trapping microorganisms in folds around the meatus.
8. Return the client's foreskin to its normal position.	8. Failure to return the foreskin to a normal position can lead to swelling of the penis and possible vascular constriction.
9. Shave any excess hair around the base of the penis if required by institutional policy.	9. Prevents discomfort from the adhesive strip when the condom catheter is removed.
10. Rinse and dry the area.	10. Moist warm environment can lead to the growth of microorganisms.
11. If a condom kit is used, open the package containing the skin preparation. Wipe and apply skin preparation solution to the shaft of the penis. If the client has an erection, wait for termination of erection before applying the catheter.	11. Preparation solution protects the client's skin from irritation. An erection may occur from manipulation of the penis while cleaning the area. This is a normal reaction and will terminate in a few minutes.
12. Apply the double-sided adhesive strip around the base of the client's penis in a spiral	12. Applying the adhesive in a spiral fashion does not compromise circulation of the penis. Encircling the

(Continues)

PROCEDURE 29-28 Applying a Condom Catheter (Continued)

ACTION | **RATIONALE**

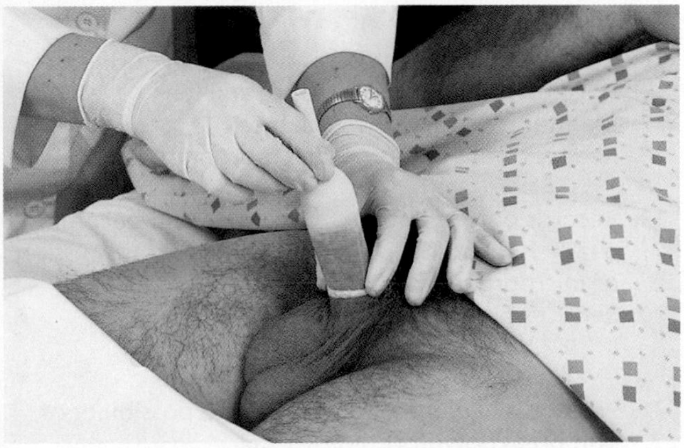

COURTESY OF DELMAR CENGAGE LEARNING

FIGURE 29-28-1 Unroll the condom from the distal portion of the penis upward to the base. Leave 1 to 2 inches between the tip of the penis and the end of the condom.

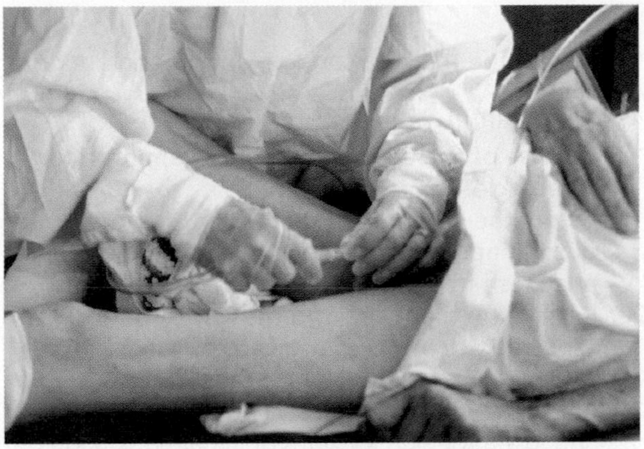

COURTESY OF DELMAR CENGAGE LEARNING

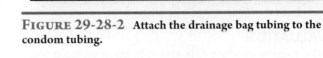

FIGURE 29-28-2 Attach the drainage bag tubing to the condom tubing.

fashion. The strip is applied 1 inch from the proximal end of the penis. Do not completely encircle the penis or tightly encompass penis.

Rationale: penis can constrict the penis, impair circulation, and cause edema.

13. Position the rolled condom at the distal portion of the penis and unroll it, covering the penis and the double-sided strip of adhesive. Leave a 1- to 2-inch space between the tip of the penis and the end of the condom (Figure 29-28-1).

    Rationale: 13. The condom sticks to the adhesive and remains in place. The extra spacing prevents pressure and erosion of the tip of the penis.

14. Gently press the condom to the adhesive strip.

    Rationale: 14. Enables the condom to adhere evenly to the adhesive strip.

15. Attach the drainage bag tubing to the catheter tubing (Figure 29-28-2). Make sure the tubing lays over the client's legs, not under (Figure 29-28-3). Secure the drainage bag to the side of the bed below the level of the client's bladder or to the drainage bag attached to the leg.

    Rationale: 15. Promotes urine flow away from the client. Constant exposure to urine and moisture can irritate the penis. Prevents reflux of the urine onto the penis and microorganisms from entering the penis.

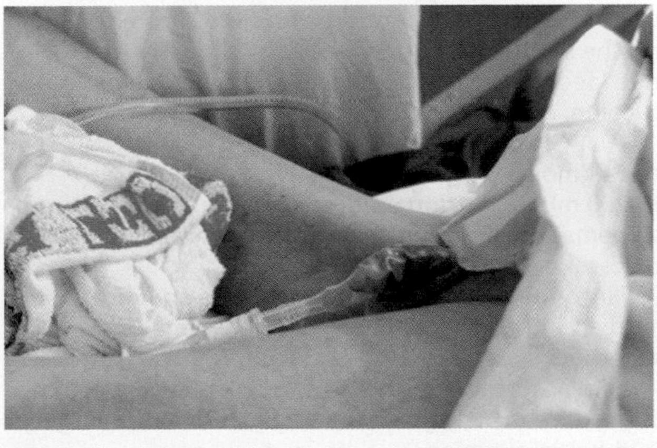

COURTESY OF DELMAR CENGAGE LEARNING

FIGURE 29-28-3 Make sure the drainage bag tubing lies over the client's leg.

(Continues)

PROCEDURE 29-28 Applying a Condom Catheter (Continued)

ACTION	RATIONALE
16. Determine that the condom and tubing are not twisted.	16. If the condom or tubing is twisted, the urine cannot flow out and the condom will leak or fall off.
17. Cover the client.	17. Maintains privacy of the client.
18. Dispose of the used equipment in appropriate receptacle.	18. Reduces transmission of microorganisms.
19. Empty the bag, measure the client's urinary output, and record every 4 hours. Remove gloves and wash hands after procedure.	19. Records output and prevents bag from becoming overly full and/or too heavy. Reduces transmission of microorganisms.
20. Return the client's bed to the lowest position and reposition client to comfortable or appropriate position.	20. Reduces potential injury from falls.
21. Remove the condom once a day to clean the area and assess the skin for signs of impaired skin integrity.	21. Promotes hygiene and reduces the possibility of skin breakdown.

EVALUATION

- The client's condom catheter is in place without leakage or discomfort.
- The client does not have any skin irritation from the condom catheter.
- The client understands the reason for, and cooperates with, the placement and retention of the condom catheter.

DOCUMENTATION

Nurses' Notes

- Time the procedure was performed
- Condition of the client's skin, recording any irritation, rashes, or open areas
- Client teaching performed

Intake and Output Record

- Amount of urine emptied from the urine drainage bag

PROCEDURE 29-29 Administering an Enema

OVERVIEW

An enema is a solution inserted into the rectum and sigmoid colon to remove feces and/or flatus. Enemas can also be used to instill medications. A cleansing enema is probably the most common type of enema. This type of enema stimulates peristalsis via irritation of the colon/rectum and by causing intestinal distention with fluid. There are two general types of cleansing enemas: the large-volume enema and the small-volume enema.

A large-volume enema is designed to clean the colon of as much feces as possible. In a large-volume enema, between 500 and 1,000 mL of fluid are instilled into the rectum/colon, and the client is asked to retain the fluid as long as possible.

Small-volume enemas are designed to clear the rectum and the sigmoid colon of fecal matter. Small-volume enemas are delivered with the traditional enema kit using 50 to 200 mL of solution, but most frequently they are administered using a prepackaged disposable kit. Prepackaged enemas are easily administered and available over-the-counter in most drugstores. This makes them ideal for home care use.

An oil retention enema is a small-volume enema that instills oil into the rectum, retained for up to an hour to soften very hard stool. It is often followed by a large-volume cleansing enema. A small-volume enema can deliver a medicated solution directly to the rectal mucosa. This method is useful when the rectum is the area to be medicated, if the client is unable to take oral medications, or if rapid absorption of the medication is required. The return-flow enema, used to remove flatus and stimulate peristalsis, is frequently given following abdominal surgery to reduce intestinal distention and to stimulate the resumption of bowel function.

Many different solutions are used for enemas, including tap water, normal saline, hypertonic solutions, soap solutions, oil, and carminative solutions. Tap water is a hypotonic solution. Because it is a less concentrated solution

(Continues)

PROCEDURE 29-29 Administering an Enema (Continued)

than the body's cells, it is drawn into the body and may cause water toxicity, electrolyte imbalance, or circulatory overload. Normal saline is an isotonic solution. It is the same concentration as the body's own fluids and is considered a safe enema solution. It is important that children and infants be given only normal saline enemas because their small size predisposes them to fluid imbalances. Prepackaged small-volume enemas use hypertonic solutions to draw fluid from the body to lubricate the stool and distend the rectum. Hypertonic solutions are contraindicated in dehydrated clients and small children. Carminative solutions are used to prevent gas from forming.

Enemas are contraindicated in clients with bowel obstruction, inflammation, or infection of the abdomen or if the client has had recent rectal or anal surgery. If there is any question regarding the advisability of administering an enema, consult the client's health care provider.

ASSESSMENT

1. Identify the type of enema ordered as well as the rationale for the enema. **Allows the nurse to verify the appropriateness of the type of enema ordered.**
2. Assess the physical condition of the client. Determine if the client has bowel sounds. Assess for a history of constipation, hemorrhoids, or diverticulitis. Determine if the client is able to hold a side-lying position or to retain the enema solution. **Allows the nurse to plan the procedure with the client's limitations in mind.**
3. Assess the client's mental state, including ability to understand and cooperate with the procedure, the client's knowledge level regarding the procedure, and any preexisting fears the client may have regarding the procedure. Knowing if the client can comprehend and cooperate with the procedure helps the nurse plan ahead. **Many clients have preexisting fears and beliefs regarding enemas and their administration.**

POSSIBLE NURSING DIAGNOSES

Constipation
Risk for Deficient Fluid Volume
Risk for Situational Low Self-Esteem

PLANNING

Expected Outcomes

1. The client's rectum will be free of feces and flatus.
2. The client will experience a minimum of trauma and embarrassment from the procedure.

Equipment Needed

Large-Volume Cleansing Enema

- Absorbent pad for the bed
- Disposable gloves
- Bedside commode or bedpan if client will not be able to ambulate to bathroom
- Lubricant
- Enema container
- Tubing with clamp and nozzle
- Toilet tissue
- Washcloth, towel, and basin

Small-Volume Prepackaged Enema

- Prescribed prepackaged enema
- Lubricant if the tip is not prelubricated
- Toilet tissue
- Bedpan or commode if the client cannot use the bathroom
- Absorbent pad for bed
- Gloves

Return-Flow Enema

- Absorbent pad for the bed
- Disposable gloves
- Bedside commode or bedpan if client will not be able to ambulate to bathroom
- Prescribed solution
- Lubricant
- Enema container
- Tubing with clamp and nozzle
- Toilet tissue

delegation tips

Administering an enema is a procedure that ancillary personnel perform after proper instruction and supervision. Instruct ancillary personnel to notify the nurse if any difficulty in administering or negative reactions such as severe cramping or inability to retain the enema occur. Results are documented and reported to the nurse.

(Continues)

PROCEDURE 29-29 Administering an Enema (Continued)

IMPLEMENTATION—ACTION/RATIONALE

ACTION	RATIONALE
* Check client's identification band * Explain procedure before beginning *	
Administering an Enema	
1. Wash hands.	1. Reduces transmission of microorganisms.
2. Assess client's understanding of procedure and provide privacy.	2. Prepares client for procedure.
3. Apply gloves.	3. Prevents contact with feces.
4. Prepare equipment.	4. Ensures a smooth procedure.
5. Place absorbent pad on bed under client. Assist client in attaining left lateral position with right leg flexed as sharply as possible. If there is a question regarding the client's ability to hold the solution, place a bedpan on the bed nearby (Figure 29-29-1).	5. Facilitates flow of solution into the rectum and colon. The flexed leg provides the best exposure of the anus.
6. Steps 6 to 12 are specific instructions for administering a large-volume cleansing enema. Enemas administered to adults are usually given at 105° to 110°F (40.5° to 43°C), and those administered to children are usually administered at 100°F (37.7°C). Solution should be at least body temperature to prevent cramping and discomfort.	6. Enemas work best when solution is warm. If enemas are too hot, damage can be done to the bowel mucosa. If enemas are too cold, spasms may occur.
7. Pour solution into the bag or bucket; add water if needed. Open clamp and allow solution to prime tubing. Clamp tubing when primed.	7. Expels air from the tubing, which could cause intestinal distention and discomfort.
8. Lubricate 5 cm (2 inches) of the rectal tube unless the tube is part of a prelubricated enema set (Figure 29-29-2).	8. Minimizes trauma to the anal sphincter during insertion of the rectal tube.
9. Hold the enema container level with the rectum. Ask the client to take a deep breath. Simultaneously, slowly and smoothly insert rectal tube into rectum approximately 7 to 10 cm (3 to 4 inches) in an adult. The rectum of an adult is usually 10 to 20 cm (4 to 6 inches). The tube	9. A deep breath helps relax the sphincter. Insertion of rectal tube toward the umbilicus guides tube along rectum.

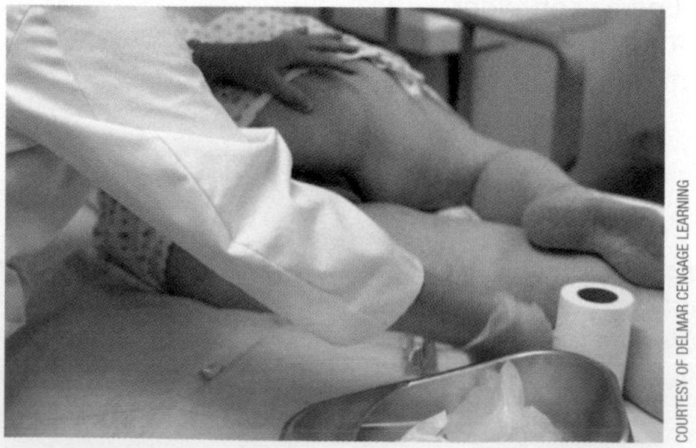

FIGURE 29-29-1 Position the client in the left lateral position with the right leg flexed.

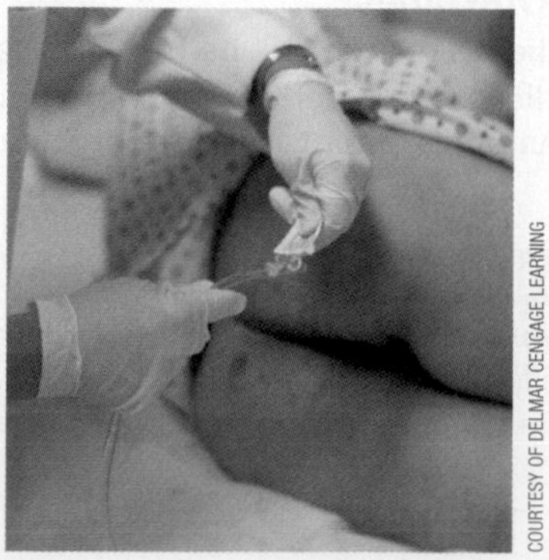

FIGURE 29-29-2 Lubricate 2 inches of the rectal tube with lubricant.

(Continues)

PROCEDURE 29-29 Administering an Enema (Continued)

ACTION	RATIONALE
should be inserted beyond the internal sphincter. Aim the rectal tube toward the client's umbilicus (Figure 29-29-3).	
10. Raise the solution container and open clamp. (If using an enema set, gently squeeze the container holding solution). The solution should be 30 to 45 cm (12 to 18 inches) (Figure 29-29-4) above the rectum for an adult and 7.5 cm (3 inches) above the rectum for an infant.	10. Solution should be at a height above rectum that allows gravity flow of solution into the rectum, but does not cause damage to the rectal lining because of a too-rapid increase in rectal pressure.
11. Slowly administer the fluid.	11. Decreases the incidence of intestinal spasms and cramps.
12. When solution has been completely administered or when the client cannot hold any more fluid, clamp the tubing, remove the rectal tube, and dispose of it properly. Steps 13 to 15 are specific instructions for administering a small-volume prepackaged enema.	12. The urge to defecate indicates that a sufficient amount of fluid has been administered.
13. Remove prepackaged enema from packaging. Be familiar with any special instructions included with the enema. The packaged enema may be stood in a basin of warm water to warm the fluid before use.	13. Prepare the enema.
14. Remove the protective cap from the nozzle and inspect the nozzle for lubrication. If the lubrication is not adequate, add more.	14. Prevents trauma to the rectal mucosa.
15. Squeeze the container gently to remove any air and prime the nozzle (Figure 29-29-5).	15. Reduces introduction of air into the rectum.
16. Have the client take a deep breath. Simultaneously, gently insert the enema nozzle into the anus, pointing the nozzle toward the umbilicus.	16. Relaxes the rectal sphincter. Pointing the nozzle toward the umbilicus positions the nozzle away from the rectal walls.
17. Squeeze the container until all the solution is instilled and remove the nozzle from the anus (Figure 29-29-6).	17. Allows the client to get the full benefit of the solution.

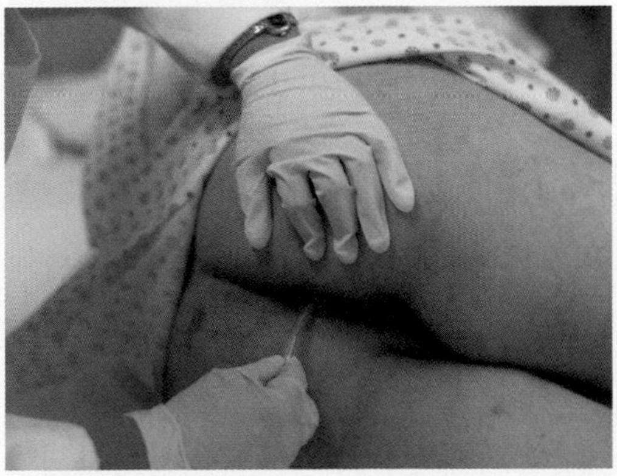

FIGURE 29-29-3 Gently and smoothly insert the rectal rube into the rectum.

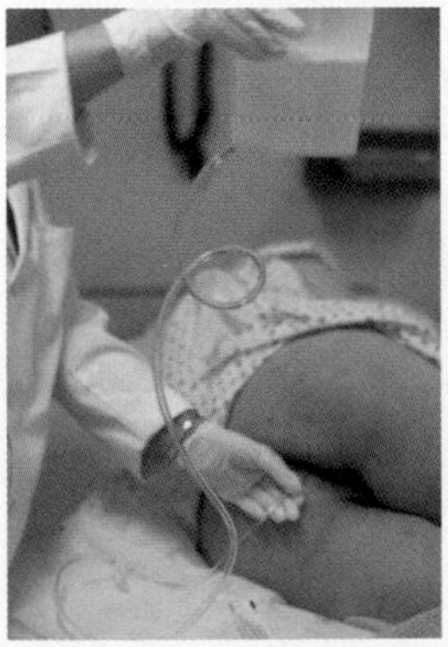

FIGURE 29-29-4 Raise the container 12 to 18 inches above the rectum and instill the solution.

(Continues)

PROCEDURE 29-29 Administering an Enema (Continued)

ACTION	RATIONALE

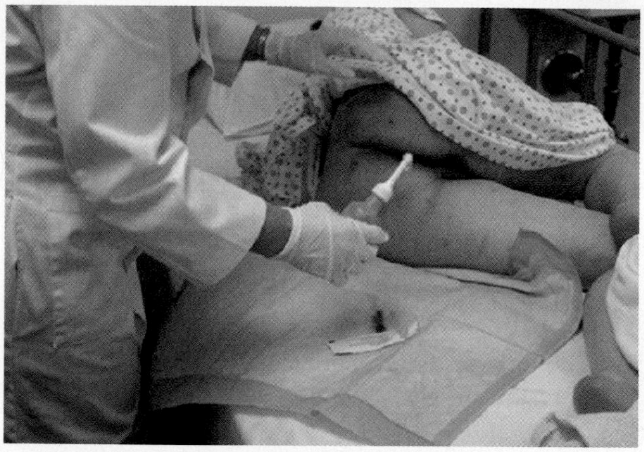

FIGURE 29-29-5 Squeeze the prepackaged enema container gently to remove any air and prime the nozzle.

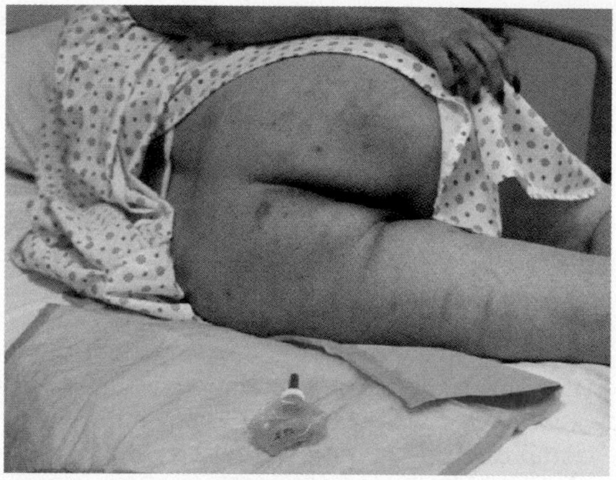

FIGURE 29-29-6 Squeeze the container until all the solution is instilled and remove the nozzle from the anus.

ACTION	RATIONALE
18. Dispose of the empty container in an appropriate receptacle.	18. Prevents the spread of microorganisms.
19. Clean lubricant, any solution, and any feces from the anus with toilet tissue.	19. Minimizes skin irritation.
20. Have the client continue to lie on the left side for the prescribed length of time. A client may need to expel a large-volume cleansing enema soon after administration. Usually, a client can hold a small-volume prepackaged enema the recommended minutes stated on the package.	20. Certain types of enemas are more effective when retained for a specified amount of time. It is easier for the client to retain the enema in a lying position, where gravity can be resisted.
21. When the client has retained the enema for the prescribed amount of time, assist to the bedside commode or toilet or onto the bedpan. If the client is using the bathroom, instruct not to flush the toilet when finished.	21. Client will be prepared to expel fluid and feces. Caregiver can see results of the enema.
22. When the client is finished expelling the enema, assist to clean the perineal area if needed.	22. Prevents skin breakdown and excoriation.
23. Return the client to a comfortable position. Place a clean, dry protective pad under the client to catch any solution or feces that may continue to be expelled.	23. Provides comfort for the client and protects the linen from potential soiling.
24. Remove gloves and wash hands.	24. Reduces transmission of microorganisms.

EVALUATION

- The client's rectum is free of feces or flatus.
- The client experienced a minimum of trauma and embarrassment from the procedure.

DOCUMENTATION

Nurses' Notes

- Time and date of the procedure
- Type of enema given, amount of fluid infused and returned, and amount and description of the feces expelled
- Client's tolerance for the procedure and any complaints or unusual findings

Medication Administration Record (MAR)

- If this is a medicated enema, be sure to note it on the MAR.

Intake and Output Record (I/O)

- If the amount of fluid returned is significantly less than the amount infused, note this on the I&O record.

PROCEDURE 29-30 Measuring Intake and Output

OVERVIEW

One of the most basic methods of monitoring a client's health is measuring intake and output, commonly called "I&O." By monitoring the amount of fluids a client takes in and comparing this to the amount of fluid a client puts out, the health care team gains valuable insights into the client's general health as well as monitors specific disease conditions.

To maintain good health, fluid intake approximately equals fluid output. Intake that exceeds output can indicate medical conditions ranging from renal failure to congestive heart failure. Output that exceeds intake can be caused by things as serious as life-threatening diarrhea or as benign as diuretic medications. An accurate record of a client's fluid balance is an important nursing function.

I&O monitoring is often ordered by the health care provider but can also be initiated by the nurse. Ideally, I&O is monitored over several days to obtain an accurate record of the client's status. In critical situations, the client's I&O is monitored and reported on an hourly basis. A urine output of less than 30 mL per hour is reported.

A daily weight is often done in conjunction with I&O because it indicates fluid retention or loss. One gallon of water weighs 8 pounds. An 8-pound weight gain over a 24- to 48-hour period indicates a life-threatening condition for the client. A significant change in a client's weight or a significant difference in a client's total I&O is reported to the client's health care provider.

Intake is any fluid consumed or infused. Generally, liquid intake is anything that is liquid at room temperature and includes water, juice, coffee, milk, ice cream, soup broth, gelatin, and popsicles. However, some facilities are including other items as liquid intake, such as oatmeal, cream of wheat, and soups. Follow the health care facility's policy when documenting. Ice is documented as one-half the total amount of mL within a container. Be sure to calculate the amount of water the client has consumed from the bedside water pitcher. Any fluids infused through IV lines, central lines, feeding tubes, or irrigant that is not returned is considered intake. Blood and blood products as well as the saline used to flush IV lines before and after the transfusion are also included in this count. IV piggybacks, fluids used to measure cardiac output, central line flushes, and TKO (to keep open) fluids are also considered in the intake total.

Urine is the largest component of output fluid volume, but diarrhea, diaphoresis, wound drainage, gastric or other fluids removed by suction, and bleeding are all fluid losses as well. These losses are measured or estimated and recorded in the total output.

Clients who are able to understand and cooperate with the I&O measurement may keep track of their fluid balance. Particularly in clients who are on a fluid restriction, client understanding and participation can greatly increase cooperation.

ASSESSMENT

1. Assess the client's risk factors for fluid overload, such as congestive heart failure, renal failure, or ascites **because edema results from excess volume in extracellular fluid spaces and transferring of fluid into tissues.**
2. Determine if the client is receiving fluids or medications that predispose to fluid overload, such as large amounts of IV fluids or steroid therapy **because steroids cause sodium and water retention and excretion of potassium.**
3. Assess the client's risk factors for fluid loss, such as diaphoresis, rapid respirations, diarrhea, gastric suction, blood loss, or wound drainage **because dehydration results from reduction of fluid within the tissues and circulatory system.**
4. Determine if the client's urine output is in excess of fluid intake **because the kidneys excrete excess fluid during periods of overhydration and conserve body water during periods of dehydration.**
5. Assess the client's ability to understand and cooperate with intake and output measurement **because cooperation in these measurements will help ensure accuracy.**

POSSIBLE NURSING DIAGNOSES

Excess Fluid Volume
Deficient Fluid Volume
Risk for Deficient Fluid Volume

PLANNING

Expected Outcomes

1. The client's fluid intake and output will be accurately measured and recorded.
2. The client will participate in the recording of fluid intake and output if possible.

Equipment Needed

- I&O form at bedside
- I&O graphic record in chart or electronic medical record
- Glass or cup
- Bedpan, urinal, or bedside commode
- Graduated container for output
- Nonsterile gloves
- Sign at bedside stating client is on I&O

(Continues)

PROCEDURE 29-30 Measuring Intake and Output (Continued)

delegation tips

Intake and output measurement may be delegated to ancillary personnel, who should be knowledgeable regarding the following:
- *Obtaining accurate measurements and reporting incontinence*
- *Observing the amount, color, and any odor from the output*
- *Protecting themselves from contamination from a body fluid and storing collection containers in designated areas*
- *Recording measurements on proper clinical records*

IMPLEMENTATION—ACTION/RATIONALE

ACTION	RATIONALE
* Check client's identification band * Explain procedure before beginning *	
1. Wash hands.	1. Reduces transmission of microorganisms.
2. Explain the rules of I&O record. All fluids taken orally are recorded on the client's intake and output form (sometimes called a fluid balance flow sheet).	2. Elicits client support.
• Client must void into bedpan, urinal, or "hat" in toilet for collecting urine, not into toilet.	• Fluid voided into the toilet cannot be measured.
• Toilet tissue is disposed of in plastic-lined container, not in bedpan.	• Liquids absorbed into toilet tissue cannot be measured by volume.
Intake	
3. Measure all oral fluids in accord with agency policy (e.g., cup =150 mL, glass = 240 mL). Record all IV fluids as they are infused.	3. Provides for consistency of measurement.
4. Record time and amount of all fluid intake in the designated space on bedside form (e.g., oral, tube feedings, IV fluids).	4. Documents fluids.
5. Transfer 8-hour total fluid intake from bedside I&O record to graphic sheet or 24-hour I&O record on client's chart or client's electronic medical record.	5. Provides for data analysis of the client's fluid status.
6. Record all fluid intake in the appropriate column of the 24-hour record or enter intake appropriately into the electronic medical record.	6. Documents intake by type and amount.
7. Complete 24-hour intake record by adding all 8-hour totals or checking that the computer has calculated data appropriately.	7. Provides consistent data for analysis of the client's fluid status over a 24-hour period.
Output	
8. Wash hands and apply nonsterile gloves.	8. Reduces potential for transmission of pathogens.
9. Empty urinal, bedpan, or Foley drainage bag (Figure 29-30-1) into graduated container or commode "hat" (Figure 29-30-2).	9. Provides accurate measurement of urine.
10. Remove gloves and wash hands.	10. Prevents cross contamination.
11. Record time and amount of output (e.g., urine, drainage from nasogastric tube, drainage tube) on I&O record.	11. Documents output.
12. Transfer 8-hour output totals to graphic sheet or 24-hour I&O record on the client's chart or client's electronic medical record.	12. Provides for data analysis of the client's fluid status.
13. Complete 24-hour output record by totaling all 8-hour totals or checking that the computer has calculated data appropriately.	13. Provides consistent data for analysis of the client's fluid status over a 24-hour period.
14. Wash hands.	14. Reduces transmission of microorganisms.

(Continues)

PROCEDURE 29-30 Measuring Intake and Output (Continued)

ACTION	RATIONALE

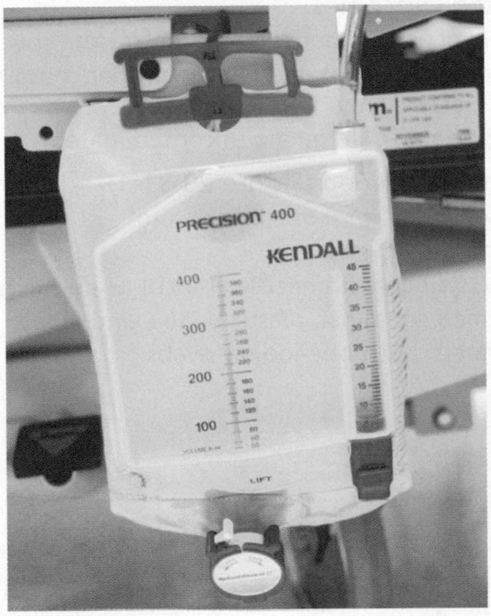

COURTESY OF DELMAR CENGAGE LEARNING

FIGURE 29-30-1 Urine in the Foley drainage bag must be measured.

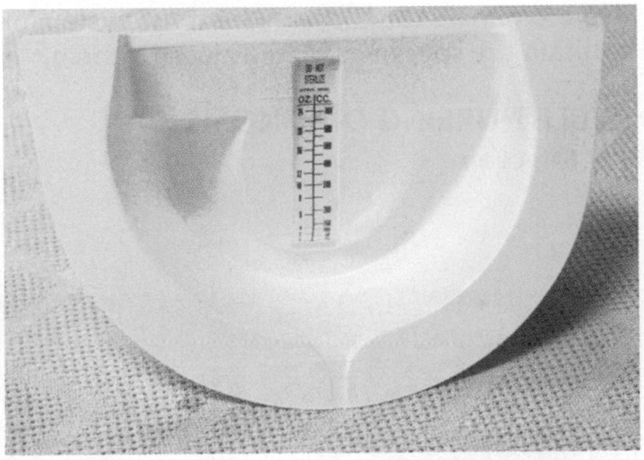

COURTESY OF DELMAR CENGAGE LEARNING

FIGURE 29-30-2 Measure urine, drainage, or other output in graduated specimen containers.

EVALUATION

- The client's fluid intake and output was accurately measured and recorded.
- Note if the client was able to participate in the recording of fluid intake and output to the best of his ability.
- Note and report any abnormal findings to the client's health care provider.

DOCUMENTATION

Intake and Output Record

- All fluid I&O
- Totals at the end of every shift
- Totals for 24 hours

Nurses' Notes

- Unusual findings, excessive intake, excessive output, or serious imbalance of intake and output and report to the client's health care provider

PROCEDURE 29-31 Urine Collection—Closed Drainage System

OVERVIEW

Indwelling catheters are used frequently in acute care settings for episodic or continuous drainage of urine. Specimens may be required to evaluate urine content, such as electrolytes, dilution, hormones, glucose, or renal function. Bacteria can be identified in urine specimens to determine if the catheter needs to be removed or if antibiotic therapy is indicated. Catheter tubing is generally designed to allow for easy access to obtain specimens without disconnecting the catheter from the tubing. Careful technique prevents contamination of the system and risk for infection.

(Continues)

PROCEDURE 29-31 Urine Collection—Closed Drainage System (Continued)

ASSESSMENT

1. Identify the purpose of the urine test **to determine the amount of urine needed and the proper container for collection.**
2. Assess the client's understanding of the test **to determine the amount of instruction needed.**
3. Identify the type of collecting tubing attached to the indwelling catheter **to determine if you need to disconnect the catheter from the system or obtain the specimen from a closed system.**

POSSIBLE NURSING DIAGNOSIS

Risk for Infection

PLANNING

Expected Outcomes

1. Client understands the reason for the specimen.
2. Specimen is obtained in the proper container in a timely manner.
3. Specimen will remain uncontaminated.

Equipment Needed (Figure 29-31-1)

- Nonserrated clamp or rubber band
- Nonsterile gloves
- 10-mL syringe with needle (1-inch) or plastic cannula
- Specimen container, plastic bag(s), and labels
- Alcohol or povidone-iodine swabs

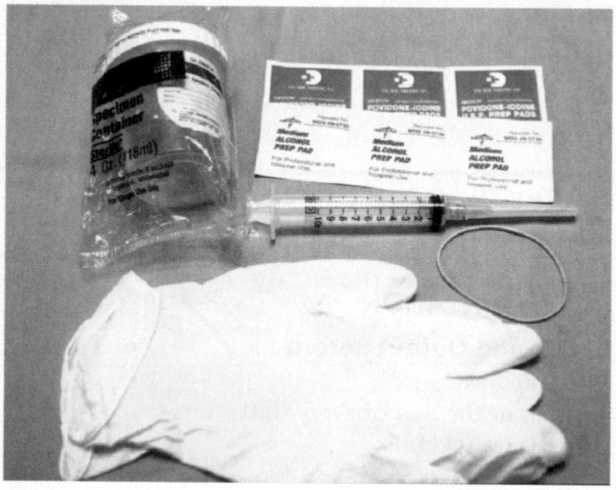

COURTESY OF DELMAR CENGAGE LEARNING

FIGURE 29-31-1 Assemble equipment to collect urine from a catheter drainage system.

delegation tips

Obtaining a urine specimen from an indwelling catheter requires the skill and problem-solving ability of a nurse. This task cannot be delegated to ancillary personnel.

IMPLEMENTATION—ACTION/RATIONALE

ACTION	RATIONALE
* Check client's identification band * Explain procedure before beginning *	
1. Wash hands.	1. Reduces transmission of microorganisms.
2. Check health care provider's order.	2. Determines test and container needed for the specimen.
3. Provide privacy.	3. Maintains client dignity.
4. Check for urine in the tubing.	4. Determines if there is sufficient urine in the collecting tubing for a specimen. *Urine from the collection bag should not be used for sterile specimens.*
5. If more urine is needed, clamp the tubing using a nonserrated clamp or a rubber band for 10 to 15 minutes (Figure 29-31-2).	5. Collects 10 mL of urine, which is needed for most urinalyses.

(Continues)

PROCEDURE 29-31 Urine Collection—Closed Drainage System (Continued)

ACTION	RATIONALE

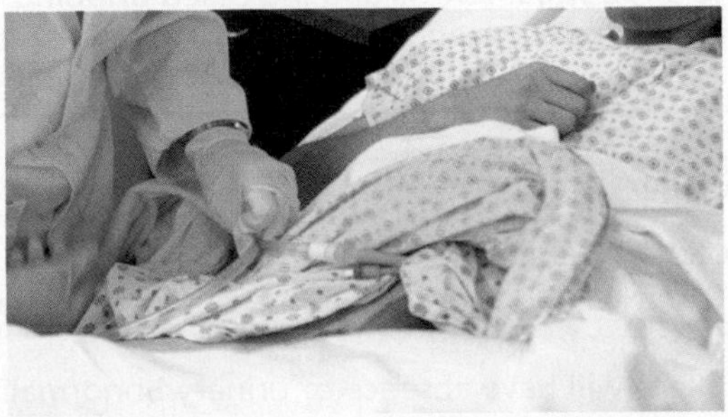

FIGURE 29-31-2 Clamp the tubing by folding it over and securing it with a rubber band to collect an adequate sample.

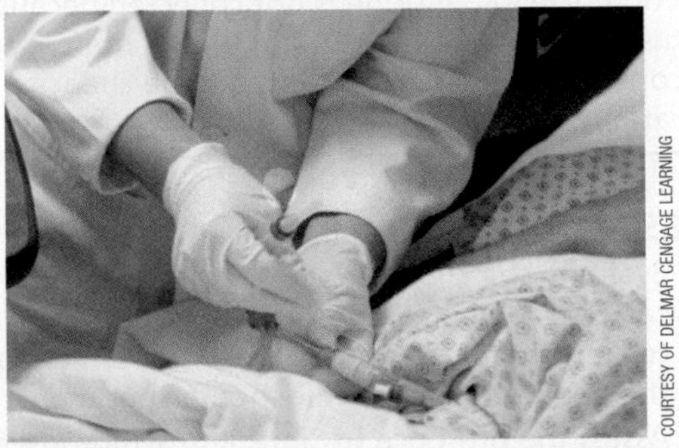

FIGURE 29-31-3 Cleanse the sample port and insert a sterile needle or sterile plastic cannula and syringe into the sample port.

ACTION	RATIONALE
6. Put on clean gloves.	6. Practices Standard Precautions.
7. Clean sample port with an alcohol or povidone-iodine swab.	7. Prevents entrance of microorganisms into the system.
8. Insert sterile needle or sterile plastic cannula of syringe into the sample port of catheter at a 45-degree angle and withdraw 10 mL of urine (Figure 29-31-3).	8. Obtains specimen with sufficient volume for most urine tests.
9. Put urine into sterile container and close tightly, taking care not to contaminate the lid of the container.	9. Prevents contamination of specimen and spill of urine.
10. Place needle and syringe into sharps container; never recap a contaminated needle.	10. Prevents accidental needlesticks.
11. Remove clamp and rearrange tubing avoiding dependent loops.	11. Reestablishes urine flow and drainage into the system.
12. Label specimen container, put it in doubled plastic bags, and send to the laboratory.	12. Ensures right test and controls transfer of pathogens.
13. Wash hands.	13. Reduces transmission of microorganisms.

EVALUATION

- Client understands the reason for the specimen.
- Specimen was obtained in the proper container in a timely manner.
- Specimen remained uncontaminated.

DOCUMENTATION

Nurses' Notes

- Date and time the specimen was sent to the laboratory
- Date, time, client name and room number, and test(s) ordered

Intake and Output Record

- Amount of urine collected for the specimen

PROCEDURE 29-32 Urine Collection—Clean Catch, Female/Male

OVERVIEW

A clean urine specimen for culture and sensitivity is collected without using an invasive method such as catheterization. This procedure is referred to as a clean-voided, clean-catch, or midstream urine specimen in that it is not a sterile procedure such as catheterization but, rather, a method of obtaining a clean specimen. This procedure is best accomplished with the client on the toilet because the use of a urinal or bedpan increases the risk of contamination. The client is asked to clean him or herself and initiate urination. After the client starts voiding,

(Continues)

PROCEDURE 29-32 Urine Collection—Clean Catch, Female/Male (Continued)

a sterile collection cup is placed under the stream of urine and a specimen collected. Hence, it is called midstream collection. The initial urine is not collected because this portion of the stream flushes the urethral opening and meatus of any bacteria. The end urine is not collected because as the urine stream slows and increased dripping and contact with the meatus occurs, the chance of contamination increases. The clean-catch specimen is sent to a laboratory for analysis.

ASSESSMENT

1. Evaluate the client's ability to obtain a clean-catch specimen **to determine if the client is able to clean himself appropriately and understands the need to obtain a midstream specimen.**
2. Assess the presence of signs and symptoms of urinary tract infections or other abnormalities **because burning or the inability to control urination may hamper the client's ability to obtain a clean specimen.**

POSSIBLE NURSING DIAGNOSES

Impaired Urinary Elimination
Acute Pain
Deficient Knowledge (collecting clean-catch urine specimen)

PLANNING

Expected Outcomes

1. Client will be able to obtain a clean, midstream specimen.
2. Client will have absence of urinary abnormalities, such as burning, tingling, pain upon urination, or inability to control stream.
3. Client will understand procedure.

Equipment Needed

- Sterile collection container with lid and label
- Sterile midstream kit, antiseptic towelettes, or cotton balls with antiseptic solution
- Toilet paper
- Nonsterile latex-free gloves

delegation tips

Collection of a clean-catch specimen may be delegated to ancillary personnel properly trained in the technique of cleaning the client and obtaining the voided specimen.

IMPLEMENTATION—ACTION/RATIONALE

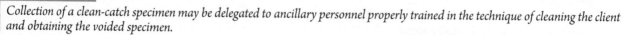

ACTION	RATIONALE
* Check client's identification band * Explain procedure before beginning *	
1. Check orders and assess need for the procedure.	1. Provides understanding of the purpose of the procedure.
2. Gather equipment.	2. Provides for organization.
3. Assess the client's ability to complete the procedure, including understanding, mobility, and balance.	3. Improves compliance and likelihood of obtaining clean specimen.
4. If the nurse is to perform the procedure: Wash hands and apply gloves. If the client performs the procedure, instruct the client to wash hands before and after the procedure. If the client wishes, provide a pair of gloves.	4. Decreases transmission of microorganisms.
5. Provide privacy.	5. Decreases embarrassment.
6. Using sterile procedure, open kit or towelettes. Open sterile container, placing the lid with sterile side up on a firm surface (Figure 29-32-1).	6. Prevents contamination of the specimen.
7. Female client: Sit with legs separated on the toilet. Use the thumb and forefinger to separate the labia, or have the client separate the labia with fingers (Figure 29-32-2). With the labia separated, use a downward stroke (from the top of the labia down toward the rectal area), and cleanse one side of the labia with the towelette (Figure 29-32-3).	7. Provides access for cleaning the labia. Cleanses area and prevents contamination of clean area. Prevents contamination by feces. Keeping labia separated avoids contamination and decreases microorganisms in specimen.

(Continues)

PROCEDURE 29-32 Urine Collection—Clean Catch, Female/Male (Continued)

ACTION	RATIONALE

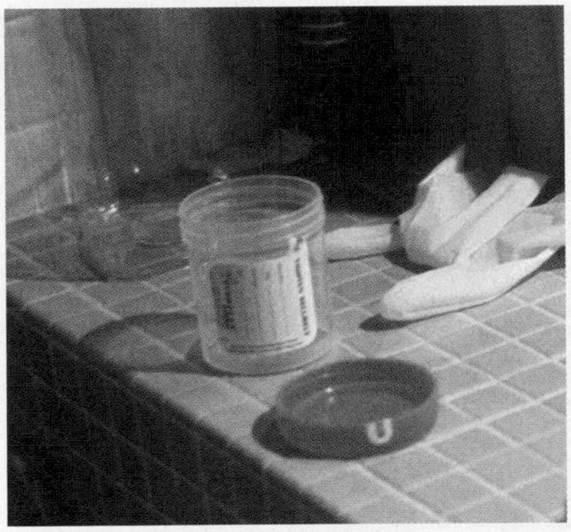

COURTESY OF DELMAR CENGAGE LEARNING

FIGURE 29-32-1 Place the lid on a firm surface, sterile side up. Do not touch the inside of the lid.

Discard the towelette and repeat the procedure on the other side with another towelette, keeping the labia separated at all times. With a third towelette, use a downward stroke from the top of the urethral opening to the bottom. Discard the towelette.

8. Male client: Stand in front of toilet. Pull back the foreskin (if present in uncircumcised male) and clean with a single stroke around meatus and glans. Use a circular motion, starting with the head of the penis at the urethral opening, moving down the glans shaft. Discard the towelette and repeat the procedure with another towelette, keeping the foreskin retracted. Wipe the head of the penis three times using a circular motion. Use a new towelette each time.

   Rationale: 8. Prevents contamination of microorganisms from foreskin. Single strokes and moving away from opening prevents contamination of the urethral opening.

9. Ask the client to begin to urinate into the toilet. After the stream starts with good flow, place the collection cup under the stream of urine (Figure 29-32-4). Avoid touching the skin with the container. Fill the container with 30 to 60 mL of urine and remove the container before urination ceases. Wipe with toilet paper.

   Rationale: 9. The specimen is collected midstream to avoid contamination of urine that touches the labia. The initial urine flushes bacteria from the orifice and the end urine may have contact with the meatus or labia and, hence, be contaminated.

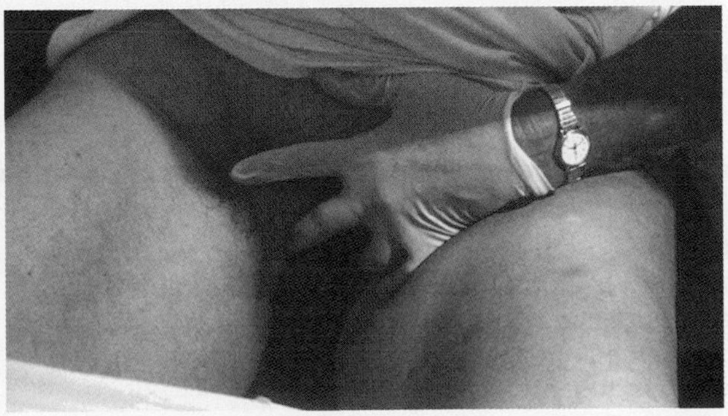

COURTESY OF DELMAR CENGAGE LEARNING

FIGURE 29-32-2 Separate the labia with the fingers of the nondominant hand.

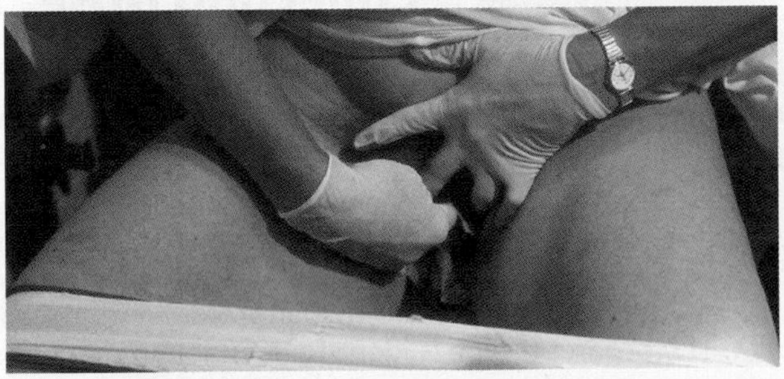

COURTESY OF DELMAR CENGAGE LEARNING

FIGURE 29-32-3 Cleanse each side and down the middle using a single downward stroke for each towelette. Keep the labia separated.

(Continues)

PROCEDURE 29-32 Urine Collection—Clean Catch, Female/Male (Continued)

ACTION	RATIONALE

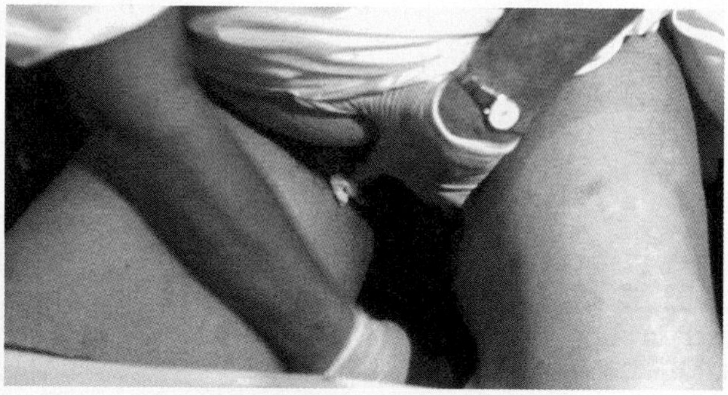

FIGURE 29-32-4 Ask the client to begin to urinate into the toilet. After the stream starts with good flow, place the collection cup under the stream of urine. Remove the cup before urination ceases.

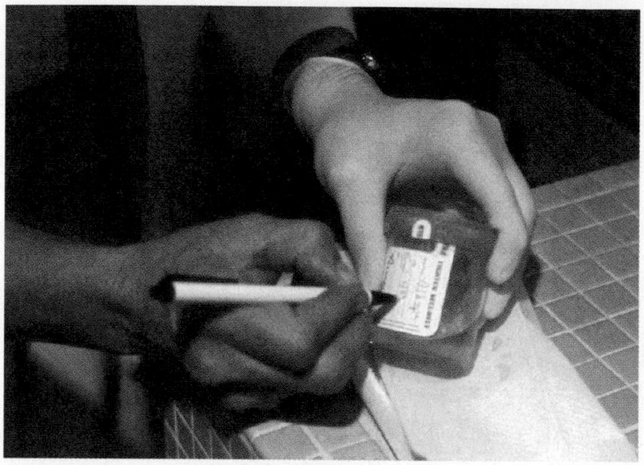

FIGURE 29-32-5 Label the container with the client's name, the date, and time specimen collected.

ACTION	RATIONALE
10. Place the sterile lid back onto the container and close tightly. Clean and dry the outside of the container with a towelette. Wash hands. Label and enclose in a double-bagged plastic biohazard bag, and follow facility policy for transporting specimen to the laboratory (Figure 29-32-5).	10. Prevents contamination of clean specimen, prevents spillage, and ensures accuracy.
11. Remove and dispose of gloves and wash hands	11. Decreases transmission of microorganisms.

EVALUATION

- Clean midstream specimen obtained.
- Client understood procedure.
- Client had no statement of burning, pain, or inability to initiate urination.

DOCUMENTATION

Nurses' Notes

- Procedure
- Date and time specimen was collected
- Characteristics of urine
- Client's signs and symptoms associated with urination
- Time urine specimen sent to lab

PROCEDURE 29-33 Collecting Nose, Throat, and Sputum Specimens

OVERVIEW

A nose, throat, or sputum specimen is a simple diagnostic tool for clients with signs or symptoms of upper respiratory or sinus infections. Nose and throat specimens are collected from the client using a sterile swab. Sputum specimens are collected in a sterile cup. Sputum specimens are also obtained via a specimen trap connected to suction. Specimens are sent to the laboratory and placed in a culture medium to allow pathogenic organisms to grow. The organism type is identified, enabling diagnosis and appropriate antimicrobial therapy.

(Continues)

PROCEDURE 29-33 Collecting Nose, Throat, and Sputum Specimens (Continued)

ASSESSMENT

1. Assess the client's understanding of the purpose of the procedure **so the client cooperates.**
2. Assess the type of nasal or sinus drainage **to determine what kind of collection equipment is needed.**
3. Review the health care provider's orders for the cultures requested **so repeat cultures are not done.**
4. Assess the client for postnasal drip, sinus headache or tenderness, nasal congestion, or sore throat **to know the purpose of the procedure.**
5. Identify whether the client has received recent antimicrobials and obtain a specimen before treatment, if possible.

POSSIBLE NURSING DIAGNOSES

Risk for Infection
Anxiety
Risk for Injury
Deficient Knowledge (regarding the procedure)

PLANNING

Expected Outcomes

1. An adequate specimen will be obtained and sent to the laboratory.
2. The procedure will be performed with a minimum of trauma to the client.

Equipment Needed

- Two sterile swabs in sterile culture tubes or a flexible wire sterile swab with cotton tip for nose or throat cultures
- Tongue blades
- Penlight
- Facial tissues
- Clean, disposable latex-free gloves
- Nasal speculum (optional)
- Emesis basin or clean container
- Sterile specimen cup, or sputum specimen collector

delegation tips

Sputum specimens are obtained by ancillary personnel. Avoiding specimen collection immediately after meals is important, as is the use of Standard Precautions when handling the specimen. Obtaining nose and throat cultures requires the problem-solving skills and techniques of a nurse, so obtaining these specimens is not delegated.

IMPLEMENTATION—ACTION/RATIONALE

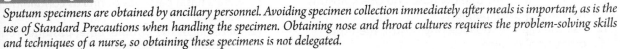

ACTION	RATIONALE
* Check client's identification band * Explain procedure before beginning *	
1. Wash hands and put on clean gloves.	1. Reduces transmission of microorganisms.
2. Ask the client to sit erect in the bed or on a chair facing the nurse.	2. Provides easy access to the nose or throat.
3. Prepare a sterile swab for use by loosening the top of the container.	3. Prevents contamination of the swab.
Collecting Throat Culture	
4. Ask the client to tilt the head backward, open the mouth, and say "ah."	4. Promotes visualization of the pharynx, relaxes the throat muscles, and minimizes the gag reflex.
5. Depress the lateral anterior one-third of the tongue with a tongue blade for better visualization.	5. Promotes visualization of the pharynx. Depressing the lateral aspect rather than the middle of the tongue decreases stimulation of the gag reflex.
6. Insert the swab without touching the cheek, lips, teeth, or tongue.	6. Prevents contamination of the specimen with oral flora.
7. Swab the tonsillar area from side to side in a quick, gentle motion (Figure 29-33-1).	7. Ensures collection of microorganisms. Retains microorganisms in the culture tube and ensures the life of bacteria for testing.
8. Withdraw the swab without touching adjacent structures and place in the culture tube. Crush ampule at bottom of tube and push swab into liquid medium (Figure 29-33-2).	8. Prevents contamination from outside microorganisms and erroneous culture results.

(Continues)

PROCEDURE 29-33 Collecting Nose, Throat, and Sputum Specimens (Continued)

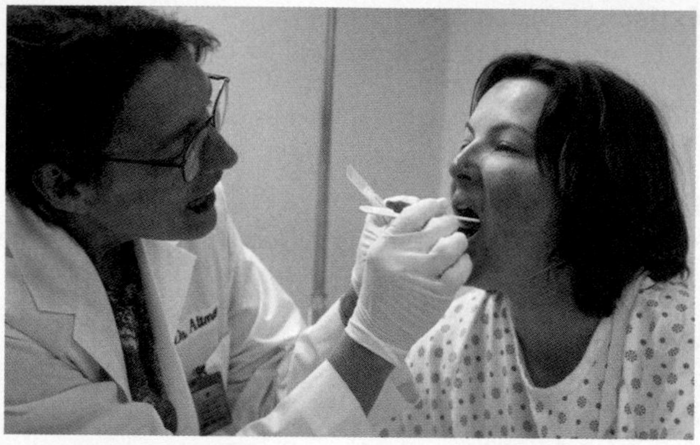

FIGURE 29-33-1 Swab the sample area using a quick, gentle motion.

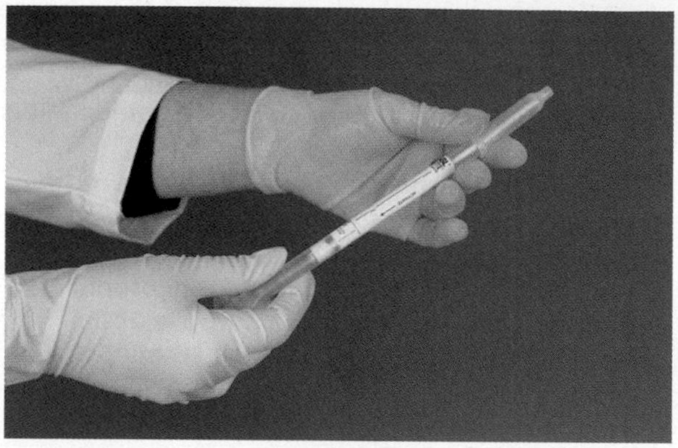

FIGURE 29-33-2 Crush ampule to release the culture medium.

ACTION	RATIONALE
9. Secure the top to the culture tube and label with the client's name.	9. Prevents identification mistakes.
10. Discard the tongue depressor. Remove gloves and discard. Wash hands.	10. Reduces transmission of microorganisms.
Collecting Nose Culture	
11. Instruct the client to blow nose and check nostrils for patency with penlight.	11. Clears nasal passages of mucus containing resident bacteria.
12. Ask the client to occlude one nostril, then the other, and exhale.	12. Determines the optimal nasal passage from which to obtain the specimen.
13. Ask the client to tilt the head back.	13. Promotes visualization of the sinuses.
14. Insert the swab into the nostril until it reaches the inflamed mucosa and rotate the swab.	14. Ensures the swab will be covered with the appropriate exudate.
15. Withdraw the swab without touching adjacent structures and place in culture tube. Crush ampule at bottom of tube and push swab into liquid medium.	15. Prevents contamination from normal nasal flora and erroneous culture results.
16. Secure the top to the culture tube and label with the client's name.	16. Prevents identification mistakes.
17. Remove gloves and discard. Wash hands.	17. Reduces transmission of microorganisms.
Collecting of Nasopharyngeal Culture	
18. Follow Actions 11 to 17, except use a swab on a flexible wire that can reach the nasopharynx via the nose.	18. Allows for access to the nasopharyngeal area.
Collecting a Sputum Culture	
19. Explain to the client that the specimen must be sputum, coughed up from the lungs.	19. Promotes client cooperation.
20. Have a sterile specimen cup ready for the sample and some tissues at hand.	20. The specimen must be collected in a sterile cup to prevent contamination.
21. Have the client take several deep breaths and then cough deeply.	21. Helps loosen secretions so the client will be able to provide a specimen.
22. Have the client expectorate the sputum into the sterile cup without touching the inside of the cup.	22. Prevents contamination of the specimen.
23. Place the lid on the specimen container without touching the inside of the lid or the container.	23. Prevents contamination of the specimen.
24. Provide the client with tissues and make him comfortable.	24. Promotes client comfort.

(Continues)

PROCEDURE 29-33 Collecting Nose, Throat, and Sputum Specimens (Continued)

ACTION	RATIONALE

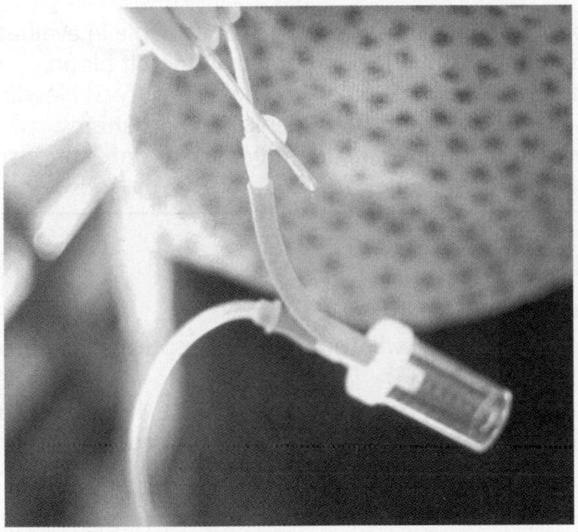

FIGURE 29-33-3 Sputum collector for use with suction.

Alternative Sputum Collection Method

* Generally used if the client is unable to expectorate an adequate sample.*

Action	Rationale
25. Obtain a sterile suction catheter and an in-line sputum collection container.	25. Prevents contamination of the specimen.
26. Provide the client with warm humidified air for about 20 minutes if it is not contraindicated by the client's condition.	26. Helps loosen secretions in the lungs.
27. Hook up the sputum collector to the suction tubing and a suction device (Figure 29-33-3). Hook up the suction catheter to the sputum collector.	27. Prepare the equipment before having the client cough.
28. If the client is able to cooperate, have him take several deep breaths and cough.	28. Loosens the secretions and brings them up to the back of the throat.
29. As the client is coughing up sputum, carefully insert the catheter either orally or nasopharyngeally into the back of the throat and suction the sputum into the specimen container.	29. Obtains a sterile specimen that is not contaminated with saliva.
30. Safely dispose of the suction catheter.	30. Prevents spread of microorganisms.
31. Close the specimen container.	31. Prevents contamination of the specimen.
32. Provide tissues or other measures for client comfort.	32. Promotes client comfort.
33. Wash hands.	33. Reduces transmission of microorganisms.
34. Label each specimen with the client's name and send to the laboratory.	34. Promotes the correct diagnosis for the client.

EVALUATION

- An adequate specimen was obtained.
- The procedure was performed with a minimum of trauma to the client.

DOCUMENTATION

Nurses' Notes

- Date, time, and site from which the specimen was obtained
- Bleeding or obvious trauma as a result of the procedure
- Description and time the specimen was collected and if the specimen is the first morning specimen, not pooled secretions

PROCEDURE 29-34 Collecting a Stool Specimen

OVERVIEW

Stool specimens are not collected as frequently as urine or blood specimens, but they are extremely valuable in evaluating and diagnosing a variety of gastrointestinal diseases. The most common tests on a stool specimen are occult blood, culture, fecal fat, fecal leukocyte, and OVA and parasite (parasite screen). A stool specimen can help identify GI bleeding; screen for carcinomas, polyps, diverticulitis, and colitis; diagnose and monitor various pathogenic microorganisms; diagnose inflammatory bowel disorders, pancreatitis, and malabsorption syndrome; and identify parasitic infestations. A single specimen is often not diagnostic, and at least three stool cultures are required for a pathogenic diagnosis.

ASSESSMENT

1. Assess the client's or family member's understanding of the need for the test **so the nurse can provide needed teaching.**
2. Assess the client's ability to cooperate with the procedure to collect the specimen **to maintain privacy while a sample is obtained.**
3. Assess the client's medical history for bleeding or GI disorders. **The nurse can initiate screening tests.**
4. Assess any medications the client receives that can cause GI bleeding, such as anticoagulants, steroids, or acetylsalicylic acid, **to help determine the need for testing and/or the possible source of bleeding.**

POSSIBLE NURSING DIAGNOSES

Constipation
Diarrhea
Deficient Knowledge (need and test procedure)

PLANNING

Expected Outcomes

1. The client will understand the purpose of the test.
2. The client will be able to collect the specimen, or allow the specimen to be collected.
3. The test will be conducted properly and results recorded.

Equipment Needed

- Paper towel
- Disposable gloves
- Wooden applicator
- Specimen container
- Gloves
- Clean, dry bedpan, bedside commode, or toilet "hat"

delegation tips

The collection of stool is delegated. Ancillary personnel are instructed to report the presence of red blood in the stool immediately to the nurse.

IMPLEMENTATION—ACTION/RATIONALE

ACTION	RATIONALE
* Check client's identification band * Explain procedure before beginning *	
1. Wash hands and apply clean gloves.	1. Reduces transmission of microorganisms from fecal specimen to nurse.
2. Depending on agency policy, assist client as needed to bedside commode or toilet. Have client void before moving bowels. Then, prepare for specimen collection. If client is not ambulatory, use a bedpan. For the toilet, use "hat" (Figure 29-34-1). Place the "hat" in the back section of the toilet to collect a stool specimen and the front section to collect a urine specimen.	2. Allows client privacy and the ability to move bowels in a more normal physiological position.
3. Instruct the client not to contaminate the specimen with urine, vaginal discharge, or toilet paper.	3. Minimizes risk of skewed laboratory results.
4. Ask the client to notify you as soon as the specimen is available.	4. Reduces the risk of contamination of specimen, allows the nurse to collect a fresh specimen, and reduces embarrassment to client.

(Continues)

PROCEDURE 29-34 Collecting a Stool Specimen (Continued)

ACTION	RATIONALE

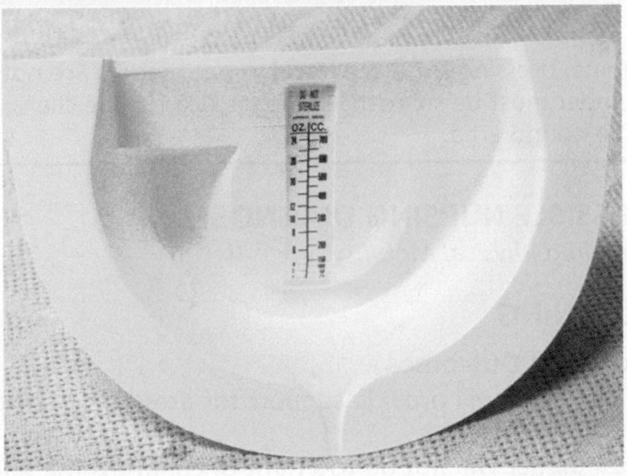

COURTESY OF DELMAR CENGAGE LEARNING

FIGURE 29-34-1 Place the commode "hat" in the back of the toilet to collect a stool specimen.

ACTION	RATIONALE
5. Assist the client with hygiene, help the client back to bed (as required), and ensure client comfort before turning attention to specimen.	5. Promotes client cleanliness and dignity.
6. Apply gloves and wear gown if client is on isolation or at risk for infectious stool, such as *vancomycin-resistant enterococcus* (VRE) or *clostridium difficile* (C. difficile or c diff).	6. Reduces the risk of transmission of microorganisms.
7. Assess the stool for color, consistency, and odor, and presence or absence of visible blood or mucus.	7. Facilitates comprehensive client assessment.
8. Using one or two tongue blades (depending on how much specimen is needed and for which test), transfer a representative sample of stool to the specimen card (Figure 29-32-2) or container, taking care not to contaminate the outside of the container (or the inside of a sterile specimen cup). If using a culture swab, swab in a representative area of stool, particularly if any purulent material is visible. Check with laboratory regarding the volume of stool needed for a particular test.	8. Provides a high-quality sample for optimal results.
9. Close the card, place the lid on the container, or place the swab in the culture tube (according to agency policy) as soon as specimen is collected.	9. Reduces the risk of spread of microorganisms and reduces odor.
10. Place the specimen container in a plastic biohazard bag for transport to the lab after proper labeling is done according to agency policy. Be careful not to contaminate the outside of bag. Provide requisition for test according to agency policy.	10. Properly identifies specimen to client; makes transport of specimen to lab more aesthetic for personnel. Provides client privacy. Reduces spread of microorganisms.
11. Dispose of rest of stool according to agency policy.	11. Reduces spread of microorganisms.
12. Remove gloves and wash hands.	12. Reduces spread of microorganisms.
13. Send specimen to laboratory immediately.	13. Maximizes quality of specimen for testing.

EVALUATION

- Note presence or absence of color change in the guaiac paper.
- Note color, character, and consistency of stool.
- Ask the client to explain the rationale and procedure for the stool test.

DOCUMENTATION

Nurses' Notes

- Date and time the collection was obtained
- Color, character, and consistency of the stool
- When the results of the test were reported to the health care provider

PROCEDURE 29-35

Applying Velcro Abdominal Binders

OVERVIEW

Abdominal Velcro binders support the abdomen and hold abdominal dressings in place. Stretch net binders are not designed for support but simply to hold dressings in place. The binder must be smooth, the right size for the client, and not interfere with circulation or put too much pressure on the bound area.

ASSESSMENT

1. Assess the reason the binder is needed **to determine the correct binder and correct placement.**
2. Assess the client's skin condition for rashes, inflammation, open areas, or dressings **to provide a baseline for future assessments.**
3. Assess and measure the client **to determine what size binder is needed.**
4. Assess for any special circumstances that may affect the placement of the binder, such as dressings, tubing, catheters or IV lines **to determine a plan for binder placement.**
5. Assess the client's understanding of the reasons for the binder and the method of placing the binder **to determine what types of client teaching is needed.**

POSSIBLE NURSING DIAGNOSES

Impaired Physical Mobility

PLANNING

Expected Outcomes

1. Binder will provide support for dressings or soft tissue.
2. Binder will not be too tight or compress the skin.
3. Client will assist in placement of the binder as much as possible.

Equipment Needed

- Correct binder (latex free if indicated)

delegation tips

Abdominal Velcro binder is applied by ancillary personnel after the nurse has assessed the client's tolerance of the binder. The client should be able to breathe effectively and move adequately. In addition, ancillary personnel should be instructed to ensure that the client's skin is intact and to report any breakdown for nurse evaluation.

IMPLEMENTATION—ACTION/RATIONALE

* Check client's identification band * Explain procedure before beginning *

Abdominal Binders

ACTION	RATIONALE
1. Wash hands.	1. Reduces transmission of microorganisms.
2. Choose correct-size binder.	2. The correct size will make the binder most effective.
3. Help the client into the proper position to place the binder. • For abdominal Velcro binders, the client should lie supine and lift the hips, or, alternatively, position the client on one side, and roll the client onto the binder.	3. Applying binders can be awkward if the client is not positioned correctly. If binders are too high, they interfere with breathing.
4. Secure binder with Velcro. Check for snug fit.	4. Velcro closure will keep binder in place.
5. Adjust if necessary. Be sure that binders are not restricting breathing or circulation. Be sure that sterile dressings are in place between the binder and any wound.	5. Binders that are too tight may make breathing difficult and may contribute to skin irritation or breakdown. Binders are generally not sterile.
6. Wash hands.	6. Reduces transmission of microorganisms.

(Continues)

PROCEDURE 29-35 Applying Velcro Abdominal Binders (Continued)

ACTION	RATIONALE

EVALUATION
- Binder provides support for dressings or soft tissue.
- Binder is not too tight and does not compress the skin.
- Client assists in placement of the binder as much as possible.

DOCUMENTATION
Nurses' Notes
- Time, date, and type of binder
- Difficulty the client experienced with the procedure

PROCEDURE 29-36 Application of Restraints

OVERVIEW
A restraint is a physical or mechanical method of involuntarily restricting movement and physical activity so that the confused, agitated, or disoriented client is protected from causing harm to self and/or to others. Restraints may be used to prevent movement during a procedure. If a client is restless or confused, a restraint may be used to prevent the client from damaging therapeutic equipment.

According to the Centers for Medicare and Medicaid Service's Final Rule for Patient Rights, effective January 8, 2007, a physician or licensed independent practitioner is required to evaluate the client within 1 hour of the initiation of restraints or seclusion within a hospital accredited for Medicare-deemed status. Registered nurses or physician assistants may evaluate the client within 1 hour of the application of restraints or seclusion if they are trained and have consulted with the attending physician or licensed independent practitioner as soon as possible after the evaluation (American Academy of Physician Assistants, 2009). Nurses or caregivers may not restrain or confine clients without documented necessity; however, the nurse or caregiver is liable if a confused client sustains injury without appropriate protection, which may include restraints. Interpretation of the Acute Medical and Surgical (Nonpsychiatric) Care restraint standards Section PC.03.03.23 requires client assessment within 15 minutes of the initiation of restraints or seclusion. After the first 15 minutes, the nurse uses clinical judgment or health care practitioner orders to establish a routine for assessing the client needs. The nurse has a legal and ethical duty to keep clients safe. The decision to restrain a client and how much are delicate balancing acts of nursing judgment.

Restraints range from a simple arm board to prevent movement of a wrist or elbow to the more commonly used soft restraints of mesh or soft canvas. They are designed to gently restrain the client without damaging the skin. According to the Joint Commission, the nature of a device does not determine if the device is a restraint but, rather, the intended device use (physical restriction), involuntary application, and/or client need that determines if the device is a restraint. If a full bed-side rail (a bed rail extending the full length of the bed) prevents a client from getting out of bed, the side rail is considered a restraint. However, if a client uses the side rail to assist in leaving the bed, it is not considered a restraint (Joint Commission, 2008).

ASSESSMENT
1. Assess the client's level of consciousness. **This helps determine the client's ability to protect himself from potential harm.**
2. Assess the client's degree of orientation. **A client who is confused regarding time, place, or person is more likely to be at risk of injuring himself. A client who is agitated or angry may be at risk of injuring others.**
3. Assess the client's physical condition. **A client who has weakness, paralysis, or impaired balance or mobility is at increased risk of injury. Impaired vision or hearing also increases the client's risk of injury.**
4. Assess the client's history for falls, accidents, confusion, agitation, or self-inflicted injury. **A client who has a history of this type is at increased risk for injury.**
5. Assess the client's intent. **A client who is verbalizing threats to harm self or others is at increased risk of injury.**
6. Assess the need for restraints. Determine if the client's treatment plan requires and allows restraints, if orders are in place, and hospital policies and laws are specified. **This will prevent**

(Continues)

PROCEDURE 29-36 Application of Restraints (Continued)

Table 29-36-1 The Joint Commision Restraint/Seclusion Standards for Nonpsychiatric Clients

To protect a client from injuring himself or others, it may be necessary to place him in seclusion or in restraints. This can be done in the absence of a licenced independent practitioner (LIP) in a crisis situation. Each organization must determine who is competent to make this decision when an LIP is not available. The Joint Commission provides the following time frames related to restraint and seclusion.

Time Frames for Restraint or Seclusion for an Adult Client	
Adult client in restrain/seclusion	Order must be obtained from LIP within 1 hour of start of restrains/seclusion.
Adult client evaluated in person by LIP	1. LIP evaluation to be completed within 1 hour of initiation of restraint/seclusion. 2. If client is released prior to expiration of original order, an LIP in-person evaluation must be conducted within 24 hours of initiation of restraints.
LIP reorders restrain after evaluation by qualified staff	Every 4 hours until adult client is released from restrain/seclusion.
In-person evaluation by LIP	Every 8 hours until adult client is released from restrain/seclusion.
Times Frames for Restraint or Seclusion for Children and Youth Clients	
Child or youth is put into restraint/seclusion	Order must be ordered from LIP within 1 hour of initiation.
Evaluation of child or youth by LIP in person	1. LIP must perform an in-person evaluation within the first 2 hours for youth 9-17 or for children under 9. 2. LIP in-person evaluation must be done within 24 hours of initiation of restraints if youth or child is released prior to expiration of original order.
Restraint and evaluation reordered by LIP by performed by qualified staff	This occurs every 2 hours for youth (9-17) and every 1 hour for children (under 9) until child is released.
Evaluation in-person by LIP	Every 4 hours for children and youth (17 or younger) until child or youth is released.

Adapted from The Joint Commission. (2005). Restraint and Seclusion, Retrieved August 3, 2008, from http://www.jointcommission.org/Accreditation-programs/BehavioralHealthCare/Standards/FAQs/Provision+of+Care+Treatment+and+Services/Restraint+and+Seclusion/Restraint_Seclusion.htm.

the inappropriate use of restraints and is necessary for legal protection in the event of an injury.

7. Assess client and family knowledge regarding the use of and rationale for restraints or protective devices. **The more the client and family understand regarding the reason for restraints, the more cooperative and understanding they will be.**

POSSIBLE NURSING DIAGNOSES

Risk for Injury
Powerlessness
Deficient Knowledge (need for restraints)
Impaired Physical Mobility

PLANNING

Expected Outcomes

1. The client will remain uninjured.
2. The client will not suffer injury or impairment from the restraints.
3. The client's therapeutic equipment will remain intact and functional.
4. Others will not be harmed by the client.
5. The client will be restrained just enough to prevent injury.

Equipment Needed

- Restraints appropriate to the client's condition and type of restraint required
- Cotton batting or foam padding

(Continues)

PROCEDURE 29-36 Application of Restraints (Continued)

delegation tips

Delegation of the application of restraints to ancillary personnel is acceptable if appropriate orders are in place and proper training has occurred. The assessment of the need for and the type of restraints required and their proper application and maintenance requires the professional nurse's observation and documentation. A physician or health care practitioner must evaluate the client within 1 hour of the application of the restraint and write an order for the restraint as deemed necessary.

IMPLEMENTATION—ACTION/RATIONALE

* Wash hands * Check client's identification band *

Chest Restraint

ACTION	RATIONALE
1. Explain that the client will be wearing a jacket attached to the bed. Explain that this is for safety.	1. Promotes client cooperation.
2. Place the restraint over the client's hospital gown or clothing.	2. Provides for client privacy and prevents the restraint from rubbing the client's skin.
3. Place the restraint on the client with the opening in the front.	3. Allows movement but restricts freedom.
4. Overlap the front pieces, threading the ties through the slot/loop on the front of the vest (Figure 29-36-1A).	4. Secures the restraint.
5. If the client is in bed, secure the ties to the movable part of the mattress frame with a half-knot or quick-release knot (Figures 29-36-2 and 29-36-3). Refer to Figure 29-36-4 for guidance in tying the half knot or quick-release knot.	5. Allows the restraint to move with the bed if the head of the bed is raised or lowered.
6. If the client is in a chair, cross the straps behind the back of the chair and secure the straps to the chair's lower legs, out of the client's reach (Figure 29-36-1B). If it is a wheelchair, be sure the straps will not get caught in the wheels.	6. Provides support for the client to sit up while restricting freedom.
7. Step back and assess the client's overall safety. Be sure the restraint is loose enough not to be a hazard to the client but tight enough to restrict the client from getting up and harming him or herself.	7. Looking at the overall picture allows one to see possible missed dangers.
8. Wash hands.	8. Prevents spread of microorganisms.

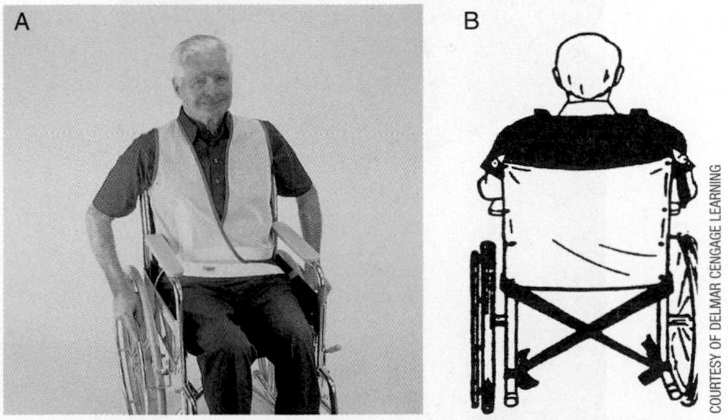

FIGURE 29-36-1 **Vest restraint; *A*, Place the restraint on the client with the opening in the front, overlapping the front pieces, and threading the ties through the slot/loop on the front of the vest. *B*, Secure the straps with a slip (easy-release) knot on the opposite side of the wheelchair kick spur.**

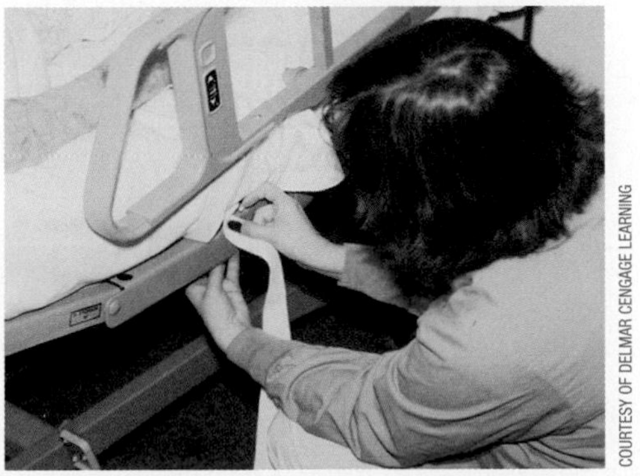

FIGURE 29-36-2 **Secure ties to the movable part of the frame with a half-knot or quick-release knot.**

(Continues)

PROCEDURE 29-36 Application of Restraints (Continued)

ACTION	RATIONALE

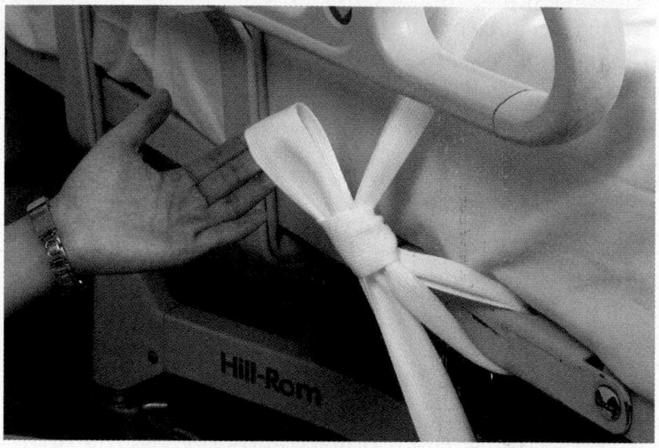

FIGURE 29-36-3 **A half-knot or quick-release knot.**

Applying Wrist or Ankle Restraints

ACTION	RATIONALE
9. Explain to the client that you are placing a wrist or ankle band that will restrict movement.	9. Promotes client cooperation.
10. Wrap the restraint around the client's wrist/ankle and fasten with Velcro grips.	10. Secures the restraint, and prevents the restraint from overtightening at the wrist.
11. Secure the restraint to the movable portion of the mattress frame with a half-knot or quick-release knot.	11. When the head or foot of the client's bed is moved, the restraint will move with it.
12. Slip two fingers under the restraint to check for tightness (Figure 29-36-5). Be sure the restraint is tight enough that the client cannot slip it off but loose enough that the neurovascular status of the client's extremity is not impaired.	12. If the restraint is too tight, the client's neurovascular status may be impaired, causing injury to the client.

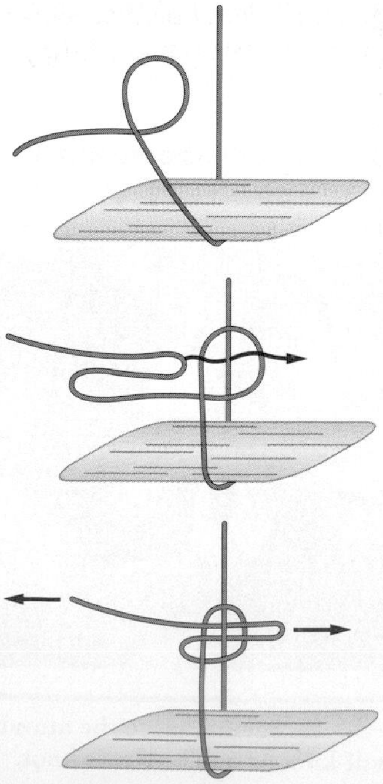

FIGURE 29-36-4 **Steps for a half-knot or quick release knot.**

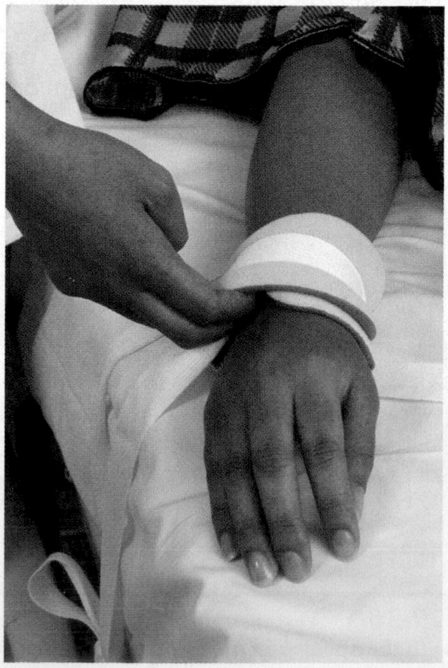

FIGURE 29-36-5 **Slip two fingers under the restraint to check for tightness.**

(Continues)

PROCEDURE 29-36 Application of Restraints (Continued)

ACTION	RATIONALE
13. Step back and assess the client's overall safety. Be sure the restraint is loose enough not to be a hazard to the client but tight enough to restrict the client from getting up and harming himself.	13. Looking at the overall picture can allow you to see dangers you might have missed.
14. Place the call light within the client's reach.	14. Allows the client to contact the nurse to have any needs met. Provides the client with an increased sense of safety.
15. Assess the client 15 minutes after the initiation of restraints or seclusion with special attention to the client's emotional status, safety of the restraint placement, and the client's neurovascular status. After the first 15 minutes, the nurse uses clinical judgment or health care practitioner orders to establish a routine for assessing the client needs. A physician or health care practitioner must evaluate the client within 1 hour of the application of the restraint and write an order for the restraint as deemed necessary.	15. Assures that the client remains safe. Clients may try to escape from restraint and injure themselves in the attempt. States, institutions, Centers for Medicare and Medicaid Services, and the Joint Commission have regulations outlining the frequency of client checks if the client is in restraints. Be aware of regulations that apply.
16. Wash hands.	16. Prevents spread of microorganisms.

EVALUATION

- The client remains uninjured.
- The client has not suffered injury or impairment from the restraints.
- The client's therapeutic equipment has remained intact and functional.
- Others have not been harmed by the client.
- The client is restrained just enough to prevent injury.

DOCUMENTATION

Nurses' Notes

- Use of restraints including reason the client was restrained, type of restraint placed, time the restraints were placed, condition of the client's skin at the site of restraint at the time of placement, and any unusual findings at the time the client was restrained.
- Nurses' notes should be made at least every 2 hours even if a flow sheet is used.
- Ongoing need for restraints
- If the client's status changes, restraints may no longer be necessary.

Flow Sheet

- Some institutions have flow sheets that are used when a client is restrained. These flow sheets document the frequency of client checks, the client's condition, and how often the restraints are released.

PROCEDURE 29-37 Performing the Heimlich Maneuver

OVERVIEW

Foreign body obstruction of the breathing passages has consistently ranked as one of the top 10 causes of accidental deaths in the United States. Complete or partial airway obstruction by a foreign body can occur in numerous settings. In adults, large, poorly chewed pieces of food are most frequently the cause of airway obstruction. Pediatric clients are at risk for choking, especially the infant and young child, and in this population, food (e.g., grapes, hot dogs, raisins, and peanuts) as well as foreign bodies (e.g., coins, beads, marbles, thumbtacks, and paper clips) often cause airway obstruction. A health care provider successfully treats a client's airway obstruction with the Heimlich maneuver or subdiaphragmatic abdominal thrusts. It is important in the pediatric population to differentiate airway obstruction as a result of infection (e.g., epiglottitis) versus a foreign body aspiration.

(Continues)

PROCEDURE 29-37 Performing the Heimlich Maneuver (Continued)

Health professionals frequently teach the Heimlich maneuver to the general public because most food/foreign body obstructions occur outside the hospital/clinic settings. It is important to have a good comfort level with this skill as well as the ability to disseminate this information in an easily understood manner to the public.

ASSESSMENT

1. Assess air exchange. A foreign body obstruction is complete or partial. Partial airway obstruction has some air exchange. If the client can cough, this should be encouraged, and do not interfere with the client's efforts. In the event of partial airway obstruction, the client will usually cough but may wheeze between coughs. **If the client has complete airway obstruction as indicated by a weak, ineffective cough, high-pitched inspiratory noises (stridor), and signs of respiratory distress (cyanosis, loss of consciousness), intervention is necessary.**
2. Establish airway obstruction. The universal sign of airway obstruction is clutching the neck with hands (Figure 29-37-1). In addition, the inability to talk or breathe as well as cyanosis and the progression to an unconscious state indicate airway obstruction. **Determine the problem.**
3. In the pediatric client, differentiate between infection and airway obstruction. Fevers, gradually increasing respiratory distress, retractions, stridor, and drooling are all signs of infection. **With an infection airway obstruction, it is important to maintain an upright position, keep the child as calm as possible, and seek immediate medical attention.** The Heimlich maneuver is not appropriate for an infection airway obstruction.

POSSIBLE NURSING DIAGNOSES

*Impaired **G**as Exchange*
*Ineffective **A**irway Clearance*
*Ineffective **B**reathing Pattern*
*Risk for **S**uffocation*
*Risk for **A**spiration*
***F**ear*

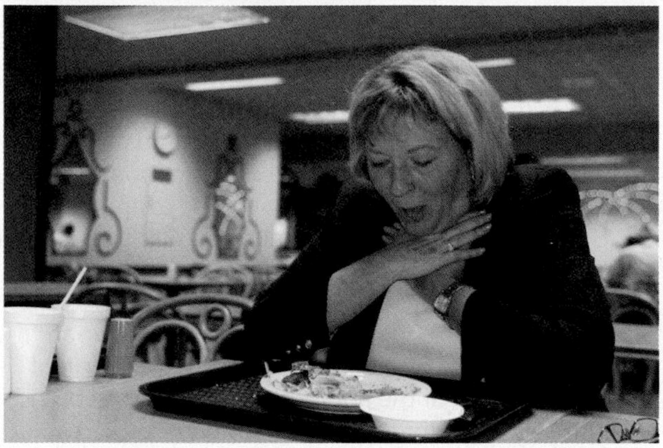

COURTESY OF DELMAR CENGAGE LEARNING

FIGURE 29-37-1 The universal sign of airway obstruction is clutching the neck with hands.

PLANNING

Expected Outcomes

1. The client will demonstrate improved clinical status as evident by airway clearance or establishment of a patent airway.
2. The client will demonstrate improved gas exchange as evident by absence of signs and symptoms of partial or complete airway obstruction (e.g., cough, wheezing, stridor, loss of consciousness, cyanosis).
3. The client will experience minimal discomfort during the Heimlich maneuver or other method of airway clearance.
4. The client will not experience complications related to airway obstruction/hypoxia.

Equipment Needed

- An individual with the training to perform this procedure

delegation tips

The Heimlich maneuver is performed by any trained individual. A technique adjustment of chest thrusts rather than subdiaphragmatic abdominal thrusts are given to choking clients with obesity and late term pregnancy (American College of Emergency Physicians Foundation, 2009).

PROCEDURE 29-37 Performing the Heimlich Maneuver (Continued)

IMPLEMENTATION—ACTION/RATIONALE

ACTION	RATIONALE
* Check client's identification band * Explain procedure before beginning *	
Foreign Body Obstruction—All Clients	
1. Assess airway for complete or partial blockage.	1. If there is good air exchange and the client is able to forcefully cough, do not intervene or interfere with the client's attempts to expel the foreign body.
2. Encourage attempts to cough and breathe.	2. Attempts to cough will provide a more forceful effort. If complete airway obstruction is apparent, the Heimlich maneuver or alternative method of subdiaphragmatic thrust is performed immediately.
3. Activate emergency response assistance if respiratory distress or complete blockage; for example, ask bystander to call 911.	3. Provides follow-up care by professionally trained personnel.
Conscious Adult Client—Sitting or Standing (Heimlich Maneuver)	
4. Stand behind the client and wrap your arms around the client's waist (Figure 29-37-2).	4. Proper positioning provides an effective subdiaphragmatic thrust.
5. Make a fist with one hand and grasp the fist with your other hand, placing the thumb side of the fist against the client's abdomen. The fist is placed midline, below the xiphoid process and lower margins of the rib cage and above the navel (Figure 29-37-3).	5. Correct hand placement is important to prevent internal organ damage.
6. Perform a quick upward thrust into the client's abdomen; each thrust is separate and distinct.	6. This subdiaphragmatic thrust produces an artificial cough by forcing air from the lungs.
7. Repeat this process 6 to 10 times until the client either expels the foreign body or loses consciousness.	7. Attempts to dislodge food or a foreign body to relieve airway obstruction is continued as long as necessary because of the serious consequences of hypoxia.

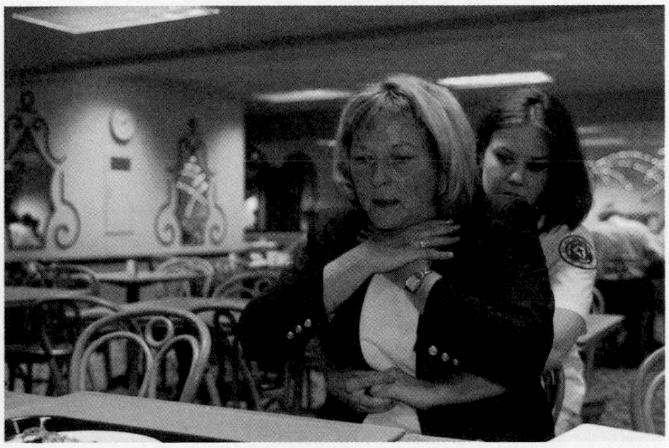
COURTESY OF DELMAR CENGAGE LEARNING

FIGURE 29-37-2 Stand behind the client and wrap your arms around the client's waist.

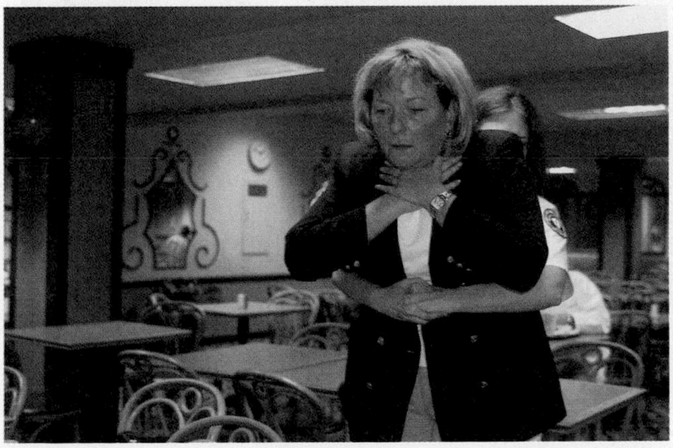
COURTESY OF DELMAR CENGAGE LEARNING

FIGURE 29-37-3 The fist is placed midline, below the xiphoid process and lower margins of the rib cage and above the navel.

(Continues)

PROCEDURE 29-37 Performing the Heimlich Maneuver (Continued)

ACTION	RATIONALE
Unconscious Adult Client or Adult Client Who Becomes Unconscious	
8. Repeat Actions 1 to 3.	8. Determines the need for intervention and summons essential help.
9. Position the client supine; kneel astride the client's abdomen.	9. Proper positioning provides an effective subdiaphragmatic thrust.
10. Place the heel of one hand midline, below the xiphoid process and lower margin of the rib cage and above the navel. Place the second hand directly on top of the first hand.	10. Proper positioning provides an effective subdiaphragmatic thrust.
11. Perform a quick upward thrust into the diaphragm, repeating 6 to 10 times.	11. A client who becomes unconscious may become more relaxed so that the previously unsuccessful Heimlich maneuver may be successful.
12. Perform a finger sweep:	12. Should only be used on the unconscious client, who will not fight the action.
a. Use one hand to grasp the lower jaw and tongue between your thumb and fingers and lift. This will open the mouth and pull the tongue away from the back of the throat.	a. Draw the tongue away from any foreign body lodged in the back of the throat.
b. Using the index finger of the other hand, do a finger sweep to remove any foreign body that can be easily seen and removed, as shown in Figure 29-37-4 (ACEP Foundation, 2009a).	
Caution must be used to prevent pushing the foreign body farther down into the airway.	
13. Open the client's airway and attempt ventilation.	13. The brain can suffer irreversible damage if it is without oxygen for more than 4 to 6 minutes.
14. Continue sequence of Heimlich maneuver, finger sweep, and rescue breathing as long as necessary.	14. Lifesaving efforts must continue until they are successful, or until the rescuer becomes exhausted and cannot go on.
Airway Obstruction—Infants and Small Children	
15. Differentiate between infection and airway obstruction.	15. Infectious complications that lead to airway obstruction require immediate medical attention, establishment of a patent airway (intubation or emergency tracheotomy), and treatment of the underlying infection. Food/foreign body airway obstruction also needs immediate attention; however, airway management differs for each scenario.

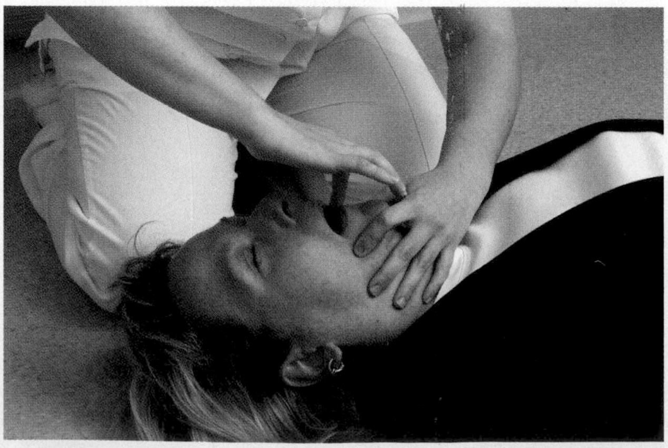

FIGURE 29-37-4 Use a sweeping motion with the index finger to remove any foreign body that can be easily seen and removed.

(Continues)

PROCEDURE 29-37 Performing the Heimlich Maneuver (Continued)

ACTION	RATIONALE
Infant Airway Obstruction	
16. Straddle infant over your forearm in the prone position with the head lower than the trunk. Support the infant's head, positioning a hand around the jaws and chest.	16. Proper positioning is essential for success of the maneuver and prevention of other organ damage.
17. Deliver five back blows between the infant's shoulder blades (Figure 29-37-5).	17. Provides correct technique for dislodging the obstruction.
18. Keeping the infant's head down, place the free hand on the infant's back and turn the infant over, supporting the back of the child with your hand and thigh.	18. Safely rotates the infant's position to continue lifesaving procedures.
19. With your free hand, deliver five thrusts in the same manner as infant external cardiac compressions (Figure 29-37-6).	19. Technique for dislodging the obstruction.
20. Assess for a foreign body in the mouth of an unconscious infant and utilize the finger sweep only if a foreign body is visualized.	20. A blind finger sweep is avoided in infants and children because a foreign object can be pushed back farther into the airway, increasing obstruction.
21. Open airway and assess for respiration. If respirations are absent, attempt rescue breathing. Assess for the rise and fall of the chest; if not seen, reposition infant and attempt rescue breathing again.	21. Many times some air can get around the foreign body causing the airway obstruction. This allows for some oxygenation of the client. Without oxygen, irreversible brain damage can occur within 4 to 6 minutes.
22. Repeat the entire sequence again: five back blows, five chest thrusts, assessment for foreign body in oral cavity, and rescue breathing as long as necessary.	22. Lifesaving efforts must continue until they are successful or until the rescuer becomes exhausted and cannot go on.
Small Child—Airway Obstruction (Conscious, Standing or Sitting)	
23. Assess air exchange and encourage coughing and breathing. Provide reassurance to the child that you are there to help.	23. Inability to breathe is a distressing event for anyone, especially a small child who may not fully understand the circumstance. Reassurance is important to gain the child's trust and cooperation with the maneuvers necessary to help him or her, especially if the child is conscious.

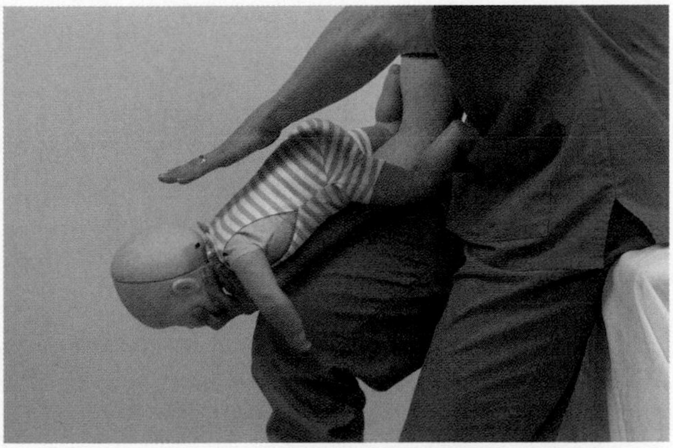

FIGURE 29-37-5 Place the infant in prone position, supporting the head with a hand around the jaws and chest, then deliver five blows between the infant's shoulder blades.

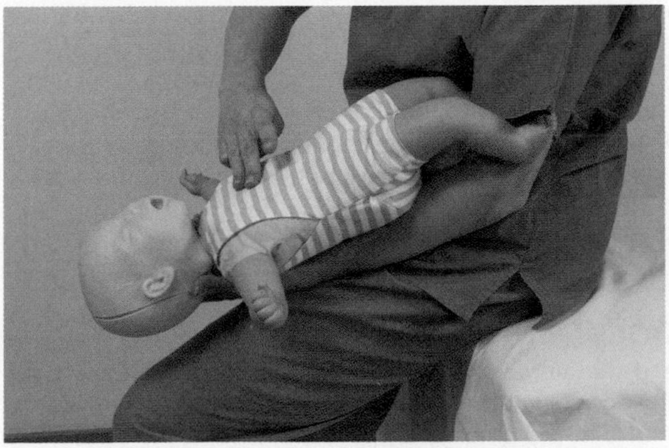

FIGURE 29-37-6 Turn the infant face up, supporting the back of the child with hand and thigh. Deliver five chest thrusts with fingers place just below the nipple line.

(Continues)

PROCEDURE 29-37 Performing the Heimlich Maneuver (Continued)

ACTION	RATIONALE
24. Ask the child if he or she is choking. If the response is affirmative, follow the steps outlined below. In addition, if the child has poor air exchange (and infection has been ruled out), initiate the following steps:	24. Many small children are capable of responding to simple questions such as "Are you choking?"
a. Stand behind the child with your arms wrapped around his or her waist and quickly administer 6 to 10 subdiaphragmatic abdominal thrusts.	a. Proper positioning is essential for success of the maneuver and prevention of other organ damage.
b. Continue until foreign object is expelled or the child becomes unconscious.	b. Lifesaving efforts must continue until they are successful or until the rescuer becomes exhausted and cannot go on.
Small Child—Airway Obstruction (Unconscious)	
25. Position the child supine and kneel at the child's feet and gently deliver five subdiaphragmatic abdominal thrusts in the same manner as for an adult but more gently.	25. This is the recommended position for small children; the astride position may be used for larger children. Proper positioning is essential for success of the maneuver and prevention of other organ damage.
26. Open airway by lifting the lower jaw and tongue forward. Perform a finger sweep only if a foreign body is visualized.	26. Opens the airway and allows visualization of the oral cavity. A blind finger sweep can cause increased obstruction by pushing a foreign object farther back into the airway.
27. If breathing is absent, begin rescue breathing. If the chest does not rise, reposition the child and attempt rescue breathing again.	27. Many times some air can get around the foreign body causing the airway obstruction. This allows for some oxygenation of the client. Without oxygen, irreversible brain damage can occur within 4 to 6 minutes.
28. Repeat this sequence as long as necessary.	28. Lifesaving efforts must continue until they are successful or until the rescuer becomes exhausted and cannot go on.
29. Wash hands.	29. Reduces transmission of microorganisms.

EVALUATION

- The client demonstrates improved clinical status as evident by airway clearance or establishment of a patent airway.
- The client demonstrates improved gas exchange as evident by absence of signs and symptoms of partial or complete airway obstruction (e.g., cough, wheezing, stridor, loss of consciousness, cyanosis).
- The client experienced minimal discomfort during the Heimlich maneuver or other method of airway clearance.
- The client did not experience complications related to airway obstruction/hypoxia.

DOCUMENTATION

- If the airway obstruction occurs in the health care setting, document the following in the narrative notes and in the emergency procedure notes if needed:
  — Time and date of onset of symptoms
  — Presentation, including onset and type of symptoms
  — Type (complete or partial) and cause of obstruction, if known
  — Interventions utilized to alleviate obstruction
  — Results of interventions
  — Other emergency support needed (e.g., emergency tracheotomy)
- If the airway obstruction occurs in an alternate setting (e.g., restaurant, home), provide the following information to the responding health care providers for documentation:
  — Presentation, including onset and type of symptoms
  — Type (complete or partial) and cause of obstruction, if known
  — Interventions utilized to alleviate obstruction
  — Length of time with airway obstruction
  — Results of interventions

PROCEDURE 29-38 Performing Cardiopulmonary Resuscitation (CPR)

OVERVIEW

Cardiac or respiratory arrest can occur at any time to individuals of all ages. It is a crisis event that can be the result of an accident (e.g., foreign body aspiration, motor vehicle accident, drowning) or a disease process (e.g., cardiac arrhythmia, epiglottitis). Cardiopulmonary resuscitation (CPR) is the basic lifesaving skill utilized in the event of cardiac, respiratory, or cardiopulmonary arrest to maintain tissue oxygenation by providing external cardiac compressions and/or artificial respiration.

This lifesaving skill is initiated in the event that an individual is found with or develops the absence of a pulse or respiration or both. The basic goals of CPR, which are often referred to as the ABCD of emergency resuscitation, are as follows:

A: Establish **A**irway
B: Initiate **B**reathing
C: Maintain **C**irculation
D: **D**efibrillate

Cardiopulmonary resuscitation must be initiated immediately once it is determined that a cardiac or pulmonary arrest has occurred. Lack of oxygen to the tissues can result in permanent cardiac and brain damage within 4 to 6 minutes.

Cardiopulmonary resuscitation is a basic lifesaving skill that nurses are expected to perform not only in the hospital and other clinical settings but in the outside environments as well. It is expected that nurses maintain certification in the administration of CPR to individuals of all ages and participate in annual review or recertification courses. In addition, this skill is frequently taught to the lay public and caregivers of medically fragile individuals.

ASSESSMENT

1. Assess responsiveness and level of consciousness by gently shaking or tapping the client while shouting, "Are you OK?" **It is important to differentiate an unconscious individual from someone who is intoxicated, hypoglycemic, sleeping, or in shock. In addition, it is important to touch clients in case they are hearing impaired.**
2. Assess the amount and abilities of any available assistance. **CPR cannot be performed indefinitely by a single individual. If in the hospital or a clinical setting, activate the appropriate "code" to signify there is an emergency situation. If outside the hospital, call for help to activate emergency assistance (e.g., call 911 or the local emergency medical service).**
3. Assess the client's position. **Proper positioning, in a supine position (flat) on a hard surface, is essential to assess respiratory and cardiac status and to adequately perform cardiopulmonary resuscitation. Care must be taken when positioning the client with a suspected neck injury.**
4. Assess respiratory status by looking for chest rise and fall, listening for air exchange, and feeling for the presence of air movement. **Presence of respirations contraindicates the initiation of artificial respiration. In addition, assessment of the respiratory status will uncover complicating factors, including foreign body obstruction and vomit or other excessive airway secretions. These complicating factors need to be resolved in order to open the airway before the initiation of artificial respirations.**
5. Assess circulatory status by using the carotid or brachial pulse points. **Presence of pulse contraindicates the initiation of external chest compressions.**

POSSIBLE NURSING DIAGNOSES

Ineffective Airway Clearance
Ineffective Breathing Pattern
Impaired Gas Exchange
Impaired Spontaneous Ventilation
Decreased Cardiac Output

PLANNING

Expected Outcomes

1. Client will experience improved clinical status, as evident by:
   - Patent airway with spontaneous respirations
   - Return of cardiac circulation
2. Client does not experience negative sequela related to hypoxic event.
3. Client does not have damage inflicted by incorrect positioning for CPR (e.g., paralysis from manipulation of neck injury, cracked ribs or sternum).
4. Cardiopulmonary resuscitation will be terminated only in the following situations:
   - Cardiopulmonary resuscitation was successful in reestablishing respirations and circulation.
   - The client is placed on advanced life support (e.g., intubated and transferred to the intensive care unit).
   - The rescuer is unassisted, fatigued, and unable to continue.

(Continues)

PROCEDURE 29-38 Performing Cardiopulmonary Resuscitation (CPR) (Continued)

- The physician or qualified practitioner pronounces the client dead and orders CPR to be discontinued.

Equipment Needed

Hospital or Clinical Setting

- Hard, flat surface (e.g., chest compression board)
- Body substance isolation items
  - — Gloves
  - — Face shield
  - — Mask/CPR oral barrier device
- Ambu®-bag
- Oral airway
- Emergency resuscitation cart (including defibrillator)
- Documentation forms

Outside: Public Environment

- Hard, flat surface (e.g., floor)
- Body substance isolation items, if available
  - — Gloves
  - — Face shield
  - — Mask/CPR oral barrier device

delegation tips

The administration of CPR to adults and children is a skill delegated to ancillary personnel and caregivers after proper instruction and CPR certification.

IMPLEMENTATION—ACTION/RATIONALE

ACTION	RATIONALE
CPR: One Rescuer—Adult, Adolescent	
1. Assess responsiveness by tapping or gently shaking client while shouting, "Are you OK?"	1. Prevents injury to a client who is not experiencing cardiac or respiratory arrest. Also assists in assessing level of consciousness and possible etiology of crisis.
2. Activate emergency medical system (EMS). In the hospital or clinical setting, follow institutional protocol. In the community or home environment, activate the local emergency response system (e.g., 911).	2. Activates assistance from personnel trained in advanced life support. Note: According to the CPR guidelines (American Heart Association [AHA], 2005), rescuers should notify the EMS or phone 911 for unresponsive adults before beginning CPR.
3. Position client in a supine position on a hard, flat surface (e.g., floor or cardiac board). Use caution when positioning a client with a possible head or neck injury.	3. Proper positioning facilitates assessment of the cardiac and respiratory status and successful external cardiac massage. Prevents further damage to a potential head or neck injury.
4. Apply appropriate body substance isolation items (e.g., gloves, face shield) if available (Figure 29-38-1).	4. Prevents transmission of disease.

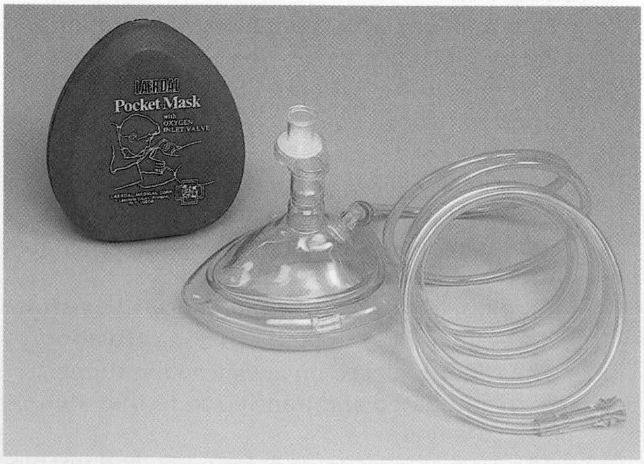

COURTESY OF DELMAR CENGAGE LEARNING

FIGURE 29-38-1 Facemask for artificial resuscitation.

(Continues)

PROCEDURE 29-38 Performing Cardiopulmonary Resuscitation (CPR) (Continued)

ACTION / **RATIONALE**

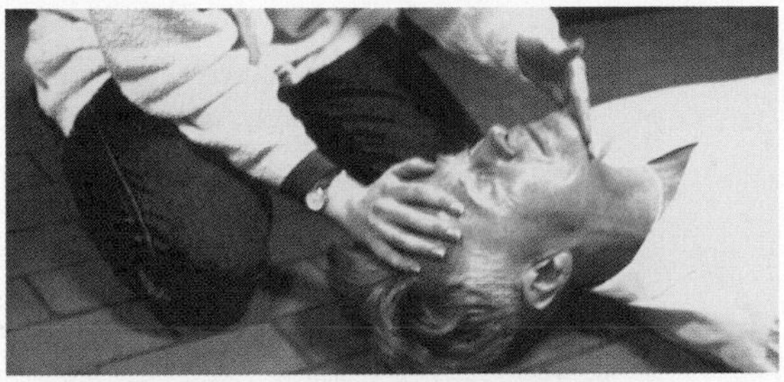

FIGURE 29-38-2 **Use the head-tilt/chin-lift method to open airway.**

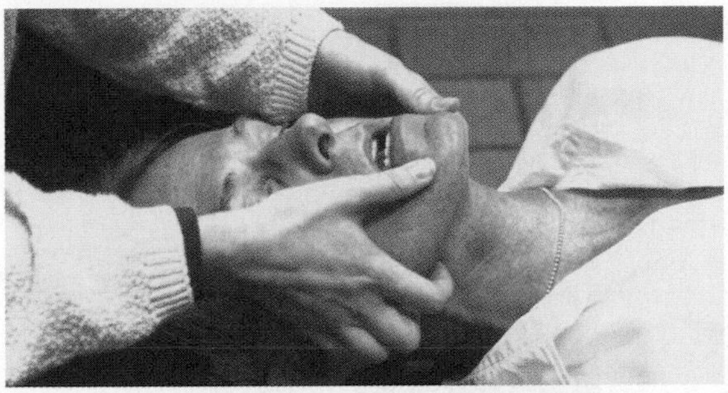

FIGURE 29-38-3 **The jaw-thrust method is used to open the airway if a neck injury is suspected.**

5. Position self. Face the client on your knees parallel to the client, next to the head, to begin to assess the airway and breathing status.

   Rationale: 5. Proper positioning prevents rescuer fatigue and facilitates CPR by allowing the rescuer to move from chest compressions to artificial breathing with minimal movement.

6. Open airway. The most commonly used method is the head-tilt/chin-lift method. This is accomplished by placing one hand on the client's forehead and applying a steady backward pressure to tilt the head back while placing the fingers of the other hand below the jaw at the location of the chin and lifting the chin (Figure 29-38-2). In the event of a suspected head or neck injury, this lift is modified and the jaw thrust is used without head extension. To perform the jaw thrust, place hands at the angles of the lower jaw and lift, displacing the mandible forward (Figure 29-38-3). Additionally, if available, insert oral airway.

   Rationale: 6. A patent airway is essential for successful artificial respirations. The head-tilt/chin-lift assists in preventing the tongue from obstructing the airway. The jaw thrust is used when a head or neck injury is suspected because it prevents extension of the neck and decreases the potential of further injury.

7. Assess for respirations. Look, listen, and feel for air movement (3 to 5 seconds).

   Rationale: 7. Cardiopulmonary resuscitation should not be administered to a client with spontaneous respirations or pulse because of the potential risk of injury.

8. If respirations are absent:
   - Occlude nostrils with the thumb and index finger of the hand on the forehead that is tilting the head back (Figure 29-38-4).
   - Form a seal over the client's face mask using either your mouth or the appropriate respiratory assist device (e.g., Ambu®-bag and mask) and give two full breaths of 1 second per breath (AHA, 2005), allowing time for both inspiration and expiration (Figure 29-38-5). The volume of each rescue breath should provide visible chest rise (AHA, 2005–2006).
   - In the event of a serious mouth or jaw injury that prevents mouth-to-mouth ventilation, mouth-to-nose ventilation may be used by tilting the head as described earlier with one hand and using the other hand to lift the jaw and close the mouth.

   Rationale: 8. Occluding the nostrils and forming a seal over the client's mouth will prevent air leakage and provide full inflation of the lungs. Excessive air volume and rapid inspiratory flow rates can create pharyngeal pressures that are greater than esophageal opening pressures. This will allow air into the stomach, resulting in gastric distention and increased risk of vomiting.

9. Assess for the rise and fall of the chest:
   - If the chest rises and falls, continue to Action 10.
   - If the chest does not move, assess for excessive oral secretions, vomit, airway obstruction, or improper positioning.

   Rationale: 9. Visual assessment of chest movement helps confirm an open airway. A volume of 800 to 1,200 mL is usually sufficient to make the chest rise in most adults.

(Continues)

PROCEDURE 29-38 Performing Cardiopulmonary Resuscitation (CPR) (Continued)

ACTION	RATIONALE

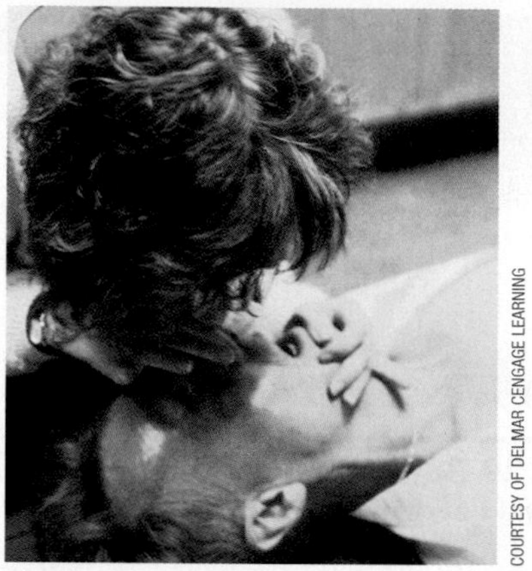

FIGURE 29-38-4 **Occlude both nostrils with fingers.**

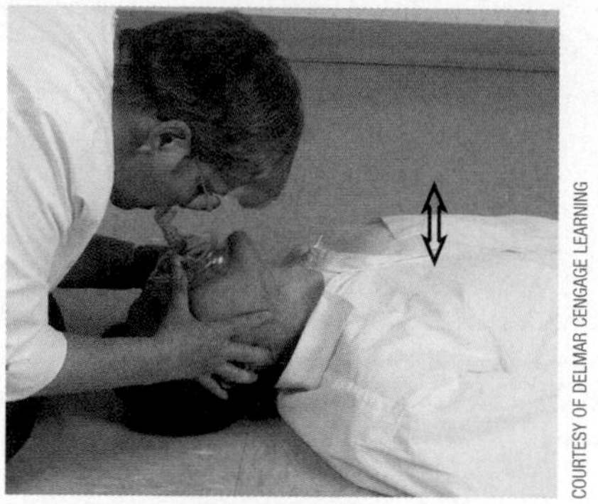

FIGURE 29-38-5 **Give two full breaths.**

Action

10. Palpate the carotid pulse (5 to 10 seconds) (Figure 29-38-6):
    - If present, continue rescue breathing, at the rate of 12 breaths per minute.
    - If absent, begin external cardiac compressions.

Rationale

10. Performing chest compressions on an individual with a pulse could result in injury. Additionally, the carotid pulse may persist when peripheral pulses are no longer palpable. Hyperventilation assists in maintaining blood oxygen levels. Additionally, a pulse may be present for approximately 6 minutes after respirations have ceased.

Action

11. Cardiac compressions are performed as follows:
    - Maintain a position on knees parallel to sternum.
    - Position the hands for compressions:

    a. Using the hand nearest to the legs, use the index finger to locate the lower rib margin and quickly move the fingers up to the location where the ribs connect to the sternum.

    b. Place the middle finger of this hand on the notch where the ribs meet the sternum and the index finger next to it.

    c. Place the heel of the opposite hand next to the index finger on the sternum (Figure 29-38-7).

Rationale

11. Irreversible brain and tissue damage can occur if a client is hypoxic for more than 4 to 6 minutes. Proper positioning is essential for the following reasons:
    - Allows for maximum compression of the heart between the sternum and vertebrae.
    - Compressions over the xiphoid process can lacerate the liver.
    - Keeping fingers off the chest during compressions reduces the risk of rib fracture.

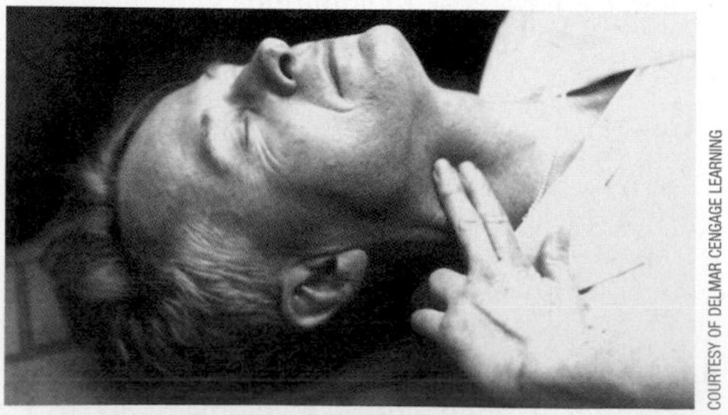

FIGURE 29-38-6 **Palpate for a carotid pulse.**

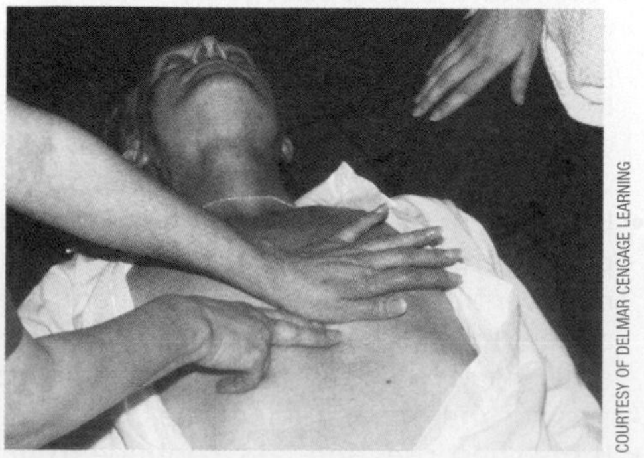

FIGURE 29-38-7 **Place the heel of one hand next to the index finger on the client's sternum.**

(Continues)

PROCEDURE 29-38 Performing Cardiopulmonary Resuscitation (CPR) (Continued)

ACTION	RATIONALE
d. Remove the first hand from the notch and place it on top of the hand that is on the sternum so they are on top of each other.	
e. Extend or interlace fingers and do not allow them to touch the chest (Figure 29-38-8).	
f. Keep arms straight with shoulders directly over hands on sternum and lock elbows (Figure 29-38-9).	
g. Compress the adult chest 3.8–5.0 cm (11/2–2 inches) at the rate of approximately 100 compressions per minute.	
h. The heel of the hand must completely release the pressure between compressions, but it should remain in constant contact with the client's skin.	
i. Use the mnemonic "one and, two and, three and . . . " to keep rhythm and timing.	
j. Ventilate client as described in Action 8.	
12. Maintain the compression rate for approximately 100 times per minute, interjecting 2 ventilations after every 30 compressions. (compression:ventilation rate at 30:2)	12. Faster rate increases blood flow to key organ tissues.
13. Reassess the client after four cycles.	13. Determines return of spontaneous pulse and respirations and need to continue CPR.
CPR: Two Rescuers—Adult, Adolescent	
14. Follow the steps above with the following changes: • One rescuer is positioned facing the client parallel to the head while the other rescuer is positioned on the opposite side facing the client parallel to the sternum next to the trunk (Figure 29-38-10). • The rescuer positioned at the client's trunk is responsible for performing cardiac compressions	14. Proper positioning allows one rescuer to perform artificial respirations while the other administers chest compressions without getting in each other's way. In addition, this facilitates ease in changing positions when one of the rescuers becomes fatigued. Palpating the carotid pulse with each chest compression during the first full minute

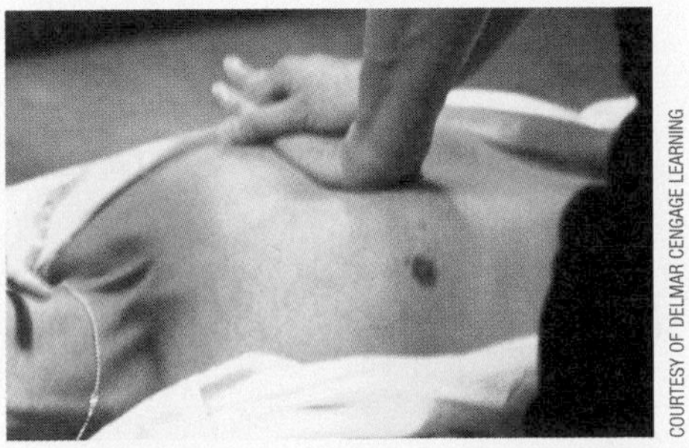

FIGURE 29-38-8 Extend or interlace the fingers.

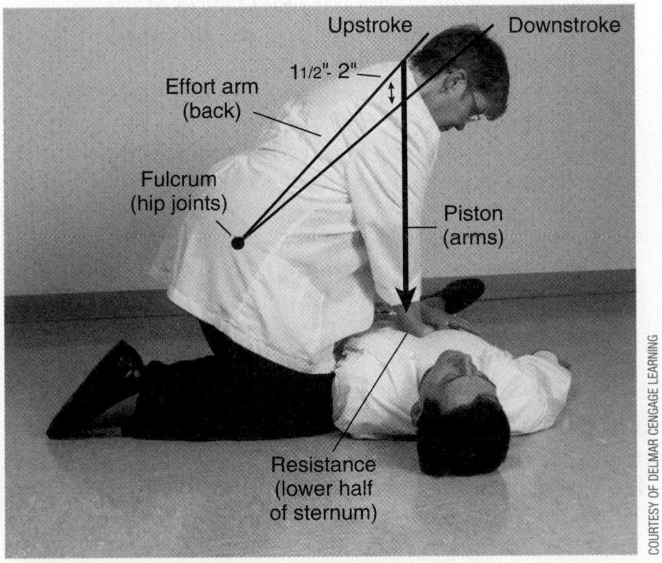

FIGURE 29-38-9 Proper position of rescuer. Keep arms straight and lock elbos.

(Continues)

PROCEDURE 29-38 Performing Cardiopulmonary Resuscitation (CPR) (Continued)

ACTION	RATIONALE

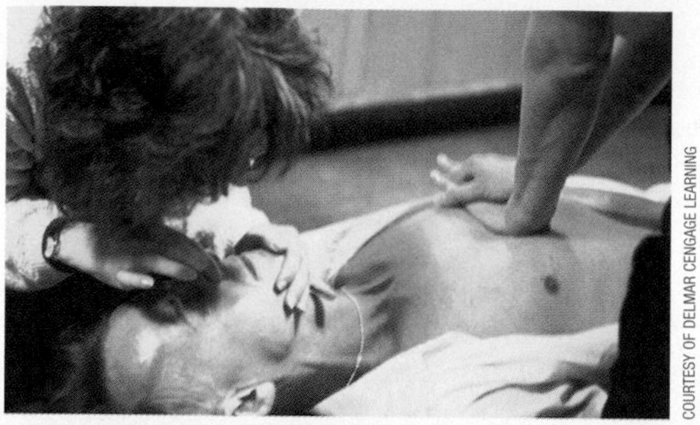

FIGURE 29-38-10 Two-rescuer positioning. One person kneels on each side of the client.

and maintaining the verbal mnemonic count. This is rescuer 1. According to the 2005 CPR guidelines, the rescuer is to make the chest compressions hard and fast and allow the chest to recoil after each compression.

- The rescuer positioned at the client's head is responsible for monitoring respirations, assessing the carotid pulse, establishing an open airway, and performing rescue breathing at the rate of 10 to 12 breaths per minute. This is rescuer 2.
- Maintain the compression rate for approximately 100 times per minute, interjecting two ventilations after every 15 compressions. (compression:ventilation rate at 15:2)
- Rescuer 2 palpates the carotid pulse with each chest compression during the first full minute.
- Rescuer 2 is responsible for calling for a change. Rescuers should change every 2 minutes or 5 cycles of CPR (1 cycle of CPR = 30 compressions: 2 rescue breaths). Rescuer 2 follows this protocol:
- Rescuer 1 calls for a change and completes the 15 chest compressions.
- Rescuer 2 administers two breaths and then moves to a position parallel to the client's sternum and assumes the proper hand position.
- Rescuer 1 moves to the rescue breathing position and checks the carotid pulse for 5 seconds. If cardiac arrest persists, rescuer 1 says, "continue CPR" and delivers one breath. Rescuer 2 resumes cardiac compressions immediately after the breath.

Rationale: assures that adequate stroke volume is delivered with each compression.

Two rescuers are needed because one person cannot maintain CPR indefinitely. According to studies, the chest compression rescuer fatigues in as little as 1 to 2 minutes (AHA, 2005–2006). When a rescuer becomes fatigued, chest compressions can become ineffective, decreasing the volume of oxygenated blood circulated to key organs and tissue.

CPR: One Rescuer—Child (1 to onset of adolescence/puberty)

ACTION	RATIONALE
15. Assess responsiveness, position the child, apply appropriate body substance isolation, position self, open airway, and assess for respirations as described in Actions 1, 3–7. Remember respiratory arrest is more common in the pediatric population.	15. See Rationales 1 and 3 to 7.

(Continues)

PROCEDURE 29-38 Performing Cardiopulmonary Resuscitation (CPR) (Continued)

ACTION	RATIONALE
16. If respirations are absent, begin rescue breathing: • Give two slow breaths (1–1 ½ sec/breath), pausing to take a breath in between. • Use only the amount of air needed to make the chest rise. When you see the chest rise and fall, you are using the right volume of air.	16. Hypoxia can cause irreversible brain and tissue damage after 4 to 6 minutes. • The volume of air in a small child's lungs is less than an adult's. Excessive air volume and rapid inspiratory rates can increase pharyngeal pressures that exceed esophageal opening pressures. This allows air to enter the stomach, causing gastric distention, increasing the risk of vomiting, and further compromising the client's respiratory status.
17. Palpate the carotid pulse (5 to 10 seconds). If present, ventilate at a rate of once every 3 to 5 seconds or 12 to 20 breaths per minute. If absent, begin cardiac compressions.	17. Performing chest compressions on a child with a pulse could result in injury. Additionally, the carotid pulse may persist when peripheral pulses are no longer palpable. Hyperventilation assists in maintaining blood oxygen levels. Additionally, a pulse may be present for approximately 6 minutes after respirations have ceased.
18. Cardiac compressions (child 1–7 years): • Maintain a position on knees parallel to child's sternum. • Position the hands for compressions: a. Locate the lower margin of the rib cage using the hand closest to the feet and find the notch where the ribs and sternum meet. b. Place the middle finger of this hand on the notch and then place the index finger next to the middle finger. c. Place the heel of the other hand next to the index finger of the first hand on the sternum with the heel parallel to the sternum (1 cm above the xiphoid process). d. Keeping the elbows locked and the shoulders over the child, compress the sternum one-third to one-half the depth of the chest at the approximate rate of 100 times per minute. e. At the end of every 30th compression, administer 2 ventilations (1 second). f. Reevaluate the child after 20 cycles. If respirations are still absent, call 911.	18. Irreversible brain and tissue damage can occur if a client is hypoxic for more than 4 to 6 minutes. Proper positioning is essential for the following reasons: • Allows for maximum compression of the heart between the sternum and vertebrae. • The backward tilt of the head lifts the back of small children. • Compressions over the xiphoid process can lacerate the liver. • Keeping fingers off the chest during compressions reduces the risk of rib fracture. • Keeping one hand on the child's forehead helps maintain an open airway. f. Guidelines published by the AHA (2005) recommend that a 1-minute CPR be performed for infants and children up to the onset of adolescence/puberty before calling 911. In institutions, follow hospital protocol.
CPR: One Rescuer—Infant (1–12 months)	
19. Assess responsiveness, activate emergency medical system, position the child, apply appropriate body substance isolation, position self, open airway, and assess for respirations as described in Actions 1, 3–7. Remember, respiratory arrest is more common in the pediatric population.	19. See Rationales 1 and 3 to 7.
20. If respirations are absent, begin rescue breathing: • Avoid overextension of the infant's neck.	20. Irreversible brain and tissue damage can occur if a client is hypoxic for more than 4 to 6 minutes. Proper positioning is essential for the following reasons: • It is believed that overextension of an infant's head can cause a closing or narrowing of the airway.

(Continues)

PROCEDURE 29-38 Performing Cardiopulmonary Resuscitation (CPR) (Continued)

ACTION	RATIONALE
• Place a small towel or diaper under the infant's shoulders or use a hand to support the neck.	• Proper positioning with support allows maximum compression of the heart between the sternum and vertebrae.
• Make a tight seal over both the infant's nose and mouth and gently administer artificial respirations.	• Making a complete seal over the infant's mouth and nose prevents air leakage.
• Give two slow breaths (1 second per breath), pausing to take a breath in between. • Use only the amount of air needed to make the chest rise.	• The volume of air in a small child's lungs is less than an adult's. Excessive air volume and rapid inspiratory rates can increase pharyngeal pressures that exceed esophageal opening pressures. This allows air to enter the stomach, causing gastric distention, increasing the risk of vomiting, and further compromising the client's respiratory status.
21. Assess circulatory status using the brachial pulse: • Locate the brachial pulse on the inside of the upper arm between the elbow and shoulder by placing your thumb on the outside of the arm and palpating the proximal side of the arm with the index finger and middle fingers. • If a pulse is palpated, continue rescue breathing 12 to 20 times per minute or once every 3 to 5 seconds. • If a pulse is absent, begin cardiac compressions.	21. The carotid pulse is often difficult to locate in the infant; therefore the brachial artery is the recommended site.
22. Cardiac compressions (infant 1–12 months): • Maintain a position parallel to the infant. Infants can easily be placed on a table or other hard surface. • Place a small towel or other support under the infant's shoulders/neck. • Position the hands for compressions: a. Using the hand closest to the infant's feet, locate the intermammary line where it intersects the sternum. b. Place the index finger 1 cm below this location on the sternum and place the middle finger next to the index finger. c. Using these two fingers, compress in a downward motion one-third to one-half the depth of the chest at the rate of 100 times per minute. d. Keep the other hand on the infant's forehead. e. At the end of every thirtieth compression, administer two ventilations (30 compressions: 2 ventilations) (1 second per breath).	22. Irreversible brain and tissue damage can occur if a client is hypoxic for more than 4 to 6 minutes. Proper positioning is essential for the following reasons: • Allows for maximum compression of the heart between the sternum and vertebrae. • A small towel, diaper roll, or some other type of support is necessary for effective cardiac compressions. • Compressions over the xiphoid process can lacerate the liver. • Keeping other fingers and hands off the chest during compressions reduces risk of rib fracture. • Keeping one hand on the infant's forehead helps maintain an open airway.
f. Reevaluate infant after 20 cycles. If respirations are still absent, call 911.	f. Guidelines published by the AHA (2005) recommend that about 5 cycles of CPR be performed for unresponsive infants and children up to the onset of adolescence/puberty before calling 911. In institutions, follow hospital protocol.
CPR: Two Rescuers—Child (1 to onset of adolescence/puberty) and Infant (1–12 months) 23. Follow Action 14 for two-rescuer CPR for adults with the following changes: • Utilize the child or infant procedure for chest compressions. • Change the ratio of compressions to ventilation to 15:2 (15 chest compressions to 2 ventilations). • Deliver the ventilation on the upstroke of the third compression.	23. Improper hand placement can cause internal organ damage or other medical complications in infants or children. Delivering ventilation during the upstroke phase allows for full lung expansion during inspiration.

(Continues)

PROCEDURE 29-38 Performing Cardiopulmonary Resuscitation (CPR) (Continued)

ACTION	RATIONALE
CPR—Neonate or Premature Infant	
24. Follow the infant guidelines with the following changes for chest compressions: • Encircle the chest with both hands. • Position thumbs over the midsternum. • Compress the midsternum with both thumbs. • Compress one-third to one-half the depth of the chest at a rate of 100 to 120 times per minute.	24. Improper hand placement can cause internal organ damage or other medical complications in infants or children.
25. If properly trained use an automated external defibrillator (AED). Use adult defibrillation pads for adults. Use the pediatric system for children 1 to 8 years of age, if available. Use AED after 5 cycles of CPR on children age 1 to the onset of adolescence/puberty. In hospital setting, use defibrillator as specified by institution protocol. Defibrillator should be placed only by properly trained personnel.	25. The use of an AED can increase the client's chances for survival by restoring rhythm and circulation. Protocol in hospital setting include the use of defibrillator with codes and can increase survival. Injury to self, staff, or the client may occur with untrained personnel.

EVALUATION

- There should be a constant evaluation for the return of spontaneous pulse and respirations.
- Successful intervention with CPR is illustrated as follows:
  - — An open airway is maintained, as evident by the visible chest rise and fall.
  - — The resistance and compliance of the client's lungs is felt.
  - — Airway movement during expiration is felt and heard.
  - — Circulation indicators, such as color, improve.
  - — The client has return of spontaneous pulse and respirations, as evidenced by a palpable carotid or brachial pulse and the presence of respiratory effort.
- Assist with transfer to hospital/advanced life-support unit.
- If CPR was unsuccessful, assist in notifying next of kin and providing psychosocial support.

DOCUMENTATION

Nurses' Notes/Code Record

- Time and condition in which the client was found
- Interventions that were implemented, including accurate times, results of the implementations, orders received from the physicians, vital signs of the client, timing of the incident, and status of the client afterward

Medication Administration Record

- Medications the client received, including time and route, during the procedure
- If the incident occurs in a noninstitutional setting, report findings and interventions to aid personnel when they arrive

PROCEDURE 29-39 Admitting a Client

OVERVIEW

The procedure for admitting a client to a health care facility is extremely important. First impressions of the facility and caregivers are lasting ones. A calm, caring approach instills confidence in the client and the belief that the client's needs are important. Orienting the client to the room, nursing unit, and facility will help the client to be comfortable in the health care environment.

ASSESSMENT

1. Assess the client's comfort level about being in a health care facility. **Identifies needed nurse–client interactions.**
2. Assess client's physical and mental state. **Provides basis for nursing care. Shows caring and concern for the client.**

(Continues)

PROCEDURE 29-39 Admitting a Client (Continued)

3. Assess client's knowledge of reason for admission. **Provides basis for nurse–client interaction and client teaching.**

POSSIBLE NURSING DIAGNOSES

Fear

Anxiety

Deficient Knowledge (health care facility)

PLANNING

Expected Outcomes

1. Client will be comfortable in health care facility.
2. Client will understand how to use call bell system, bed controls, television, and telephone.
3. The client will adjust to facility routine.

Equipment Needed

- Admission kit: wash basin, emesis basin, pitcher, glass, etc.
- Client orientation materials
- Valuables envelope (if needed)
- Belongings checklist
- Admission Nursing Assessment form
- Sphygmomanometer, stethoscope, thermometer

delegation tips

Admitting a client may be delegated to ancillary personnel after proper instruction. The nursing assessment must be performed by the nurse and may not be delegated.

IMPLEMENTATION—ACTION/RATIONALE

ACTION	RATIONALE
* Wash hands *	
1. Welcome client to unit. Introduce yourself by name and title. Ask client to state his or her name.	1. Verifies identification.
2. Orient client to room and nursing unit. Describe items such as nurse call bell system, location of bathroom, place for clothing, bed controls, television, telephone, visiting hours, meal times, Standard Precautions, and review items in client education materials such as client rights and other written information about the facility.	2. Reduces client anxiety; allows fuller participation in care.
3. Provide privacy for client to change into pajamas or hospital gown, if not already done.	3. Respects client privacy.
4. Show client ID bracelet to double-check proper identification. Attach bracelet to wrist. (This may have been done in Admitting Department.) Review drug allergies and attach allergy bracelet to same wrist, according to agency policy.	4. Confirms client identification; promotes client safety.
5. Document and store client's belongings and valuables according to agency policy.	5. Reduces the risk of loss.
6. Begin nursing assessment, according to agency policy.	6. Starts development of client database.
7. Perform any other actions, as directed by agency policy.	7. Different facilities have different needs, regulations, and guidelines for client admission.

EVALUATION

- The client is comfortable in the health care facility.
- The client uses call bell system, bed controls, television, and telephone.
- The client has adjusted to facility routing.

DOCUMENTATION

- Complete admitting nursing assessment record
- Time and condition of client on admission
- All valuables sent to the safe
- Client's belongings
- Client's comfort level

PROCEDURE 29-40 Transferring a Client

OVERVIEW

Transferring a client to a different unit in a health care facility can be very stressful to the client. It may mean that the client's condition has deteriorated (transferring to ICU) or improved (transferring to a rehabilitation unit after a hip replacement), thus requiring different treatments.

However short the stay before a transfer, the client has a sense of knowing the environment and the health care personnel on that unit. Explaining the reason for transfer to the client and family, as well as gathering all equipment, medications, and assisting in collecting client's personal belongings, help ease the stress of a transfer.

Introducing the client and family to health care personnel working on the new unit and sharing some of the client's personal preferences in the client's presence (i.e., prefers one pillow and an extra blanket) shows caring and concern for the client and helps ensure continuity of care.

ASSESSMENT

1. Assess client's knowledge and feelings about the transfer. **Allows for explanations and discussion about the situation.**
2. Assess which equipment is to be transferred with the client and that those medications and client's personal belongings are ready to move. **Provides organization to the transfer and encourages completeness.**
3. Assess readiness of new unit to accept client. **Allows transfer to proceed smoothly with no waiting.**

POSSIBLE NURSING DIAGNOSES

Anxiety
Fear
Hopelessness

PLANNING

Expected Outcomes

1. Client will understand reason for transfer.
2. Client will be safely moved with needed equipment and medications and all personal belongings.
3. Client's move will be communicated to appropriate department for continuity of care (i.e., Dietary, Pharmacy).

Equipment Needed

- Client's medical record (if not electronic)
- Client's imprint card
- Client's medications
- Stretcher or wheelchair
- Cart to carry client's belongings

delegation tips

Ancillary personnel may assist with transferring a client. The nurse is responsible for transferring the client's medical record and medications and for giving a thorough report to the accepting nurse on the new unit.

IMPLEMENTATION—ACTION/RATIONALE

ACTION	RATIONALE
* Wash hands * Check client's identification band *	
1. Check to see if order is needed to initiate transfer according to agency policy.	1. Policies differ among facilities.
2. Call nursing unit of new location to see if bed is ready and to give report.	2. Provides continuity of care.
3. Explain the transfer to the client (and family, if appropriate). Answer any questions. Allay anxieties about moving.	3. Keeps client informed and promotes cooperation.
4. Review the valuables and belongings checklist completed on admission. Compare with belongings.	4. Ensures all of client's belongings are transferred with the client. Prevents loss.
5. Gather records and any other equipment that is transferred with the client, according to agency policy, such as eyedrops, other medications, IV pump, and respiratory therapy equipment.	5. Helps make transfer more efficient and reduces multiple trips to new area.

(Continues)

PROCEDURE 29-40 Transferring a Client (Continued)

ACTION	RATIONALE
6. Transfer client by appropriate vehicle (wheelchair, stretcher). Accompany client to new unit. Transfer care to another staff member in person. Ensure that call bell is within reach or staff member is in room before leaving client.	6. Enhances continuity of care. Promotes safety.
7. Document time of transfer and any other information required by agency policy.	7. Promotes communication among members of the health care team.
8. Upon return to unit, notify appropriate personnel according to agency policy that client has left the unit. Arrange for personnel to clean the bed and surroundings the client left.	8. Prepares bed for new admission. Reduces transfer of microorganisms.

EVALUATION

- The client understands the reason for transferring to a new unit.
- The client is safely moved with needed equipment and medications and all personal belongings.
- The client's move was communicated to appropriate departments for continuity of care.

DOCUMENTATION

- Client's condition when leaving unit
- Equipment and medications transferred with the client
- Personal belongings sent with client.
- Report on client given to receiving nurse
- Departments notified of client's transfer

PROCEDURE 29-41 Discharging a Client

OVERVIEW

A client may be discharged from a health care facility to another facility or to home. This can be a frightening experience depending on the level of recuperation the client has achieved, the amount and type of medications prescribed, dietary needs or restrictions, and other treatments to be conducted. Being transferred from one facility to another is seen either as improvement or as a lack of progress in recovery.

Discuss with the client and family the discharge process. Complete all paperwork and all discharge teaching. Collect the client's belongings and valuables (as documented on admission) so they accompany the client. These things make the discharge process pleasant and effective.

ASSESSMENT

1. Assess client's feelings about being discharged. **Opens communication about the discharge.**
2. Assess that family and home or the other facility is prepared to receive the client. **Provides a smooth process with less stress for the client.**
3. Assess client's or family's knowledge of care at home. **Ensures continuity of care.**

POSSIBLE NURSING DIAGNOSES

Anxiety

PLANNING

Expected Outcomes

1. Client will complete discharge to another facility with no problems.
2. Client will feel confident about care at home.

Equipment Needed

- Required facility paperwork
- Stretcher or wheelchair
- Cart for client's belongings

For Discharge to Home

- Prescriptions
- Instructions—care, diet, medications, follow-up appointment

(Continues)

PROCEDURE 29-41 Discharging a Client (Continued)

delegation tips

Ancillary personnel assist with the physical movements of discharging a client. The nurse reviews with the client prescriptions and instructions on care, diet, medications, and making a follow-up appointment.

IMPLEMENTATION—ACTION/RATIONALE

ACTION	RATIONALE
* Wash hands * Check client's identification band *	
1. Check order for discharge.	1. Most agency policies require order for discharge.
Discharge to Another Facility	
2. Explain discharge to client, and family, if appropriate.	2. Includes client in care. Promotes cooperation.
3. Complete intra-agency transfer form, according to policy. Be sure to note last time of medication doses. Complete nursing discharge summary. Prepare transfer paperwork, according to policy.	3. Facilitates continuity of care. Promotes client safety.
4. Notify receiving agency of impending transfer. Provide report and confirm ability to receive client.	4. Facilitates continuity of care. Ensures that new facility will accept client before client leaves current facility.
5. Arrange for transportation to new facility. Call transportation company according to agency policy.	5. Reduces waiting time; facilitates continuity of care.
6. Review the valuables and belongings checklist completed on admission. Compare with belongings.	6. Ensures all of client's belongings leave with the client. Prevents loss.
7. When personnel from transportation company arrive, assist client transfer to stretcher or wheelchair. Provide transportation personnel with required information, such as client's DNR status, for transfer. See that client's belongings accompany client, along with any required paperwork or equipment.	7. Provides continuity of care.
Discharge to Home	
8. Discuss discharge with client, and family, if appropriate. Confirm that discharge teaching has been done. Ask client if there are any questions about self-care at home. If so, follow up with appropriate personnel (typically, RN).	8. Promotes client cooperation. Allays anxiety.
9. LP/VN or RN (according to agency policy) reviews with client: prescriptions to be filled, including telling client when next dose is due based on medications administered in the facility; food and drug interactions and any other essential medication information; care of incision or dressings, if indicated; dietary needs or restrictions or other pertinent information; and when client should make appointment for follow-up with private physician.	9. Promotes continuity of care.
10. Have client/family provide return demonstration of skills required for self-care at home.	10. Demonstrates that learning has occurred.
11. Check that transportation to home is available. Check client room area for any personal belongings.	11. Reduces waiting time.

(Continues)

PROCEDURE 29-41 Discharging a Client (Continued)

ACTION	RATIONALE
12. Complete any paperwork with client, as required by agency policy.	12. Meets regulatory requirements.
13. Escort client to transportation vehicle.	13. Promotes client safety.
For Any Discharge	
14. Notify appropriate personnel according to agency policy that client left the unit. Arrange for personnel to clean the bed and surroundings the client left.	14. Prepares bed for new admission. Reduces transfer of microorganisms.

EVALUATION

- The client encountered no problems in discharge to another facility.
- The client, with the assistance of family, is confident about care at home.

DOCUMENTATION

- Date and time of discharge
- Belongings and valuables with client

Discharge to Another Facility

- Person receiving report on client
- Company transporting client

Discharge to Home

- Mode of taking client to transportation vehicle
- Person taking client home
- Prescriptions and instructions given to client

PROCEDURE 29-42 Initiating Strict Isolation Precautions

OVERVIEW

Occasionally, a client is placed in isolation to prevent the spread of an infectious process. Barrier protective equipment is put on outside the room before providing any client care. All linens and trash are double-bagged, according to agency policy, before he is removed from an isolation room. Meals are served on disposable dishes.

Visitors may be limited because everyone entering the room must wear barrier protective equipment. Some clients feel the isolation very profoundly. Paperback books (to be discarded later), TV, and other diversional activities help the client pass the time.

ASSESSMENT

1. Review physician's orders for isolation to ensure proper setup.
2. Assess client's and family's understanding of client's condition and reason for isolation to identify required teaching needed.

POSSIBLE NURSING DIAGNOSES

Social Isolation
Impaired Social Interaction
Deficient Knowledge (disease process, isolation)
Risk for Powerlessness
Risk for Loneliness

PLANNING

Expected Outcomes

1. The room will be set up for the appropriate type of isolation.
2. The client and family will understand the client's condition and the reason for isolation.

Equipment Needed

- Isolation sign
- Disposable gowns
- Gloves (nonsterile and sterile)
- Goggles or face shield
- Disposable masks
- Impermeable bags (for linen and trash)
- Tape or bag ties and labels
- Disposable vital signs equipment (single-use thermometers, stethoscope, and sphygmomanometer) if available
- Disposable water pitcher and cups
- Linen
- Room with sink and running water
- Other supplies relative to client's condition

(Continues)

PROCEDURE 29-42 Initiating Strict Isolation Precautions (Continued)

delegation tips

Initiating strict isolation precautions is a nursing responsibility. Properly trained ancillary personnel may provide some client care according to agency policy.

IMPLEMENTATION—ACTION/RATIONALE

* Check client's identification band * Explain procedure before beginning *
* Note: Barrier protection must be on before checking client's ID *

ACTION	RATIONALE
1. Review physician orders and agency protocols relative to the type of isolation precautions: a. Implement protocol related to the type of disinfectants needed to eliminate specific microorganisms. b. Alert housekeeping regarding the room number and type of isolation supplies needed in the room. c. Make sure the room has proper ventilation (the door remains closed at all times) and that the bed and other electrical equipment are functioning properly.	1. Ensures compliance without unnecessary stress being placed on the client and family. Allows housekeeping to have the necessary supplies on their cleaning carts. Provides for client comfort and decreases the spread of microorganisms. Limits the number of personnel coming into the client's room and the client's exposure to microorganisms.
2. Place appropriate isolation supplies outside the client's room and place isolation sign on the door.	2. Ensures staff follows isolation protocol and alerts visitors to check with the nurses' station before entering the room.
3. Gather appropriate supplies to take in the room: a. Linen b. Impermeable bags c. Disposable vital signs equipment, if available d. Wound care supplies, if appropriate	3. Provides for organized care, hand hygiene, proper isolation, and client care materials. Decreases the spread of microorganisms and the number of times caregivers go into and out of the room.
4. Remove jewelry, lab coat, and other items not necessary for providing client care.	4. Decreases the spread of resident and transient microorganisms.
5. Wash hands and don disposable clothing: a. Apply mask by placing the top of the mask over the bridge of your nose (top part of mask has a lightweight metal strip) and pinch the metal strip to fit snugly against your skin. b. Apply cap to cover hair and ears completely, if policy requires cap. c. Apply gown to cover outer garments completely: Hold gown in front of body and place arms through sleeves (Figure 29-42-1A). Pull sleeves down to wrist. Tie gown securely at neck and waist (Figure 29-42-1B, C). d. Don nonsterile gloves and pull gloves to cover gown's cuff. e. Don goggles or face shield.	5. Disposable garments act as a barrier protecting from contact with pathogens. e. Eyeglasses do not offer adequate protection.
6. Enter client's room with all gathered supplies; if client is to receive medications, bring them at this time.	6. Prevents trips into and out of client room and keeps supplies clean.
7. Assess client and family knowledge relative to client's diagnosis and isolation: a. Reason isolation initiated b. Type of isolation c. Duration of isolation d. How to apply barrier protection	7. Client's and family's understanding of isolation procedures will increase their participation in care.

(Continues)

PROCEDURE 29-42 Initiating Strict Isolation Precautions (Continued)

ACTION	RATIONALE

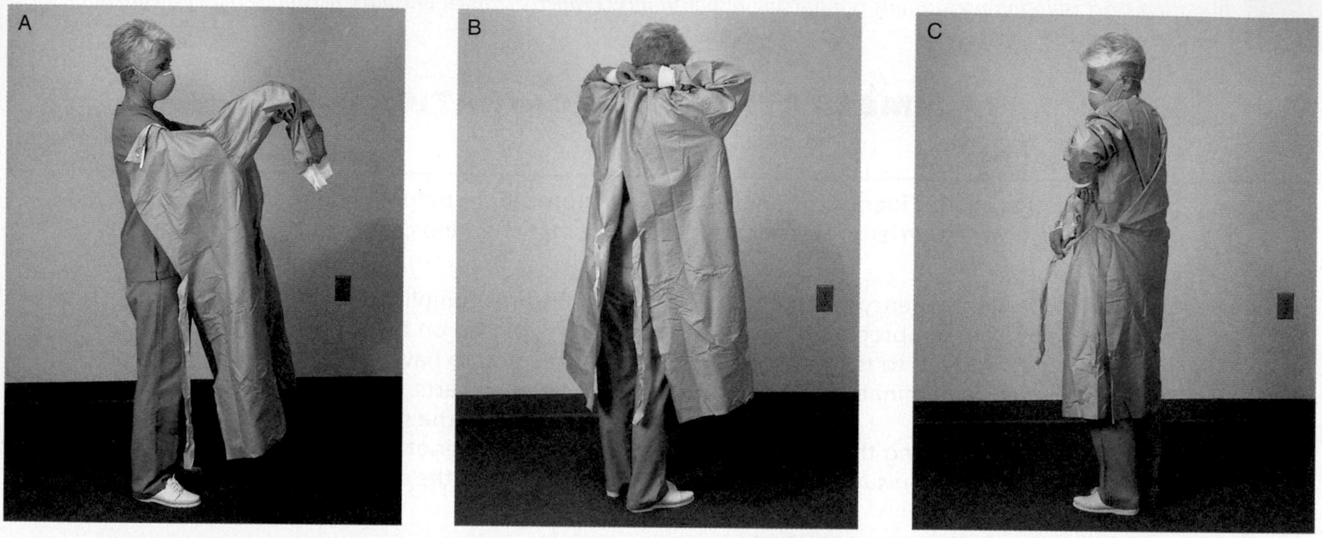

COURTESY OF DELMAR CENGAGE LEARNING

FIGURE 29-42-1 Donning disposable gowns; *A*, Hold gown in front of the body and place arms through the sleeves. *B*, Fasten neck ties. *C*, Fasten waist ties.

ACTION	RATIONALE
8. Assess vital signs, administer medications if appropriate, and perform other functions of nursing care to meet client needs. Record assessment data on a piece of paper, avoiding contact with any articles in the client's room.	8. Allows for data collection and the performance of client care measures.
9. Dispose of soiled articles in the impermeable bags, which should be labeled correctly according to contents. If soiled reusable equipment is removed from the room, label bag accordingly.	9. Impermeable bags prevent the leakage of contaminated materials, thereby preventing the spread of infection. Labeling is a warning to other personnel that the contents are infectious.
10. Double-bag soiled linen according to agency policy in an impermeable bag or in plastic linen bag.	10. Double-bagging allows the washing of soiled linen without human contact. When linen is double-bagged, the first bag is removed before washing and the second bag goes into the machine with the dirty linen and dissolves.
11. Replenish supplies before leaving the client's room by having another staff member bring the clean supplies and transfer at the door. Ask client if anything is needed (e.g., juice or personal care items).	11. Decreases the number of times staff members go in and out of the room.
12. Before leaving, let the client know when you will return and make sure call light is accessible.	12. Decreases a feeling of abandonment; provides client with a means of communication.
13. Exiting the isolation room: a. Untie gown at waist. b. Remove one glove by grasping the glove's cuff and pulling down so that the glove turns inside out (glove on glove) and dispose of it. With your ungloved hand, slip your fingers inside the cuff of the other glove, pull it off, inside out, and dispose of it.	13. Gloves are removed inside out to avoid contact with skin. The gown is removed and folded with hands touching only the inside of the garment. Only the ties and the inside of the cap are touched with your hands. All articles are disposed of as soon as they are removed.
c. Grasp and release the ties of the mask, and dispose of it.	c. If a client has an airborne-spread disease, the mask may be removed last.
d. Release neck ties of the gown and allow the gown to fall forward. Place fingers of dominant	

(Continues)

PROCEDURE 29-42 Initiating Strict Isolation Precautions (Continued)

ACTION	RATIONALE

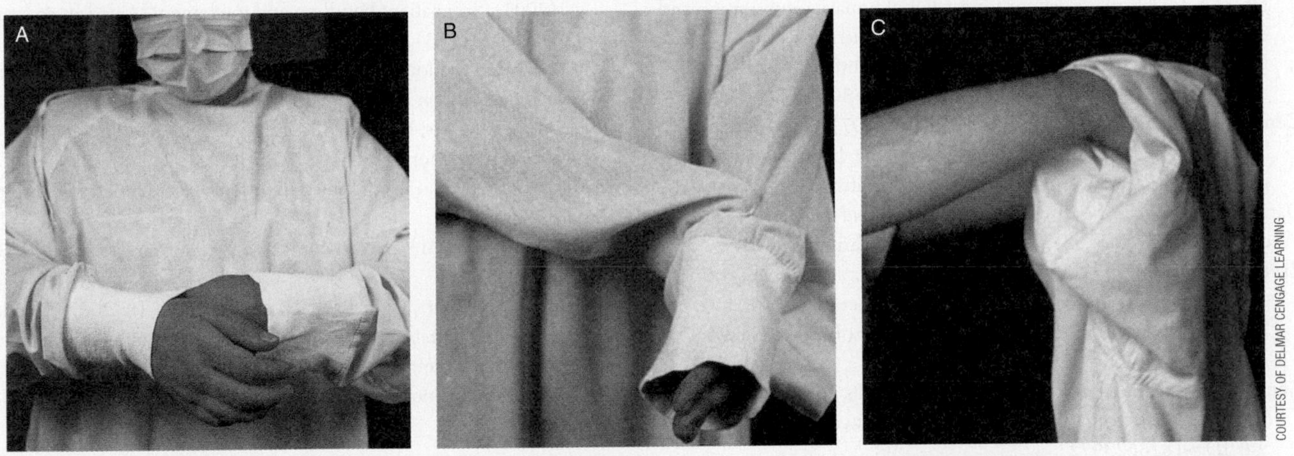

FIGURE 29-42-2 Removing disposable gown: *A*, Place fingers of dominant hand inside the cuff of the other hand and pull gown down over other hand; *B*, With the gown-covered hand, pull gown down over the dominant hand. C, As the gown is removed, fold the outside of the gown together and dispose of it.

ACTION	RATIONALE
hand inside cuff of other hand and pull down over other hand (Figure 29-42-2A). With gown-covered hand, pull gown over the dominant hand (Figure 29-42-2B). While gown is still on arm, fold outside of gown together, remove, and dispose of it (Figure 29-42-2C).	
e. Remove cap by slipping your finger under the cap and removing from the front to back and dispose of it.	
14. Wash hands. Don nonsterile gloves and remove bags from the client's room. Exit room and close door. Dispose of bags according to agency protocol. Remove gloves and wash hands.	14. Reduces transmission of microorganisms.

EVALUATION

- The appropriate type of isolation was instituted.
- The client and family express understanding of the client's condition and the reason for isolation.

DOCUMENTATION

Nurses' Notes

- Date, time, and type of isolation instituted
- Client response to isolation
- Client and family teaching regarding isolation
- Document on appropriate electronic medical record or flow sheet

REFERENCES/SUGGESTED READING

American Academy of Physician Assistants (AAPA). (2009). Joint Commission Standards-restraint and seclusion. Retrieved March 15, 2009 from http://www.aapa.org/gandp/joint-commission-restraint.html

American College of Emergency Physicians Foundation. (2009a). What to do in a medical emergency. Retrieved March 15, 2009, from http://www.emergencycareforyou.org/EmergencyManual/WhatToDoInMedical Emergency

American College of Emergency Physicians Foundation. (2009b). How to perform CPR. Retrieved March 15, 2009, from http://www.emergencycareforyou.org/EmergencyManual/HowToPerformCPR/Default/aspx

American Heart Association. (2005). 2005 American Heart Association guidelines for cardiopulmonary resuscitation and emergency cardiovascular care (Part 3: Overview of CPR). *Circulation, 112*, IV-12–IV-18. Retrieved March 15, 2009, from http://circ.ahajournals.org/cgi/content/full/112/24_suppl/IV-12

American Heart Association. (2005–2006). Highlights of the American Heart Association guidelines for cardiopulmonary resuscitation and emergency cardiovascular care. *Currents in Emergency Cardiovascular Care, 16*(4). Retrieved March 15, 2009, from http://www.americanheart.org/presenter.jhtml?identifier+3012268

Centers for Disease Control and Prevention. (2007). Guideline for hand hygiene in health-care settings. Available: http://www.cdc.gov/mmwr/preview/mmwrhtml/ rr5116a1.htm

Daniels, R. (2010). *Delmar's guide to laboratory and diagnostic tests, 2nd edition.* Clifton Park, NY: Delmar Cengage Learning.

Exergen Corporation. (2009). *Exergen temporal artery thermometry: Changing the way the world take temperature.* Retrieved March 8, 2009 from http://exergencorporations.web.officelive.com/Thermal.aspx

General Practice Notebook. (2009). Dorsalis pedis pulse. Retrieved on March 4, 2009, from http://www.gpnotebook.co.uk/simplepage.cfm?ID=-1818623972

Infection Control. (2002). "Hand hygiene" news. *Nursing2002, 32*(5), 32hn6.

Joint Commission. (2008). Provision of care, treatment, and services. Retrieved March 9, 2009 from HYPERLINK "http://www.jointcommission.org/AccreditationPrograms/BehavioralHealthCare/Standards/O" http://www.jointcommission.org/AccreditationPrograms/BehavioralHealthCare/Standards/09_FAQs/PC/Restraint+_Seclusion.htm

Martin, P. (2003). CPR when the patient's pregnant. *RN, 66*(8), 34–39.

National Institutes of Health. (2008). NIH policy manual (OD/OM/ORFDO/DEP 301-496-3537). Retrieved March 3, 2009, from http://www1.od.nih.gov/oma/manualchapters/intramural/3033/main.html

Nelson, A., Owen, B., Lloyd, J., Fragala, G., Matz, M., Amato, M., et al. (2003). Safe patient handling and movement. *American Journal of Nursing, 103*(3), 32–43.

NANDA International. (2009). *NANDA-I nursing diagnoses: Definitions and classification 2009–2011.* Ames, IA: Wiley-Blackwell.

Parini, S., & Myers, F. (2003). Keeping up with hand hygiene recommendations. *Nursing2003, 33*(2), 17.

Pullen, R. (2003). Caring for a patient on pulse oximetry. *Nursing2003, 33*(9), 30.

Ramponi, D. (2001). Eye on contact lens removal. *Nursing2001, 31*(8), 56–57.

Siegel, J., Rhinehart, E., Jackson, M., & Chiarello, L. (2007). Guideline for isolation precations: Preventing transmission of infectious agents in healthcare settings. Retrieved December 5, 2009 from http://www.cdc.gov/ncidod/dhqp/pdf/guidelines/Isolation2007.pdf

CHAPTER 30
Intermediate Procedures

PROCEDURE 30-1 Surgical Asepsis: Preparing and Maintaining a Sterile Field

OVERVIEW

Preparing and maintaining a sterile field is basic to many nursing procedures, such as inserting a urinary catheter and changing surgical dressings. It takes practice to develop a "sterile conscience," a consistent awareness of what is sterile, and to maintain the sterility.

ASSESSMENT

1. Assess all packages to determine that they are dry and intact. **Assesses the sterility of packages.**
2. Assess the local environment for a dry, horizontal, stable area. **A dry, flat workspace is best for a sterile field.**

POSSIBLE NURSING DIAGNOSIS

Risk for Infection

PLANNING

Expected Outcomes

1. Sterility of the field and all packages, while being opened, will be maintained.
2. Sterility of the procedure will be maintained.

Equipment Needed

- Sterile kit as needed for procedure
- Sterile gloves (if not in kit)
- Sterile drape (if needed)
- Sterile solution (if needed)
- Other sterile items as required

delegation tips

Only nurses should prepare and maintain a sterile field, with the exception of surgical technicians in the OR.

IMPLEMENTATION—ACTION/RATIONALE

ACTION	RATIONALE
* Wash hands * Check client's identification band*	
1. Gather equipment for the type of procedure: a. Select only clean, dry packages marked sterile, and read listing of contents. b. Check the package for integrity and expiration date.	1. Prevents break in technique during procedure. If the package is moist or outdated, it is considered contaminated and cannot be used.
2. Select a clean area in the client's environment to establish the sterile field.	2. Promotes access to the sterile field during the procedure.
3. Explain procedure to the client; provide specific instructions if client assistance is required during the procedure.	3. Gains client's understanding and cooperation during the procedure.

(Continues)

PROCEDURE 30-1 Surgical Asepsis: Preparing and Maintaining a Sterile Field (Continued)

ACTION	RATIONALE
4. Inquire about and attend to the client's toileting needs.	4. Prevents break in technique during the procedure.
5. Hospital environment: If the procedure is to be performed at the client's bedside, the client should be in a private room or moved to a clean treatment room if available.	5. Minimizes microorganisms in the environment.
6. Home environment: Secure privacy and remove pets from the room.	6. Puts the client at ease and promotes a clean environment.
7. Position client and attend to comfort measures; the client's position should provide easy access to the area and facilitate good body mechanics during the procedure.	7. Helps the client relax and prevents movement during the procedure; prevents reaching, decreasing the risk of contamination and back strain.
8. Wash hands.	8. Reduces transmission of microorganisms.
9. Place sterile package (drape or tray) in the center of the clean, dry work area.	9. Prevents reaching over exposed sterile items when wrapper is removed.
Drape	
10. Open the wrapper, pulling away from the body first.	10. Prevents contamination.
11. Grasp the top edge of the drape with fingertips of one hand.	11. Edges are considered unsterile.
12. Remove the drape by lifting up and away from all objects while it unfolds; discard the outer wrapper with other hand.	12. If the drape touches an unsterile object, it is contaminated and must be discarded.
13. With free hand, grasp the other drape corner, keeping it away from all objects.	13. Avoids contamination.
14. Lay the drape on the surface, with the drape bottom first touching the surface farthest from you; step back and allow the drape to cover the surface.	14. Prevents you from reaching over the sterile field; stepping back decreases risk that drape will touch your uniform.
Tray	
15. Remove outer wrapping and place the tray on the work surface so that the top flap of the sterile wrapper opens away from you.	15. Prevents reaching over the sterile items.
16. Reach around the tray, not over it. With thumb and index fingertips grasping the wrapper's top flap, gently pull up, then down to open over the surface.	16. Only the edges of the field can be contaminated, pulling up frees the top folded flap.
17. Repeat the same steps to open the side flaps.	17. Keeps the arm from reaching over the sterile field.
18. Grasp the corner of the bottom flap with fingertips, step back, and pull flap down (Figure 30-1-1).	18. Creates a sterile work surface.

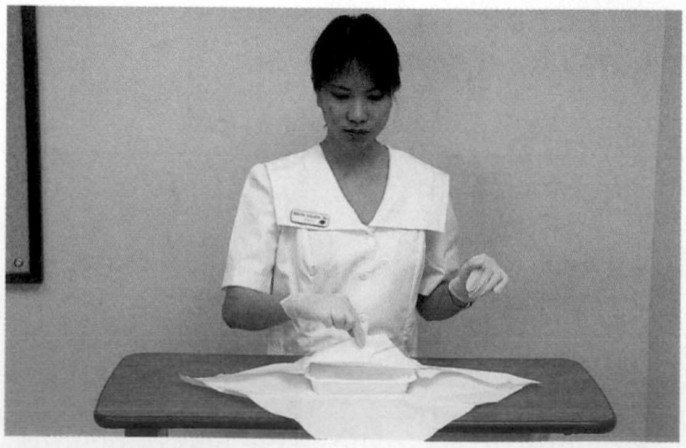

FIGURE 30-1-1 Grasp the corner of the bottom flap with fingertips, step back, and pull flap down (gloves not required for this procedure).

(Continues)

PROCEDURE 30-1 Surgical Asepsis: Preparing and Maintaining a Sterile Field (Continued)

ACTION	RATIONALE
Adding Additional Sterile Items to Sterile Field	
19. While facing the sterile field, step back, remove the outer wrapper, and grasp the item in your nondominant hand so that the top flap will open away from you.	19. Keeps your dominant hand free, item remains sterile.
20. With your dominant hand, open the flaps as previously described.	20. Prevents reaching over the sterile item.
21. With your dominant hand, pull the wrapper back and away from the sterile field (toward your nondominant arm holding the item) and place the item onto the field.	21. Prevents the wrapper from touching the sterile field.
22. When adding additional gauze or dressings to the sterile field, open the package as directed, grasp the top flaps of the wrapper and pull downward (Figure 30-1-2), then drop the contents onto the center of the field (Figure 30-1-3).	22. Prevents contamination of item and sterile field.

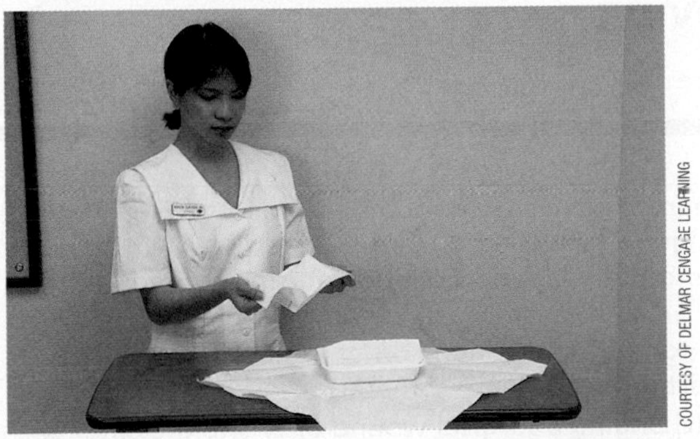

FIGURE 30-1-2 Grasp the flaps of the wrapped supply and pull downward.

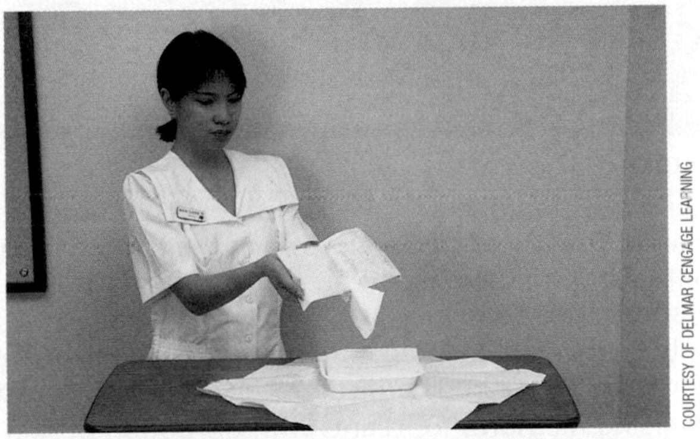

FIGURE 30-1-3 Add contents to the sterile field by holding the package 6 inches (15 cm) above the field and allowing the contents to drop onto the field.

ACTION	RATIONALE
Adding Solutions to Sterile Field	
23. Read the labels and strengths of all solutions three times before pouring.	23. Ensures proper solution and strength.
24. Remove the lid from the bottle of solution and invert the lid onto a clean surface.	24. Inverting the lid prevents contamination of the inner surface.
25. Hold the bottle, label facing ceiling, 4 to 6 inches (10 to 15 cm) over the container on the sterile field; slowly pour the solution into the container to avoid splashing. Pour from the side of the sterile field. Do not reach over it.	25. Prevents the label from getting wet. If the solution splashes onto the label, the field is contaminated because moisture conducts microorganisms from the nonsterile surface. Prevents contamination. If the solution splashes out of the container and the drape becomes wet, the field is contaminated.
26. Replace the lid on the container, label the container with the date and time, and initial the container.	26. Sterility of the solution will be lost if exposed to air for an extended period.
Using Sterile Gloves	
27. Wash hands and perform open gloving (see Procedure 30-2).	27. Prevents transmission of microorganisms.
28. Continue with procedure, keeping gloved hands above waist level at all times, touching only items on the sterile field.	28. Decreases chance of contamination.
29. If using a solution to cleanse a site, use the sterile forceps to prevent contamination of gloves; dispose of forceps after use or process instruments according to agency policy.	29. Prevents field contamination.

(Continues)

PROCEDURE 30-1 Surgical Asepsis: Preparing and Maintaining a Sterile Field (Continued)

ACTION	RATIONALE
30. Postprocedure, dispose of all contaminated items in appropriate receptacle.	30. Decreases risk of transmission of microorganisms to all health care workers.
31. Remove gloves as shown in Procedure 30-2.	31. Minimizes risk of contact with infectious wastes on the gloves.
32. Reposition the client.	32. Promotes client comfort.
33. Clean the environment; wash hands.	33. Prevents transmission of microorganisms.

EVALUATION
- Sterility of field was maintained.
- Sterility of procedure was maintained.

DOCUMENTATION
- Procedure completed following sterile technique.

PROCEDURE 30-2 Performing Open Gloving

OVERVIEW
Asepsis, or sterile technique, consists of those practices that eliminate all microorganisms and spores from an object or area. The use of sterile gloves is at the heart of aseptic technique. The ability to manipulate sterile items without contaminating them is critical to many diagnostic and therapeutic interventions. Common nursing procedures that require sterile technique are:
- All invasive procedures, either intentional perforation of the skin (injection, insertion of IV needles or catheters) or entry into a body orifice (tracheobronchial suctioning, insertion of a urinary catheter)
- Nursing measures for clients with disruption of skin surfaces (changing a surgical wound or IV site dressing) or destruction of skin layers (trauma and burns)

There are two methods for applying sterile gloves: open and closed. The open method is used most frequently when performing procedures that require the sterile technique, such as dressing changes, but that do not require donning a sterile gown.

ASSESSMENT
1. Assess the glove package. Is it intact? Is it wet or otherwise contaminated? **Assesses the sterility of the glove.**
2. Assess the local environment. Is there an area suitable for opening the package and applying the gloves? Is it dry? Is it reasonably stable and horizontal? Are there obvious airborne contaminants? **A flat, clear workspace is necessary to successfully carry out the procedure.**
3. Assess the correct glove size for proper fit. **Gloves come in many sizes, and proper fit is conducive to maintaining asepsis.**

POSSIBLE NURSING DIAGNOSIS
Risk for Infection

PLANNING

Expected Outcomes
1. Sterility of the gloves will be maintained while they are being applied.
2. Sterility of the procedure will be maintained.

Equipment Needed (Figure 30-2-1)
- Package of proper-sized sterile gloves

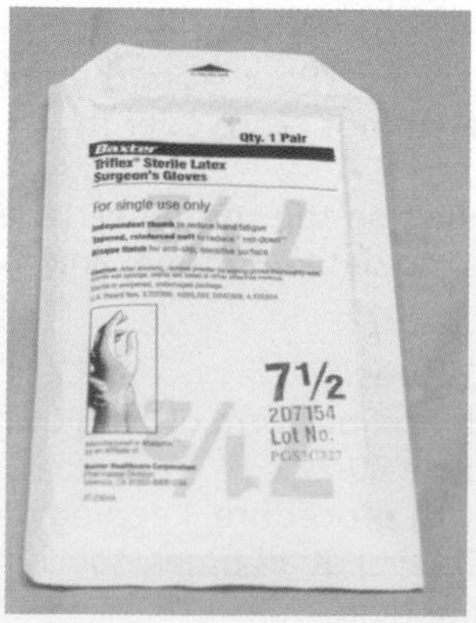

COURTESY OF DELMAR CENGAGE LEARNING

FIGURE 30-2-1 Sterile Gloves

(Continues)

PROCEDURE 30-2 Performing Open Gloving (Continued)

delegation tips

Sterile gloving is only delegated if the personnel are specifically trained, such as in a surgical suite or a testing laboratory setting.

IMPLEMENTATION—ACTION/RATIONALE

ACTION	RATIONALE
1. Wash hands.	1. Reduces transmission of microorganisms.
2. Read the manufacturer's instructions on the package of sterile gloves; proceed as directed in removing the outer wrapper from the package (Figure 30-2-2), placing the inner wrapper onto a clean, dry surface (Figure 30-2-3). Open inner wrapper to expose gloves (Figure 30-2-4).	2. Different manufacturers package gloves differently; the instructions will tell you how to open properly to avoid contamination of the inner wrapper; any moisture on the surface will contaminate the gloves.

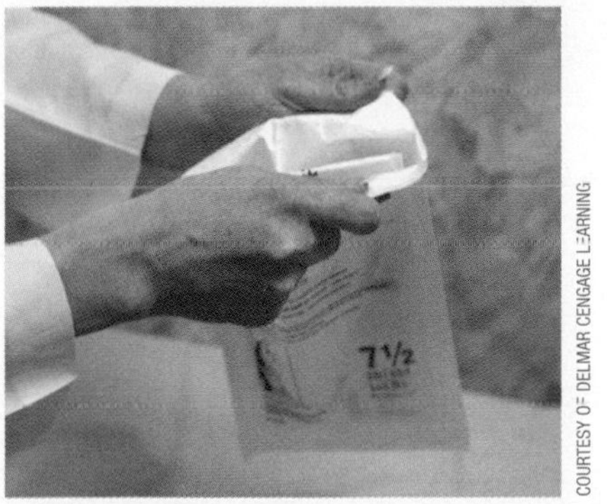

FIGURE 30-2-2 Remove the outer wrapper of the sterile glove package.

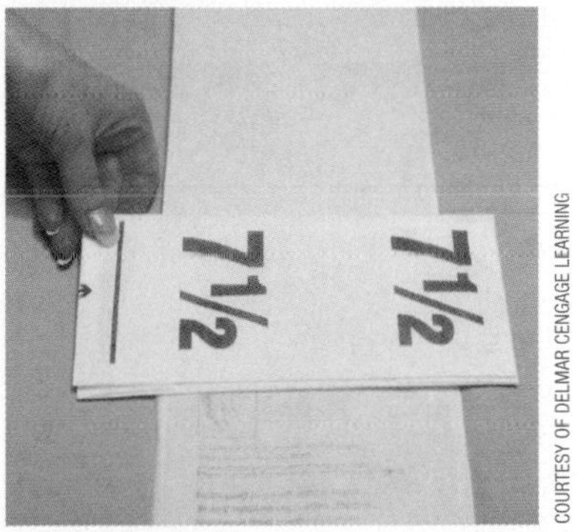

FIGURE 30-2-3 Place the gloves in the inner wrapper on a clean dry surface.

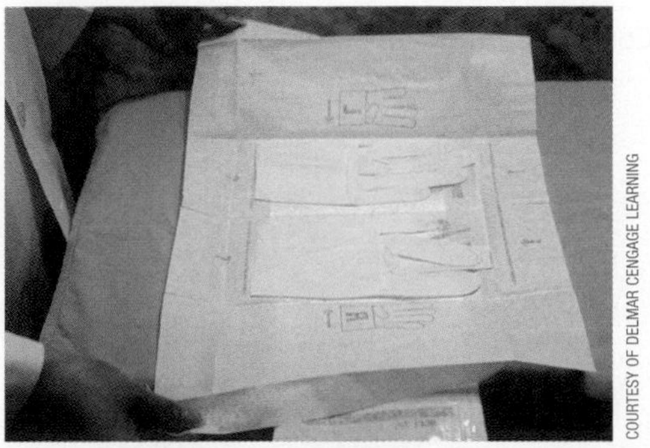

FIGURE 30-2-4 Open the inner wrapper to expose the gloves.

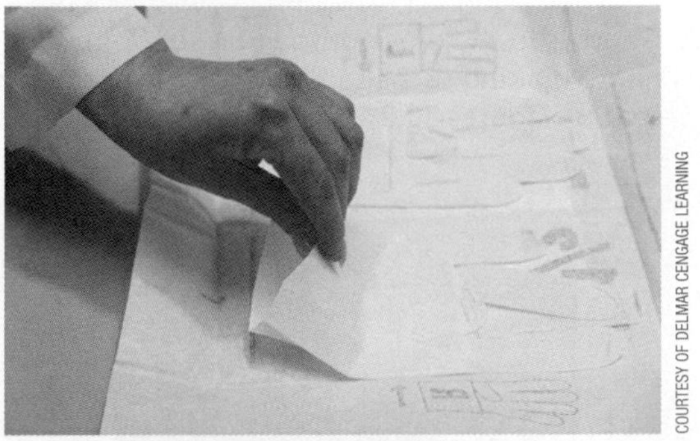

FIGURE 30-2-5 Grasp first cuff with the nondominant hand.

ACTION	RATIONALE
3. Identify right and left hand; glove dominant hand first.	3. Dominant hand should facilitate motor dexterity during gloving.
4. Grasp the 2-inch (5-cm) wide cuff with the thumb and first two fingers of the nondominant hand, touching only the inside of the cuff (Figure 30-2-5).	4. Maintains sterility of the outer surfaces of the sterile glove.
5. Gently pull the glove over the dominant hand, making sure the thumb and fingers fit into the proper spaces of the glove (Figure 30-2-6).	5. Prevents tearing the glove material; guiding the fingers into proper places facilitates gloving.

(Continues)

PROCEDURE 30-2 Performing Open Gloving (Continued)

ACTION | **RATIONALE**

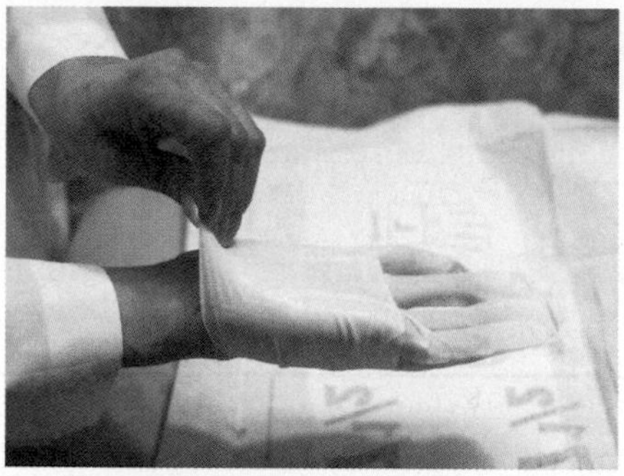

COURTESY OF DELMAR CENGAGE LEARNING

FIGURE 30-2-6 **Pull the glove over the dominant hand.**

6. With the gloved dominant hand, slip your fingers under the cuff of the other glove, gloved thumb abducted, making sure it does not touch any part on your nondominant hand (Figure 30-2-7).

6. Cuff protects gloved fingers, maintaining sterility.

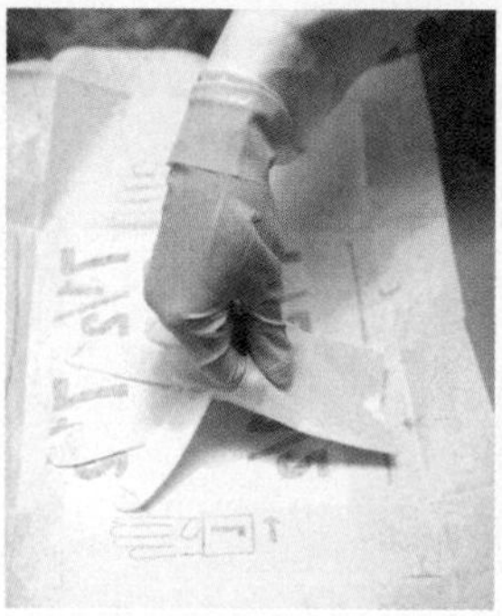

COURTESY OF DELMAR CENGAGE LEARNING

FIGURE 30-2-7 **Slip fingers under the cuff of the second glove.**

7. Gently slip the glove onto your nondominant hand, making sure the fingers slip into the proper spaces (Figures 30-2-8 and 30-2-9).

7. Contact is made with two sterile gloves.

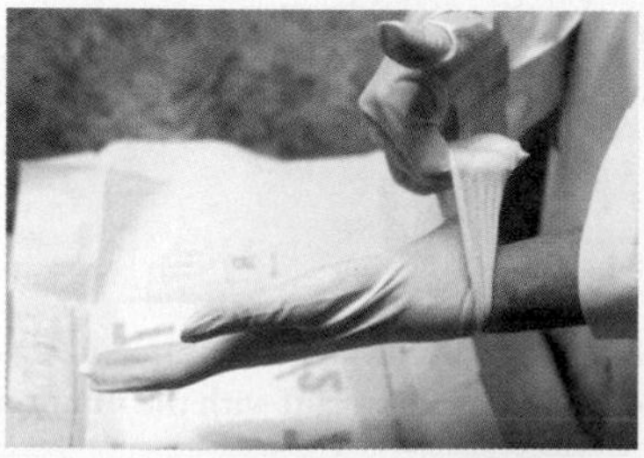

COURTESY OF DELMAR CENGAGE LEARNING

FIGURE 30-2-8 **Pull on the second glove.**

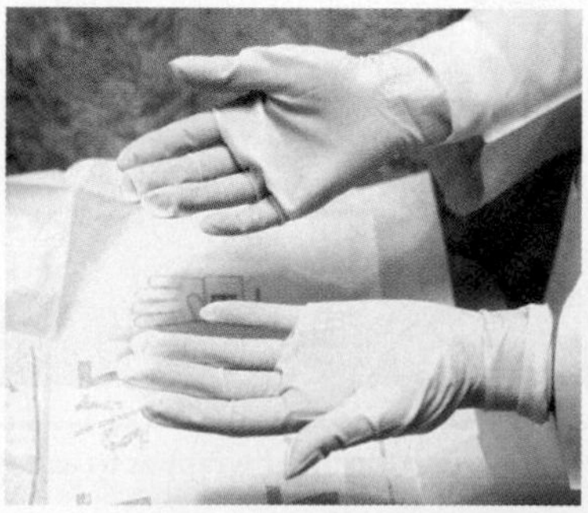

COURTESY OF DELMAR CENGAGE LEARNING

FIGURE 30-2-9 **Make sure all fingers are in the proper spaces.**

8. With gloved hands, interlock fingers to fit the gloves onto each finger. If the gloves are soiled, remove by turning inside out as follows:

8. Promotes proper fit over the fingers.

(Continues)

PROCEDURE 30-2 Performing Open Gloving (Continued)

ACTION	RATIONALE

Removing Gloves

If the gloves are soiled, remove them by turning inside out as follows:

9. With your dominant hand, grasp the other glove at the wrist. Avoid touching the skin of your wrist with the fingers of the glove. Pull the glove off, turning it inside out. (Figure 30-2-10).
   - Rationale: 9. Prevents the transfer of microorganisms.
10. Place removed glove in palm of gloved hand.
    - Rationale: 10. Prevents the transmission of microorganisms.
11. Place thumb of ungloved hand inside the cuff of the gloved hand touching only the inside of the glove (Figure 30-2-11).
    - Rationale: 11. Reduces the transmission of microorganisms.

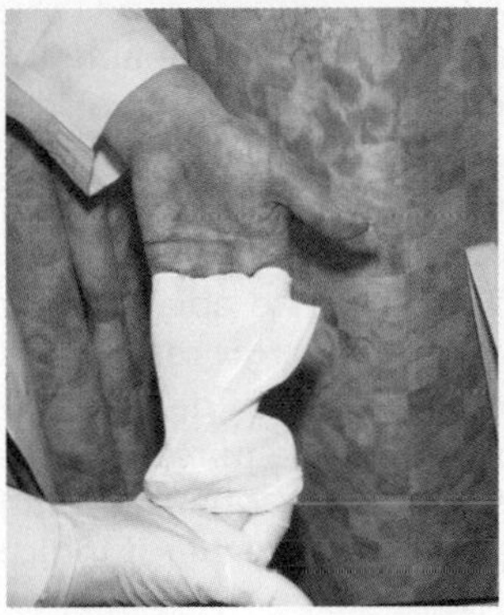

FIGURE 30-2-10 Pull glove off, turning it inside out.

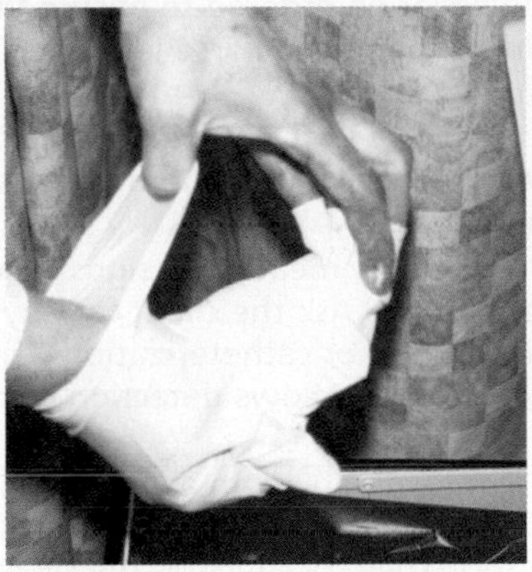

FIGURE 30-2-11 Slip uncovered thumb into the opposite glove.

12. Pull glove off, turning it inside out and over the other glove (Figure 30-2-12).
    - Rationale: 12. Reduces the transmission of microorganisms.
13. Dispose of soiled gloves according to institutional policy and wash hands (Figure 30-2-13).
    - Rationale: 13. Prevents the transfer of microorganisms.

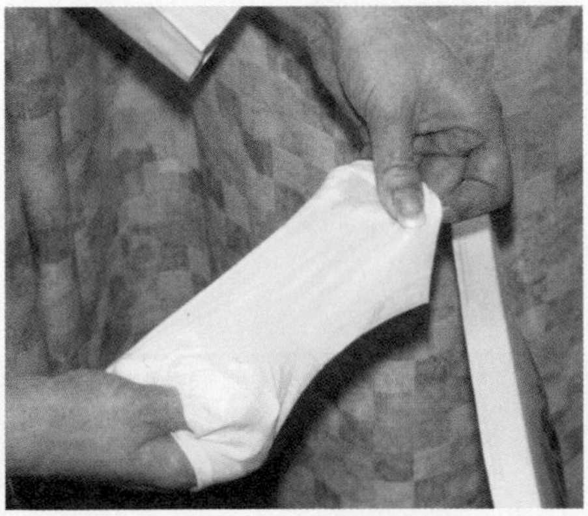

FIGURE 30-2-12 When soiled gloves are removed correctly, only the inside, clean surface of one glove is exposed.

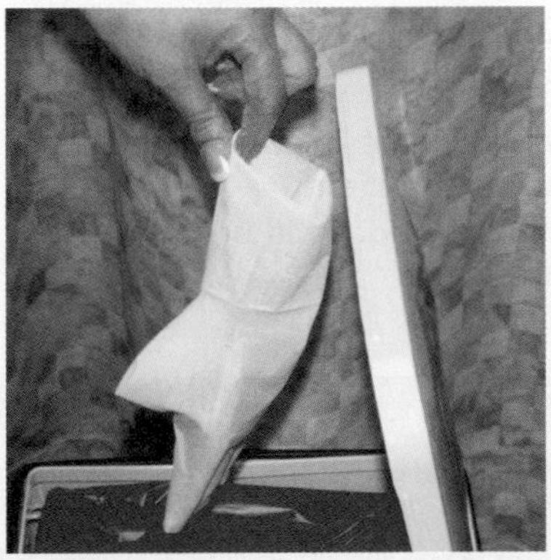

FIGURE 30-2-13 Dispose of gloves in appropriate receptacle.

EVALUATION

- Sterility of the gloves, sterile field, and procedure was maintained without breaks.

DOCUMENTATION

Nurses' Notes

- Procedure was performed using sterile technique.
- Document on appropriate electronic medical record or flow sheet.

PROCEDURE 30-3 Performing Urinary Catheterization: Female/Male

OVERVIEW

Catheterization involves passing a rubber or plastic tube into the bladder via the urethra to drain urine from the bladder or to obtain a urine specimen. Intermittent catheterization may be used to obtain a sample or to relieve bladder distention. Indwelling catheters may be used short-term to keep the bladder empty, prevent urinary retention, or allow precise measurement of urine. Long-term indwelling, or retention, catheters are used to control incontinence, prevent retention, or prevent the leakage of urine. Catheterization is a sterile procedure.

ASSESSMENT

1. Assess the need for catheterization and the type of catheterization ordered **to ensure the proper procedure is performed.** Use latex-free catheter if client has latex allergy.
2. Assess for the need for perineal care before catheterization **to reduce the transmission of microorganisms.**
3. Assess the urinary meatus for signs of infection or inflammation. Ask the client for any history of difficulty with prior catheterizations, anxiety, or urinary strictures. **Allows detection of potential complications.**
4. Assess the client's ability to assist with the procedure. Can she maintain the proper position while you perform the procedure? Is the client agitated, and could she contaminate the sterile field? Will you need assistance to hold her legs in position? **Determines how the procedure is to be carried out.**
5. Assess the light. Will you be able to see well enough to place the catheter, or do you need a secondary light source? **Determines what preparation needs to be done to ensure a successful procedure.**
6. Assess for an allergy to povidone-iodine and/or latex **to avoid an allergic reaction.**
7. Watch for indications of distress or embarrassment, especially if the nurse is of the opposite gender, **to determine what teaching and support are needed.** Explore further if indicated.

POSSIBLE NURSING DIAGNOSES

*Impaired **U**rinary Elimination*
Urinary Retention
*Risk for **I**nfection*
*Risk for **I**mpaired Skin Integrity*
*Deficient **K**nowledge* (insertion of a catheter)

PLANNING

Expected Outcomes

1. A catheter will be inserted without pain, trauma, or injury to the client.
2. The client's bladder will be emptied without complication.
3. The nurse will maintain the sterility of the catheter during insertion.

Equipment Needed

- Straight or indwelling catheter with drainage system (Figure 30-3-1)
- Sterile catheterization kit (Figure 30-3-2)
- Adequate lighting source
- Nonsterile latex-free gloves
- Blanket or drape
- Soap and washcloth
- Warm water
- Towel

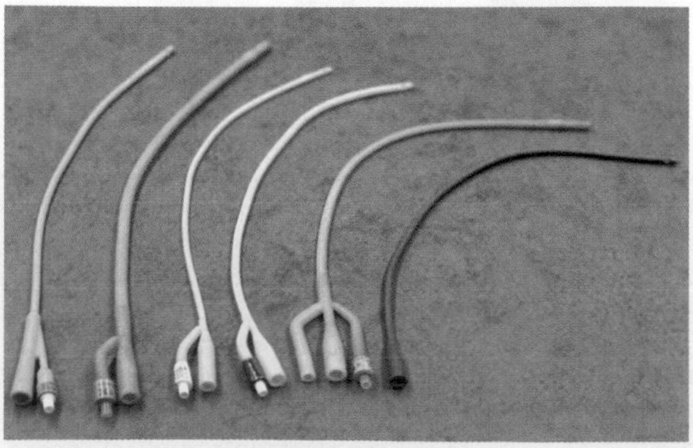

COURTESY OF DELMAR CENGAGE LEARNING

FIGURE 30-3-1 Indwelling and Straight Catheters

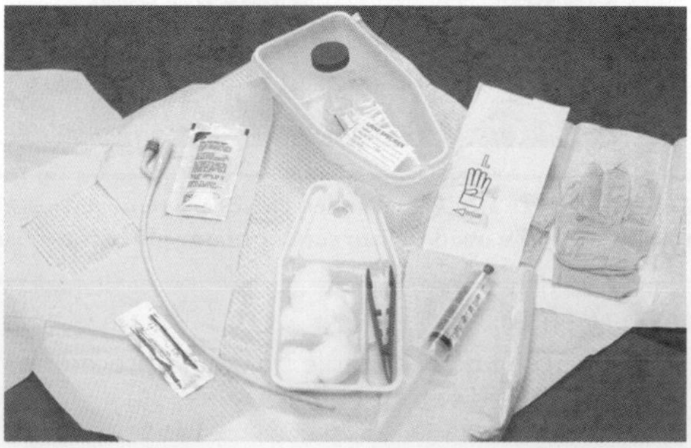

COURTESY OF DELMAR CENGAGE LEARNING

FIGURE 30-3-2 Catheterization Kit

(Continues)

PROCEDURE 30-3 Performing Urinary Catheterization: Female/Male (Continued)

delegation tips

Insertion of an indwelling catheter in a female client is generally not delegated to ancillary personnel. The delegation of this skill depends on institution policy and the availability of licensed staff versus properly trained ancillary personnel. Male urinary catheterization may be delegated to properly trained ancillary personnel depending on institution policies. The nurse is responsible to evaluate the client for contraindications to delegating this procedure, such as the risk for a difficult or traumatic insertion. The nurse may then decide to perform the procedure or to defer to the health care practitioner.

IMPLEMENTATION—ACTION/RATIONALE

* Check client's identification band * Explain procedure before beginning *

Performing Female Urinary Catheterization

ACTION	RATIONALE
1. Gather the equipment needed. Read the label on the catheterization kit. Note if the catheter is included in the kit and, if so, what type it is. Gather any supplies you will need that are not in the prepackaged kit.	1. Promotes efficiency in the procedure. Kits from various manufacturers come with different equipment. The catheter may or may not be packaged in the kit. Sterile gloves and the urine drainage bag may also need to be gathered separately.
2. Identify client by reading arm band assessing two client identifiers.	2. Verifies correct client.
3. Provide for privacy. Assess for allergy to povidone-iodine.	3. Promotes client dignity. Prevents known allergic reactions.
4. Set the bed to a comfortable height to work, and raise the side rail on the side opposite to you.	4. Promotes proper body mechanics and ensures client safety.
5. Assist the client to a supine position with legs spread and feet together (Figure 30-3-3).	5. Relaxes muscles and allows visualization of the area to facilitate insertion of the catheter.
6. Drape the client's abdomen and thighs for warmth if needed.	6. Promotes client comfort and warmth.
7. Ensure adequate lighting of the perineal area.	7. Facilitates proper execution of technique.
8. Wash hands and apply nonsterile latex-free gloves.	8. Reduces transfer of microorganisms.
9. Wash perineal area.	9. Reduces transfer of microorganisms.
10. Remove gloves and wash hands.	10. Reduces transfer of microorganisms.
11. Remove plastic wrap from catheterization kit. Place catheterization kit between client's legs and open the catheterization kit, using aseptic technique (Figure 30-3-4).	11. Provides an area for the sterile equipment to be laid out and assembled. Establish the sterile field close to the client. If the client is able to cooperate, the sterile field can sometimes be established in the open area between the client's legs. Plastic wrap may be used as receptacle for contaminated supplies.

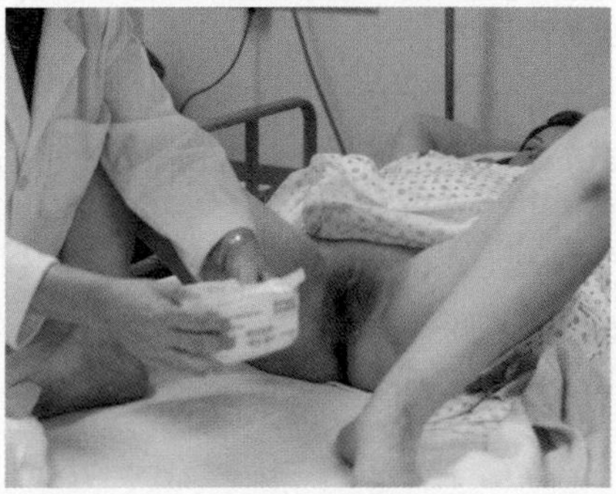
COURTESY OF DELMAR CENGAGE LEARNING

FIGURE 30-3-3 Position the client supine with legs spread.

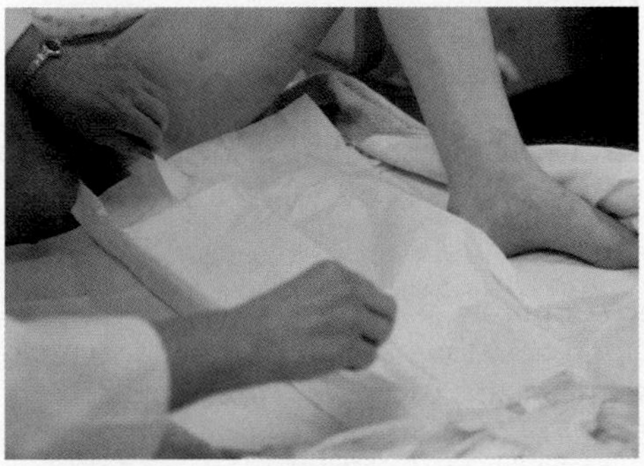
COURTESY OF DELMAR CENGAGE LEARNING

FIGURE 30-3-4 Open the catheterization kit, using the wrapper to establish a sterile field between the client's legs.

(Continues)

PROCEDURE 30-3 Performing Urinary Catheterization: Female/Male (Continued)

ACTION	RATIONALE
a. Open the top flap away from your body by grasping the corner of the outer surface between your thumb and finger only.	a. Outer surface is considered contaminated.
b. Grasp the outer surface of the left and right flaps and open.	b. Maintains sterile technique.
c. Grasp the proximal (closest) flap and open towards you. Avoid touching the inside of the flap or package with your hands or clothing.	c. Opening the proximal flap last prevents reaching over the sterile field.
12. If the catheter is not included in the kit, drop the sterile catheter onto the field using aseptic technique. Add any other items needed.	12. Prevents contamination of the sterile equipment and the sterile field.
13. Apply sterile gloves. These may be included in the kit.	13. Prevents contamination of the sterile equipment and the sterile field.
14. Place the sterile drape from the catheterization kit between the client's thighs, close to the perineum, and be careful not to touch nonsterile areas with sterile gloves.	14. Provides a sterile field at the procedural site.
15. If inserting a retention catheter, attach the syringe filled with sterile water to the Luerlock tail of the catheter. Inflate and deflate the retention balloon. Keep water-filled syringe attached to the port. (Figure 30-3-5).	15. Tests the patency of the retention balloon. A new catheter must be obtained if the balloon leaks or does not inflate.

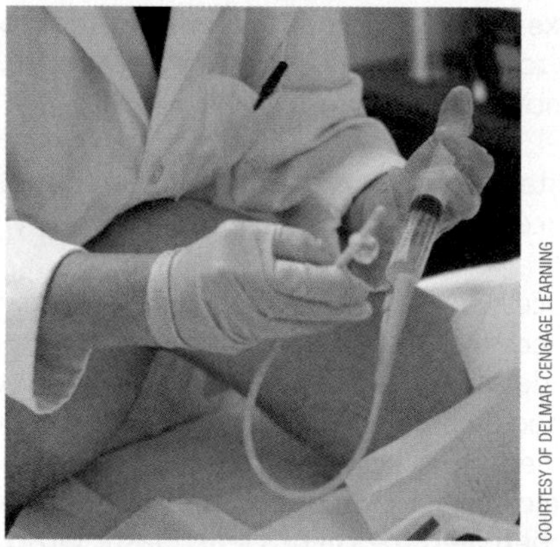

FIGURE 30-3-5 Inflate and deflate the retention balloon to test its patency.

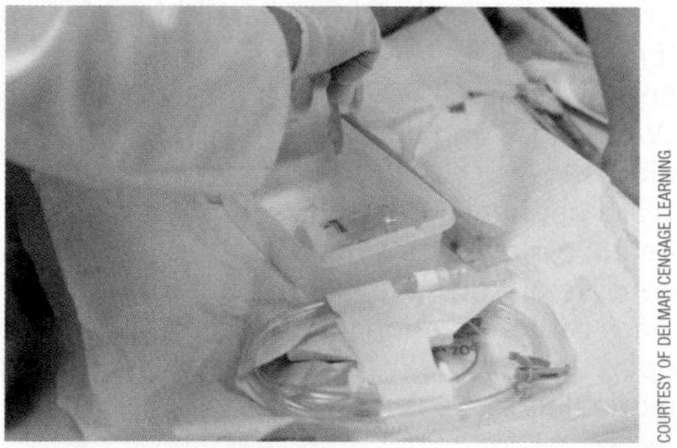

FIGURE 30-3-6 Open the lubrication package and squeeze lubricant onto the sterile field where it will be used to lubricate the catheter.

ACTION	RATIONALE
16. Attach the catheter to the urine drainage bag if it is not preconnected.	16. The catheter and drainage system may be preconnected; otherwise, connect it before catheterization to avoid exposing the client to ascending infection from an open-ended catheter.
17. Open supplies: a. Open povidone-iodine or other antimicrobial solution and pour over cotton balls. b. Squeeze lubrication package onto sterile field.	17. Maintains sterile technique and facilitates execution of the procedure.
18. Generously coat the distal portion of the catheter with water-soluble, sterile lubricant and place it nearby on the sterile field (Figure 30-3-6).	18. Facilitates catheter insertion.

(Continues)

PROCEDURE 30-3 Performing Urinary Catheterization: Female/Male (Continued)

ACTION	RATIONALE
19. Place the fenestrated drape from the catheterization kit over the client's perineal area with the labia visible through the opening.	19. Provides a sterile field at the procedural site. Prevents accidental contamination from adjacent areas.
20. Gently spread the labia minora with the fingers of your nondominant hand and visualize the urinary meatus (Figure 30-3-7).	20. Helps locate the meatus, so the catheter can be placed in the correct spot.
21. Holding the labia apart with your nondominant hand, use the forceps to pick up a cotton ball soaked in povidone-iodine, and cleanse the periurethral mucosa. Use one downward stroke for each cotton ball and dispose. Keep the labia separated with your nondominant hand until you insert the catheter (Figure 30-3-8).	21. Cleans the area and minimizes the risk of urinary tract infection by removing surface pathogens.

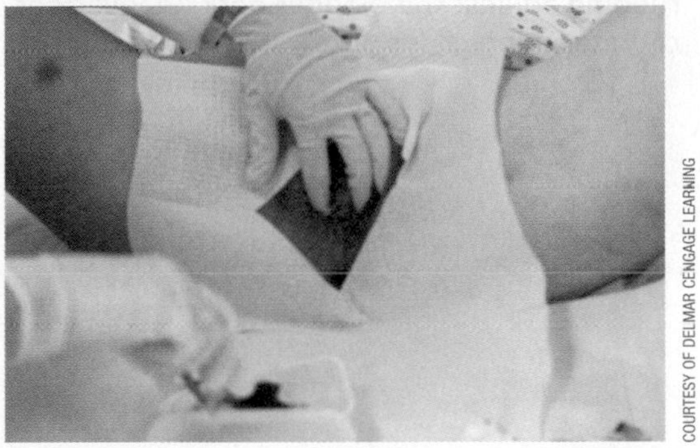

FIGURE 30-3-7 Spread the labia minora and visualize the urinary meatus.

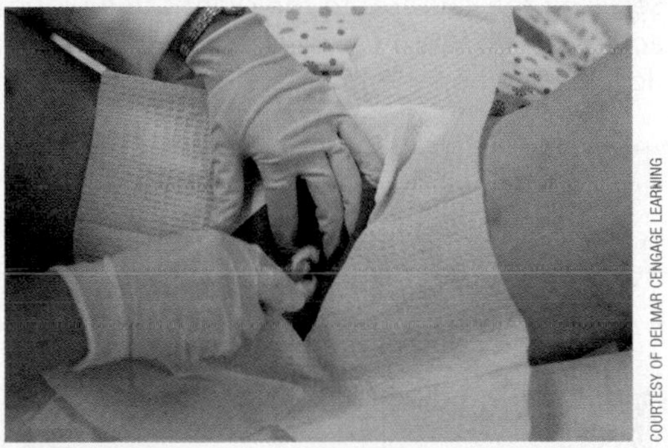

FIGURE 30-3-8 Using forceps, pick up a cotton ball soaked in povidone-iodine. Cleanse the periurethral mucosa.

ACTION	RATIONALE
22. Holding the catheter in the dominant hand, steadily insert the catheter into the meatus until urine is noted in the drainage bag or tubing (Figure 30-3-9).	22. Provides a visual confirmation that the catheter tip is in the bladder.

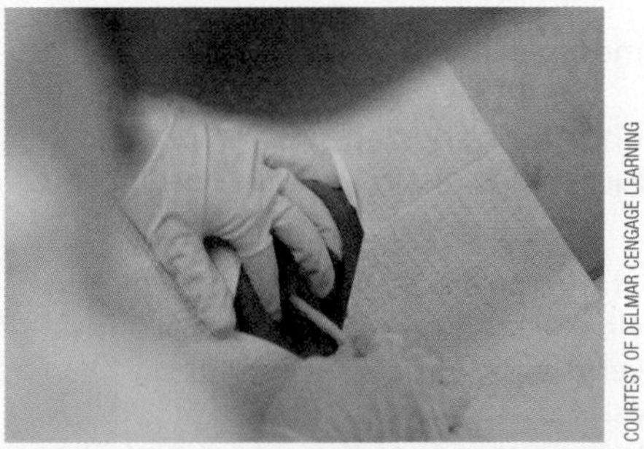

FIGURE 30-3-9 Steadily insert the catheter into the meatus.

ACTION	RATIONALE
23. If the catheter will be removed as soon as the client's bladder is empty, insert the catheter another inch and hold the catheter in place as the bladder drains.	23. The catheter needs to be inserted far enough to allow complete bladder drainage, but not so far as to possibly irritate the bladder, causing spasms.
24. If the catheter will be indwelling with a retention balloon, continue inserting another 1 to 3 inches.	24. Ensures adequate catheter insertion before retention balloon is inflated.

(Continues)

PROCEDURE 30-3 Performing Urinary Catheterization: Female/Male (Continued)

ACTION	RATIONALE
25. Inflate the retention balloon using the manufacturer's recommendations or according to the health care provider's instructions.	25. Ensures retention of the balloon. Retention catheters are available with a variety of balloon sizes. Use a catheter with the appropriate-size balloon.
26. Instruct the client to immediately report discomfort or pressure during balloon inflation; if pain occurs, discontinue the procedure, deflate the balloon, and insert the catheter farther into the urethra. If the client continues to complain of pain with balloon inflation, remove the catheter and notify the client's health care provider.	26. Pain or pressure indicates inflation of the balloon in the urethra; further insertion will prevent misplacement and further pain or bleeding.
27. Once the balloon has been inflated, gently pull the catheter until the retention balloon is resting snugly against the bladder neck (resistance will be felt when the balloon is properly seated).	27. Maximizes continuous bladder drainage and prevents urine leakage around the catheter.
28. Secure the catheter according to institutional policy. Securing the catheter to the client's thigh is usually acceptable; be sure to leave enough slack so that it does not pull on the bladder (Figure 30-3-10).	28. Prevents excessive traction from the balloon rubbing against the bladder neck, inadvertent catheter removal, or urethral erosion.

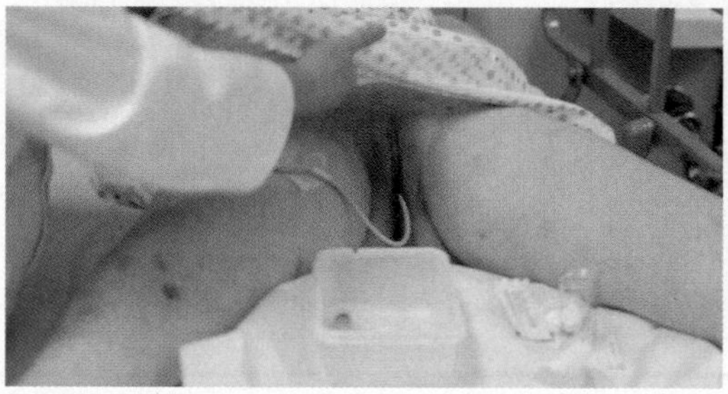

FIGURE 30-3-10 Tape the catheter to the client's thigh.

ACTION	RATIONALE
29. Place the drainage bag below the level of the bladder. Do not let it rest on the floor. Make sure the tubing lies over, not under, the leg.	29. Maximizes continuous drainage of urine from the bladder (drainage is prevented when the drainage bag is placed above the abdomen).
30. Wash the perineal area with soap and water.	30. Removes antiseptic solution to prevent skin irritation.
31. Dispose of equipment, remove gloves, and wash hands.	31. Prevents transfer of microorganisms
32. Assist client to a comfortable position and lower the bed.	32. Promotes client comfort and safety.
33. Assess the color, odor, quality, and amount of urine.	33. Monitors urinary status.
34. Wash hands.	34. Reduces transmission of microorganisms.
Performing Male Urinary Catheterization	
35. Repeat Actions 1 to 14.	35. See Rationales 1 to 14.
36. Place the fenestrated drape from the catheterization kit over the client's perineal area with the penis extending through the opening.	36. Provides a sterile field at the procedural site. Prevents accidental contamination from adjacent areas.
37. If inserting a retention catheter, attach the syringe filled with sterile water to the Luerlock tail of the catheter. Inflate and deflate the retention balloon. Keep water-filled syringe attached to the port.	37. Tests the patency of the retention balloon. A new catheter must be obtained if the balloon leaks or does not inflate.
38. Attach the catheter to the urine drainage bag if it is not preconnected.	38. The catheter and drainage system may be preconnected; otherwise it is connected before catheterization to avoid exposing the client to ascending infection from an open-ended catheter.
39. Open povidone-iodine or other antimicrobial solution and pour over cotton balls. Remove the cap from the water-soluble lubricant syringe.	39. Maintains sterile technique.

(Continues)

PROCEDURE 30-3 Performing Urinary Catheterization: Female/Male (Continued)

ACTION	RATIONALE
40. With your nondominant hand, gently grasp the penis and retract the foreskin (if present). With your dominant hand, use the forceps to pick up a saturated cotton ball. Place the cotton ball on the meatus. Using a circular motion and cleanse from the meatus to the base of the penis. Discard cotton ball. Cleanse the meatus three times using a new saturated cotton ball each time (Figure 30-3-11).	40. Removes microorganisms and minimizes the risk of urinary tract infection.

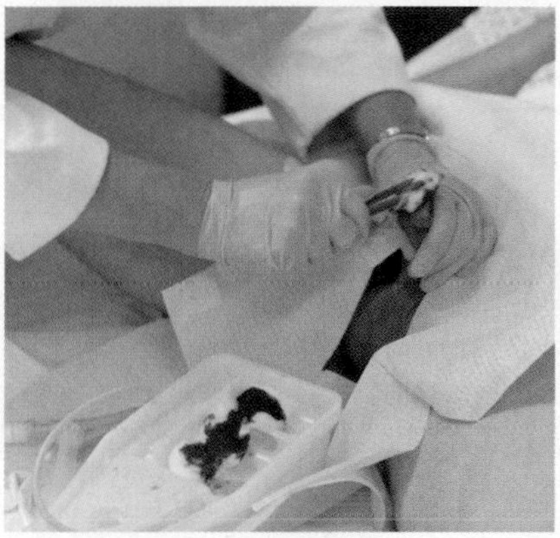

FIGURE 30-3-11 Cleanse the glans penis with a povidone-iodine solution.

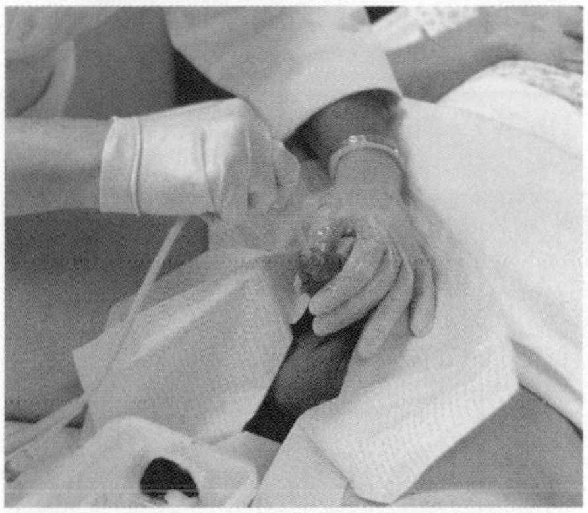

FIGURE 30-3-12 Steadily insert the catheter.

ACTION	RATIONALE
41. Hold the penis perpendicular to the body and pull up gently.	41. Facilitates catheter insertion by straightening urethra.
42. Inject 10 mL sterile, water-soluble lubricant (use a 2% Xylocaine lubricant whenever feasible) into the urethra.	42. Avoids urethral trauma and discomfort during catheter insertion and facilitates insertion.
43. Holding the catheter in the dominant hand, steadily insert the catheter about 8 inches until urine is noted in the drainage bag or tubing (Figure 30-3-12).	43. Provides a visual confirmation that the catheter tip is in the bladder.
44. If the catheter will be removed as soon as the client's bladder is empty, insert the catheter another inch, place the penis in a comfortable position, and hold the catheter in place as the bladder drains.	44. The catheter needs to be inserted far enough to allow complete bladder drainage, but not so far as to possibly irritate the bladder, causing spasms.
45. If the catheter will be indwelling with a retention balloon, continue inserting until the hub of the catheter (bifurcation between drainage port and retention balloon arm) is met.	45. Ensures adequate catheter insertion before retention balloon is inflated.
46. Inflate the retention balloon with sterile water per manufacturer's recommendations or according to the health care provider's orders (Figure 30-3-13).	46. Ensures retention of the balloon. Retention catheters are available with a variety of balloon sizes. Use a catheter with the appropriate size balloon.
47. Instruct the client to immediately report discomfort or pressure during balloon inflation; if pain occurs, discontinue the procedure, deflate the balloon, and insert the catheter farther into the bladder. If the client continues to complain of pain with balloon inflation, remove the catheter and notify the client's health care provider.	47. Pain or pressure indicates inflation of the balloon in the urethra; further insertion will prevent misplacement and further pain or bleeding.
48. Once the balloon has been inflated, gently pull the catheter until the retention balloon is resting snugly against the bladder neck (resistance will be felt when the balloon is properly seated).	48. Maximizes continuous bladder drainage and prevents urine leakage around the catheter.

(Continues)

PROCEDURE 30-3 Performing Urinary Catheterization: Female/Male (Continued)

ACTION	RATIONALE

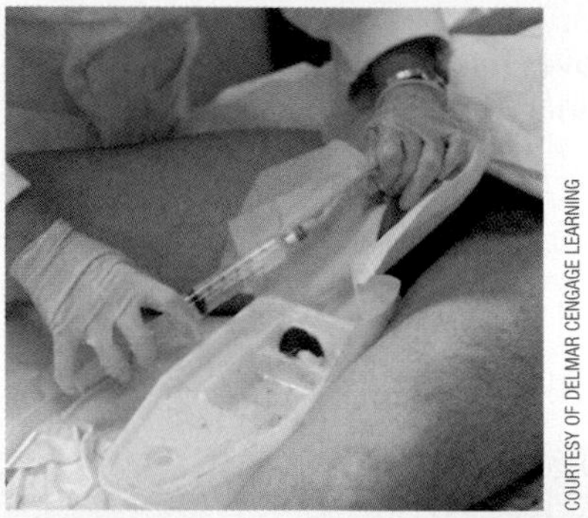

FIGURE 30-3-13 Inflate the retention balloon.

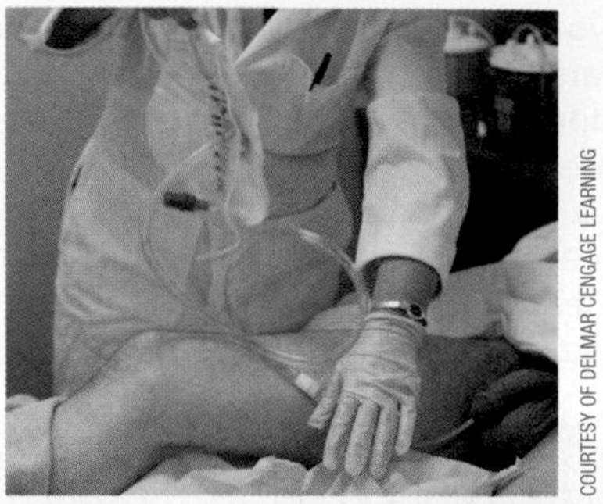

FIGURE 30-3-14 Place the drainage bag tubing over the leg.

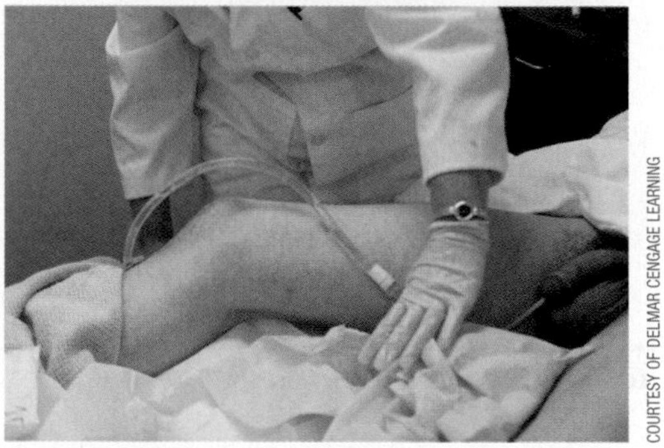

FIGURE 30-3-15 Place the drainage bag below the level of the bladder, but do not rest it on the floor.

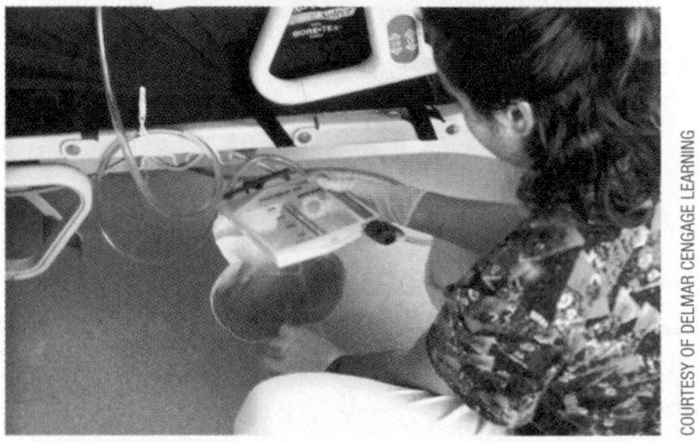

FIGURE 30-3-16 Monitor the urinary status. Assess and document the amount, color, and quality of urine.

ACTION	RATIONALE
49. Secure the catheter to the client's thigh according to institutional policy. Allow enough slack in the catheter so that it will not pull on the bladder when the client moves.	49. Prevents excessive traction from the balloon rubbing against the bladder neck, inadvertent catheter removal, or urethral erosion.
50. Place the drainage bag below the level of the bladder. Do not let it rest on the floor. Make sure the tubing lies over, not under, the leg (Figures 30-3-14 and 30-3-15).	50. Maximizes continuous drainage of urine from the bladder (drainage is prevented when the drainage bag is placed above the abdomen).
51. Clean perineal area with soap and water, and dry the area.	51. Removes antiseptic solution to prevent skin irritation.
52. Dispose of equipment, remove gloves, and wash hands.	52. Prevents transfer of microorganisms.
53. Assist client to a comfortable position. Lower the bed.	53. Promotes client comfort and safety.
54. Assess and document the amount, color, odor, and quality of urine (Figure 30-3-16).	54. Monitors urinary status.
55. Wash hands.	55. Reduces transmission of microorganisms.

EVALUATION

- The catheter was inserted without pain, trauma, or injury to the client.
- The client's bladder was emptied without complication.
- The nurse maintained the sterility of the catheter during insertion.

DOCUMENTATION

Nurses' Notes

- Time and date the catheter was inserted
- Size and type of catheter used, including the size of the retention balloon and the amount of sterile water used to inflate the balloon
- Client's response to the procedure and the amount, color, and quality of urine returned
- Document on appropriate electronic medical record or flow sheet.

Intake and Output Record

- Amount of urine returned

PROCEDURE 30-4 Irrigating a Urinary Catheter

OVERVIEW

Open intermittent irrigation of a urinary catheter is generally done for one of two reasons: either to instill medication into the bladder or to irrigate the catheter itself, which may be blocked by either blood clots or urinary sediment. This irrigation is referred to as "open" because the closed bladder drainage system is opened where the drainage tubing inserts into the urinary catheter; the catheter is generally indwelling. Maintaining sterility of the system is paramount in this type of irrigation.

ASSESSMENT

1. Identify the following items in the health care provider's orders: type of irrigation (bladder or catheter); purpose of the irrigation; type and amount of solution to irrigate with; any premedication ordered; and any other details of the order. **Allows the nurse to anticipate responses to the procedure and assess pertinent features of the client's condition.**
2. Assess the condition of the client as it relates to the procedure: patency of the catheter, characteristics of urinary drainage, and total intake and output status of the client. **Establishes a baseline of the client's condition as it relates to elimination and in the case of PRN catheterization, which may indicate whether there is a need for the procedure.**
3. Assess for current pain or bladder spasms. **Even when medication is not specifically ordered, medicating for pain before the procedure can increase client comfort, and if irrigation does not relieve spasms, the client may need medication afterward.**
4. Assess client's knowledge about the procedure **to determine need for education and reduce anxiety about the procedure.**
5. If this is a repeat of the procedure, read the charting from previous times. **Provides a history of how this client tolerates the procedure and of any teaching done.**

POSSIBLE NURSING DIAGNOSES

Risk for Infection
Impaired Urinary Elimination
Acute Pain
Urinary Retention

PLANNING

Expected Outcomes

1. Urinary catheter will be patent.
2. Sediment/blood clots will be passed through the catheter.
3. Bladder will be free of sources of local irritation.
4. Urinary pH will be lowered to a more acidic state.

Equipment Needed

- Sterile gloves
- Nonsterile latex-free gloves
- Sterile cover for the end of the drainage tubing
- Disposable, water-resistant drape or towel
- Sterile Asepto or Toomey syringe with container for irrigant
- Sterile antiseptic swabs
- Sterile irrigating solution (labeled with date and time of opening, if opened)

delegation tips

The procedure of irrigating a urinary catheter cannot be delegated because it requires the skills and problem-solving abilities of a nurse.

IMPLEMENTATION—ACTION/RATIONALE

ACTION	RATIONALE
* Check client's identification band * Explain procedure before beginning *	
1. Verify the need for bladder or catheter irrigation.	1. Ensures that procedure is being applied correctly, to reduce unnecessary opening of the system and risk of infection.
2. For prn catheter irrigation, palpate for full bladder and check current output against previous totals.	2. If irrigation is on an as-needed basis, it may not be needed at this time.

(Continues)

PROCEDURE 30-4 Irrigating a Urinary Catheter (Continued)

ACTION	RATIONALE
3. Check health care provider's orders for type of irrigation, irrigant, and the amount.	3. Ensures procedural accuracy.
4. If this is a repeat procedure, read previous documentation in the record.	4. Establishes prior client response to procedure.
5. Assemble all supplies.	5. Having all supplies in room enables the nurse to maintain sterility of supplies once they are opened and laid out.
6. Premedicate client if ordered or needed.	6. Increases comfort for the procedure.
7. Educate client as needed based on what the client already knows.	7. Knowledge will increase client compliance and decrease anxiety.
8. Provide for client privacy with a closed door or curtain.	8. Decreases client anxiety.
9. Assist the client to a dorsal recumbent position.	9. Facilitates the flow of irrigant into the bladder.
10. Wash hands.	10. Decreases transmission of microorganisms.
11. Apply nonsterile latex-free gloves and empty the collection bag of urine.	11. Starting with an empty collection bag makes it easier to identify clots or sediment passed as a result of irrigation.
12. Remove gloves and wash hands.	12. Reduces transmission of microorganisms.
13. Expose the indwelling catheter and place the water-resistant drape underneath it.	13. Protects the bedclothes and client from urine and body fluids.
14. Open the sterile syringe and container. Stand it up carefully in or on the wrapper and add 100 to 200 mL sterile diluent without touching or contaminating the tip of the syringe or the inside of the receptacle.	14. Enables nurse to maintain sterility of gloves once they are applied.
15. Open the end of the antiseptic swab package, exposing the swab sticks, and the sterile cover for drainage tube.	15. Enables nurse to maintain sterility of gloves once they are applied.
16. Apply the sterile gloves.	16. Maintains sterility of the procedure.
17. Using the antiseptic swab sticks, disinfect the connection between the catheter and the drainage tubing.	17. Minimizes risk of contaminating the system.
18. After the disinfectant dries, loosen the ends of the connection.	18. Enables the nurse to open the connection without accidentally contaminating either end.
19. Grasp the catheter and tubing 1 to 2 inches from their ends, with catheter in the nondominant hand.	19. Maintains sterility of the procedure and allows the nurse to be positioned to use the dominant hand for the syringe.
20. Fold the catheter to pinch it closed between the palm and last three fingers; use the thumb and first finger to hold the sterile cap for the drainage tube.	20. Allows for one nurse to handle all equipment simultaneously, thus maintaining sterility.
21. Separate the catheter and tube, covering the tube tightly with the sterile cap.	21. Maintains sterility of equipment.
22. Fill the syringe with 30 mL for catheter irrigation, 60 mL for bladder irrigation. Insert the tip of the syringe into the catheter and gently instill the solution into the catheter (Figures 30-4-1 and 30-4-2).	22. Catheter can be irrigated with 30 mL of solution, minimizing bladder discomfort, while irrigating a bladder takes 60 mL.
23. Clamp catheter if ordered (medicated solution). If not clamped, irrigant may be released into a collection container or aspirated back into the syringe (Figure 30-4-3).	23. Fine sediment or clear irrigant with medication can run freely; material with more solids (sediment or clots) may need gentle aspiration.
24. If the bladder or catheter is being irrigated to clear solid material, repeat irrigation until return is clear.	24. Clearing the catheter completely in this irrigation means a lower total number of irrigations and less opening of the system, thus decreasing the risk of infection.

(Continues)

PROCEDURE 30-4 Irrigating a Urinary Catheter (Continued)

ACTION	RATIONALE

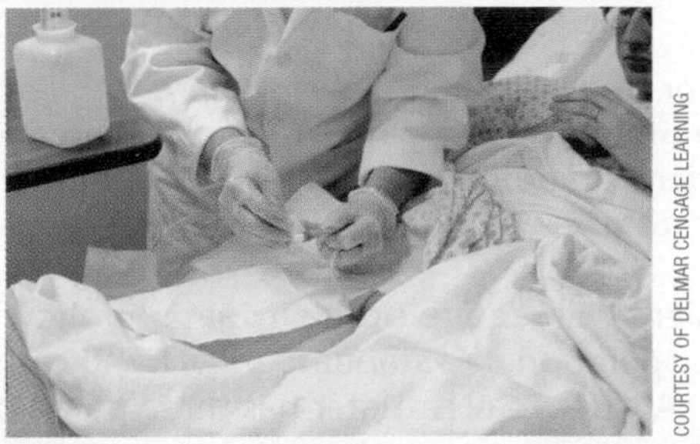

FIGURE 30-4-1 Separate the catheter and tube.

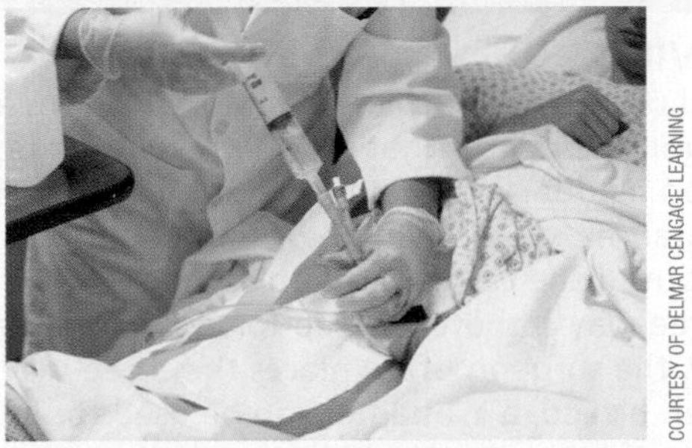

FIGURE 30-4-2 Insert the tip of the syringe into the catheter and gently instill the solution.

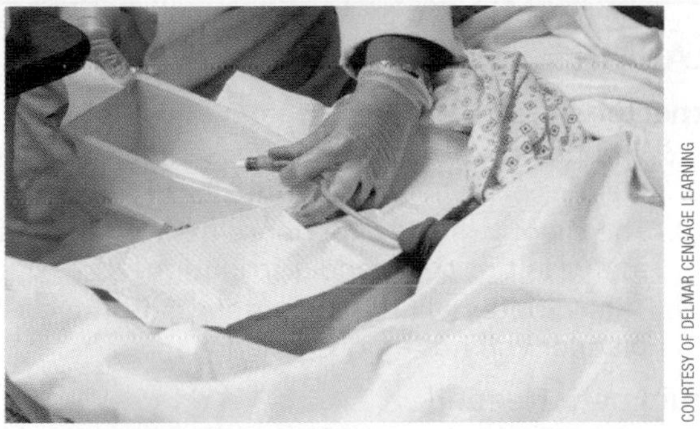

FIGURE 30-4-3 Irrigant is released into a collection container.

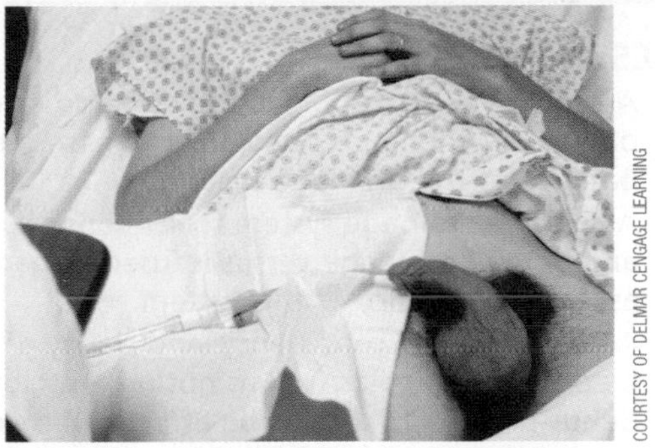

FIGURE 30-4-4 Reconnect the tubing to the catheter.

ACTION	RATIONALE
25. Reconnect system and remove sterile gloves. Wash your hands (Figure 30-4-4).	25. Maintains sterility of system and reduces transmission of microorganisms.
26. Record the type of irrigation, total amount of irrigant used, and the color and quality of return.	26. Evaluation of the urinary tract status and catheter.
27. Monitor client for pain, urine color and clarity, any solid material passed, and total intake and output.	27. Monitoring output after irrigation evaluates the efficacy of the treatment.
28. Wash hands.	28. Reduces transmission of microorganisms.

EVALUATION

- Urinary catheter remains patent.
- Any sediment/blood clots were passed through the catheter.
- Bladder is free of local irritation.
- Urinary pH was more acidic.

DOCUMENTATION

Nurses' Notes

- Assessment indicating need for irrigation, such as decreased output, increased sediment, clots, bladder spasms/pain, or palpation of a full bladder
- Type of irrigant and amount in each instillation
- Amount and quality of returns (returns often include urine trapped in the bladder)
- Medication given before or after the procedure and response to same
- Urine output, color, and clarity and any solids passed 30 to 60 minutes after procedure
- Client response, especially changes in pain, spasms, or discomfort
- Document on appropriate electronic medical record or flow sheet.

Medication Administration Record

Record:

- Type of irrigant, if medicated, and amount in each instillation
- Any medication given before or after the procedure

Intake and Output Record

Document:

- Amount of urine emptied from the drainage bag prior to and following the procedure
- Amount of irrigant instilled

PROCEDURE 30-5 Irrigating the Bladder Using a Closed-System Catheter

OVERVIEW

Surgical procedures such as prostate resections and bladder surgery or traumatic injury may require frequent or continuous bladder irrigation. To prevent the potential introduction of infectious organisms, and as a practical matter, open bladder irrigation is not used in these cases. A closed bladder irrigation system is preferable under these circumstances. Closed bladder irrigation may be used to instill medication, encourage hemostasis, or flush clots and debris out of the catheter and bladder.

A three-way catheter is used for closed bladder irrigation. If the client will require closed irrigation following surgery, the surgeon often places the three-way catheter during the operation. If a standard indwelling catheter has been placed, a Y adapter can be used for intermittent irrigation. A three-way catheter has three ports: one for inflation of the retention balloon, one for urine drainage, and one for instilling irrigant.

As with open bladder irrigation, closed bladder irrigation is a sterile procedure. The irrigant, tubing, and drainage systems must be maintained as a closed sterile system to decrease the risk of infection. Because of the risk of blockage from clots and debris, the system must also be monitored closely for equal amounts of irrigant instilled and irrigant returned.

ASSESSMENT

1. Assess the client for bladder distention or complaints of fullness or discomfort **to assess the patency of the drainage system.**
2. Assess the drainage system for equal or larger amounts of drainage versus infused irrigant **to assess the patency of the system.**
3. Assess the color, consistency, and clarity of the bladder drainage as well as noting any clots or debris present **to assess the effectiveness of the irrigation.**

POSSIBLE NURSING DIAGNOSES

Risk for Infection
Impaired Urinary Elimination
Urinary Retention
Acute Pain

PLANNING

Expected Outcomes

1. The client will not exhibit signs or symptoms of bladder or urinary tract infection.
2. The client will not experience pain or discomfort as a result of the bladder irrigation.
3. The catheter will remain patent, and the client's bladder will not be distended.

Equipment Needed

- Three-way indwelling catheter or Y adapter
- IV pole
- Ordered irrigation solution
- Sterile gloves
- Closed-irrigation tubing
- Large urine collection bag
- Antiseptic swabs

delegation tips

This procedure cannot be delegated. Bladder irrigation using a closed-system catheter requires the skills of a nurse.

IMPLEMENTATION—ACTION/RATIONALE

ACTION	RATIONALE
* Check client's identification band * Explain procedure before beginning *	
Intermittent Bladder Irrigation Using a Standard Indwelling Catheter and a Y Adapter	
1. Wash hands.	1. Prevents spread of microorganisms.
2. Close privacy curtain or door.	2. Provides privacy.
3. Hang the prescribed irrigation solution from an IV pole.	3. Different solutions may be ordered depending on the results the health care provider desires. Bladder irrigant is generally packaged in 2,000- to 4,000-mL bottles.
4. Insert the clamped irrigation tubing into the bottle of irrigant and prime the tubing with fluid, expel all air and reclamp the tube (Figure 30-5-1).	4. Prevents introduction of air into the bladder.

(Continues)

PROCEDURE 30-5 Irrigating the Bladder Using a Closed-System Catheter (Continued)

ACTION	RATIONALE

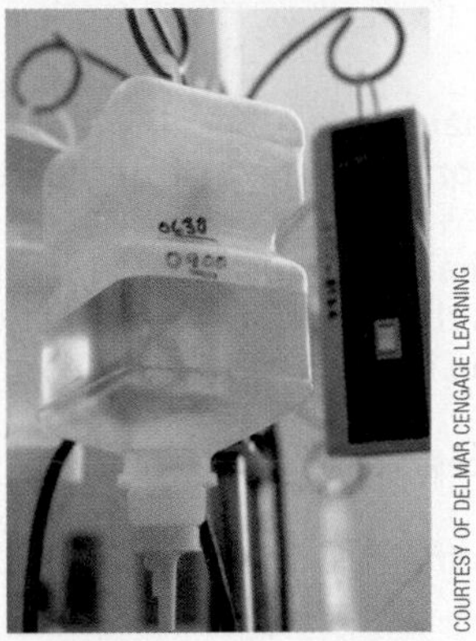

FIGURE 30-5-1 Insert the clamped irrigation tubing into the bottle of irrigant.

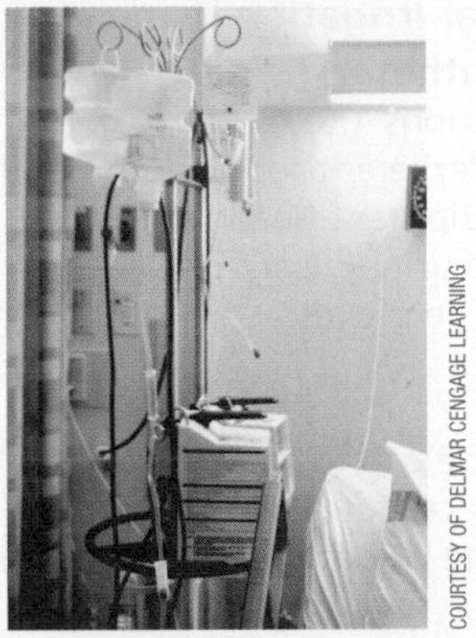

FIGURE 30-5-2 Clamp the irrigant tubing.

ACTION	RATIONALE
5. Prepare sterile antiseptic swabs and sterile Y connector if one will be used.	5. Prevents contamination of sterile gloves and field.
6. Clamp the urinary catheter.	6. Prevents urine leakage onto the bed linens.
7. Apply sterile gloves.	7. Minimizes the client's risk of infection.
8. Unhook the drainage bag from the indwelling catheter.	8. Allows the Y adapter to be inserted into the system.
9. While holding the drainage tubing and the drainage port of the catheter in your nondominant hand, cleanse both the tubing and the port with antiseptic swabs.	9. Reduces risk of contamination and infection.
10. Connect one port of the Y connector to the drainage port of the catheter.	10. Provides a bifurcation for irrigant to instill as well as urine to drain.
11. Connect another port of the Y adapter to the drainage tubing.	11. Collects the urine and drained irrigant. This may be the established urine collection bag or a new, sterile bag that is large enough to hold the increased volume of drainage.
12. Attach the third port of the Y adapter to the irrigant tubing.	12. Instills the irrigant into the closed system.
13. Unclamp the urinary catheter and establish that urine is draining through the catheter into the drainage bag.	13. If the urine does not flow freely after unclamping, the catheter may have become clogged with a clot or debris. Notify the client's health care provider of the lack of urine drainage.
14. To irrigate the catheter and bladder, clamp the drainage tubing distal to the Y adapter.	14. Prevents the irrigant from bypassing the bladder and flowing directly into the drainage bag.
15. Unclamp irrigation tubing and instill the prescribed amount of irrigant.	15. The bladder normally feels full when it contains approximately 300 mL of urine. If a prescribed amount of irrigant was not ordered, do not instill more than 150 mL of irrigant. If the client has undergone bladder surgery, do not instill irrigant without knowing the specific amount ordered.
16. Clamp the irrigant tubing (Figure 30-5-2).	16. Prevents further instillation of irrigant.
17. If the health care provider has ordered the irrigant to remain in the bladder for a measured length of time, wait the prescribed length of time.	17. Some irrigation solutions contain medication and are meant to remain in contact with the bladder wall for a prescribed length of time.
18. Unclamp the drainage tubing and monitor the drainage as it flows into the drainage bag.	18. Assess the drainage for volume, color, clarity, and the presence of any clots or debris.

(Continues)

PROCEDURE 30-5 Irrigating the Bladder Using a Closed-System Catheter (Continued)

ACTION	RATIONALE
Closed Bladder Irrigation Using a Three-Way Catheter	
19. Follow Actions 1 to 4.	19. See Rationales 1 to 4.
20. Prepare sterile antiseptic swabs and any other sterile equipment needed.	20. Prevents contamination of sterile gloves and field.
21. Clamp the urinary catheter.	21. Prevents leakage of urine onto the bedclothes.
22. Apply sterile gloves.	22. Minimizes the client's risk of infection when connecting the irrigant to the catheter and drainage system.
23. Remove the cap from the irrigation port of the three-way catheter (Figure 30-5-3).	23. Allows access for the irrigant tubing.
24. Cleanse the irrigation port with the sterile antiseptic swabs.	24. Minimizes the risk of infection.
25. Attach the irrigation tubing to the irrigation port of the three-way catheter.	25. Connects irrigant to the system.
26. Remove the clamp from the catheter and observe for urine drainage (Figure 30-5-4).	26. Ensures catheter remains patent after being clamped. Some surgical procedures can cause bleeding and clotting of the catheter.
If intermittent irrigation has been ordered:	
27. Follow Actions 15 to 16.	27. See Rationales 15 to 16.
28. If the health care provider has ordered the irrigant to remain in the bladder for a measured length of time, clamp the drainage tube before instilling the irrigant and wait the prescribed length of time.	28. Some irrigation solutions contain medication and are meant to remain in contact with the bladder wall for a prescribed length of time.
29. Monitor the drainage as it flows into the drainage bag.	29. Assesses the drainage for volume, color, clarity, and the presence of any clots or debris.
If continuous bladder irrigation has been ordered:	
30. Adjust the clamp on the irrigation tubing to allow the prescribed rate of irrigant to flow into the catheter and bladder.	30. Regulates the amount of irrigant flowing in and out of the bladder to prevent distention or damage to any surgical site.
31. Monitor the drainage for color, clarity, debris, and volume as it flows back into the drainage bag.	31. Assesses for bleeding, clotting, and blockage of urine drainage or other complications.
32. Tape the catheter securely to the thigh (Figure 30-5-5).	32. Prevents the catheter from becoming dislodged.
33. Remove gloves and wash hands.	33. Reduces transmission of microorganisms.

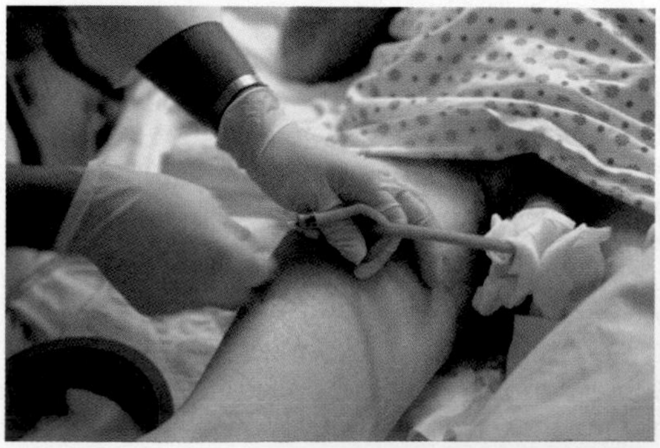

FIGURE 30-5-3 Remove the cap from the irrigation port of the three-way catheter.

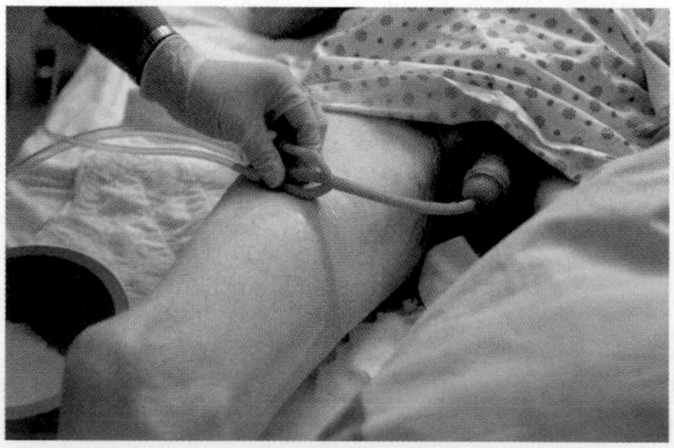

FIGURE 30-5-4 Attach the irrigation tubing, remove the clamp from the catheter, and observe for urine drainage. Carefully observe the drainage for color, clarity, and the presence of debris.

(Continues)

PROCEDURE 30-5 Irrigating the Bladder Using a Closed-System Catheter (Continued)

ACTION	RATIONALE

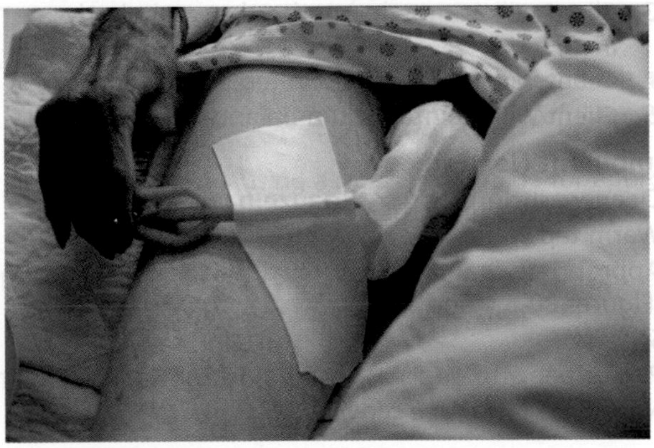

FIGURE 30-5-5 Securely tape the catheter to the thigh to prevent it from becoming dislodged.

EVALUATION

- The client does not exhibit signs or symptoms of bladder or urinary tract infection.
- The client has not experienced pain or discomfort as a result of the bladder irrigation.
- The catheter remains patent, and the client's bladder is not distended.

DOCUMENTATION

Intake and Output Record

- Amount of irrigant instilled and amount of drainage measured. Subtracting the used irrigant from the drainage total will leave the amount of the client's urine output.

Nurses' Notes

- Client's tolerance for the procedure
- Color, clarity, volume, and debris in the drainage
- Document on appropriate electronic medical record or flow sheet.

PROCEDURE 30-6 Changing a Bowel Diversion Ostomy Appliance: Pouching a Stoma

OVERVIEW

A colostomy is an opening surgically created from the ascending, transverse, or descending colon to the abdominal wall. An ileostomy is an opening from the ileum to the abdominal wall. Colostomies and ileostomies function to discharge waste (liquids, solids, and gases) to the outside of the body. Pouching a fecal diversion ensures that the client's peristomal skin remains intact and provides the client with artificial continence.

The purpose of creating ileostomies and colostomies is to improve survival and the quality of life. Anger, grief, body image disturbances, socialization disturbances, depression, and helplessness often accompany these procedures.

ASSESSMENT

1. Inspect the stoma for color and texture. **Allows the nurse to determine the viability and turgor of the stoma.**
2. Inspect the condition of the skin surrounding the stoma. **Alterations in skin integrity prohibit a closed drainage system from adhering to the skin.**
3. Measure the dimensions of the stoma before obtaining an ostomy appliance system from central supply. **Alleviates the problem of obtaining the wrong size equipment.**

(Continues)

PROCEDURE 30-6 Changing a Bowel Diversion Ostomy Appliance: Pouching a Stoma (Continued)

ACTION	RATIONALE
16. Tape the wafer edges down with hypoallergenic tape (optional).	16. Ensures that the edges of the wafer will not adhere to client's clothing.
17. Dispose of used materials, remove gloves, and wash hands.	17. Reduces transmission of microorganisms.

EVALUATION

- Peristomal skin integrity remains intact.
- Irritated or denuded peristomal skin integrity is healed.
- Client acknowledges the change in body image.
- Client expresses positive feelings about self.
- Client maintains fluid balance.

DOCUMENTATION

Nurses' Notes

- Assessment of peristomal skin
- Assessment of stoma
- Stoma measurements (length, width, height)
- Color and amount of drainage
- Peristomal skin care if alteration in skin integrity was noted
- Type of ostomy pouch applied
- Document on appropriate electronic medical record or flow sheet.

PROCEDURE 30-7 Application of Heat and Cold

OVERVIEW

Heat application is used to promote vasodilatation, increase capillary permeability, decrease blood viscosity, increase tissue metabolism, and reduce muscle tension. Moist heat can be in the form of immersion of a body part in a warmed solution or water. It can also be accomplished by wrapping body parts in dressings that are saturated with warmed solution.

Dry heat can be used to enhance circulation, promote healing, reduce swelling and inflammation, reduce pain, reduce muscle spasms, and increase systemic temperature.

Cold therapy is used to decrease blood flow to an area by promoting vasoconstriction and increased blood viscosity. These changes facilitate clotting and control bleeding. Cold decreases tissue metabolism, reduces oxygen consumption, and decreases inflammation and edema formation. Cold therapy has a local anesthetic effect by raising the threshold of pain receptors. It causes a decrease in muscle tension. Cold is used to reduce fever.

ASSESSMENT

1. Assess the area to receive heat or cold treatment for circulation. **Heat increases circulation; adequate vasculature must be present to be effective. Cold decreases circulation; adequate circulation must be present to prevent further tissue damage.**
2. Assess the skin sensation and integrity around the area to be treated. **Heat treatment cannot be used over areas of blisters, burns, or redness indicative of burning.**
3. Assess for open wounds that may be affected by the treatment. **Moist heat provides an ideal climate for the growth of microorganisms. Moist heat should be applied to open wounds only with orders from a physician or qualified practitioner.**
4. Check the client's systemic temperature. **If large areas are exposed to heat or cold, the total body temperature may be increased or decreased.**
5. Assess age. **Tolerance to heat and cold varies with individuals and is related to age, thinner layers of skin, or general sensitivity to heat and cold.**

POSSIBLE NURSING DIAGNOSES

Ineffective Tissue Perfusion
Acute Pain
Risk for Impaired Skin Integrity
Risk for Imbalanced Body Temperature
Ineffective Thermoregulation
Risk for Injury

(Continues)

PROCEDURE 30-7 Application of Heat and Cold (Continued)

PLANNING

Expected Outcomes

1. The client will derive the intended benefits of the heat or cold treatment.
2. The client will not experience any injury to skin integrity.

Equipment Needed

- Aquathermia pad
- Commercial heat or cold pack
- Solution for heat or cold treatment
- 4 × 4 gauze and waterproof pads
- Nonsterile latex-free gloves
- Sterile gloves if open wounds
- Towels
- Heat cradle
- Portable sitz bath
- Peri-care equipment
- Timer or clock

delegation tips

These procedures are routinely delegated to properly trained ancillary personnel. Reassessment of the client after application to maintain proper temperature and to evaluate the client response is essential.

IMPLEMENTATION—ACTION/RATIONALE

ACTION	RATIONALE
* Check client's identification band * Explain procedure before beginning *	
Moist Heat	
1. Check the physician's order and the reason for warm compress.	1. A physician's or nurse practitioner's order is generally required.
2. Wash hands.	2. Reduces transmission of microorganisms.
3. Assess the client's skin for areas of redness, breakdown, or scar tissue. If open wounds are involved, carefully assess the open wounds. Explain to client the reason for the compress.	3. Provides baseline information for comparison assessments. Because scar tissue may be heat sensitive or insensitive, this area should be avoided, if possible, when the compress is applied. Any open wounds should be avoided unless the treatment is specific for these areas. Client understanding of reason for compress may improve compliance.
4. Review the client's condition, medical diagnosis, and any history of diabetes mellitus or impairments in sensation.	4. Sensation is often impaired in peripheral vascular disease, diabetes, and especially in peripheral neuropathy. People with impairments in sensation may not be able to identify when the compresses are too hot. The risk of burns is greater with moist heat than with dry heat. The client's history and medical diagnosis may alert you to other problems.
5. Warm the container of sterile saline or tap water by placing it in a bath basin filled with hot tap water. Sterile saline should be warmed to 105°–113°F. If you are using a commercial compress, follow the manufacturer's directions for heating the compress.	5. Sterile saline is used to prevent any contamination of the wound. A temperature above 113°F will cause further injury.
6. Place a waterproof pad under the body area that needs the warm compress (Figure 30-7-1).	6. Protects the client's bed and clothing.
7. Pour the sterile saline into the sterile basin. Soak an appropriate-size piece of gauze or a towel, wring out the excess saline, and place it on the affected area (Figure 30-7-2). Wear gloves if there is any drainage of the client's body fluids. Wear sterile gloves if there is an open wound.	7. A sterile basin is used to prevent further contamination. Excess saline may increase the chance of burns.

(Continues)

PROCEDURE 30-7 Application of Heat and Cold (Continued)

ACTION | **RATIONALE**

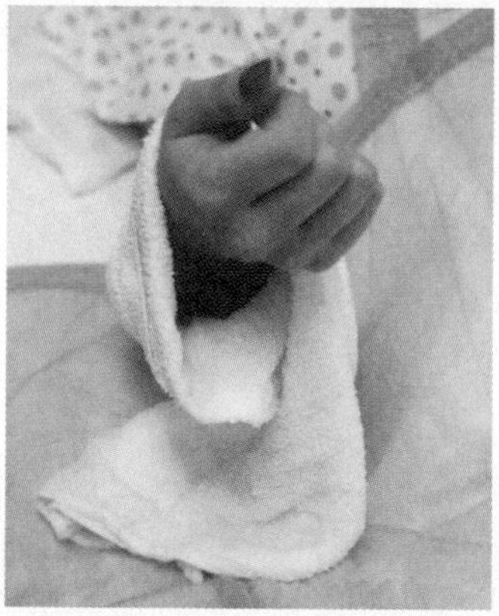

FIGURE 30-7-1 Place a waterproof pad under the body area to protect the client's bed and clothing.

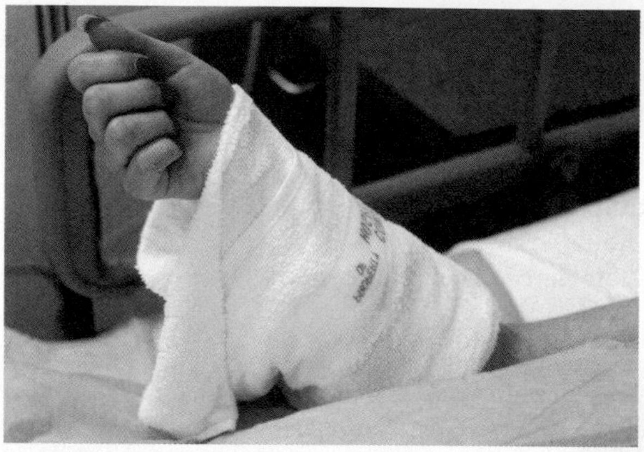

FIGURE 30-7-2 Place the moist towel on the area being treated.

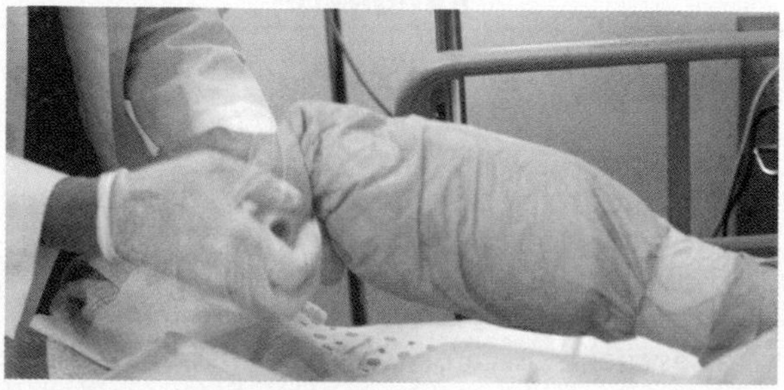

FIGURE 30-7-3 Wrap the hot, moist towel with a waterproof pad and secure the pad.

ACTION	RATIONALE
8. Wrap the area with a waterproof pad or apply a disposable heat or Aquathermia pad (Figure 30-7-3).	8. Maintains or holds in the heat.
9. Check the client's skin periodically for signs of heat intolerance. Tell the client to report any signs of discomfort immediately.	9. Signs of intolerance may include redness or further swelling.
10. If it is tolerated, leave the compress in place for approximately 20 minutes and then remove it.	10. Application of moist heat for a longer period of time may damage the client's skin and predispose the client to edema formation from circulatory congestion.
11. Dry the affected area with sterile towels if there is an open wound and with clean towels if there is no open wound.	11. The client may feel chilled when the warm compress is removed. Dry the area completely to prevent chilling.
12. Properly dispose of all single-use equipment according to hospital protocol.	12. Proper disposal of all other equipment reduces transmission of microorganisms.
13. Remove gloves, if they were worn, and wash hands.	13. Reduces transmission of microorganisms.
14. Reassess the condition of the client's skin.	14. The condition of the client's skin and any signs of heat sensitivity should be assessed and documented.

(Continues)

PROCEDURE 30-7 Application of Heat and Cold (Continued)

ACTION	RATIONALE
15. Record the procedure: condition of the client's skin and length of time of moist heat application. Report any abnormal findings to the physician.	15. Communicates procedure and findings to other members of the health care team and legally documents the care provided.
Sitz Bath	
16. Wash hands and assemble equipment (Figure 30-7-4).	16. Reduces transmission of microorganisms and organizes time.
17. Run tap water to preferred temperature (between 100°F and 110°F). Have client test the temperature on the dorsal surface of the wrist.	17. Prevents burn injury.
18. For toilet insert model, raise the seat of the toilet. Set the basin on the rim of the toilet bowel. Fill water bag and prime tubing. Close the clamp. Hang the water bag above the toilet. Thread the tubing through the front of the basin. Secure the tubing in the notch in the bottom of the basin.	18. Basin will rest on the bowl. Water bag will create a gentle swirling of water. The higher the bag, the more forceful the flow and the faster the water will run out.
19. For stand-alone model, fill basin with water (Figure 30-7-5).	19. Allows client to sit in the water.
20. Pad the seat with a towel (Figure 30-7-6).	20. Provides client comfort.
21. Always use Standard Precautions when assisting with perineal care treatments. Have client remove and dispose of peri-pad in a biohazard receptacle.	21. Prevents infection. Dressings that contain blood are disposed of in a biohazard container to prevent the spread of microorganisms.

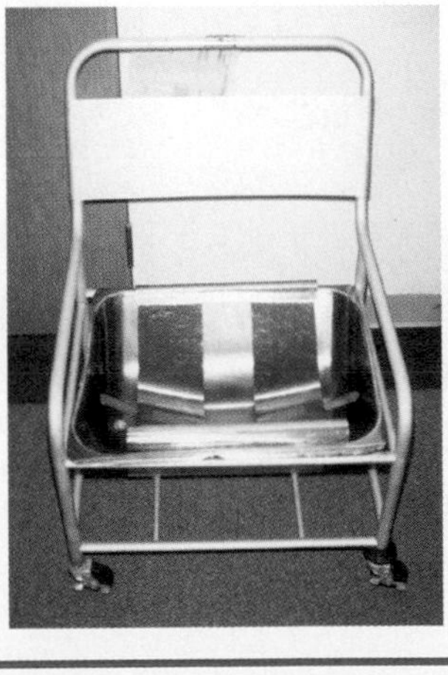

COURTESY OF DELMAR CENGAGE LEARNING

FIGURE 30-7-4 Portable Sitz Bath

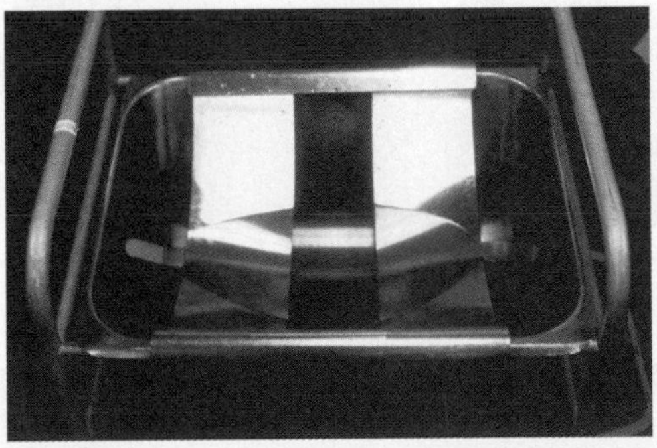

COURTESY OF DELMAR CENGAGE LEARNING

FIGURE 30-7-5 Fill the sitz bath basin with warm water.

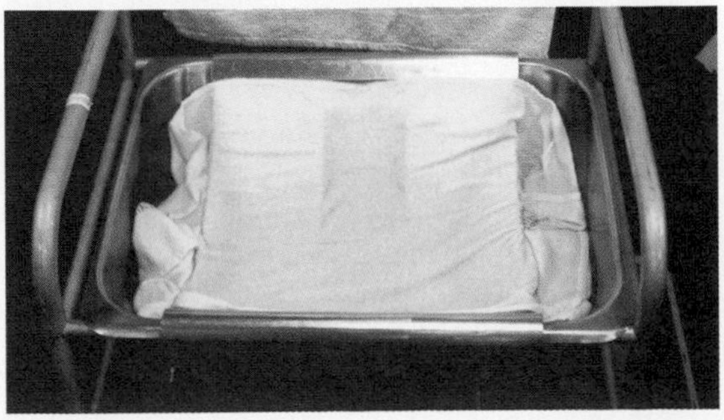

COURTESY OF DELMAR CENGAGE LEARNING

FIGURE 30-7-6 Pad the seat of the sitz bath with a towel for comfort.

(Continues)

PROCEDURE 30-7 Application of Heat and Cold (Continued)

ACTION	RATIONALE
22. Ensure that the floor is dry. Assist client to the bathroom if necessary.	22. Prevents injury from falling.
23. Have client sit in the basin (Figure 30-7-7). For toilet insert model, demonstrate how to unclamp the tubing to start the water flow.	23. Water flow is soothing and helps cleanse the area.
24. Cover client's lap for warmth and modesty (Figure 30-7-8).	24. Provides client comfort and privacy.
25. Ensure that the client can reach the call button. Instruct the client to call before standing up.	25. Water may splash over the floor, creating a slipping hazard.
26. After 20 minutes (or sooner if client is finished), help the client dry the area by gently patting with clean towels.	26. Warm soaks should last no longer than 20 minutes to prevent rebound vasoconstriction.
27. Assist client to bed. Encourage client to lie flat or elevate hips for 20 minutes.	27. Prevents congestion and decreases swelling.
28. For toilet insert model, empty remaining water into toilet. Rinse basin and bag. Clean according to institutional policy. For stand-alone model, empty water from drain trap into basin (Figure 30-7-9). Clean according to institutional policy.	28. Prepares equipment for the next use.

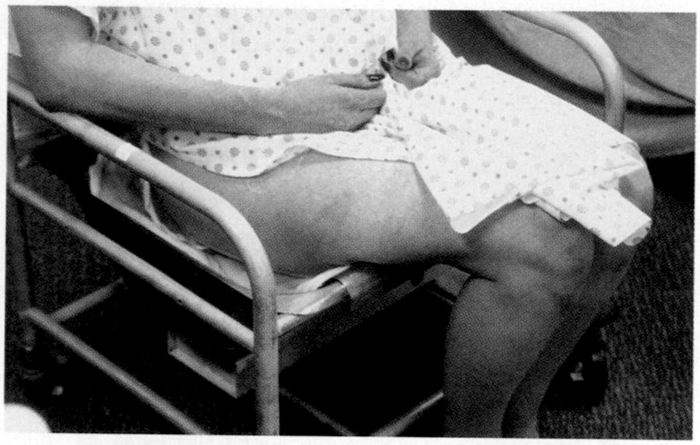
COURTESY OF DELMAR CENGAGE LEARNING

FIGURE 30-7-7 Have the client sit in the basin.

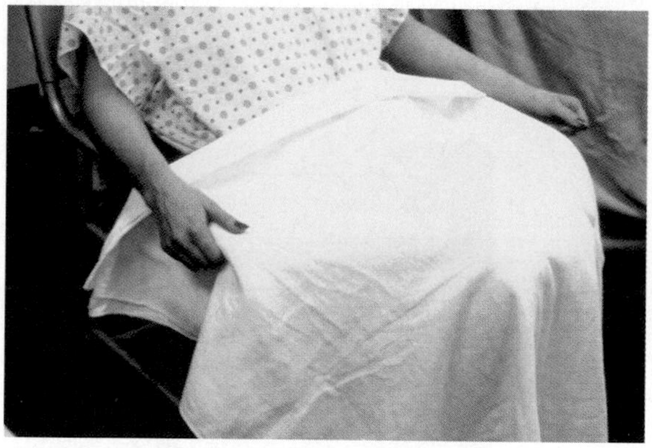
COURTESY OF DELMAR CENGAGE LEARNING

FIGURE 30-7-8 Cover the client's lap with a blanket or towel for modesty.

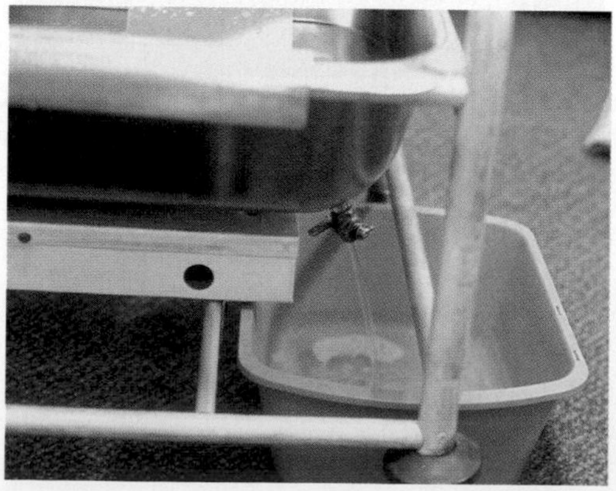
COURTESY OF DELMAR CENGAGE LEARNING

FIGURE 30-7-9 Empty water from drain tap into a basin for disposal.

Dry Heat

ACTION	RATIONALE
29. Check the physician's or qualified practitioner's order and the purpose of the heat treatment.	29. An order is required. Because there are many purposes of heat treatment, it is helpful to know what outcomes are expected and the site/sites to be treated.

(Continues)

PROCEDURE 30-7 Application of Heat and Cold (Continued)

ACTION	RATIONALE
30. Determine if there are any underlying problems that may affect the use of heat treatment, such as decreased sensation; decreased mentation; or a history of diabetes mellitus, bleeding disorders, peripheral vascular disease, or peripheral neuropathy. Heat should not be used over areas of scarring.	30. If the client has decreased sensation or mental status, heat treatment should be used only if the client can be observed closely. Heat should not be applied over areas where the client cannot alert the nurse about the sensation of burning.
31. Wash hands.	31. Reduces transmission of microorganisms.
32. Check the skin for lotions or ointments and remove if present.	32. Lotions and ointments retain heat and can lead to an increased risk of burning.
33. Gather equipment and complete as follows:	33.
For a disposable heat pack:	
• Activate the pack according to the manufacturer's directions. Some packs must be heated in boiling water, others can be heated by microwave, and some require bending and chemical activation (Figure 30-7-10).	• Manufacturer's directions should be followed because activation differs. If a microwave is used to heat a pack that should be heated in boiling water, the bag might break.
• Wrap the pack in a towel or protective covering (some manufacturers include cover). Do not use pins. Use tape if needed to secure the towel.	• A barrier between the client's skin and the heat source is necessary to avoid burns.
• Discard after use.	• Chemically activated packs will not reactivate once activated. In medical facilities, gel packs cannot be reheated in common areas without causing the transmission of microorganisms. In the home setting, packs activated by boiling or the microwave can be used on the same client again.
For an Aquathermia pad:	
• Follow manufacturer's directions.	• There are various brands of Aquathermia pads and each one may have slight differences in operating instructions.
• Fill the control unit with distilled water or as indicated by manufacturer's directions.	• Distilled water prevents the accumulation of mineral deposits that will damage equipment.
• Check the control unit and tubing for leaks. Turn on the unit and check the temperature of the water with a thermometer after several minutes. The proper temperature of the water is 105°F. Some units require that the control unit is level with the pad to function because overcoming gravity can put undue strain on the motor (Figure 30-7-11).	• This will ensure that the control unit is properly functioning. If there is a leak in the tubing, another pad should be obtained because this presents an electrical danger to the client and the staff.
34. Wash hands.	34. Reduces transmission of microorganisms.

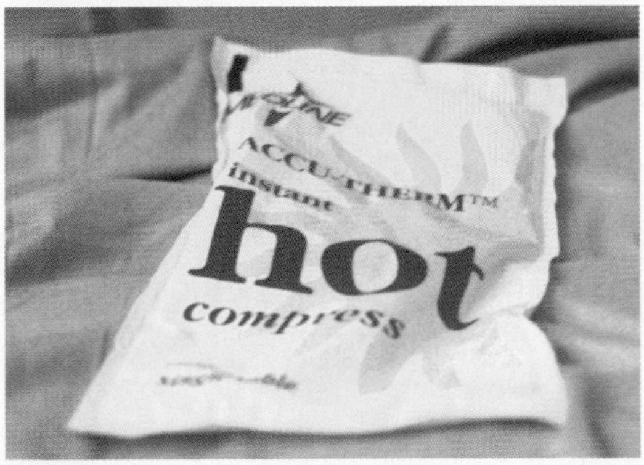

COURTESY OF DELMAR CENGAGE LEARNING

FIGURE 30-7-10 Disposable Hot Pack

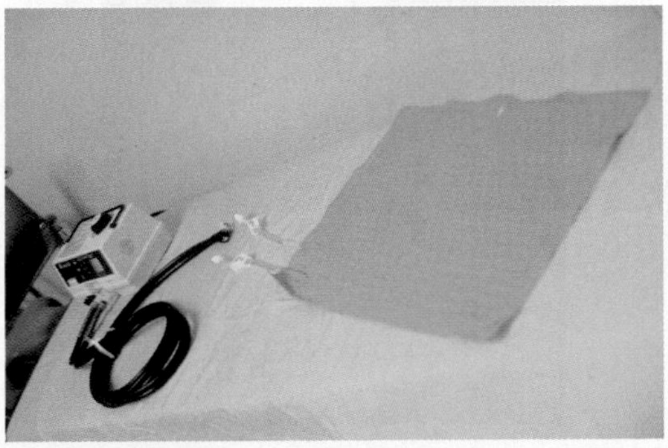

COURTESY OF DELMAR CENGAGE LEARNING

FIGURE 30-7-11 Aquathermia Pad

(Continues)

PROCEDURE 30-7 Application of Heat and Cold (Continued)

ACTION	RATIONALE
Application of Cold	
35. Wash hands.	35. Reduces transmission of microorganisms.
36. Assess the client's sensation and skin color at the site of planned application. Determine if any tissue damage is present. Assess for bleeding or wound drainage (Figure 30-7-12).	36. Provides baseline data for post-treatment comparison.
37. Identify whether the client has a history of circulatory impairment or neuropathy (Figure 30-7-13).	37. Cold causes vasoconstriction and decreased metabolism and can cause tissue damage in people with impaired circulation and sensation.
38. Check the physician's or qualified practitioner's order and the reason for the application of cold.	38. A physician's or qualified practitioner's order is needed in most situations of cold treatment. The reason for application of cold should be taught to the client.
39. If using an ice bag with moist gauze or towels, fill the bag three-fourths full with ice and remove the remaining air from the bag. Close the bag. Check for leaks. Wrap the bag in a towel or protective cover and place it on the affected area. If cold soaks are being applied, use the appropriate-size basin for the body part to be soaked.	39. If air is removed from the bag, the bag will be easier to mold to the client's body. The bag is wrapped to prevent injury to the client's skin or exposed tissue because direct cold can cause damage.
40. If an ice collar is used, fill the collar three-fourths full with ice and remove the remaining air from the collar before closing the collar. Check for leaks. Place the collar in a protective cover and around the client's neck.	40. Easier to mold to the client's body. The collar is wrapped to prevent injury to the client's skin.

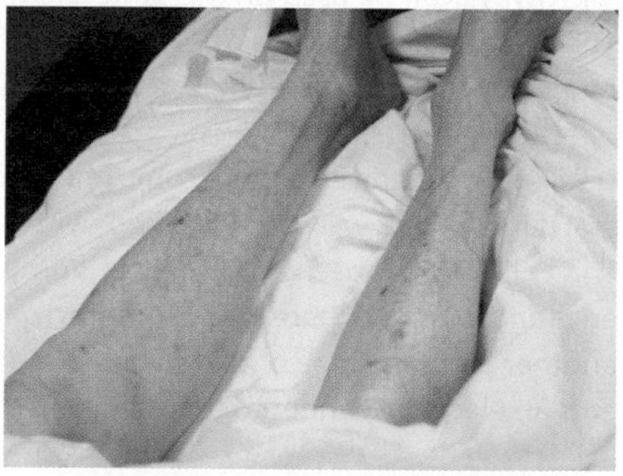

FIGURE 30-7-12 Assess the skin at the site of planned cold application for color, sensation, wounds, or skin irritation.

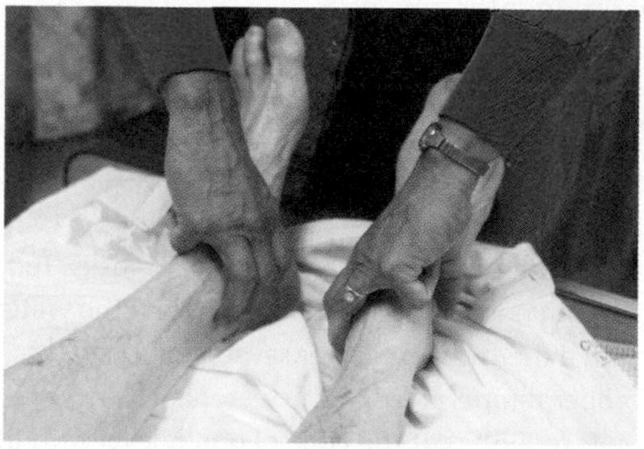

FIGURE 30-7-13 Assess for circulatory or neuropathy before beginning the procedure.

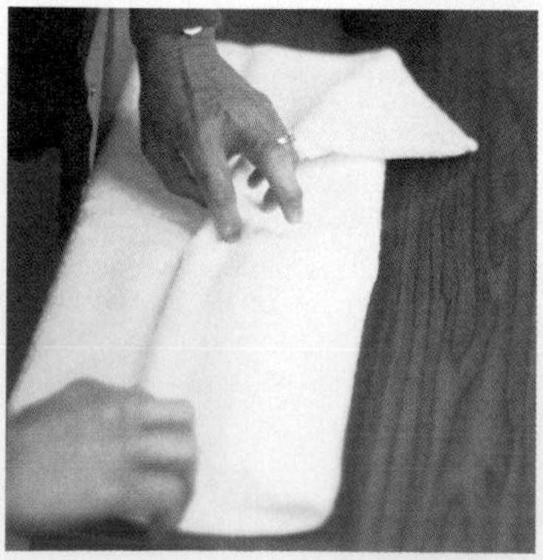

FIGURE 30-7-14 Wrap the cold pack in a towel.

(Continues)

PROCEDURE 30-7 Application of Heat and Cold (Continued)

ACTION	RATIONALE
41. If a disposable cold pack is used, activate the pack according to the manufacturer's directions, wrap the pack in a towel (Figure 30-7-14), and place it on the affected area (Figure 30-7-15). Some packs come with covers. Secure the pack in place with tape, elastic wrap, or bandage (Figures 30-7-16, 30-7-17, and 30-7-18). Dispose of the pack after the treatment.	41. When the pack is squeezed or kneaded, an alcohol-based solution is released, creating the cold temperature. The pack cannot be used again.
42. Assess the client's skin periodically for signs of cold intolerance or tissue damage.	42. Signs of intolerance to cold are pallor, blanching, mottling, or numbness of the skin.
43. If the client can tolerate the cold, leave the cold application in place for approximately 20 minutes at approximately 15°C (59°F).	43. Longer application can cause tissue damage, especially because the client's pain sensation is decreased in the presence of cold. A reflex vasodilation occurs after 20 minutes, thereby negating the therapeutic effect of the cold treatment.
44. Dispose of equipment according to agency policy.	44. Reduces transmission of microorganisms.
45. Reassess the condition of the client's skin or exposed tissue.	45. The client's skin should be assessed, and any signs of cold changes and intolerance should be documented.
46. Wash hands.	46. Reduces transmission of microorganisms.

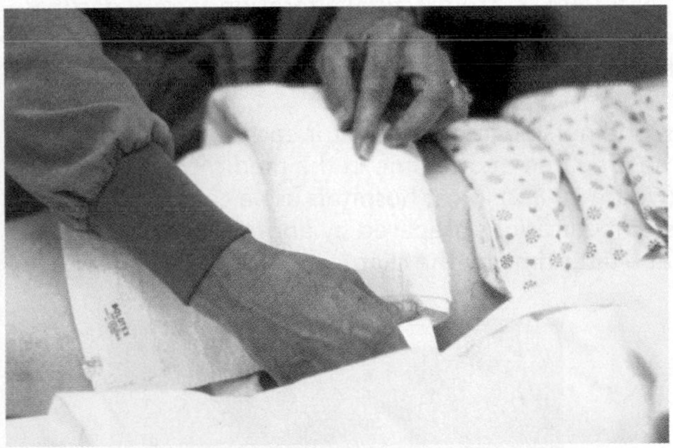

COURTESY OF DELMAR CENGAGE LEARNING

FIGURE 30-7-15 Place the cold pack on the affected body area.

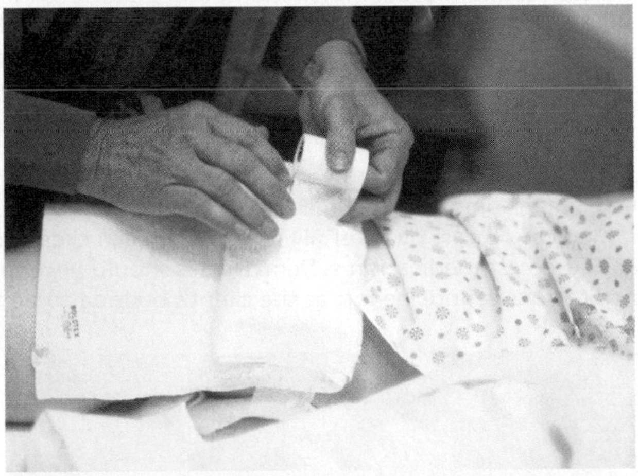

COURTESY OF DELMAR CENGAGE LEARNING

FIGURE 30-7-16 Secure the cold pack to the area with tape.

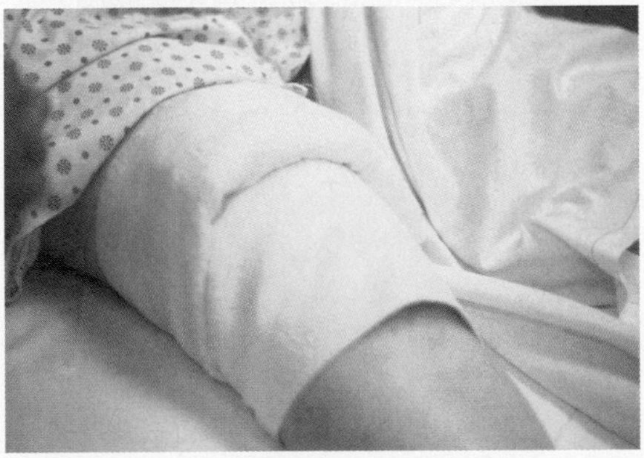

COURTESY OF DELMAR CENGAGE LEARNING

FIGURE 30-7-17 Cold pack properly wrapped in a towel and secured with tape.

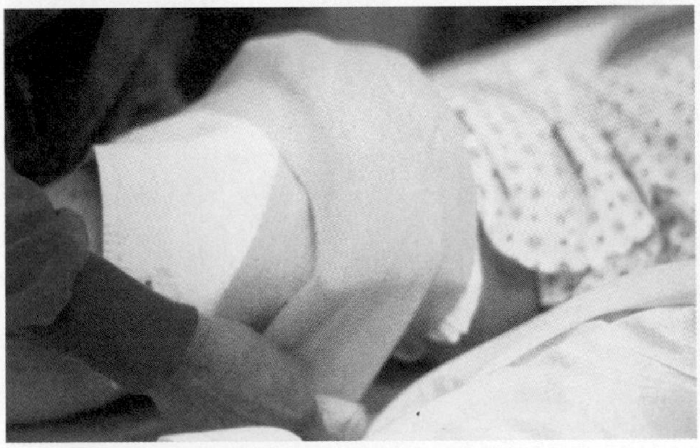

COURTESY OF DELMAR CENGAGE LEARNING

FIGURE 30-7-18 Elastic wrap may be used to hold bulky cold wraps in place.

(Continues)

PROCEDURE 30-7 Application of Heat and Cold (Continued)

EVALUATION

- The client derived the intended benefits of the heat or cold treatment.
- The client had no injury to skin integrity.

DOCUMENTATION

Nurses' Notes

- Document the procedure and the client's response to the procedure
- Record the equipment used
- Record the length of time of application
- Record the client's skin condition after the procedure

PROCEDURE 30-8 Administering Oral, Sublingual, and Buccal Medications

OVERVIEW

The easiest and most common method of administering a medication is usually by mouth (Figure 30-8-1). Clients may be taught to administer the medication by themselves at home, or a nurse can prepare the medications and dispense to clients. Oral medications are contraindicated for clients with gastrointestinal alterations, using nasogastric tube or gastrostomy tube, or who have a poor gag reflex. Clients with an inability to swallow because of neuromuscular disorder, esophageal stricture, or lesion of the mouth or those who are unresponsive or comatose are also ineligible to receive oral administration of medication.

Nurses need to know the action, normal dosage, side effects, and nursing implications for each drug they administer. In some settings, medications for several clients may be prepared at one time in the medication room or medication cart by carefully identifying each client's doses (Figure 30-8-2). Most hospitals use a computerized, limited-access medication system. Nurses should never administer medications prepared by another individual, and medications cannot be left at the client's bedside to be taken at a later time by the client.

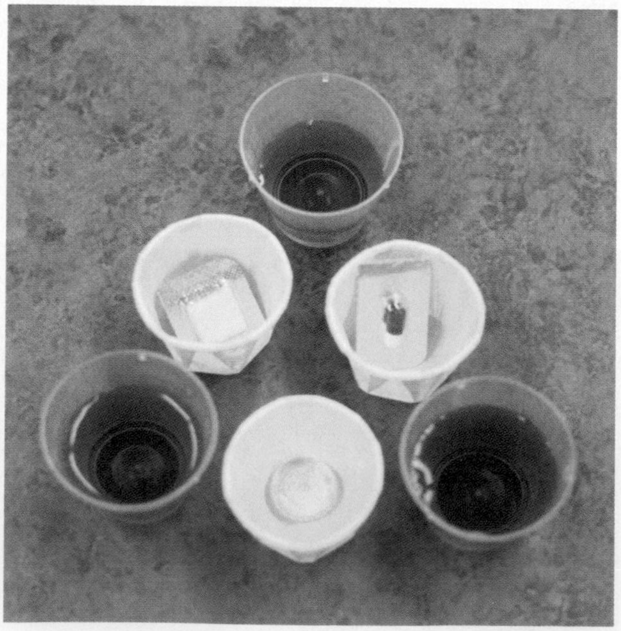

FIGURE 30-8-1 Oral, Sublingual, and Buccal Medications

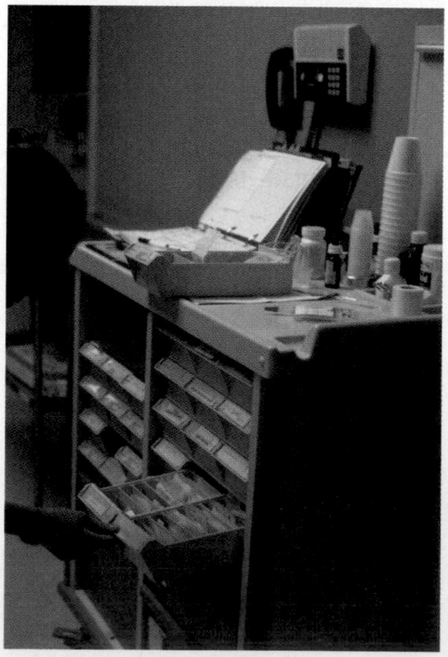

FIGURE 30-8-2 In some settings, medications for several clients are prepared at the medication cart at the same time.

(Continues)

PROCEDURE 30-8 Administering Oral, Sublingual, and Buccal Medications (Continued)

ASSESSMENT

1. Assess the seven rights: right client, right medication, right route, right dose, right time, right to refuse, and right documentation. **Prevents errors in medication administration.**
2. Review the action, purpose, normal dosage and route, common side effects, time of onset and peak action, and nursing implications of each drug **so the client's response to the medication may be monitored.**
3. Assess the client's condition to be sure the order of the health care provider is appropriate **because the client's condition may have changed since the order was written.**
4. Assess the client's ability to swallow food and fluid **because an alternate route for medication may be needed if unable to swallow a pill.**
5. Assess for any contraindications for administering an oral medication such as nausea and vomiting, gastric suction, or gastric surgery resulting in decreased peristalsis **because alterations in gastrointestinal function may interfere with drug absorption and excretion.**
6. Assess the client's medical record for a history of allergies to food or medications **so these medications can be avoided.**
7. Assess the client's knowledge about the use of medications **so client teaching can be tailored to client's needs. This may also assess compliance for taking the drugs at home or reveal drug dependence or abuse.**
8. Assess the client's age **because pediatric or geriatric clients may have special needs according to their ability to swallow a pill.**
9. Assess the client's need for fluids **because swallowing a pill is usually easier with fluid and promotes fluid intake; however, fluid restrictions are sometimes necessary.**
10. Assess the client's ability to sit or turn to the side. **The client must be able to swallow the pill without aspiration.**

POSSIBLE NURSING DIAGNOSES

Noncompliance
Impaired Swallowing
Deficient Knowledge (medication regimen)

PLANNING

Expected Outcomes

1. The client will swallow the prescribed medication.
2. The client will be able to explain the purpose and schedule for taking the medication.
3. The client will have no gastrointestinal discomfort or alterations in function.
4. The client will show the desired response to the medication such as pain relief, regular heart rate, or stable blood pressure.
5. The client will not have an allergic reaction.

Equipment Needed

- Health care provider's order for the medication
- Medication administration record (MAR)
- Medication cart or dispensing computer
- Medication tray
- Disposable medication cups
- Glass of water, juice, or other liquid
- Drinking straw
- Mortar and pestle, if needed
- Pill-cutting device, if needed
- Paper towels

delegation tips

The procedure of medication administration and assessment of effects is not delegated to ancillary personnel in acute care settings. This may vary in state or federal institutions. Ancillary personnel are generally informed about the medications the client is receiving if adverse effects are anticipated or are being monitored.

IMPLEMENTATION—ACTION/RATIONALE

ACTION	RATIONALE
1. Wash hands.	1. Reduces the number of microorganisms.
2. Arrange the medication tray and cups in the medication room or on the medication cart outside the client's room. Most hospitals use a computerized limited-access medication cart. Follow institutional protocol.	2. Organizing medications and equipment saves time and reduces the possibility of error.

(Continues)

PROCEDURE 30-8 Administering Oral, Sublingual, and Buccal Medications (Continued)

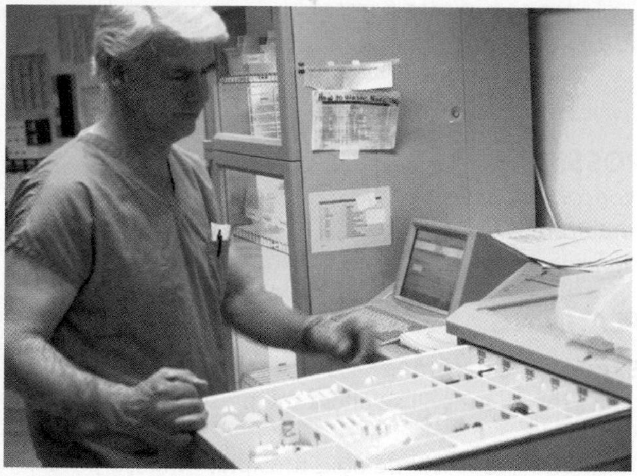

FIGURE 30-8-3 Prepare oral medication following the five rights: right client, time, medication, dose, and route.

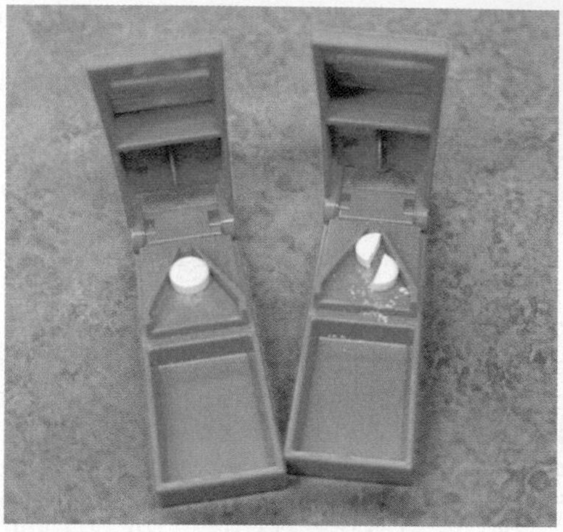

FIGURE 30-8-4 Scored tablets may be broken, if necessary.

ACTION	RATIONALE
3. Unlock the medication cart or log on to the computer.	3. Medications need to be safeguarded.
4. Prepare the medication for one client at a time following the first five rights. Select the correct drug from the medication drawer according to the MAR (Figure 30-8-3). Calculate the drug dosage if needed.	4. The first five rights are right client, right time, right medication, right dose, and right route. Comparing the MAR with the label reduces error. Double-checking reduces error in calculation.
5. To prepare a tablet or capsule: Pour the required number of tablets or capsules into the bottle cap and transfer the medication to a medication cup without touching them.	5. Avoids wasting expensive medications and avoids contamination of medication.
• Scored tablets may be broken, if necessary, using gloved hands or with a pill-cutting device (Figure 30-8-4).	• Tablets that are not scored are not meant to be broken. The medication's effectiveness would be diminished if the tablet were broken or crushed.
• A unit-dose tablet should be placed directly into the medicine cup *without* opening it until it is administered to the client.	• The wrapper maintains cleanliness and identification until it is administered.
• For clients with difficulty in swallowing, some tablets may be crushed into a powder using a mortar and pestle or by being placed between two paper medication cups and ground with a blunt object, then mixed in a small amount of applesauce. *Time-released or specially coated medications must not be crushed.* Check with the pharmacy if you are uncertain (Figure 30-8-5).	• A large tablet is usually easier to swallow if it is ground and mixed with soft food.
6. To prepare a liquid medication: Remove the bottle cap from the container and place cap upside down on the cart. Hold the bottle with the label up and place the medication cup at eye level on a level surface while pouring (Figure 30-8-6). Fill the cup to the desired level using the surface or base of the meniscus as the scale, not the edge of the liquid on the cup. Wipe lip of bottle with paper towel.	6. Placing the bottle cap upside down on the cart prevents contamination of the inside of the container. Holding the bottle with the label up keeps spilled liquid from obliterating the label. Holding the medication cup at eye level ensures an accurate dose. Wiping the lip of the bottle prevents the bottle cap from sticking.

(Continues)

PROCEDURE 30-8 Administering Oral, Sublingual, and Buccal Medications (Continued)

ACTION	RATIONALE

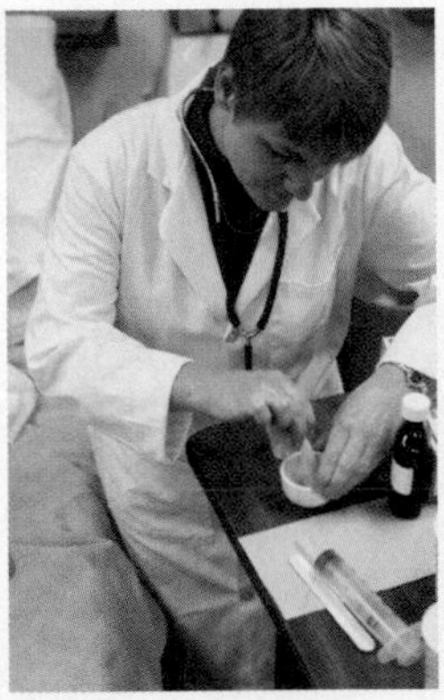

COURTESY OF DELMAR CENGAGE LEARNING

FIGURE 30-8-5 Some medications may be crushed and mixed with a soft food, such as applesauce, for clients who have difficulty in swallowing.

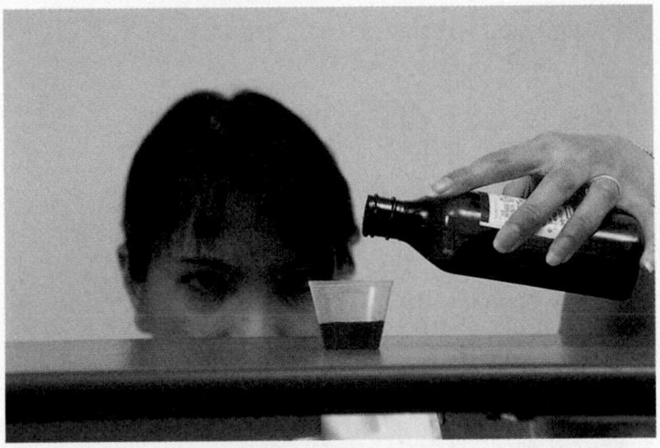

COURTESY OF DELMAR CENGAGE LEARNING

FIGURE 30-8-6 Measure liquid medications at eye level on a level surface.

ACTION	RATIONALE
7. To prepare a narcotic, obtain the key to the narcotic drawer and check the narcotic record for the drug count when signing out the dose. If the drug count does not agree with records, report to charge nurse immediately.	7. Controlled substance laws require records of each dose dispensed. Early identification of errors assists in corrective action. Facility may require an incident report be filed.
8. Check expiration date on all medications.	8. Expired medications may lose their effectiveness.
• Double-check the MAR with the prepared drugs.	• Reduces risk of error.
• Return stock medications to their shelf or drawer.	• Ensures safety of stock medications.
• Place MARs with the client's medications.	• Ensures identification of medications.
• Do not leave drugs unattended.	• Drugs are safeguarded by nurse.
9. Administer medications to client: Observe the correct time to give the medication.	9. Ensures the therapeutic effect of the drug when given within 30 minutes of the prescribed time. (*Right time.*)
• Identify the client using two identifiers by reading the client's name bracelet, repeating the name, and/or asking the client to state his or her name (Figure 30-8-7). Additionally, check the hospital number if name alert or client is not reliable.	• Identification bracelets made at the time of admission are the most reliable source of identification even if the client is unable to state his or her name. (*Right client.*)
• Check the drug packaging if it is present to ensure the medication type and dosage.	• Prevents giving the wrong medication or wrong dose. (*Right medication, right dose.*)
• Assess the client's condition and the form of the medication.	• Allows you to assess the route of the medication and if this route is appropriate. (*Right route.*)
• Perform any assessment required for specific medications such as a pulse or blood pressure.	• Determines whether the medication should be given at that time or not.
• Explain the purpose of the drug and ask if the client has any questions, assessing the client's sixth right to refuse the medications.	• Improves compliance with drug therapy.
• Assist the client to a sitting or lateral position.	• Prevents aspiration during swallowing.
• Allow client to hold the tablet or medication cup.	• Client becomes familiar with medications.
• Give a glass of water or other liquid, and straw if needed, to help the client swallow the medication (Figure 30-8-8).	• Promotes client comfort in swallowing and can improve fluid intake.
• For *sublingual* medications, instruct client to place medication under the tongue and allow it to dissolve completely.	• Drug is absorbed through the mucous membranes into the blood vessels. If swallowed, the drug may be destroyed by gastric juices or detoxified in the liver too quickly so that its intended effects will not occur.

(Continues)

PROCEDURE 30-8 Administering Oral, Sublingual, and Buccal Medications (Continued)

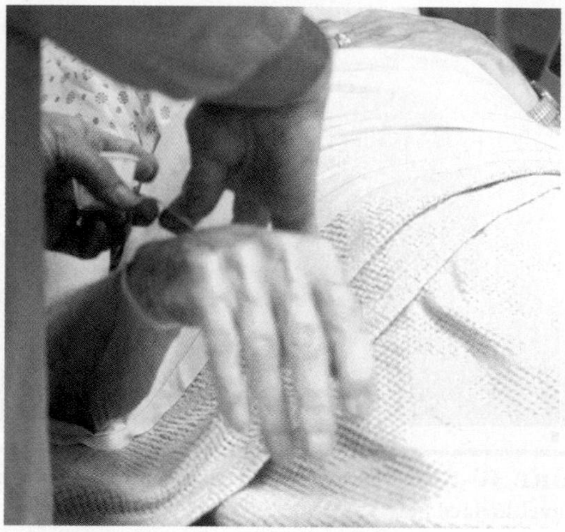

FIGURE 30-8-7 Identify the client using two identifiers by reading the client's name bracelet and asking his or her name before administering medication.

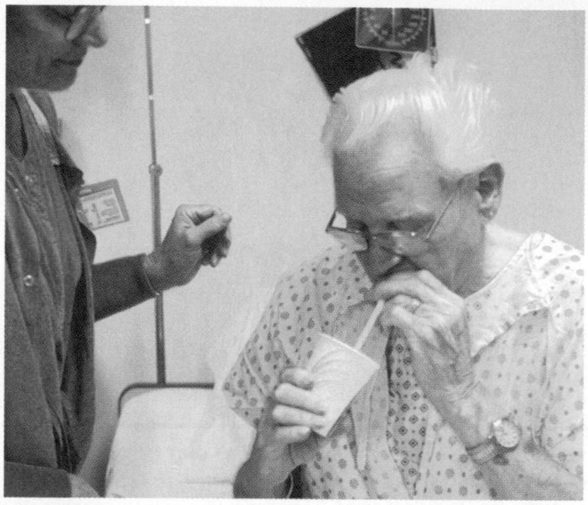

FIGURE 30-8-8 Allow the client to hold the tablet, and give water or juice to help him swallow the medication.

ACTION	RATIONALE
• For *buccal* administration of drugs, instruct the client to place the medication in the mouth against the cheek until it dissolves completely.	• Promotes local activity on mucous membranes.
• For oral medications given through a *nasogastric tube*, crush tablets or open capsules and dissolve powder with 20 to 30 mL of warm water in a cup. Be sure medication will still be properly absorbed if crushed and dissolved. Check placement of the feeding tube or nasogastric tube before instilling anything but air into the tube.	• Allows medication administration via nasogastric or feeding tube. Ensures that the medication is absorbed and utilized correctly.
• Remain with the client until each medication has been swallowed or dissolved.	• Ensures that the client receives the dose and does not save it or discard it.
• Assist the client into a comfortable position.	• Maintains client's comfort.
10. Dispose of soiled supplies and wash hands.	10. Reduces transmission of microorganisms.
11. Document (seventh right) the time and route of medication administration on the MAR and return it to the client's file.	11. Prevents administration error.
12. Return the cart to the medicine room; restock the supplies as needed. Clean the work area.	12. Assists other staff in completing duties efficiently.

EVALUATION

- Evaluate the client's response to the drug within 30 minutes of administration or sooner if an allergic reaction is anticipated.
- Ask client or caregiver to discuss the purpose, action, dosage schedule, and side effects of the drug.

DOCUMENTATION

Medication Administration Record

- Date and time each drug was administered, including initials and signature
- If drug is withheld, circle the time the drug was scheduled on the MAR.
- Document on appropriate electronic medical record or flow sheet.

Nurses' Notes

Document:

- Date, time, and reason a drug was withheld
- Response to drug administered

PROCEDURE 30-9 Withdrawing Medication from an Ampule

OVERVIEW

Ampules are containers that hold a single dose of medication. The ampules are made of clear glass and have a distinctive shape with a constricted neck. The head of the ampule is broken off at the neck, and the medication is withdrawn with a filter needle and syringe (Figure 30-9-1).

The neck of the ampule is often colored and usually scored. This scoring allows the neck to be broken off easily from the body to obtain the medication. Place a sterile piece of gauze around the neck of the ampule and break the neck in an outward motion. The gauze protects the nurse's fingers from the glass.

Medication can become trapped in the uppermost portion of the ampule. Before opening the ampule, flick the upper portion of the ampule with a fingernail to drop the medication from the upper segment down into the body of the ampule. This step may need to be repeated several times.

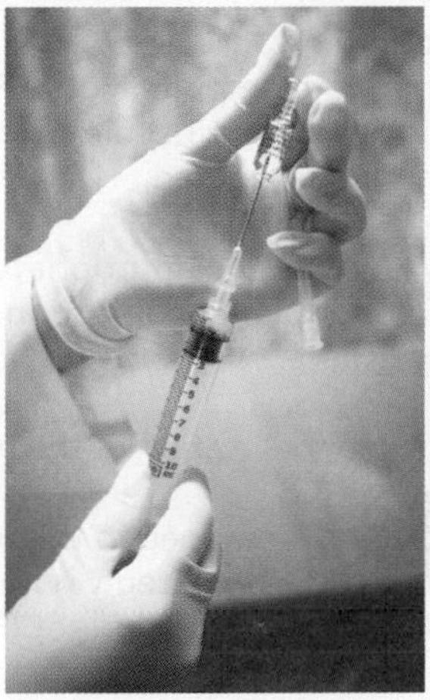

FIGURE 30-9-1 Withdrawing medication from an ampule.

ASSESSMENT

1. Identify the correct ampule, including medication, dosage strength, dosage volume, dosage route, and expiration date **to avoid medication errors.**
2. Assess the syringe, filter needle, and injection needle for expiration date and package intactness **to evaluate the sterility of the equipment.**
3. Assess the fluid in the ampule for cloudiness, particulate matter, or color changes **to evaluate for usability of the medication.**
4. Identify the medication's intended action, purpose, normal dosage range, time of action, common side effects, and nursing implications **to avoid medication errors.**

POSSIBLE NURSING DIAGNOSES

Risk for Impaired Skin Integrity
Risk for Infection

PLANNING

Expected Outcomes

1. The correct medication ampule will be selected.
2. The medication will be drawn into an appropriate syringe.
3. Microorganisms will not be introduced into the sterile system.
4. Foreign objects will not be introduced into the sterile system.

Equipment Needed (Figure 30-9-2)

- Medication ampule
- Sterile gauze pad or alcohol pad
- Syringe with filter needle
- Replacement needle
- Clean work space
- Medication administration record (MAR)

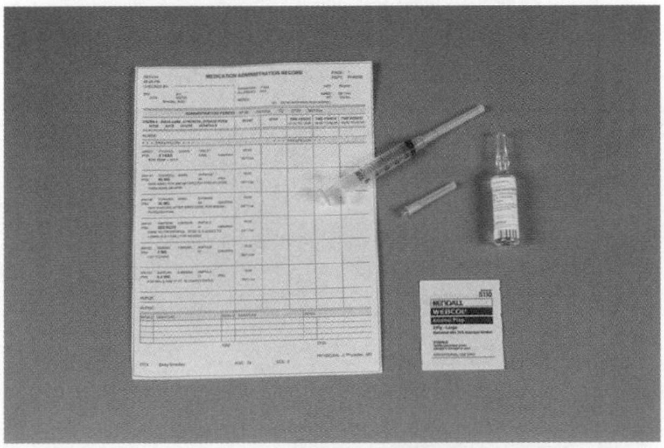

FIGURE 30-9-2 Syringes, needles, medication ampules, and alcohol wipes are used to withdraw medication from an ampule.

delegation tips

The procedure of medication administration is not delegated to ancillary personnel in acute care settings. This may vary in state or federal institutions. Ancillary personnel are generally informed about the medications the client is receiving if adverse effects are anticipated or are being monitored.

(Continues)

PROCEDURE 30-9 Withdrawing Medication from an Ampule (Continued)

IMPLEMENTATION—ACTION/RATIONALE

ACTION	RATIONALE
1. Wash hands.	1. Decreases transmission of microorganisms.
2. Select appropriate ampule (Figure 30-9-3).	2. Ensures client receives correct medication.
3. Select syringe with filter needle (Figure 30-9-4).	3. Filter needle entraps any glass fragments.
4. Obtain a sterile gauze pad.	4. Using a gauze pad prevents cuts on the jagged edge of the broken ampule.
5. Select and set aside the appropriate length of safety needle for planned injection.	5. Accurate needle length ensures the medication is administered where it is intended.
6. Clear a work space.	6. Prevents contamination with microdroplets that may spill when the ampule is broken.
7. Observe ampule for location of the medication.	7. The medication frequently becomes trapped in the top of the ampule.
8. If the medication is trapped in the top, flick the neck of the ampule repeatedly with your fingernail while holding the ampule upright (Figure 30-9-5).	8. Flicking the neck and top of the ampule moves the medication into the body of the ampule.

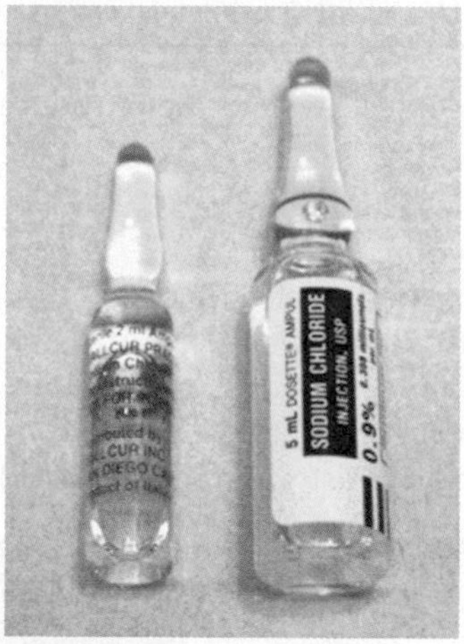

FIGURE 30-9-3 Medication Ampules

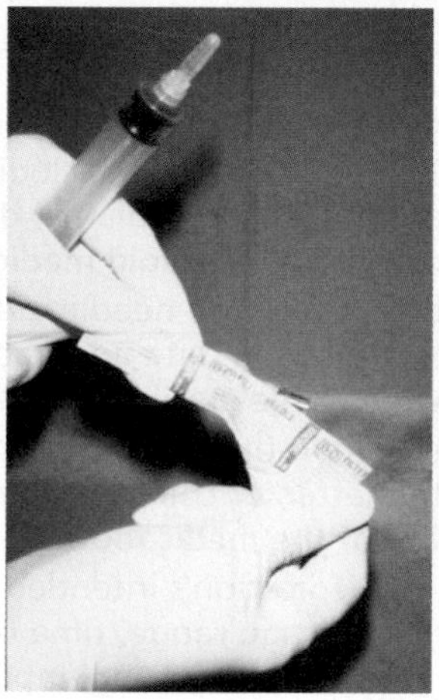

FIGURE 30-9-4 Select a syringe and filter needle.

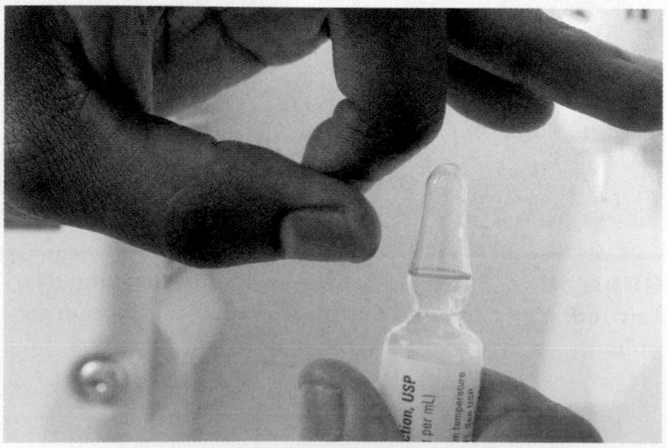

FIGURE 30-9-5 Flick the neck of the upright ampule to dislodge medication from the top of the vial.

(Continues)

PROCEDURE 30-9 Withdrawing Medication from an Ampule (Continued)

ACTION	RATIONALE
9. Wrap the sterile gauze pad around the neck and snap off the top in an outward motion directed away from self (Figures 30-9-6 and 30-9-7).	9. The gauze prevents the nurse from being cut by the jagged edge of the broken ampule. The outward motion provides added safety for the nurse.
10. Invert ampule and place the filter needle into the liquid. Gently withdraw medication into the syringe (Figure 30-9-8).	10. Inverting the ampule allows all of the medication to be withdrawn into the syringe. Surface tension will hold the medication in the ampule until the negative pressure of the syringe barrel draws it into the syringe.
11. Alternately, place the ampule on the counter, hold and tilt slightly with the nondominant hand. Insert the needle below the level of liquid and gently draw liquid into the syringe, tilting the ampule as needed to reach all the liquid.	11. While it is more difficult to read the syringe calibrations, it is easier to hold the ampule steady. Choose the method most comfortable for you.
12. Remove the filter needle and replace with the safety injection needle.	12. The filter needle is designed to trap glass particles and must not be used for client injections.
13. Dispose of filter needle and glass ampule (including lid) in appropriate sharps container.	13. Needles or sharp glass objects must always be disposed of in puncture and leak-proof containers to provide safety for clients and health care workers.
14. Label the syringe with drug, dose, date, and time.	14. Prevents medication errors from taking place.
15. Wash hands.	15. Decreases transmission of microorganisms.

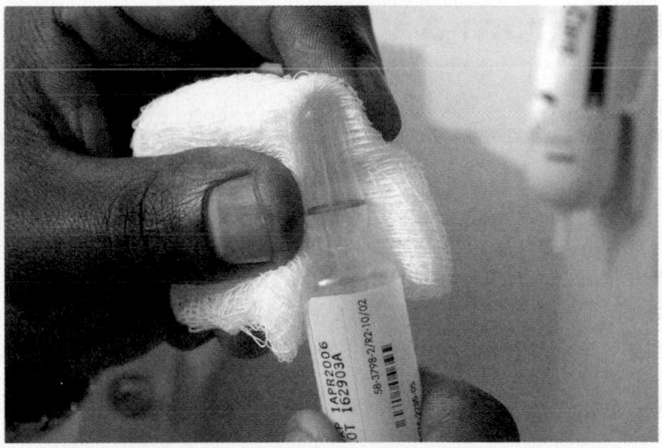

FIGURE 30-9-6 Wrap gauze or alcohol pad around the neck to protect fingers.

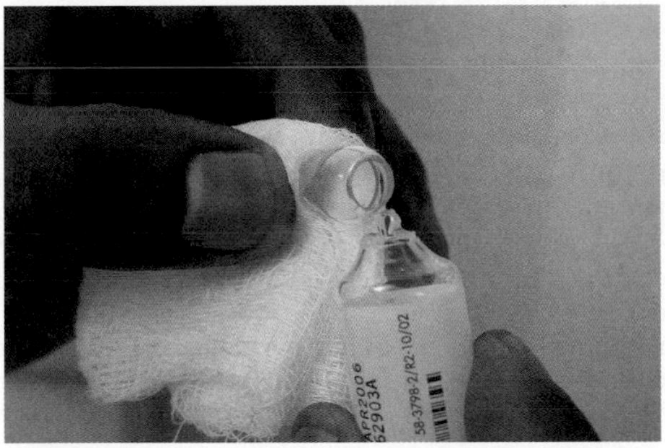

FIGURE 30-9-7 Snap the top of the ampule off in an outward motion away from self.

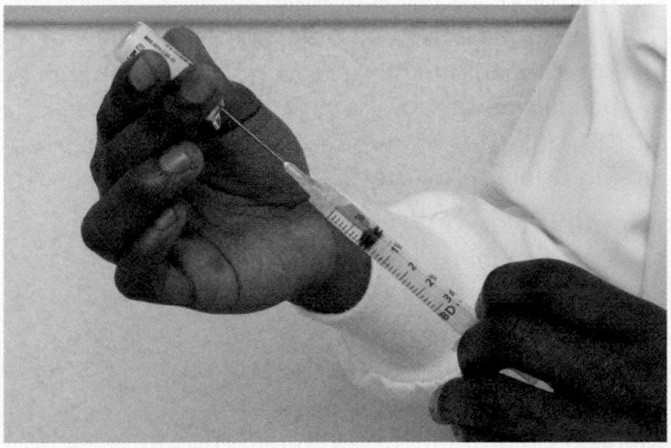

FIGURE 30-9-8 Invert ampule and gently draw the liquid into the syringe. Remove the filter and replace with the injection needle.

(Continues)

PROCEDURE 30-9 Withdrawing Medication from an Ampule (Continued)

EVALUATION
- The correct medication ampule was selected.
- The medication was drawn into an appropriate syringe.
- Microorganisms were not introduced into the sterile system.
- Foreign objects were not introduced into the sterile system.

DOCUMENTATION

Medication Administration Record

Document:
- Name of the medication
- Dosage drawn up
- Date and time the medication was drawn up

If the medication drawn up is a controlled substance, document in the Controlled Substances Record Book:
- Name of the medication
- Dosage drawn up
- Date and time the medication was drawn up
- Any controlled substance that was wasted
- Name of nurse drawing up the controlled substance

Controlled substances must be documented at the time they are removed from the locked cabinet. Documentation on the MAR is done after the medication is administered.

PROCEDURE 30-10 Withdrawing Medication from a Vial

OVERVIEW
Vials are often used to package multidose or single-dose parenteral medication. A vial is a small glass or plastic bottle with a rubber seal at the top. Vials come with a protective plastic or metal cap that prevents the rubber from being punctured before use. The rubber top must be cleaned with 70% alcohol with every usage of the medication. In order to aspirate the medication from the vial, an equal amount of air must be injected into the vial before attempting to withdraw any medication. In order to draw the medication out of the vial, the entire vial should be turned upside down. The syringe should be held at eye level to ensure an accurate amount of medication is drawn into the syringe.

ASSESSMENT
1. Assess the expiration date on the vial to be sure it is current **to avoid administering outdated medications.**
2. Assess the contents of the medication vial you are about to use for the correct medication in the correct dosage strength **to avoid medication error.**
3. Assess the contents of the vial for color, consistency, and debris **to avoid administering contaminated medication.**
4. Assess the integrity of the vial and its stopper **to avoid using a vial that may be contaminated.**
5. Assess the integrity of the syringe and needle that will be used to withdraw the medication **to avoid using equipment that may be contaminated.**

POSSIBLE NURSING DIAGNOSES
Risk for Infection
Risk for Injury

PLANNING

Expected Outcomes
1. The correct medication will be drawn from the vial using sterile technique.
2. The correct dose will be drawn from the vial.
3. The remaining contents of multiuse vials will not be contaminated.
4. The date will be marked on the vial after opening using an ink pen.

Equipment Needed (Figure 30-10-1)
- Medication vial
- Syringe with needle
- Alcohol sponge pad
- Nonsterile latex-free gloves (optional)
- Clean work space
- Medication administration record (MAR)

(Continues)

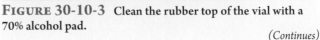

PROCEDURE 30-10 Withdrawing Medication from a Vial (Continued)

ACTION	RATIONALE

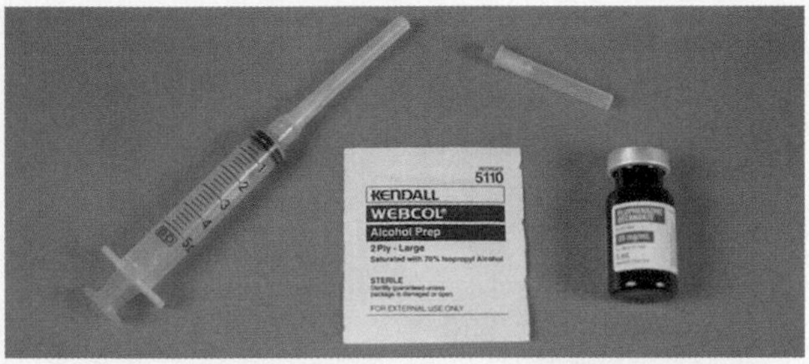

COURTESY OF DELMAR CENGAGE LEARNING

FIGURE 30-10-1 Syringe, needle, vial of medication, and alcohol wipes are used to withdraw medication from a vial.

delegation tips

The procedure of medication administration is not delegated to ancillary personnel in acute care settings. This may vary in state or federal institutions. Ancillary personnel are generally informed about the medications the client is receiving if adverse effects are anticipated or are being monitored.

IMPLEMENTATION—ACTION/RATIONALE

ACTION	RATIONALE
1. Wash hands. Apply nonsterile latex-free gloves (optional).	1. Decreases transmission of microorganisms.
2. Select the appropriate vial (Figure 30-10-2).	2. Prevents medication errors.
3. Verify health care provider's orders.	3. Prevents medication errors.
4. Check expiration date on vial.	4. Avoids giving expired medication, which may have altered potency.
5. Determine the route of medication delivery and select the appropriate size syringe and needle.	5. The route of medication delivery is essential to selecting the appropriate size syringe and needle.
6. While holding the syringe at eye level, withdraw the plunger to the desired volume of medication.	6. Holding the syringe at eye level makes it easier to read the syringe calibrations and increases accuracy.
7. Clean the rubber top of the vial with a 70% alcohol pad. Use a circular motion starting at the center and working out (Figure 30-10-3).	7. Ensures that the center of the rubber top is the cleanest area for needle entry. Reduces potential contamination with microorganisms.
8. Using sterile technique, uncap the needle and lay the needle cap on a clean surface.	8. Prevents spread of microorganisms.

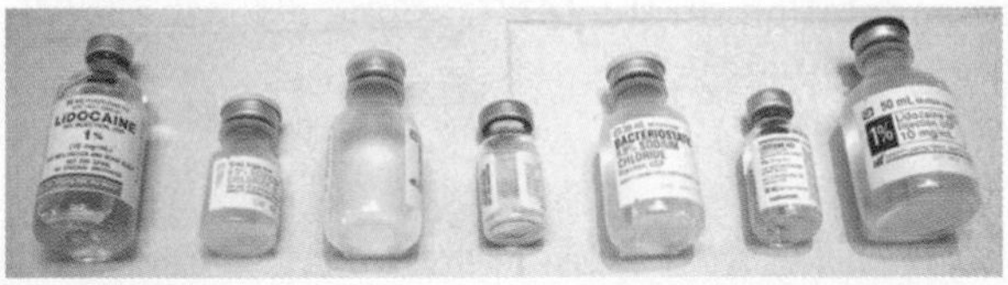

COURTESY OF DELMAR CENGAGE LEARNING

FIGURE 30-10-2 Carefully select the ordered medication.

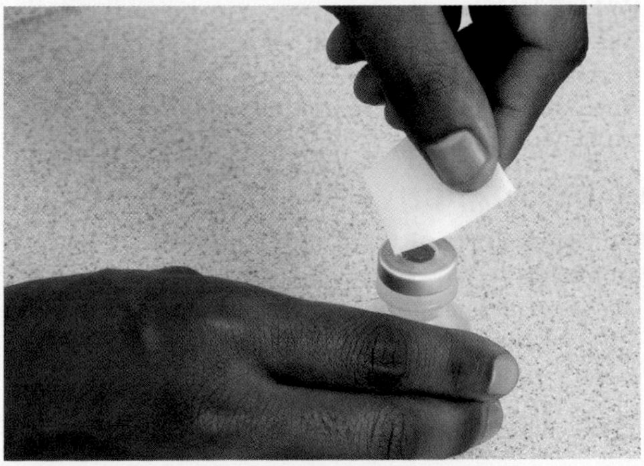

COURTESY OF DELMAR CENGAGE LEARNING

FIGURE 30-10-3 Clean the rubber top of the vial with a 70% alcohol pad.

(Continues)

PROCEDURE 30-10 Withdrawing Medication from a Vial (Continued)

ACTION	RATIONALE

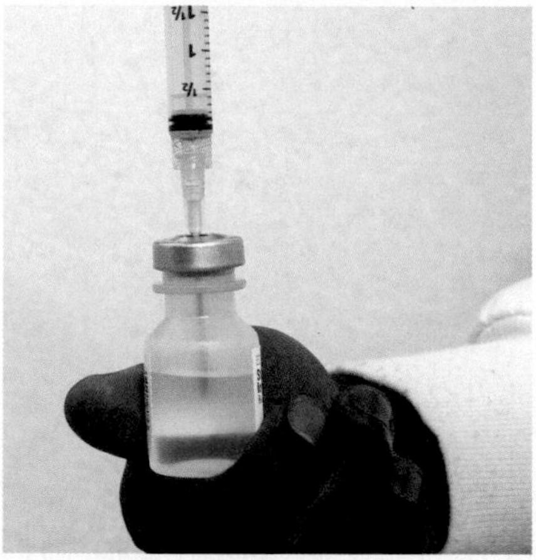

COURTESY OF DELMAR CENGAGE LEARNING

FIGURE 30-10-4 Place the needle into the vial through the center of the rubber top.

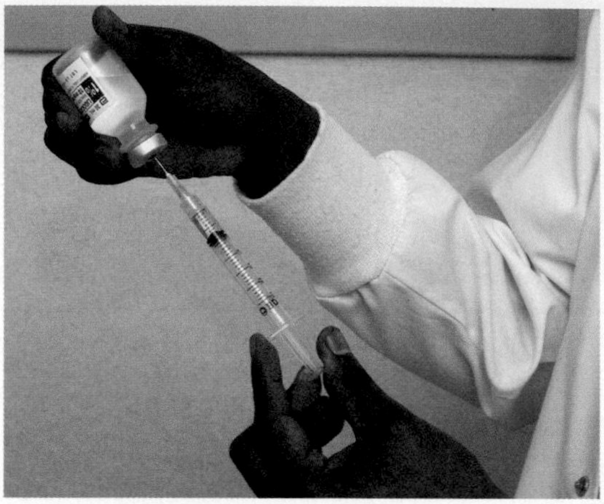

COURTESY OF DELMAR CENGAGE LEARNING

FIGURE 30-10-5 Invert the vial and slowly withdraw the medication until the appropriate dosage has been reached.

ACTION	RATIONALE
9. Placing the needle in the center of the vial, inject the air slowly. Do not cause turbulence (Figure 30-10-4).	9. Adding air prevents the buildup of negative pressure in the vial. Turbulence, which can result in air bubbles forming within the vial, can affect the accuracy of the volume of liquid being withdrawn.
10. Invert the vial and slowly, using gentle negative pressure, withdraw the medication. Keep the needle tip in the liquid (Figure 30-10-5).	10. Decreases the number of air bubbles that tend to form with unsteady, fast, jerky motions. Keeping the needle tip in the liquid prevents drawing in air.
11. With the syringe at eye level, determine that the appropriate dose has been reached by volume.	11. Ensures client receives the ordered dose of medication.
12. Slowly withdraw the needle from the vial. Follow the institution's policy regarding recapping and changing needles.	12. Avoids splatter of medication and potential contamination of nearby supplies. Keeps the needle sterile.
13. Using ink, mark the current date and time and initials on the vial.	13. Prevents using a medication that has been opened too long per institutional protocol.
14. Label the syringe with drug, dose, date, and time.	14. Prevents medication errors.
15. Wash hands.	15. Decreases transmission of microorganisms.

EVALUATION

- The vial was current and the rubber seal intact.
- The correct amount of medication was withdrawn.
- The needle did not become contaminated or damaged.

DOCUMENTATION

Medication Administration Record

Document:

- Name of the medication
- Dosage drawn up
- Date and time the medication was drawn up

If the medication drawn up is a controlled substance, document in the Controlled Substances Record Book:

- Name of the medication
- Dosage drawn up
- Date and time the medication was drawn up
- Any controlled substance that was wasted
- Name of nurse drawing up the controlled substance

Controlled substances must be documented at the time they are removed from the locked cabinet. Documentation on the MAR is done after the medication is administered.

PROCEDURE 30-11 Administering an Intradermal Injection

OVERVIEW

An intradermal injection is a method used to administer medications just below the skin. Potent medications that should be absorbed slowly are given intradermally because of the less richly supplied blood vessels of this layer; however, the client may respond rapidly and should be monitored for allergic reactions.

The most common reason for an intradermal injection is skin testing such as tuberculin screening or allergy testing. Only small amounts (0.01 to 0.10 mL) of fluid are given intradermally.

The most common sites for injections are forearms, upper chest, and upper back. The site should be lightly pigmented, free of lesions, and hairless. Because these areas are easily accessible, the nurse can monitor the reaction (Figure 30-11-1).

A tuberculin or small hypodermic syringe is used with a short (¼ to ½ inch), fine (26 to 27) gauge needle.

As of April 2001, a Federal Needle Stick Safety and Prevention Law requires safe medical devices. The position of the Occupational and Safety Health Act (OSHA) provides that whenever exposure to bloodborne pathogens is anticipated, controls to eliminate employee exposure should be used, hence, safe devices. Examples of such devices are needle-protected or needleless systems. In the case of intradermal injections, safety syringes or needles should be used. These can be safety-glide needles or safety-retraction or slide syringes. Instruction should be provided appropriate to manufacturers' specifications.

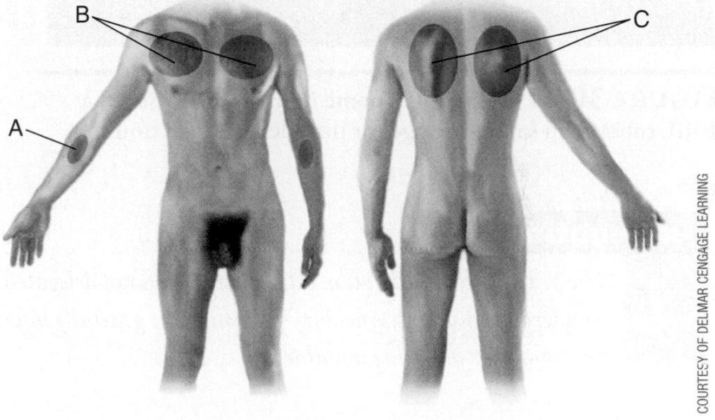

FIGURE 30-11-1 Common Intradermal Injection Sites: *A*, Inner Aspect of the Forearm; *B*, Upper Chest; *C*, Upper Back

ASSESSMENT

1. Assess the seven rights: right client, right medication, right route, right dose, right time, right to refuse, and right documentation. **Prevents errors in medication administration.**
2. Review health care provider's order **so the drug is administered safely and correctly.**
3. Review information regarding the expected reaction to the allergen **to anticipate the type of reaction a client may have.**
4. Assess for the indications for intradermal injection, including the client's allergy history, **so the nurse will not administer a substance to which the client is known to be sensitive.**
5. Check the expiration date of the medication vial **because the drug loses its potency over time.**
6. Assess client's knowledge regarding the medication to be received **so client education may be tailored according to need.**
7. Assess the client's response to discussion about an injection **because some clients may express anticipatory anxiety, which may increase pain.**

POSSIBLE NURSING DIAGNOSES

Risk for Infection
Impaired Skin Integrity
Deficient Knowledge (procedure)
Anxiety
Fear

PLANNING

Expected Outcomes

1. The client will experience only minimal pain or burning at the injection site.
2. The client will experience no allergic reaction or other side effects from the injection.
3. The client will be able to explain the significance of the presence or absence of a skin reaction.
4. The client will keep follow-up appointments within the recommended time frame to have responses to the medication evaluated.

(Continues)

PROCEDURE 30-11 Administering an Intradermal Injection (Continued)

Equipment Needed
- Tuberculin syringe, 1 mL (Figure 30-11-2)
- Needle (25- to 27-gauge, ¼- to ⅝-inch)
- Antiseptic or alcohol swabs
- Medication ampule or vial
- Medication card or medication administration record
- Nonsterile latex-free gloves

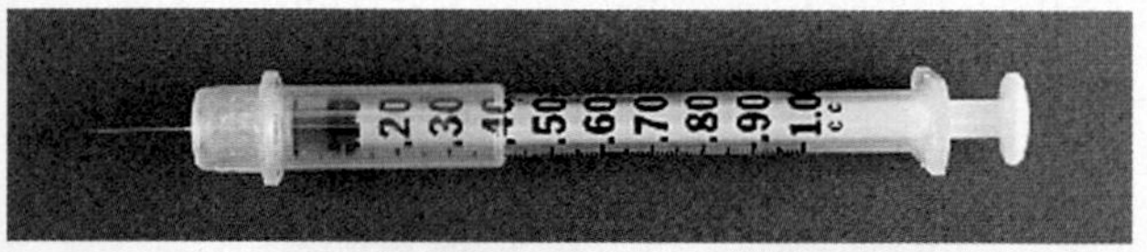

FIGURE 30-11-2 Syringes come in many sizes. Select a 1-mL tuberculin safety-syringe for intradermal injections.

delegation tips

The procedure of medication administration is not delegated to ancillary personnel in acute care settings. This may vary in state or federal institutions. Ancillary personnel are generally informed about the medications the client is receiving if adverse effects are anticipated or are being monitored.

IMPLEMENTATION—ACTION/RATIONALE

* Check client's identification band * Explain procedure before beginning *

ACTION	RATIONALE
1. Wash hands and put on nonsterile latex-free gloves.	1. Reduces transmission of microorganisms.
2. In the inpatient setting, close door or curtains around bed and keep gown or sheet draped over body. In the outpatient setting, close door to exam or treatment room. Identify client and assess right to refuse (sixth right).	2. Provides privacy. Ensures that medication is given to right client.
3. Select injection site (Figure 30-10-1). • Inspect skin for bruises, inflammation, edema, masses, tenderness, and sites of previous injections. • Forearm site should be 3 to 4 finger widths below antecubital space and one hand width above wrists on inner aspect of forearm.	3. Injection site should be free of lesions. Repeated daily injections should be rotated. Ensures a clear site for interpreting results.
4. Select 1 mL tuberculin syringe and ¼- to ⅝-inch 25- to 27-gauge needle.	4. Ensures that needle will be inserted into the dermis.
5. Assist client into a comfortable position. Forearm site: Relax the arm with elbow and forearm extended on a flat surface. Distract client by talking about an interesting subject.	5. Relaxation minimizes discomfort. Distraction reduces anxiety.
6. Use alcohol pad or antiseptic swab in a circular motion to clean skin at site.	6. Circular motion and mechanical action of swab remove secretions containing microorganisms.

(Continues)

PROCEDURE 30-11 Administering an Intradermal Injection (Continued)

ACTION	RATIONALE
7. While holding the swab between fingers of nondominant hand, pull the cap from needle.	7. Swab remains accessible during procedure. Prevents contamination of needle.
8. Administer injection:	8.
• With nondominant hand, stretch skin over site with forefinger and thumb.	• Needle penetrates tight skin easier than loose skin.
• Insert needle slowly at a 5- to 15-degree angle, bevel up, until resistance is felt; then advance to no more than ⅛ inch below the skin. The needle tip should be seen through the skin.	• Ensures needle tip is in the dermis.
• Slowly inject the medication. Resistance will be felt.	• Dermal layer is tight and does not expand easily when fluid is injected.
• Note a small bleb, like a mosquito bite, forming under the skin surface (Figure 30-11-3).	• Indicates the medication was deposited in the dermis.
9. Withdraw the needle while applying gentle pressure with the antiseptic swab.	9. Supporting tissue around injection site minimizes discomfort.
10. Do not massage the site.	10. Prevents medication from being dispersed into the tissue and altering test results.
11. Assist the client to a comfortable position.	11. Promotes comfort.
12. Discard the uncapped needle and syringe in a sharps container.	12. Decreases risk of needlestick.
13. Remove gloves and wash hands.	13. Reduces transmission of microorganisms.
14. Document (seventh right).	14. Maintains legal record and prevents medication errors.

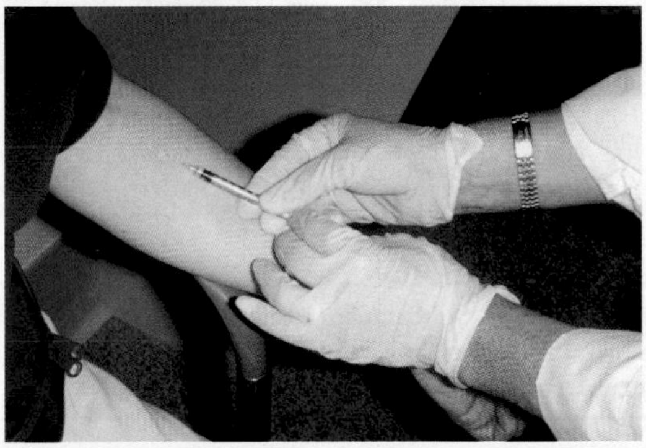

FIGURE 30-11-3 Note a small bleb, like a mosquito bite, forming under the skin surface as the medication is injected.

EVALUATION

- The client experienced only minimal pain or burning at the injection site.
- The client experienced no allergic reaction or other side effects from the injection.
- The client was able to explain the significance of the presence or absence of a skin reaction.
- The client kept all follow-up appointments within the recommended time frame to have responses to the medication evaluated.

DOCUMENTATION

Medication Administration Record

- Date, time, medication, dose, route, site, and signature or initials.

Nurses' Notes

Document:

- Date and time of skin reaction
- Date and time of any systemic side effects of the medication. Report to health care provider.

PROCEDURE 30-12 Administering a Subcutaneous Injection

OVERVIEW

A subcutaneous injection is a method used to administer medications into the loose connective tissues just below the dermis of the skin. Medications that do not need to be absorbed as quickly as those given intramuscularly are given subcutaneously because of the less richly supplied blood vessels in the subcutaneous tissue; however, the client may respond more rapidly to a subcutaneous injection than to oral medication and should be monitored for potential side effects, allergic reactions, the risk of infection, or bleeding.

Only small (0.5- to 1-mL) doses of isotonic, nonirritating, nonviscous, and water-soluble medications should be given subcutaneously, such as anticoagulants, insulin, tetanus toxoid, allergy medications, epinephrine, and vitamin B_{12}. If larger volumes of medications remain in these sensitive tissues, a sterile abscess could form, causing a hard, painful lump.

The most common sites for subcutaneous injections are the vascular areas around the outer aspect of the upper arms, the abdomen, and the anterior aspect of the thighs (Figure 30-12-1). Because these areas are easily accessible, the client may learn how to self-administer medications. Rotation of sites of injections should be observed so that no site is used more often than every 6 to 7 weeks.

For a subcutaneous injection, a 2- to 3-mL syringe or a 1-mL syringe is recommended. U-100 insulin syringes in 30-, 50-, and 100-unit sizes are used for subcutaneous insulin injections. The most commonly used needle for a subcutaneous injection is a ⅝-inch 25-gauge needle. Adjustments need to be made for pediatric, obese, or cachectic clients.

As of April 2001, a Federal Needle Stick Safety and Prevention Law requires safe medical devices. The position of the Occupational and Safety Health Act (OSHA) provides that whenever exposure to blood-borne pathogens is anticipated, controls to eliminate employee exposure should be used, hence, safe devices. Failure to comply with using safe devices and safe disposal can result in fines. Examples of safe devices are needle-protected or needleless systems with proper disposal in clearly marked sharps containers. In the case of subcutaneous injections, safety syringes or needles should be used. These can be safety-glide or retraction needles or slide syringes. Instruction should be provided appropriate to manufacturers' specifications.

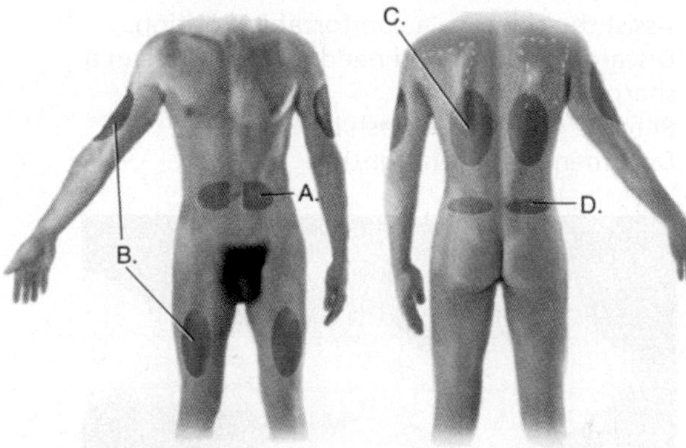

COURTESY OF DELMAR CENGAGE LEARNING

FIGURE 30-12-1 Subcutaneous Injection Sites: *A*, Abdomen; *B*, Lateral and Anterior Aspects of Upper Arm and Thigh; *C*, Scapular Area of Back; *D*, Upper Ventrodorsal Gluteal Area.

ASSESSMENT

1. Assess the seven rights: right client, right medication, right route, right dose, right time, right to refuse, and right documentation. **Prevents errors in medication administration.**
2. Review health care provider's order **so the drug is administered safely and correctly.**
3. Review information regarding the drug ordered, such as action, purpose, time of onset and peak action, normal dosage, common side effects, and nursing implications **to anticipate the drug's effects and anticipate a reaction.**
4. Assess client for factors that may influence an injection such as circulatory shock or reduced local tissue perfusion **because reduced tissue perfusion will interfere with the absorption and distribution of the drug.**
5. Assess for previous subcutaneous injections **in order to rotate sites and avoid repeating a dose in the same site.**
6. Assess for the indications for subcutaneous injection **because an injection is preferred for clients who are confused or unconscious, are unable to swallow a tablet, or have a gastrointestinal disturbance, including the use of nasogastric suction.**
7. Assess the client's age **because older clients or pediatric clients have special needs based on their physiologic status.**
8. Assess client's knowledge regarding the medication to be received **so client education may be tailored according to need.**
9. Assess the client's response to discussion about an injection **because some clients may express anticipatory anxiety, which may increase pain.**
10. Check the client's drug allergy, history **as an allergic reaction could occur.**

(Continues)

PROCEDURE 30-12 Administering a Subcutaneous Injection (Continued)

POSSIBLE NURSING DIAGNOSES

Risk for Infection
Impaired Skin Integrity
Anxiety
Deficient Knowledge (procedure)
Fear

PLANNING

Expected Outcomes

1. The client will experience only minimal pain or burning at the injection site.
2. The client will experience no allergic reaction or other side effects from the injection.
3. The client will be able to explain the action, side effects, dosage and schedule of the medication, and rationale for rotation of sites.

Equipment Needed (Figures 30-12-2 and 30-12-3)

- Syringe appropriate for the medication being given
- Needle (25- to 27-gauge, ⅜- to ⅝-inch)
- Antiseptic or alcohol swabs
- Medication ampule or vial
- Medication record
- Nonsterile latex-free gloves

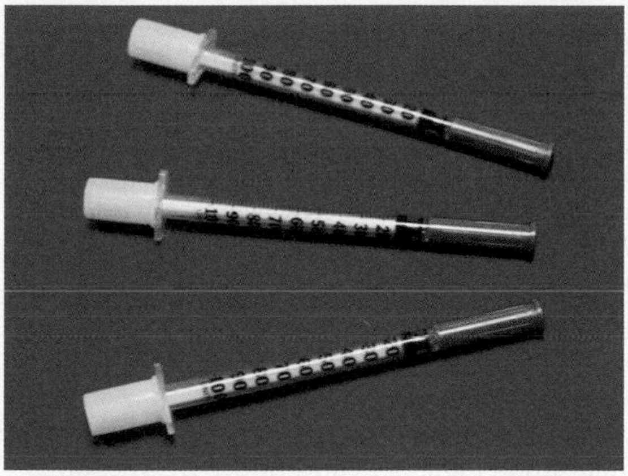

COURTESY OF DELMAR CENGAGE LEARNING

FIGURE 30-12-2 100-unit insulin syringes are used to administer insulin subcutaneously.

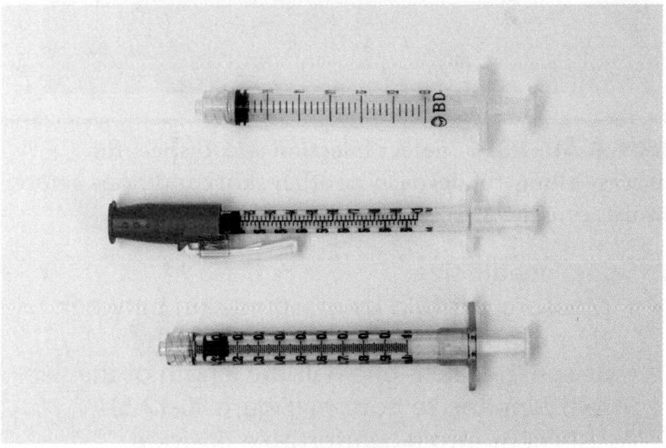

COURTESY OF DELMAR CENGAGE LEARNING

FIGURE 30-12-3 Syringes that are used for a subcutaneous injection include a 3-mL syringe, and insulin syringe, and a tuberculin syringe.

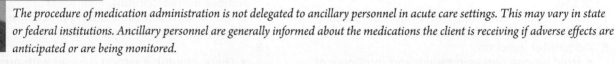

delegation tips

The procedure of medication administration is not delegated to ancillary personnel in acute care settings. This may vary in state or federal institutions. Ancillary personnel are generally informed about the medications the client is receiving if adverse effects are anticipated or are being monitored.

IMPLEMENTATION—ACTION/RATIONALE

ACTION	RATIONALE
* Check client's identification band * Explain procedure before beginning *	
1. Wash hands and put on nonsterile latex-free gloves.	1. Reduces the number of microorganisms.
2. Close door or curtains around bed and keep gown or sheet draped over client. Identify client using two different identifiers.	2. Provides privacy. Ensures that medication is given to the right client.
3. Select injection site (Figure 30-12-1).	3. Injection site should be free of lesions.
• Inspect skin for bruises, inflammation, edema, masses, tenderness, and sites of previous injections and avoid these areas (Figure 30-12-4).	• Repeated daily injections should be rotated.
• Use subcutaneous tissue around the abdomen, lateral aspects of upper arm or thigh, or scapular area.	• Avoids injury to underlying nerves, bone, or blood vessels.

(Continues)

PROCEDURE 30-12 Administering a Subcutaneous Injection (Continued)

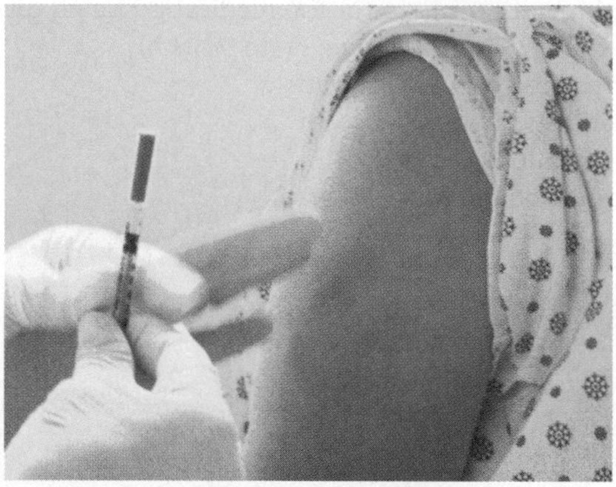

FIGURE 30-12-4 Select injection site. Inspect for bruises, swelling, tenderness, or other skin conditions before administering the injection.

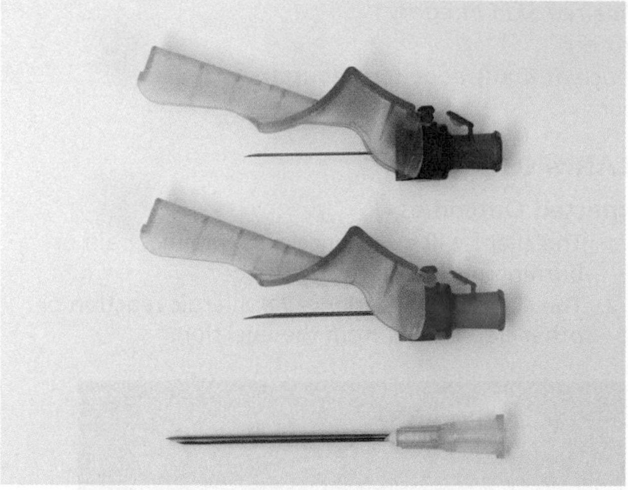

FIGURE 30-12-5 Shown are different types of needles used for an injection that have safety shields to protect against accidental needle sticks after the injection is given.

ACTION	RATIONALE
4. Select needle size: • Measure skinfold by grasping skin between thumb and forefinger. • Be sure needle is one-half the length of the skinfold from top to bottom (Figure 30-12-5).	4. Ensures that needle will be inserted into subcutaneous tissue.
5. Assist client into a comfortable position: • Relax the arm, leg, or abdomen. • Distract client by talking about an interesting subject or explaining what you are doing step by step.	5. Relaxation minimizes discomfort. Distraction reduces anxiety.
6. Use alcohol swab or antiseptic swab to clean skin at site.	6. Circular motion and mechanical action of swab remove microorganisms.
7. While holding swab between fingers of nondominant hand, pull cap from needle.	7. Swab remains accessible during procedure. Prevents contamination of needle.
8. Administer injection:	8.
• Hold syringe between thumb and forefinger of dominant hand like a dart.	• Quick, smooth injection is easier with proper position of syringe.
• Pinch skin with nondominant hand (Figure 30-12-6).	• Needle penetrates tight skin easier than loose skin. Pinching skin elevates subcutaneous tissue.
• Inject needle quickly and firmly (like a dart) at a 45- to 90-degree angle (Figure 30-12-7).	• Quick, firm injection minimizes discomfort. Angle depends on amount of subcutaneous tissue present and the site used.
• Release the skin.	
• Grasp the lower end of the syringe with nondominant hand and position dominant hand to the end of the plunger. Do not move the syringe.	• Injection requires smooth manipulation of syringe parts. Movement of syringe may cause discomfort.
• Pull back on the plunger to ascertain that the needle is not in a vein. If no blood appears, slowly inject the medication. (Aspiration is contraindicated with some medications; check with the pharmacy if you are unclear.)	• Aspiration of blood indicates intravenous placement of needle so procedure may have to be abandoned.

(Continues)

PROCEDURE 30-12 Administering a Subcutaneous Injection (Continued)

ACTION	RATIONALE

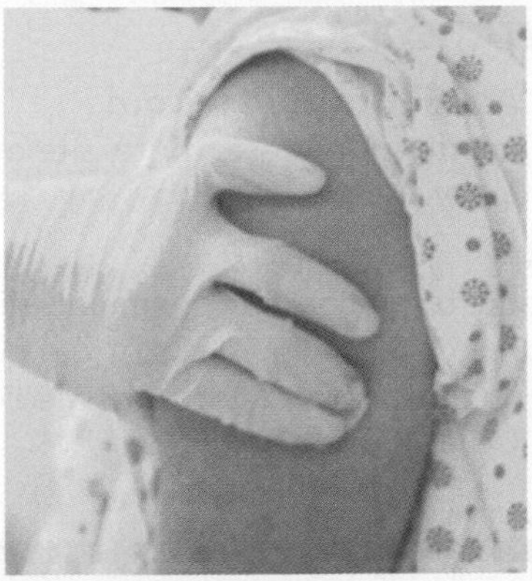

FIGURE 30-12-6 Pinch the skin with the nondominant hand.

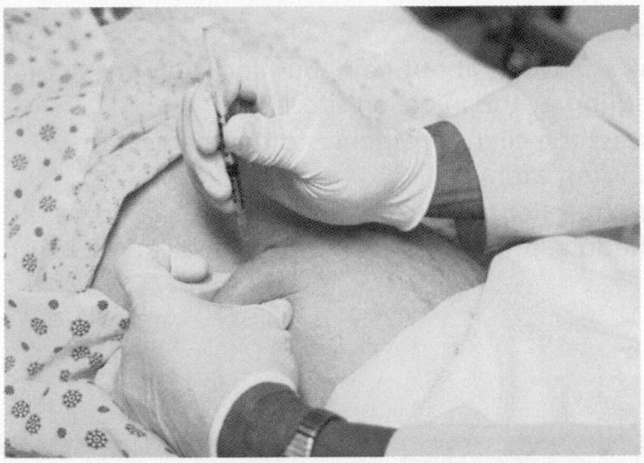

FIGURE 30-12-7 When injecting at a 90° angle, hold the syringe like a dart and pierce the skin quickly and firmly.

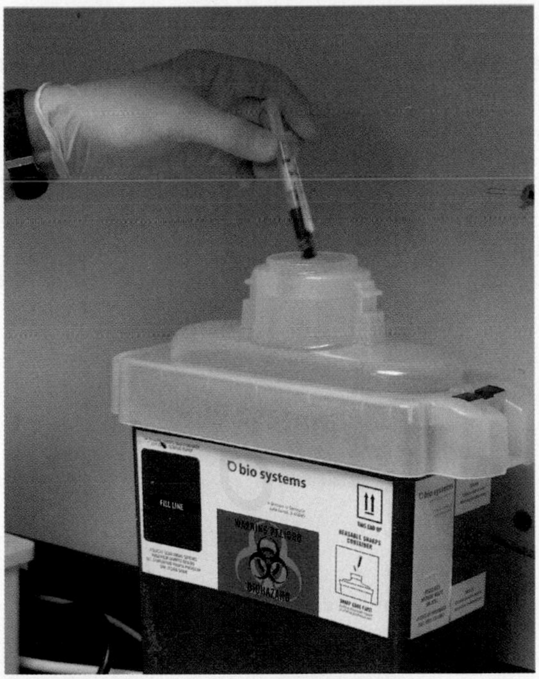

FIGURE 30-12-8 Dispose the uncapped needle in a specified biohazard sharps container.

ACTION	RATIONALE
9. Remove hand from injection site and quickly withdraw the needle. Apply pressure with the antiseptic swab. Do not push down on the needle with the swab while withdrawing it, because this will cause more pain.	9. Supporting tissue around injection site minimizes discomfort. Removing hand before withdrawing needle reduces chance of needlestick.
10. Apply pressure. Some medications should not be massaged. Ask the pharmacy if you are unclear.	10. Stimulates circulation and improves drug distribution and absorption.
11. Discard the uncapped needle and syringe in a disposable needle receptacle (Figure 30-12-8).	11. Decreases risk of needlestick.
12. Assist the client to a comfortable position.	12. Promotes comfort and encourages client to remain still.
13. Remove gloves and wash hands.	13. Reduces transmission of microorganisms.

(Continues)

PROCEDURE 30-12 Administering a Subcutaneous Injection (Continued)

ACTION	RATIONALE

EVALUATION

- Ask the client about pain, burning, numbness, or tingling at the injection site.
- Assess the client's response to the medication 30 minutes later.
- Ask the client to discuss the purpose, action, schedule, and side effects of the medication.

DOCUMENTATION

Medication Administration Record

- Date, time, medication, dose, route, site of injection, and signature or initials

Nurses' Notes

- Date and time of response to the medication
- Date and time of any side effects of the medication
- Document on appropriate electronic medical record or flow sheet (seventh right).

PROCEDURE 30-13 Administering an Intramuscular Injection

OVERVIEW

An intramuscular injection is a method used to administer medications into the deep muscle tissue. Medications will be absorbed quickly because of the richly supplied blood vessels in the muscle. Most aqueous medications are absorbed in 10 to 30 minutes. Average-sized adults can tolerate up to 3 mL of medication injected into a large muscle because muscle is less sensitive to irritating and viscous drugs than subcutaneous tissue.

The most common sites for intramuscular injections are the vastus lateralis, the ventrogluteal, the dorsogluteal, and the deltoid muscles (Figure 30-13-1). The *vastus lateralis* muscle is located on the anterior lateral aspect of the

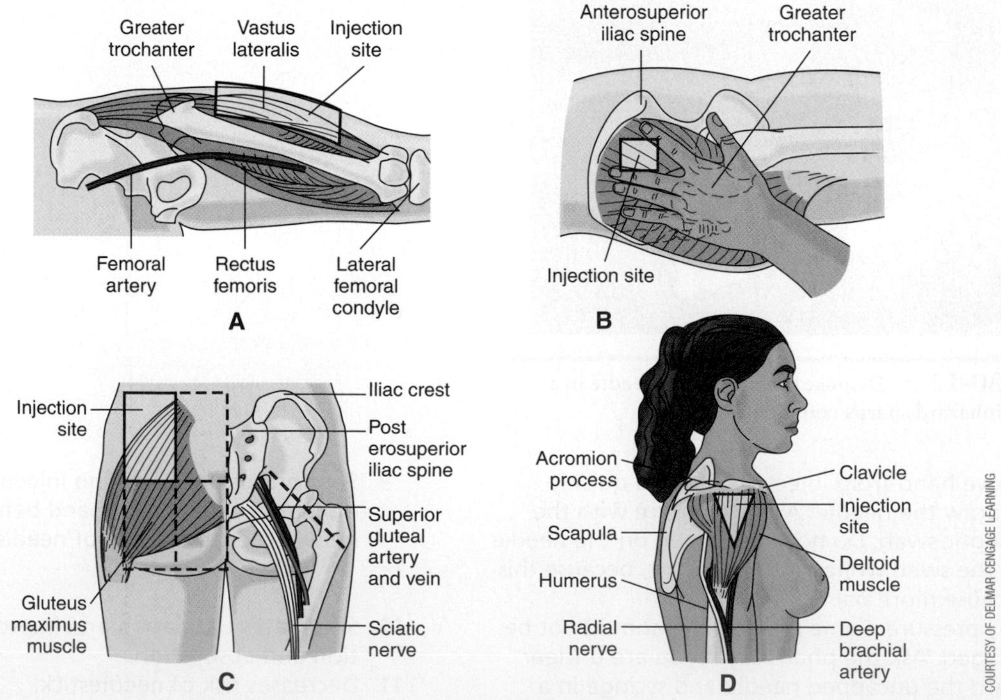

FIGURE 30-13-1 Intramuscular injection sites. *A*, Vastus lateralis: Identify greater trochanter; place hand at lateral femoral condyle; injection site is middle third of anterior lateral aspect. *B*, Ventrogluteal: Place palm of left hand on right greater trochanter so that index finger points toward anterosuperior iliac spine; spread first and middle fingers to form a V; injection site is the middle of the V angle. *C*, Dorsogluteal: Place hand on iliac crest and locate the posterosuperior iliac spine. Draw an imaginary line between the trochanter and the iliac spine; the injection site is the outer quadrant. *D*, Deltoid: Locate the lateral side of the humerus from two to three finger widths below the acromion process in adults or one finger width below the acromion process in children.

(Continues)

PROCEDURE 30-13 Administering an Intramuscular Injection (Continued)

ACTION | **RATIONALE**

thigh. This easily accessible site is the preferred site for clients of all ages because it has no major blood vessels or nerves nearby. The *ventrogluteal* site is the preferred site in adults because it is located deep and away from major blood vessels and nerves. It is preferred over the dorsogluteal for the following reasons: There is less risk of damage to the sciatic nerve and blood vessels; this site is less painful because the muscle is most often not tense even in an anxious client. The *dorsogluteal* muscle in the upper outer quadrant of the buttock poses greater risk of damage to the sciatic nerve, major blood vessels, and the greater trochanter bone. It should not be used in children younger than 5 years of age because this muscle is not developed. The *deltoid* muscle is found on the upper arm about 1 to 2 inches below the acromion process. Major nerves and blood vessels are beneath this site, and only small volumes of medication should be injected.

Originally the Z-track method of intramuscular injections was used as a special procedure for only certain medications. Medications such as iron dextran and hydralazine hydrochloride can be irritating to the tissues and stain the skin. Using the Z-track method prevents potentially irritating medications from being tracked up through the tissues by interrupting the injection tract. This method can help reduce pain also with nonstaining or irritating substances.

There are many different types and sizes of syringes. Prefilled syringes that consist of a prefilled barrel and needle assembly placed in a reusable plunger are often used (Figure 30-13-2). For an intramuscular injection, a 2- to 3-mL syringe is recommended with a 1¼- to 1½-inch, 19- to 23-gauge needle. Adjustments need to be made for pediatric, obese, or cachectic clients.

As of April 2001, a Federal Needle Stick Safety and Prevention Law requires safe medical devices. The position of the Occupational and Safety Health Act (OSHA) provides that whenever exposure to blood-borne pathogens is anticipated, controls to eliminate employee exposure should be used, hence, safe devices. Failure to comply with using safe devices and safe disposal can result in fines. Examples of safe devices are needle-protected or needleless systems with proper disposal in sharps containers clearly marked. With intramuscular injections, safety syringes or needles should be used. These can be safety-glide or retraction needles or slide syringes. Instruction should be provided appropriate to manufacturers' specifications.

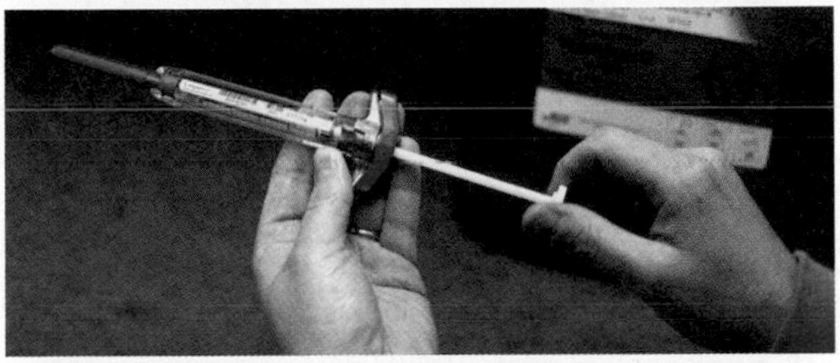

FIGURE 30-13-2 **A prefilled syringe consists of a prefilled barrel and needle assembly placed in a reusable plunger.**

ASSESSMENT

1. Assess the seven rights: right client, right medication, right route, right dose, right time, right to refuse, and right documentation. **Prevents errors in medication administration.**
2. Review health care provider's order **so the drug is administered safely and correctly.**
3. Review information regarding the drug ordered, such as action, purpose, time of onset and peak action, normal dosage, common side effects, and nursing implications **to anticipate the drug's effects and anticipate a reaction.**
4. Assess client for factors that may influence an injection, such as circulatory shock, reduced local tissue perfusion, or muscle atrophy **because reduced tissue perfusion will interfere with the absorption and distribution of the drug.**
5. Assess for previous intramuscular injections **to rotate sites and avoid repeating a dose in the same site.**
6. Assess for the indications for intramuscular injection **because an injection is preferred for clients who require the fast action of the medication, are confused or unconscious, are unable to swallow a tablet, or have a gastrointestinal disturbance, including the use of nasogastric suction.**
7. Assess the client's age **because older clients or pediatric clients have special needs based on their physiologic status.**
8. Assess client's knowledge regarding the medication to be received **so client education may be tailored according to need.**
9. Assess the client's response to discussion about an injection **because some clients may express anticipatory anxiety, which may increase pain.**
10. Assess the client's size and muscle development. **Assists in identification of appropriate site, needle size, angle to be used, and amount of medication that can be administered in the site.**
11. Check the client's allergy history, **as an allergic reaction could occur.**

(Continues)

PROCEDURE 30-13 Administering an Intramuscular Injection (Continued)

POSSIBLE NURSING DIAGNOSES

Risk for Infection
Impaired Skin Integrity
Anxiety
Deficient Knowledge (injection)
Fear

PLANNING

Expected Outcomes

1. The correct client will receive the correct medication.
2. The client will experience only minimal pain or burning at the injection site.
3. The client will experience no allergic reaction or other side effects from the injection.
4. The client will be able to explain the action, side effects, dosage, and schedule of the medication.
5. The client will obtain the expected benefit from the medication.
6. The client will not experience pain or skin staining secondary to the medication when Z-track injection is given.

Equipment Needed (Figures 30-13-3 and 30-13-4)

- Safety-syringe (1- to 3-mL)
- Safety-needle (19- to 23-gauge, 1¼ to 1½ inches)
- Antiseptic or alcohol swabs
- Medication ampule or vial
- Medication record
- Nonsterile latex-free gloves

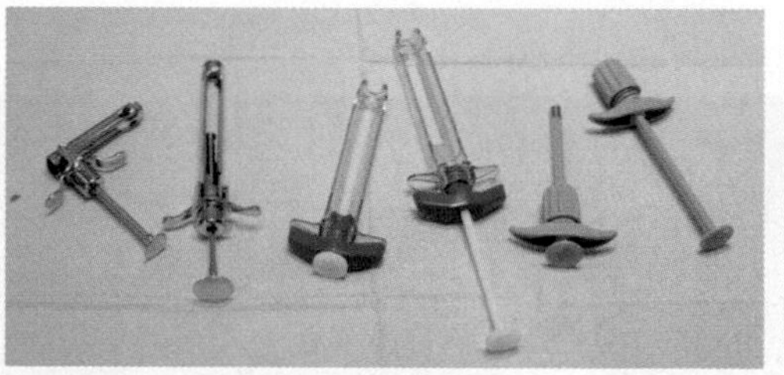

FIGURE 30-13-3 Shown are various types of prefilled syringe plungers.

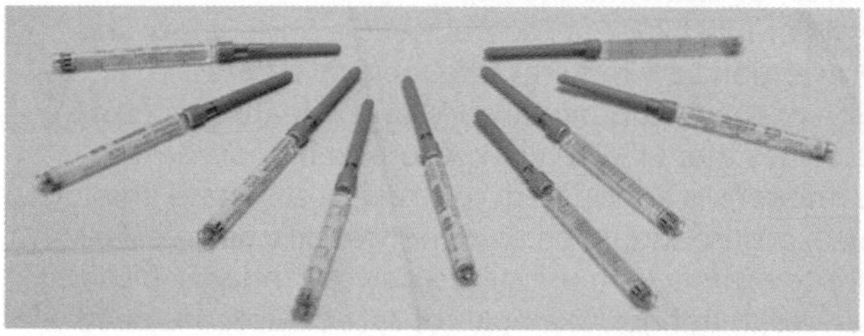

FIGURE 30-13-4 Prefilled Barrel and Needle Cartridges

delegation tips

The procedure of medication administration is not delegated to ancillary personnel in acute care settings. This may vary in state or federal institutions. Ancillary personnel are generally informed about the medications the client is receiving if adverse affects are anticipated or are being monitored.

IMPLEMENTATION—ACTION/RATIONALE

ACTION	RATIONALE
* Check client's identification band * Explain procedure before beginning *	
1. Wash hands and put on nonsterile latex-free gloves.	1. Reduces the number of microorganisms.
2. Close door or curtains around bed and keep gown or sheet draped over client. Identify client using two different identifiers.	2. Provides privacy. Ensures that medication is given to the right client.
3. Select injection site (Figure 30-13-1). • Inspect skin for bruises, inflammation, edema, masses, tenderness, and sites of previous injections.	3. Injection site should be free of lesions. • Repeated daily injections should be rotated.

(Continues)

PROCEDURE 30-13 Administering an Intramuscular Injection (Continued)

• Use anatomic landmarks.	• Avoids injury to underlying nerves, bone, or blood vessels. Site should be selected based on muscle development, type, and amount of medication, and comfortable access to site.
4. Select needle size: Assess size and weight of client and site to be used.	4. Ensures that needle will be inserted into the muscle.
5. Assist client into a comfortable position: • For vastus lateralis, lying flat or supine with knee slightly flexed. • For ventrogluteal, lying on side or back with knee and hip slightly flexed. • For dorsogluteal, lying prone with feet turned inward or on side with upper knee and hip flexed and placed in front of lower leg. • For deltoid, standing with arm relaxed at side or sitting with lower arm relaxed on lap or lying flat with lower arm relaxed across abdomen (Figure 30-13-5). • Distract client by talking about an interesting subject.	5. Relaxation minimizes discomfort. Distraction reduces anxiety.
6. Use antiseptic swab or alcohol swab to clean skin at site.	6. Circular motion and mechanical action of swab remove secretions containing microorganisms.
7. While holding swab between fingers of nondominant hand, pull cap from needle.	7. Swab remains accessible during procedure. Prevents contamination of needle.
8. Administer injection: • Hold syringe between thumb and forefinger of dominant hand like a dart. • Spread skin tightly or pinch a generous section of tissue firmly—for cachectic clients. • Inject needle quickly and firmly (like a dart) at a 90-degree angle (Figure 30-13-6). • Release the skin.	8. • Quick, smooth injection is easier with proper position of syringe. • Needle penetrates tight skin more easily than loose skin. • Quick, firm injection minimizes discomfort. • Injection requires smooth manipulation of syringe parts. Movement of syringe may cause discomfort.

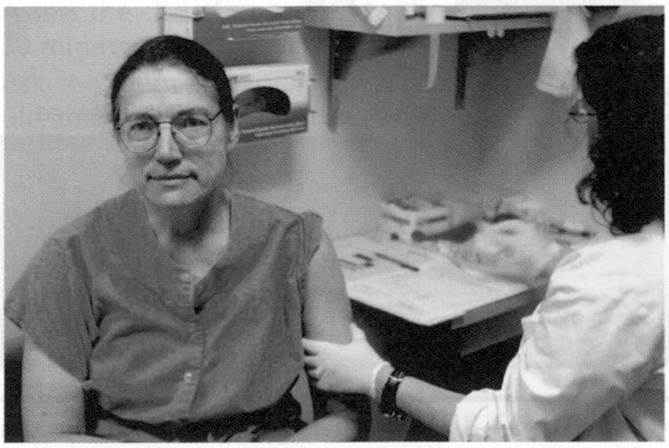

FIGURE 30-13-5 Have the client stand or sit with arm relaxed at side.

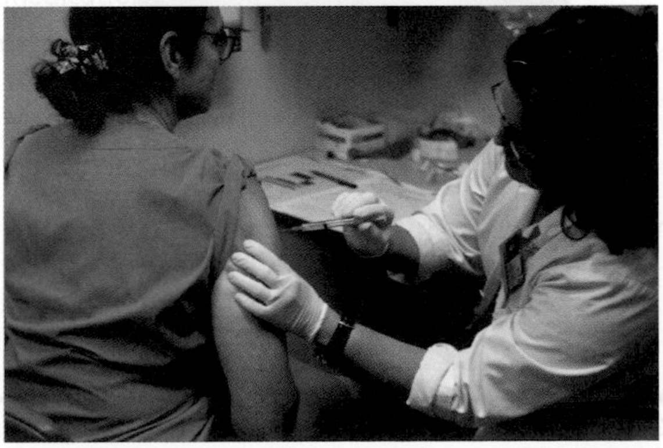

FIGURE 30-13-6 Inject needle quickly and firmly at a 90° angle.

(Continues)

PROCEDURE 30-14 Administering Eye and Ear Medications

OVERVIEW

Eye Medications

Eye medications refer to drops, ointment, and disks. These drugs are used for diagnostic and therapeutic purposes—to lubricate the eye or socket for a prosthetic eye and to prevent or treat eye conditions such as glaucoma (elevated pressure within the eye) and infection. Diagnostically, eyedrops can be used to anesthetize the eye, dilate the pupil, and stain the cornea to identify abrasions and scars.

Review the abbreviations used in medication orders to ensure that the medication is instilled in the correct eye. Cross contamination is a potential problem with eyedrops. Adhere to the following safety measures to prevent cross contamination:

- Each client should have his or her own bottle of eyedrops.
- Discard any solution remaining in the dropper after instillation.
- Discard the dropper if the tip is accidentally contaminated by touching the bottle or any part of the client's eye.

Ear Medications

Solutions ordered to treat the ear are often referred to as otic (pertaining to the ear) drops or irrigation. Eardrops may be instilled to soften ear wax, to produce anesthesia, to treat infection or inflammation, or to facilitate removal of a foreign body, such as an insect. External auditory canal irrigations are usually performed for cleaning purposes and less frequently for applying heat and antiseptic solutions.

Before instilling a solution into the ear, inspect the ear for signs of drainage, which is an indication of a perforated tympanic membrane. Eardrops are usually contraindicated when the tympanic membrane is perforated. If the tympanic membrane is damaged, all procedures must be performed using sterile technique; otherwise, medical asepsis is used when instilling medication into the ear.

Certain conditions have contraindications for specific drugs (e.g., hydrocortisone eardrops are contraindicated in clients with a fungal infection or a viral infection such as herpes).

ASSESSMENT

1. Assess the seven rights: right client, right medication, right route, right dose, right time, right to refuse, and right documentation. **Prevents errors in medication administration.**
2. Assess the condition of the client's eyes and/or ears. Are there any contraindications to administering this medication present? Is there drainage from the ear indicating a possible tympanic rupture? If so, the medication administration must be done using sterile technique. **Reassessing the client before every medication dose prevents possibly injuring the client.**
3. Assess the medication order. Is the medication for only one eye/ear or both? With eye medications be sure to understand the abbreviations used for right eye (OD), left eye (OS), and both eyes (OU). **Prevents errors in medication administration.**

POSSIBLE NURSING DIAGNOSES

Risk for Injury
Deficient Knowledge (medication regime)
Disturbed Sensory Perception (visual or auditory)

PLANNING

Expected Outcomes

1. The right client will receive the right dose of the right medication via the right route at the right time.
2. The client will encounter minimum discomfort during the medication administration procedure.
3. The client will receive maximum benefit from the medication.

Equipment Needed (Figure 30-14-1)

Eye Medication

- Medication administration record (MAR)
- Eye medication
- Tissue or cotton ball
- Nonsterile latex-free gloves (if needed)

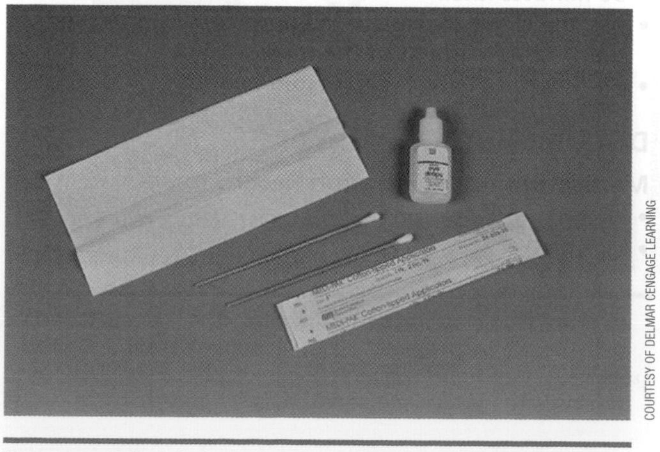

FIGURE 30-14-1 Supplies needed for administering eye and ear drops.

(Continues)

PROCEDURE 30-14 Administering Eye and Ear Medications (Continued)

Ear Medication

- Medication administration record (MAR)
- Medication
- Nonsterile latex-free gloves
- Cotton-tipped applicator
- Tissue

delegation tips

The procedure of medication administration is not delegated to ancillary personnel in acute care settings. This may vary in state or federal institutions. Ancillary personnel are generally informed about the medications the client is receiving if adverse effects are anticipated or are being monitored.

IMPLEMENTATION—ACTION/RATIONALE

* Check client's identification band * Explain procedure before beginning *

ACTION	RATIONALE
Eye Medication	
1. Check with the client and the chart for any known allergies or medical conditions that would contraindicate use of the drug.	1. Prevents occurrence of adverse reactions.
2. Gather the necessary equipment.	2. Promotes efficiency.
3. Follow the seven rights of drug administration.	3. Promotes safety.
4. Take the medication to the client's room and place on a clean surface.	4. Decreases risk of contamination of bottle cap.
5. Identify client using two different identifiers.	5. Accurately identifies the client.
6. Inquire if the client wants to instill medication. If so, assess the client's ability to do so.	6. Some clients are used to instilling their own medication.
7. Wash hands, and don nonsterile latex-free gloves if needed.	7. Reduces transmission of microorganisms. Decreases contact with bodily fluids.
8. Place client in a supine position with the head slightly hyperextended.	8. Minimizes drainage of medication through the tear duct.
Instilling Eyedrops	
9. Remove cap from eye bottle and place cap on its side.	9. Prevents contamination of the bottle cap.
10. Place a tissue below the lower lid.	10. Absorbs the medication that flows from the eye.
11. With dominant hand, hold eyedropper ½–¾ inch above the eyeball; rest hand on client's forehead to stabilize.	11. Reduces risk of dropper touching eye structure, and prevents injury to the eye.
12. Place hand on cheekbone and expose lower conjunctival sac by pulling down on cheek.	12. Stabilizes hand and prevents systemic absorption of eye medication.
13. Instruct the client to look up and drop prescribed number of drops into center of conjunctival sac (Figure 30-14-2).	13. Reduces stimulation of the blink reflex; prevents injury to the cornea.
14. Instruct client to gently close eyes and move eyes. Briefly place fingers on either side of the client's nose to close the tear ducts and prevent the medication from draining out of the eye (Figure 30-14-3).	14. Distributes solution over conjunctival surface and anterior eyeball.
15. Remove gloves; wash hands.	15. Reduces transmission of microorganisms.
16. Document (seventh right) on the MAR the route, site (which eye), and the time administered.	16. Provides documentation that the medication was given.

(Continues)

PROCEDURE 30-14 Administering Eye and Ear Medications (Continued)

ACTION	RATIONALE

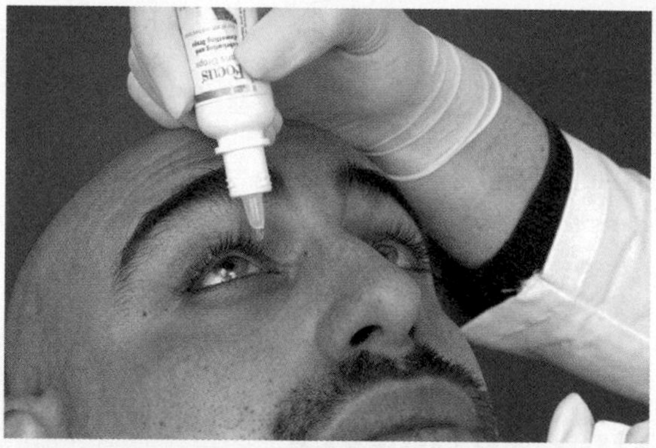

FIGURE 30-14-2 Have the client look upward while instilling drops into the lower conjunctival sac.

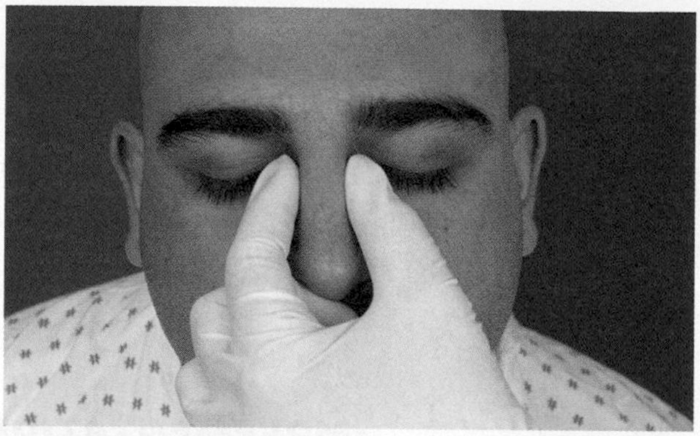

FIGURE 30-14-3 Placing the fingers on the sides of the client's nose closes the tear ducts and prevents the medication from draining out of the eye.

Eye Ointment Application

ACTION	RATIONALE
17. Repeat Actions 1 to 8.	17. See Rationales 1 to 8.
18. Lower lid:	18.
• With nondominant hand, gently separate client's eyelids with thumb and finger and grasp lower lid near margin immediately below the lashes; exert pressure downward over the bony prominence of the cheek.	• Provides access to the lower lid.
• Instruct the client to look up.	• Reduces stimulation of the blink reflex and keeps cornea out of the way of the medication.
• Apply eye ointment along inside edge of the entire lower eyelid, from inner to outer canthus.	• Ensures drug is applied to entire lid
19. Upper lid:	19.
• Instruct client to look down.	• Keeps cornea out of the way of the medication.
• With nondominant hand, gently grasp client's lashes near center of upper lid with thumb and index finger, and draw lid up and away from eyeball.	
• Squeeze ointment along upper lid starting at inner canthus.	• Ensures that medication is applied to entire length of lid.
20. Repeat actions 15 to 16.	20. See Rationales 15 to 16.

Medication Disk

ACTION	RATIONALE
21. Repeat Actions 1 to 8.	21. See Rationales 1 to 8.
22. Open sterile package and press dominant, sterile gloved finger against the oval disk so that it lies lengthwise across fingertip.	22. Promotes sticking of disk to fingertip.
23. Instruct the client to look up.	23. Reduces stimulation of the blink reflex and keeps cornea out of the way of the medication.
24. With nondominant hand, gently pull the client's lower eyelid down and place the disk horizontally in the conjunctival sac.	24. Allows the disk to automatically adhere to the eye.
• Then pull the lower eyelid out, up, and over the disk.	• Secures the disk in the conjunctival sac.
• Instruct the client to blink several times.	• Allows the disk to settle into place.
• If disk is still visible, repeat steps.	• Ensures correct placement of the disk.

(Continues)

PROCEDURE 30-14 Administering Eye and Ear Medications (Continued)

ACTION	RATIONALE
• Once the disk is in place, instruct the client to gently press the fingers against the closed lids; do not rub eyes or move the disk across the cornea.	• Secures disk placement. Prevents corneal scratches.
• If the disk falls out, pick it up, rinse under cool water, and reinsert.	• Preserves medication. This is not a sterile procedure. Health care provider must wear gloves to pick up disk.
25. If the disk is prescribed for both eyes (OU), repeat Actions 22 to 24.	25. Ensures both eyes are treated at the same time.
26. Repeat Actions 14 to 16.	26. See Rationales 14 to 16.
Removing an Eye Medication Disk	
27. Repeat Actions 3 and 5 to 8.	27. See Rationales 3 and 5 to 8.
28. Remove the disk:	28.
• With nondominant hand, invert the lower eyelid and identify the disk.	• Exposes the disk for removal.
• If the disk is located in the upper eye, instruct the client to close the eye, and place your finger on the closed eyelid. Apply gentle, long, circular strokes; instruct client to open the eye. Disk should be located in corner of eye. With your fingertip, slide the disk to the lower lid, then proceed.	• Safely moves the disk to the lower conjunctival sac.
• With dominant hand, use the forefinger to slide the disk onto the lid and out of the client's eye.	• Safely removes the disk without scratching the cornea.
29. Remove gloves; wash hands.	29. Reduces transmission of microorganisms.
30. Record on the MAR the removal of the disk.	30. Provides documentation that the disk was removed.
Ear Medication	
31. Check with client and chart for any known allergies.	31. Prevents the occurrence of hypersensitivity reactions.
32. Check the MAR against the health care provider's written orders.	32. Ensures accuracy in identification of the medication.
33. Wash hands.	33. Reduces transfer of microorganisms.
34. Place the client in a side-lying position with the affected ear facing up.	34. Facilitates the administration of the medication.
35. Straighten the ear canal by pulling the pinna down and back for children less than 3 years of age or upward and outward in adults and older children.	35. Opens the canal and facilitates introduction of the medication.
36. Instill the drops into the ear canal by holding the dropper at least ½ inch above the ear canal (Figure 30-14-4).	36. Prevents injury to the ear canal.
37. Ask the client to maintain the position for 2 to 3 minutes.	37. Allows for distribution of the medication.
38. Place a cotton ball on the outermost part of the canal, if approved by the health care prescriber.	38. Prevents the medication from escaping when the client changes to a sitting or standing position.
39. Wash hands.	39. Reduces the transmission of microorganisms.

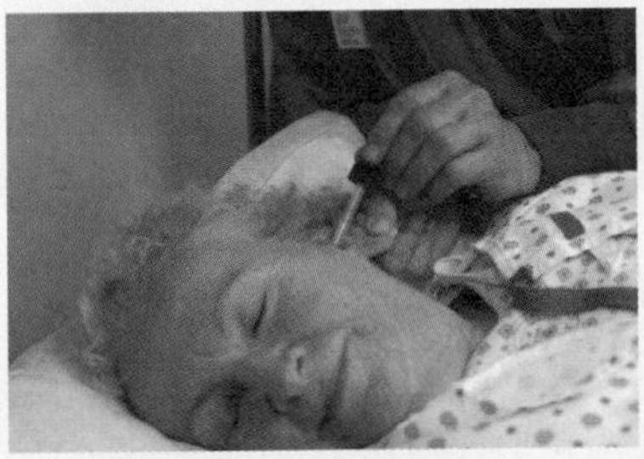

COURTESY OF DELMAR CENGAGE LEARNING

FIGURE 30-14-4 Slowly instill the drops, holding the dropper at least ½ inch above the ear canal.

(Continues)

PROCEDURE 30-14 Administering Eye and Ear Medications (Continued)

EVALUATION

- The right client received the right dose of the right medication via the right route at the right time.
- The procedure was performed with minimum trauma and/or discomfort to the client.
- The client received maximum benefit from the medication.
- All the prescribed medication went into the eye or ear, and none was spilled.

DOCUMENTATION

Medication Administration Record (MAR)

- Date, time, medication, location, and dosage administered
- If an ordered medication was not given, note this, usually by circling the time of the missed medication.

NURSES' NOTES

- If an ordered medication was not given, record the reason.
- If an as-needed medication was given, note the reason for giving the medication and the client's response.
- Document on appropriate electronic medical record or flow sheet (seventh right).

PROCEDURE 30-15 Administering Skin/Topical Medications

OVERVIEW

Topical medications are applied directly to the skin or mucous membranes. These types of medications are used for their local effect or to produce systemic effects by absorption from percutaneous routes. Topical medications include creams, ointments, and lotions. Topical medications applied to the skin are commonly used to relieve itching, prevent local infections, moisten the skin, or for vasodilation. Most topical medications are used for local effects; however, certain medications can be absorbed percutaneously to provide systemic effects, such as topical nitroglycerin, nicotine patches, or certain estrogen products.

ASSESSMENT

1. Assess the seven rights: right client, right medication, right route, right dose, right time, right to refuse, and right documentation. **Prevents errors in medication administration.**
2. Assess the area where treatment will be applied **to establish a baseline condition of the skin for future comparison.**
3. If drug is being used for systemic effect, assess for area free of scars, moles, or other skin aberrations **to facilitate selection of a site with no barriers to absorption.**
4. Check the client's allergy history, **as an allergic reaction could occur.**

POSSIBLE NURSING DIAGNOSIS

Risk for Impaired Skin Integrity

PLANNING

Expected Outcomes

1. Good skin integrity
2. Relief of itching, irritation, or pain
3. Improved circulation

Equipment Needed (Figure 30-15-1)

- Correct medication
- Correct applicator (cotton balls, sterile gauze pad, tongue blades, or cotton applicator)
- Nonsterile latex-free gloves (sterile gloves if broken skin integrity)
- Basin with warm water
- Mild soap (if appropriate and not contraindicated by skin condition or interaction with medication)
- Washcloth and towel
- Gauze dressing, tape as indicated
- Disposable waterproof pad
- Chart or medication sheet for medication verification
- Nonsterile latex-free gloves

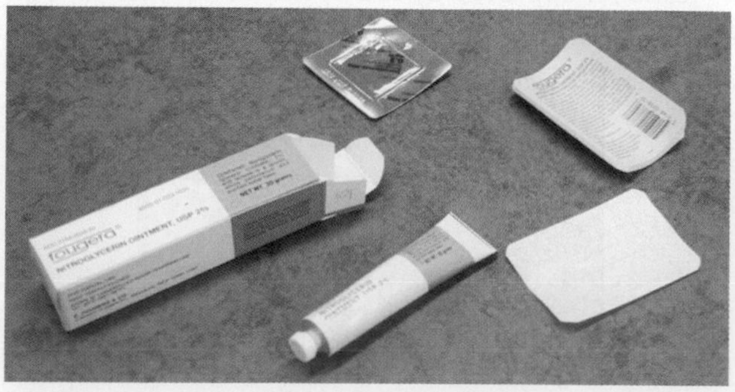

COURTESY OF DELMAR CENGAGE LEARNING

FIGURE 30-15-1 Lotions, creams, ointments, and patches are used to dispense topical medications.

(Continues)

PROCEDURE 30-15 Administering Skin/Topical Medications (Continued)

delegation tips

The application of some creams, lotions, and ointments may be delegated to properly trained ancillary personnel, but these are generally over-the-counter preparations and not prescription medications.

IMPLEMENTATION—ACTION/RATIONALE

* Check client's identification band * Explain procedure before beginning *

ACTION	RATIONALE
1. Wash hands.	1. Reduces transmission of microorganisms.
2. Obtain order for medication from health care provider.	2. Prevents inappropriate medication administration. An order is needed for any medication.
3. Ascertain client's allergic status.	3. Avoids allergic reactions. Nurses are responsible for medication errors including reactions. Charts may not always be current regarding allergies or an oversight might have occurred.
4. If unfamiliar with medication, read label and insert or seek appropriate information.	4. Prevents inappropriate medication administration and errors. Medications should never be administered without knowledge about the medication.
5. Select medication and verify medication with orders (**first medication verification**).	5. Prevents medication errors.
6. Check medication expiration date.	6. Outdated medications may not be effective.
7. Read medication label again before leaving medication room or cart as available in facilities (**second medication verification**).	7. Avoids medication errors.
8. Take the medication to the client's room and introduce yourself to the client. In some facilities, topical medications used for skin irritations are kept in the client's room, so verification must be done at the bedside.	8. Identifies appropriate medication with right client.
9. Ask the client if he or she has had the medication before and to describe its effect. Ascertain client's allergy status.	9. Provides another verification for the medication. Prevents allergic reaction.
10. Explain the purpose of the medication.	10. Helps to inform and involve the client in his or her care and promotes learning more about condition.
11. Read the label for the third time (**third medication verification**) and check the client's identification band.	11. Avoids medication errors.
12. Position the client appropriately for administration of medication. Keep client draped for privacy.	12. Keeps the client in a comfortable position for medication administration. Protects privacy.
13. Put on gloves. If dressing is over area to be treated, remove, discard, and change gloves.	13. Decreases contact with microorganisms.
14. If an open wound, clean area to be treated with mild soap (if no allergies or reactions to soap) and water. If skin is irritated, use only warm water. If administering a systemically absorbed topical medication, clean the skin surface thoroughly and pat skin dry, leaving no residues of soap. Do not rub vigorously because absorption can be altered (Figure 30-15-2).	14. Soap can irritate an open wound. If skin is already irritated, soap may cause more irritation. Systemically absorbed medication can be effected by residue on the skin or rubbing, which causes vasodilation.
15. Assess the client's skin condition, making notation of circulation, drainage, color, temperature, or any altered skin integrity.	15. Information can be compared with future assessment and effect of medication.

(Continues)

PROCEDURE 30-15 Administering Skin/Topical Medications (Continued)

ACTION	RATIONALE

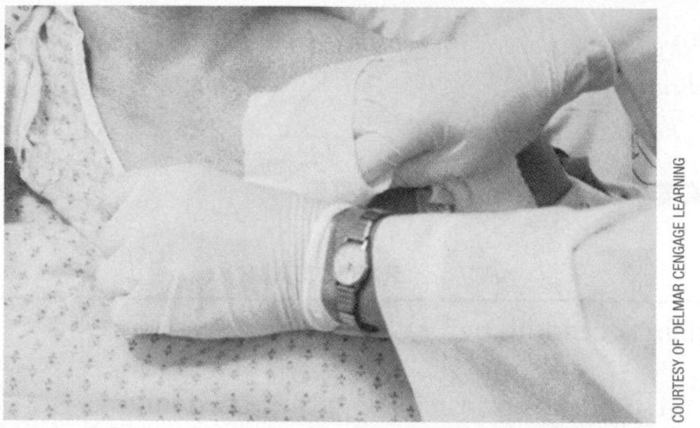

FIGURE 30-15-2 Cleanse the skin before applying topical medication.

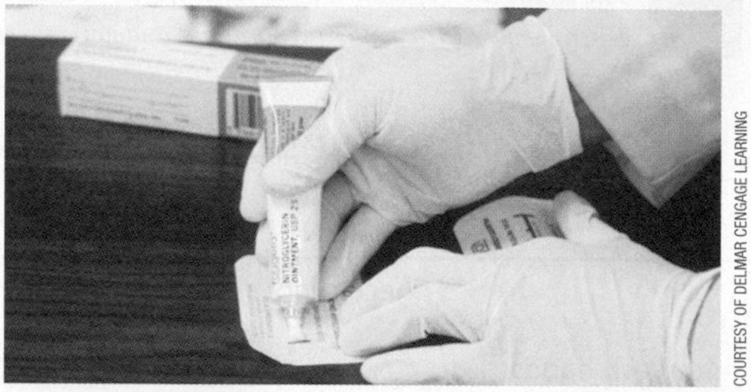

FIGURE 30-15-3 Squeeze the correct dose out onto the enclosed medication measuring strip.

ACTION	RATIONALE
16. Change gloves.	16. Prevents spread of microorganisms and avoids absorption of medication by caregivers. (This is especially important with systemically absorbed medication.)
17. Apply medication according to label. If lotion or ointment, apply a thin layer and smooth into skin as indicated.	17. Medication dosages have been studied and are recommended according to certain standards.
18. If an aerosol spray is used, shake the container and administer according to direction. Spray evenly over affected area and avoid spraying close to client's or caregiver's face.	18. Aerosol may need to be mixed to be effective. Avoid inhalation because it may have adverse effects on the mucous membranes and lungs.
19. If gels or pastes are used, applicators may be needed. Apply evenly. If applying over an area with hair growth, follow direction of hair.	19. Apply evenly to affected areas. Excess gel or paste will be wasted because absorption can only occur at skin level. The client will experience less discomfort if hair growth pattern is followed.
20. If powders are used, dust lightly and avoid inhalation by client and caregiver.	20. Excess powder will be wasted because absorption can only occur at skin level. Inhalation can cause untoward effects on the lungs and mucous membranes.
21. If nitroglycerin ointment or paste are used, follow instructions and orders carefully to administer correct dosage.	21. Nitroglycerin is systemically absorbed and accurate dosing is essential. If thick lines of ointment are applied, the dose will be different; therefore, the manufacturer's suggestions must be followed carefully for safe use of this drug.
• Remove the old ointment strip and clean the old site thoroughly. New ointment will be applied in a different area.	• If areas of ointment from previous doses are not removed, the client will be receiving more than one dose at a time.
• Cleanse the new site with the appropriate cleaner.	• Ensures proper absorption of the medication.
• Squeeze the dose out onto the enclosed medication measuring strip (Figure 30-15-3). Nitroglycerin paste dosages are measured in inches and applied to the paper measuring strip before being applied to the client.	• Use care not to over- or undermedicate by squeezing out a line of ointment that is too thick or too thin.
• Flatten the roll of nitroglycerin so the ointment will be spread over a wider area when applied to the client.	• The wider area of contact and thinner coating of ointment increases absorption.

(Continues)

PROCEDURE 30-15 Administering Skin/Topical Medications (Continued)

ACTION	RATIONALE
• Apply the measuring paper, ointment side down, to a portion of the client's body without hair.	• Using a nonhairy area increases the absorption of the medication.
• Tape the paper in place.	• Keeps the medication in place.
22. If a transdermal patch is used, follow the manufacturer's directions and apply the patch to a smooth, cleaned skin surface.	22. Patches offer a more reliable means of controlling dosage; however, patches are generally more expensive than ointments.
• Remove the old patch and wash the site of the old patch.	• Prevents overdose.
• Wash and prepare the skin at a new site.	• Allows for maximal medication absorption.
• Remove the protective covering over the transdermal portion of the patch and apply the new patch (Figure 30-15-4).	• Removing the protective covering allows the medication to be absorbed.
• Write the date and time on the patch.	• Alerts caregivers of when the patch was applied.
23. Remove gloves; wash hands.	23. Reduces transmission of microorganisms.
24. Document (seventh right) the medication given, the site it was applied to, and the client's response to the medication.	24. Proper documentation is essential for safe client care.

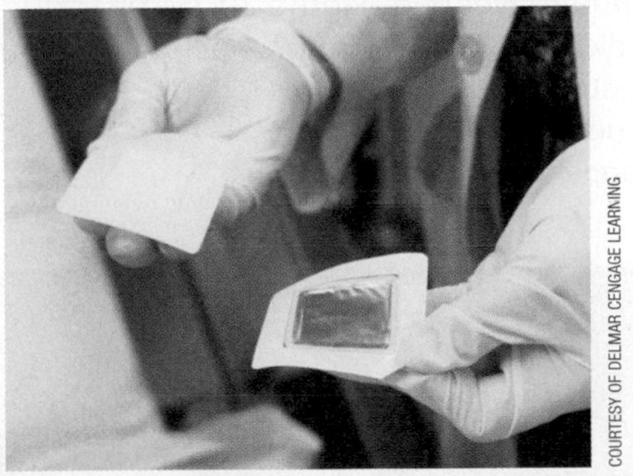

FIGURE 30-15-4 When applying a transdermal patch, remove the protective covering and apply the patch.

EVALUATION

- The client's skin integrity was maintained.
- The client experienced relief of itching, irritation, or pain if this was the intent of the medication.
- The client experienced maximum effect from the topical medication.
- The client experienced no allergic reaction.

DOCUMENTATION

Medication Administration Record

- Date, time, and site of application of the topical medication.

Nurses' Notes

- Changes in the client's skin integrity, coloration, or sensation
- If medication was for irritation, itching, or rash, document any improvement or change
- Unusual findings or client complaints
- Document on appropriate electronic medical record or flow sheet.

PROCEDURE 30-16 Administering Nasal Medications

OVERVIEW

Nasal medications may be administered by drops or sprays. Sprays may be packaged as pump sprays, sprays in aerosolized containers (pressurized containers, sometimes called nasal nebulizers), or powdered turbo inhalers. Prescribed medications are generally available in pump sprays or aerosolized sprays, whereby sprays and nasal drops are available in over-the-counter medications. Nasal medications may be used to achieve local effects on the nasal mucosa, indirect effects on the sinuses, or a systemic effect. Examples of medications that have systemic effects and are available in nasal sprays are insulin, agents to suppress nicotine use, and agents to treat migraine headaches. The four groups of sinuses (frontal, ethmoid, sphenoid, and maxillary) communicate with the nasal fossae and are lined with mucous membranes similar to those that line the nose. Even though it is unlikely that nasal medications penetrate the sinuses, positioning may aid in decreasing inflammation and congestion in the mucous membranes adjacent to the sinuses, thereby indirectly decreasing pressure in the sinuses. To medicate the mucous membranes adjacent to the frontal sinuses, the client will assume a supine position with the head turned to the affected side to be treated. To medicate the mucous membranes adjacent to the ethmoid sinuses, the client will lie supine with his or her head leaning back over the side of the bed with the client's head supported by the nurse's hand to avoid muscle strain on the client's neck. Although the nose is not considered a clean or sterile cavity, because of its connection with the sinuses, employ medical asepsis when performing nasal instillation.

ASSESSMENT

1. Assess the seven rights: right client, right medication, right route, right dose, right time, right to refuse, and right documentation. **Prevents errors in medication administration.**
2. Assess the client's nasal congestion and nasal obstruction **to determine if the medicine can be inhaled to reach the nasal mucosa and to determine the effectiveness of the medication.**
3. Assess the color, quantity, and odor of the client's discharge and the color and moistness of the nasal mucosa **to check for signs and symptoms of infection, to discern tissue damage, and to establish a baseline for future assessments.**
4. Assess the client's pain and/or discomfort level in the areas of sinuses **because this is another symptom of infection. May determine if the client can use the inhaler or drops.**
5. Assess the client for systemic conditions that may be adversely affected by nasal medications (see manufacturer's information). **Clients with cardiovascular conditions and hypertension may need to use caution with medications containing sympathomimetic** ingredients.

POSSIBLE NURSING DIAGNOSES

Impaired Oral Mucous Membrane
Impaired Tissue Integrity

PLANNING

Expected Outcomes

1. The client will be free of nasal congestion.
2. The client will be free of nasal discharge and odor.
3. The client will breathe freely through the nasal passages.
4. The client will be free of sinus pain and nasal pain.
5. The client's nasal passages will be moist and pink.

Equipment Needed (Figure 30-16-1)

- Medication in spray, drops, or aerosolized form
- Nonsterile latex-free gloves
- Tissue as needed
- Dropper as needed

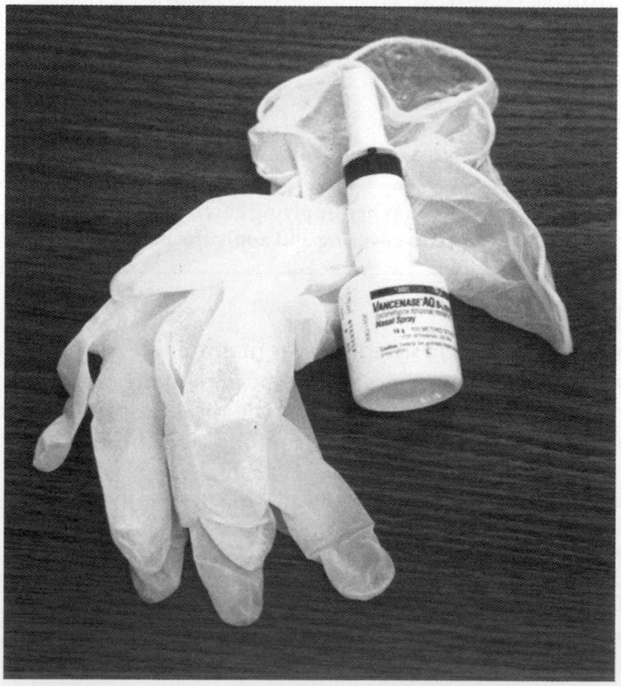

COURTESY OF DELMAR CENGAGE LEARNING

FIGURE 30-16-1 Nasal medication spray and latex-free gloves are needed when administering nasal medication to a client.

(Continues)

PROCEDURE 30-16 Administering Nasal Medications (Continued)

delegation tips

The procedure of medication administration is not delegated to ancillary personnel in acute care settings. This may vary in state or federal institutions. Ancillary personnel are generally informed about the medications the client is receiving if adverse effects are anticipated or are being monitored.

IMPLEMENTATION—ACTION/RATIONALE

ACTION	RATIONALE
* Check client's identification band * Explain procedure before beginning *	
1. Wash hands. Wear a mask if the client is coughing or sneezing. Don nonsterile latex-free gloves.	1. Reduces transmission of microorganisms. Respiratory-related microorganisms are easily transferred by the hands and air droplets. Gloves prevent absorption of medication through the skin of health care worker.
2. Explain the purpose of the medication and the position desired for the client.	2. Ensures nose drops will reach the area of treatment by gravity with the client assuming a dependent position.
3. Explain to the client the sensation of the local effects of the medications, such as burning, tingling, and effect on taste buds. If drops are used, explain to the client that a sensation of medications may be felt in the posterior oral pharynx.	3. Some nasal medications cause undesirable tastes. If this occurs, the health care provider may order other medications or encourage mouthwashes after treatment. Prepares the client for sensation that may be felt.
4. Have the client clear the nostrils by blowing the nose.	4. Removes discharge that would prevent medication from contacting the mucous membrane.
Nose Drops	
5. Follow the seven rights and three checks of safe medication administration.	5. Prevents medication error.
6. Ask client to lie supine and hyperextend the neck (Figure 30-16-2). Turn head to the appropriate position described in the Overview.	6. Allows the nose drops to reach the appropriate area.
7. Squeeze some medication into dropper.	7. Makes medication ready to administer.
8. Have client exhale and occlude one nostril with a finger.	8. Readies client to inhale as medication is administered.
9. Insert dropper about 3⁄8 inch into the nostril, keeping it away from the sides of the nostril. Ask client to inhale as prescribed dosage of medication is administered.	9. Prevents getting microorganisms back into medication bottle. Medication is distributed better during inhalation.
10. Discard any unused medication remaining in the dropper.	10. Prevents contamination of medication.
11. Client may blot excess drainage but may not blow the nose and should remain in position for 5 minutes.	11. Removes discomfort of drainage on face. Allows time for medication to be absorbed.
12. Repeat on other nostril if ordered.	12. Generally, both nostrils are treated.
Nasal Inhalers	
13. Repeat Actions 1 to 5.	13. See Rationales 1 to 5.
14. Explain the manufacturer's directions and how inhalers work.	14. Clients will be more compliant if they understand the use of the inhalers and that a fine cold mist will be released into the nasal passage via a pressurized container.
15. Have the client assume an upright position. Squeeze nose drops into dropper.	15. The client should be as comfortable as possible. Makes medication ready to administer.
16. Have the client exhale and occlude one nostril with a finger.	16. Readies the client to inhale as medication is administered.

(Continues)

PROCEDURE 30-16 Administering Nasal Medications (Continued)

ACTION	RATIONALE

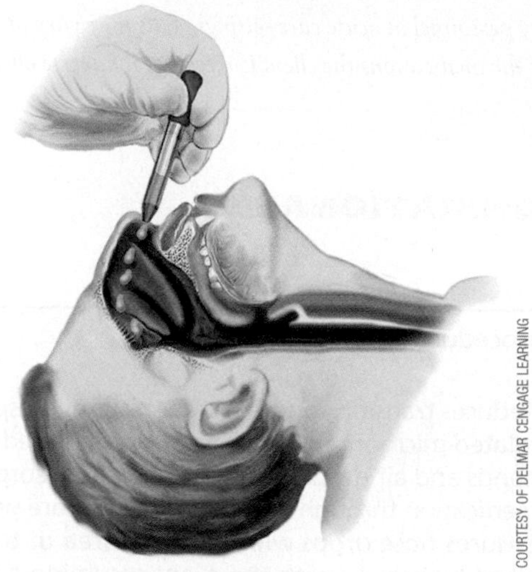

FIGURE 30-16-2 Positioning a client for nose drop instillation.

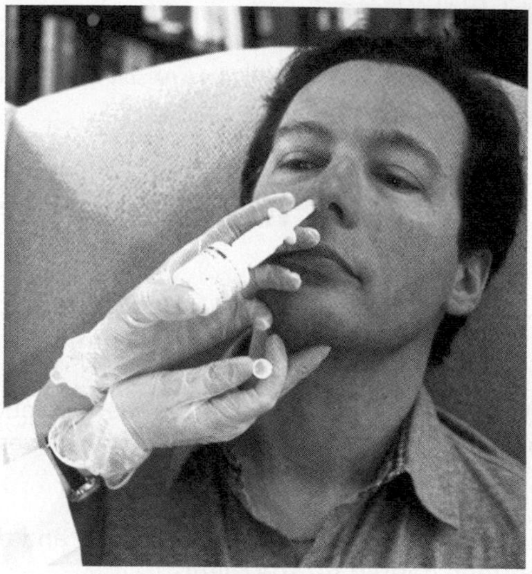

FIGURE 30-16-3 Ask the client to inhale while the spray is administered.

ACTION	RATIONALE
17. Ask the client to inhale while the spray is administered (Figure 30-16-3).	17. Nasal medications are more effective if instilled during inhalation.
18. Repeat the procedure on the other nostril.	18. Most often, both nostrils are treated.
19. Remove all soiled supplies and dispose of them according to Standard Precautions. Remove gloves. Wash hands carefully.	19. Decreases the chance of transmission of microorganisms. Respiratory diseases are especially easily transmitted.
20. Evaluate the effect of the medication in 15 to 20 minutes.	20. Identifies if the medication is effective without adverse side effects.

EVALUATION

- The client is free of nasal congestion.
- The client is free of nasal discharge and odor.
- The client breathes freely through the nasal passages.
- The client is free of sinus pain and nasal pain.
- The client's nasal passages are moist and pink.
- The client is free of adverse side effects secondary to the nasal medication.

DOCUMENTATION

Medication Administration Record

- Time and date medication was given, amount (number of drops may be necessary), and nostril medicated.

Nurses' Notes

- Results of the treatment
- Adverse or unpleasant side effects
- Document (seventh right) on appropriate electronic medical record or flow sheet

PROCEDURE 30-17 Administering Rectal Medications

OVERVIEW

The administration of rectal medications is an important responsibility for nurses in numerous health care settings. Rectal suppositories include medications that produce both local and systemic effects. Suppositories that produce a local effect include laxatives, which promote defecation. Medications to help relieve nausea, fever, or bladder spasms can also be administered via rectal suppository but produce a systemic effect.

(Continues)

PROCEDURE 30-17 Administering Rectal Medications (Continued)

ASSESSMENT

1. Assess the seven rights: right client, right medication, right route, right dose, right time, right to refuse, and right documentation. **Prevents errors in medication administration.**
2. Review the health care provider's order and identify the medication to be delivered, verifying dosage, route, time, and correct client. **This ensures safe and correct administration of medications.**
3. Assess the client's need and appropriateness for rectal medication administration and review the client's history for contraindications. **A history of rectal surgery or bleeding may contraindicate use of a suppository.**
4. Consider any adjustments that may need to be taken in delivery of medications resulting from the age of the client. **This allows the nurse to deliver the medication in a correct manner if the client is an infant, child, or adult.**
5. Observe the client for the desired therapeutic effects or any adverse reactions, and document this response appropriately **to determine the effectiveness of the treatment.**
6. Assess the client's knowledge and understanding of the procedure. **Explaining the procedure will decrease client fear and anxiety and will promote understanding and cooperation. If physically able, the client may wish to self-administer the medication.**
7. Assess the client's rectal area to determine condition of skin, mucosa, and presence of hemorrhoids or other rectal conditions. **Preventive action can be taken to protect injured skin and ensure client comfort.**

POSSIBLE NURSING DIAGNOSES

Dysfunctional Gastrointestinal Motility
Constipation
Nausea
Chronic Pain

PLANNING

Expected Outcomes

1. The medication will be delivered appropriately and safely following the seven rights of medication administration.
2. The desired outcome will be verbalized by the client and documented appropriately by the nurse.
3. The treatment will be completed as quickly and efficiently as possible to decrease discomfort and anxiety.
4. Client will state relief of complaint after medication administration.

Equipment Needed (Figure 30-17-1)

- Medication (suppository or medicated enema)
- Water-soluble lubricant
- Nonsterile latex-free gloves
- Tissue or washcloth
- Bedpan if client physically immobile
- Medication administration record
- Towels or pads (such as disposable "Blue pads")

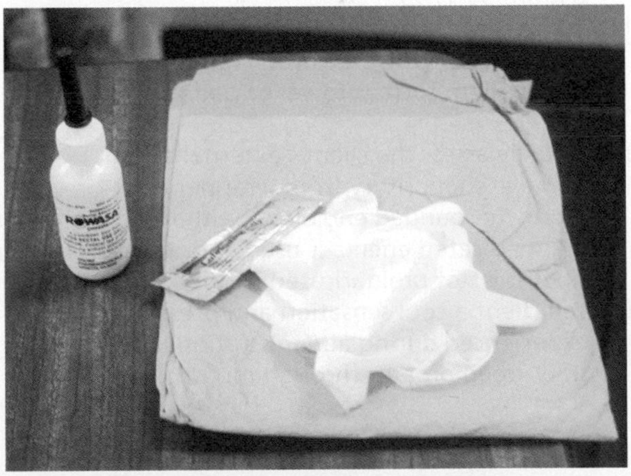

COURTESY OF DELMAR CENGAGE LEARNING

FIGURE 30-17-1 Latex-Free Gloves, Protective Pad, Water Based Lubricant, and Rectal Medication

delegation tips

The procedure of medication administration is not delegated to ancillary personnel in acute care settings. This may vary in state or federal institutions. Ancillary personnel are generally informed about the medications the client is receiving if adverse effects are anticipated or are being monitored.

(Continues)

PROCEDURE 30-17 Administering Rectal Medications (Continued)

IMPLEMENTATION—ACTION/RATIONALE

* Check client's identification band * Explain procedure before beginning *

ACTION	RATIONALE
1. Assess the client's need for the medication.	1. Allows the nurse to determine the need and effectiveness of the medication.
2. Check the health care provider's written order.	2. Ensures safe and accurate administration of medication.
3. Check the medication administration record against the written order to verify the correct client, medication, route, time, and dosage.	3. Decreases the chance of a medication error and ensures accuracy (right dosage, right route, right time, right client, right medication, right to refuse, and right documentation).
4. Assess client for any drug allergies.	4. Decreases the risk for an allergic reaction.
5. Review the client's history for any previous surgeries or bleeding.	5. Contraindications for rectal administration may be discovered.
6. Gather the equipment needed for the procedure before entering the client's room.	6. Prevents numerous trips to gather supplies and helps the procedure flow smoothly.
7. Provide privacy for client.	7. Maintains dignity and self-image.
8. Wash hands.	8. Reduces transmission of microorganisms.
9. Ask the client to state his or her full name and check his or her identification band.	9. Ensures correct client (right client).
10. Apply nonsterile latex-free gloves (Figure 30-17-2).	10. Prevents contact with fecal material.
11. Assist client into Sims' (left) position with upper leg drawn up toward chest. Provide protection under client such as towel or pad.	11. The descending colon is on the left side; this is a more anatomically correct position. Exposes the anus to identify placement. Provides comfort to client who may fear soiling linen.
12. Visually assess the client's external anus.	12. Determines presence of any active bleeding.
13. Remove suppository from wrapper and lubricate rounded end along with insertion finger. If a medicated enema is used, lubricate the enema tip if it is not prelubricated (Figure 30-17-3).	13. Lubrication decreases friction and decreases discomfort.
14. Tell client a cool sensation and pressure will be experienced during administration. Encourage slow, deep breaths through mouth.	14. Prepares the client for administration. Relaxes the rectal sphincter.

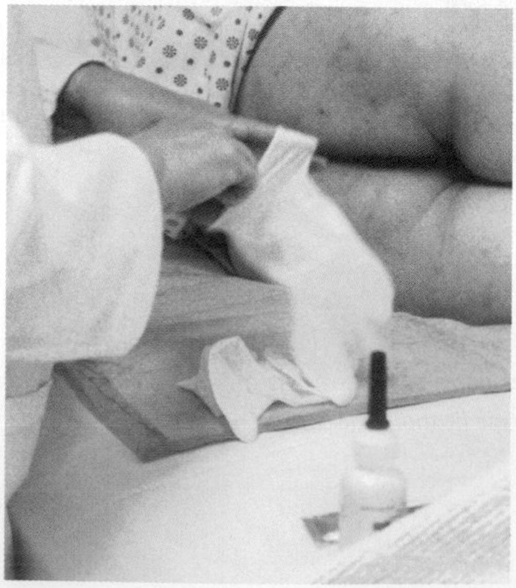

COURTESY OF DELMAR CENGAGE LEARNING

FIGURE 30-17-2 Apply latex-free gloves before administering rectal medications.

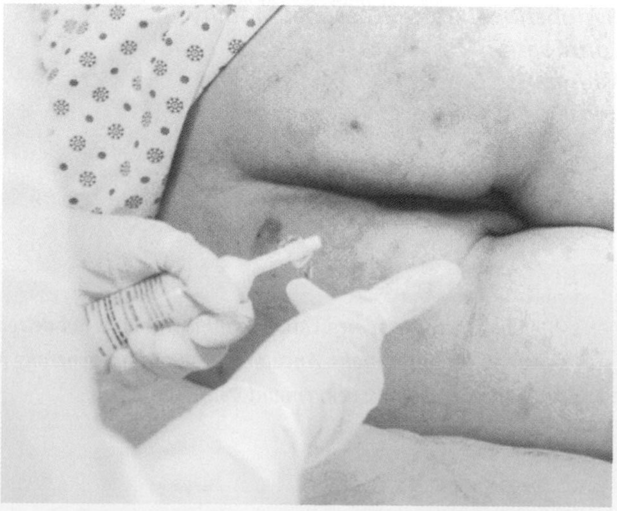

COURTESY OF DELMAR CENGAGE LEARNING

FIGURE 30-17-3 The enema needs to be lubricated with water soluble lubricant.

(Continues)

PROCEDURE 30-17 Administering Rectal Medications (Continued)

ACTION	RATIONALE
15. Retract buttocks with nondominant hand, visualizing the anus (Figure 30-17-4). Using the dominant index finger, slowly and gently insert the suppository through the anus, past the internal sphincter, and against the rectal wall (Figure 30-17-5). Depth of insertion will differ if client is a child or infant. If instilling a medicated enema, gently insert the enema tip past the internal sphincter and instill the contents by slowly squeezing (Figure 30-17-6).	15. Slow insertion minimizes pain. Correct placement ensures adequate absorption and less chance for expulsion of medication.
16. Remove finger or enema tip and wipe client's anal area with a washcloth or tissue.	16. Removes lubricant externally. Promotes cleanliness and comfort.
17. Remove and discard gloves.	17. Reduces transfer of microorganisms.
18. Wash hands.	18. Reduces transfer of microorganisms.
19. Have client remain in position for 10 to 15 minutes.	19. Keeps suppository or medicated fluid in place for better absorption.
20. Place call light in client's reach.	20. Gives client control over situation.
21. Document administration of medication (seventh right).	21. Provides documentation of medication administration.
22. Document effectiveness or any side effects on nursing notes.	22. Communicates effectiveness of treatment with other caregivers.

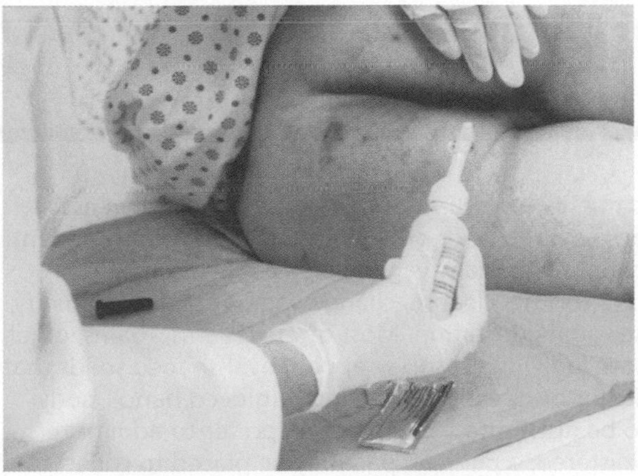

COURTESY OF DELMAR CENGAGE LEARNING

FIGURE 30-17-4 Retract the buttocks and visualize the anus.

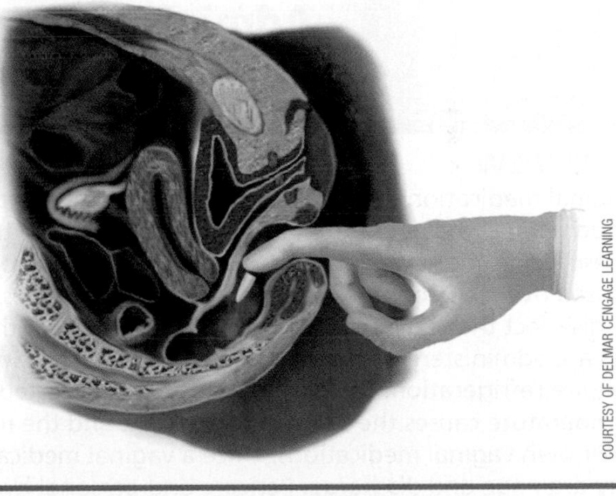

COURTESY OF DELMAR CENGAGE LEARNING

FIGURE 30-17-5 Inserting a Rectal Suppository

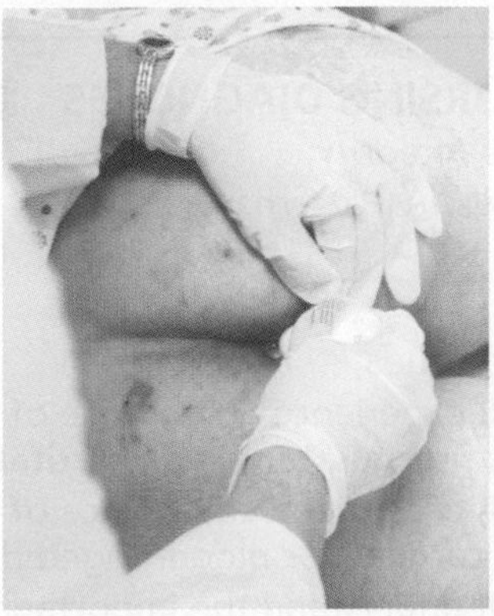

COURTESY OF DELMAR CENGAGE LEARNING

FIGURE 30-17-6 When administering an enema, gently insert the enema tip and instill the contents by slowly squeezing the bottle.

(Continues)

PROCEDURE 30-17 Administering Rectal Medications (Continued)

EVALUATION

- The medication was delivered appropriately and safely, following the seven rights of medication administration.
- The desired outcome was verbalized by the client and documented appropriately by the nurse.
- The treatment was completed as quickly and efficiently as possible to decrease discomfort and anxiety.
- Client stated relief of complaint after medication administration.

DOCUMENTATION

Medication Administration Record

- Name of medication
- Dosage
- Route of administration
- Time administered
- Initials and signature of nurse administering medication

Nurses' Notes

- Time and type of client complaint
- Medication administered
- Outcome of treatment (client response)
- Health care provider notified, if needed
- Nurse's signature
- Document on appropriate electronic medical record or flow sheet.

PROCEDURE 30-18 Administering Vaginal Medications

OVERVIEW

Vaginal medications come in the form of creams, suppositories, foams, jellies, or irrigations (commonly known as douches). Vaginal medications are generally used to treat infections, irritations, or pruritis requiring topical treatment. These medications may be prescribed by a physician or nurse practitioner, or many vaginal medications can be purchased over-the-counter (OTC). Irrigations or douches can be used to soothe, cleanse, change vaginal acidity/alkalinity, or disinfect the vagina; however, if used excessively, they can cause vaginal irritation. Most often, creams, foams, or jellies are administered with an applicator or inserter. Suppositories are individually foil-wrapped, oval-shaped solids that require refrigeration. Once the suppository is inserted by an applicator or directly with a finger (gloved hand), body temperature causes the suppository to melt and the medication to be distributed. Clients often prefer to administer their own vaginal medications. Once a vaginal medication is administered, a perineal pad may be placed to collect any drainage and discharge. Pericare and personal hygiene are essential because many vaginal infections cause foul-smelling discharge and irritation. Assess the client's level of pain, pruritis, burning, or general discomfort to establish a baseline for future assessment.

ASSESSMENT

1. Assess the client's comfort level. Evaluate the level of burning, irritation, pruritis, pain, and odor **to establish a baseline for assessment of treatment.**
2. Assess the client's knowledge of the purpose of the medication and treatment. **Enables client to understand and monitor effects of medication.**
3. If the client prefers to self-administer the medication, assess the client's ability to do so, such as ability to manipulate the applicator or insert a suppository the appropriate distance. **Clients may prefer to self-administer vaginal medications for privacy, but if medication is not properly inserted, it will not be effective.**

POSSIBLE NURSING DIAGNOSES

Impaired Tissue Integrity
Ineffective Sexuality Patterns

PLANNING

Expected Outcomes

1. Client will experience an absence of vaginal infection, pruritus, burning, or irritation.
2. Client will experience an absence of foul-smelling, curdlike, or blood-tinged discharge.
3. Client will understand the importance of continued treatment until infection is absent.
4. Client will understand the importance of personal hygiene in combination with medication.

(Continues)

PROCEDURE 30-18 Administering Vaginal Medications (Continued)

5. Client will understand the need to properly clean and store equipment.

Equipment Needed (Figure 30-18-1)

- Vaginal medication: cream, foam, jelly, or suppository
- Applicator (if needed)
- Water-soluble lubricating jelly (for suppository)
- Nonsterile latex-free gloves
- Perineal pad
- Paper towel, toilet tissue, or tissue paper
- Washcloth and warm water (optional)

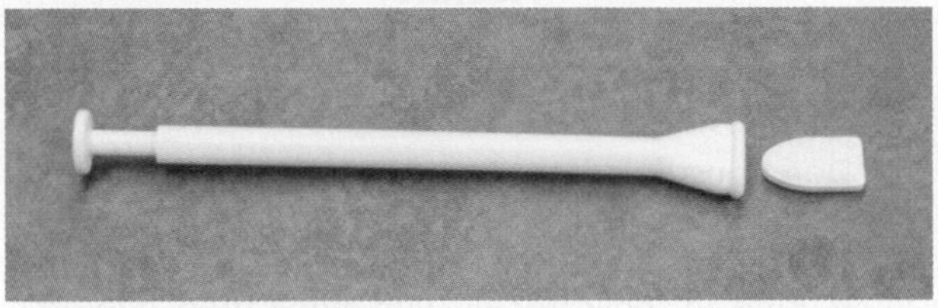

FIGURE 30-18-1 Vaginal Medication and Applicator

delegation tips

The procedure of medication administration is not delegated to ancillary personnel in acute care settings. This may vary in state or federal institutions. Ancillary personnel are generally informed about the medications the client is receiving if adverse effects are anticipated or are being monitored.

IMPLEMENTATION—ACTION/RATIONALE

ACTION	RATIONALE
* Check client's identification band * Explain procedure before beginning *	
1. Check the medication administration record against the health care provider's orders to verify the correct client, medication, route, time, and dosage.	1. Decreases the chance of a medication error and ensures accuracy (right dosage, right route, right time, right client, and the right medication).
2. Assess the client for any drug allergies.	2. Decreases the risk for an allergic reaction.
3. Ask the client to void.	3. Provides for client comfort during the procedure.
4. Wash hands.	4. Reduces transmission of microorganisms.
5. Arrange equipment at client's bedside.	5. Promotes organization.
6. Provide privacy by closing door and curtains.	6. Protects the client's privacy.
7. Assist the client into a dorsal-recumbent or Sims' position (Figure 30-18-2).	7. Allows for administration and for medication to remain in vagina.
8. Drape the client as appropriate, such as over the client's abdomen and lower extremities. Provide towel or protective pad on bed.	8. Provides privacy. Prevents linen from becoming soiled.

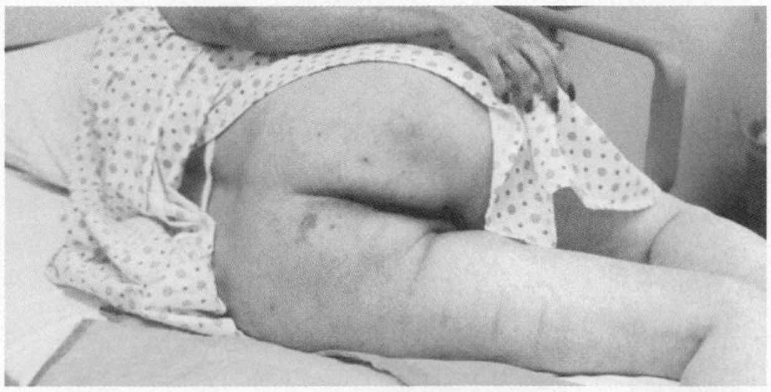

FIGURE 30-18-2 The client is placed in Sim's position for administering vaginal medication.

(Continues)

PROCEDURE 30-18 Administering Vaginal Medications (Continued)

ACTION	RATIONALE
9. Position lighting to illuminate vaginal orifice.	9. Assists in visualization of vagina and proper administration of medication.
10. Don nonsterile latex-free gloves and assess the perineal area for redness, inflammation, discharge, or foul odor.	10. Decreases transmission of microorganisms and risk of reaction to latex. Provides baseline data.
11. If using an applicator, fill with medication. If inserting a suppository, remove the suppository from the foil and position in the applicator (applicator is optional) (Figure 30-18-3). An applicator may be used for suppositories, or a gloved finger may be used. The foil is discarded. Apply water-soluble lubricant to suppository or applicator (optional for applicator).	11. Prepares medication for insertion. Lubricant provides comfort and ease of insertion.
12. For suppository, with nondominant hand, retract the labia (Figure 30-18-4).	12. Allows visualization of the vaginal orifice and eases insertion of medication.
13. With dominant hand, insert the applicator 2 to 3 inches into the vagina, sliding the applicator posteriorly (Figure 30-18-5). Push the plunger to administer the medication (Figure 30-18-6). With a suppository, insert the tapered end first with the index finger or applicator along the posterior wall of the vagina (approximately 3 inches) (Figure 30-18-7).	13. Medication must be inserted completely to provide coverage of the entire vagina. When medication is deposited at the posterior end of the vagina, gravity will allow medication to move toward the orifice.

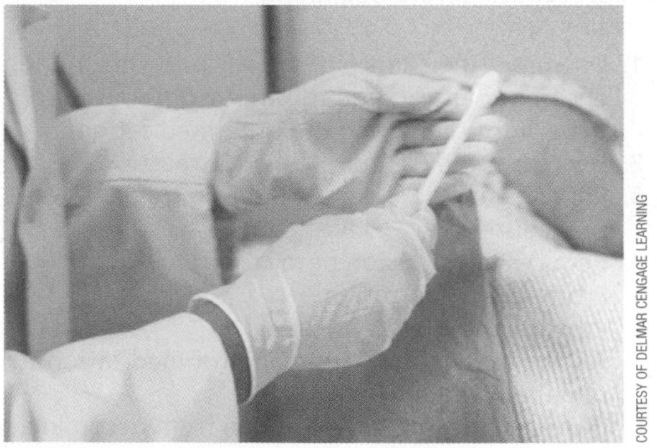

FIGURE 30-18-3 Place the vaginal suppository in the applicator.

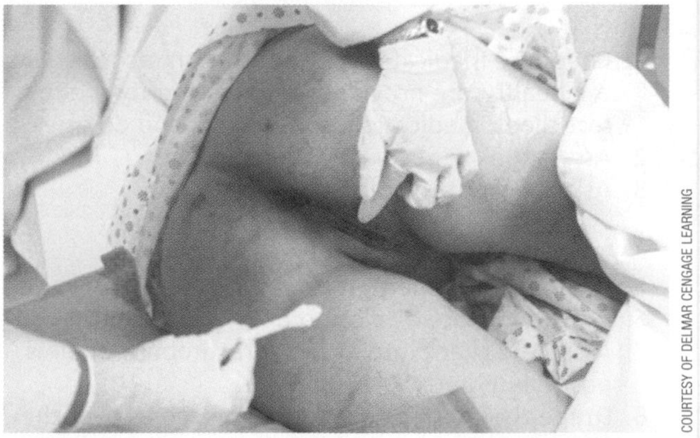

FIGURE 30-18-4 Retract the labia with the nondominant hand.

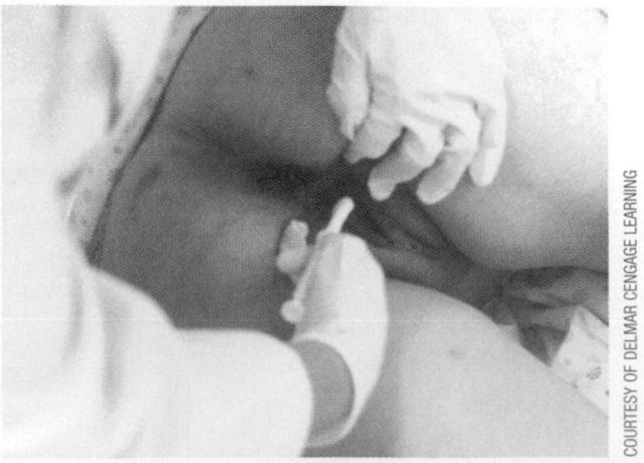

FIGURE 30-18-5 Slide the applicator 2 to 3 inches into the vagina.

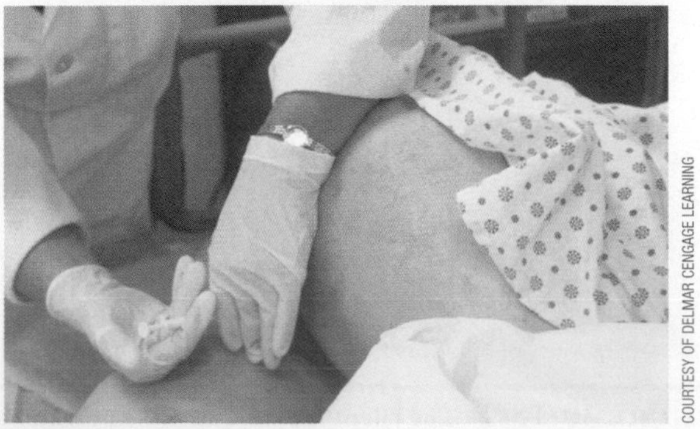

FIGURE 30-18-6 Push the plunger to administer the medication.

(Continues)

PROCEDURE 30-18 Administering Vaginal Medications (Continued)

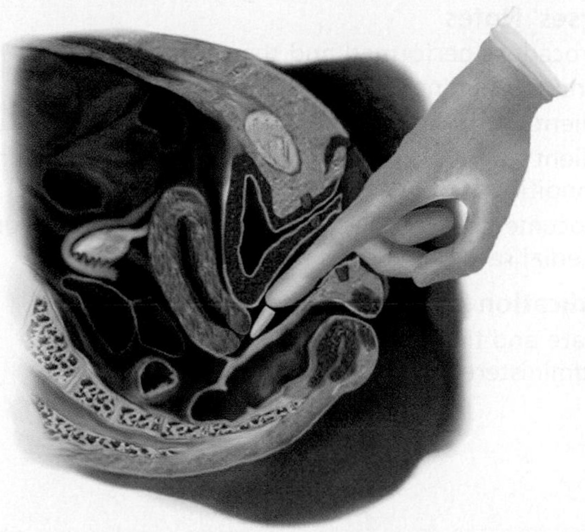

FIGURE 30-18-7 Inserting a vaginal suppository along the posterior wall of the vagina.

ACTION	RATIONALE
14. Withdraw the applicator and place on a towel.	14. Reduces transmission of microorganisms.
15. If administering a douche or irrigation:	15.
• Warm solution to slightly above body temperature (105° to 110°F). Check using the back of the hand or the wrist.	• Avoids burning the client. The mucous membranes of the vagina are sensitive.
• Position the client in a semirecumbent position on a bedpan, on a toilet seat, or in a tub.	• Provides comfort during procedure and allows for appropriate drainage of irrigation solution.
• Apply lubricant to the irrigation nozzle and insert approximately 3 inches into the vagina.	• Provides comfort.
• Hang the irrigant container approximately 2 feet above the client's vaginal area.	• Height is necessary for drainage by gravity. If the container is too high, the flow will be too forceful and uncomfortable.
• Open the clamp and allow a small amount of solution to flow into the vagina.	• Allows the client to evaluate the temperature.
• Move the nozzle and rotate around the entire vaginal area. If the labia are inflamed, allow the solution to flow over the labia as well. If the client is on the toilet seat, alternate between closing off the labia and allowing solution to be expelled.	• Rotation allows for irrigation throughout vagina. Closing off labia allows medication to stay in and flush total vagina.
16. Wipe and clean the client's perineal area, including the labia, from the front to the back with toilet tissue. Some clients may prefer that the perineal area is also cleaned with a washcloth and warm water.	16. Provides comfort for client and avoids spread of infective agents to perineal area.
17. Apply a perineal pad.	17. Protects client from discomfort of drainage and spread of infection or irritation to perineal area.
18. Wash the applicator (if reusable) with soap and warm water and store in appropriate container in client's room.	18. Applicator can only be used for individual clients; however, some applicators and inducers are reusable and must be appropriately cleaned and stored to prevent reinsertion of infective agents.
19. Remove gloves and wash hands.	19. Reduces transmission of microorganisms.
20. Instruct the client to remain flat for at least 30 minutes.	20. Allows maximum contact between the medication and the vaginal mucous membranes.
21. Raise side rails and place the call light in reach.	21. Provides for client comfort and safety.

(Continues)

PROCEDURE 30-18 Administering Vaginal Medications (Continued)

EVALUATION
- Client experiences an absence of vaginal infection, pruritus, burning, or irritation.
- Client experiences an absence of foul-smelling, curd-like, or blood-tinged discharge.
- Client understands the importance of continued treatment until infection is absent.
- Client understands the importance of personal hygiene in combination with medication.
- Client understands the need to properly clean and store equipment.

DOCUMENTATION
Nurses' Notes
- Procedure performed and the results
- Unusual findings or client complaints
- Client's response to treatment
- Client's signs and symptoms associated with vaginal condition
- Document (seventh right) on appropriate electronic medial record or flow sheet.

Medication Administration Record
- Date and time the medication/treatment was administered

PROCEDURE 31-19 Administering Nebulized Medications

OVERVIEW
A nebulizer is a device that is used to aerosolize medications into a mist for delivery directly into the lungs. Medication that is inhaled in the form of small droplets is absorbed immediately into the mucosa and bloodstream and is available to the body within minutes. This method of medication delivery is one of the fastest noninvasive methods of medication delivery. Many medications can be delivered by inhalation, but currently this delivery method is used primarily for medications designed to ease respiratory distress symptoms such as those seen with asthma.

There are two types of nebulizers: the single-dose nebulizer, which is driven by an air compressor, wall air, or wall oxygen, and the portable metered-dose inhaler. The single-dose, compressor-driven nebulizer delivers smaller droplets, allowing faster, more complete assimilation of the medication. The single-dose nebulizer can be filled with any type of medication that is ordered and can be used by clients who cannot coordinate use of the metered-dose inhaler. The primary drawback of the single-dose nebulizer is its lack of portability. The nebulizer must also be loaded with medication for each use, thus delaying the client's relief.

The metered-dose inhaler has the benefit of being small and portable. It can be carried in the client's pocket. Because the meter dispenses measured doses of the preloaded medication, no special training is needed to prime the inhaler. The primary drawback of a metered-dose inhaler is the need to coordinate dispensing the dose and inhalation. A spacer or extender chamber may be attached to the mouthpiece of the inhaler to hold the medication in suspension and provide the client an opportunity to inhale all the medication so that the dose is not lost during exhalation.

ASSESSMENT
1. Assess the seven rights: right client, right medication, right route, right dose, right time, right to refuse, and right documentation. **Prevents errors in medication administration.**
2. Assess the client's respiratory status. Note if the client is using accessory muscles for respiration or if there is flaring of the nares. Auscultate the client's chest for wheezes and crackles. **Respiratory distress is the primary reason to administer nebulized medications.**
3. Evaluate the history of this episode of the client's distress. Take a complete history from the client or a reliable informant about the symptoms and length of time the client has had them. Respiratory distress can have many causes. Asthma, bronchitis, a foreign object in the airways, and chronic obstructive pulmonary disease can all cause respiratory distress. **Assessing the client's current symptoms provides more accurate diagnosis and care. The client's history of asthma does not mean that this episode of distress is asthma.**

(Continues)

PROCEDURE 30-19 Administering Nebulized Medications (Continued)

4. Assess the client's ability to use the nebulizer or metered-dose inhaler. Determine the client's ability to understand and follow the directions, to hold and manipulate the equipment, and to coordinate the release of the medication with inhalation. **Determines the type of equipment used for the client. Very young children may need a mask instead of a mouthpiece on the nebulizer. The elderly may need specialized dispensers for their metered-dose inhalers.**
5. Assess the medication(s) currently ordered by the health care provider: action, purpose, common side effects, time of onset, and peak of action. **Permits the nurse to anticipate what to observe from the client.**
6. Assess the medications the client is currently taking, including over-the-counter drugs. **Some medications can interact. Beta-blockers (propranolol, atenolol, and betalol) can antagonize the beta agonists and cause or increase asthma symptoms.**
7. Assess the client's knowledge regarding the medications and use of the nebulizer or metered-dose inhaler. **Allows the nurse to determine the need for client education to promote compliance.**
8. Verify the client's drug allergy history, **as an allergic reaction could occur.**

POSSIBLE NURSING DIAGNOSES

*Impaired **G**as Exchange*
*Ineffective **B**reathing Pattern*
*Deficient **K**nowledge* (proper use of the nebulizer or metered-dose inhaler)
Anxiety
Fear

PLANNING

Expected Outcomes

1. The client will experience improved gas exchange.
2. The client's breathing pattern will become effective.
3. The client will demonstrate understanding of the need for the medication and use of the nebulizer or metered-dose inhaler.
4. The client will not experience any adverse effects secondary to medication interactions.
5. The client's anxiety level will decrease following treatment.

Equipment Needed (Figures 30-19-1 and 30-19-2)

Handheld Nebulizer
- Medication administration record
- Nebulizer set (cup, tubing, cap, T-shaped tube, mouthpiece, or mask) or prepackaged nebulizer and applicator
- Medication(s)
- Saline
- Air compressor, wall air, or wall oxygen

Metered-Dose Inhaler
- Metered-dose inhaler
- AeroChamber, if appropriate

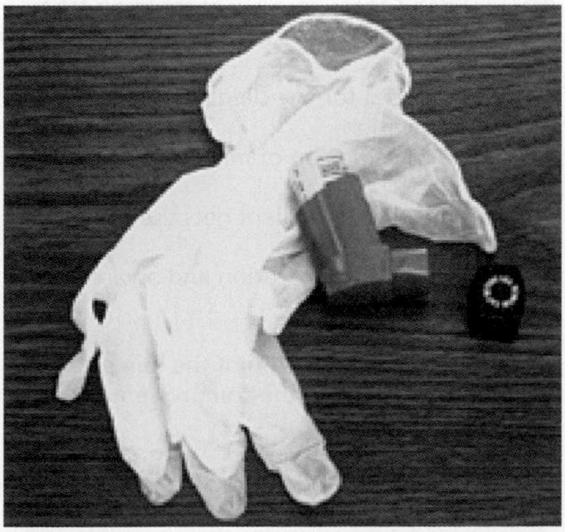
COURTESY OF DELMAR CENGAGE LEARNING

FIGURE 30-19-1 Handheld Metered-Dose Inhaler

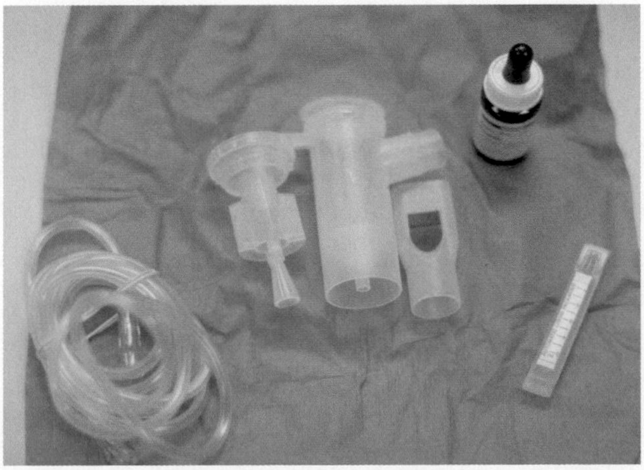
COURTESY OF DELMAR CENGAGE LEARNING

FIGURE 30-19-2 Nebulizer Cup, Tubing, Cap, T-Shaped Tube, Mouthpiece, and Medication

(Continues)

PROCEDURE 30-19 Administering Nebulized Medications (Continued)

delegation tips

The procedure of medication administration is not delegated to ancillary personnel in acute care settings. This may vary in state or federal institutions. Ancillary personnel are generally informed about the medications the client is receiving if adverse effects are anticipated or are being monitored.

IMPLEMENTATION—ACTION/RATIONALE

ACTION	RATIONALE
* Check client's identification band * Explain procedure before beginning *	
Single-Dose Handheld Nebulizer	
1. Assess the client's ability to use the nebulizer.	1. Ensures client compliance and accurate use of the nebulizer.
2. Check the medication administration record against the health care provider's written order to verify the correct client, medication, route, time, and dosage.	2. Decreases the chance of a medication error and ensures accuracy (right dosage, right route, right time, right client, and the right medication).
3. Assess the client for any drug allergies.	3. Decreases the risk for an allergic reaction.
4. Wash hands.	4. Reduces transmission of microorganisms
5. Set up and prepare the medication(s) for one client at a time.	5. Ensures the client receives the right medication(s).
6. Look at the medication at eye level if using a dropper to dispense the solution into the nebulizer.	6. Ensures accuracy.
7. Carefully pour the entire amount of the drug(s) into the nebulizer cup.	7. Determines the correct amount of medicine and ensures accurate dosage.
• Avoid touching the drug while pouring into the nebulizer cup.	• Reduces the transmission of microorganisms.
8. Cover the cup with the cap and fasten.	8. Prevents spillage of the medication.
9. Fasten the T-piece to the top of the cap.	9. Provides a connector for the mouthpiece.
10. Fasten a short length of tubing to one end of the T-piece.	10. Provides dead space to prevent room air from entering the system and medicated aerosol from escaping.
11. Fasten the mouthpiece or mask to the other end of the T-piece.	11. Provides a portal for the client to inhale the aerosolized medication.
• Avoid touching the nebulizer mouthpiece or the interior part of the mask.	• Reduces transmission of microorganisms.
12. Identify the client prior to the administration of the medication(s).	12. Ensures that the right client gets the medication.
13. Identify the medication(s) to the client and clearly explain the therapeutic purpose(s) of the medication.	13. Promotes client's cooperation and awareness of the medication's effects.
14. Advise the client to sit in an upright position.	14. Promotes better expansion of the lungs.
15. Attach tubing to the bottom of the nebulizer cup and attach the other end to the air compressor or wall air.	15. Provides a conduit for the compressed air.
• Before turning it on, adjust the wall oxygen valve to 6 liters/min (or less per health care provider's orders).	• Drives the medication into a mist or wet aerosol form.
• Leave the air on for about 6 to 7 minutes until the medications are used up.	• Allows the client to receive the entire dose of medication.

(Continues)

PROCEDURE 30-19 Administering Nebulized Medications (Continued)

ACTION	RATIONALE
16. Instruct the client to breathe in and out slowly and deeply through the mouthpiece/mask.	16. Promotes better deposition and efficacy of the medication in the airways.
• The client's lips should be sealed tightly around the mouthpiece.	
17. Remain with the client long enough to observe the proper inhalation-exhalation technique.	17. Ensures the correct use of the nebulizer to get the full effects from the medications administered.
18. Wash hands.	18. Reduces transmission of microorganisms.
19. When the nebulizer cup is empty, turn off the compressor or wall air.	19. Stops the aerosolization.
• Detach the tubing from the compressor and the nebulizer cup.	• Prepares components for cleaning or disposal.
• If the nebulizer is disposable, dispose of the nebulizer in the appropriate container.	• Prevents transmission of microorganisms.
• If the nebulizer is to be reused for this client, carefully wash, rinse, and dry the nebulizer components.	• Prevents transmission of microorganisms.
20. Assess the client immediately following the treatment for results or adverse effects from the treatment.	20. Determines the effectiveness of the treatment.
21. Reassess the client 5 to 10 minutes following the treatment.	21. Some effects may be delayed.
22. Wash hands.	22. Reduces transmission of microorganisms.
Metered-Dose Nebulizer	
23. Assess the client for ability to use the metered-dose nebulizer.	23. Ensures client compliance.
24. Check the medication administration record against the health care provider's order to verify the correct client, medication, route, time, and dosage.	24. Decreases the chance of a medication error and ensures accuracy (right dosage, right route, right time, right client, and the right medication).
25. Assess the client for any drug allergies.	25. Decreases the risk for an allergic reaction.
26. Wash hands.	26. Decreases transmission of microorganisms.
27. Shake the prepackaged nebulizer.	27. Thoroughly mixes the medication.
28. Place the nebulizer into the applicator.	28. Allows for proper administration of the medication.
29. Place the AeroChamber onto the nebulizer if needed (Figure 30-19-3).	29. The AeroChamber provides dead space for the medicated mist while the client inhales.

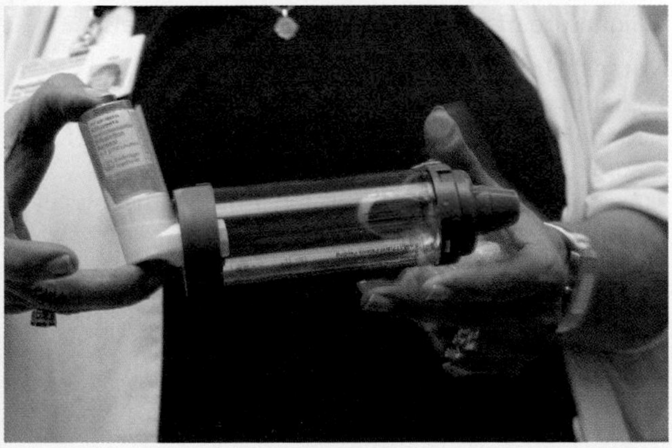

FIGURE 30-19-3 Preparing a Metered-Dose Inhaler and Medication

(Continues)

PROCEDURE 30-19 Administering Nebulized Medications (Continued)

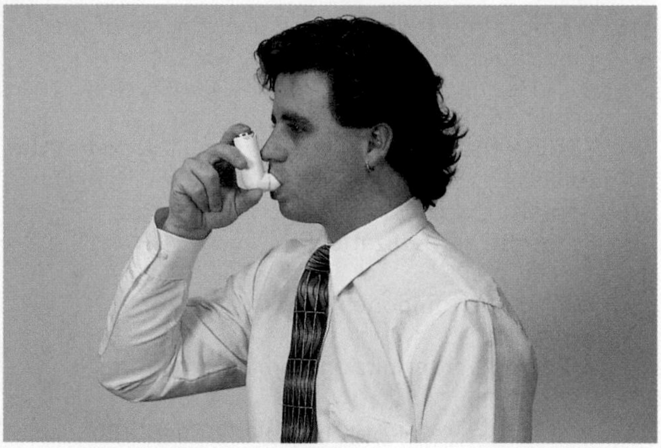

FIGURE 30-19-4 Self-Administration with a Metered-Dose Inhaler

ACTION	RATIONALE
30. Have the client exhale and place the mouthpiece in his or her mouth (Figure 30-19-4).	30. Prepares for delivery of the medication to the lungs.
31. Have the client press down on the prepackaged dispenser and simultaneously inhale slowly until lungs feel full. Hold breath for 10 seconds and exhale slowly.	31. Draws medication into the lungs. Allows medication to reach alveoli.
32. If there is an AeroChamber attached to the nebulizer, have the client inhale slowly and deeply.	32. Allows for proper delivery of the medication.
33. Observe the client for several minutes to assess for possible adverse effects from the medication.	33. Reactions can occur right away.
34. Have the client rinse his or her mouth.	34. The medication may leave a metallic taste.
35. Wash hands.	35. Prevents transmission of microorganisms.
36. Document the medication administration (seventh right).	36. Provides a record of medication administration.

EVALUATION

- The client experienced improved gas exchange.
- The client's breathing pattern became effective.
- The client demonstrates understanding of the need for the medication and the use of the nebulizer or metered-dose inhaler.
- The client did not experience any adverse effects secondary to medication interactions.
- The client's anxiety level decreased following treatment.

DOCUMENTATION

Medication Administration Record

- Name of medication(s)
- Dosage
- Route
- Site
- Time of administration
- Initials of the nurse who administered the medication(s)
- Signature of the nurse identifying the initials

Nurses' Notes

- Client's assessment parameters
- Name of medication, dosage, route, and time of administration
- Amount of oxygen delivered per minute from wall oxygen or air compressor machine
- Signature and initials of the nurse
- Client's response
- Document on appropriate electronic medical record or flow sheet.

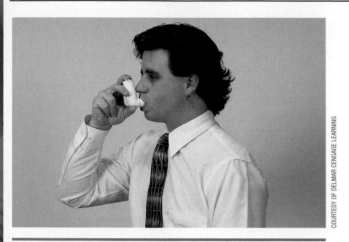

PROCEDURE 30-20 Applying a Dry Dressing

OVERVIEW

A closed surgical wound can be described as a wound that was caused, revised, or debrided by a surgical intervention. Closed wounds are generally categorized as clean. They may be closed with sutures, staples, or tapes. The general purpose of the closed wound dressing is to cover and protect as well as absorb the minimal drainage that may occur with this type of wound. Dressing care may vary according to the surgeon's preference and institutional policy. General guidelines for the closed surgical wound dressing is covered in this procedure.

There are different approaches to wound care. Cleaning solutions can dry the wound and interfere with wound healing at the cellular level. Furthermore, clients may be allergic or sensitive to these solutions. Although they reduce the risk of infection, frequent application may not be necessary. In many cases, sterile normal saline, sterile water, or pH-neutral solutions will be adequate to cleanse the wound. It is standard for the surgeon to do the first postoperative dressing change. The initial dressing is maintained for 24 to 48 hours postoperatively, unless conditions of the dressing call for contacting the health care provider for a dressing change order. Until the removal of the initial dressing, reinforce the dressing as needed.

The frequency of the dressing change depends on the needs of the wound and the preference of the health care provider. This will usually be specified in the orders. It is important to follow agency guidelines and observe the preferences of the health care provider.

ASSESSMENT

1. Assess the client's comfort level postoperatively upon arrival from the operating room, before wound care, and as needed throughout the postoperative course. **Surgical wounds are painful. If clients are made comfortable with appropriate pain medications and positioning, there will be better tissue gas exchange from deep breathing, coughing, and early ambulation, thereby promoting healing of tissues. Clients will be more cooperative and less anxious during dressing changes if they are comfortable.**
2. Assess the external appearance of the initial postoperative dressing and subsequent dressings. **The initial dressing may need to be reinforced. Excess saturation with drainage, blood, or other bodily fluids, dislodgement, or anything unusual about the dressing should be brought to the attention of the health care provider. The appearance of the external portion of the dressing provides information about needed supplies.**
3. Assess the appearance of the wound and drains once the dressing is removed. **Inspection of the wound is important for assessment of the skin and tissues and for determining dressing supply needs. Assessment includes noting signs of infection as evident by redness, swelling, foul odor, amount of drainage, color of wound exudate (yellow and viscous would indicate purulent), or unusual pain or tenderness; signs of tissue trauma as evident by swelling or ecchymosis; evidence of bleeding or leakage of tissue fluids from the site; and the position of indwelling catheters, drainage tubes, and the sutures or stabilizing devices closing the wound and supporting the drains.**
4. Assess the client's understanding about the postoperative care of the surgical wound site. **It is important to take into consideration the client's ability to understand verbal and written instructions and the cultural and social variations that may affect the delivery of health care and client/family education.**
5. If solutions are to be used on the wound, assess the client's allergy status and test a drop of solution on the skin. **This prevents an adverse reaction.**

POSSIBLE NURSING DIAGNOSES

Impaired Skin Integrity
Impaired Tissue Integrity
Risk for Infection

PLANNING

Expected Outcomes

1. The site will be inspected for signs of infection, drainage, drainage tubes, and position of sutures or staples.
2. The initial postoperative dressing will be reinforced until changed by the health care provider.
3. The site will have the appropriate dressing applied.
4. The client/family will verbalize and/or demonstrate understanding and the ability, if indicated, to perform the dressing change and associated wound care of the surgical wound site.

Equipment Needed (Figure 30-20-1)

- Nonsterile latex-free gloves
- Container for proper disposal of soiled dressing
- Sterile 4 × 4 gauze pads
- Washcloth (optional)
- ABD pads (optional)
- 2-inch tape (foam or paper)
- Cleaning solution (if ordered)

(Continues)

PROCEDURE 30-20 Applying a Dry Dressing (Continued)

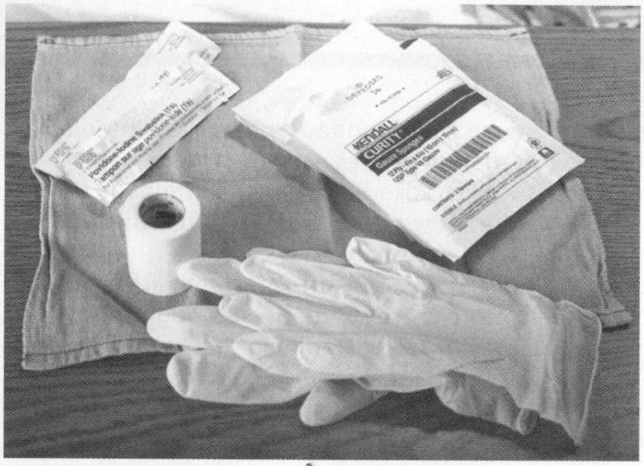

FIGURE 30-20-1 Clean gloves, gauze sponges, tape, and antiseptic solution are used to change a dry dressing.

delegation tips

The application of bandages is not delegated to ancillary personnel. Family members may be taught this before the client's discharge. Occasionally, ancillary personnel will be delegated the task of applying a clean dry gauze as skin protection, but the nurse is responsible for assessing the integrity of the client's skin.

IMPLEMENTATION—ACTION/RATIONALE

ACTION	RATIONALE
* Check client's identification band * Explain procedure before beginning *	
1. Gather supplies.	1. Promotes a smooth work flow.
2. Provide privacy; draw curtains; close door.	2. Maintains client comfort and privacy while body is exposed during procedure.
3. Wash hands.	3. Reduces transmission of microorganisms.
4. Apply nonsterile latex-free gloves.	4. Promotes infection control and protection from body fluids.
5. Remove dressing and place in appropriate receptacle. Remove soiled gloves with contaminated surfaces inward and discard in appropriate receptacle; apply nonsterile latex-free gloves.	5. Dressings and gloves soiled with body fluids are considered contaminated and subject to biohazard disposal in the correct manner per institution protocol.
6. Assess the undressed wound for signs of redness, foul odor, swelling, irritation, drainage, dehiscence, bleeding, or skin breakdown.	6. These may be signs of infection or inadequate wound healing.
7. Remove used exam gloves.	7. Exam gloves that are used to remove the old dressing are considered contaminated and should be removed and discarded appropriately.
8. Wash hands.	8. Reduces transmission of microorganisms.
9. Set up supplies. Open 4 × 4 gauze packages. • If incision requires cleaning, pour cleaning solution on 4 × 4 gauze pads (consult health care provider's orders and institution policy regarding cleaning incisions).	9. Following the removal of the dressing, you will have a better idea of what supplies are needed.
10. Apply a new pair of clean gloves.	10. This is considered to be a clean procedure after the initial dressing is removed if the skin margins are approximated with the skin closures.

(Continues)

PROCEDURE 30-20 Applying a Dry Dressing (Continued)

ACTION	RATIONALE

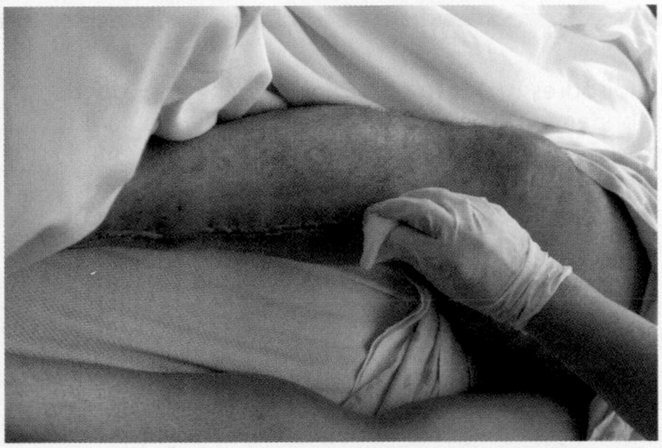

FIGURE 30-20-2 Clean the suture lines gently.

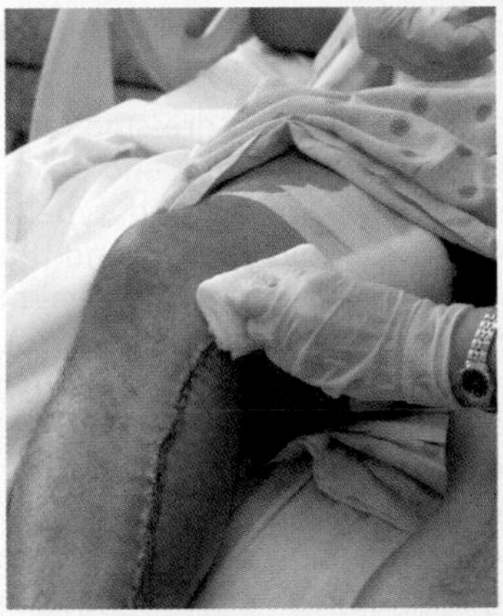

FIGURE 30-20-3 Apply 4 × 4 gauze pads, folded in half. Tape the gauze in place.

ACTION	RATIONALE
11. Cleanse wound if indicated. Grasp the edges of the gauze that contains cleaning solution. • **Incision:** Moving from top to bottom, clean the incision line first (Figure 30-20-2). Clean each side of incision using a new gauze for each swipe. • **Drain:** Using a circular motion, begin at the drain site and move outward. If additional cleaning is required, obtain a new gauze and clean from drain site outward.	11. Wounds are cleansed from least contaminated to most contaminated.
12. Remove gloves and wash hands.	12. Reduces transmission of microorganisms.
13. Apply nonsterile latex-free gloves.	13. Promotes infection control.
14. Apply a new dressing using 4 × 4 gauze pads folded in half to the 2 × 4 size. Place the folded gauze pad lengthwise on wound and tape lightly or apply tubular mesh for those with sensitive skin (Figure 30-20-3). Initial the dressing, citing date and time it was changed. • **Optional:** An ABD pad may be applied on top of the dressing for added protection over sutures or for client comfort.	14. A light dressing of 4 × 4 pads may be the only dressing that is needed to protect the incision from clothing or to collect a small amount of tissue drainage. This maintains a record of the dressing change for the next nurse.
15. Dispose of dressings appropriately, remove gloves, and then wash hands.	15. Reduces transmission of microorganisms.
16. Conduct client/family education about the dressing, which may include teaching the dressing technique to the client/family.	16. Educates the client/family and prepares for discharge.

EVALUATION

- Assess client comfort level during dressing change procedure.
- Determine whether the client's privacy was protected during the dressing change.
- Assess whether the correct supplies were brought in for the dressing change and whether any modifications need to be made to the dressing change.
- Determine the effectiveness of client/family education by having the client/family return-demonstrate the dressing or verbally review the steps of the dressing.

DOCUMENTATION

Nurses' Notes

- Date and time dressing done
- Brief description of the wound site
- Brief description of the site care done and dressing applied
- Client comfort before and after dressing change
- Client/family education done and evaluation of the teaching
- Document on appropriate electronic medical record or flow sheet.

(Continues)

PROCEDURE 30-21

Applying a Wet to Damp Dressing

OVERVIEW

The purpose of a wet to damp dressing (also known as wet to moist dressing) is to cover and protect the wound, collect exudate, promote healing, and promote light surface debridement. The decision to apply a wet to damp dressing depends on the wound bed, type of tissue and presence of eschar, amount of exudate, stage of wound healing, state of surrounding tissue, and the presence of infection.

Wound healing is promoted by a warm, moist environment; however, it is imperative to avoid moisture on the surface of the dressing. A wet external dressing can act as a wick with the external environment and draw contamination into the wound. Gentle debridement of a red wound is accomplished with a wet to damp dressing. One must be careful not to apply a dressing so wet that it ends up macerating the surrounding good tissue. Wet dressings are contraindicated in black eschar wounds, where the eschar represents full-thickness tissue destruction, because bacteria will multiply under such a dressing.

The wet to damp dressing consists of gauze, applied wet and allowed to become "near dry" before the next dressing change. Specifics of the wet to damp dressings vary according to the preferences of the surgeon and wound specialist, institutional policy, and outcome measurement standards used to evaluate the effectiveness of the dressing. General guidelines for a simple wet to damp dressing are covered.

ASSESSMENT

1. Assess the client's comfort level **to assess the need for medication before the dressing change**. Clients will be more cooperative and less anxious during dressing changes if they are comfortable.
2. Assess the external appearance of the dressing **to evaluate dressing adequacy as well as needed supplies.**
3. Assess the appearance of the wound and drains once the dressing is removed, noting redness, swelling, purulent drainage, or ecchymosis **to determine the condition of the wound and the effectiveness of the wet to damp dressing**.
4. Assess the client's understanding regarding the dressing changes and wound care **to determine any client teaching needed**.
5. Assess the client's healing response to previous treatments. The effectiveness of the wet to moist application should be routinely reassessed and the treatment modified if healing is not occurring.

POSSIBLE NURSING DIAGNOSES

Impaired Skin Integrity
Impaired Tissue Integrity
Risk for Infection
Acute Pain

PLANNING

Expected Outcomes

1. The site will be inspected for healing, signs of infection, and drainage.
2. The site will have the appropriate dressing applied.
3. The client/family will verbalize and/or demonstrate understanding and the ability, if indicated, to perform the dressing change and associated wound care of the surgical wound site.
4. The client will experience minimal discomfort during the procedure.

Equipment Needed (see Figure 30-21-1)

- Nonsterile latex-free gloves
- Container for proper disposal of soiled dressing
- Sterile gloves
- Moisture-proof gown (optional)
- Sterile towel
- Normal saline or ordered solution
- Sterile bowl
- Sterile 4 × 4 gauze pads, multiple
- Cover sponges or fluffs (optional)
- ABD dressing pads
- 2-inch tape (foam or paper)
- Tubular mesh (optional)
- Montgomery straps (optional)

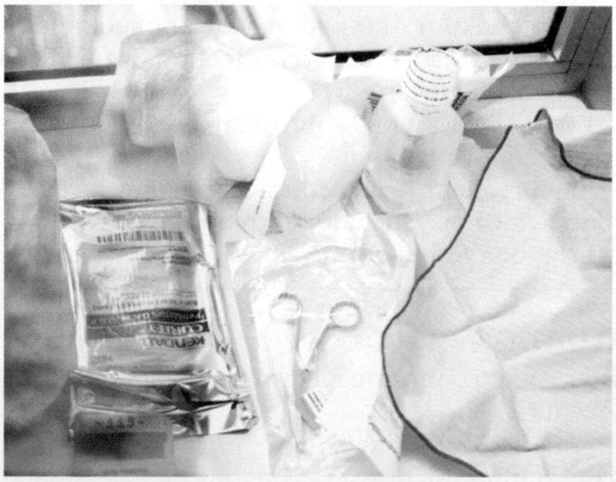

FIGURE 30-21-1 Sterile bandages, sterile saline, sterile scissors, and a sterile field are necessary to create a wet-to-damp dressing.

(Continues)

PROCEDURE 30-21 Applying a Wet to Damp Dressing (Continued)

delegation tips

Applying a wet to damp dressing requires sterile technique and professional assessment skills and cannot be delegated to ancillary personnel.

IMPLEMENTATION—ACTION/RATIONALE

ACTION	RATIONALE
* Check client's identification band * Explain procedure before beginning *	
1. Review order of health care provider for wound care and gather supplies.	1. Promotes a smooth work flow.
2. Provide privacy; draw curtains; close door.	2. Maintains client comfort and privacy while body is exposed during procedure.
3. Assess need for pain medication. Pain is rated on a scale from 0 (lowest) to 10 (greatest). Assess need based on quality, pain pattern, location, and last pain medication received.	3. Removal of a wet to damp or moist dressing may be painful to the client, so careful assessment of pain medication needs before the dressing change is important.
4. Wash hands.	4. Reduces transmission of microorganisms.
5. Apply nonsterile latex-free gloves. If there is copious drainage or the wound is infected, wear a gown, a mask, and eye protection.	5. Provides infection control and protection from body fluids.
6. Remove dressing, noting number of gauze pads used and place them in appropriate receptacle (Figure 30-21-2). If it is found that the dressing is extremely dry and removal will result in injury, a small amount of saline to loosen that portion of the dressing is indicated (Figure 30-21-3).	6. To counteract the problem of an extremely dry dressing, increase the wetness of the dressing or increase the frequency of dressing changes. Provides number of gauze pads needed to replace the dressing.
7. Observe the undressed wound for healing (granulation and approximation of edges), signs of infection (inflammation, edema, warmth, pain), and drainage.	7. Allows for evaluation of effectiveness of treatment.
8. Cleanse the skin around the incision if necessary with a clean, warm, wet washcloth.	8. Dried blood or drainage on the surrounding skin can be an irritant and a medium for microbes.

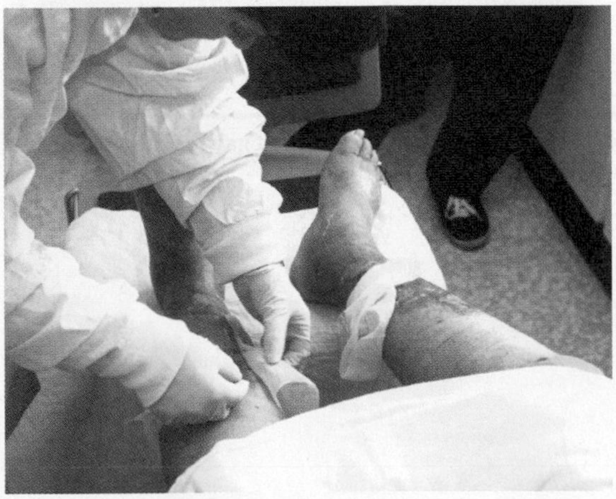

COURTESY OF DELMAR CENGAGE LEARNING

FIGURE 30-21-2 Carefully remove the old dressing, allowing the old dressing to debride the wound as you pull it away.

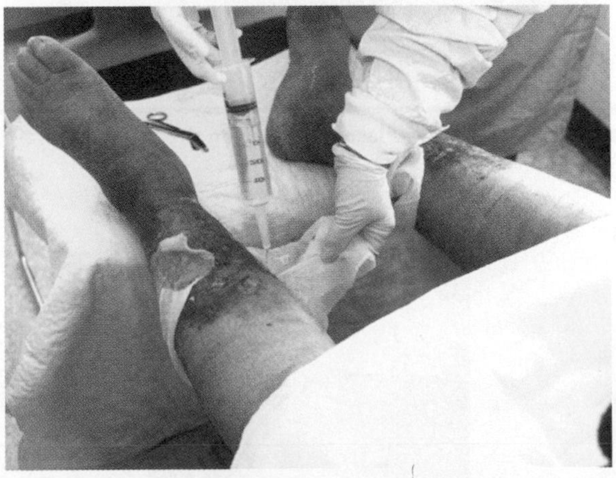

COURTESY OF DELMAR CENGAGE LEARNING

FIGURE 30-21-3 If the dressing is too dry and removing it will cause injury, use a small amount of saline to loosen the portion of the dressing that adheres too tightly to the wound.

(Continues)

PROCEDURE 30-21 Applying a Wet to Damp Dressing (Continued)

ACTION	RATIONALE
9. Remove gloves and wash hands.	9. Reduces transmission of microorganisms.
10. Set up supplies in a sterile field, including pouring ordered solutions into appropriate containers if indicated for the dressing.	10. Maintains sterility.
11. Apply sterile gloves.	11. This is a sterile dressing change.
12. Place gauze or packing material in the bowl with the normal saline or specified solution.	12. Wets gauze or packing material for dressing.
• Wring excess solution from gauze or packing. Avoid overwringing the dressing to prevent excessive drying.	• If too wet, wound bed can get soupy, increasing chance of bacterial growth.
• Gently place wet gauze over the area (Figure 30-21-4).	• Dresses the wound.
13. Apply external dressing of dry 4 3 4 gauze pads, cover sponges, fluffs, or ABD pads (Figure 30-21-5).	13. Prevents excess drying and protects wound.
• Secure dressing in place with tape, Montgomery straps, or tubular mesh (Figure 30-21-6).	• Tape for short-term dressings in clients who are not sensitive to adhesives. For long-term dressings or for those who are sensitive to tape, use Montgomery straps or tubular mesh to prevent skin irritation.
14. Remove gloves and wash hands.	14. Reduces transmission of microorganisms.
15. Mark the dressing with the date and time it was changed. Initial the dressing.	15. Maintains a record of the dressing change and provides for continuity of care.
16. Conduct client/family education about the dressing, which may include teaching the dressing technique to the client/family.	16. Educates the client/family and prepares for discharge.

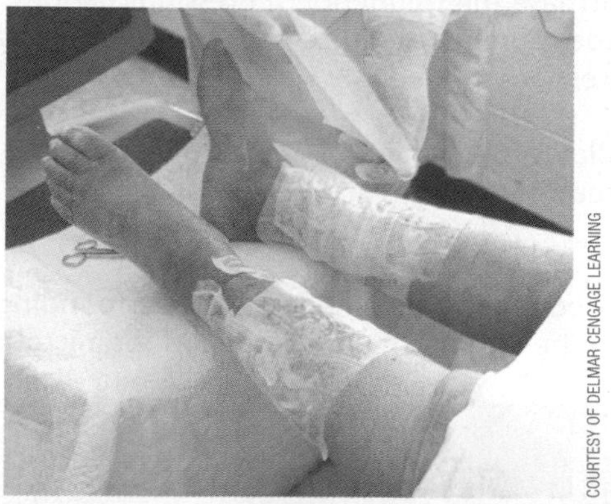

FIGURE 30-21-4 Place the gauze on the wound.

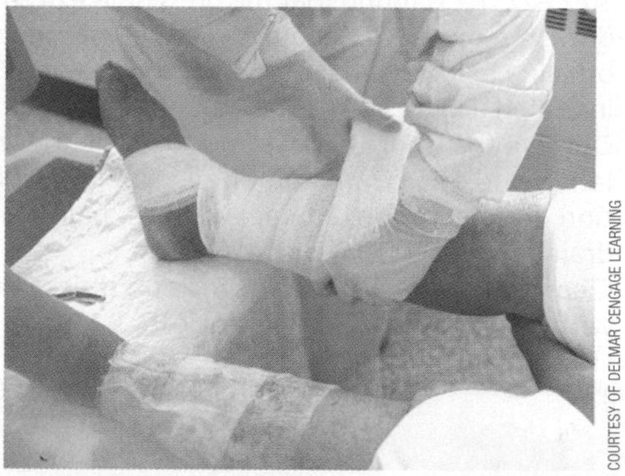

FIGURE 30-21-5 Wrap the wet gauze with an external dressing of dry gauze bandages.

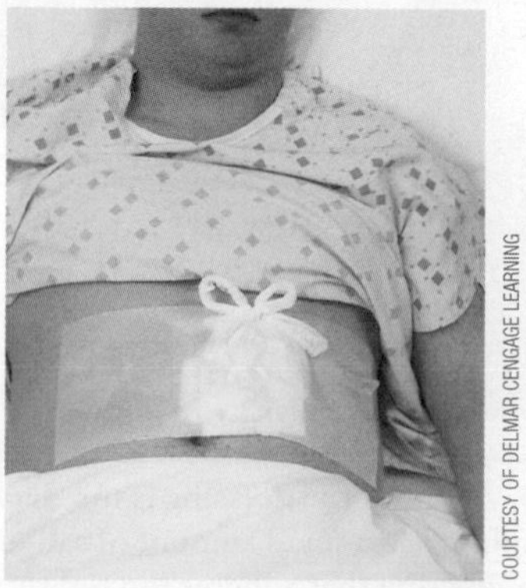

FIGURE 30-21-6 Montgomery Straps

(Continues)

PROCEDURE 30-21 Applying a Wet to Damp Dressing (Continued)

EVALUATION

- The site was inspected for healing, signs of infection, and drainage.
- The site had the appropriate dressing applied.
- The client/family verbalized or demonstrated understanding and the ability, if necessary, to perform the dressing change and associated wound care of the surgical wound site.
- The procedure was performed with minimal discomfort to the client.

DOCUMENTATION

Nurses' Notes

- Administration of pain medication before dressing change
- Date and time dressing done
- Brief description of the wound site
- Brief description of the site care done and dressing applied
- Client comfort before and after dressing change
- Client/family education done and evaluation of the teaching
- Document on appropriate electronic medical record or flow sheet.

PROCEDURE 30-22 Culturing a Wound

OVERVIEW

Bacterial wound contamination is one of the most common causes of altered wound healing. A surgical wound can become infected preoperatively, intraoperatively, or postoperatively. Nicks or abrasions created during preoperative shaving may be a source of pathogens. The risk for intraoperative exposure to pathogens increases when the respiratory, gastrointestinal, genitourinary, and oropharyngeal tracts are opened. Nonsurgical wounds from trauma, pressure ulcers, or disease can become infected as well.

If the amount of bacteria in the wound is sufficient or the client's immune defenses are compromised, clinical infection may become apparent 2 to 11 days postoperatively. Infection slows healing by prolonging the inflammatory phase of healing, competing for nutrients, and producing chemicals and enzymes that are damaging to the tissues. Identifying the infectious agent in a wound is an important step in wound healing.

ASSESSMENT

1. Assess the wound and the surrounding tissues for signs of infection. Check for heat, redness, inflammation, and drainage. Check the color and consistency of the drainage. Check the smell and color of the wound. **Allows for intervention to detect and treat infection.**
2. Assess the client's overall status, including vital signs, for signs of infection such as fever, chills, or elevated white blood cell count (WBC). **Allows for intervention to detect and treat infection.**

POSSIBLE NURSING DIAGNOSES

Risk for Infection
Impaired Skin Integrity
Disturbed Body Image

PLANNING

Expected Outcomes

1. The wound culture will be collected with a minimum of pain and trauma to the client.
2. The wound culture will be representative of the flora present in the wound, without contamination by flora outside the wound.

Equipment Needed (see Figure 30-22-1)

- Nonsterile latex-free gloves
- Sterile gloves and dressing supplies
- Normal saline and irrigation tray
- Culture tube and swab
- Moisture-proof container or bag

(Continues)

PROCEDURE 30-22 Culturing a Wound (Continued)

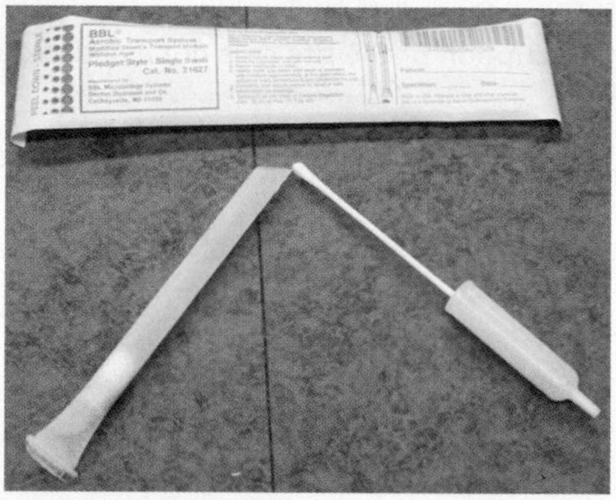

COURTESY OF DELMAR CENGAGE LEARNING

FIGURE 30-22-1 Sterile Culture Tube and Swab

delegation tips

Obtaining a wound culture requires nursing assessment and aseptic technique, and is potentially an invasive procedure; therefore, delegation to ancillary personnel is not appropriate.

IMPLEMENTATION—ACTION/RATIONALE

ACTION	RATIONALE
* Check client's identification band * Explain procedure before beginning *	
1. Wash hands, apply nonsterile latex-free gloves, and remove old dressing. Place old dressing in moisture-proof container and remove and discard gloves. Wash hands again.	1. Reduces transmission of microorganisms. Makes the wound accessible for obtaining the culture.
2. Open the dressing supplies using sterile technique and apply sterile gloves.	2. Maintains sterile environment.
3. Assess the wound's appearance; note quality, quantity, color, and odor of discharge.	3. Provides assessment of the amount and character of the wound's drainage before irrigation. Reddened areas and heavy drainage suggest infection.
4. Irrigate the wound with normal saline before culturing the wound; do not irrigate with antiseptic.	4. Decreases the risk of culturing normal flora and other exudates such as protein; an antiseptic may destroy the bacteria.
5. Using a sterile gauze pad, absorb the excess saline, then discard the pad.	5. Prevents maceration of tissue caused by excess moisture.
6. Remove the culture tube from the packaging (Figure 30-22-2). Remove the culture swab from the culture tube and gently roll the swab over the granulation tissue. Avoid eschar and wound edges (Figure 30-22-3).	6. Decreases the chance of collecting superficial skin microorganisms.
7. Replace the swab into the culture tube, being careful not to touch the swab to the outside of the tube. Recap the tube. Crush the ampule of medium located in the bottom or cap of the tube (Figure 30-22-4).	7. Avoids contamination with microorganisms. Releases the medium to surround the swab.
8. Remove gloves, wash hands, and apply sterile gloves. Dress the wound with sterile dressing.	8. Reduces transmission of microorganisms. Prevents contamination of the wound.

(Continues)

PROCEDURE 30-22 Culturing a Wound (Continued)

ACTION	RATIONALE

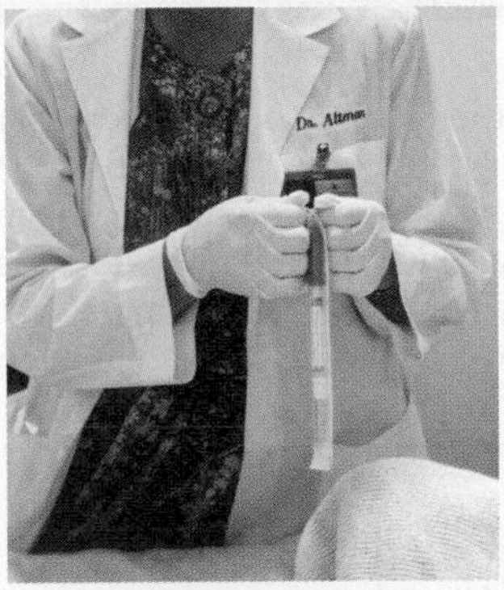

FIGURE 30-22-2 Remove the culture tube from the packaging.

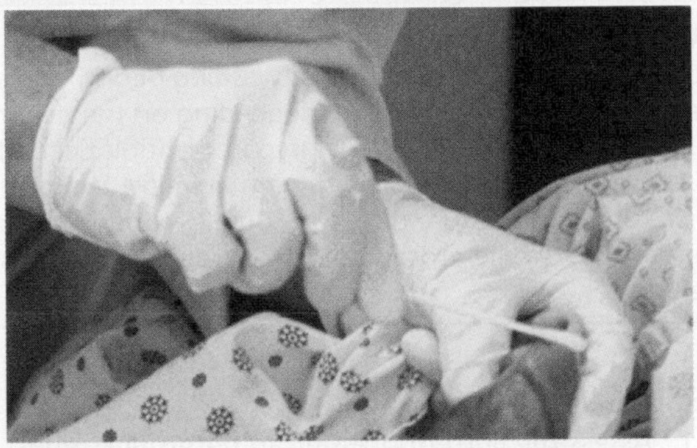

FIGURE 30-22-3 Roll the swab over the area to be cultured.

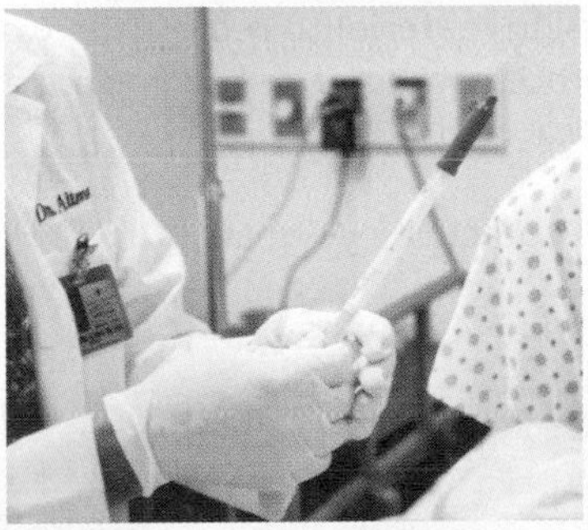

FIGURE 30-22-4 Crush the ampule to release the medium inside the culture tube.

ACTION	RATIONALE
9. Label the specimen, place in biohazard transport bag, and arrange to transport the specimen to the laboratory according to institutional policy.	9. Ensures proper handling of specimen.
10. Remove gloves and wash hands.	10. Reduces transmission of microorganisms.
11. Document assessment findings, actions taken, and that specimen was obtained.	11. Promotes continuity of care and records information for evaluation.

EVALUATION

- Assess whether the wound culture was collected with a minimum of pain and trauma to the client.
- Determine whether the wound culture is representative of the flora present in the wound, without contamination by other bacteria.

DOCUMENTATION

Nurses' Notes

- Time and method of collection of the culture, and what was done with the specimen
- Fill out the lab requisition form with the client's information as well as time and date specimen was collected, location of the culture, and requested tests. Often there are duplicate numbered or coded labels on the lab slips. One copy is placed in the chart.
- Document on appropriate electronic medical record or flow sheet.

(Continues)

PROCEDURE 30-23 Irrigating a Wound

OVERVIEW

Wound irrigation is the process of washing debris, drainage, or exudate out of the wound to promote healing. The fluid used to irrigate a wound varies depending on the health care provider's orders. Fluids commonly used include normal saline, acetic acid, and specially prepared antibiotic solutions. If cytotoxic solutions are used, then the area must be flushed/irrigated afterward with normal saline. Wounds that require irrigation also vary. They may be simple open lacerations; tunneled pressure ulcers; or complex, open abdominal wounds extending down to the abdominal fascia. Wound irrigation is a sterile procedure. Take care not to contaminate the wound and not to become contaminated with wound drainage.

ASSESSMENT

1. Assess the current dressing **to determine what equipment will be needed to replace it with a clean dressing and whether the dressing has been adequate to protect the wound and contain any drainage or exudate.**
2. Assess the client to determine if able **to understand the need for the wound irrigation and cooperate with the procedure.**
3. Assess whether the client has concerns about pain or body image regarding this wound and the irrigation **to determine what client teaching and support will be most effective.**
4. Assess the client's environment **to plan if the necessary equipment and supplies are available, including irrigant, hand hygiene facilities, and an adequate work area to lay out supplies and establish a sterile field.**

POSSIBLE NURSING DIAGNOSES

*Impaired **S**kin Integrity*
*Risk for **I**nfection*
*Acute **P**ain*

PLANNING

Expected Outcomes

1. The wound will be free of exudate, drainage, and debris.
2. The wound will be free of signs and symptoms of infection.
3. The procedure will be performed with a minimum of trauma and pain to the client.

Equipment Needed (see Figure 30-23-1)

- Sterile latex-free gloves
- Nonsterile latex-free gloves
- Sterile irrigation kit (basin, piston irrigation syringe, solution container)
- Irrigation solution (per health care provider's order)
- Waterproof pad
- Sterile dressing material to redress the wound
- Moisture-proof container or bag for use after the irrigation procedure
- Gown
- Mask with protective eye gear

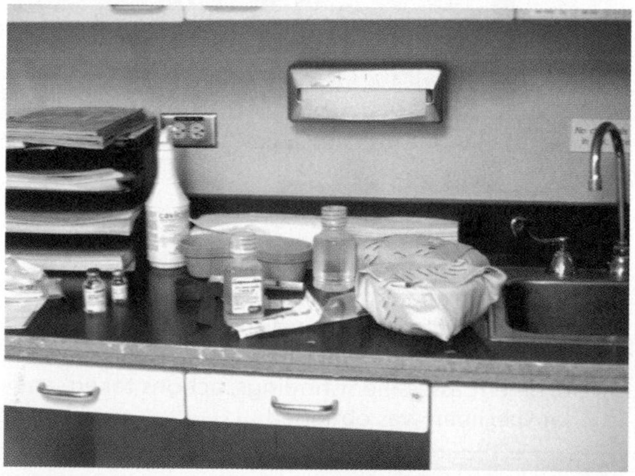

FIGURE 30-23-1 Sterile solution, sterile syringes, and a sterile basin are used to irrigate a wound.

delegation tips

Wound irrigation requires nursing assessment, aseptic technique, and monitoring of wound healing. This procedure is not delegated to ancillary personnel.

(Continues)

PROCEDURE 30-23 Irrigating a Wound (Continued)

IMPLEMENTATION—ACTION/RATIONALE

ACTION	RATIONALE
* Check client's identification band * Explain procedure before beginning *	
1. Confirm the health care provider's order for wound irrigation and note the type and strength of the ordered irrigation solution.	1. Wound irrigation is a dependent nursing action that requires a medical order stating the type of solution to be used.
2. Assess the client's pain level and medicate if needed with analgesic 60 minutes before procedure if the medication is to be given orally (PO) or intramuscularly (IM).	2. Allows time for medication to be absorbed to increase the analgesic effect.
3. Place a waterproof pad on the bed. Assist the client onto the pad. Then assist the client into a position that will allow the irrigant to flow through the wound and into the basin from the cleanest to dirtiest area of the wound.	3. Positioning of the client and placement of a waterproof pad will decrease contamination of bed linen.
4. Wash hands and apply nonsterile latex-free gloves, gown, and mask with protective eye gear if splashes from wound fluid or blood are anticipated. Remove and discard old dressing in appropriate receptacle.	4. Reduces transmission of microorganisms.
5. Assess the wound's appearance and note quality, quantity, color, and odor of drainage.	5. Provides assessment of wound status.
6. Remove gloves and wash hands.	6. Reduces transmission of microorganisms.
7. Prepare the sterile irrigation tray and dressing supplies. Pour the room-temperature irrigation solution into the solution container.	7. Prevents introduction of microorganisms into the wound. Reduces client discomfort.
8. Apply sterile gloves (new gown and goggles if needed).	8. Promotes sterile environment. Follows Standard Precautions.
9. Position the sterile basin below the wound so the irrigant will flow from the cleanest area to the dirtiest area and into the basin.	9. Decreases possibility of wound contamination.
10. Fill the piston or bulb syringe with irrigant and gently flush the wound. Hold the syringe approximately 1 inch above the wound bed to irrigate. Refill the syringe and continue to flush the wound until the solution returns clear and no exudate is noted or until the prescribed amount of fluid has been used (Figures 30-23-2 and 30-23-3).	10. Decreases trauma to granulation tissue, yet provides the ideal pressure for cleansing and removal of debris.

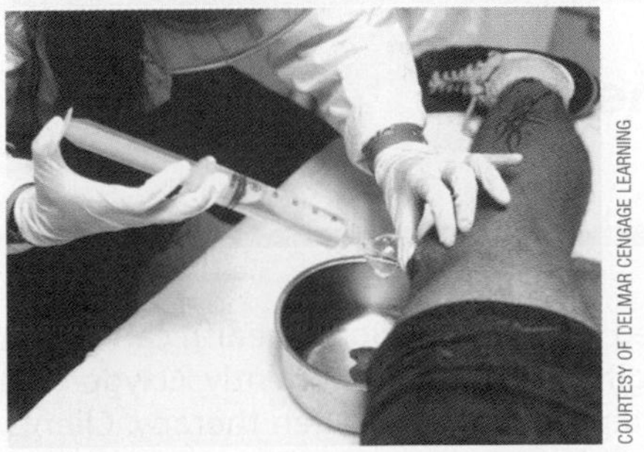

FIGURE 30-23-2 Gently flush the wound.

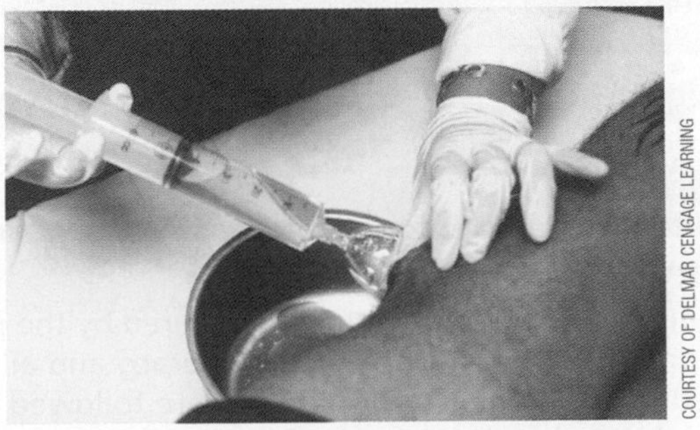

FIGURE 30-23-3 Hold the syringe close to the wound, but be careful not to touch the wound with the syringe.

(Continues)

PROCEDURE 30-23 Irrigating a Wound (Continued)

ACTION	RATIONALE

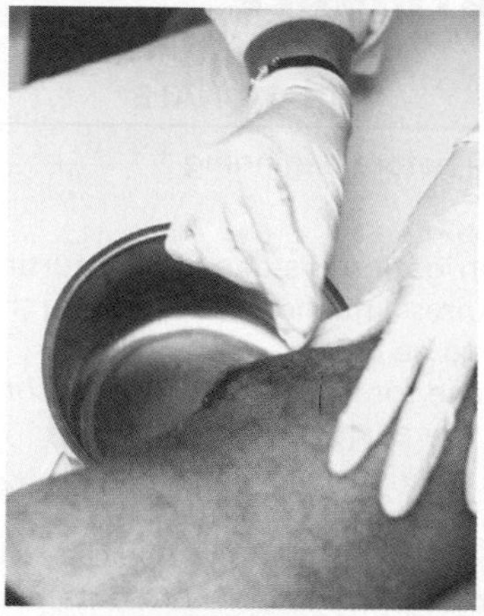

FIGURE 30-23-4 Dry the edges of the wound with sterile gauze.

ACTION	RATIONALE
11. Dry the edges of the wound with sterile gauze (Figure 30-23-4).	11. Prevents maceration of tissues caused by excess moisture.
12. Assess the wound's appearance and drainage.	12. Provides indication of change in wound status.
13. Apply a sterile dressing.	13. Protects the wound from microorganisms.
14. Dispose of dressings and equipment. Remove gown, mask with protective eye gear, and gloves. Wash hands.	14. Reduces transmission of microorganisms.
15. Document all assessment findings and actions taken.	15. Records information for evaluation.

EVALUATION

- Assess whether the wound is free of exudate, drainage, and debris.
- Assess whether the wound is free of signs and symptoms of infection.
- Evaluate whether the procedure was performed with a minimum of trauma and pain to the client.

DOCUMENTATION

Nurses' Notes

- Wound's appearance and quality, quantity, color, and odor of drainage
- Client's tolerance of the procedure and any observations regarding the client's body image
- Document on appropriate electronic medical record or flow sheet.

Kardex

- Special equipment or techniques required with the client to provide the information to other staff members

PROCEDURE 30-24 Administering Oxygen Therapy

OVERVIEW

Administration of oxygen must be ordered by the physician or qualified practitioner. Some health care facilities will have protocols that govern oxygen therapy and allow the nurse to begin therapy independently. Oxygen is a drug, so medication administration criteria are followed in addition to the steps unique to oxygen therapy. Clients unable to maintain adequate PO_2 and O_2 saturation levels on room air are candidates for oxygen therapy. An adequate airway is essential to effectiveness of the treatment. It is best to treat the hypoxia with the lowest oxygen dose possible. Some clients with a normal oxygen level are also given oxygen if they are at risk for complications related to hypoxia; for example, the myocardial infarction client often receives oxygen therapy to prevent dysrhythmias.

(Continues)

PROCEDURE 30-24 Administering Oxygen Therapy (Continued)

The health care provider orders the oxygen delivery system and flow rate, and the nurse monitors client response to the therapy. The dosage of oxygen may be ordered as an FIO_2 (fraction of inspired oxygen), which is expressed as a percentage or as liters per minute (L/min). Respiratory therapists may be available to assist in the administration of oxygen therapy and client assessment.

ASSESSMENT

1. Determine client history and acute and chronic health problems. **Clients with carbon dioxide retaining chronic obstructive pulmonary disease (COPD) will need lower amounts of oxygen so as not to obliterate their hypoxic respiratory drive. They may already be on oxygen and need long-term continuous therapy.**
2. Assess the client's baseline respiratory signs, including airway, respiratory pattern, rate, depth, and rhythm, noting indications of increased work of breathing. **Helps determine the client's need for oxygen as well as response to the therapy.**
3. Check the extremities and mucous membranes closely for color. **Gives some indication of oxygenation, although problems with circulation and tissue perfusion can also alter these factors.**
4. Review arterial blood gas (ABG) and pulse oximetry results. **These are the most important determinants of the effectiveness of the pulmonary system and determine the need for therapy as well as changes in therapy.**
5. Note lung sounds for wheezes/crackles. **Secretions will interfere with airway patency and diffusion of oxygen and carbon dioxide across the alveolar-capillary bed.**
6. Assess the nares, behind the earlobes, cheek, tracheostomy site, or other places where oxygen tubing or equipment is in constant contact with the skin **to look for signs of skin irritation or breakdown.**

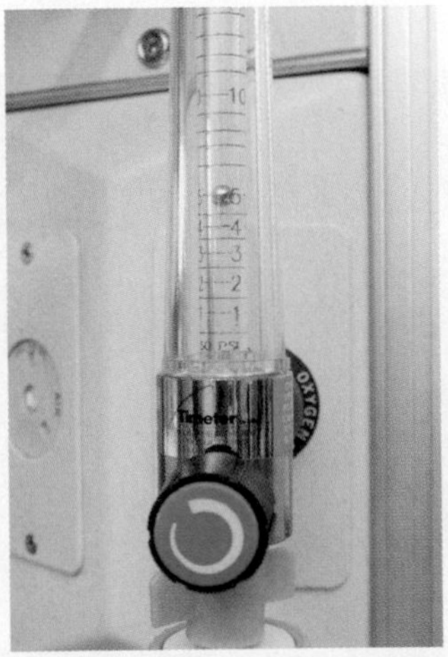

COURTESY OF DELMAR CENGAGE LEARNING

FIGURE 30-24-1 In-Line Oxygen and Flow Meter

POSSIBLE NURSING DIAGNOSES

*Impaired **G**as Exchange*
*Ineffective **B**reathing Pattern*
*Risk for **I**njury*
*Ineffective **A**irway Clearance*
*Risk for Impaired **S**kin Integrity*
Activity Intolerance

PLANNING

Expected Outcomes

1. Oxygen level will return to normal in blood and tissues as evident by oxygen saturation greater than or equal to 92%, skin color normal.
2. Respiratory rate, pattern, and depth will be within the normal range for client.
3. The client will not develop any skin or tissue irritation or breakdown.
4. The client will demonstrate methods to clear secretions and maintain optimal oxygenation.
5. Breathing efficiency and activity tolerance will be increased.
6. The client will understand the rationale for the therapy.

Equipment Needed (see Figures 30-24-1 and 30-24-2)

- Stethoscope
- Oxygen source—portable or in-line
- Oxygen flow meter
- Oxygen delivery device: nasal cannula, mask, tent, or T-tube with adapter for artificial airway
- Oxygen tubing
- Pulse oximeter
- Humidifier and distilled or sterile water (not needed with low flow rates per nasal cannula)

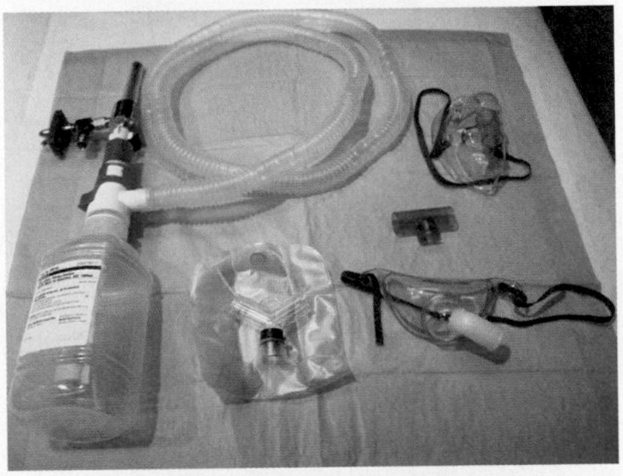

COURTESY OF DELMAR CENGAGE LEARNING

FIGURE 30-24-2 Humidifier, reservoir bag, tracheostomy mask, T-tube, and a simple face mask are used when administering oxygen therapy.

(Continues)

PROCEDURE 30-24 Administering Oxygen Therapy (Continued)

delegation tips

The initiation of oxygen therapy requires assessment by a nurse or respiratory care practitioner. All personnel are responsible to maintain fire/safety precautions when oxygen is in use. Ancillary personnel should be instructed to report dyspnea, tachycardia, any changes in the client's activity tolerance, a respiratory rate less than 12 or greater than 20 breaths per minute in the adult client, or changes in mental status. Ancillary personnel should be instructed how to properly reapply respiratory therapy equipment, how to initiate assistance with activities of daily living for the client requiring oxygen therapy, and to report any abnormal client responses.

IMPLEMENTATION—ACTION/RATIONALE

* Check client's identification band * Explain procedure before beginning *

Nasal Cannula (see Figure 30-24-3)

ACTION	RATIONALE
1. Wash hands.	1. Reduces transmission of microorganisms.
2. Verify the health care provider's order.	2. Ensures correct dosage and route.
3. Remind clients who smoke of the reasons for not smoking while O_2 is in use.	3. Increases compliance with procedures. Oxygen supports combustion.
4. If using humidity, fill humidifier to fill line with distilled water and close container.	4. Prevents drying of the client's airway and thins any secretions.
5. Attach humidifier to oxygen flow meter.	5. Allows the oxygen to pass through the water and become humidified.
6. Insert humidifier and flow meter into oxygen source in wall or portable unit.	6. Gives access to oxygen. Reduces possibility of inserting into wrong outlet. Many institutions also have compressed air available from outlets very similar in appearance to oxygen outlets. Green always stands for oxygen. Be sure to plug the flow meter into the green outlet.
7. Attach the oxygen tubing and nasal cannula to the flow meter and turn it on to the prescribed flow rate (1 to 5 L/min). Use extension tubing for ambulatory clients so they can get up to go to the bathroom.	7. Rates above 6 L/min are not efficacious and can dry the nasal mucosa.
8. Check for bubbling in the humidifier.	8. Ensures proper functioning.
9. Place the nasal prongs in the client's nostrils (Figure 30-24-4). Secure the cannula in place by adjusting the tubing around the client's ears and using the slip ring to stabilize it under the client's chin (Figure 30-24-5).	9. Keeps delivery system in place so client receives the amount of oxygen ordered.

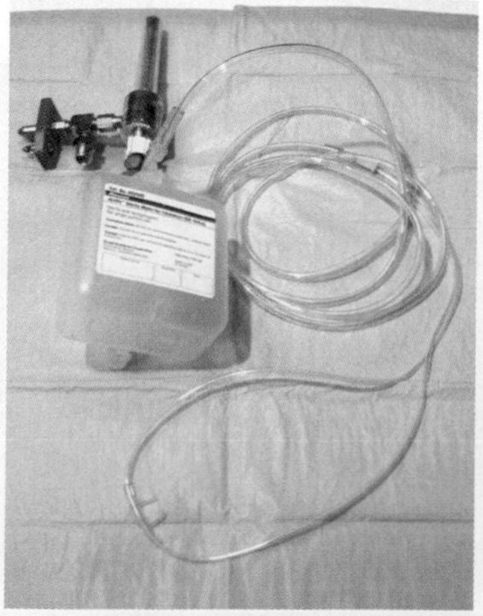

COURTESY OF DELMAR CENGAGE LEARNING

FIGURE 30-24-3 Nasal cannula and oxygen attached to a humidifier.

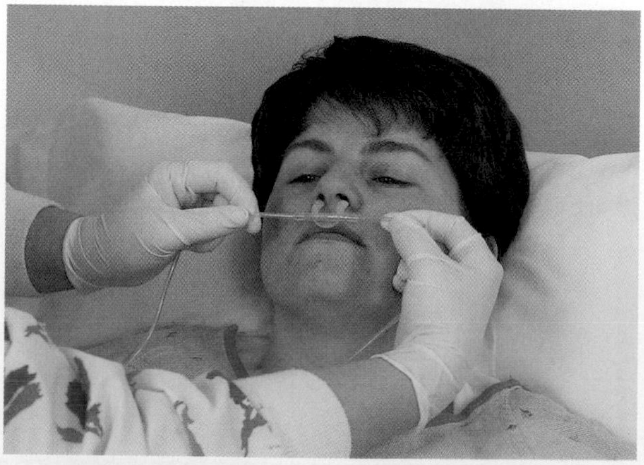

COURTESY OF DELMAR CENGAGE LEARNING

FIGURE 30-24-4 Insert cannula prong into nostrils (gloves are optional).

(Continues)

PROCEDURE 30-24 Administering Oxygen Therapy (Continued)

ACTION	RATIONALE
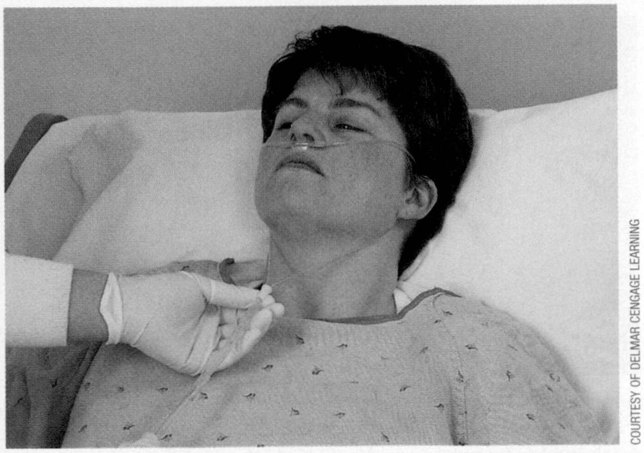 FIGURE 30-24-5 Adjust Tubing	
10. Check for proper flow rate every 4 hours and when the client returns from procedures.	10. Ensures that client receives proper dose. The nasal cannula is a low-flow system because it administers oxygen while the client also inspires room air. The actual dose of oxygen received by the client will vary depending on the client's respiratory pattern.
11. Assess client's nostrils every 8 hours. If the client complains of dryness or has signs of irritation, use sterile lubricant to keep mucous membranes moist. Add humidifier if not already in place.	11. Dry membranes are more prone to breakdown by friction or pressure from nasal cannula.
12. Monitor vital signs, oxygen saturation, and client condition every 4 to 8 hours (or as indicated or ordered) for signs and symptoms of hypoxia.	12. Detects any untoward effects from therapy.
13. Wean client from oxygen as soon as possible using standard protocols.	13. Oxygen is not without side effects and should be used only as long as needed. Problems with reimbursement may develop if criteria for therapy are not met.
Mask: Venturi (high-flow device), simple mask (low flow), partial rebreather mask, nonrebreather mask, and face tent	
14. Repeat Actions 1 to 6.	14. See Rationales 1 to 6.
15. Attach appropriately sized mask (Figure 30-24-6 and Figure 30-24-7) or face tent to oxygen tubing and turn on flow meter to prescribed flow rate. The Venturi mask will have color-coded inserts that list the flow rate necessary to obtain the desired percentage of oxygen. Allow the reservoir bag of the nonrebreathing or partial rebreathing mask to fill completely.	15. Ensures proper fit; size needed is based on the client's size. Checks the oxygen source and primes the tubing and mask or tent.
16. Check for bubbling in the humidifier.	16. Ensures proper functioning.
17. Place the mask or tent on the client's face, fasten the elastic band around the client's ears, and tighten until the mask fits snugly.	17. Prevents loss of oxygen from the sides of the mask.
18. Check for proper flow rate every 4 hours.	18. Ensures that client is receiving the proper dose.

(Continues)

PROCEDURE 30-24 Administering Oxygen Therapy (Continued)

ACTION	RATIONALE

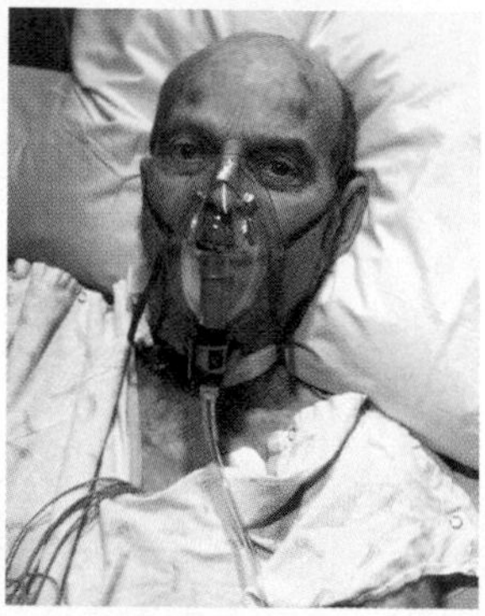

COURTESY OF DELMAR CENGAGE LEARNING

FIGURE 30-24-6 Make sure that the mask is the appropriate size for the client.

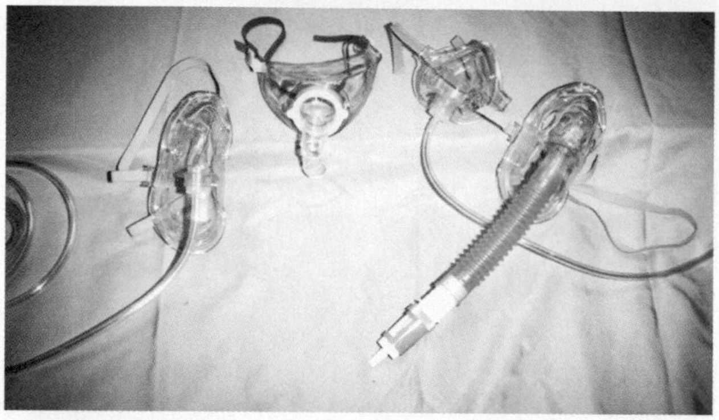

COURTESY OF DELMAR CENGAGE LEARNING

FIGURE 30-24-7 Simple oxygen mask, tracheostomy mask, pediatric mask, and Venturi mask are different types of oxygen masks.

ACTION	RATIONALE
19. Ensure that the ports of the Venturi mask are not under covers or impeded by any other source.	19. Air must be entrained to mix room air and oxygen coming from source to ensure proper oxygen percentage (FIO_2).
20. Assess client's face and ears for pressure from the mask and use padding as needed.	20. Provides client comfort and prevents skin breakdown.
21. Wean client to nasal cannula and then wean off oxygen per protocol.	21. Oxygen is not without side effects and should be used only as long as needed. The nasal cannula provides a lower FIO_2 than the mask. Problems with reimbursement may develop if criteria for therapy are not met.

EVALUATION

- Oxygen level returned to normal in blood and tissues as evident by oxygen saturation ≥92%; skin color normal for client.
- Respiratory rate, pattern, and depth are within the normal range.
- The client did not develop any skin or tissue irritation or breakdown.
- Breathing efficiency and activity tolerance are increased.
- The client understands the rationale for the therapy.

DOCUMENTATION

Nurses' Notes

- O_2 saturation and respiratory status
- Method of oxygen delivery and rate
- Client's assessment parameters and response to treatment
- Changes in mental status
- Document on appropriate electronic medical record or flow sheet.

PROCEDURE 30-25 Performing Nasopharyngeal and Oropharyngeal Suctioning

OVERVIEW

Suctioning secretions is necessary to maintain a patent airway for a client who is unable to effectively clear secretions by coughing. It is considered a sterile procedure, thereby preventing the introduction of microorganisms into the client's airway and lungs.

Suctioning is performed as often as necessary to remove excess secretions, depending on the amount of secretions the client is generating and the client's ability to clear the airway. The client's airway and oxygenation are evaluated to determine the need for suctioning.

(Continues)

PROCEDURE 30-25 Performing Nasopharyngeal and Oropharyngeal Suctioning (Continued)

Wall suction should be set at 100 to 120 mm Hg for adults, 50 to 100 mm Hg for children, and 40 to 60 mm Hg for infants. Portable suction should be set at 8 to 15 mm Hg for adults, 5 to 8 mm Hg for children, and 3 to 5 mm Hg for infants.

ASSESSMENT

1. Assess respirations for rate, rhythm, depth, and bubbling or gurgling noises **to evaluate airway.**
2. Auscultate lung fields **to evaluate airway and determine need for suctioning.**
3. Monitor arterial blood gases and/or pulse oximetry values **to determine oxygen level and adequate air exchange.**
4. Assess for anxiety and restlessness, **which may be signs of airway distress and/or hypoxia.**
5. Assess the client's understanding of the suctioning procedure **to decrease the client's anxiety.**

POSSIBLE NURSING DIAGNOSES

Ineffective Airway Clearance
Impaired Gas Exchange
Anxiety

PLANNING

Expected Outcomes

1. The client will have no coarse bubbling or gurgling noises with respirations.
2. The client will report breathing comfortably.
3. The client will have no apparent anxiety or restlessness.
4. The client will have arterial blood gases and pulse oximetry values within normal limits.
5. The client will express understanding of the suctioning process.

Equipment Needed

- Suction source (wall or portable with collection bottle)
- Sterile suction kit
- Sterile gloves (if not in kit)
- Sterile water-soluble lubricant
- Small bottle of sterile water or normal saline (if not in kit)
- Tubing connected to suction source
- Personal protective equipment: gown, mask, and goggles or face shield

delegation tips

Nasopharyngeal and oropharyngeal suctioning is generally performed by the nurse. Properly trained ancillary personnel may perform oropharyngeal suctioning in some situations.

IMPLEMENTATION—ACTION/RATIONALE

ACTION	RATIONALE
* Check client's identification band * Explain procedure before beginning *	
1. Choose the most appropriate route (nasopharyngeal or oropharyngeal) for your client. If nasopharyngeal approach is considered, inspect the nares with a penlight to determine patency. Alternately, you may assess patency by occluding each nare in turn with finger pressure while asking the client to breathe through the remaining nare.	1. The oropharyngeal approach is easier but requires that the client cooperate; it may also produce gagging more readily. The nasopharyngeal route is more effective for reaching the posterior oropharynx but is contraindicated in clients with a deviated nasal septum, nasal polyps, or any tendency toward excessive bleeding (low platelet count, use of anticoagulants, recent history of epistaxis or nasal trauma).
2. Advise the client that suctioning may cause coughing or gagging but emphasize the importance of clearing the airway.	2. Promotes cooperation and reduces anxiety.
3. Wash hands.	3. Reduces transmission of microorganisms.
4. Position the client in a high Fowler's or semi-Fowler's position.	4. Maximizes lung expansion and effective coughing.

(Continues)

PROCEDURE 30-25 Performing Nasopharyngeal and Oropharyngeal Suctioning (Continued)

ACTION	RATIONALE
5. If the client is unconscious or otherwise unable to protect his or her airway, place in a side-lying position.	5. Protects the client from aspiration in the event of vomiting.
6. Connect extension tubing to suction device if not already in place, and adjust suction control to between 100 and 120 mm Hg for adult.	6. Excessive negative pressure can cause tissue trauma, whereas insufficient pressure will be ineffective.
7. Put on gown and mask and goggles or face shield.	7. Protects nurse from splattering of body fluids.
8. Using sterile technique, open the suction kit. Consider the inside wrapper of the kit to be sterile, and spread the wrapper out carefully to create a small sterile field.	8. Produces an area in which to place sterile items without contaminating them.
9. Open a packet of sterile water-soluble lubricant and squeeze out the contents of the packet onto the sterile field.	9. Lubricant will be used to further lubricate the catheter tip if the nasopharyngeal route is used.
10. If sterile solution (water or saline) is not included in the kit, pour about 100 mL of solution into the sterile container provided in the kit.	10. Will be used to lubricate the catheter and to rinse the inside of the catheter to clear secretions.
11. If gloves are wrapped, carefully lift the wrapped gloves from the kit without touching the inside of the kit or the gloves themselves. Lay the wrapped gloves next to the suction kit, and open the wrapper. Put on the gloves using sterile gloving technique (Procedure 30-2).	11. Keeps gloves sterile for handling the sterile suction catheter to avoid introducing pathogens into the client's airway.
12. If a cup of sterile solution is included in the suction kit, open it.	12. Will be used to lubricate the catheter and to rinse the inside of the catheter to clear secretions.
13. Designate one hand as *sterile* (able to touch only sterile items) and the other as clean (able to touch only unsterile items).	13. Usually, the dominant hand is the sterile hand, while the nondominant hand is clean. This prevents contamination of sterile supplies while allowing unsterile items to be handled.
14. *Using your sterile hand*, pick up the suction catheter. Grasp the plastic connector end between your thumb and forefinger and coil the tip around your remaining fingers.	14. Prevents accidental contamination of the catheter tip.
15. Pick up the extension tubing *with your clean hand*. Connect the suction catheter to the extension tubing, taking care not to contaminate the catheter (Figure 30-25-1).	15. The extension tubing is not sterile.
16. Position your clean hand with the thumb over the catheter's suction port.	16. Suction is activated by occluding this port with the thumb. Releasing the port deactivates the suction.
17. Dip the catheter tip into the sterile solution, and activate the suction. Observe as the solution is drawn into the catheter.	17. Tests the suction device as well as lubricates the interior of the catheter to enhance clearance of secretions.

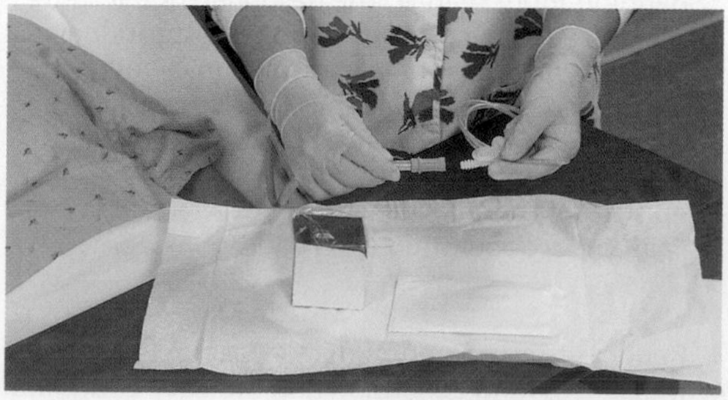

FIGURE 30-25-1 Attach catheter to tubing.

(Continues)

PROCEDURE 30-25 Performing Nasopharyngeal and Oropharyngeal Suctioning (Continued)

ACTION	RATIONALE
18. For oropharyngeal suctioning, ask the client to open his or her mouth. Without activating the suction, use sterile hand to gently insert the catheter and advance it until you reach the pool of secretions or until the client coughs. Do not poke catheter in oropharynx.	18. To minimize trauma, do not apply suction while the catheter is being advanced.
19. For nasopharyngeal suctioning, estimate the distance from the tip of the client's nose to the earlobe and grasp the catheter between your thumb and forefinger at a point equal to this distance from the catheter's tip.	19. Ensures placement of the catheter tip in the oropharynx and not in the trachea.
20. Dip the tip of the suction catheter into the water-soluble lubricant to coat catheter tip liberally.	20. Promotes the client's comfort and minimizes trauma to nasal mucosa.
21. Use *sterile* hand to insert the catheter tip into the nostril with the suction control port uncovered. Advance the catheter gently with a slight downward slant. Slight rotation of the catheter may be used to ease insertion (Figure 30-25-2). Advance the catheter to the point marked by your thumb and forefinger.	21. Guides the catheter toward the posterior oropharynx along the floor of the nasal cavity.
22. If resistance is met, *do not force the catheter.* Withdraw it and attempt insertion via the opposite nostril.	22. Forceful insertion may cause tissue damage and bleeding.
23. With *clean* hand, apply suction by occluding the suction control port with your thumb; at the same time, slowly rotate the catheter by rolling it between your thumb and fingers while slowly withdrawing it. Apply suction for no longer than 15 seconds at a time.	23. Prolonged suction applied to a single area of tissue can cause tissue damage.
24. Repeat step 23 until secretions have been cleared, allowing for brief rest periods between suctioning episodes.	24. Promotes complete clearance of the airway.
25. Withdraw the catheter by looping it around your fingers as you pull it out.	25. Allows you to maintain control over the catheter tip as it is withdrawn.
26. Dip the catheter tip into the sterile solution and apply suction.	26. Clears the extension tubing of secretions that would promote bacterial growth and could block tubing.

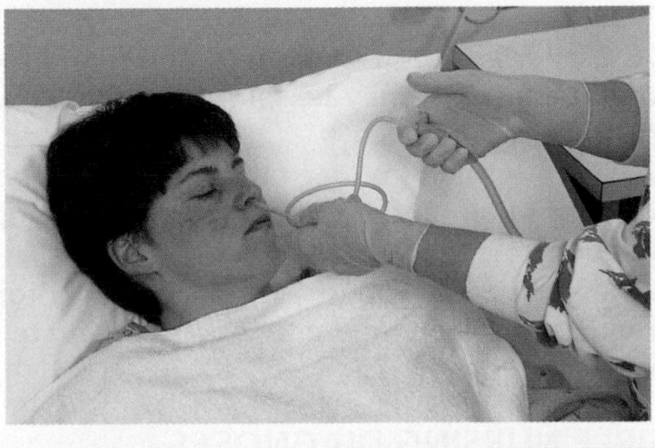

COURTESY OF DELMAR CENGAGE LEARNING

FIGURE 30-25-2 Insert catheter into nostril. (This nurse is left-handed.)

(Continues)

PROCEDURE 30-25 Performing Nasopharyngeal and Oropharyngeal Suctioning (Continued)

ACTION	RATIONALE
27. Disconnect the catheter from the extension tubing. Holding the coiled catheter in your gloved hand, remove the glove by pulling it over the catheter. Discard catheter and gloves in an a ppropriate container.	27. Contains the catheter and secretions in the glove for disposal.
28. Discard remaining supplies in the appropriate container and wash your hands.	28. Prevents transmission of microorganisms. Suctioning and coughing may produce an unpleasant taste.
29. Provide the client with oral hygiene if indicated or desired.	29. Suctioning and coughing may produce an unpleasant taste.

EVALUATION

- Check breath sounds for a patent airway.
- Ask client if breathing is easier.
- Assess client for signs of dyspnea.
- Review arterial blood gases and/or pulse oximetry results.
- Assess consistency, color, amount, and odor of secretions.

DOCUMENTATION

Nurses' Notes

- Date and time of suctioning procedure
- Client's tolerance of the procedure
- Amount, consistency, color, and odor or secretions
- Arterial blood gases and/or pulse oximetry results
- Document on appropriate electronic medical record or flow sheet.

PROCEDURE 30-26 Performing Tracheostomy Care

OVERVIEW

A tracheotomy is an incision made into the trachea with insertion of a cannula for airway management. Tracheostomy is the creation of an opening into the trachea through the neck. The two terms can be used interchangeably. A tracheostomy is performed for the client with potential or present airway obstruction, for ventilatory assistance, to provide pulmonary hygiene, to decrease the anatomic dead space in the client with chronic obstructive pulmonary disease, to avoid prolonged endotracheal intubation, and to provide an airway for clients with severe obstructive sleep apnea syndrome. The tracheostomy is performed below the level of the vocal cords and allows air to enter and exit the tracheostomy rather than through the upper airway. The tracheostomy tube can have a single or double cannula. The determination of the tube design used is based on the needs of the client. The double cannula tube allows for the tube to be cleaned to prevent obstruction caused by dried secretions. During the acute phase after a tracheostomy has been performed, all care must be performed using sterile technique. Once care of the tracheostomy tube becomes a client procedure, a clean technique is used.

ASSESSMENT

1. Assess respirations for rate, rhythm, and depth **to evaluate the airway.**
2. Assess the client's lung sounds **to determine the need for suctioning.**
3. Assess the client's arterial blood gases and/or pulse oximetry values **to evaluate air exchange and blood oxygen levels.**
4. Assess the movement of air through the tracheostomy tube **to evaluate the air exchange through the tube and determine whether there is any obstruction.**
5. Assess the amount and color of tracheal secretions **to evaluate for bleeding, infection, and the need for suctioning.**
6. Assess for anxiety, restlessness, and fear. **Anxiety and restlessness may be symptoms of airway distress and hypoxia.**
7. Assess the client's understanding of the procedure **to determine client education and support needed.**
8. Assess the area around the tracheostomy for redness, swelling, and drainage **to evaluate skin integrity.**

POSSIBLE NURSING DIAGNOSES

Ineffective Airway Clearance
Risk for Infection
Risk for Suffocation
Impaired Skin Integrity

(Continues)

PROCEDURE 30-26 Performing Tracheostomy Care (Continued)

Impaired Verbal Communication
Deficient Knowledge (Tracheostomy Care)
Anxiety
Impaired Gas Exchange

PLANNING

Expected Outcomes

1. The client's airway will be free of obstruction.
2. The procedure will be performed with a minimum of client anxiety.
3. The client's skin will remain intact and free of redness and excoriation.
4. The client will remain free of signs and symptoms of infection.
5. The client will have cannulas free of secretions and clean, secure ties.

Equipment Needed

Cleaning the Inner Cannula

- Sterile latex-free gloves
- Nonsterile latex-free gloves
- Disposable inner cannula (if available)
- Tracheostomy care kit: 2 basins, tracheostomy brush, tracheostomy ties (twill tape, commercially available Velcro ties)
- Hydrogen peroxide
- Sterile water or sterile saline
- Cotton-tip applicators
- Tracheostomy dressing (4 × 4 gauze without cotton lining)

delegation tips

Tracheostomy care cannot be delegated by the nurse. Ancillary personnel may assist the nurse in providing care to clients receiving this treatment and should be instructed to report a client experiencing increased secretions, dyspnea, or the need for suctioning to the nurse.

IMPLEMENTATION—ACTION/RATIONALE

ACTION	RATIONALE
* Check client's identification band * Explain procedure before beginning *	
1. Wash hands and apply nonsterile latex-free gloves.	1. Reduces transmission of microorganisms.
2. Remove soiled dressing and discard. Remove gloves and discard. Wash hands.	2. Prevents contamination of other areas.
Conventional/Reusable Inner Cannula	
3. Open tracheostomy care set (Figure 30-26-1).	3. Provides sterile equipment for use in the procedure.
4. Place hydrogen peroxide solution in one basin and sterile water or saline in a second basin.	4. Prepare solutions prior to applying gloves.
5. Apply sterile gloves.	5. Uses aseptic technique.
6. Dip the applicator in the basin of hydrogen peroxide.	6. Prevents contamination of the applicator.
7. Remove inner cannula.	7. Allows for cleaning.
8. Place inner cannula in basin of hydrogen peroxide.	8. Loosens secretions.
9. Clean the area under the neck plate of the tracheostomy tube using a cotton applicator moistened with hydrogen peroxide (Figure 30-26-2).	9. Decreases microorganisms and removes crusting.
10. Rinse area under neck plate with cotton applicator moistened with sterile water or saline.	10. Removes hydrogen peroxide from the skin.
11. Dry skin under neck plate with cotton-tip applicator.	11. Prevents skin excoriation from moisture.

(Continues)

PROCEDURE 30-26 Performing Tracheostomy Care (Continued)

ACTION | **RATIONALE**

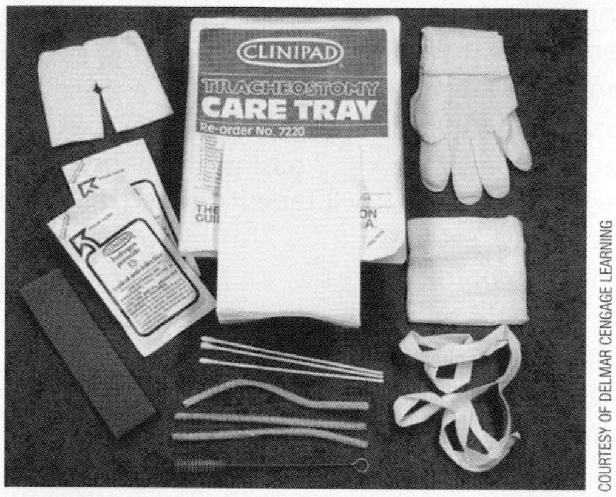

FIGURE 30-26-1 Tracheostomy Care Kit and Supplies

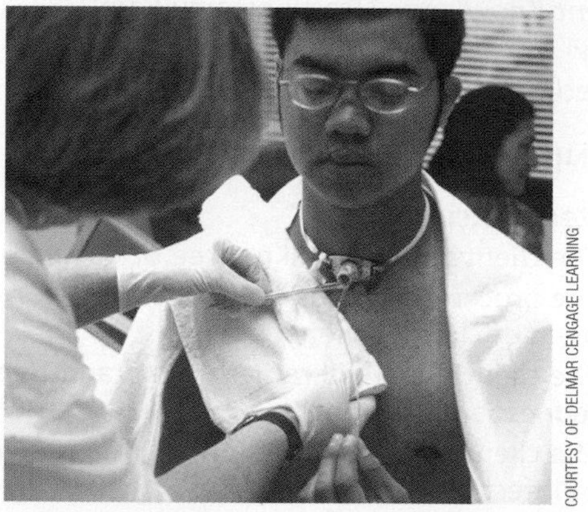

FIGURE 30-26-2 Clean the area under the neck plate with a cotton applicator moistened with hydrogen peroxide.

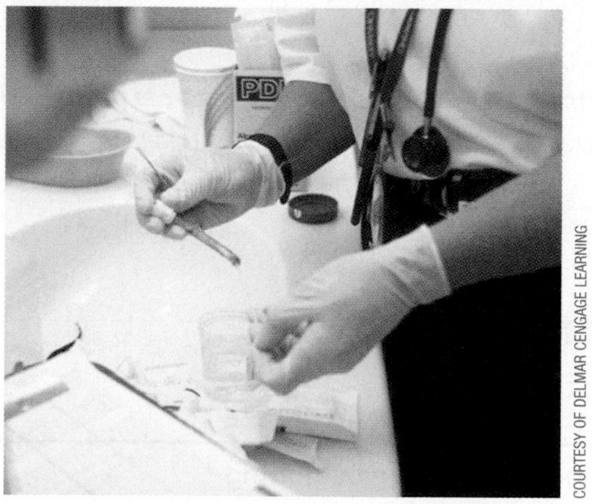

FIGURE 30-26-3 Use a sterile cotton-tipped applicator to clean the inner cannula area and remove crusted secretions.

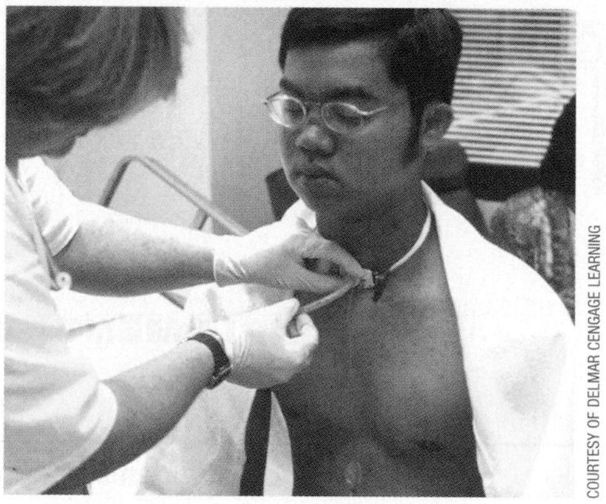

FIGURE 30-26-4 Carefully reinsert inner cannula and lock into place.

ACTION	RATIONALE
12. Apply tracheostomy gauze under neck plate of tube. Note: if using tracheostomy gauze under neck plate of tube, change gauze frequently to prevent infection and skin breakdown.	12. Prevents rubbing and irritation of the skin.
13. Use a tracheostomy brush or sterile cotton-tip applicator to clean inner cannula (Figure 30-26-3).	13. Removes crusted secretions.
14. Rinse inner cannula with sterile water or sterile saline.	14. Removes hydrogen peroxide from inner cannula.
15. Dry inner cannula.	15. Prevents introduction of solutions into the trachea.
16. Reinsert inner cannula and lock it into place (Figure 30-26-4).	16. Prevents accidental removal of the inner cannula during coughing.
17. Remove gloves and wash hands.	17. Reduces transmission of microorganisms.
Disposable Inner Cannula	
18. Wash hands. Open disposable cannula container without touching cannula.	18. Reduces transmission of microorganisms.

(Continues)

PROCEDURE 30-26 Performing Tracheostomy Care (Continued)

ACTION	RATIONALE
19. Apply sterile gloves.	19. Uses aseptic technique.
20. Remove inner cannula and discard.	20. Disposable inner cannulas are not to be reused.
21. Replace inner cannula with new disposable cannula.	21. Provides a clean open cannula.
22. Remove gloves and wash hands.	22. Prevents transmission of microorganisms.
Two-Person Technique of Changing Tracheostomy Ties	
23. Cut two pieces of twill tape about 12 to 14 inches in length.	23. Prepares equipment before beginning procedure.
24. Make a fold about 1 inch below the end of each piece of twill tape and cut a half-inch slit lengthwise in the center of the fold.	24. Prepares tape for insertion.
25. Have a second person gently hold the tracheostomy tube in place with fingers on both sides of the neck plate.	25. Prevents accidental movement of the tracheostomy tube resulting in coughing and accidental decannulation.
26. Untie old tracheostomy ties and discard.	26. Removes tracheostomy ties.
27. Insert the split end of the tracheostomy tape through the opening on one side of the tracheostomy tube neck plate. Pull the distal end of the tracheostomy tie through the cut end and pull tightly.	27. Secures tracheostomy tie within neck plate.
28. Repeat procedure with second piece of twill tape.	28. Secures tracheostomy tube.
29. Tie tracheostomy tapes with a double knot at the side of the neck.	29. Secures tracheostomy tube.
30. Insert one finger under tracheostomy tapes.	30. Ensures that tube has been tied securely.
31. Insert tracheostomy gauze under neck plate of tube.	31. Prevents irritation of skin from secretions and rubbing of tracheostomy tube.
32. Discard all used materials and wash hands.	32. Reduces transmission of microorganisms.
One-Person Technique of Changing Tracheostomy Ties	
33. Follow Actions 23 to 24 and 27 to 29.	33. See Rationales 23 to 24 and 27 to 29.
34. Hold the neck plate firmly with one hand; untie and remove old tracheostomy tapes and discard.	34. Prevents dislodgment while untying and removing old tracheostomy tapes.
35. Place one finger under tracheostomy ties.	35. Checks for tightness and security.
36. Discard all used materials and wash hands.	36. Reduces transmission of microorganisms.

EVALUATION

- Airway is free of obstruction.
- Client anxiety was minimal during procedure.
- There is no evidence of infection.
- Airway is patent.
- Cannulas free of secretions, and clean, secured ties.
- Client's skin intact and free of redness and excoriation.

DOCUMENTATION

Nurses' Notes

- Date, time, procedure performed, and client's tolerance of the procedure
- Size and type of tracheostomy tube in place
- Amount and consistency of any secretions
- Condition of the client's skin
- Client teaching and participation
- Document on appropriate electronic medical record or flow sheet.

PROCEDURE 30-27 Performing Tracheostomy Suctioning

OVERVIEW

Suctioning secretions is necessary to maintain the airway of a client who is unable to clear his or her own secretions by coughing. Some clients may be able to cough but not effectively enough to expel the secretions. Suctioning the client's airway is considered a sterile procedure. Using sterile technique prevents the introduction of contagion into the client's airway and lungs.

Suctioning is performed as often as necessary to remove excess secretions. The procedure may be performed as often as every 5 minutes or as infrequently as every few hours, depending on the amount of secretions the client is generating and the client's ability to clear his or her own airway. Evaluate the client's airway and oxygenation to determine the need for suctioning. Wall suction should be set at 100 to 120 mm Hg for adults, 50 to 100 mm Hg for children, and 40 to 60 mm Hg for infants. Portable suction set at 8 to 15 mm Hg for adults, 5 to 8 mm Hg for children, and 3 to 5 mm Hg for infants.

ASSESSMENT

1. Assess respirations for rate, rhythm, and depth **to evaluate airway.**
2. Auscultate lung fields **to evaluate airway and determine need for suctioning.**
3. Monitor arterial blood gases and/or pulse oximetry values **to determine oxygen levels and adequate air exchange.**
4. Assess passage of air through the tracheostomy tube **to determine air exchange and obstruction of the tube.**
5. Monitor tracheal secretions for amount, color, consistency, and odor **to assess for evidence of bleeding or signs of infection and need for suctioning.**
6. Assess for anxiety and restlessness, **which may be signs of airway distress and/or hypoxia.**
7. Assess the client's understanding of the suctioning procedure **to decrease the client's anxiety.**

POSSIBLE NURSING DIAGNOSES

Impaired Gas Exchange
Anxiety
Ineffective Airway Clearance
Risk for Infection

PLANNING

Expected Outcomes

1. The client will have no crackles or wheezes in large airways and the absence of cyanosis.
2. The client will report breathing comfortably and will have no apparent anxiety or restlessness.
3. The client will have minimal amount of thin, normal-colored secretions.
4. The client will maintain a patent airway.
5. The client will maintain adequate pulse oximetry.

Equipment Needed

- Sterile latex-free gloves
- Mask, eye protection, and gown if appropriate
- Source of negative pressure (suction machine or wall suction)
- Sterile suction catheter
- Oxygen or Ambu-bag
- Equipment for tracheostomy care or tracheostomy care tray

delegation tips

Suctioning a tracheostomy is not delegated by the nurse. Ancillary personnel may assist the nurse in providing care to clients receiving this treatment and should be instructed to report a client experiencing increased secretions, dyspnea, or the need for suctioning to the nurse.

IMPLEMENTATION—ACTION/RATIONALE

ACTION	RATIONALE
* Check client's identification band * Explain procedure before beginning *	
1. Assess depth and rate of respirations; auscultate breath sounds.	1. Determines need for suctioning.
2. Assemble supplies on bedside table.	2. Organizes work.
3. Wash hands.	3. Reduces transmission of microorganisms.

(Continues)

PROCEDURE 30-27 Performing Tracheostomy Suctioning (Continued)

ACTION	RATIONALE
4. Position the client in a high Fowler's or semi-Fowler's position.	4. Maximizes lung expansion and effective coughing.
5. Connect extension tubing to suction device, if not already in place, and adjust suction control to between 100 and 120 mm Hg.	5. Excessive negative pressure can cause tissue trauma, hypoxemia, and atelectasis, whereas insufficient pressure will be ineffective.
6. Put on gown and mask and goggles or face shield.	6. Protects from splattering body fluids.
7. Using sterile technique, open tracheostomy care kit. Consider the inside wrapper of the kit to be sterile, and spread the wrapper out carefully to create a small sterile field. Add sterile suction catheter if not in kit.	7. Produces an area in which to place sterile items without contaminating them.
8. If gloves are wrapped, carefully lift the wrapped gloves from the kit without touching the inside of the kit or the gloves themselves. Lay the wrapped gloves down and open the wrapper. Put on the gloves using sterile gloving technique.	8. Reduces introduction of pathogens into the client's airway.
9. Pour hydrogen peroxide in one basin and sterile water or saline in the other.	9. Provides solution to clean inner cannula and to lubricate the catheter and rinse the inside of the catheter to clear secretions.
10. Designate one hand as *sterile* (able to touch only sterile items), usually the dominant hand, and the other as *clean* (able to touch only nonsterile items), the nondominant hand.	10. Prevents contamination of sterile supplies while allowing you to handle unsterile items.
11. *Using your sterile hand*, pick up the suction catheter. Grasp the plastic connector end between your thumb and forefinger and coil the tip around your remaining fingers.	11. Prevents accidental contamination of the catheter tip.
12. Pick up the extension tubing *with your clean hand*. Connect the suction catheter to the extension tubing, taking care not to contaminate the catheter.	12. The extension tubing is not sterile.
13. If client is not receiving oxygen, administer oxygen or use Ambu-bag with *clean* hand before beginning procedure.	13. Hyperoxygenates client and prevents hypoxia during suctioning.
14. Remove inner cannula and place in basin of hydrogen peroxide to loosen secretions, if reusable, or set aside if disposable. Do not dispose of disposable cannula until new inner cannula is securely in place.	14. Allows easier passage of the suction catheter. Retain old cannula until you are sure the new cannula fits correctly.
15. Position your clean hand with the thumb over the catheter's suction port, dip the catheter tip into the sterile solution, and activate the suction. Observe as the solution is drawn into the catheter.	15. Tests the suction device as well as lubricating the interior of the catheter to enhance clearance of secretions.
16. Remove thumb from suction port.	16. Deactivates the suction.
17. Using your *clean* hand, remove the oxygen delivery device from the tracheostomy tube and place it on a clean surface.	17. Permits access to the tracheostomy tube. Placing the oxygen device on a clean surface reduces contamination (the sterile glove wrapper may be used for this purpose).
18. Without occluding the suction control port, insert the catheter tip into the tracheostomy tube and advance it until the client coughs or resistance is met (Figure 30-27-1) and withdraw slightly.	18. Minimizes trauma when suction not applied while the catheter is being advanced.
19. Apply suction by occluding the suction control port with your thumb, while slowly rotating the	19. Prolonged suction can cause tissue damage, atelectasis, and hypoxemia.

(Continues)

PROCEDURE 30-27 Performing Tracheostomy Suctioning (Continued)

ACTION	RATIONALE

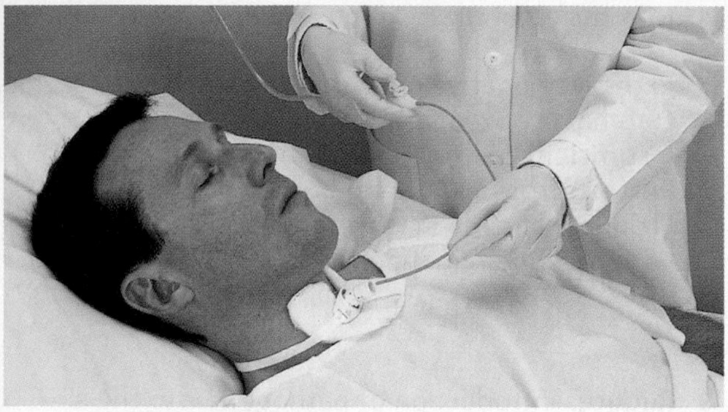

FIGURE 30-27-1 Suction Tracheostomy

ACTION	RATIONALE
catheter between your thumb and finger and slowly withdrawing it. Apply suction for no longer than 15 seconds at a time.	
20. Repeat step 19 until all secretions have been cleared, allowing brief rest periods between suctioning episodes. Encourage client to breathe deeply between suctioning episodes. Provide oxygen between passes of the suction catheter.	20. Promotes complete clearance of the airway.
21. Withdraw the catheter and dip it into the cup of sterile saline, applying suction.	21. Cleans suction catheter of secretions.
22. Clean inner cannula using tracheostomy brush and rinse well in sterile water or sterile saline. Dry (or open new disposable inner cannula).	22. Removes secretions and maintains patent inner cannula.
23. Reinsert inner cannula and lock into place.	23. Prevents secretions from obstructing outer cannula.
24. Reapply oxygen delivery device.	24. Reoxygenates the client and restores supplemental oxygen and humidification.
25. Dip the catheter tip into the sterile solution and apply suction.	25. Clears the extension tubing of secretions, which would promote bacterial growth.
26. Disconnect the catheter from the extension tubing. Holding the coiled catheter in your gloved hand, remove the glove by pulling it over the catheter. Discard catheter and gloves in an appropriate container.	26. Contains the catheter and secretions in the glove for disposal.
27. Discard remaining supplies in the appropriate container.	27. Follow institutional policy regarding disposal of client care supplies.
28. Wash hands.	28. Reduces transmission of pathogens.
29. Provide the client with oral hygiene if indicated/desired.	29. Suctioning and coughing may produce an unpleasant taste.

EVALUATION

- Ask client whether breathing is easier.
- Auscultate breath sounds for a patent airway.
- Review arterial blood gases and/or pulse oximetry values.
- Assess client for signs of dyspnea.
- Evaluate consistency, color, amount, and odor of secretions.

DOCUMENTATION

Nurses' Notes

- Date and time of suctioning procedure
- Client's tolerance of the suctioning procedure
- Amount, consistency, color, and odor of secretions
- Arterial blood gases and/or pulse oximetry values
- Document on appropriate electronic medical record or flow sheet.

PROCEDURE 30-28

Postoperative Exercise Instruction

OVERVIEW

Preoperative teaching of postoperative exercises prepares the client physically and emotionally for the impending surgery. The goal of instruction is to have the client demonstrate the performance of exercises while verbalizing why the exercises are used during the postoperative phase.

Several postoperative exercises help speed recovery from surgery. Turning, deep breathing, and coughing facilitate removal of accumulated pulmonary secretions. Clients may experience their worst postoperative pain while doing these exercises. Inhaled gases and oxygen have a drying effect on the respiratory mucosa, which increases the viscosity of secretions, making them difficult to raise with coughing.

To prevent respiratory complications, teach clients to breathe deeply to achieve sustained maximum inspiration (SMI). SMI promotes the reinflation of the alveoli and the removal of mucus secretions.

Several devices help encourage clients to perform SMI exercises. The breathing devices, called incentive spirometers, measure the client's ventilatory volume and provide the user with a tangible reward for generating an adequate respiratory flow. When the client takes a deep breath, the ball moves upward and the amount of air is measured, thereby making the results visible to the client.

Turning, deep breathing, coughing, and using spirometry prevent respiratory complications by doing the following:

- Promoting pulmonary circulation
- Promoting the exchange of gases by increasing lung compliance
- Facilitating the removal of mucus secretions from the tracheobronchial tree

Postoperatively the client is encouraged to move in bed and perform leg exercises. These exercises assist in preventing circulatory complications that can arise from anesthetic agents that depress the metabolic and heart rates. Early ambulation also increases respiratory function and the return of peristalsis.

ASSESSMENT

1. Assess the client's current understanding of postoperative procedures. **Establishes baseline for teaching.**
2. Assess the client's ability to understand the postoperative exercise instructions. **Establishes baseline for teaching. Affects how the teaching and procedures will be performed.**
3. Assess any preoperative limitations the client may have that would prevent or impair the ability to perform the postoperative exercises accordingly. **Establishes baseline for teaching. Affects how the teaching and procedures will be performed. Allows modification of the exercises.**

POSSIBLE NURSING DIAGNOSES

*Acute **P**ain*
*Impaired Physical **M**obility*
*Impaired **G**as Exchange*
*Risk for Impaired **S**kin Integrity*

PLANNING

Expected Outcomes

1. The client will be able to successfully demonstrate postoperative exercises, deep breathing, coughing, pillow splinting, turning and proper body alignment, leg and foot exercises, and out-of-bed transfers.
2. The client will be able to successfully demonstrate proper use of the incentive spirometer.

Equipment Needed (see Figure 30-28-1)

- Educational materials
- Pillow
- Tissue
- Nonsterile latex-free gloves
- Disposable, volume-oriented incentive spirometer

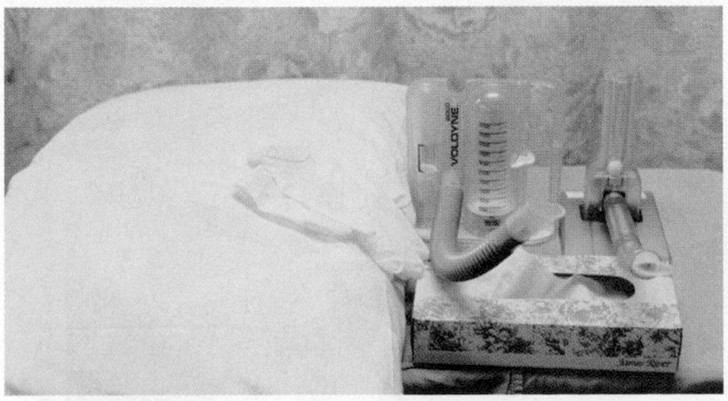

COURTESY OF DELMAR CENGAGE LEARNING

FIGURE 30-28-1 Incentive spirometers encourage deep breathing. A pillow may be used to splint the incision site. Tissues are used to cover the mouth when coughing.

(Continues)

PROCEDURE 30-28 Postoperative Exercise Instruction (Continued)

delegation tips

Postoperative instruction requires the assessment and intervention of a nurse. Ancillary staff may reinforce the information and directions taught to the client.

IMPLEMENTATION—ACTION/RATIONALE

ACTION	RATIONALE
* Check client's identification band * Explain procedure before beginning *	
1. Wash hands and organize equipment.	1. Reduces the transmission of microorganisms and promotes efficiency.
2. Apply nonsterile latex-free gloves.	2. Reduces the transmission of microorganisms.
3. Place client in a sitting position.	3. Promotes full chest expansion.
4. Demonstrate deep breathing exercises.	4. Shows the client how to breathe deeply.
• Place one hand on abdomen (umbilical area) during inhalation.	• Exerts counterpressure during inhalation.
• Expand the abdomen and rib cage on inspiration.	• Promotes maximum chest expansion.
• Inhale slowly and evenly through your nose until you achieve maximum chest expansion.	• Maintains full expansion of the alveoli.
• Hold breath for 2 to 3 seconds.	• Increases the pressure, thereby preventing immediate collapse of the alveoli.
• Slowly exhale through your mouth until maximum chest contraction has been achieved.	• Promotes maximum chest contraction.
5. Have the client return-demonstrate deep breathing and repeat 3 to 4 times.	5. Reinforces learning. Promotes increased air exchange.
6. Instruct the client on the use of an incentive spirometer (Figure 30-28-2).	6. Reinflates the alveoli and removes mucus secretions.
• Hold the volume-oriented spirometer upright.	• Promotes proper functioning of the device.
• Take a normal breath and exhale, then seal lips tightly around the mouthpiece; take a slow, deep breath to elevate the balls in the plastic tube, hold the inspiration for at least 3 seconds.	• Allows for greater lung expansion; holding the inspiration increases the pressure, preventing the immediate collapse of the alveoli.
• The client simultaneously measures the amount of inspired air volume on the calibrated plastic tube.	• Encourages the client to do respiratory exercises.
• Remove the mouthpiece, exhale normally.	• Allows normal expiration.
• Take several normal breaths.	• Provides the client the opportunity to relax.
7. Have the client repeat the procedure 4 to 5 times.	7. Encourages sustained maximal inspiration and loosens secretions.

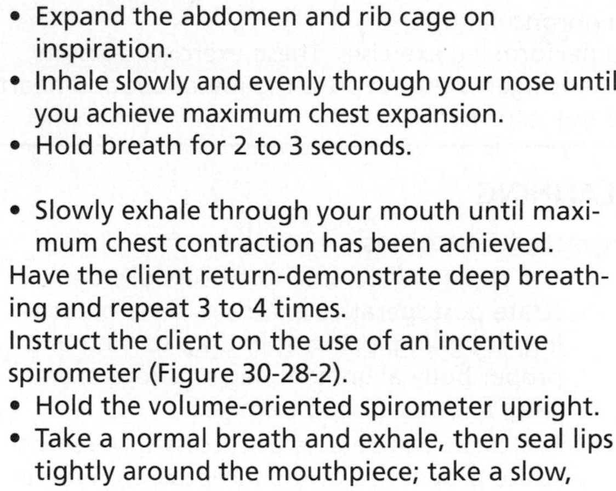

FIGURE 30-28-2 **Instruct the client to take a slow, deep breath to elevate the ball in the tube.**

(Continues)

PROCEDURE 30-28 Postoperative Exercise Instruction (Continued)

ACTION	RATIONALE
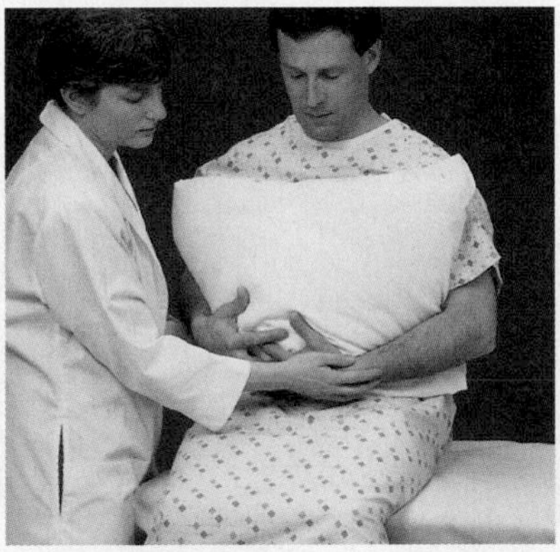 COURTESY OF DELMAR CENGAGE LEARNING FIGURE 30-28-3 Use a pillow to support the abdominal muscles when coughing.	
8. Have the client cough after the incentive effort. See the following section.	8. Facilitates the removal of secretions.
9. Demonstrate splinting and coughing.	9. Shows the client how to raise mucus secretions from the tracheobronchial tree.
• Have the client slowly raise head and sniff the air.	• Increases the amount of air and helps aerate the base of the lungs.
• Have the client slowly bend forward and exhale slowly through pursed lips.	• Dries the tracheal mucosa as air flows over it. There is a slight increase in carbon dioxide level, which stimulates deeper breathing.
• Repeat breathing 2 to 3 times.	• Loosens mucus plugs and moves secretions to the main bronchus.
• When the client is ready to cough, have client place a folded pillow against the abdomen with clasped hands (Figure 30-28-3).	• Elevates the diaphragm and expels air in a more forceful cough; supports the abdominal muscles and reduces pain while coughing, if the client has an abdominal incision.
• Have client take a deep breath and begin coughing immediately after inspiration is completed by bending forward slightly and producing a series of soft, staccato coughs.	• Removes secretions from the main bronchus.
• Have a tissue ready.	• Preparation for sputum disposal.
10. Have the client return-demonstrate splinting and coughing.	10. Fosters learning.
11. Wash the incentive spirometer mouthpiece under running water and store in a clean container. Disposable mouthpieces should be changed every 24 hours.	11. Reduces transmission of microorganisms.
12. Teach the client leg and foot exercises (Figure 30-28-4).	12. To improve venous blood return from the legs.
• Have the client, with heels on bed, push the toes of both feet toward the foot of the bed until the calf muscles tighten, then relax feet. Pull the toes toward the chin, until calf muscles tighten; then relax feet (Figure 30-28-4A).	• Causes contraction and relaxation of the calf muscles.
• With heels on bed, lift and circle each ankle, first to the right and then to the left; repeat three times, relax (Figure 30-28-4B).	• Causes contraction and relaxation of the quadriceps muscles.
• Flex and extend each knee alternately, sliding foot up along the bed; relax (Figure 30-28-4C).	• Causes contraction and relaxation of the quadriceps muscles.
13. Have the client return-demonstrate the leg and foot exercises.	13. Fosters learning of how to improve venous blood return.

(Continues)

PROCEDURE 30-28 Postoperative Exercise Instruction (Continued)

ACTION	RATIONALE

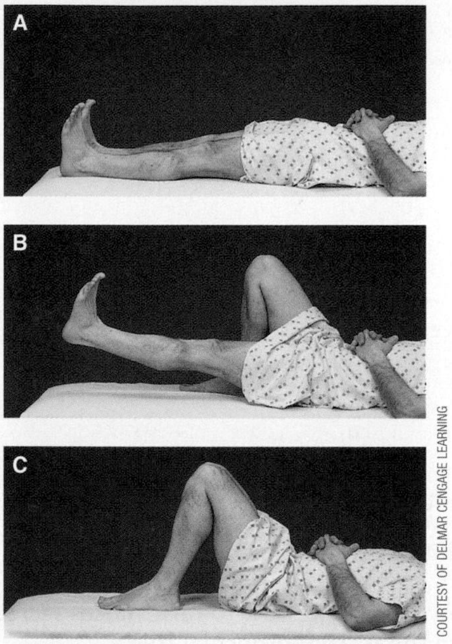

FIGURE 30-28-4 **Leg exercises improve venous blood return. *A,* Flex foot forward; *B,* Lift leg up and flex foot forward; *C,* Bend the knee.**

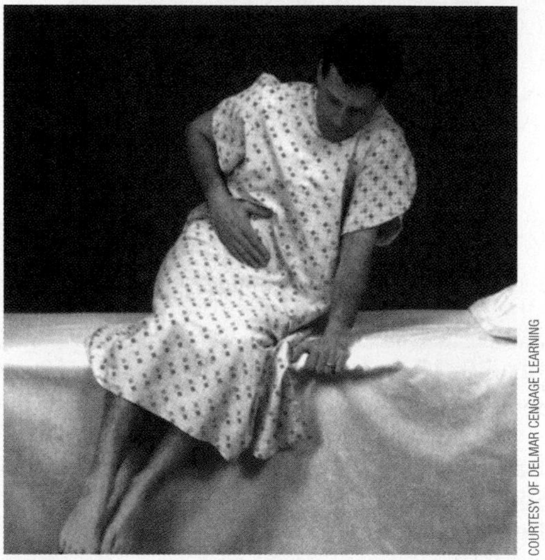

FIGURE 30-28-5 **Using the hand to splint the incision site when sitting up in bed will reduce the pain and pressure at the incision site.**

ACTION	RATIONALE
14. Explain how to turn in bed and get out of bed.	14. Elicits client cooperation.
15. Instruct the client who has a left-sided abdominal or chest incision to turn to the right side of bed and sit up as follows: • Flex the knees. • With the right hand, splint the incision with hand or small pillow. • Turn toward right side by pushing with the left foot and grasping the shoulder of the nurse or partial side rail of the bed with the left hand. • Rise up to a sitting position on the side of the bed by using the left arm and hand to push down against the mattress or side rail.	15. Fosters learning how to turn and get out of bed without putting pressure on the incision line.
16. Reverse instructions (use left side instead of right) for the client with a right-sided incision according to Action 15 (Figure 30-28-5).	16. Same as Rationale 15.
17. Instruct clients with orthopedic surgery (e.g., hip surgery) how to use a trapeze bar.	17. Facilitates movement in bed without putting pressure on a leg or hip joint.
18. Wash hands.	18. Reduces transmission of microorganisms.

EVALUATION

- The client is able to successfully demonstrate postoperative exercises, deep breathing, coughing, pillow splinting, turning and proper body alignment, leg and foot exercises, and out-of-bed transfers.
- The client is able to successfully demonstrate proper use of the incentive spirometer.

DOCUMENTATION

Nurses' Notes

- Document teaching the client postoperative exercises.
- Note the client's level of understanding and cooperation with the teaching.
- Document on appropriate electronic medical record or flow sheet.

Preoperative Checklist

- Initial the check-off area for documentation of preoperative teaching.

PROCEDURE 30-29 Performing a Skin Puncture

OVERVIEW

Skin punctures are performed when small quantities of capillary blood are needed for analysis or when the client has poor veins. Capillary puncture is also commonly performed for blood-glucose analysis. The common sites for capillary punctures are:

- Heel—most common site for neonates and infants
- Fingertip—the inner aspect of palmar fingertip used most commonly in children and adults
- Earlobe—used when the client is in shock or the extremities are edematous

ASSESSMENT

1. Assess the condition of the client's skin at the potential puncture site **to determine whether it is intact, free of bruising, and can be used without causing undue trauma to the site.**
2. Assess the circulation at the potential puncture site **to determine whether it is a good site to obtain a sample, and to determine if healing at the site might be compromised.**
3. Assess the client's comfort level regarding the procedure **to determine client education and support needed.**
4. Assess the cleanliness of the client's skin **to determine how much cleansing is needed before the skin puncture.**

POSSIBLE NURSING DIAGNOSES

Risk for Impaired Skin Integrity
Acute Pain
Anxiety

PLANNING

Expected Outcomes

1. An adequate blood specimen will be obtained.
2. The client will suffer minimal trauma during the specimen collection.
3. The specimen will be collected and stored in a manner compatible with the ordered tests.

Equipment Needed

- Antiseptic 70% isopropanol or povidone-iodine
- Microhematocrit tubes or micropipette (collection tubes)
- Sterile 2×2 gauze
- Sterile lancet
- Nonsterile latex-free gloves
- Hand towel or absorbent pad

delegation tips

Properly trained ancillary personnel may perform skin puncture. Agency policy usually dictates certification and recertification requirements for this skill. Proper client and specimen identification are of the utmost importance and must be consistently demonstrated by the ancillary personnel.

IMPLEMENTATION—ACTION/RATIONALE

ACTION	RATIONALE
* Check client's identification band * Explain procedure before beginning *	
1. Wash hands.	1. Reduces transmission of microorganisms.
2. Check the client's identification band if appropriate.	2. Ensures the correct client.
3. Explain the procedure to the client.	3. Allays anxiety and encourages cooperation.
4. Prepare supplies: • Open sterile packages. • Label specimen collection tubes. • Place in easy reach.	4. Ensures efficiency.
5. Apply nonsterile latex-free gloves.	5. Follows Standard Precautions.

(Continues)

PROCEDURE 30-29 Performing a Skin Puncture (Continued)

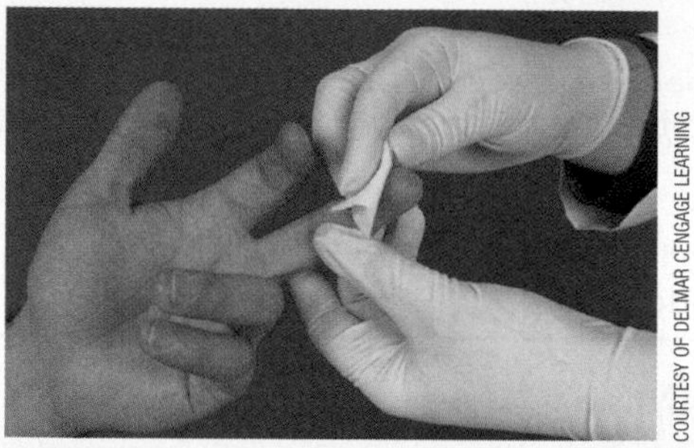

FIGURE 30-29-1 Cleanse the puncture site and allow it to dry.

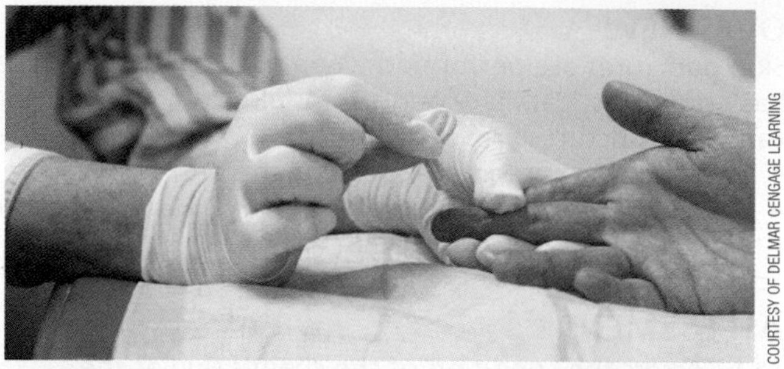

FIGURE 30-29-2 Use a quick stab to puncture the skin.

ACTION	RATIONALE
6. Select site: lateral aspect of the fingertips in adults/children; heel for neonates and infants.	6. Avoids damage to nerve endings and calloused areas of the skin.
7. Place the hand or heel in a dependent position; apply warm compresses if fingers or heel are cool to touch.	7. Increases the blood supply to the puncture site.
8. Place hand towel or absorbent pad under the extremity.	8. Prevents soiling the bed linen.
9. Cleanse puncture site with an antiseptic and allow it to dry. Use 70% isopropanol if the client is allergic to iodine (Figure 30-29-1).	9. Reduces skin surface bacteria; povidone-iodine must dry to be effective.
10. With nondominant hand, apply gentle milking pressure above or around the puncture site. Do not touch the puncture site.	10. Increases blood to puncture site and maintains asepsis.
11. Read directions carefully before using the lancet. • With the sterile lancet at a 90-degree angle to the skin, use a quick stab to puncture the skin (about 2 mm deep) (Figure 30-29-2). • With the automatic unistik, push the lancet into the body of unistik until it clicks. Hold the body of the unistik and twist off the lancet cap. Place the end of the unistik tightly against the client's finger and press the lever. The needle automatically retracts after use.	11. Provides a blood sample with minimal discomfort to the client.
12. Wipe off the first drop of blood with sterile 2 × 2 gauze; allow the blood to flow freely (Figure 30-29-3).	12. The first drop may contain a large amount of serous fluid, which could affect the results. Pressure at the puncture site can cause hemolysis.
13. Collect the blood into the tube(s). If blood for a platelet count is to be collected, obtain this specimen first (Figure 30-29-4).	13. Allows blood collection; avoids aggregation of platelets at the puncture site.
14. Apply pressure to the puncture site with a sterile 2 × 2 gauze.	14. Controls bleeding.
15. Place contaminated articles into a sharps container.	15. Reduces the risk of needlestick.
16. Remove gloves; wash hands.	16. Reduces transmission of microorganisms.
17. Position client for comfort with call light in reach.	17. Provides for comfort and communication.
18. Wash hands.	18. Reduces transmission of microorganisms.

(Continues)

PROCEDURE 30-29 Performing a Skin Puncture (Continued)

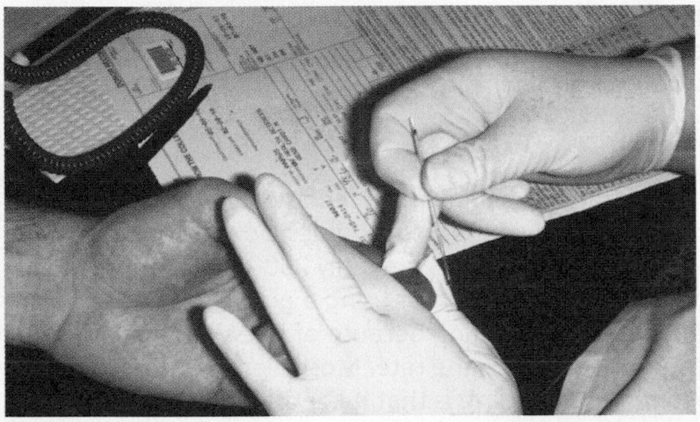

FIGURE 30-29-3 Allow the blood to flow from the puncture site to ensure that an adequate amount can be obtained.

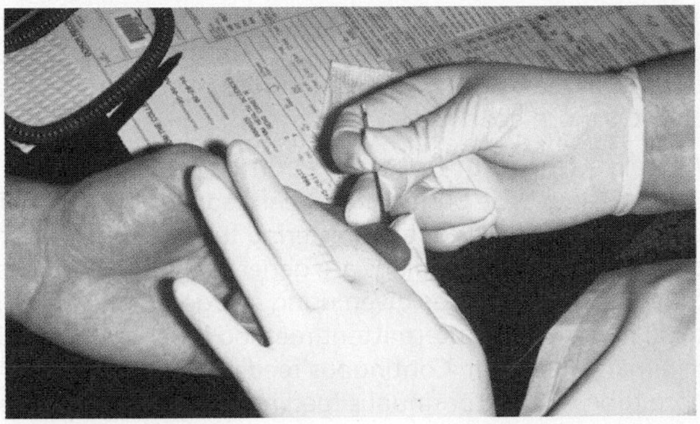

FIGURE 30-29-4 Collect a small sample of blood.

EVALUATION

- Specimen is adequate.
- No trauma to client.

DOCUMENTATION

Nurses' Notes

- Puncture site and the reason for the puncture.
- Report test results if the testing is performed at the time of the puncture.

PROCEDURE 30-30 Feeding and Medicating via Enteral Tube

OVERVIEW

Enteral nutrition is a procedure whereby liquid food (formula) is instilled directly into the stomach or small intestines using a tube. Other names for this procedure are tube feedings and gastric gavage. Candidates for tube feedings are clients who have a functional gastrointestinal (GI) tract and will not, should not, or cannot eat. Tube feedings are used for clients who are (or may become) malnourished and in whom oral feedings are insufficient to maintain adequate nutritional status.

Enteral tube feedings maintain the structural and functional integrity of the GI tract, enhance the utilization of nutrients, and provide a safe and economic method of feeding.

Enteral tube feedings are contraindicated in clients with the following:

- Diffused peritonitis
- Intestinal obstruction that prohibits normal bowel functioning
- Intractable vomiting; paralytic ileus
- Severe diarrhea

Enteral tube feedings are used with caution in clients with the following:

- Severe pancreatitis
- GI ischemia
- Enterocutaneous fistula

Feeding Tubes

Most feeding tubes are made of silicone or polyurethane, which are durable and biocompatible with formulas. They vary in diameter (8–12 French) and length in accord with the route and formula. The health care provider selects the route and type of feeding tube on the basis of the anticipated duration of feeding, the condition of the GI tract, and the potential for aspiration.

A nasogastric, small-bore feeding tube is generally used when the anticipated duration of use is short.

The gastrostomy tube is placed through an opening in the abdominal wall into the intestines. This is done via an enterostomy, the surgical creation of an artificial fistula into the intestines. Tube enterostomies can be placed at various points along the GI tract and are performed when long-term tube feeding is anticipated or when obstruction makes nasoenteral tube feeding impossible.

(Continues)

PROCEDURE 30-30 Feeding and Medicating via Enteral Tube (Continued)

Percutaneous endoscopic gastrostomy (PEG) tube placement is performed by the health care provider at the bedside or in the endoscopy room; insertion of a PEG tube does not require general anesthesia surgery. This method of enteral feeding is more common than conventional enterostomies; it is less risky because surgery is not required, and it is more economic.

Administration of Enteral Feedings

Once feeding tube position has been radiographically verified, the formula can be administered as prescribed. There are two typical methods of administering tube feedings. Intermittent feeding is given four to six times a day in the form of a bolus. Intermittent feedings are generally given through a large-bore tube. The bolus (generally 250–400 mL of formula for adult clients) can be given using a large syringe fit into the end of the feeding tube or using a gravity drip over 20 to 30 minutes. The intermittent method is generally practiced in the home care setting because of its ease and need for minimal equipment. Continuous feeding delivers formula with a pump to regulate the rate. Most clients with a small-bore tube receive continuous feeding. One of the advantages of continuous feeding is that it keeps gastric volume small, minimizing residual volume and reducing the risk of aspiration pneumonia; the client is less likely to experience bloating, nausea, abdominal distention, and diarrhea. Continuous feeding is recommended for the seriously ill or comatose client.

Safety Considerations

Clients receiving enteral nutrition through a tube feeding are at risk for aspiration. Auscultate for bowel sounds to determine gastric motility. If the bowel sounds are hypoactive or absent, stop or withhold additional feeding and notify the health care provider.

Always assess placement of the feeding tube before administering any liquids. Clients who are receiving continuous gastric feeding should be assessed every 4 hours for tube placement and residual gastric contents. Aspirate gastric contents with a syringe. Observe and check the pH of the aspirate. If less than 100 mL, replace stomach contents after checking the residual to prevent fluid and electrolyte imbalance.

Client safety and comfort require daily cleansing of the feeding tube exit site. Cleanse the skin with a clean washcloth, soap, and water. Enterostomy tubes require surgical asepsis of the exit site until the incision heals; rotate the tubes within the stoma to promote healing. Report any observations of redness, irritation, or gastric leakage at the site. Between feedings, a prosthetic device may be used to cover the ostomy opening.

The PEG tubes require daily rotation to relieve pressure on the skin. Notify the health care provider if unable to rotate the PEG; it may be an indication of internal embedding of the tube into the gastric wall. When the tube is internally embedded, it can cause gastric acid reflux, which results in skin breakdown, sepsis, and cellulitis. Care must be taken to avoid dislodgment of the tube. Keep it secured to the client's abdomen with tape, being careful not to use excessive tension. The PEG tubes require frequent flushing to prevent clogging. These tubes have small lumens. If a tube becomes clogged, flush it with 60 mL of lukewarm tap water.

ASSESSMENT

1. Assess the client for signs of gastric distress, such as nausea, vomiting, and cramping, **to determine the client's tolerance for the tube feeding.**
2. Assess the feeding tube placement every 4 hours **to confirm tube placement in the intestines.**
3. Assess the client's respiratory status **to evaluate for pulmonary aspiration of gastric contents.**
4. Assess the client's ongoing nutritional status **to evaluate the effectiveness of the tube feeding.**
5. Assess the client's intake and output **to evaluate for fluid deficit or excess.**

POSSIBLE NURSING DIAGNOSES

*Risk for Imbalanced **N**utrition: Less Than Body Requirements*
*Risk for Deficient **F**luid Volume*
*Risk for **A**spiration*
*Risk for Impaired **S**kin Integrity*
*Impaired **O**ral Mucous Membrane*

PLANNING

Expected Outcomes

1. The client will receive the correct feeding formula and the correct volume of formula over the correct time period.
2. The client will not experience any undesirable effects: aspiration, nausea, vomiting, abdominal distention, cramping, diarrhea, or constipation.
3. The client's weight and nutritional status will remain stable or improve.
4. The client will not experience any adverse skin or gastrointestinal effects from the gastrostomy or PEG tube.

Equipment Needed

- Asepto syringe or 20- to 50-mL syringe
- Emesis basin
- Clean towel
- Disposable gavage bag and tubing
- Formula
- Infusion pump for feeding tube (if needed)
- Water to follow feeding
- Nonsterile latex-free gloves

(Continues)

PROCEDURE 30-30 Feeding and Medicating via Enteral Tube (Continued)

delegation tips

Feedings via gastrostomy tubes may be given by properly trained ancillary personnel if the facility and the state permit. The ancillary personnel must be properly trained in assessing tube placement, proper positioning of the client, and in the administration of the correct type and rate of feeding. All medications must be administered by a nurse.

IMPLEMENTATION—ACTION/RATIONALE

* Check client's identification band * Explain procedure before beginning *

ACTION	RATIONALE
1. Review client's medical record for formula, amount, and time.	1. Verifies health care provider's prescription for appropriate formula and amount.
2. Wash hands and gather equipment and formula.	2. Reduces transmission of microorganisms and promotes efficiency during procedure.
3. Identify client by checking armband.	3. Verifies correct client.
4. Explain procedure to client.	4. Increases client compliance and reduces anxiety.
5. Assemble equipment. Add color to formula per institutional policy. If using a bag, fill with prescribed amount of formula (Figure 30-30-1).	5. Ensures efficiency when initiating feeding. Color will distinguish formula aspirate.
6. Place client on right side in high Fowler's position.	6. Reduces risk of pulmonary aspiration in the event client vomits or regurgitates formula.
7. Provide for privacy.	7. Places client at ease.
8. Wash hands and don nonsterile latex-free gloves.	8. Reduces transmission of pathogens.
9. Observe for abdominal distention; auscultate for bowel sounds.	9. Assesses for delayed gastric emptying; indicates presence of peristalsis and ability of GI tract to digest nutrients.
10. Check feeding residuals (Figure 30-30-2). Insert syringe into adapter port, aspirate stomach contents, and determine amount of gastric residual. If residual is greater than 50 to 100 mL (or in accordance with agency protocol), hold feeding until residual diminishes. Instill aspirated contents back into feeding tube.	10. Indicates whether gastric emptying is delayed. Reduces risk of regurgitation and pulmonary aspiration related to gastric distention. Prevents electrolyte imbalance.
11. Administer tube feeding.	11. Provides nutrients as prescribed.

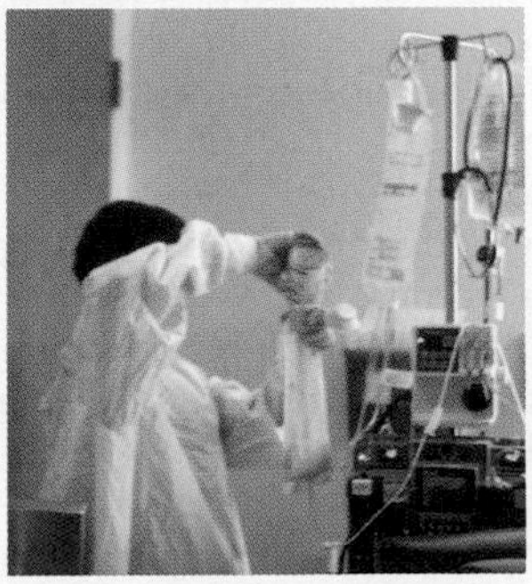

COURTESY OF DELMAR CENGAGE LEARNING

FIGURE 30-30-1 Fill the bag with the prescribed amount of formula.

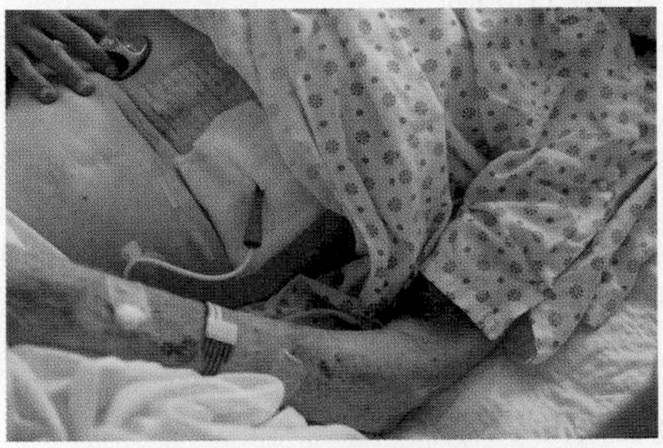

COURTESY OF DELMAR CENGAGE LEARNING

FIGURE 30-30-2 Check that the feeding tube is intact and in place, auscultate for bowel sounds, and look for abdominal distention.

(Continues)

PROCEDURE 30-30 Feeding and Medicating via Enteral Tube (Continued)

ACTION	RATIONALE
Intermittent Bolus	
12. Pinch the tubing.	12. Prevents air from entering tubing.
13. Remove plunger from barrel of syringe and attach to adapter.	13. Provides system to delivery feeding.
14. Fill syringe with formula (Figure 30-30-3).	14. Allows gravity to control flow rate, reducing risk of diarrhea from bolus feeding.
15. Allow formula to infuse slowly; continue adding formula to syringe until prescribed amount has been administered.	15. Prevents air from entering stomach. Decreases risk of diarrhea.
16. Flush tubing with 30 to 60 mL or prescribed amount of water.	16. Ensures that remaining formula in tubing is administered and maintains patency of tube; prevents air from entering the stomach.
17. Remove syringe and replace cap into adaptor port	17. Prevents airs from entering the stomach and prevents gastric contents from leaving the stomach.

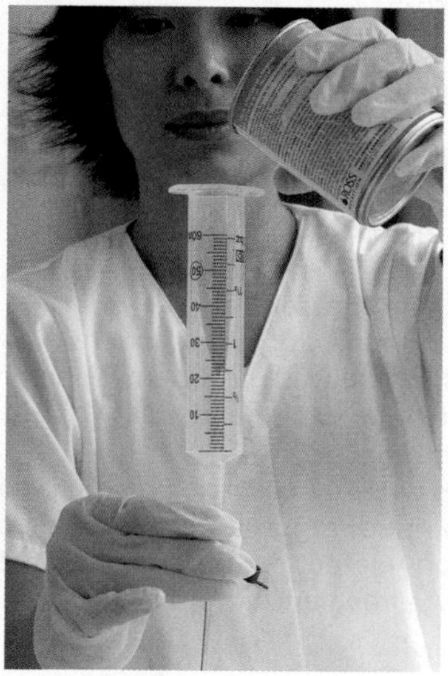

FIGURE 30-30-3 Fill syringe with formula.

ACTION	RATIONALE
Intermittent Gavage Feeding	
18. Hang bag on IV pole so that it is 18 inches above the client's head.	18. Allows gravity to promote infusion of formula.
19. Fill bag with ordered amount of feeding. Remove air from tubing by opening clamp on tubing and allow feeding to flow through tubing.	19. Prevents air from entering stomach. Decreases risk of diarrhea.
20. Attach distal end of tubing to feeding tube adapter and adjust drip to infuse over prescribed time.	20. Allows gravity to control flow rate, reducing risk of diarrhea from bolus feeding.
21. When bag empties of formula, add 30 to 60 mL or prescribed amount of water; close clamp.	21. Prevents air from entering stomach and reduces risk for gas accumulation. Maintains patency of feeding tube.
22. Remove tubing from adaptor port and cap adaptor port.	22. Prevents air from entering stomach and prevents gastric contents from leaving the stomach.
23. Change bags every 24 hours.	23. Decreases risk of microorganism multiplication in bag and tubing.

(Continues)

PROCEDURE 30-30 Feeding and Medicating via Enteral Tube (Continued)

ACTION	RATIONALE
Continuous Gavage	
24. Check tube placement at least every 4 hours.	24. Ensures that feeding tube remains in stomach.
25. Check residual at least every 4 hours.	25. Indicates ability of GI tract to digest and absorb nutrients.
26. If residual is above 100 mL, stop feeding.	26. Reduces risk of regurgitation and pulmonary aspiration related to gastric distention.
27. Add prescribed amount of formula to bag for a 4-hour period; dilute with water if prescribed.	27. Provides client with prescribed nutrients and prevents bacterial growth (formula is easily contaminated).
28. Hang gavage bag on IV pole. Prime tubing.	28. Removes air from tubing.
29. Thread tubing through feeding pump and attach distal end of tubing to feeding tube adapter; keep tubing straight between bag and pump.	29. Provides for controlled flow rate; prevents loops in tubing.
30. Program rate.	30. Infuses formula over prescribed time.
31. Monitor infusion rate and signs of respiratory distress or diarrhea.	31. Prevents complications associated with continuous gavage.
32. Flush tube with water every 4 hours as prescribed or following administration of medications.	32. Maintains patency of tube.
33. Replace disposable feeding bag at least every 24 hours, in accord with institution protocol.	33. Decreases transmission of microorganisms.
34. Elevate head of bed at least 30 degrees at all times and turn client every 2 hours.	34. Prevents aspiration and promotes digestion and reduces skin breakdown.
35. Provide oral hygiene every 2 to 4 hours.	35. Provides comfort and maintains the integrity of buccal cavity.
36. Administer water as prescribed with and between feedings.	36. Ensures adequate hydration.
37. Remove gloves and wash hands.	37. Reduces transmission of microorganisms.
Instilling Medications into Enteral Tubes	
38. Wash hands and don nonsterile gloves.	38. Reduces spread of microorganisms.
39. Assist the client to high or semi-Fowler's position.	39. Gravity assists to keep medications down.
40. Place linen saver over bed linens.	40. Prevents soiling during procedure.
41. Verify nasogastric (NG) tube placement.	41. Ensures tube placement is correct.
42. Attach syringe to tube and pour 30 mL of prepared medication into syringe.	42. Readies medication to be given.
43. Open clamp on tube.	43. Allows medication into tube.
44. Hold syringe at a slight angle; add more medication before syringe empties.	44. Allows medication to flow at a slow, steady rate.
45. For two or more medications, give each separately, with 5-mL water rinse between medications.	45. Ensures each medication is given.
46. As syringe empties with the last of the medication, slowly add 30 to 50 mL water.	46. Clears medication from the sides and distal end of tube to prevent clogging.
47. Before tube empties of water, clamp the tube, detach and dispose of the syringe.	47. Prevents air from getting into the stomach. Disposes of used equipment.
48. Place clients with an NG tube on the right side with head slightly elevated for 30 minutes.	48. Prevents regurgitation.
49. Remove gloves and wash hands.	49. Reduces spread of microorganisms.

EVALUATION

- The client received the correct feeding formula and the correct volume of formula over the correct time period.
- Client did not experience any undesirable effects such as aspiration, nausea, vomiting, abdominal distention, cramping, diarrhea, or constipation.
- Client's weight and nutritional status remained stable or improved.

(Continues)

PROCEDURE 30-30 Feeding and Medicating via Enteral Tube (Continued)

- Client did not experience any adverse skin or gastrointestinal effects from the gastrostomy or PEG tube.

DOCUMENTATION

Nurses' Notes

- Time, date, formula, and amount of feeding, and client's response
- Amount of residual aspirated before the feeding
- Tube placement checked and method used
- If the dressing at the tube insertion site was changed and the condition of the client's skin
- If the tube was rotated or adjusted
- Any client complaints or adverse effects such as bloating, nausea, vomiting, diarrhea, or constipation
- Document on appropriate electronic medical record or flow sheet.

Medication Administration Record

- Date and time the feeding was instilled (per institution specifications)

Intake and Output Record

- Amount of tube feeding instilled and the amount of water used to flush the feeding tube

REFERENCES/SUGGESTED READINGS

Altman, G. (2010). *Fundamental and advanced nursing skills 3rd edition.* Clifton Park, New York: Delmar, Cengage Learning.

Gray, M. (2008). Securing the indwelling catheter. *AJN,* 108(12), 44–50.

Lord, L. (2001). How to insert a large-bore nasogastric tube. *Nursing2001, 31*(9), 46–48.

Metheny, N., & Titler, M. (2001). Assessing placement of feeding tubes, *AJN, 101*(5), 36–45.

Metules, T. (2007). Hands-on help hot and cold packs. *RN,* 70(1), 45–48.

North American Nursing Diagnosis Association International. (2010). *NANDA-I nursing diagnoses: Definitions and classification 2009–2011.* Ames, IA: Wiley-Blackwell.

Raymond, M. (2008). Piercing ears to test glucose. *RN,* 71(12), 23.

CHAPTER 31
Advanced Procedures

PROCEDURE 31-1 Inserting and Maintaining a Nasogastric Tube

OVERVIEW

Nasogastric (NG) tubes are used for several purposes, including feeding for nutrition when the client is comatose, semiconscious, or unable to consume sufficient nutrition orally. Nasogastric suction tubes are used for decompression of gastric content after gastrointestinal surgery and to obtain gastric specimens for diagnosis of peptic ulcer. Tubes are used for irrigation to clean and flush the stomach after oral ingestion of poisonous substances. Finally, NG tubes are used to document the presence of blood in the stomach, monitor the amount of bleeding from the stomach, and identify the recurrence of bleeding in the stomach.

The two most commonly used NG tubes are the single-lumen Levin's tube and the double-lumen Salem sump tube.

The gastrointestinal tract is considered to be a clean area rather than a sterile one. The procedure to place an NG tube is performed using clean technique unless it is performed in conjunction with gastrointestinal surgery.

ASSESSMENT

1. Assess client's consciousness level **to determine the ability of the client to cooperate during the procedure.**
2. Check the client's chart for any previous medical history of nostril surgery or injury or unusual nostril bleeding. **Reduces risk of injury from the tube.**
3. Use a penlight to assess nostrils for a deviated septum. **Facilitates choice of nostril and size of tube.**
4. Ask the client to breathe through each nostril, occluding the other with a finger. **Facilitates choice of nostril and decreases chance that tube will interfere with respirations.**
5. Assess for latex allergy. **Prevents reaction to latex and determines need to use latex-free tubes and gloves.**

POSSIBLE NURSING DIAGNOSES

Imbalanced ***N****utrition: Less Than Body Requirement*
Impaired ***S****wallowing*
Risk for ***A****spiration*
Risk for ***D****iarrhea*
Impaired ***O****ral Mucous Membrane*
Risk for Deficient ***F****luid Volume*
Acute ***P****ain*
Impaired ***S****kin Integrity*

PLANNING

Expected Outcomes

1. Client's nutritional status will improve, as indicated by increased body weight, physical strength, and mental status.
2. Client's nutritional needs will be met with the assistance of tube feeding.
3. Client will maintain a patent airway, as evident by absence of coughing, no shortness of breath, and no aspiration.
4. Client will not have diarrhea caused by nasogastric feeding.
5. Mouth mucous membranes will remain moist and intact.
6. Client will maintain a normal fluid volume, as evident by good skin texture, muscle tone, and blood volume.
7. Client's comfort level will increase.
8. Skin around the tube will remain intact, with no redness or blisters.

Equipment Needed

- Nasogastric tube: adult, 14 to 18 French; child/infant, 5 to 10 French; single-lumen (Levin's tube): feeding; double-lumen (Salem sump tube): feeding, suction, irrigation
- Water-soluble lubricant
- Syringe with catheter tip or adapter, 50 mL

PROCEDURE 31-1 Inserting and Maintaining a Nasogastric Tube (Continued)

- Glass of tap water with straw, or ice
- Towel or tissue
- Emesis basin with ice chips
- Tongue blade
- pH chemstrip
- Stethoscope
- Hypoallergenic tape, rubber band, and safety pin
- Personal protective equipment: gown; disposable, nonsterile latex-free gloves; face shield or goggles; and mask
- Penlight or flashlight
- Disposable irrigation set (if needed)
- Wall mount or portable suction equipment (if needed)
- Administration set with pump or controller for feeding tube

delegation tips

Inserting and maintaining a nasogastric tube is the responsibility of a nurse. Oral hygiene for the client may be delegated.

IMPLEMENTATION—ACTION/RATIONALE

ACTION	RATIONALE
* Check client's identification band * Explain procedure before beginning *	
1. Review client's medical history for conditions that have resulted in a loss of the gag reflex.	1. To assess for any nostril surgery and abnormal bleeding. A client without a gag reflex is at risk for aspiration.
2. Identify client by checking armband. Assess client's consciousness and ability to understand. Develop a hand signal.	2. Verifies correct client. Decreases anxiety and promotes cooperation.
3. Provide privacy. Prepare the equipment, putting tissues, a cup of water, and an emesis basin nearby.	3. Provides privacy. Facilitates an efficient procedure.
4. Prepare the environment; raise the bed and place it in a high Fowler's position (45 to 60 degrees). Cover the chest with a towel.	4. Prevents back strain and facilitates insertion.
5. Wash hands and then put on gloves and personal protective equipment.	5. Reduces transmission of microorganisms. Protects from body fluids.
6. Assess client's nostrils with penlight and have the client blow nose one nostril at a time.	6. Decreases discomfort and unnecessary trauma by choosing the more patent nostril for insertion.
7. Using the NG tube, measure the distance from the tip of the nose to the earlobe and then to the xiphoid process of the sternum and mark this distance on the tube with a piece of tape (Figure 31-1-1).	7. Determines the approximate amount of tube needed to reach the stomach.
8. Lubricate first 4 inches of the tube with water-soluble lubricant.	8. Facilitates passage into the naris.
9. Ask the client to slightly flex the neck backward.	9. Makes insertion easier.
10. Gently insert the tube into a naris (Figure 31-1-2).	10. Promotes passage of tube with minimal trauma to mucosa.
11. Ask the client to tip the head forward once the tube reaches the nasopharynx—this is usually where the client starts to gag. If the client continues to gag, stop for a moment.	11. Tipping the head forward facilitates passage of the tube into the esophagus instead of the trachea. Tube may stimulate gag reflex. Allows the client to rest, reduces anxiety, and prevents vomiting.
12. Advance the tube several inches at a time as the client swallows. If gag reflex is present, have the client swallow water or ice chips as tube is advanced.	12. Assists in advancing the tube past the oropharynx. The action of swallowing facilitates the insertion process. With each swallow, the tracheal opening is closed to prevent inspiration. Clients who do not have a gag reflex are at risk for aspiration.

(Continues)

PROCEDURE 31-1 Inserting and Maintaining a Nasogastric Tube (Continued)

ACTION	RATIONALE

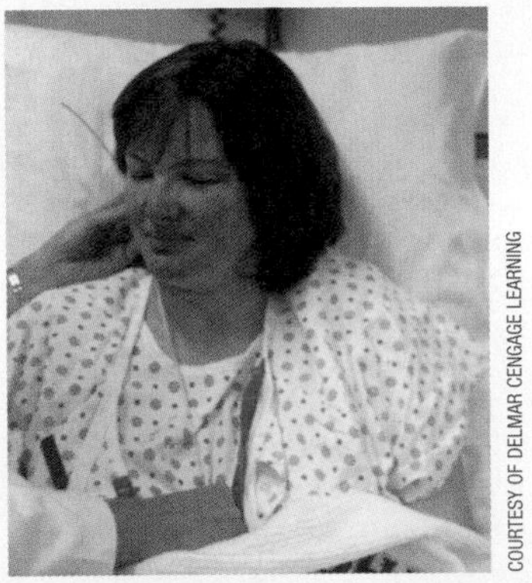

FIGURE 31-1-1 Measure the distance from the nose to earlobe to the xiphoid process to determine how much tube will need to be inserted to reach the stomach.

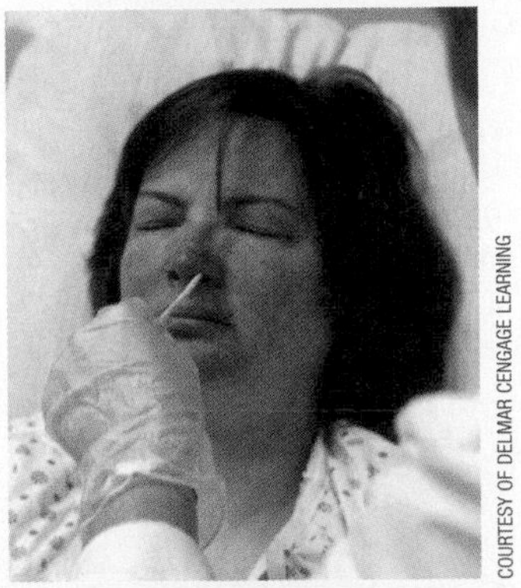

FIGURE 31-1-2 Gently insert the tube into the naris.

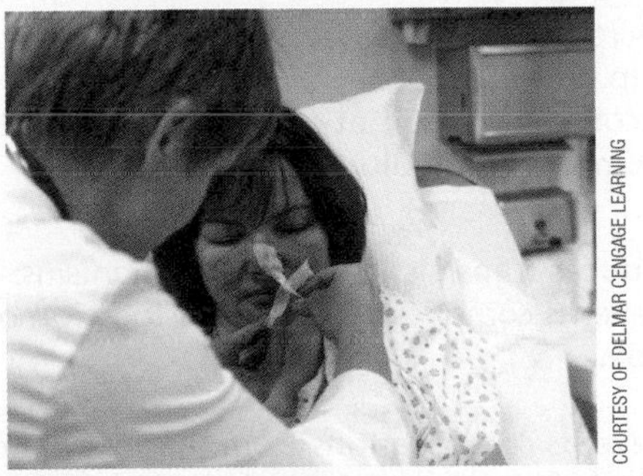

FIGURE 31-1-3 Secure the tube to the nose.

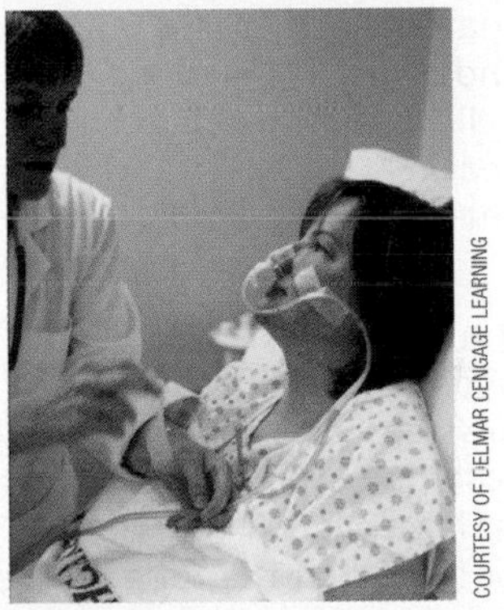

FIGURE 31-1-4 Tape the tube to the cheek as well, if desired, to provide extra support.

13. Withdraw the tube immediately if there are signs of respiratory distress.
    - 13. Prevents trauma to bronchus or lung.
14. Advance the tube until the taped mark is reached.
    - 14. Enables the tube to reach the stomach.
15. Wipe or wash body oils off tip of nose and allow to dry. Split a 4-inch strip of tape lengthwise 2 inches. Secure the tube with the tape by placing the wide portion of the tape on the bridge of the nose and wrapping the split ends around the tube (Figure 31-1-3). Tape to cheek as well if desired (Figure 31-1-4).
    - 15. Prevents tube displacement.
16. Check the placement of the tube:
    - Aspirate for gastric content, assess the color and quality of the content. If required, measure with pH indicator strip (Figure 31-1-5). Follow protocol regarding reinsertion of contents versus discarding.
    - Prepare the client for x-ray checkup, if prescribed.
    - 16. Ensures correct placement. A pH below 5 indicates the tube is in the stomach.
17. Connect the distal end of the tube to suction, draining bag, or adapter according to the purpose of this nursing intervention.
    - 17. Establishes an appropriate pathway for intervention.
18. Secure the tube with tape, or with rubber band and safety pin, to client's gown.
    - 18. Enhances the level of comfort and secures the tubing system.

(Continues)

PROCEDURE 31-1 Inserting and Maintaining a Nasogastric Tube (Continued)

ACTION	RATIONALE
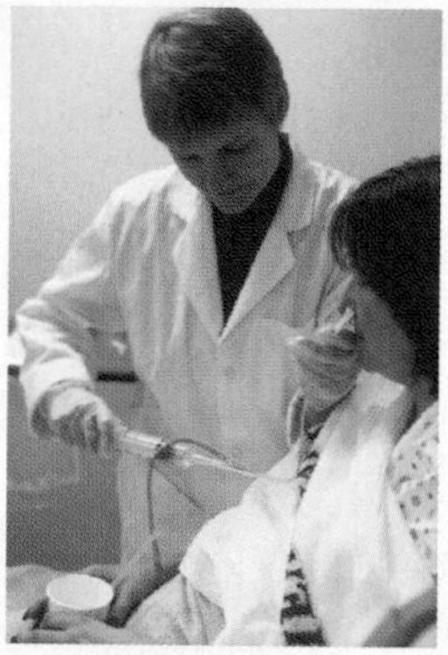 COURTESY OF DELMAR CENGAGE LEARNING FIGURE 31-1-5 Aspirate a sample of gastric content to check for pH.	
19. Remove protective equipment, dispose of contaminated materials in proper container, and wash hands.	19. Implements Standard Precautions.
20. Position client comfortably and place the call light in easy reach.	20. Decreases client's anxiety and provides access to help if needed.
21. Document procedure.	21. Records implementation of intervention and promotes continuity of care.
Maintaining a Nasogastric Tube	
22. Wash hands and apply gloves.	22. Reduces transmission of microorganisms.
23. Follow the steps in Action 16 to check the proper tubing position before instilling anything per NG tube or at least every 8 hours.	23. Prevents complications from dislocation of the tube.
24. Assess for signs that the tube has become blocked, including epigastric pain and vomiting, and/or the inability to pass medications or feedings through the tube.	24. Prevents complications from the loss of beneficial effects from the tube.
25. Remember never to irrigate or rotate a tube that has been placed by the health care provider during gastric or esophageal surgery.	25. Rotation or irrigation may disturb incisions.
26. Provide oral hygiene and assist client to clean nares daily.	26. Enhances client's comfort and the integrity of skin and nose mucosa.
27. Remove gloves, dispose of contaminated materials in proper container, and wash hands.	27. Reduces transmission of microorganisms.

EVALUATION

- Client's nutritional status improves, as indicated by increased body weight, physical strength, and mental status.
- Client's nutritional needs are met with the assistance of tube feeding.
- Client maintains a patent airway, as evident by absence of coughing, no shortness of breath, and no aspiration.
- Client does not have diarrhea caused by nasogastric feeding.
- Mouth mucous membranes remain moist and intact.
- Client maintains a normal fluid volume, as evident by good skin texture, muscle tone, and blood volume.
- Client's stomach decompressed and comfort level increases.
- Skin around the tube remains intact, with no redness or blisters.

DOCUMENTATION

Nurses' Notes

- Type of NG tube inserted, the naris used, how the client tolerated the procedure, and the methods used to verify placement
- Care provided to the client to increase comfort of the NG insertion naris
- Any unusual findings

(Continues)

PROCEDURE 31-1 Inserting and Maintaining a Nasogastric Tube (Continued)

- Document on appropriate electronic medical record or flow sheet

Intake and Output Record

- Amount of fluid the client drank to aid insertion of the NG tube
- Amount of gastric contents removed for testing
- Amount of gastric suctioning

PROCEDURE 31-2 Performing Venipuncture (Blood Drawing)

OVERVIEW

Obtaining a sample of blood through venipuncture is a commonly used procedure for many diagnostic tests. Blood test results are a source of valuable information to screen for disease, to evaluate the progress of therapy, and to monitor the well-being of the client. The nurse is often required to obtain a variety of specimens. Because some specimens require special handling, it is important to be familiar with the particular test that is ordered.

There are three primary methods of obtaining blood specimens: venipuncture, skin puncture, and arterial stick. Venipuncture is the most common method and involves inserting a large-bore needle into a vein. The nurse attaches either a syringe or a vacutainer tube for the collection of the blood specimen. Skin puncture is the easiest way to obtain a small specimen from the finger, toe, or heel. A lancet is used for the puncture, and a drop of blood is collected through a capillary tube. An arterial stick is the most complicated and requires special assessment skills and techniques.

As with any procedure, it is important to review the employer's policies and procedures as well as their state's nurse practice act.

ASSESSMENT

1. Determine which test(s) is ordered and be familiar with any special conditions associated with the timing of the collection or the handling of the specimen. Many specimens may be collected at very specific times (i.e., before or after administration of a drug, while the client is NPO, or after fasting). Other specimens may require special handling (i.e., ice is used to transport for ammonia level; heparinized collection containers are needed for platelet count; and so on). A blood specimen drawn at the incorrect time or put into an incorrect collection container cannot be used. Test results will be delayed and the client has to be stuck again.
2. Assess the integrity of the veins that may be used in the procedure. Identify any conditions that may contraindicate venipuncture. Avoid veins injured by infiltration or phlebitis or compromised by surgery (i.e., modified radical mastectomy). **Using a damaged vein may cause further injury to the vein. A compromised site may not provide an adequate amount of blood for the specimen and may lead to another venipuncture for the client. In addition, drawing samples from sites near IV infusion solutions may alter the composition of the blood sample.**
3. Review the client's medical history to determine if there are any expected complications from the venipuncture. **Clients with a history of abnormal clotting disorders, low platelets, or related disorders (hemophilia) may be at risk for increased bleeding at the site or hematoma formation.**
4. Determine the client's ability to cooperate with the procedure. **Many clients are fearful of needles—especially children—and additional help may be needed. Very young children may need to have the extremity restrained during the procedure.**
5. Review the physician's or qualified practitioner's order. Check for appropriateness of the test as well as the frequency of the test. Critically ill clients may require frequent blood tests and venipuncture. **Combining tests and carefully evaluating frequency may reduce unnecessary blood loss for the client.**

POSSIBLE NURSING DIAGNOSES

Deficient Knowledge (purpose of blood sample and procedure)
Risk for Infection
Impaired Tissue Integrity
Anxiety
Fear
Risk for Injury

(Continues)

PROCEDURE 31-2 Performing Venipuncture (Blood Drawing) (Continued)

PLANNING

Expected Outcomes

1. Venipuncture site will show no evidence of continued bleeding or hematoma.
2. The venipuncture site will show no evidence of signs and symptoms of infection.
3. The laboratory test will be properly acquired and appropriately handled after collection.
4. The client will be able to discuss the purpose of the test and describe the procedure.
5. The client will report minimal anxiety associated with the procedure.

Equipment Needed

- Disposable gloves
- Alcohol swabs
- Rubber tourniquet
- Sterile 2 × 2 gauze pads
- Band-Aid or adhesive tape (precut)Assessment
- Band-Aid or adhesive tape (precut)
- Appropriate blood collection tubes
- Labels for each collection tube with the appropriate client information included
- Completed laboratory requisition forms
- Needle/equipment disposal container
- Small pillow or folded towel to support the extremity if needed
- Syringe method: sterile needles: 20- to 21-gauge for adults, 23- to 25-gauge butterfly for older adults, 23- to 25-gauge butterfly for children
- Vacutainer method: Vacutainer tube with needle holder; sterile double needles (20- to 21-gauge for adults, 23- to 25-gauge for children)

delegation tips

The procedure of performing a venipuncture for the purposes of blood drawing is frequently delegated to properly trained ancillary personnel. Documentation of their competency and skill should be available to the nurse, and periodic reevaluation should occur according to agency and state policy. The ancillary personnel should be reminded to not obtain blood specimens from an extremity above the site of infusing fluids and to report to the nurse any complications or concerns the client might express postprocedure.

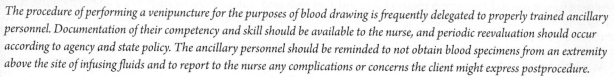

IMPLEMENTATION—ACTION/RATIONALE

* Check client's identification band * Explain procedure before beginning *

ACTION	RATIONALE
1. Validate client's identification.	1. Verifies correct client.
2. Wash hands.	2. Reduces transmission of microorganisms.
3. Bring equipment to bedside or exam room. Transfer client to the exam room, especially small children.	3. Provides an organized approach to the procedure. Keeps their hospital room a "safe haven."
4. Close curtain or door.	4. Provides privacy.
5. Raise or lower bed/table to comfortable working height.	5. Maintains good body mechanics during the procedure.
6. Before selecting an appropriate site for the venipuncture, assess the extremities for the presence of an arteriovenous shunt used for dialysis or history of a mastectomy.	6. Extremities with a shunt or on the same side of the body as a mastectomy should not be used.
7. Position client's arm; extend arm to form a straight line from shoulder to wrist. Place pillow or towel under upper arm to enhance extension. Client should be in a supine or semi-Fowler's position.	7. Helps stabilize the arm. The bed should support the client's body (when possible) in case the client feels faint during the procedure.
8. Apply disposable gloves.	8. Reduces the risk of infection to both the client and the nurse (Standard Precautions).
9. Apply the tourniquet 3 to 4 inches above the venipuncture site. Most often, the antecubital fossa site is used. The tourniquet should be able to be removed by pulling the end with a single motion.	9. Provides improved visibility of the veins as they dilate in response to decreased venous return of blood flow from the extremity to the heart.

(Continues)

PROCEDURE 31-2 Performing Venipuncture (Blood Drawing) (Continued)

ACTION	RATIONALE
10. Check for the distal pulse. If there is no pulse felt, then the tourniquet is applied too tightly and must be reapplied more loosely.	10. Impedes arterial flow, preventing venous filling.
11. Have client open and close fist several times, leaving fist clenched before venipuncture.	11. Increases the venous distension and enhances visibility of the vein.
12. Maintain tourniquet for only 1 to 2 minutes.	12. Prolonged time may increase client discomfort and alter some laboratory results (falsely elevated serum potassium).
13. Identify the best venipuncture site through palpation; the ideal site is a straight, prominent vein that feels firm and slightly rebounds when palpated. Palpate potential site.	13. Straight, intact veins are easier to puncture. A thrombosed vein is rigid, or rolls easily, and is difficult to stick.
14. Select the vein for venipuncture. (If the tourniquet has been on too long, release it and let the client rest for 1 to 2 minutes before reapplying the tourniquet.)	14. Increases client comfort and ensures accurate laboratory results.
15. Prepare to obtain the blood sample. Technique varies depending on equipment used:	15.
• *Syringe method:* Have syringe with appropriate needle attached.	• A needle with a very small bore can damage the red cells as the blood is drawn and lead to inaccurate test results.
• *Vacutainer method:* Attach double-ended needle to vacutainer tube and have the proper blood specimen tube resting inside the vacutainer. Do not puncture the rubber stopper yet.	• The long end of the needle is used to puncture the vein, and the short end enters the blood tube.
16. Cleanse the venipuncture site according to agency policy using a circular method at the site and extending 2 inches beyond the site. Allow to dry.	16. Cleans the skin surface of bacteria that may cause infection at the site. Allowing the alcohol to dry reduces stinging. Povidone-iodine must dry to be effective.
17. Remove the needle cover and warn that client will feel the needlestick.	17. Clients will be better able to control their reaction if they know what to expect.
18. Place the thumb or forefinger of the nondominant hand 1 inch below the site and pull the skin taut.	18. Helps stabilize the vein during insertion.
19. Hold syringe needle or vacutainer at a 15- to 30-degree angle from the skin with the bevel up.	19. This angle reduces the chance of penetrating through the vein during insertion. The needle causes less trauma to the skin and vein when the bevel is up during insertion.
20. Slowly insert needle/vacutainer.	20. Prevents puncture through the other side of the vein.
21. Technique varies depending on equipment used:	21.
• *Syringe method:* Gently pull back on syringe plunger and look for blood return. Obtain desired amount of blood into the syringe.	• If blood does not appear, the needle is not in the vein.
• *Vacutainer method:* Hold vacutainer securely and advance specimen tube into needle of holder. Be careful not to advance the needle into the vein. The blood should flow into the collection tube. After the collection tube is full, grasp the vacutainer firmly, remove the tube, and insert additional specimen collection tubes as indicated (Figure 31-2-1).	• Pushing the needle through the stopper breaks the vacuum and causes the flow of blood into the collection tube. Failure of blood to appear in the collection tube indicates the vacuum in the tube has been lost or the needle is not in the vein.
22. After the specimen collection is completed, release the tourniquet.	22. Reduces bleeding from pressure when the needle is removed.
23. Apply 2 × 2 gauze over the puncture site without applying pressure and quickly withdraw the needle from the vein.	23. Helps prevent the skin from pulling with the needle removal.

(Continues)

PROCEDURE 31-2 Performing Venipuncture (Blood Drawing) (Continued)

ACTION	RATIONALE
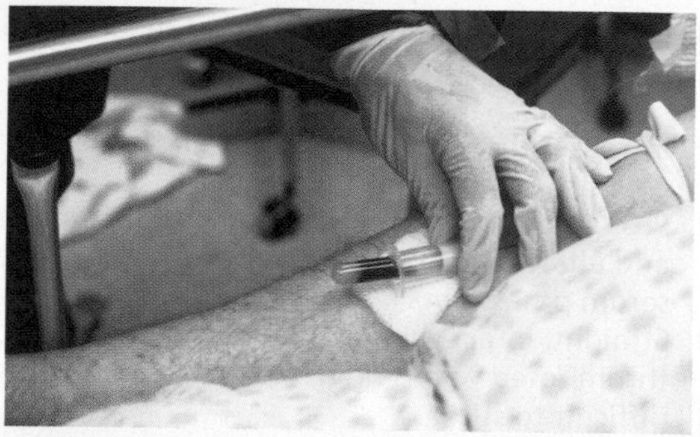 COURTESY OF DELMAR CENGAGE LEARNING **FIGURE 31-2-1 Allow the tube to fill with blood. When it is full, remove the tube and insert additional tubes if needed.**	
24. Immediately apply pressure over the venipuncture site with the gauze for 2 to 3 minutes or until the bleeding has stopped. Tape the gauze dressing over the site (or apply the Band-Aid).	24. Direct pressure stops the bleeding and minimizes formation of a hematoma. You may avoid using tape or a Band-Aid if, after applying pressure, no bleeding is present. Many clients are sensitive to tape, and its removal can be painful.
25. Syringe method: • Using one hand, insert the syringe needle into the appropriate collection tube and allow vacuum to fill. You may also remove the stopper from each vacutainer collection tube, remove the needle from the syringe, fill the tube, and replace the stopper.	25. Using a one-handed method to fill the syringe helps reduce the chance of needlestick injury. • This alternative method allows you to control the speed and amount of fill in the collection tubes.
26. If any of the blood tubes contain additives, gently rotate back and forth 8 to 10 times.	26. Ensures that the additive is properly mixed throughout the specimen.
27. Inspect the client's puncture site for bleeding. Reapply clean gauze and tape, if necessary.	27. Keeps site clean and dry.
28. Assist client into a comfortable position. Return bed to low position with side rails up, if appropriate.	28. Provides comfort and safety for the client.
29. Check tubes for any external blood and decontaminate with alcohol as appropriate.	29. Prevents contamination to other equipment and personnel.
30. Check tubes for proper labeling. Place tubes into appropriate bags/containers for transport to the laboratory.	30. Ensure the specimens are properly identified. Follows Standard Precautions.
31. Dispose of needles, syringes, and soiled equipment into proper container.	31. Prevents spread of disease and needlestick injury.
32. Remove and dispose of gloves.	32. Reduces transmission of microorganisms.
33. Wash hands.	33. Reduces transmission of microorganisms.
34. Send specimens to the laboratory.	34. Facilitates timely handling of specimens and accurate results.

EVALUATION

- Venipuncture site shows no evidence of continued bleeding or hematoma.
- Venipuncture site shows no signs or symptoms of infection.
- The blood specimen is properly acquired and appropriately handled after collection.
- The client is able to discuss the purpose of the test and describe the procedure.
- The client reports minimal anxiety associated with the procedure.

DOCUMENTATION

Nurses' Notes

- Date and time of the venipuncture, the site used for the procedure, any complications, the tests to be run, and the disposition of the specimens
- Client's reaction to the procedure and the condition in which the client was left (i.e., bed lowered with side rails up)
- Document on appropriate electronic medical record or flow sheet

PROCEDURE 31-3 Preparing an IV Solution and Starting an IV

OVERVIEW

An intravenous solution is a method of correcting or preventing a fluid and electrolyte disturbance. Clients who are acutely ill, are NPO after surgery, or have severe burns are examples of those who require IV therapy.

The solution in an IV bag is ordered by the health care provider according to the client's needs and is changed at least every 24 hours, or per the institution's policy, to decrease the risk of infection. Tubing is used to connect the solution in the IV bag with the client's IV catheter or needle. Use needleless systems if available. OSHA requires safe devices.

Performing venipuncture in order to establish venous access is a priority for clients with fluid and electrolyte disturbances, clients who are critically ill, clients who are NPO after surgery, or clients who, for other reasons, are not able to take fluids or food by mouth. Venous access can be used for infusions of IV fluids, emergency medications, parenteral nutrition, blood products, and routine IV medications.

There are a variety of IV needles and catheters. They vary in gauge from small bore to large bore. A 20- to 22-gauge flexible catheter is used for adults, and a 22- to 24-gauge catheter is used for pediatric clients. If large volumes of fluid or blood products are anticipated to be given, a larger bore (18- or 19-gauge) is recommended.

A commonly used angiocatheter has an over-the-needle catheter (ONC) made of plastic, Teflon, or other materials. These flexible catheters have a metal stylet that is used to pierce the skin and vein and a plastic catheter that is threaded into the vein and attached to the IV tubing after the stylet has been removed.

The other type of IV needle is a straight steel needle that is inserted into the vein and secured after being attached to an IV tubing. With an increased emphasis on safety, many health care facilities use a safety-shielded intravenous catheter or retractable needle system when placing a peripheral IV line. This consists of a traditional metal stylet used for the skin puncture covered by the plastic or Teflon angiocatheter. Once the IV line is successfully placed, the person initiating the IV pushes a button and the stylet retracts completely into a protective casing, thereby reducing the risk of needlestick injury.

The Centers for Disease Control and Prevention (CDC) guidelines must be followed to decrease the risk of infection for the client by changing the IV solution every 24 hours, changing the IV site and catheter every 48 to 72 hours, and changing the IV tubing every 72 hours. Occupational Safety and Health Administration (OSHA) standards are necessary to prevent exposure to blood-borne pathogens through the use of gloves, sharps containers, and special training for health care workers.

ASSESSMENT

1. Check the health care provider's order for the IV solution to be infused and rate of flow **to determine the optimal needle size and type to use and ensure accurate administration.**
2. Review information regarding the solution and insertion of the IV and nursing implications **in order to insert the catheter and administer the solution safely.**
3. Know the agency's policy regarding who may start an IV **because many agencies require that nurses have special training before they can perform this procedure.**
4. Check all additives in the solution and other medications **so that there will be no incompatibilities of additives with the solution.**
5. Assess the client's veins to **optimize planning of the IV site.**
6. Check the client's fluid, electrolyte, and nutritional status **to provide baseline data for comparison with the client's response to IV therapy.**
7. Assess the client's understanding of the purpose of the procedure **so that client teaching can be used to decrease anxiety.**

POSSIBLE NURSING DIAGNOSES

Deficient Knowledge (need for IV)
Risk for Infection
Excess Fluid Volume
Deficient Fluid Volume
Impaired Skin Integrity
Risk for Injury

PLANNING

Expected Outcomes

1. The appropriate fluids at the ordered dosages will be available for IV infusion.
2. The IV infusion will be sterile, without precipitate or contamination.
3. The IV will be inserted into the vein without complications and will remain patent.
4. Fluid and electrolyte balance will be restored.
5. Nutrition will be restored or maintained.
6. The IV site will remain free of swelling and inflammation.

(Continues)

PROCEDURE 31-3 Preparing an IV Solution and Starting an IV (Continued)

Equipment Needed

- Appropriate safety needle or catheter for venipuncture
- Tourniquet
- Povidone-iodine swabs (3) or chlorhexidine alcohol (chloroprep)
- Alcohol swab sticks (3) (not needed if using chlorhexidine alcohol)
- Disposable gloves
- Arm board, if needed
- Towel or absorbent drape
- Povidone-iodine ointment (not used in all institutions)
- Gauze dressing
- Tape
- Scissors
- IV solution and tubing

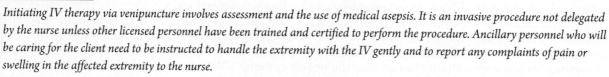

delegation tips

Initiating IV therapy via venipuncture involves assessment and the use of medical asepsis. It is an invasive procedure not delegated by the nurse unless other licensed personnel have been trained and certified to perform the procedure. Ancillary personnel who will be caring for the client need to be instructed to handle the extremity with the IV gently and to report any complaints of pain or swelling in the affected extremity to the nurse.

IMPLEMENTATION—ACTION/RATIONALE

ACTION	RATIONALE
* Check client's identification band * Explain procedure before beginning *	
1. Check health care provider's order for an IV and the solution. Identify client.	1. Ensures accurate insertion of catheter and administration of the solution to the correct client.
2. Wash hands.	2. Reduces transmission of microorganisms.
3. Prepare solution bag by removing protective cover from bag.	3. Allows for access to the solution container.
4. Inspect the bag for leaks, tears, or cracks. Inspect the fluid for clarity, particulate matter, and color. Check expiration date.	4. Prevents infusing contaminated or outdated solution.
5. Prepare a label for the IV bag: • On the label, note date, time, and your initials. • Attach the label to the bag. Keep in mind that the bag will be inverted when it is hanging. Make sure the label can be read when the IV is hanging.	5. • Communicates when the bag was opened. • Labeling the bag upside-down makes identification easier when the bag is hanging.
6. Open new infusion set. Unroll tubing and close roller clamp.	6. Prevents fluid from leaking after IV bag is spiked.
7. Grasp the port of the IV bag with your nondominant hand, remove the plastic tab covering the port (Figure 31-3-1), and insert the full length of the spike into the bag's port (Figure 31-3-2).	7. Promotes rapid flow of solution through new tubing without air bubbles.
8. Compress drip chamber to fill halfway.	8. Allows the chamber to provide a clear measurement of drip rate when the IV is flowing.
9. Loosen protective cap from the end of the IV tubing, open roller clamp, and flush tubing with solution (Figure 31-3-3 A and B).	9. Removes air from tubing.
10. Close roller clamp and replace cap protector.	10. Prevents fluid from leaking and maintains sterility.
11. Take prepared fluid and needed equipment to bedside.	11. Ensures smooth procedure without accidents or contamination.
12. Check client's identification band and explain procedure.	12. Ensures correct client and decreases anxiety.
13. Wash hands and put on mask and gown if needed.	13. Reduces transmission of microorganisms.

(Continues)

PROCEDURE 31-3 Preparing an IV Solution and Starting an IV (Continued)

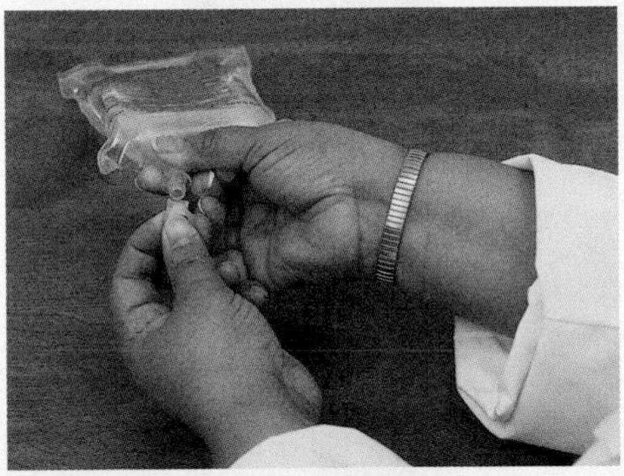

COURTESY OF DELMAR CENGAGE LEARNING

FIGURE 31-3-1 Open the IV plastic bag and pull down the plastic tab covering the port with one hand while pinching the port with the other hand.

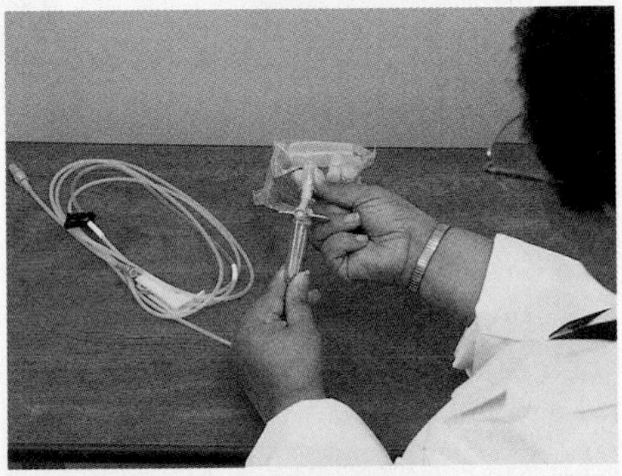

COURTESY OF DELMAR CENGAGE LEARNING

FIGURE 31-3-2 Remove the cap from the spike and spike the IV port.

A B

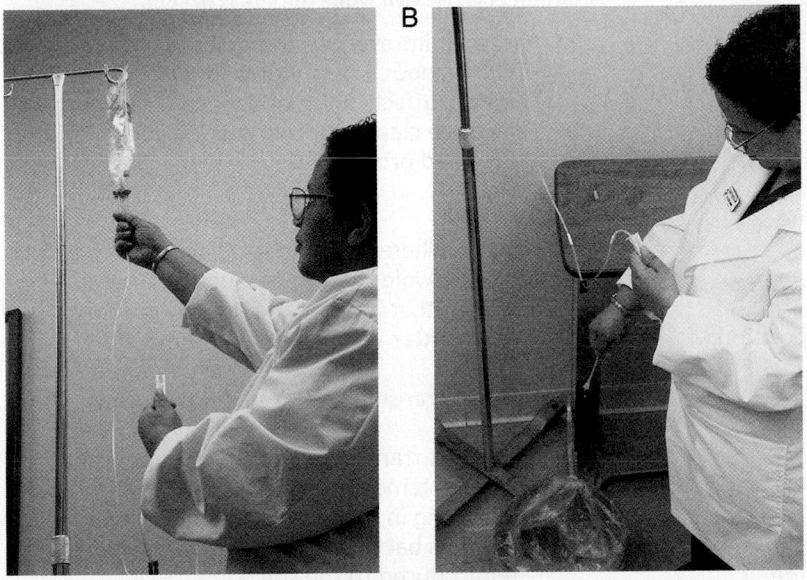

COURTESY OF DELMAR CENGAGE LEARNING

FIGURE 31-3-3 Priming the IV tubing. Open the roller clamp on the tubing to allow the fluid to enter the tube and expel the air.

ACTION	RATIONALE
14. Assess the extremities for the presence of an arteriovenous shunt used for dialysis or history of mastectomy before selecting an appropriate site for the IV.	14. Extremities with a shunt or on the same side as the mastectomy should not be used for an IV site.
15. Inspect potential veins to be used:	15. Promotes ease of placement of catheter.
• Place a tourniquet around the upper arm, close to the axilla.	• Distends vein to allow visual and tactile examination.
• Examine the veins as they dilate.	• Evaluates viability of the veins.
• Palpate the vein to test for firmness (Figure 31-3-4).	• Determines best site for venipuncture and IV placement.
• Release the tourniquet.	• Prevents engorgement of vein.
16. Select vein for venipuncture:	16.
• Use most distal part of the vein first.	• If the vein is later damaged, the proximal part can be used.
• Avoid bony prominences.	• Increases client comfort.
• Avoid client's wrist or hand.	• Bending increases risk of infiltration or phlebitis.
• Avoid client's dominant hand and arm.	• Allows freedom of movement.
• Avoid an extremity with decreased sensation.	• Promotes earlier detection of infiltration.
• Avoid an area of skin affected by a rash or infection.	• Decreases risk of infection.

(Continues)

PROCEDURE 31-3 Preparing an IV Solution and Starting an IV (Continued)

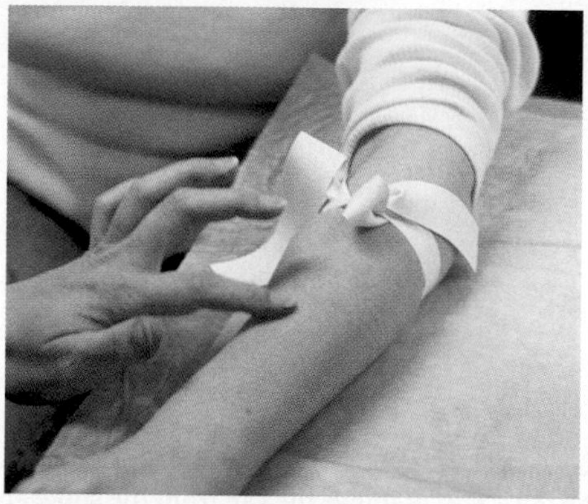

FIGURE 31-3-4 Inspect the site for potential veins to use, and palpate to further locate a vein and test for firmness.

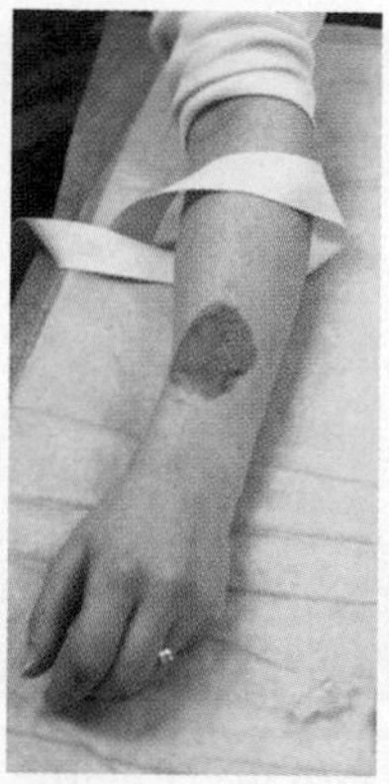

FIGURE 31-3-5 After scrubbing the insertion site with alcohol and povidone-iodine, allow it to dry. *Note:* The tourniquet is released while the site is drying.

ACTION	RATIONALE
17. Select safety shield or angiocatheter that is appropriate for ordered IV fluid. Select the correct size (gauge and length) of catheter.	17. Particular intravenous therapies require specific sizes of intravenous access. Age and quality or location of veins can affect choice of size.
18. Prepare supplies: • Place towel or drape on table for supplies. • Place supplies on towel. • Open needle adapter end of IV tubing set.	18. Provides a clean working surface for an efficiently performed procedure.
19. Shave hair on skin at site if necessary.	19. Ensures adherence of dressing and a less painful removal. Avoid shaving because it causes small abrasions that increase the risk of infection.
20. Ask client to rest arm in a dependent position, if possible.	20. Allows better venous dilation and visibility.
21. Put on disposable gloves.	21. Reduces transmission of microorganisms.
22. Prepare insertion site (Figure 31-3-5):	22.
• Place absorbent drape under the arm.	• Reduces transmission of microorganisms.
• Scrub the insertion site with 3 alcohol swabs then 3 povidone-iodine swabs. • Follow institution protocol. Some facilities use chlorhexidine alcohol instead of iodine. • Use separate swab and start in the middle of the site and work outward.	• Alcohol removes fat on the skin and vigorous scrubbing in circular motion with povidone-iodine removes bacteria. Prevents bacteria from being reintroduced to the site.
• Allow the antiseptic solution to air dry.	• Povidone-iodine or chlorhexidine alcohol must be dry to be effective.
23. Apply tourniquet 5 to 6 inches above the insertion site.	23. Allows the vein to engorge for easier venipuncture.
• Secure it tightly enough to occlude venous flow, not arterial flow.	• Decreased arterial flow prevents venous filling.
• Check presence of distal pulse.	• Ensures arterial flow is present.
24. Perform the venipuncture:	24.
• Anchor the vein by placing thumb over vein and stretching the skin against the direction of insertion 2 to 3 inches distal to the site.	• Stabilizes the vein for ease of venipuncture.
• Insert the stylet needle at a 10- to 30-degree angle with the bevel up (Figure 31-3-6).	• Prevents puncture of posterior wall of vein.
• Watch for a quick blood return through the flashback chamber of the ONC.	• Venous pressure from tourniquet causes backflow of blood into catheter or tubing.
• Verify needle placement in a vein, not an artery.	• Some veins are close to an artery. Arterial blood is bright red and pulses.
• Advance ONC ¼ inch into the vein while it is parallel to the skin.	• Ensures the catheter is in the vein.

(Continues)

PROCEDURE 31-3 Preparing an IV Solution and Starting an IV (Continued)

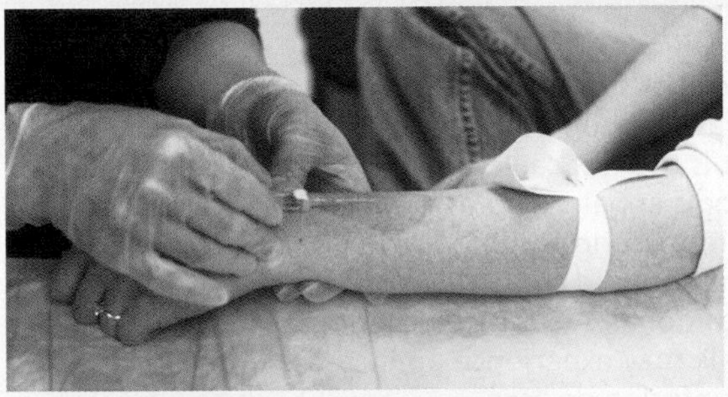

COURTESY OF DELMAR CENGAGE LEARNING

FIGURE 31-3-6 Insert the needle with the beveled side up. Keep the angle low, 10 to 30°.

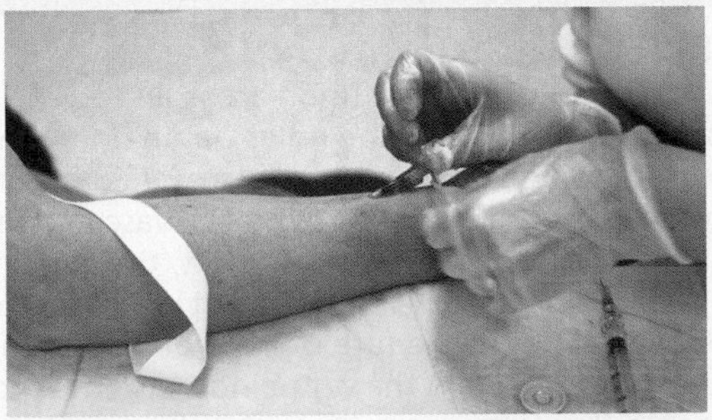

COURTESY OF DELMAR CENGAGE LEARNING

FIGURE 31-3-7 Loosen the stylet and advance the catheter into the vein until the hub rests on the skin at the venipuncture site.

ACTION	RATIONALE
• Loosen stylet and advance catheter into vein until hub rests at venipuncture site (Figure 31-3-7).	• Ensures proper placement of the catheter.
• Do not reinsert stylet.	• Prevents the catheter from being punctured by the stylet.
• Hold thumb over vein above catheter tip.	• Prevents blood from leaking out of vein until IV tubing is connected.
• Release the tourniquet.	• Reestablishes venous blood flow.
25. Attach IV tubing to ONC.	25.
• Stabilize the catheter with one hand.	• Maintains catheter placement.
• Remove the stylet from ONC or, if using a safety catheter, push the button on the protective casing and stylet will fully retract into the casing.	• Provides entry portal for IV fluids. Reduces risk of inadvertent needlestick injury.
• Quickly release pressure over vein and quickly connect needle adapter of IV set to hub of ONC.	• Reduces blood loss.
• Begin infusion at slow rate to keep vein open.	• Prompt initiation of infusion maintains patency of IV.
26. Secure catheter in place:	26.
• Place tape over the hub of the catheter.	• Ensures catheter's safe position.
• Place transparent dressing over the site and secure.	• Controls bleeding and prevents infection. Allows visualization of site through transparent dressing.
• Secure tubing in loop fashion with tape.	• Prevents dislodgement of IV if tubing is pulled.
27. Regulate flow or, if applicable, attach tubing to infusion device or rate controller if used. Turn on pump and set flow rate (see Procedure 31-4, Setting the IV Flow Rate).	27. Sets flow rate at prescribed rate.
28. Remove gloves and dispose with all used materials.	28. Reduces transmission of microorganisms.
29. Place label with date and time of insertion and size and gauge of catheter on the dressing. Follow protocol for scheduled dressing change.	29. Provides information to schedule next dressing change.
30. Wash hands.	30. Reduces transmission of microorganisms.

EVALUATION

- The appropriate fluids at the ordered dosages were available for IV infusion.
- The IV infusion was sterile, without precipitate or contamination.
- The IV was inserted into the vein without complications and remains patent.
- Fluid and electrolyte balance were restored.
- Nutrition was restored or maintained.
- The IV site remains free of swelling and inflammation.

DOCUMENTATION

Nurses' Notes

- Date and time the IV was inserted
- Type and gauge of catheter
- Date of dressing placement
- Fluid to be infused or if a saline or heparin lock
- Client's reaction to the procedure
- Document on appropriate electronic medical record or flow sheet

PROCEDURE 31-4 Setting the IV Flow Rate

OVERVIEW

Setting the rate of an IV infusion according to the health care provider's order is a nursing responsibility. The flow rate can be controlled by the roller clamp on the IV tubing or by an infusion pump. It is important for the rate to be accurate to prevent complications in fluid balance. A rate that is too fast can result in fluid overload, which is potentially serious in clients with cardiovascular, renal, or neurologic impairment, as well as in very young or very old clients. If an infusion is set too slow, the vein may clot or the more serious complication of circulatory collapse in a dehydrated or severely injured client who required large volumes of fluid could develop.

Sudden changes in the rate of infusion may be accidental or positional. A confused client may loosen the roller clamp or get tangled in the IV tubing. A client who gets up to walk may experience an increase in the IV rate. Changes in flow rate can occur with tubing and a roller clamp or infusion devices.

An infusion pump is an electronic device used to deliver a prescribed amount of fluid over a period of time in milliliters per hour. Pumps may have a drop sensor that counts each drop of fluid and sounds an alarm if the flow rate differs from what is programmed. An alarm sounds when the bag is empty or when pressure increases in the system, as in the case of an infiltrated IV.

An IV controller delivers fluid by gravity, so the bag must be at least 36 inches above the IV site. The number of drops per minute, as well as the IV tubing size and viscosity of the fluid, are necessary to calculate the actual volume delivered per hour. The controller cannot force fluid into the vein like a pump, so infiltrations are detected more quickly; however, the sensitivity of the pump system increases the number of alarms caused by client movement.

A volume-control device is a calibrated chamber placed between the IV bag and the drip chamber so that a small volume of IV fluid (<200 mL) can flow into the chamber and then infuse without the danger that the whole bag will be infused into the client.

ASSESSMENT

1. Check the health care provider's order for the IV to be infused and rate of flow **to ensure accurate administration.**
2. Review information regarding the solution and nursing implications **in order to administer the solution safely.**
3. Assess the patency of the IV **to ensure that the solution will enter the vein and not the surrounding tissue.**
4. Assess the skin at the IV site **so that the solution will not be administered into an inflamed or edematous site, which could cause injury to the tissue.**
5. Assess the client's understanding of the purpose of the IV infusion **so that client teaching can be tailored to his needs.**

POSSIBLE NURSING DIAGNOSES

Excess Fluid Volume
Risk for Deficient Fluid Volume
Deficient Knowledge (IV infusion)

PLANNING

Expected Outcomes

1. The fluid will be infused into the vein without complications.
2. The IV catheter will remain patent.
3. The fluid and electrolyte balance will return to normal.
4. The client will be able to discuss the purpose of the IV therapy.

Equipment Needed

- Watch with a second hand
- IV solution in a bag
- IV tubing
- IV infusion pump (optional)
- Volume control device (optional)
- Paper and pencil

delegation tips

Setting the rate of the IV after establishing the infusion is the responsibility of the nurse. This procedure is not delegated unless other licensed personnel have been trained and certified to perform the procedure. Ancillary personnel may be instructed to report an infusion that is dripping too fast or an IV bag that is almost empty. It is the nurse's responsibility to monitor the infusion, but ancillary personnel may also be instructed to report observations such as swelling, leaking, or client concerns about pain, numbness, or tingling at the site or in the extremity used for the infusion.

PROCEDURE 31-4 Setting the IV Flow Rate (Continued)

IMPLEMENTATION—ACTION/RATIONALE

ACTION	RATIONALE
* Check client's identification band * Explain procedure before beginning *	
1. Check health care provider's order for the IV solution and rate of infusion. Check client's identification armband.	1. Ensures accurate administration of the solution to the correct client.
2. Wash hands.	2. Reduces transmission of microorganisms.
3. Prepare to set flow rate:	3.
• Have paper and pencil ready to calculate flow rate.	• A nurse unfamiliar with IV fluid rates should calculate the rate at first.
• Review calibration in drops per milliliter (gtt/mL) of each infusion set.	• Drops per milliliter vary with manufacturer and tubing type. Macrodrip tubing varies from 10 to 15 gtt/mL. Microdrip tubing generally delivers 60 gtt/mL.
4. Determine hourly rate by dividing total volume by total hours. *Example 1:* The order reads 1000 mL D_5W with 20 mEq KCl over 8 hours: $\frac{1000\text{ mL}}{8\text{ hr}} = 125\text{ mL/hr}$ *Example 2:* Three liters are ordered for 24 hours: $\frac{3000\text{ mL}}{24\text{ hr}} = 125\text{ mL/hr}$	4. Provides a prescribed hourly rate.
5. Mark a length of tape placed on the IV bag with the hourly time periods according to the rate.	5. Provides a visual check of the fluid infused to be sure the rate is correct.
6. Calculate the minute rate based on the drop factor of the infusion set: $\frac{\text{mL/ hr}}{60\text{ min}} = \text{mL/min}$ Drop factor × mL/min = gtt/min $\frac{\text{mL hr} \times \text{drop factor}}{60\text{ min}} = \text{gtt/min}$ $\frac{\text{hourly rate} \times \text{drop factor}}{60\text{ min}} = \text{gtt/min}$ • Microdrip example: $\frac{125\text{ mL} \times 60\text{ gtt/mL}}{60\text{ min}} = \frac{7500\text{ gtt}}{60\text{ min}} = 125\text{ gtt/min}$ • Macrodrip example: $\frac{125\text{ mL} \times 15\text{ gtt/mL}}{60\text{ min}} = 31\text{ gtt/min}$	6. Formulas calculate how many drops per minute to be infused.
7. Set flow rate:	7.
• *For regular tubing without a device:* Count drops in drip chamber for 1 minute while watching second hand of watch and adjust the roller clamp as necessary (Figure 31-4-1).	• Ensures that infusion is administered as ordered.
• *For an infusion pump:* Insert the tubing into the flow control chamber, select the desired rate (generally calibrated in milliliters per minute), open the roller clamp, and push start button.	• Pumps the solution through the tubing at the rate set.
• *For a controller:* Place IV bag 36 inches above the IV site, select the desired drops per minute, open the roller clamp, and count drops for 1 minute to verify rate.	• The controller works by gravity.

(Continues)

PROCEDURE 31-4 Setting the IV Flow Rate (Continued)

ACTION	RATIONALE

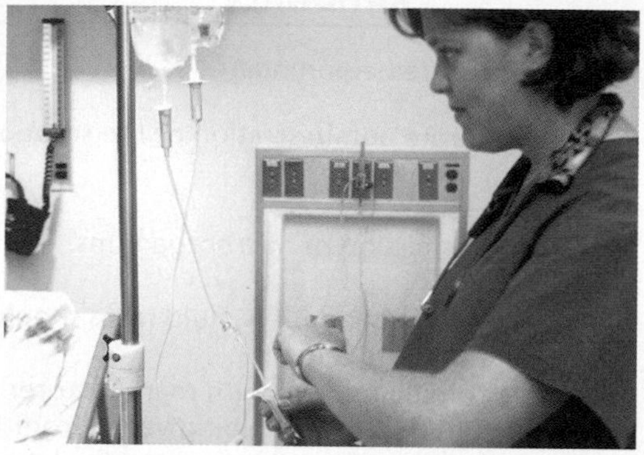

COURTESY OF DELMAR CENGAGE LEARNING

FIGURE 31-4-1 Count the drips in the drip chamber for 1 minute.

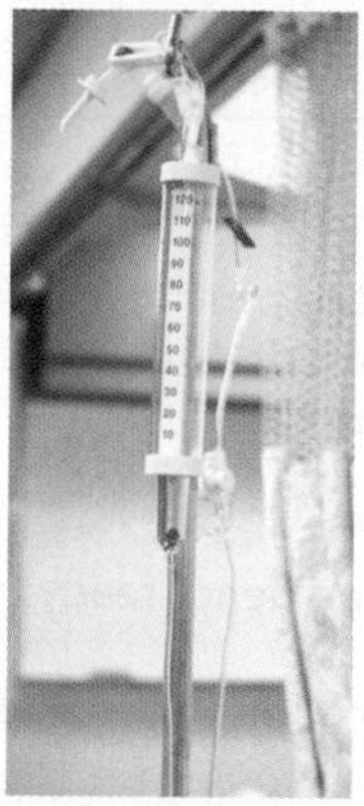

COURTESY OF DELMAR CENGAGE LEARNING

FIGURE 31-4-2 The volume-control device is placed between the IV bag and the client. It is filled with 1 to 2 hours worth of IV fluid.

ACTION	RATIONALE
• *For volume-control device:* Place device between IV bag and insertion spike of IV tubing, fill with 1 to 2 hours amount of IV fluid, and count drops for 1 minute (Figure 31-4-2).	• The amount of fluid in the volume control chamber depends on the amount of fluid to be infused per hour: 50 mL/hour = 50 to 100 mL of fluid 100 mL/hour = 100 to 200 mL of fluid
8. Monitor infusion rate and IV site for infiltration.	8. Infusion devices may fail.
9. Assess infusion when alarm sounds.	9. Sounds when a drip has not been sensed. It can be caused by an empty IV bag, a kink in the tubing, a clotted needle, an infiltrated IV, or another malfunction of the device.
10. Wash hands.	10. Reduces transmission of microorganisms.

EVALUATION

- The fluid is infusing into the vein without complications.
- The IV catheter remains patent.
- The fluid and electrolyte balance returned to normal.
- The client is able to discuss the purpose of IV therapy.
- The client receives the correct amount of IV fluid.

DOCUMENTATION

Flow Sheet

- Date and time IV solution was started
- Rate of infusion in drops per minute and milliliters per hour
- Any changes in the IV rate

Nurses' Notes

- Client's response to the IV therapy
- Changes in condition caused by a complication in the IV infusion
- Document on appropriate electronic medical record or flow sheet

PROCEDURE 31-5 Administering Medications via Secondary Administration Sets (Piggyback)

OVERVIEW

A medication is given intravenously when a rapid response to a drug is required or when several medications need to be given IV on a regular schedule. This is best accomplished by using an existing IV as the basic infusion and adding medications by "piggyback" when they are ordered. It also carries the highest risk of side effects because of the immediate response of the medication and the inability to correct a medication administration error.

(Continues)

PROCEDURE 31-5 Administering Medications via Secondary Administration Sets (Piggyback) (Continued)

The drug is diluted and mixed with a small volume (50 to 100 mL) of compatible solution and then joined to the primary IV line for infusion. The bag is connected to the upper Y-port of the primary infusion line and hung higher than the primary IV bag, thus the name piggyback. The piggyback infusion works because of the backflow valve. When the piggyback infusion starts flowing, the valve stops the flow of the primary infusion. After the piggyback infusion is complete and the solution within the tubing falls below the level of the primary infusion drip chamber, the valve opens and the primary infusion flows.

It is important to note that some medications can be irritating to the lining of blood vessels. Other medications, when injected into a vein that is beginning to infiltrate, will injure the tissue to such an extent that tissue could slough, become abscessed, or become necrotic. No IV medication should be administered through IV sites that are suspected to be inflamed or infiltrated. Use needleless systems if available. Safety needles and syringes are required by OSHA standards.

ASSESSMENT

1. Check the health care provider's order or the medication administration record (MAR) for the medication, dosage, and time and route of administration **to ensure accurate administration.**
2. Review information regarding the drug, including action, purpose, side effects, normal dose, peak onset, and nursing implications, **in order to administer the drug safely.**
3. Determine additives in the solution of an existing IV line **so that the medication will be compatible with the solution.**
4. Assess the placement of the IV catheter in the vein **to ensure that the medication will enter the vein and not the surrounding tissue.**
5. Assess the skin at the IV site **so that the medication will not be administered into an inflamed or edematous site, which could cause injury to the tissue.**
6. Check the client's drug allergy history, **because an allergic reaction could occur rapidly and be fatal.**
7. Assess the client's understanding of the purpose of the medication **so that client teaching can be tailored to needs.**
8. Assess the compatibility of the piggyback IV medication with the primary IV solution **to avoid an adverse reaction such as the formation of precipitate in the IV tubing.**

POSSIBLE NURSING DIAGNOSES

Risk for Infection
Risk for Injury
Impaired Skin Integrity
Deficient Knowledge (medication)

PLANNING

Expected Outcomes

1. The drug is infused into the vein without complications.
2. The IV site remains free of swelling and inflammation.
3. The client will be able to discuss the purpose of the drug.
4. The client is free from allergic reaction.

Equipment Needed

- Disposable gloves
- Medication prepared in a labeled infusion bag
- Short microdrip or macrodrip tubing set for piggyback (needleless system preferred)
- Safety sterile needles, 21- or 23-gauge, if needleless system is not available
- Antiseptic swab
- Adhesive tape
- IV pole
- Medication administration record (MAR)

delegation tips

The skill of medication administration is not delegated to ancillary personnel in acute care settings. This may vary in state or federal institutions. Ancillary personnel are generally informed about the medications the client is receiving if adverse effects are anticipated or are being monitored.

IMPLEMENTATION—ACTION/RATIONALE

ACTION	RATIONALE
* Check client's identification band * Explain procedure before beginning *	
1. Check health care provider's order.	1. Ensures accurate administration of medication.
2. Wash hands. *Gloves are not necessary if you are adding fluids to an existing infusion line.*	2. Reduces transmission of microorganisms.
3. Check client's identification armband.	3. Ensures medication is given to the correct client.

(Continues)

PROCEDURE 31-5 Administering Medications via Secondary Administration Sets (Piggyback) (Continued)

ACTION	RATIONALE
4. Prepare medication bag:	4.
• Close clamp on tubing of infusion set.	• Prevents leakage of solution.
• Spike medication bag with infusion tubing.	• Provides a method of infusing the medication into the system.
• Open clamp.	• Allows the solution to fill the tubing.
• Allow tubing to be filled with solution to evacuate air from tubing.	• Prevents air embolus.
5. Hang piggyback medication bag above level of primary IV bag. Use extender found in the piggyback tubing package to lower the primary bag (Figure 31-5-1).	5. Relationship between height of the bags affects the flow rate to the client.
6. Connect piggyback tubing to primary tubing at Y-port:	6. Ensures medication in piggyback bag is infused.
• For needleless system, remove cap on port and connect tubing (Figure 31-5-2).	• A needleless system is preferred to prevent accidental needlesticks.
• If a needle is used, clean port with antiseptic swab and insert small-gauge needle into center of port.	• A small-gauge needle does less damage to the rubber stopper on the port.
• Secure tubing with adhesive tape.	• Prevents accidental removal of tubing.
7. Administer the medication:	7.
• Check the prescribed length of time for the infusion.	• Each medication has a recommended rate for IV piggyback administration.
• Regulate flow rate of piggyback by adjusting regulator clamp (Figure 31-5-3).	• Medication infuses through primary line.
• Observe whether backflow valve on piggyback has stopped flow of primary infusion during drug administration (Figure 31-5-4).	• Prevents backup of medication into primary infusion line.
8. Check primary infusion line when medication is finished:	8.
• Regulate primary infusion rate.	• Reestablishes primary infusion.
• Leave secondary bag and tubing in place for next drug administration.	• Reduces risk for entry of microorganisms by repeated changes of tubing.

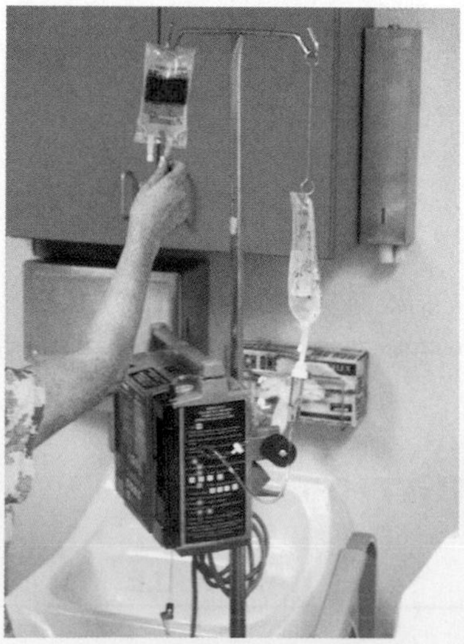

COURTESY OF DELMAR CENGAGE LEARNING

FIGURE 31-5-1 Hang the piggyback bag higher than the primary IV bag.

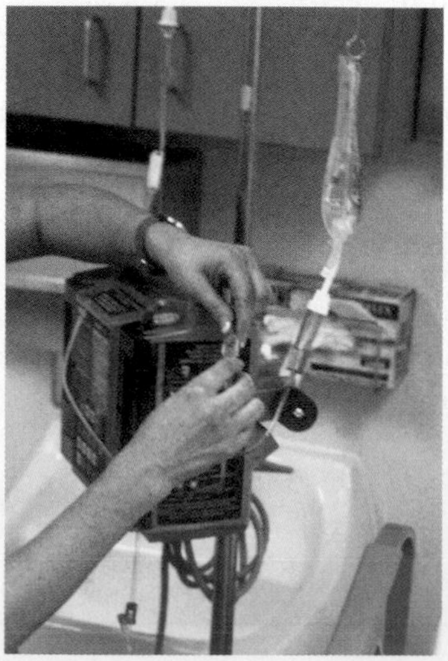

COURTESY OF DELMAR CENGAGE LEARNING

FIGURE 31-5-2 Connect the needleless system tubing.

(Continues)

PROCEDURE 31-5 Administering Medications via Secondary Administration Sets (Piggyback) (Continued)

ACTION	RATIONALE

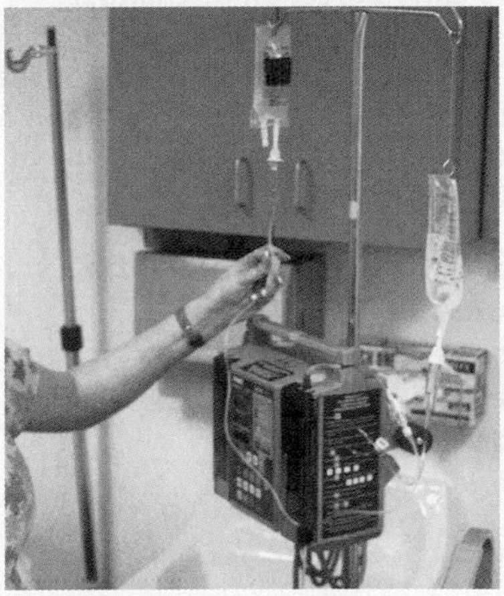

FIGURE 31-5-3 Regulate the flow rate of the piggyback by adjusting the regulator clamp.

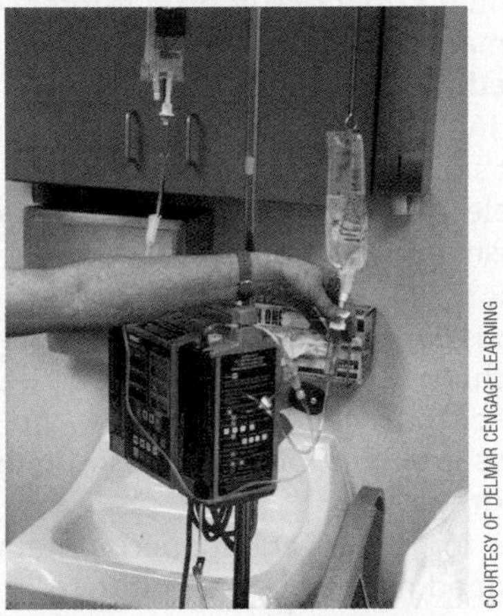

FIGURE 31-5-4 Double-check that the primary infusion has stopped flowing.

ACTION	RATIONALE
9. Dispose of all used materials and place needles in needle biohazard sharps container.	9. Reduces transmission of microorganisms.
10. Wash hands.	10. Reduces transmission of microorganisms.

EVALUATION

- The drug was infused into the vein without complications.
- The IV site remained free of swelling and inflammation.
- The client was able to discuss the purpose of the drug.

DOCUMENTATION

Medication Administration Record

- Date, time, dose, and route of medication

Flow Sheet

- Date, time, and volume of fluid infused IV piggyback

Nurses' Notes

- Client's response to the medication
- Any serious side effects and report them to the health care provider immediately
- Document on appropriate electronic medical record or flow sheet

Intake and Output Record

- Amount of fluid infused

PROCEDURE 31-6 Assessing and Maintaining an IV Insertion Site

OVERVIEW

Assessing an established IV site requires knowledge about the length of time since the insertion, the condition of the dressing, and the site itself. The site should be without redness, swelling, pain, or discharge. When palpating the vein, it should have the characteristics of a healthy vein without signs of infection or phlebitis. Knowledge of both the IV solution and medications to be given and their potential side effects on the veins should be included in the assessment. Intravenous solutions with electrolytes and medications can have irritant properties that would require more frequent IV monitoring.

PROCEDURE 31-6 Assessing and Maintaining an IV Insertion Site (Continued)

ASSESSMENT

1. Review the order for IV therapy: Identify potential side effects from medication actions, and fluid rate. Consult drug reference books or pharmacists for information. **Decreases the risk of medication errors.**
2. Identify potential risk factors for your client's condition that might indicate fluid and electrolyte imbalances. **Allows targeted assessment and monitoring.**
3. Assess for dehydration: sunken eyes, dry skin, mucous membranes, flattened neck veins, vital sign changes, inelastic skin turgor, decreased urine output, behavior changes, and confusion. **Allows intervention to increase fluids and reduce dehydration.**
4. Assess for fluid overload: periorbital edema, distended neck veins, auscultation of crackles or wheezes in lungs, changes in vital signs, and level of consciousness. **Allows intervention to decrease fluids.**
5. Determine the client's risk for developing complications from IV therapy: very young or very old, heart or renal failure. **Allows the procedure to be modified if needed, and promotes targeted assessment to look for signs of risk-related problems.**
6. Observe IV site for complications, that is, signs of infection, phlebitis, or infiltration: redness, swelling, pallor, or warmth at the IV site and surrounding tissue, and bleeding or drainage. **Allows interventions to reduce further damage.**
7. Observe IV site for patency by briefly compressing the IV cannulated vein above the site. Note slowing or momentary cessation of IV rate with a positive blood return. **Provides ongoing assessment of current patency status. Allows early detection of changes.**
8. Assess the client's knowledge regarding the need for the IV therapy. **Allows for teaching, including information and education regarding medications, fluid needs, and signs of IV site irritation or phlebitis.**

POSSIBLE NURSING DIAGNOSES

Impaired Tissue Integrity
Risk for Impaired Skin Integrity
Risk for Infection
Excess Fluid Volume
Deficient Fluid Volume

PLANNING

Expected Outcomes

1. The client will have a patent IV, without signs of infection or inflammation.
2. The client's fluid and electrolyte imbalance will return to normal and will be maintained.
3. The client will be able to report signs of inflammation or infiltration.
4. The client's IV rate will be administered and maintained per order.
5. The client's IV dressing will remain intact, clean, and dry.

Equipment Needed

- Clean gloves
- Gauze dressing
- Tape

delegation tips

Assessing and maintaining the IV after establishing the infusion is the responsibility of the nurse. This procedure is not delegated unless other licensed personnel have been trained and certified to perform the procedure. Ancillary personnel may be instructed to report an infusion that is dripping too fast or an IV bag that is almost empty. It is the nurse's responsibility to monitor the infusion, but ancillary personnel may also be instructed to report any observations, such as swelling, leaking, client concerns about pain, numbness, or tingling at the site or in the extremity used for the infusion. Ancillary personnel may also be involved in monitoring the client's daily weight, if ordered, along with intake and output. Ancillary personnel should be instructed not to obtain vital signs on an extremity with solutions infusing.

IMPLEMENTATION—ACTION/RATIONALE

ACTION	RATIONALE
* Check client's identification band * Explain procedure before beginning *	
1. Review health care provider's order for IV therapy.	1. Ensures accuracy in the administration of IV therapy.
2. Review client's history for medical conditions or allergies.	2. Decreases risk of fluid overload and allergic reactions.
3. Review client's IV site record and intake and output record.	3. Assesses for potential problems with fragile IV sites and fluid balance.

(Continues)

PROCEDURE 31-6 Assessing and Maintaining an IV Insertion Site (Continued)

ACTION	RATIONALE

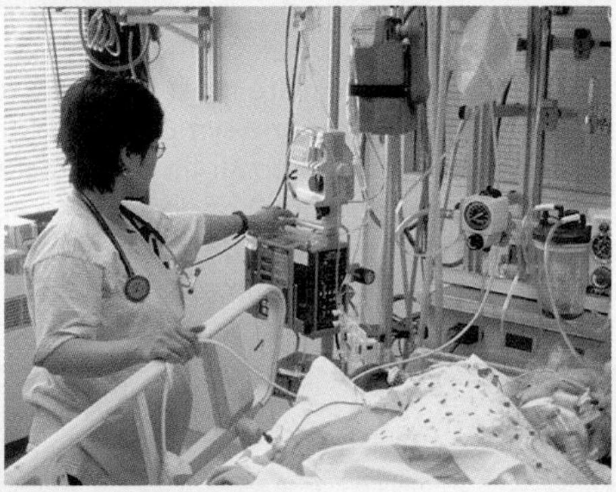

FIGURE 31-6-1 **Check the IV fluid rate, volume, tubing, and additives at the beginning of the shift.**

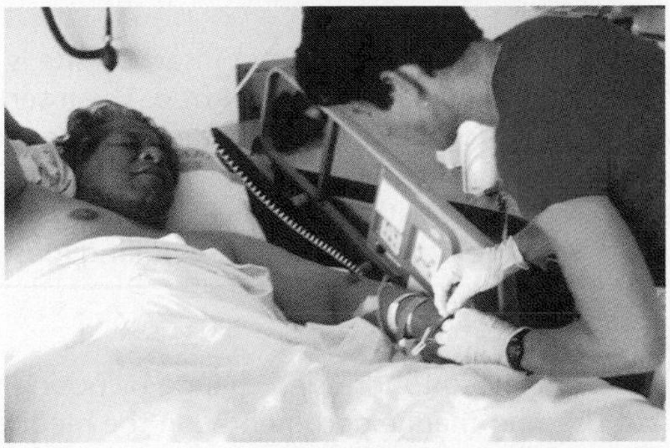

FIGURE 31-6-2 **Check the IV dressing site every hour.**

ACTION	RATIONALE
4. Wash hands.	4. Decreases transmission of microorganisms.
5. Obtain client's vital signs.	5. Assesses for changes in cardiovascular system.
6. Check IV fluid for correct fluid, additives, rate, and volume at the beginning of your shift (Figure 31-6-1).	6. Ensures client is receiving correct therapy.
7. Check IV tubing for tight connections every 4 hours.	7. Ensures that no fluid leaks from tubing and connections.
8. Check gauze IV dressing hourly to be sure it is dry and intact (Figure 31-6-2).	8. Ensures there is no sign of infiltration or infection at IV insertion site.
9. If the gauze is not dry and intact, remove the dressing and observe site for redness, swelling, or drainage.	9. Ensures there is no sign of inflammation or infection at IV site.
10. Replace with new dry sterile gauze dressing if site is okay.	10. Protects IV insertion site.
11. If an occlusive dressing is used, do not remove the dressing when assessing the site.	11. Ensures there is no sign of inflammation or infection at IV site.
12. Observe vein track for redness, swelling, warmth, or pain hourly.	12. These are early signs of phlebitis or infiltration.
13. Document IV site findings on appropriate electronic medical record or IV flow sheet.	13. Provides documentation of frequent IV site observation.
14. Wash hands.	14. Decreases transmission of microorganisms.

EVALUATION

- IV site observed on an hourly basis to avoid complications of phlebitis and infiltration.
- Client reported no signs or symptoms of redness, swelling, and pain.

DOCUMENTATION

Flow Sheet

- Name of IV solution with additives
- Hourly rate of fluids
- IV site condition
- Time checked
- Initials/signature of nurse

PROCEDURE 31-7 Changing the Central Venous Dressing

OVERVIEW

Because the central venous catheter insertion site is a direct route to the circulatory system, care must be taken to keep the insertion site clean and infection-free. The insertion site is inspected frequently for signs and symptoms of infection, such as inflammation, heat, or drainage. Regular, aseptic dressing changes help decrease the possibility of infection at the insertion site and systemically. Policies vary from institution to institution regarding the type of dressing to apply as well as the frequency with which they are changed. Be aware of the policy at your institution and the rationale for it. Dressings that have become wet or are pulling loose from the insertion site must be changed immediately.

ASSESSMENT

1. Assess the need for dressing change by noting the last dressing change documented in the medical record and standard of care recommended by the manufacturer and the institution. **This decreases the risk of infection by following the standard of care.**
2. Assess the timing of the dressing change as it relates to medication, IV fluid and transfusion schedules, and as well as the time of the client's daily shower or bath. **This allows the nurse to avoid simultaneous administration of medication and the need for two dressing changes in one day.**
3. Assess the type of central venous access in place **in order to obtain the appropriate supplies.**
4. Assess the integrity of the skin at the site **for signs of infection or bleeding.**
5. Assess the client and caregiver's knowledge of the purpose and care of the catheter **so a teaching plan can be developed.**

POSSIBLE NURSING DIAGNOSES

Risk for Infection
Impaired Skin Integrity
Deficient Knowledge

PLANNING

Expected Outcomes

1. Skin is intact at catheter site, has normal color, is not edematous, and has no drainage.
2. Client has no signs of systemic infection such as fever, malaise, or chills.

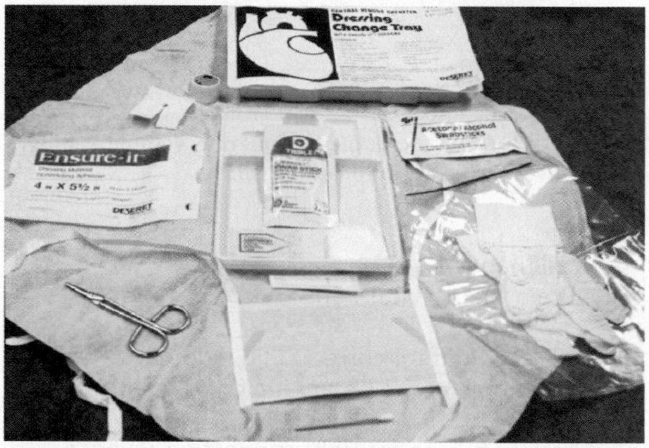

COURTESY OF DELMAR CENGAGE LEARNING

FIGURE 31-7-1 Central venous catheter dressing change supplies.

3. Catheter and tubing are intact.
4. Client and caregiver are able to perform skin care and dressing change.

Equipment Needed: (see Figure 31-7-1)

- Povidone-iodine swabs, chlorhexidine or agency-approved antiseptic solution
- Povidone-iodine ointment
- Sterile gauze, tape, or moisture transparent dressing
- Label with date and time of dressing change
- Latex-free clean gloves
- Mask
- Latex-free sterile gloves

delegation tips

Changing the central venous catheter dressing is a skill involving assessment and the use of sterile technique. It is a procedure not delegated by the nurse unless other licensed personnel have been trained and certified to assist with the procedure. Ancillary personnel who will be caring for the client need to be instructed to report any disruption of the closed dressing, along with complaints of pain, redness, or swelling at the insertion site.

(Continues)

PROCEDURE 31-7 Changing the Central Venous Dressing (Continued)

IMPLEMENTATION—ACTION/RATIONALE

* Check client's identification band * Explain procedure before beginning *

ACTION	RATIONALE
1. Wash hands and put on latex-free clean gloves.	1. Reduces the number of microorganisms.
2. Put on mask.	2. Reduces the number of microorganisms.
3. Remove old dressing carefully (see Figures 31-7-2 and 31-7-3), being careful not to dislodge the central catheter.	3. Skin integrity may be impaired.
4. Note drainage on dressing for color, odor, consistency, and amount.	4. Potential for bleeding or infectious material.
5. Inspect skin at insertion site for redness, tenderness, or swelling (see Figure 31-7-4).	5. Assesses for infection.
6. Palpate tunneled catheter for presence of Dacron cuff, using care not to palpate close to the exit site.	6. Documents proper placement of catheter.
7. Visually inspect catheter from hub to skin.	7. Checks whether catheter has a crack or is split or cut.
8. Remove gloves and put on latex-free sterile gloves.	8. Prevents transmission of microorganisms from skin to exit site.
9. Clean exit site according to institution protocol. Most use alcohol wipes first, then povidone-iodine swab beginning at the catheter and moving out in a circular manner for 3 cm to maintain aseptic technique (see Figure 31-7-5).	9. Eliminates microorganisms by chemical and mechanical means.
10. Some institutions use povidone-iodine ointment to exit site (check agency policy).	10. Reduces growth of bacteria at exit site.
11. Apply transparent dressing (see Figures 31-7-6, 31-7-7, and 31-7-8). Some institutions prefer to omit the gauze dressing to allow visualization of the site; in this case, only apply the transparent dressing.	11. Prevents bacteria from entering exit site.
12. Label with date and time of dressing change (see Figure 31-7-9).	12. Documents time to plan for next change.
13. Secure tubing to client's clothing.	13. Prevents accidental displacement.
14. Remove gloves and dispose of all used materials according to agency policy.	14. Reduces transmission of microorganisms.
15. Wash hands.	15. Reduces transmission of microorganisms.

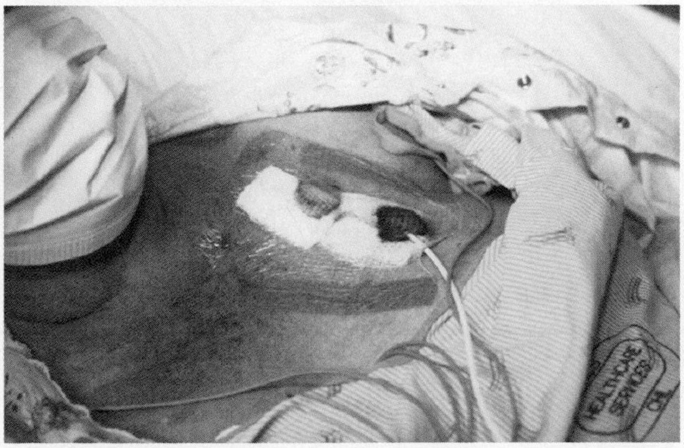

FIGURE 31-7-2 Inspect the dressing.

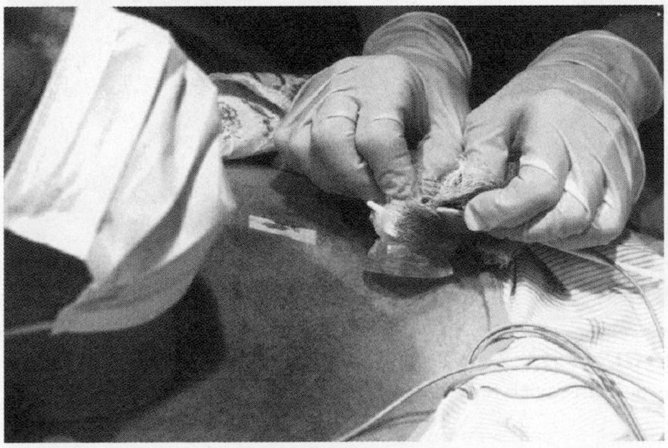

FIGURE 31-7-3 Be careful not to dislodge the catheter when removing the old dressing.

(Continues)

PROCEDURE 31-7 Changing the Central Venous Dressing (Continued)

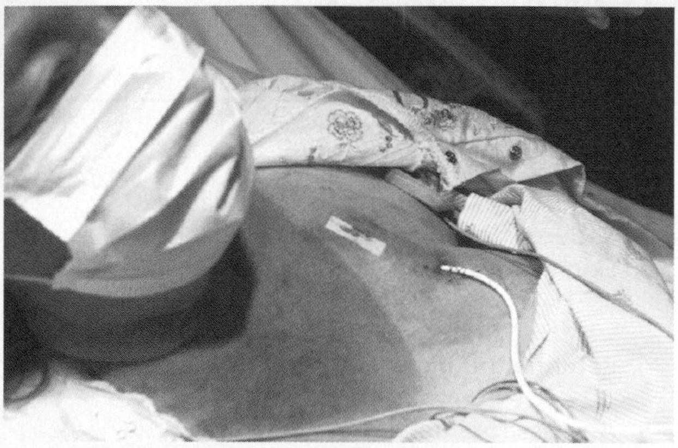

COURTESY OF DELMAR CENGAGE LEARNING

FIGURE 31-7-4 Inspect the site for redness, tenderness, and swelling.

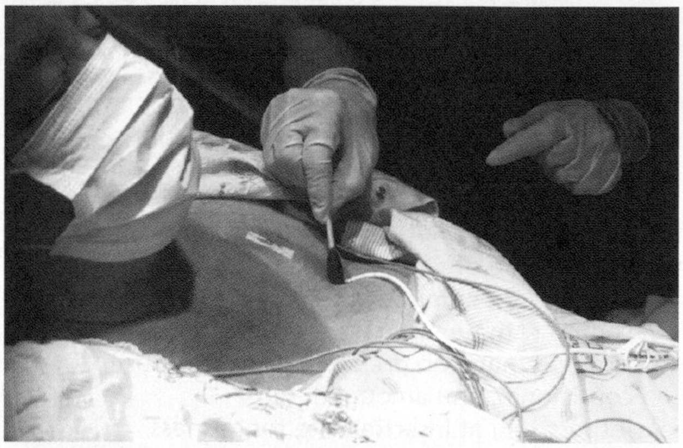

COURTESY OF DELMAR CENGAGE LEARNING

FIGURE 31-7-5 Clean the site with povidone-iodine swab.

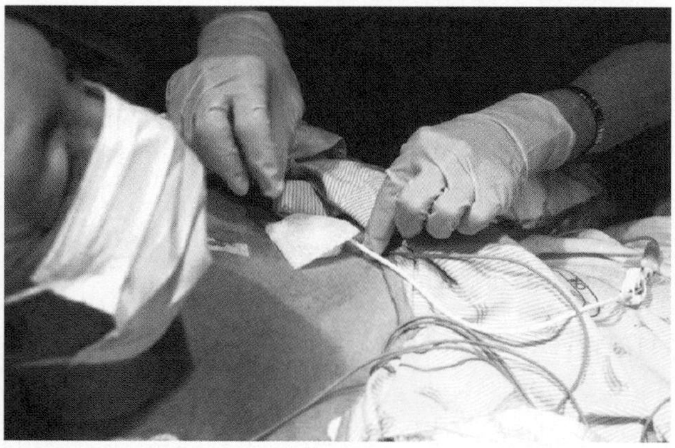

COURTESY OF DELMAR CENGAGE LEARNING

FIGURE 31-7-6 Slide the first piece of gauze directly over and under the catheter.

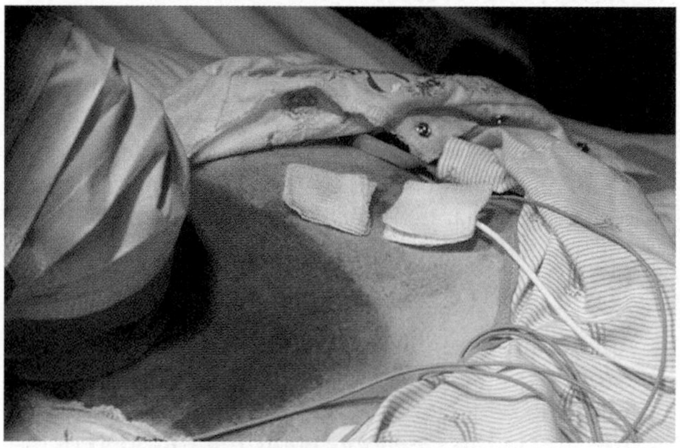

COURTESY OF DELMAR CENGAGE LEARNING

FIGURE 31-7-7 Place the next piece of gauze directly over the insertion site.

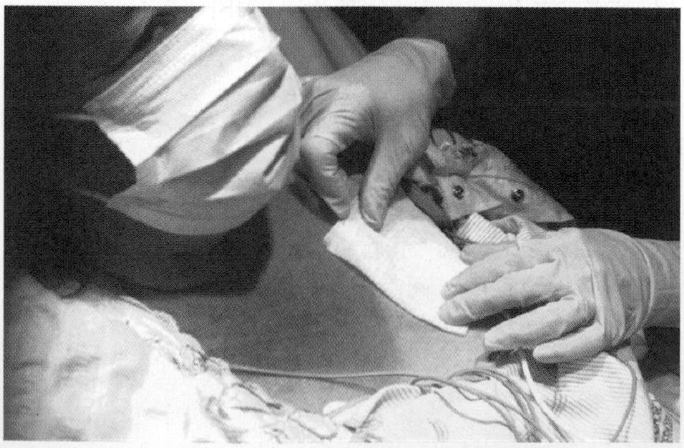

COURTESY OF DELMAR CENGAGE LEARNING

FIGURE 31-7-8 Place a larger piece of gauze over the area and secure with tape or transparent dressing.

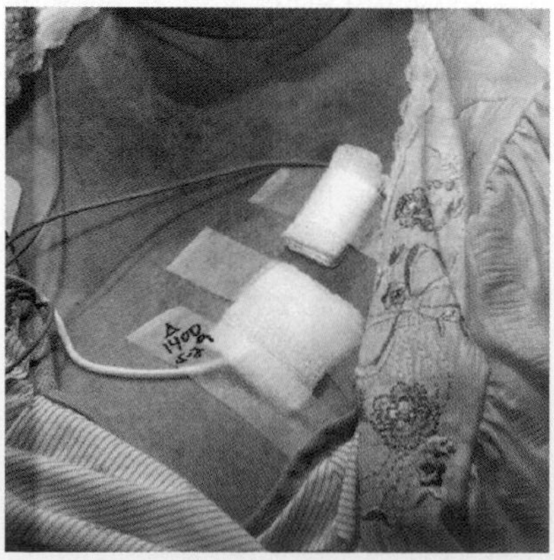

COURTESY OF DELMAR CENGAGE LEARNING

FIGURE 31-7-9 Write the date and time of the dressing change on the dressing.

(Continues)

PROCEDURE 31-7 Changing the Central Venous Dressing (Continued)

EVALUATION

- The client's skin is intact at catheter site, has normal color, and is not edematous.
- The client has no signs of systemic infection such as fever or malaise.
- The central venous catheter and tubing are intact.
- Client and caregiver are able to perform skin care and dressing change.

DOCUMENTATION

Nurses' Notes

- The date and time the dressing was changed
- The type of ointment and dressing applied
- The condition of the skin at the site
- The presence of any exudate or bleeding at the site
- The client or caregiver's ability to perform the dressing change
- Document on appropriate flow sheet or electronic medical record (EMR)

PROCEDURE 31-8 Removing Skin Sutures and Staples

OVERVIEW

Sutures and staples are a surgical means of closing a wound by sewing, wiring, or stapling the edges of the wound together. Most wounds are sutured in layers to maintain alignment of the tissues and reduce scarring. Sutures are generally removed 7 to 10 days after surgery, depending on where the wound is located and how well it is healing. Suture removal requires a health care provider's orders. Timing is important because sutures left in too long can increase the risk of infection and irritation from a foreign substance.

Sutures placed deep within the tissue layers are made of absorbable materials. Surface sutures are made of wire, nylon, or cotton. Continuous sutures are made with one thread, tied at the beginning and end of the suture line. Interrupted sutures are tied individually. Staples are used for large incision areas where the risk of dehiscence is greater, such as in sterneotomies, in clients with increased adipose tissue, abdominal areas, and wounds that fail to heal or adhere.

ASSESSMENT

1. Assess the wound **to determine whether the edges are approximate and healing.** In deep wounds, palpate around the suture site for edema or any evidence of failure of tissue to adhere below the skin's surface.
2. Assess **for any signs of infection**, such as increased warmth, redness, exudate or drainage, and pain.
3. Assess for any conditions **that impede the healing process**, such as age, immunosuppression, diabetes, obesity, smoking, radiation, poor cellular nutrition, infection, and deep wounds.

POSSIBLE NURSING DIAGNOSES

*Impaired **S**kin Integrity*
*Risk for **I**nfection*
*Acute **P**ain*
*Deficient **K**nowledge* (fear of dehiscence)
*Impaired Physical **M**obility*

PLANNING

Expected Outcomes

1. The wound is healing, with the edges of the wound well-approximated.
2. There is no redness or signs of infection.
3. The procedure is performed with a minimum of pain and trauma to the client.

Equipment Needed

- Suture removal kit or sterile forceps with sterile suture removal scissors
- Gauze size as appropriate for wound area to be covered
- Biohazard bag or appropriate waterproof disposable bag
- Sterile saline, prepackaged antiseptic swabs, or gauze for cleaning if appropriate
- Examination gloves
- Sterile gloves if dressings are to be applied

(Continues)

PROCEDURE 31-8 Removing Skin Sutures and Staples (Continued)

- Adhesive strips or butterfly adhesive tape as needed
- Sterile gauze to wipe stitches or sutures from forceps and scissors
- Tincture of benzoin as indicated

delegation tips

Suture removal is a skill requiring aseptic technique and wound assessment by a nurse and, therefore, is not delegated to ancillary personnel.

IMPLEMENTATION—ACTION/RATIONALE

* Check client's identification band * Explain procedure before beginning *

ACTION	RATIONALE
1. Wash hands.	1. Reduces transmission of microorganisms.
2. Assess the wound to determine whether the edges of the wound are well-approximated and healing has occurred.	2. Health care providers often have standing orders for sutures to be removed at a specified date. If the wound is not well-healed, sutures should be left in place longer and the health care provider notified.
3. Close the door and curtains around the client's bed.	3. Provides for privacy.
4. Raise the bed to a comfortable level.	4. Provides for proper body mechanics.
5. Position the client for comfort with easy access and visibility of the suture line.	5. Facilitates removal of the sutures and allows for careful observation of suture line.
6. Drape the client so that only the suture area is exposed.	6. Provides for privacy.
7. Open the suture removal kit on a clean surface and assemble any supplies needed within easy access.	7. Facilitates removal of sutures.
8. Apply clean gloves to remove the old dressing and place it in a disposable bag.	8. Follows Standard Precautions protocol.
9. Remove gloves and wash hands.	9. Reduces transmission of microorganisms.
10. If dressings are to be used, assemble equipment and supplies on sterile field.	10. Protects client from microorganisms.
11. Apply sterile gloves according to institutional policy. Clean the incision with saline-soaked gauze pads, antiseptic swabs, or per institutional policy.	11. Protects the incision from microorganisms on the nurse's hands. Protects the nurse from possible contact with bodily fluids. Various opinions exist regarding use of cleansing solutions for wound care.
12. When removing an interrupted suture, hold forceps in your nondominant hand and grasp the suture near the knot (Figure 31-8-1).	12. Pulls the suture up and away from the client's skin.
13. Place the curved edge of the scissors under the suture or near the knot (Figure 31-8-2).	13. Facilitates clipping of the suture.
14. Cut the suture close to the skin where the suture emerges from the skin (not in the middle). Pull the long end and remove it in one piece.	14. Facilitates suture removal. Avoids pulling large amounts of contaminated suture through tissue.
15. If the client has a continuous suture, cut both the first and second suture before removing them.	15. Facilitates suture removal without traumatizing the incision line.
16. Some policies require the removal of every other suture, with the remaining sutures removed at a later time. Assess the suture line to ensure that the edges remain approximated.	16. Any dehiscence should be detected early, and every other suture can be left in place.
17. Discard the sutures onto the gauze squares as they are removed and place the gauze squares in the disposable bag when all the sutures have been removed.	17. Decreases transmission of microorganisms and follows Standard Precaution protocol.
18. Assess the suture line to ensure that the edges remain approximated and that all sutures have been removed.	18. Detects early signs of dehiscence. Ensures that sutures do not remain in the skin when they are no longer needed.

(Continues)

PROCEDURE 31-8 Removing Skin Sutures and Staples (Continued)

ACTION	RATIONALE
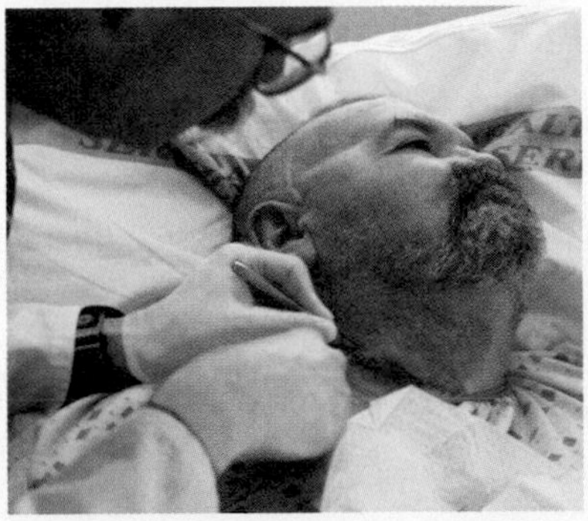 **FIGURE 31-8-1** Hold forceps in your nondominant hand and grasp the suture near the knot.	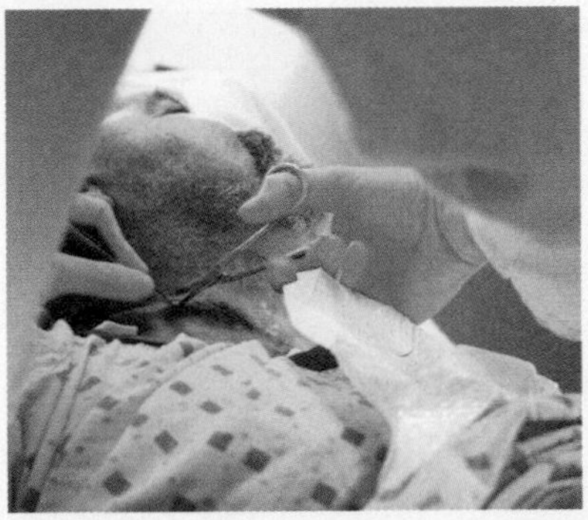 **FIGURE 31-8-2** Hold the scissors in your dominant hand. Place the curved edge of the scissors under the suture.
19. Apply adhesive strips or butterfly tape adhesive strips across the suture line to secure the edges. The amount of reinforcement varies depending on the adherence of the suture line and the length of the suture line. Adhesive skin closures may be placed 1 inch apart or closer together. Tincture of benzoin may be applied to skin adjacent to the incision.	19. If the suture line pulls apart a little after the sutures are removed, adhesive skin closures can be used to reinforce the suture line. Helps adhesive adhere to skin.
20. Dispose of the soiled equipment.	20. Reduces odors in the client's room and reduces transmission of microorganisms.
21. Remove gloves and wash hands.	21. Reduces transmission of microorganisms.
22. If removing staples:	22.
• Repeat Actions 2–11.	• Prepares for staple removal.
• Use a staple extractor to remove every other staple. Place the lower tip of staple remover under the staple and squeeze the handles together. The ends of the staple will extract from the skin. Move the staple away from the skin surface and release the staple into a disposal container. Assess the wound for adherence. Move on to the next staple if the skin has adhered well.	• When removing staples, it is best to remove every other staple and assess wound adherence before removing all staples. A staple extractor is designed to remove the staple with a minimum of discomfort and trauma to the surrounding skin and tissue.
• Repeat Actions 19 to 21.	• See Rationales 19 to 21.

EVALUATION

- The wound is intact, edges are adhered, and there are no signs of infection or drainage.
- Sutures/staples removed with a minimum of pain and trauma to the client.

DOCUMENTATION

Nurses' Notes

- Procedure and findings at wound site, such as redness, pain, or drainage
- Time sutures/staples were removed
- Follow-up instructions and client teaching provided
- Document on appropriate electronic medical record or flow sheet

REFERENCE/SUGGESTED READING

Altman, G. (2010). *Fundamental and advanced nursing skills.* (3rd ed.). Clifton Park, NY: Delmar Cengage Learning.

APPENDIX A NANDA-I Nursing Diagnoses 2009–2011

Domain 1
Health Promotion
Ineffective **Health** Maintenance
Ineffective Self **Health** Management
Impaired **Home** Maintenance
Readiness for Enhanced **Immunization** Status
Self **Neglect**
Readiness for Enhanced **Nutrition**
Ineffective Family **Therapeutic** Regimen Management
Readiness for Enhanced **Self Health** Management

Domain 2
Nutrition
Ineffective Infant **Feeding** Pattern
Imbalanced **Nutrition**: Less Than Body Requirements
Imbalanced **Nutrition**: More Than Body Requirements
Risk for Imbalanced **Nutrition**: More Than Body Requirements
Impaired **Swallowing**
Risk for Unstable Blood **Glucose** Level
Neonatal **Jaundice**
Risk for Impaired **Liver** Function
Risk for **Electrolyte** Imbalance
Readiness for Enhanced **Fluid** Balance
Deficient **Fluid** Volume
Excess **Fluid** Volume
Risk for Deficient **Fluid** Volume
Risk for Imbalanced **Fluid** Volume

Domain 3
Elimination and Exchange
Functional Urinary **Incontinence**
Overflow Urinary **Incontinence**
Reflex Urinary **Incontinence**
Stress Urinary **Incontinence**
Urge Urinary **Incontinence**
Risk for Urge urinary **Incontinence**
Impaired **Urinary** Elimination
Readiness for Enhanced **Urinary** Elimination
Urinary Retention
Bowel Incontinence
Constipation
Perceived **Constipation**
Risk for **Constipation**
Diarrhea
Dysfunctional Gastrointenstinal **Motility**
Risk for Dysfunctional Gastrointestinal **Motility**
Impaired **Gas** Exchange

Domain 4
Activity Rest
Insomnia
Disturbed **Sleep** Pattern
Sleep Deprivation
Readiness for Enhanced **Sleep**
Risk for **Disuse** Syndrome
Deficient **Diversional** Activity
Sedentary **Lifestyle**
Impaired Bed **Mobility**
Impaired Physical **Mobility**
Impaired Wheelchair **Mobility**
Delayed **Surgical** Recovery
Impaired **Transfer** Ability
Impaired **Walking**
Disturbed **Energy** Field
Fatigue
Activity Intolerance
Risk for **Activity** Intolerance
Risk for **Bleeding**
Ineffective **Breathing** Pattern
Decreased **Cardiac** Output
Ineffective Peripheral Tissue **Perfusion**
Risk for Decreased Cardiac Tissue **Perfusion**
Risk for Ineffective Cerebral Tissue **Perfusion**
Risk for Ineffective Gastrointestinal

Perfusion
Risk for **Ineffective Renal Perfusion**
Risk for **Shock**
Impaired Spontaneous **Ventilation**
Dysfunctional **Ventilatory** Weaning Response
Readiness for Enhanced **Self-Care**
Bathing **Self-Care** Deficit
Dressing **Self-Care** Deficit
Feeding **Self-Care** Deficit
Toileting **Self-Care** Deficit

Domain 5
Perception/Cognition
Unilateral **Neglect**
Impaired **Environmental** Interpretation Syndrome
Wandering
Disturbed **Sensory** Perception (Specify: Visual, Auditory, Kinesthetic, Gustatory, Tactile, Olfactory)
Acute **Confusion**
Chronic **Confusion**
Risk for Acute **Confusion**
Deficient **Knowledge**
Readiness for Enhanced **Knowledge**
Impaired **Memory**
Readiness for Enhanced **Decision-Making**
Ineffective **Activity** Planning
Impaired Verbal **Communication**
Readiness for Enhanced **Communication**

Domain 6
Self-Perception
Risk for Compromised Human **Dignity**
Hopelessness
Disturbed Personal **Identity**
Risk for **Loneliness**
Readiness for Enhanced **Power**
Powerlessness
Risk for **Powerlessness**
Readiness for Enhanced **Self-Concept**
Situational Low **Self-Esteem**
Chronic Low **Self-Esteem**
Risk for Situational Low **Self-Esteem**
Disturbed **Body** Image

Domain 7
Role Relationships
Caregiver Role Strain
Risk for **Caregiver** Role Strain
Impaired **Parenting**
Readiness for Enhanced **Parenting**
Risk for Impaired **Parenting**
Risk for Impaired **Attachment**
Dysfunctional **Family** Processes
Interrupted **Family** Processes
Readiness for Enhanced **Family** Processes
Effective **Breastfeeding**
Ineffective **Breastfeeding**
Interrupted **Breastfeeding**
Parental Role **Conflict**
Readiness for Enhanced **Relationship**
Ineffective **Role** Performance
Impaired **Social** Interaction

Domain 8
Sexuality
Sexual Dysfunction
Ineffective **Sexuality** Pattern
Readiness for Enhanced **Childbearing** Process
Risk for Disturbed **Maternal/Fetal** Dyad

Domain 9
Coping/Stress Tolerance
Post-Trauma Syndrome
Risk for **Post-Trauma** Syndrome
Rape-Trauma Syndrome
Relocation Stress Syndrome
Risk for **Relocation** Stress Syndrome
Anxiety
Death **Anxiety**
Risk-Prone Health **Behavior**
Compromised Family **Coping**
Defensive **Coping**
Disabled Family **Coping**
Ineffective **Coping**
Ineffective Community **Coping**
Readiness for Enhanced **Coping**
Readiness for Enhanced Community **Coping**
Readiness for Enhanced Family **Coping**
Ineffective **Denial**
Fear
Grieving
Complicated **Grieving**
Risk for Complicated **Grieving**
Impaired Individual **Resilience**
Readiness for Enhanced **Resilience**
Risk for Compromised **Resilience**
Chronic **Sorrow**
Stress Overload

Autonomic Dysreflexia
Risk for **Autonomic** Dysreflexia
Disorganized **Infant** Behavior
Risk for Disorganized **Infant** Behavior
Readiness for Enhanced Organized **Infant** Behavior
Decreased **Intracranial** Adaptive Capacity

Domain 10
Life Principles
Readiness for Enhanced **Hope**
Readiness for Enhanced **Spiritual** Well-Being
Decisional **Conflict**
Moral **Distress**
Noncompliance
Impaired **Religiosity**
Readiness for Enhanced **Religiosity**
Risk for Impaired **Religiosity**
Spiritual Distress
Risk for **Spiritual** Distress

Domain 11
Safety/Protection
Risk for **Infection**
Ineffective **Airway** Clearance
Risk for **Aspiration**
Risk for Sudden Infant **Death** Syndrome
Impaired **Dentition**
Risk for **Falls**
Risk for **Injury**
Risk for Perioperative-Positioning **Injury**
Impaired **Oral** Mucous Membrane
Risk for **Peripheral** Neurovascular Dysfunction
Ineffective **Protection**
Impaired **Skin** Integrity
Risk for Impaired **Skin** Integrity
Risk for **Suffocation**
Impaired **Tissue** Integrity
Risk for **Trauma**
Risk for Vascular **Trauma**
Self-Mutilation
Risk for **Suicide**
Risk for Other-Directed **Violence**
Risk for Self-Directed **Violence**
Contamination
Risk for **Contamination**
Risk for **Poisoning**
Latex **Allergy** Response
Risk for Latex **Allergy** Response
Risk for Imbalanced **Body** Temperature
Hyperthermia
Hypothermia
Ineffective **Thermoregulation**

Domain 12
Comfort
Readiness for Enhanced **Comfort**
Impaired **Comfort**
Nausea
Acute **Pain**
Chronic **Pain**
Social Isolation

Domain 13
Growth/Development
Adult **Failure** to Thrive
Delayed **Growth** and Development
Risk for Disproportionate **Growth**
Risk for Delayed **Development**

APPENDIX B
Recommended Immunization Schedules

Recommended Immunization Schedule for Persons Aged 0 Through 6 Years—United States • 2009

For those who fall behind or start late, see the catch-up schedule

<table>
<tr><th>Vaccine ▼ Age ▶</th><th>Birth</th><th>1 month</th><th>2 months</th><th>4 months</th><th>6 months</th><th>12 months</th><th>15 months</th><th>18 months</th><th>19–23 months</th><th>2–3 years</th><th>4–6 years</th></tr>
<tr><td>Hepatitis B[1]</td><td>HepB</td><td colspan="2">HepB</td><td>see footnote 1</td><td colspan="4">HepB</td><td></td><td></td><td></td></tr>
<tr><td>Rotavirus[2]</td><td></td><td></td><td>RV</td><td>RV</td><td>RV[2]</td><td></td><td></td><td></td><td></td><td></td><td></td></tr>
<tr><td>Diphtheria, Tetanus, Pertussis[3]</td><td></td><td></td><td>DTaP</td><td>DTaP</td><td>DTaP</td><td>see footnote 3</td><td colspan="2">DTaP</td><td></td><td></td><td>DTaP</td></tr>
<tr><td>Haemophilus influenzae type b[4]</td><td></td><td></td><td>Hib</td><td>Hib</td><td>Hib[4]</td><td colspan="2">Hib</td><td></td><td></td><td></td><td></td></tr>
<tr><td>Pneumococcal[5]</td><td></td><td></td><td>PCV</td><td>PCV</td><td>PCV</td><td colspan="2">PCV</td><td></td><td></td><td colspan="2">PPSV</td></tr>
<tr><td>Inactivated Poliovirus</td><td></td><td></td><td>IPV</td><td>IPV</td><td colspan="4">IPV</td><td></td><td></td><td>IPV</td></tr>
<tr><td>Influenza[6]</td><td></td><td></td><td></td><td></td><td colspan="7">Influenza (Yearly)</td></tr>
<tr><td>Measles, Mumps, Rubella[7]</td><td></td><td></td><td></td><td></td><td></td><td colspan="2">MMR</td><td colspan="3">see footnote 7</td><td>MMR</td></tr>
<tr><td>Varicella[8]</td><td></td><td></td><td></td><td></td><td></td><td colspan="2">Varicella</td><td colspan="3">see footnote 8</td><td>Varicella</td></tr>
<tr><td>Hepatitis A[9]</td><td></td><td></td><td></td><td></td><td></td><td colspan="4">HepA (2 doses)</td><td colspan="2">HepA Series</td></tr>
<tr><td>Meningococcal[10]</td><td></td><td></td><td></td><td></td><td></td><td></td><td></td><td></td><td></td><td colspan="2">MCV</td></tr>
</table>

Range of recommended ages

Certain high-risk groups

This schedule indicates the recommended ages for routine administration of currently licensed vaccines, as of December 1, 2008, for children aged 0 through 6 years. Any dose not administered at the recommended age should be administered at a subsequent visit, when indicated and feasible. Licensed combination vaccines may be used whenever any component of the combination is indicated and other components are not contraindicated and if approved by the Food and Drug Administration for that dose of the series. Providers should consult the relevant Advisory Committee on Immunization Practices statement for detailed recommendations, including high-risk conditions: http://www.cdc.gov/vaccines/pubs/acip-list.htm. Clinically significant adverse events that follow immunization should be reported to the Vaccine Adverse Event Reporting System (VAERS). Guidance about how to obtain and complete a VAERS form is available at http://www.vaers.hhs.gov or by telephone, 800-822-7967.

1. **Hepatitis B vaccine (HepB).** ***(Minimum age: birth)***

At birth:
- Administer monovalent HepB to all newborns before hospital discharge.
- If mother is hepatitis B surface antigen (HBsAg)-positive, administer HepB and 0.5 mL of hepatitis B immune globulin (HBIG) within 12 hours of birth.
- If mother's HBsAg status is unknown, administer HepB within 12 hours of birth. Determine mother's HBsAg status as soon as possible and, if HBsAg-positive, administer HBIG (no later than age 1 week).

After the birth dose:
- The HepB series should be completed with either monovalent HepB or a combination vaccine containing HepB. The second dose should be administered at age 1 or 2 months. The final dose should be administered no earlier than age 24 weeks.
- Infants born to HBsAg-positive mothers should be tested for HBsAg and antibody to HBsAg (anti-HBs) after completion of at least 3 doses of the HepB series, at age 9 through 18 months (generally at the next well-child visit).

4-month dose:
- Administration of 4 doses of HepB to infants is permissible when combination vaccines containing HepB are administered after the birth dose.

2. **Rotavirus vaccine (RV).** ***(Minimum age: 6 weeks)***
- Administer the first dose at age 6 through 14 weeks (maximum age: 14 weeks 6 days). Vaccination should not be initiated for infants aged 15 weeks or older (i.e., 15 weeks 0 days or older).
- Administer the final dose in the series by age 8 months 0 days.
- If Rotarix® is administered at ages 2 and 4 months, a dose at 6 months is not indicated.

3. **Diphtheria and tetanus toxoids and acellular pertussis vaccine (DTaP).** ***(Minimum age: 6 weeks)***
- The fourth dose may be administered as early as age 12 months, provided at least 6 months have elapsed since the third dose.
- Administer the final dose in the series at age 4 through 6 years.

4. ***Haemophilus influenzae*** **type b conjugate vaccine (Hib).** ***(Minimum age: 6 weeks)***
- If PRP-OMP (PedvaxHIB® or Comvax® [HepB-Hib]) is administered at ages 2 and 4 months, a dose at age 6 months is not indicated.
- TriHiBit® (DTaP/Hib) should not be used for doses at ages 2, 4, or 6 months but can be used as the final dose in children aged 12 months or older.

5. **Pneumococcal vaccine.** ***(Minimum age: 6 weeks for pneumococcal conjugate vaccine [PCV]; 2 years for pneumococcal polysaccharide vaccine [PPSV])***
- PCV is recommended for all children aged younger than 5 years. Administer 1 dose of PCV to all healthy children aged 24 through 59 months who are not completely vaccinated for their age.
- Administer PPSV to children aged 2 years or older with certain underlying medical conditions (see *MMWR* 2000;49[No. RR-9]), including a cochlear implant.

6. **Influenza vaccine.** ***(Minimum age: 6 months for trivalent inactivated influenza vaccine [TIV]; 2 years for live, attenuated influenza vaccine [LAIV])***
- Administer annually to children aged 6 months through 18 years.
- For healthy nonpregnant persons (i.e., those who do not have underlying medical conditions that predispose them to influenza complications) aged 2 through 49 years, either LAIV or TIV may be used.
- Children receiving TIV should receive 0.25 mL if aged 6 through 35 months or 0.5 mL if aged 3 years or older.
- Administer 2 doses (separated by at least 4 weeks) to children aged younger than 9 years who are receiving influenza vaccine for the first time or who were vaccinated for the first time during the previous influenza season but only received 1 dose.

7. **Measles, mumps, and rubella vaccine (MMR).** ***(Minimum age: 12 months)***
- Administer the second dose at age 4 through 6 years. However, the second dose may be administered before age 4, provided at least 28 days have elapsed since the first dose.

8. **Varicella vaccine.** ***(Minimum age: 12 months)***
- Administer the second dose at age 4 through 6 years. However, the second dose may be administered before age 4, provided at least 3 months have elapsed since the first dose.
- For children aged 12 months through 12 years the minimum interval between doses is 3 months. However, if the second dose was administered at least 28 days after the first dose, it can be accepted as valid.

9. **Hepatitis A vaccine (HepA).** ***(Minimum age: 12 months)***
- Administer to all children aged 1 year (i.e., aged 12 through 23 months). Administer 2 doses at least 6 months apart.
- Children not fully vaccinated by age 2 years can be vaccinated at subsequent visits.
- HepA also is recommended for children older than 1 year who live in areas where vaccination programs target older children or who are at increased risk of infection. See *MMWR* 2006;55(No. RR-7).

10. **Meningococcal vaccine.** ***(Minimum age: 2 years for meningococcal conjugate vaccine [MCV] and for meningococcal polysaccharide vaccine [MPSV])***
- Administer MCV to children aged 2 through 10 years with terminal complement component deficiency, anatomic or functional asplenia, and certain other high-risk groups. See *MMWR* 2005;54(No. RR-7).
- Persons who received MPSV 3 or more years previously and who remain at increased risk for meningococcal disease should be revaccinated with MCV.

The Recommended Immunization Schedules for Persons Aged 0 Through 18 Years are approved by the Advisory Committee on Immunization Practices (www.cdc.gov/vaccines/recs/acip), the American Academy of Pediatrics (http://www.aap.org), and the American Academy of Family Physicians (http://www.aafp.org).

DEPARTMENT OF HEALTH AND HUMAN SERVICES • CENTERS FOR DISEASE CONTROL AND PREVENTION

Recommended Immunization Schedule for Persons Aged 7 Through 18 Years—United States • 2009

For those who fall behind or start late, see the schedule below and the catch-up schedule

Vaccine ▼ Age ▶	7–10 years	11–12 years	13–18 years
Tetanus, Diphtheria, Pertussis[1]	*see footnote 1*	Tdap	Tdap
Human Papillomavirus[2]	*see footnote 2*	HPV (3 doses)	HPV Series
Meningococcal[3]	MCV	MCV	MCV
Influenza[4]	Influenza (Yearly)		
Pneumococcal[5]	PPSV		
Hepatitis A[6]	HepA Series		
Hepatitis B[7]	HepB Series		
Inactivated Poliovirus[8]	IPV Series		
Measles, Mumps, Rubella[9]	MMR Series		
Varicella[10]	Varicella Series		

Range of recommended ages

Catch-up immunization

Certain high-risk groups

This schedule indicates the recommended ages for routine administration of currently licensed vaccines, as of December 1, 2008, for children aged 7 through 18 years. Any dose not administered at the recommended age should be administered at a subsequent visit, when indicated and feasible. Licensed combination vaccines may be used whenever any component of the combination is indicated and other components are not contraindicated and if approved by the Food and Drug Administration for that dose of the series. Providers should consult the relevant Advisory Committee on Immunization Practices statement for detailed recommendations, including high-risk conditions: http://www.cdc.gov/vaccines/pubs/acip-list.htm. Clinically significant adverse events that follow immunization should be reported to the Vaccine Adverse Event Reporting System (VAERS). Guidance about how to obtain and complete a VAERS form is available at http://www.vaers.hhs.gov or by telephone, 800-822-7967.

1. Tetanus and diphtheria toxoids and acellular pertussis vaccine (Tdap). ***(Minimum age: 10 years for BOOSTRIX® and 11 years for ADACEL®)***
- Administer at age 11 or 12 years for those who have completed the recommended childhood DTP/DTaP vaccination series and have not received a tetanus and diphtheria toxoid (Td) booster dose.
- Persons aged 13 through 18 years who have not received Tdap should receive a dose.
- A 5-year interval from the last Td dose is encouraged when Tdap is used as a booster dose; however, a shorter interval may be used if pertussis immunity is needed.

2. Human papillomavirus vaccine (HPV). ***(Minimum age: 9 years)***
- Administer the first dose to females at age 11 or 12 years.
- Administer the second dose 2 months after the first dose and the third dose 6 months after the first dose (at least 24 weeks after the first dose).
- Administer the series to females at age 13 through 18 years if not previously vaccinated.

3. Meningococcal conjugate vaccine (MCV).
- Administer at age 11 or 12 years, or at age 13 through 18 years if not previously vaccinated.
- Administer to previously unvaccinated college freshmen living in a dormitory.
- MCV is recommended for children aged 2 through 10 years with terminal complement component deficiency, anatomic or functional asplenia, and certain other groups at high risk. See *MMWR* 2005;54(No. RR-7).
- Persons who received MPSV 5 or more years previously and remain at increased risk for meningococcal disease should be revaccinated with MCV.

4. Influenza vaccine.
- Administer annually to children aged 6 months through 18 years.
- For healthy nonpregnant persons (i.e., those who do not have underlying medical conditions that predispose them to influenza complications) aged 2 through 49 years, either LAIV or TIV may be used.
- Administer 2 doses (separated by at least 4 weeks) to children aged younger than 9 years who are receiving influenza vaccine for the first time or who were vaccinated for the first time during the previous influenza season but only received 1 dose.

5. Pneumococcal polysaccharide vaccine (PPSV).
- Administer to children with certain underlying medical conditions (see *MMWR* 1997;46[No. RR-8]), including a cochlear implant. A single revaccination should be administered to children with functional or anatomic asplenia or other immunocompromising condition after 5 years.

6. Hepatitis A vaccine (HepA).
- Administer 2 doses at least 6 months apart.
- HepA is recommended for children older than 1 year who live in areas where vaccination programs target older children or who are at increased risk of infection. See *MMWR* 2006;55(No. RR-7).

7. Hepatitis B vaccine (HepB).
- Administer the 3-dose series to those not previously vaccinated.
- A 2-dose series (separated by at least 4 months) of adult formulation Recombivax HB® is licensed for children aged 11 through 15 years.

8. Inactivated poliovirus vaccine (IPV).
- For children who received an all-IPV or all-oral poliovirus (OPV) series, a fourth dose is not necessary if the third dose was administered at age 4 years or older.
- If both OPV and IPV were administered as part of a series, a total of 4 doses should be administered, regardless of the child's current age.

9. Measles, mumps, and rubella vaccine (MMR).
- If not previously vaccinated, administer 2 doses or the second dose for those who have received only 1 dose, with at least 28 days between doses.

10. Varicella vaccine.
- For persons aged 7 through 18 years without evidence of immunity (see *MMWR* 2007;56[No. RR-4]), administer 2 doses if not previously vaccinated or the second dose if they have received only 1 dose.
- For persons aged 7 through 12 years, the minimum interval between doses is 3 months. However, if the second dose was administered at least 28 days after the first dose, it can be accepted as valid.
- For persons aged 13 years and older, the minimum interval between doses is 28 days.

The Recommended Immunization Schedules for Persons Aged 0 Through 18 Years are approved by the Advisory Committee on Immunization Practices (www.cdc.gov/vaccines/recs/acip), the American Academy of Pediatrics (http://www.aap.org), and the American Academy of Family Physicians (http://www.aafp.org).

DEPARTMENT OF HEALTH AND HUMAN SERVICES • CENTERS FOR DISEASE CONTROL AND PREVENTION

Recommended Adult Immunization Schedule

UNITED STATES · 2009

Note: These recommendations *must* be read with the footnotes that follow containing number of doses, intervals between doses, and other important information.

Figure 1. Recommended adult immunization schedule, by vaccine and age group

VACCINE ▼ / AGE GROUP ▶	19–26 years	27–49 years	50–59 years	60–64 years	≥65 years
Tetanus, diphtheria, pertussis (Td/Tdap)[1,*]	Substitute 1-time dose of Tdap for Td booster; then boost with Td every 10 yrs				Td booster every 10 yrs
Human papillomavirus (HPV)[2,*]	3 doses (females)				
Varicella[3,*]	2 doses				
Zoster[4]				1 dose	
Measles, mumps, rubella (MMR)[5,*]	1 or 2 doses		1 dose		
Influenza[6,*]	1 dose annually				
Pneumococcal (polysaccharide)[7,8]	1 or 2 doses				1 dose
Hepatitis A[9,*]	2 doses				
Hepatitis B[10,*]	3 doses				
Meningococcal[11,*]	1 or more doses				

*Covered by the Vaccine Injury Compensation Program.

- For all persons in this category who meet the age requirements and who lack evidence of immunity (e.g., lack documentation of vaccination or have no evidence of prior infection)
- Recommended if some other risk factor is present (e.g., on the basis of medical, occupational, lifestyle, or other indications)
- No recommendation

Report all clinically significant postvaccination reactions to the Vaccine Adverse Event Reporting System (VAERS). Reporting forms and instructions on filing a VAERS report are available at www.vaers.hhs.gov or by telephone, 800-822-7967.

Information on how to file a Vaccine Injury Compensation Program claim is available at www.hrsa.gov/vaccinecompensation or by telephone, 800-338-2382. To file a claim for vaccine injury, contact the U.S. Court of Federal Claims, 717 Madison Place, N.W., Washington, D.C. 20005; telephone, 202-357-6400.

Additional information about the vaccines in this schedule, extent of available data, and contraindications for vaccination is also available at www.cdc.gov/vaccines or from the CDC-INFO Contact Center at 800-CDC-INFO (800-232-4636) in English and Spanish, 24 hours a day, 7 days a week.

Use of trade names and commercial sources is for identification only and does not imply endorsement by the U.S. Department of Health and Human Services.

Figure 2. Vaccines that might be indicated for adults based on medical and other indications

VACCINE ▼ / INDICATION ▶	Pregnancy	Immuno-compromising conditions (excluding human immunodeficiency virus [HIV])[13]	HIV infection[3,12,13] CD4+ T lymphocyte count <200 cells/µL	HIV infection[3,12,13] CD4+ T lymphocyte count ≥200 cells/µL	Diabetes, heart disease, chronic lung disease, chronic alcoholism	Asplenia[12] (including elective splenectomy and terminal complement component deficiencies)	Chronic liver disease	Kidney failure, end-stage renal disease, receipt of hemodialysis	Health-care personnel
Tetanus, diphtheria, pertussis (Td/Tdap)[1,*]	Td	Substitute 1-time dose of Tdap for Td booster; then boost with Td every 10 yrs	Substitute 1-time dose of Tdap for Td booster; then boost with Td every 10 yrs	Substitute 1-time dose of Tdap for Td booster; then boost with Td every 10 yrs	Substitute 1-time dose of Tdap for Td booster; then boost with Td every 10 yrs	Substitute 1-time dose of Tdap for Td booster; then boost with Td every 10 yrs	Substitute 1-time dose of Tdap for Td booster; then boost with Td every 10 yrs	Substitute 1-time dose of Tdap for Td booster; then boost with Td every 10 yrs	Substitute 1-time dose of Tdap for Td booster; then boost with Td every 10 yrs
Human papillomavirus (HPV)[2,*]		3 doses for females through age 26 yrs	3 doses for females through age 26 yrs	3 doses for females through age 26 yrs	3 doses for females through age 26 yrs	3 doses for females through age 26 yrs	3 doses for females through age 26 yrs	3 doses for females through age 26 yrs	3 doses for females through age 26 yrs
Varicella[3,*]	Contraindicated	Contraindicated	Contraindicated	2 doses	2 doses	2 doses	2 doses	2 doses	2 doses
Zoster[4]	Contraindicated	Contraindicated	Contraindicated		1 dose	1 dose	1 dose	1 dose	1 dose
Measles, mumps, rubella (MMR)[5,*]	Contraindicated	Contraindicated	Contraindicated	1 or 2 doses	1 or 2 doses	1 or 2 doses	1 or 2 doses	1 or 2 doses	1 or 2 doses
Influenza[6,*]	1 dose TIV annually	1 dose TIV annually	1 dose TIV annually	1 dose TIV annually	1 dose TIV annually	1 dose TIV annually	1 dose TIV annually	1 dose TIV annually	1 dose TIV or LAIV annually
Pneumococcal (polysaccharide)[7,8]	1 or 2 doses	1 or 2 doses	1 or 2 doses	1 or 2 doses	1 or 2 doses	1 or 2 doses	1 or 2 doses	1 or 2 doses	1 or 2 doses
Hepatitis A[9,*]	2 doses	2 doses	2 doses	2 doses	2 doses	2 doses	2 doses	2 doses	2 doses
Hepatitis B[10,*]	3 doses	3 doses	3 doses	3 doses	3 doses	3 doses	3 doses	3 doses	3 doses
Meningococcal[11,*]	1 or more doses	1 or more doses	1 or more doses	1 or more doses	1 or more doses	1 or more doses	1 or more doses	1 or more doses	1 or more doses

*Covered by the Vaccine Injury Compensation Program.

- (light shading) For all persons in this category who meet the age requirements and who lack evidence of immunity (e.g., lack documentation of vaccination or have no evidence of prior infection)
- (dark shading) Recommended if some other risk factor is present (e.g., on the basis of medical, occupational, lifestyle, or other indications)
- (blank) No recommendation

These schedules indicate the recommended age groups and medical indications for which administration of currently licensed vaccines is commonly indicated for adults ages 19 years and older, as of January 1, 2009. Licensed combination vaccines may be used whenever any components of the combination are indicated and when the vaccine's other components are not contraindicated. For detailed recommendations on all vaccines, including those used primarily for travelers or that are issued during the year, consult the manufacturers' package inserts and the complete statements from the Advisory Committee on Immunization Practices (www.cdc.gov/vaccines/pubs/acip-list.htm).

The recommendations in this schedule were approved by the Centers for Disease Control and Prevention's (CDC) Advisory Committee on Immunization Practices (ACIP), the American Academy of Family Physicians (AAFP), the American College of Obstetricians and Gynecologists (ACOG), and the American College of Physicians (ACP).

DEPARTMENT OF HEALTH AND HUMAN SERVICES
CENTERS FOR DISEASE CONTROL AND PREVENTION

CS200484-A

Footnotes

Recommended Adult Immunization Schedule—UNITED STATES · 2009

For complete statements by the Advisory Committee on Immunization Practices (ACIP), visit www.cdc.gov/vaccines/pubs/ACIP-list.htm.

1. Tetanus, diphtheria, and acellular pertussis (Td/Tdap) vaccination

Tdap should replace a single dose of Td for adults aged 19 through 64 years who have not received a dose of Tdap previously.

Adults with uncertain or incomplete history of primary vaccination series with tetanus and diphtheria toxoid-containing vaccines should begin or complete a primary vaccination series. A primary series for adults is 3 doses of tetanus and diphtheria toxoid-containing vaccines; administer the first 2 doses at least 4 weeks apart and the third dose 6–12 months after the second. However, Tdap can substitute for any one of the doses of Td in the 3-dose primary series. The booster dose of tetanus and diphtheria toxoid-containing vaccine should be administered to adults who have completed a primary series and if the last vaccination was received 10 or more years previously. Tdap or Td vaccine may be used, as indicated.

If a woman is pregnant and received the last Td vaccination 10 or more years previously, administer Td during the second or third trimester. If the woman received the last Td vaccination less than 10 years previously, administer Tdap during the immediate postpartum period. A dose of Tdap is recommended for postpartum women, close contacts of infants aged less than 12 months, and all health-care personnel with direct patient contact if they have not previously received Tdap. An interval as short as 2 years from the last Td is suggested; shorter intervals can be used. Td may be deferred during pregnancy and Tdap substituted in the immediate postpartum period, or Tdap may be administered instead of Td to a pregnant woman after an informed discussion with the woman.

Consult the ACIP statement for recommendations for administering Td as prophylaxis in wound management.

2. Human papillomavirus (HPV) vaccination

HPV vaccination is recommended for all females aged 11 through 26 years (and may begin at 9 years) who have not completed the vaccine series. History of genital warts, abnormal Papanicolaou test, or positive HPV DNA test is not evidence of prior infection with all vaccine HPV types; HPV vaccination is recommended for persons with such histories.

Ideally, vaccine should be administered before potential exposure to HPV through sexual activity; however, females who are sexually active should still be vaccinated consistent with age-based recommendations. Sexually active females who have not been infected with any of the four HPV vaccine types receive the full benefit of the vaccination. Vaccination is less beneficial for females who have already been infected with one or more of the HPV vaccine types.

A complete series consists of 3 doses. The second dose should be administered 2 months after the first dose; the third dose should be administered 6 months after the first dose.

HPV vaccination is not specifically recommended for females with the medical indications described in Figure 2, "Vaccines that might be indicated for adults based on medical and other indications." Because HPV vaccine is not a live-virus vaccine, it may be administered to persons with the medical indications described in Figure 2. However, the immune response and vaccine efficacy might be less for persons with the medical indications described in Figure 2 than in persons who do not have the medical indications described or who are immunocompetent. Health-care personnel are not at increased risk because of occupational exposure, and should be vaccinated consistent with age-based recommendations.

3. Varicella vaccination

All adults without evidence of immunity to varicella should receive 2 doses of single-antigen varicella vaccine if not previously vaccinated or the second dose if they have received only one dose unless they have a medical contraindication. Special consideration should be given to those who 1) have close contact with persons at high risk for severe disease (e.g., health-care personnel and family contacts of persons with immunocompromising conditions) or 2) are at high risk for exposure or transmission (e.g., teachers; child care employees; residents and staff members of institutional settings, including correctional institutions; college students; military personnel; adolescents and adults living in households with children; nonpregnant women of childbearing age; and international travelers).

Evidence of immunity to varicella in adults includes any of the following: 1) documentation of 2 doses of varicella vaccine at least 4 weeks apart; 2) U.S.-born before 1980 (although for health-care personnel and pregnant women, birth before 1980 should not be considered evidence of immunity); 3) history of varicella based on diagnosis or verification of varicella by a health-care provider (for a patient reporting a history of or presenting with an atypical case, a mild case, or both, health-care providers should seek either an epidemiologic link with a typical varicella case or to a laboratory-confirmed case or evidence of laboratory confirmation, if it was performed at the time of acute disease); 4) history of herpes zoster based on health-care provider diagnosis or verification of herpes zoster by a health-care provider; or 5) laboratory evidence of immunity or laboratory confirmation of disease.

Pregnant women should be assessed for evidence of varicella immunity. Women who do not have evidence of immunity should receive the first dose of varicella vaccine upon completion or termination of pregnancy and before discharge from the health-care facility. The second dose should be administered 4–8 weeks after the first dose.

4. Herpes zoster vaccination

A single dose of zoster vaccine is recommended for adults aged 60 years and older regardless of whether they report a prior episode of herpes zoster. Persons with chronic medical conditions may be vaccinated unless their condition constitutes a contraindication.

5. Measles, mumps, rubella (MMR) vaccination

Measles component: Adults born before 1957 generally are considered immune to measles. Adults born during or after 1957 should receive 1 or more doses of MMR unless they have a medical contraindication, documentation of 1 or more doses, history of measles based on health-care provider diagnosis, or laboratory evidence of immunity.

A second dose of MMR is recommended for adults who 1) have been recently exposed to measles or are in an outbreak setting; 2) have been vaccinated previously with killed measles vaccine; 3) have been vaccinated with an unknown type of measles vaccine during 1963–1967; 4) are students in postsecondary educational institutions; 5) work in a health-care facility; or 6) plan to travel internationally.

Mumps component: Adults born before 1957 generally are considered immune to mumps. Adults born during or after 1957 should receive 1 dose of MMR unless they have a medical contraindication, history of mumps based on health-care provider diagnosis, or laboratory evidence of immunity.

A second dose of MMR is recommended for adults who 1) live in a community experiencing a mumps outbreak and are in an affected age group; 2) are students in postsecondary educational institutions; 3) work in a health-care facility; or 4) plan to travel internationally. For unvaccinated health-care personnel born before 1957 who do not have other evidence of mumps immunity, administering 1 dose on a routine basis should be considered and administering a second dose during an outbreak should be strongly considered.

Rubella component: 1 dose of MMR vaccine is recommended for women whose rubella vaccination history is unreliable or who lack laboratory evidence of immunity. For women of childbearing age, regardless of birth year, rubella immunity should be determined and women should be counseled regarding congenital rubella syndrome. Women who do not have evidence of immunity should receive MMR upon completion or termination of pregnancy and before discharge from the health-care facility.

6. Influenza vaccination

Medical indications: Chronic disorders of the cardiovascular or pulmonary systems, including asthma; chronic metabolic diseases, including diabetes mellitus, renal or hepatic dysfunction, hemoglobinopathies, or immunocompromising conditions (including immunocompromising conditions caused by medications or human immunodeficiency virus [HIV]); any condition that compromises respiratory function or the handling of respiratory secretions or that can increase the risk of aspiration (e.g., cognitive dysfunction, spinal cord injury, or seizure disorder or other neuromuscular disorder); and pregnancy during the influenza season. No data exist on the risk for severe or complicated influenza disease among persons with asplenia; however, influenza is a risk factor for secondary bacterial infections that can cause severe disease among persons with asplenia.

Occupational indications: All health-care personnel, including those employed by long-term care and assisted-living facilities, and caregivers of children less than 5 years old.

Other indications: Residents of nursing homes and other long-term care and assisted-living facilities; persons likely to transmit influenza to persons at high risk (e.g., in-home household contacts and caregivers of children aged less than 5 years old, persons 65 years old and older and persons of all ages with high-risk condition[s]); and anyone who would like to decrease their risk of getting influenza. Healthy, nonpregnant adults aged less than 50 years without high-risk medical conditions who are not contacts of severely immunocompromised persons in special care units can receive either intranasally administered live, attenuated influenza vaccine (FluMist®) or inactivated vaccine. Other persons should receive the inactivated vaccine.

7. Pneumococcal polysaccharide (PPSV) vaccination

Medical indications: Chronic lung disease (including asthma); chronic cardiovascular diseases; diabetes mellitus; chronic liver diseases, cirrhosis; chronic alcoholism, chronic renal failure or nephrotic syndrome; functional or anatomic asplenia (e.g., sickle cell disease or splenectomy [if elective splenectomy is planned, vaccinate at least 2 weeks before surgery]); immunocompromising conditions; and cochlear implants and cerebrospinal fluid leaks. Vaccinate as close to HIV diagnosis as possible.

Other indications: Residents of nursing homes or long-term care facilities and persons who smoke cigarettes. Routine use of PPSV is not recommended for Alaska Native or American Indian persons younger than 65 years unless they have underlying medical conditions that are PPSV indications. However, public health authorities may consider recommending PPSV for Alaska Natives and American Indians aged 50 through 64 years who are living in areas in which the risk of invasive pneumococcal disease is increased.

8. Revaccination with PPSV

One-time revaccination after 5 years for persons with chronic renal failure or nephrotic syndrome; functional or anatomic asplenia (e.g., sickle cell disease or splenectomy); and for persons with immunocompromising conditions. For persons aged 65 years and older, one-time revaccination if they were vaccinated 5 or more years previously and were aged less than 65 years at the time of primary vaccination.

9. Hepatitis A vaccination

Medical indications: Persons with chronic liver disease and persons who receive clotting factor concentrates.

Behavioral indications: Men who have sex with men and persons who use illegal drugs.

Occupational indications: Persons working with hepatitis A virus (HAV)-infected primates or with HAV in a research laboratory setting.

Other indications: Persons traveling to or working in countries that have high or intermediate endemicity of hepatitis A (a list of countries is available at wwwn.cdc.gov/travel/contentdiseases.aspx) and any person seeking protection from HAV infection.

Single-antigen vaccine formulations should be administered in a 2-dose schedule at either 0 and 6–12 months (Havrix®), or 0 and 6–18 months (Vaqta®). If the combined hepatitis A and hepatitis B vaccine (Twinrix®) is used, administer 3 doses at 0, 1, and 6 months; alternatively, a 4-dose schedule, administered on days 0, 7 and 21 to 30 followed by a booster dose at month 12 may be used.

10. Hepatitis B vaccination

Medical indications: Persons with end-stage renal disease, including patients receiving hemodialysis; persons with HIV infection; and persons with chronic liver disease.

Occupational indications: Health-care personnel and public-safety workers who are exposed to blood or other potentially infectious body fluids.

Behavioral indications: Sexually active persons who are not in a long-term, mutually monogamous relationship (e.g., persons with more than 1 sex partner during the previous 6 months); persons seeking evaluation or treatment for a sexually transmitted disease (STD); current or recent injection-drug users; and men who have sex with men.

Other indications: Household contacts and sex partners of persons with chronic hepatitis B virus (HBV) infection; clients and staff members of institutions for persons with developmental disabilities; international travelers to countries with high or intermediate prevalence of chronic HBV infection (a list of countries is available at wwwn.cdc.gov/travel/contentdiseases.aspx); and any adult seeking protection from HBV infection.

Hepatitis B vaccination is recommended for all adults in the following settings: STD treatment facilities; HIV testing and treatment facilities; facilities providing drug-abuse treatment and prevention services; health-care settings targeting services to injection-drug users or men who have sex with men; correctional facilities; end-stage renal disease programs and facilities for chronic hemodialysis patients; and institutions and nonresidential daycare facilities for persons with developmental disabilities.

If the combined hepatitis A and hepatitis B vaccine (Twinrix®) is used, administer 3 doses at

0, 1, and 6 months; alternatively, a 4-dose schedule, administered on days 0, 7 and 21 to 30 followed by a booster dose at month 12 may be used.

Special formulation indications: For adult patients receiving hemodialysis or with other immunocompromising conditions, 1 dose of 40 µg/mL (Recombivax HB®) administered on a 3-dose schedule or 2 doses of 20 µg/mL (Engerix-B®) administered simultaneously on a 4-dose schedule at
0, 1, 2 and 6 months.

11. Meningococcal vaccination

Medical indications: Adults with anatomic or functional asplenia, or terminal complement component deficiencies.

Other indications: First-year college students living in dormitories; microbiologists who are routinely exposed to isolates of *Neisseria meningitidis*; military recruits; and persons who travel to or live in countries in which meningococcal disease is hyperendemic or epidemic (e.g., the "meningitis belt" of sub-Saharan Africa during the dry season [December–June]), particularly if their contact with local populations will be prolonged. Vaccination is required by the government of Saudi Arabia for all travelers to Mecca during the annual Hajj.

Meningococcal conjugate (MCV) vaccine is preferred for adults with any of the preceding indications who are aged 55 years or younger, although meningococcal polysaccharide vaccine (MPSV) is an acceptable alternative. Revaccination with MCV after 5 years might be indicated for adults previously vaccinated with MPSV who remain at increased risk for infection (e.g., persons residing in areas in which disease is epidemic).

12. Selected conditions for which *Haemophilus influenzae* type b (Hib) vaccine may be used

Hib vaccine generally is not recommended for persons aged 5 years and older. No efficacy data are available on which to base a recommendation concerning use of Hib vaccine for older children and adults. However, studies suggest good immunogenicity in persons who have sickle cell disease, leukemia, or HIV infection or who have had a splenectomy; administering 1 dose of vaccine to these persons is not contraindicated.

13. Immunocompromising conditions

Inactivated vaccines generally are acceptable (e.g., pneumococcal, meningococcal, and influenza [trivalent inactivated influenza vaccine]), and live vaccines generally are avoided in persons with immune deficiencies or immunocompromising conditions. Information on specific conditions is available at www.cdc.gov/vaccines/pubs/acip-list.htm.

APPENDIX C
Abbreviations, Acronyms, and Symbols

>	greater than
<	less than
ʒ	dram
℥	ounce
♏	minum
ā	before
AAPB	Association of Applied Psychophysiology and Biofeedback
AARP	American Association of Retired Persons
AASM	American Academy of Sleep Medicine
AAT	animal-assisted therapy
AATH	American Association for Therapeutic Humor
ABC	airway, breathing, circulation
ABD	abdominal
ABG	arterial blood gases
ABO	blood types
a.c.	before meals
ACIP	Advisory Committee on Immunization Practices
ACS	American Cancer Society
ACTH	adrenocorticotropic hormone
AD	Alzheimer's disease
AD	right ear
ad lib	freely, as desired
ADA	Americans with Disabilities Act
ADH	antidiuretic hormone
ADLs	activities of daily living
ADN	associate degree nurse (nursing)
AEB	as evidenced by
AFP	alpha-fetoprotein
AHA	American Hospital Association
AHCA	American Health Care Association
AHCPR	Agency for Health Care Policy and Research
AHNA	American Holistic Nurses' Association
AHRQ	Agency for Healthcare Research and Quality
AI	adequate intake
AIDS	acquired immunodeficiency syndrome
AJN	*American Journal of Nursing*
ALFA	Assisted Living Federation of America
ALT	alanine aminotransferase
AMA	against medical advice
AMA	American Medical Association
ANA	American Nurses Association
ANA	antinuclear antibody
AoA	Administration on Aging
AP	anterior/posterior
AP	apical pulse
APIC	Association for Practitioners in Infection Control and Epidemiology
APRN	advance practice registered nurse
APS	Adult Protective Services
APS	American Pain Society
APTT	activated partial thromboplastin time
AROM	active range of motion
AS	left ear
ASA	acetylsalicylic acid
ASO	antireptolysin-O
AST	aspartate aminotransferase
AT	axillary temperature
ATC	around the clock
ATP	adenosine triphosphatase
AU	both ears
B_1	thiamine
B_2	riboflavin
B_6	pyridoxine
B_{12}	cobolomine
BBA	Balanced Budget Act
BE	base excess
bid	twice a day
BMD	bone mineral density
BMI	body mass index
BMR	basal metabolic rate

BP	blood pressure
BPH	benign prostatic hypertrophy
BPM	beats per minute
BSA	body surface area
BSE	breast self-examination
BSI	body substance isolation
BSN	bachelor of science in nursing
BUN	blood urea nitrogen
c	cup
c̄	with
C	Celsius
Ca	calcium
Ca^{++}	calcium ion
$CaCl_2$	calcium chloride
C/A	complementary/alternative
CAD	coronary artery disease
CAI	computer-assisted instruction
CAM	complementary/alternative medicine
C & S	culture and sensitivity
cap	capsule
CARF	Commission on Accreditation of Rehabilitation Facilities
CAT	computed axial tomography
CAT	computerized adaptive testing
CBC	complete blood count
CBD	common bile duct
CBE	charting by exception
cc	cubic centimeter
CCRC	continuing care retirement community
CCU	coronary care unit
CDC	Centers for Disease Control and Prevention
CEA	carcinoembryonic antigen
CEPN-LTC™	Certification Examination for Practical and Vocational Nurses in Long-Term Care
CEU	continuing education unit
CHAP	Community Health Accreditation Program
CHD	coronary heart disease
CHF	congestive heart failure
CHIP	Children's Health Insurance Program
CHO	carbohydrate (carbon, hydrogen, oxygen)
CHON	protein (carbon, hydrogen, oxygen, nitrogen)
CK or CPK	creatine kinase or creatine phosphokinase
Cl	chlorine, chloride
Cl^-	chloride ion
CLTC	certified in long-term care
cm	centimeter
CMS	Centers for Medicare and Medicaid Services
CN	cranial nerve
CNA	certified nursing assistant
CNM	certified nurse midwife
CNO	community nursing organization
CNS	central nervous system
CNS	clinical nurse specialist
Co	cobalt
CO_2	carbon dioxide
CO_2^-	carbon dioxide ion
COBRA	Comprehensive Omnibus Budget Reconciliation Act
COOH	carboxyl group
COPD	chronic obstructive pulmonary disease
CPAP	continuous positive airway pressure
CPNP	Council of Practical Nursing Programs
CPR	cardiopulmonary resuscitation
CPR	computerized patient record
Cr	chromium
CRNA	Certified Registered Nurse Anesthetist
CRP	C-reactive protein
C&S	culture and sensitivity
CSF	cerebrospinal fluid
CSM	circulation, sensation, motion
CT	computed tomography
Cu	copper
CVA	cerebrovascular accident
CVC	central venous catheter
D_5W	dextrose 5% in water
D & C	dilatation and curettage
DAR	document, action, response
dc	discontinue
DDB	Disciplinary Data Bank
DDS	doctor of dental surgery
DEA	Drug Enforcement Agency
DHHS	Department of Health and Human Services
DIC	disseminated intravascular coagulation
DICC	dynamic infusion cavernosometry and cavernosography
dL	deciliter
DMD	doctor of dental medicine
DNA	deoxyribonucleic acid
DNR	do not resuscitate
DO	doctor of osteopathy
DPAHC	durable power of attorney for health care
dr	dram, or ʒ
DRG	diagnosis-related group
DRI	dietary reference intake
DSM-IV	*Diagnostic and Statistical Manual of Mental Disorders,* 4th edition
DST	dexamethasone suppression test
DT	delirium tremens
DTaP	diphtheria, tetanus, acellular pertussis
DTP	diphtheria, tetanus, pertussis
DVT	deep vein thrombosis
EAR	estimated average requirement
ECF	extended care facility
ECF	extracellular fluid
ED	emergency department
EDTA	ethylenediaminetetraacetic acid
EEG	electroencephalograph
EGD	esophagogastroduodenoscopy
EKG (ECG)	electrocardiogram
ELISA	enzyme-linked immunosorbent assay
elix	elixir
EMG	electromyogram
EMLA	eutectic (cream) mixture of local anesthetics
EMS	emergency medical services

EMT	emergency medical technician
EMT-P	emergency medical technician-paramedic
EPA	Environmental Protection Agency
EPO	exclusive provider organization
ER	emergency room
ERCP	endoscopic retrograde cholangiopancreatogram
ERG	electroretinogram
ERT	estrogen replacement therapy
ESR	erythrocyte sedimentation rate
ET	ear (tympanic) temperature
EVAD	explantable venous access device
F	fahrenheit
FAS	fetal alcohol syndrome
FBS	fasting blood sugar
FCA	False Claims Act
FDA	Food and Drug Administration
Fe	iron
$FeSO_4$	iron sulfate
fl	fluid
Fl	fluorine
FOBT	fecal occult blood test
FSH	follicle-stimulating hormone
ft	foot or feet
FVD	fluid volume deficit
g	gram
GAO	General Accounting Office
GAS	general adaptation syndrome
GCS	Glasgow Coma Scale
g/dL	grams per deciliter
GED	general education development
GER	gastroesophageal reflux
GFR	glomerular filtration rate
GGT (GGTP)	gammaglutamy transpeptidase
GH	growth hormone
GHB	glycosylated hemoglobin
GI	gastrointestinal
gr	grain
gtt	drop
GTT	glucose tolerance test
gtt/min	drops per minute
GU	genitourinary
h	hour(s)
H^+	hydrogen ion
H_2CO_3	carbonic acid
H_2O	water
H&H	hemoglobin and hematocrit
HB_sAG	hepatitis B surface antigen
HBV	hepatitis B virus
HCFA	Health Care Financing Administration
hCG	human chorionic gonadotropin
HCl	hydrochloric acid, hydrochloride
HCO_3^-	bicarbonate ion
Hct	hematocrit
HCV	hepatitis C virus
HDL	high density lipoprotein
HDV	hepatitis D virus
Hep B	hepatitis B
HFA	Hospice Foundation of America
Hg	mercury
Hgb	hemoglobin
Hgbs	hemoglobins
HICPAC	Hospital Infection Control Practices Advisory Committee
HIS	hospital information system
HIV	human immunodeficiency virus
HLA	human leukocyte antigen
HMO	health maintenance organization
HPO_4	phosphate
HR	heart rate
HRSA	Health Resources and Services Administration
h.s.	hour of sleep
I	iodine
IADLs	instrumental activities of daily living
I&O	intake and output
IASP	International Association for the Study of Pain
ICF	intermediate care facility
ICF	intracellular fluid
ICN	International Council of Nurses
ICU	intensive care unit
ID	identification
ID	intradermal
IgG	immunoglobulin G
IgM	immunoglobulin M
IHCT	interdisciplinary health care team
IM	intramuscular
in	inch
INR	International Normalized Ratio
I&O	intake and output
IOL	intraocular lens
IOM	Institute of Medicine
ITT	insulin tolerance test
IV	intravenous
IVAD	implantable vascular access device
IVP	intravenous push, intravenous pyelogram
IVPB	intravenous piggyback
JCAHO	Joint Commission on Accreditation of Healthcare Organizations
K	potassium
K^+	potassium ion
kcal	kilocalorie
KCl	potassium chloride
kg	kilogram
KS	ketosteroids
KUB	kidneys/ureters/bladder
KVO	keep vein open
L	liter
LAS	local adaptation syndrome
lb	pound
LDH	lactic dehydrogenase
LDL	low density lipoprotein
LE	lupus erythematosus
LES	lower esophageal sphincter
LFT	liver function test

LH	luteinizing hormone
LLQ	left lower quadrant
LMP	last menstrual period
L/min	liters per minute
LOC	level of consciousness
LP	lumbar puncture
LP/VN	licensed practical/vocational nurse
LPN	licensed practical nurse
LUQ	left upper quadrant
LVN	licensed vocational nurse
m	meter
m^2	square meter
MAO	monoamine oxidase
MAOI	monoamine oxidase inhibitor
MAR	medication administration record
mcg (or μg)	microgram
MD	doctor of medicine
MDI	metered-dose inhaler
MDR	multidrug-resistant
MDR-TB	multidrug-resistant tuberculosis
MDS	minimum data set
mEq	milliequivalent
mEq/L	milliequivalents per liter
mg	milligram
mg/dL	milligrams per deciliter
Mg	magnesium
Mg^{++}	magnesium ion
MgCl	magnesium chloride
$MgSO_4$	magnesium sulfate
MI	myocardial infarction
min	minute
mL	milliliter
mm^3	cubic millimeter
mm Hg	millimeters of mercury
mmol/L	millimoles per liter
MMR	measles, mumps, rubella
Mn	manganese
Mo	molybdenum
MOM	Milk of Magnesia
mOsm/kg	milliosmoles/kilogram
MRI	magnetic resonance imaging
MRSA	methicillin-resistant *staphylococcus aureus*
MS	morphine sulfate
MSDS	material safety data sheet
MUGA	multi-gated acquisition
N_2	nitrogen
Na	sodium
Na^+	sodium ion
Na_2SO_4	sodium sulfate
NaCl	sodium chloride
NA	not applicable
NADSA	National Adult Day Services Associations
NaH_2PO_4	sodium dihydrogen phosphate
Na_2HPO_4	disodium phosphate
NAHC	National Association for Home Care
$NaHCO_3$	sodium bicarbonate
$NaHPO_4$	sodium monohydrogen phosphate
NANDA	North American Nursing Diagnosis Association
NaOH	sodium hydroxide
NAPNE	Natonal Association of Practical Nurse Education
NAPNES	National Association for Practical Nurse Education and Services
NCCAM	National Center for Complementary and Alternative Medicine
NCHS	National Center for Health Statistics
NCLEX®	National Council Licensure Examination
NCLEX-PN®	National Council Licensure Examination—Practical Nurse
NCLEX-RN®	National Council Licensure Examination—Registered Nurse
NCLD	National Center for Learning Disabilities
NCOA	National Council on Aging
NCSBN	National Council of State Boards of Nursing
NCVHS	National Committee on Vital and Health Statistics
NF	*National Formulary*
NFLPN	National Federation of Licensed Practical Nurses, Inc.
NG	nasogastric
NH_2	amino group
NHO	National Hospice Organization
NIA	National Institute on Aging
NIC	Nursing Interventions Classification
NIH	National Institutes of Health
NIOSH	National Institute of Occupational Safety and Health
NIS	nursing information system
NLEA	Nutrition, Labeling, and Education Act
NLN	National League for Nursing
NLNAC	National League for Nursing Accrediting Commission
NMDS	nursing minimum data set
NOC	Nursing Outcomes Classification
NP	nurse practitioner
NPDB	National Practitioner Data Bank
NPO	*nil per os,* Latin for "nothing by mouth"
NREM	non-rapid eye movement
NS	normal saline
NSAID	nonsteroidal anti-inflammatory drug
NSF	National Sleep Foundation
O_2	oxygen
OAM	Office of Alternative Medicine
O&P	ova and parasite
OBRA	Omnibus Budget Reconciliation Act
OD	right eye
OH^-	hydroxyl
OR	operating room
ORIF	open reduction/internal fixation
OS	left eye
OSHA	Occupational Safety and Health Administration
OT	occupational therapist
OT	oral temperature

OTC	over-the-counter
OU	both eyes
oz	ounce
p̄	after
P	phosphorus
P	pulse
PA	physician's assistant
PA	posterioanterior
$PaCO_2$	partial pressure of carbon dioxide
PaO_2	partial pressure of oxygen
Pap	Papanicolaou test
p.c.	after meals
PCA	patient-controlled analgesia
PCO_2 ($PaCO_2$)	partial pressure of carbon dioxide
PCP	primary care provider
PCR	polymerase chain reaction
PCV	pneumococcal conjugate vaccine
PDPH	postdural puncture headache
PEG	percutaneous endoscopic gastrostomy
PERRLA	pupils equal, round, reactive to light and accommodation
PET	positron emission tomography
PFT	pulmonary function test
pH	potential hydrogen
PICC	peripherally inserted central catheter
PIE	problem, implementation, evaluation
PKU	phenylketonuria
PLMS	periodic limb movements in sleep
PMI	point of maximum intensity
PMR	progressive muscle relaxation
PMS	premenstrual syndrome
PNI	psychoneuroimmunology
PNS	peripheral nervous system
po	*per os,* Latin for "by mouth"
PO_2 (PaO_2)	partial pressure of oxygen
PO_4^{--}	phosphate ion
POMR	problem-oriented medical record
POR	problem-oriented record
PPBS	post prandial blood sugar
PPE	personal protective equipment
PPG	post prandial glucose
PPO	preferred provider organization
PPS	prospective payment system
PRA	plama renin activity
PRL	prolactin level
PRN	*pro re nata,* Latin for "as required"
PRO	peer review organization
PROM	passive range of motion
PSA	prostate specific antigen
PSDA	Patient Self-Determination Act
PSP	phenolsulfonphtalein
pt	pint
PT	physical therapist
PT	prothrombin time
PTH	parathyroid hormone
PTSD	post-traumatic stress disorder
PTT	partial thromboplastin time
PVD	peripheral vascular disease
q	*quaque,* Latin for "every"
qd	every day
qh	every hour
qid	four times a day
qod	every other day
qs	quantity sufficient
q2h	every 2 hours
qt	quart
R (Resp)	respiration
RAIU	radioactive iodine uptake
RAST	radio allergosorbent test
RBC	red blood count, red blood cell
RD	registered dietician
RDA	recommended dietary allowance
REM	rapid eye movement
RF	rheumatoid factor
RLQ	right lower quadrant
RLS	restless leg syndrome
RN	registered nurse
RNA	ribonucleic acid
RNFA	registered nurse first assistant
ROM	range of motion
ROS	review of systems
RPCH	rural primary care hospital
RPh	registered pharmacist
RPR	rapid plasma reagin
RR	recovery room
RSV	respiratory syncytial virus
R/T	related to
RT	rectal temperature
RT	respiratory therapist
RTI	respiratory tract infection
RUGS	resource utilization group system
RUQ	right upper quadrant
RWJF	Robert Wood Johnson Foundation
s̄	without
S	sulfur
SAMe	S-adenosylmethionine
SaO_2	oxygen saturation
SBC	school-based clinic
SC/SQ	subcutaneous
SCHIP	State Children's Health Insurance Program
Se	selenium
SGOT	serum glutamate oxaloacetate transaminase
SGPT	serum glutamic pyruvic transaminase
SL	sublingual
SNF	skilled nursing facility
SOAP	subjective data, objective data, assessment, plan
SOAPIE	subjective data, objective data, assessment, plan, implementation, evaluation
SOAPIER	subjective data, objective data, assessment, plan, implementation, evaluation, revision
SPF	sun protection factor
s̄s̄	one half
SSA	Social Security Administration
STAT	*statim,* Latin for "immediately"
STD	sexually transmitted disease

supp	suppository
susp	suspension
SW	social worker
T	temperature
T_3	triiodothyronine
T_4	thyroxine
tab	tablet
TAC	tetracaine, adrenaline, cocaine
TB	tuberculosis
Tbsp	tablespoon
Td	tetanus/diphtheria
TDD	telecommunication device for the deaf
TEFRA	Tax Equity Fiscal Responsibility Act
TENS	transcutaneous electrical nerve stimulation
TF	tube feeding
THA	total hip arthroplasty
TIA	transient ischemic attack
TIBC	total iron binding capacity
t.i.d.	three times a day
TMJ	temporomandibular joint
t.o.	telephone order
TPN	total parenteral nutrition
TPR	temperature, pulse, respirations
Tr or tinct	tincture
TRH	thyrotropin-releasing hormone
TSE	testicular self examination
TSH	thyroid-stimulating hormone
tsp	teaspoon
U	unit
U/L	unit per liter
UA	routine urinalysis
UAP	unlicensed assistive personnel
UIS	Universal Intellectual Standards
UL	upper intake level
UMLS	Universal Medical Language System
UNOS	United Network for Organ Sharing
U-100	100 units insulin per cc
UPP	urethra pressure profile
URQ	upper right quadrant
USDHHS	United States Department of Health and Human Services
USP	*United States Pharmacopeia*
USPHS	United States Public Health Service
UTI	urinary tract infection
VA	Veterans Administration, Veterans Affairs
VAD	ventricular assist device, vascular access device
VAS	Visual Analog Scale
VDRL	venereal disease research laboratory
VLDL	very low-density lipoprotein
VMA	vanilymandelic acid
VRE	vancomycin-resistant enterococci
VS	vital signs
WASP	white, Anglo-Saxon, Protestant
WBC	white blood cell, white blood count
WHO	World Health Organization
WNL	within normal limits
WPM	words per minute
wt	weight
YWCA	Young Women's Christian Association
Zn	Zinc

APPENDIX D
English/Spanish Words and Phrases

Being able to say a few words or phrases in the client's language is one way to show that you care. It lets the client know that you as a nurse are interested in the individual. There are three rules to keep in mind regarding the pronunciation of Spanish words.

- If a word ends in a vowel, or in *n* or *s*, the accent is on the next to the last syllable.
- If the word ends in a consonant other than *n* or *s*, the accent is on the last syllable.
- If the word does not follow these rules, it has a written accent over the vowel of the accented syllable.

Courtesy phrases, names of body parts, and expressions of time and numbers are included in this section for quick reference. The English version will appear first, followed by the Spanish translation and Spanish pronunciation.

Courtesy Phrases

Please	Por favor	Por fah-**vor**
Thank-you	Grácias	**Grah**-the-as
Good morning	Buénos dias	Boo-**ay**-nos **dee**-as
Good afternoon	Buénas tardes	Boo-**ay**-nas **tar**-days
Good evening	Buénas noches	Boo-**ay**-nas **no**-chays
Yes/No	Si/no	See/no
Good	Bien	Be-en
Bad	Mal	Mahl
How many?	¿Cuántos?	¿Coo-**ahn**-tos?
Where?	¿Dónde?	¿**Don**-day?
When?	¿Cuándo?	¿Coo**ahn**-do?

Body Parts

abdomen	el abdomen	el ab-doh-men
ankle	el tobillo	el to-**beel**-lyo
anus	el ano	el **ah**-no
anvil (incus)	el yunque	el **yoon**-kay
appendix	el apéndice	el ah-**pen**-de-thay
aqueous humor	el humor acuoso	el oo-**mor** ah-coo-**o**-so
bladder	la vejiga	lah vay-**nee**-gah
brain	el cerebro	el thay-**ray**-bro
breast	el pecho	el **pay**-cho
buttock	la nalga	lah **nahl**-gah
calf	la pantorrilla	lah pan-tor-**reel**-lyah
cervix	la cerviz	lah ther-**veth**
cheek	la mejilla	lah may-**heel**-lyah

chin	la barbilla	lah bar-**beel**-lyah
choroid	la coroidea	lah co-ro-e-**day**-ah
ciliary body	el cuerpo ciliar	el coo-**err**-po the-le-**ar**
clitoris	el clítoris	el **clee**-to-ris
coccyx	el coxis	el **coc**-sees
conjunctiva	la conjuntiva	lah con-hoon-**tee**vah
cornea	la córnea	lah **cor**-nay-ah
penis	el pene	el **pay**-nay
prostate gland	la próstata	lah **pros**-ta-tah
pupil	la pupila	lah poo-**pee**-lah
rectum	el recto	el **rec**-to
retina	la retina	lah ray-**tee**-nah
sclera	la esclerótica	lah es-clay-**ro**-te-cah
scrotum	el escroto	el es-**cro**-to
seminal vesicle	la vesícula seminal	lah vay-**see**-coo-lah say-me-**nahl**
shoulder	el hombro	el **om**-bro
small intestine	el intestino delgado	el in-tes-**tee**-no del-**gah**-do
spinal cord	la médula espinal	lah **may**-doo-lah es-pe-**nahl**
spleen	el bazo	el **bah**-tho
stirrup (stapes)	el estribo	el es-**tree**-bo
stomach	el estómago	el es-**toh**-mah-go
temple	la sien	lah se-**ayn**
testis	el testículo	el tes-**tee**-coo-lo
thigh	el muslo	el **moos**-lo
thorax	el tórax	el **to**-rax
tongue	la lengua	lah **len**-goo-ah
trachea	la tráquea	lah **trah**-kay-ah
upper extremities	las extremidades superiores	las ex-tray-me-**dahd**-es soo-pay-re-**or**-es
ureter	el uréter	el oo-**ray**-ter
uterus	el útero	el **oo**-tay-ro
vagina	el vagina	lah vah-**hee**-nah
vitreous humor	el humor vítreo	el oo-**mor vee**-tray-o
wrist	la muñeca	lah moo-**nyay**-cah

Expressions of Time, Calendar, and Numbers

after meals	después de comer	des-poo-**es** day co-**merr**
at bedtime	al acostarse	al ah-cos-**tar**-say
before meals	antes de comer	**ahn**-tes day co-**merr**
daily	el diario	el de-**ah**-re-o
date	la fecha	lah **fay**-chah
day	el dia	el **dee**-ah
every hour	a cada hora	ah **cah**-dah **o**-rah
hour (time)	la hora	lah **o**-rah
how often	cada cuánto tiempo	**cah**-dah coo-**ahn**-to te-**em**-po
noon	el mediodia	el may-de-o-**dee**-ah
now	ahora	ah-**o**-rah
once	una vez	**oo**-nah veth
today	hoy	**oh**-e
tomorrow	mañana	mah-**nyah**-nah
tonight	esta noche	**es**-tah **no**-chay
week	la semana	lah say-**mah**-nah
year	año	**a**-nyo
Sunday	el domingo	el do-**meen**-go
Monday	el lunes	el **loo**-nes
Tuesday	el martes	el **mar**-tes
Wednesday	el miércoles	el me-**err**-co-les
Thursday	el jueves	el hoo-**ay**ves
Friday	el viernes	el ve-**err**-nes

Saturday	el sábado	el **sah**-bah-do
zero	cero	**thay**-ro
one	uno	**oo**-no
two	dos	dose
three	tres	trays
four	cuatro	coo-**ah**-tro
five	cinco	**theen**-co
six	seis	**say**-ees
seven	siete	se-**ay**-tay
eight	ocho	**o**-cho
nine	nueve	noo-**ay**-vay
ten	diez	de-**eth**

Nursing Care Sentences and Questions

What is your name?
¿Como se llama usted?
¿**Co**-mo say **lyah**-mah oos-**ted?**

I am a student nurse.
Soy estudiente enfermera(o).
Soy es-too-de-**ahn**-tay en-fer-**may**-ra(o).

My name is . . .
Mi nombre es . . .
Mee **nom**-bray es . . .

Do you need a wheelchair?
¿Necesita usted una silla de rueda?
¿Nay-thay-**se**-ta oos-**ted** **oo**-nah **seel**-lyah day roo-**ay**-dah?

How do you feel?
¿Como se siente?
¿**Co**-mo say se-**ayn**-tah?

When is your family coming?
¿Cuándo viene su familia?
¿Coo-**ahn**-do vee-**en**-nah soo fah-**mee**-le-ah?

This is the call light.
Esta es la luz para llamar a la enfermera.
Es-tah es lah looth **pah**-ra lyah-**mar** a lah en-fer-**may**-ra.

If you need anything, press the button.
Si usted necesita algo, oprima el botón.
See oos-**ted** nay-thay-**se**-ta **ahl**-go o-pre-**ma** el bo-**tone.**

Do not turn without calling the nurse.
No se voltee sin llamar a la enfermera.
No say **vol**-tay seen lyah-**mar** a lah en-fer-**may**-ra.

The side rails on your bed are for your protection.
Los rieles del costado están para su protección.
Los re-**el**-es del cos-**tah**-do es-**tahn** **pah**-ra soo pro-tec-the-**on.**

Please do not try to lower or climb over the side rail.
Por favor no pretenda bajarlos (barjarlas) o treparse sobre ellos.
Por fah-**vor** no pray-**ten**-dah ba-**har**-los o tray-**par**-say **so**-bray **ayl**-lyos.

The head nurse is . . .
La jefa de enfermeras es . . .
La **hay**-fay day en-fer-**may**-ras es . . .

Do you need more blankets or another pillow?
¿Necesita usted más frazadas u orta almohada?
¿Nay-thay-**si**-ta oos-**ted** mahs frah-**thad**-dahs oo **o**-trah al-mo-**ah**-dah?

You may not smoke in the room.
No se puede fumar en el cuarto.
No say poo-**ay**-day foo-**mar** en el coo-**ar**-to.

Do you want me to turn on (turn off) the lights?
¿Quiere usted que encienda (apague) la luz?
¿Ke-**ay**-ray oos-**ted** day en-the-**en**-dah (a-**pah**-gay) lah looth?

Are you thirsty?
¿Tiene usted sed?
¿Tee-**en**-nah oos-**ted** sayd?

Are you allergic to any medication?
¿Es usted alérgico(a) a alguna medicina?
¿Es oos-**ted** ah-**lehr**-hee-co(a) ah ah-**goo**-nah nay-de-**thee**-nah?

You may take a bath.
Usted puede bañarse.
Oos-**ted** poo-**ay**-day bah-**nyar**-say.

Do not lock the door, please.
No cierre usted la puerta con llave, por favor.
No the-**err**-ray oos-**ted** lah poo-**err**-tah con **lyah**-vay por fah-**vor.**

Call if you feel faint or in need of help.
Llame si usted se siente débil o si necesita ayuda.
Lyah-mah see oos-**ted** say se-**ayn**-tah **day**-bil o see nay-thay-**se**-ta ah-**yoo**-dah.

Call when you have to go to the toilet.
Llame cuando tenga que ir al inodoro.
Lyah-mah coo-**ahn**-do **ten**-gah kay eer al in-o-**do**-ro.

I will give you an enema.
Le pondré una enema.
Lay pon-**dray oo**-nah ay-**nay**-mah.

Turn on your left (right) side.
Voltese a su lado izquierdo (derecho).
Vol-**tay**-say ah soo **lah**-do ith-ke-**er**-do(dah) (day-**ray**-cho[cha]).

Here is an appointment card.
Aqui tiene usted una tarjeta con la información escrito.
Ah-**kee** tee-**en**-nah oos-**ted oo**-nah tar-**hay**-tah con lah in-for-mah-the-**on** es-**cree**-to.

You are going to be discharged (released) today.
A usted le van a dar de alta hoy.
Ah oos-**ted** lay vahn ah dar day **ahl**-tah **oh**-e.

How did this illness begin?
¿Como empezó esta enfermedad?
¿**Co**-mo em-pa-**tho es**-tah en-fer-may-**dahd**?

Is the pain better after the medicine?
¿Siente usted alivio depués de tomar la medicina?
¿Se-**ayn**-tah oos-**ted** al-**lee**-ve-o des-poo-**es** day to-**mar** lah may-de-**thee**-nah?

Where is the pain?
¿Que la duele? (or) Dónde le duele?
¿Kay lah doo-**ay**-le? (or) **Don**-day lay doo-**ay**-le?

Do you have pains in your chest?
¿Tiene usted dolores in el pecho?
¿Tee-**en**-nah oos-**ted** do-**lor**-es en el **pay**-cho?

Are you in pain now?
¿Tiene usted dolores ahora?
¿Tee-**en**-nah oos-**ted** do-**lor**-es ah-**o**-rah?

Is it constant pain or does it come and go?
¿Es un dolor constante o va y vuelve?
¿Es oon do-**lor** cons-**tahn**-tay o vah ee voo-**el**-vah?

Is there anything that makes the pain better?
¿Hay algo que lo alivie?
¿**Ah**-ee **ahl**-go kay lo al-**le**-ve?

Is there anything that makes the pain worse?
¿Hay algo que lo aumente?
¿**Ah**-ee **ahl**-go kay lo ah-oo-**men**-tay?

Where do you feel the pain?
¿Dónde siente usted el dolor?
¿**Don**-day se-**ayn**-tah oos-**ted** el do-**lor**?

Point to where it hurts.
Apunte usted por favor, adonde le duele.
Ah-**poon**-tay oos-**ted** por fah-**vor** ah-**don**-day lay doo-**ay**-le.

Show me where it hurts.
Enséñeme usted donde le duele.
En-**say**-nah-may oos-**ted don**-day lay doo-**ay**-le.

Is the pain sharp or dull?
¿Es agudo o sordo el dolor?
¿Es ah-**goo**-do o **sor**-do el do-**lor**?

Do you know where you are?
¿Sabe usted donde esta?
¿Sah-**bay** oos-**ted don**-day es-**tah**?

You are in the hospital.
Usted está en el hospital.
Oos-**ted** es-**tah** en el os-pee-**tahl**.

You will be okay.
Usted va a estar bien.
Oos-**ted** vah a es-**tar be**-en.

Do you have any drug reactions?
¿Tiene usted alguna sensibilidad a productos químicos?
¿Te-**en**-nah oos-**ted** al-**goo**-nah sen-se-be-le-**dahd** a pro-**dooc**-tos **kee**-me-cos?

Have you seen another doctor or native healer for this problem?
¿Ha visto usted a otro médico o curandero tocante a este problema?
¿Ah **vees**-to oos-**ted** a **o**-tro **may**-de-co o coo-ran-**day**-ro to-**cahn**-tay a **es**-ah pro-**blay**-mah?

Have you vomited?
¿Ha vomitado usted?
¿Ah vo-me-**tah**-do oos-**ted**?

Do you have any difficulty in breathing?
¿Tiene usted alguna dificultad para respirar?
¿Te-**en**-nah oos-**ted** ah-**goo**-nah de-fe-cool-**tahd pah**-ra res-pe-**rar**?

Do you smoke?
¿Fuma usted?
¿Foo-**mar** oos-**ted**?

How many per day?
¿Cuántos al dia?
¿Coo-**ahn**-tos al **dee**-ah?

For how many years?
¿Por cuántos años?
¿por coo-**ahn**-tos **a**-nyos?

Do you awaken in the night because of shortness of breath?
¿Se despierta usted por la noche por falta de respiración?
¿Say des-pee-**err**-tah oos-**ted** por lah **no**-chay por **fahl**-tah day res-pe-rah-the-**on**?

Is any part of your body swollen?
¿Tiene usted alguna parte del cuerpo hinchada?
¿Te-**en**-nah oos-**ted** ah-**goo**-nah **par**-tay del coo-**err**-po in-**chah**-da?

How much water do you drink daily?
¿Cuántos vasos de agua bebe usted diariamente?
¿Coo-**ahn**-tos **vah**-sos day **ah**-goo-ah **bay**-be oos-**ted** de-ah-re-ah-**men**-tay?

Are you nauseated?
¿Tiene náusea?
¿Te-**en**-nah **nah**-oo-say-ah?

Are you going to vomit?
¿Va a vomitar?
¿Vah a vo-me-**tar**?

When was your last bowel movement?
¿Cuánto tiempo hace que evacúa usted?
¿Coo-**ahn**-to te-**em**-po **ah**-the kay ay-vah-**coo**-ah oos-**ted**?

Do you have diarrhea?
¿Tiene usted diarrea?
¿Te-**en**-nah oos-**ted** der-ar-**ray**-ah?

How much do you urinate?
¿Cuánto orina usted?
¿Coo-**ahn**-to o-**re**-nah oos-**ted**?

Did you urinate?
¿Orinó usted?
¿O-re-**no** oos-**ted**?

What color is your urine?
¿De qué color es la orina?
¿Day kay co-**lor** es lah o-**re**-nah?

Call when you have to go to the toilet.
Llame usted cuando tenga que ir al inodoro.
Lyah-mah oos-**ted** coo-**ahn**-do **ten**-gah kay eer al in-o-**do**-ro.

I need a urine specimen from you.
Necesito una muestra de orina de usted.
Nay-thay-**se**-to **oo**-nah moo-**ays**-trah day o-**re**-nah day oos-**ted**.

We will put a tube in your bladder so that you can urinate.
Le pondremos un tubo en la vejiga para que puede orinar.
Lay pon-**dray**-mos un **too**-be en lah vay-**hee**-gah **pah**-rah kay poo-**ay**-day o-re **nar.**

When was your last menstrual period?
¿Cuándo fue se última menstruación?
¿Coo-**ahn**-do foo-**ay** soo **ool**-te-mah mens-troo-ah-the-**on?**

Are you bleeding heavily?
¿Está sangrando mucho?
¿Es-**tah** san-**grahn**-do **moo**-cho?

Take off your clothes, please
Desvístase usted, por favor.
Des-**ves**-tah-say oos-**ted** por-fah-**vor.**

Just relax.
Relaje usted el cuerpo.
Ray-**lah**-he oos-**ted** el coo-**err**-po.

I am going to listen to your chest.
Voy a escucharle el pecho.
Voye a es-coo-**char**-lay el **pay**-cho.

Let me feel your pulse.
Déjeme tomarle el pulso.
Day-ha-me to-**bar**-lay el **pool**-so.

I am going to take your temperature.
Voy a tomarle la temperatura.
Voye a to-**mar**-lay lah tem-pay-rah-**too**-rah.

Lie down, please.
Acuéstese, por favor.
Ah-coo-**es**-tah-say por fah-**vor.**

Do you understand?
¿Me comprende usted?
¿May com-**pren**-day oos-**ted?**

That's right.
Así. Bien.
Ah-**see. Be**-en.

You are doing very well.
Usted va muy bien.
Oos-**ted** vah **moo**-e **be**-en.

Do not take any medicine from home.
No tome usted ninguna medicina traída de su casa.
No **to**-may oos-**ted** nin-**goon**-ay may-de-**thee**-nah trah-**ee**-dah day soo **cah**-sah.

I am going to give you an injection.
Voy a ponerle ana inyección.
Voye a po-**nerr**-lay **oo**-nah in-yec-the-**on.**

Take a sip of water.
Tome usted un traguito de agua.
To-may oos-**ted** un trah-**gee**-to day **ah**-goo-ah.

Very good. That was fine.
Muy bien. Excelente.
Moo-e **be**-en. Ex-thay-**len**-tay.

Don't be nervous.
No se ponga nervioso(a).
No say **pon**-gah ner-ve-**o**-so(ah).

Do you feel dizzy?
¿Se siente vertigo?
¿Say see-**ayn**-tah **verr**-to-go?

Please lie still.
Quédese inmóvil, por favor.
Kay-day-say in-**mo**-veel por fah-**vor.**

You must drink lots of liquids.
Usted debe tomar muchos líquidos.
Oos-**ted day**-bay to-**mar moo**-chos **lee**-ke-dos.

References

Kelz, R. K. (1982.) *Conversational Spanish for Medical Personnel.* Clifton Park, NY: Delmar Cengage Learning.

Velazquez de la Cadena, M., Gray, E., & Iribas, J. (1985). *New Revised Velazquez Spanish and English Dictionary*. Clinton, NJ: New Win Publishing, Inc.

GLOSSARY

A

abduction Lateral movement away from the body
ability Competence in an activity
abortion Termination of pregnancy before the age of fetal viability, usually 24 weeks
abruptio placenta Premature separation, from the wall of the uterus, of normally implanted placenta
absorption Passage of a drug from the site of administration into the bloodstream; process whereby the end products of digestion pass through the epithelial membranes in the small and large intestines and into the blood or lymph system
abuse Incident involving some type of violation to the client; misuse, excessive, or improper use of a substance, the absence of which does not cause withdrawal symptoms
acanthosis nigricans A velvety hyperpigmented patch on the back of neck, in axilla, or anticubital area found in children with type 2 diabetes
accreditation Process by which a voluntary, nongovernmental agency or organization appraises and grants accredited status to institutions, programs, services, or any combination of these that meet predetermined structure, process, and outcome criteria
acculturation Process of learning beliefs, norms, and behavioral expectations of a group
acid Any substance that in a solution yields hydrogen ions bearing a positive charge
acidosis Condition characterized by an excessive number of hydrogen ions in a solution
acme Peak of a contraction
acquired immunity Formation of antibodies (memory B cells) to protect against future invasions of an already experienced antigen
acquired immunodeficiency syndrome (AIDS) Progressively fatal disease that destroys the immune system and the body's ability to fight infection; caused by the human immunodeficiency virus (HIV)
acrocyanosis Blue coloring of hands and feet
actively suicidal Descriptor of an individual intent upon hurting or killing him- or herself and who is in imminent danger of doing so
activities of daily living Basic care activities that include mobility, bathing, hygiene, grooming, dressing, eating, and toileting
acupressure Technique of releasing blocked energy within an individual when specific points (tsubas) along the meridians are pressed or massaged by the practitioner's fingers, thumbs, and heel of the hands
acupuncture Technique of application of needles and heat to various points on the body to alter the energy flow
acute pain Has a sudden onset, relatively short duration, mild to severe intensity, with a steady decrease in intensity over several days or weeks
adaptation Ongoing process whereby individuals use various responses to adjust to stressors and change; change resulting from assimilation and accommodation
adaptive energy Inner forces that an individual uses to adapt to stress (phrase coined by Selye)
adaptive measure Measure for coping with stress that requires a minimal amount of energy
addiction Overwhelming preoccupation with obtaining and using a drug for its psychic effects; used interchangeably with dependence
adhesion Internal scar tissue from previous surgeries or disease processes

adjuvant medication Drug used to enhance the analgesic efficacy of opioids, treat concurrent symptoms that exacerbate pain, and provide independent analgesia for specific types of pain
adult day care Centers that provide a variety of services in a protective setting for adults who are unable to stay alone but who do not need 24-hour care; the centers are located in a separate unit of a long-term care facility, in a private home, or are freestanding
adventitious breath sound Abnormal sound, including sibilant wheezes (formerly wheezes), sonorous wheezes (formerly rhonchi), fine and course crackles (formerly rales), pleural friction rubs, and stridor
affect Outward expression of mood or emotions
affective domain Area of learning that involves attitudes, beliefs, and emotions
afferent nerve pathway Ascending spinal cord pathway that transmits sensory impulses to the brain
afferent pain pathway Ascending spinal cord
afterpains Discomfort caused by the contracting uterus after the infant's birth
age appropriate care Nursing care that takes into consideration the client's physical, mental, emotional, and spiritual developmental levels
age of viability Gestational age at which a fetus could live outside the uterus, generally considered to be 24 weeks
agent Entity capable of causing disease
agglutination Clumping together of red blood cells
agglutinin Specific kind of antibody whose interaction with antigens is manifested as agglutination
agglutinogen Any antigenic substance that causes agglutination by the production of agglutinin
agnosia Inability to recognize, either by sight or sound, familiar objects such as a hairbrush
agnostic Individual who believes that the existence of God cannot be proved or disproved
agranulocytosis Acute condition causing a severe reduction in the number of granulocytes (basophils, eosinophils, and neutrophils)
Airborne Precautions Measures taken in addition to Standard Precautions and for clients known to have or suspected of having illnesses spread by airborne droplet nuclei
airborne transmission Transfer of an agent to a susceptible host through droplet nuclei or dust particles suspended in the air
Aldrete Score Scoring system for objectively assessing the physical status of clients recovering from anesthesia; serves as a basis for dismissal from the postanesthesia care unit (PACU) and ambulatory surgery; also known as the postanesthetic recovery score
algor mortis Decrease in body temperature after death, resulting in lack of skin elasticity
alkalosis Condition characterized by an excessive loss of hydrogen ions from a solution
allergen Type of antigen commonly found in the environment
allogeneic From a donor of the same species
alopecia Partial or complete baldness or loss of hair
alternative therapy Therapy used instead of conventional or mainstream medical practices
ambulatory care A facility that provides clients diagnostic treatment, medical treatment, preventive care, and rehabilitative care on an outpatient basis
ambulatory surgery Surgical operation performed under general, regional, or local anesthesia, involving less than 24 hours of hospitalization
amenorrhea Absence of menstruation
amnesia Inability to remember things
amniocentesis Withdrawal of amniotic fluid to obtain a sample for specimen examination
amnion Inner fetal membrane originating in the blastocyst
amniotomy Artificial rupture of the membranes
amphiarthrosis Articulation of slightly movable joints such as the vertebrae
amputation Removal of all or part of an extremity
anabolism Constructive process of metabolism whereby new molecules are synthesized and new tissues are formed, as in growth and repair
analgesia Pain relief without producing anesthesia
analgesic Substance that relieves pain
analyte Substance that is measured
anaphylaxis Type I systemic reaction to allergens
anasarca Generalized edema
anesthesia Absence of normal sensation
anesthesiologist Licensed physician educated and skilled in the delivery of anesthesia who also adds to the knowledge of anesthesia through research or other scholarly pursuits
anesthetist Qualified RN, dentist, or medical doctor who administers anesthetics
aneurysm Weakness in the wall of a blood vessel
anger control assistance Nursing intervention aimed at facilitating the expression of anger in an adaptive and nonviolent manner
angina pectoris Chest pain caused by a narrowing of the coronary arteries
angiocatheter Intracatheter with a metal stylet
angioedema Allergic reaction consisting of edema of subcutaneous tissue, mucous membranes, or viscera
angiogenesis Formation of new blood vessels
angiography Visualization of the vascular structures through the use of fluoroscopy with a contrast medium
angioma Benign vascular tumor involving skin and subcutaneous tissue; most are congenital
anion Ion bearing a negative charge

annulus Valvular ring in the heart
anorexia Loss of appetite
anosognosia Lack of awareness of own neurological deficits
anthrax An acute, infectious disease caused by the bacterium Bacillus anthracis, which has an incubation period of 2-60 days; it is an Important potential agent for bioterrorism
anthropometric measurements Measurements of the size, weight, and proportions of the body
antibody Immunoglobulin produced by the body in response to bacteria, viruses, or other antigenic substances; destroys antigens
anticipatory grief Occurrence of grief before an expected loss actually occurs
anticipatory guidance Information, teaching, and guidance given to a client in anticipation of an expected event
antigen Any substance identified by the body as nonself
antineoplastic Agent that inhibits the growth and reproduction of malignant cells
antioxidant Substance that prevents or inhibits oxidation, a chemical process wherein a substance is joined to oxygen
antipyretic Drug used to reduce an abnormally high temperature
anxiety Subjective response that occurs when a person experiences a real or perceived threat to well-being; a diverse feeling of dread or apprehension
anxiolytic Antianxiety medication
aphasia Absence of speech; often the result of a brain lesion
apheresis Removal of unwanted blood components
appendicitis Inflammation of the vermiform appendix
appropriate for gestational age Infant's weight falls between the 90th and 10th percentile for gestational age
areflexia Absence of reflexes
aromatherapy Therapeutic use of concentrated essences or essential oils extracted from plants and flowers
arousal State of wakefulness and alertness
arterial blood gases Measurement of levels of oxygen, carbon dioxide, pH, partial pressure of oxygen ($PO2$ or $PaO2$), partial pressure of carbon dioxide ($PCO2$ or $PaCO2$), saturation of oxygen ($SaO2$), and bicarbonate ($HCO3$) in arterial blood
arteriography Radiographic study of the vascular system following the injection of a radiopaque dye through a catheter
arteriosclerosis Cardiovascular disease wherein plaque forms on the inside of artery walls, reducing the space for blood flow
arthroplasty Replacement of both articular surfaces within a joint capsule
ascites Abnormal accumulation of fluid in the peritoneal cavity
asepsis Absence of pathogenic microorganisms
aseptic technique Collection of principles used to control and/or prevent the transfer of pathogenic microorganisms from sources within (endogenous) and outside (exogenous) the client
aspiration Procedure performed to withdraw fluid that has abnormally collected or to obtain a specimen; also inhalation of secretion or fluids into the pulmonary system
assent Voluntary agreement to participate in a research project or to accept treatment
assisted living A facility that combines housing and services for persons who require assistance with activities of daily living
asthma Condition characterized by intermittent airway obstruction due to antigen antibody reaction
astigmatism Asymmetric focus of light rays on the retina
ataxia Inability to coordinate voluntary muscle action
atelectasis Collapse of a lung or a portion of a lung
atheist Individual who does not believe in God or any other deity
atherosclerosis Cardiovascular disease of fatty deposits on the inner lining, the tunica intima, of vessel walls
atom Smallest unit of an element that still retains the properties of that element and that cannot be altered by any chemical change
atresia Absence or closure of a body orifice
attachment Long-term process that begins during pregnancy and intensifies during the postpartum period, which establishes an enduring bond between parent and child, and develops through reciprocal (parent-to-child and child-to-parent) behaviors
attitude Manner, feeling, or position toward a person or thing
attribute Characteristic that belongs to an individual
audible wheeze Wheeze that can be heard without the aid of a stethoscope
auditory hallucination Perception by an individual that someone is talking when no one in fact is there
auditory learner Person who learns by processing information through hearing
augmentation of labor Stimulation of uterine contractions after spontaneously beginning but having unsatisfactory progress of labor
aura Peculiar sensation preceding a seizure or migraine; may be a taste, smell, sight, sound, dizziness, or just a "funny feeling"

auscultation Physical examination technique that involves listening to sounds in the body that are created by movement of air or fluid
autoimmune disorder Disease wherein the body identifies its own cells as foreign and activates mechanisms to destroy them
autologous From the same organism (person)
automatism Mechanical, repetitive motor behavior performed unconsciously
autonomic nervous system That part of the peripheral nervous system consisting of the sympathetic and parasympathetic nervous systems and controlling unconscious activities
autonomy Self-direction; ethical principle based on the individual's right to choose and the individual's ability to act on that choice
autopsy Examination of a body after death by a pathologist to determine cause of death
autosomal Pertaining to a condition transmitted by a nonsex chromosome
awareness Capacity to perceive sensory impressions through thoughts and actions
azotemia Nitrogenous wastes present in the blood

B

bacteremia Condition of bacteria in the blood
bactericide Bacteria-killing chemicals; found in tears
ballottement Rebounding of the floating fetus when pushed upward through the vagina or abdomen
bands Immature neutrophils
barium Chalky-white contrast medium
Barrier Precautions Use of personal protective equipment, such as masks, gowns, and gloves, to create a barrier between the person and the microorganisms and thus prevent transmission of the microorganism
basal metabolism Energy needed to maintain essential physiologic functions when a person is at complete rest; the lowest level of energy expenditure
base Substance that when dissociated produces ions that will combine with hydrogen ions
baseline level Lab value that serves as a reference point for future value levels
behavioral tolerance Compensatory adjustments of behavior made under the influence of a particular substance
benign Not progressive; favorable for recovery
bereavement Period of grief that follows the death of a loved one
bioavailability Readiness to produce a drug effect
biofeedback Measures physiologic responses that assist individuals to improve their health by using signals from their own bodies
biologic response modifier Agent that destroys malignant cells by stimulating the body's immune system
biological agent Living organism that invades a host, causing disease
biological clock Internal mechanism in a living organism capable of measuring time
biopsy Excision of a small amount of tissue
bioterrorism the purposeful use of a biological preparation for the purposes of harming, killing large numbers of people, and/or instilling fear in large numbers of people
blanching White color of the skin when pressure is applied
blastic phase Intensified phase of leukemia that resembles an acute phase in which there is an increased production of white blood cells
blastocyst Cluster of cells that will develop into the embryo
bloody show Expulsion of cervical secretions, blood-tinged mucus, and the mucus plug that blocked the cervix during pregnancy
body image Individual's perception of physical self, including appearance, function, and ability
body mass index Measurement used to ascertain whether a person's weight is appropriate for height; calculated by dividing the weight in kilograms by the height in meters squared
body mechanics Use of the body to safely and efficiently move or lift objects
bodymind Inseparable connection and operation of thoughts, feelings, and physiologic functions
bonding Rapid process of attachment, parent to infant, that takes place during the sensitive period, the first 30 to 60 minutes after birth
borborygmi High-pitched, loud, rushing sounds produced by the movement of gas in the liquid contents of the intestine
bradycardia Heart rate less than 60 beats per minute in an adult
bradykinesia Slowness of voluntary movement and speech
bradypnea Respiratory rate of 10 or fewer breaths per minute
Braxton-Hicks contractions Irregular, intermittent contractions felt by the pregnant woman toward the end of pregnancy
breakthrough pain Sudden, acute, temporary pain that is usually precipitated by a treatment, a procedure, or unusual activity of the client
brief dynamic therapy Short-term psychotherapy that focuses on resolving core conflicts deriving from personality and living situations

bronchial sound Loud, high-pitched, hollow-sounding breath sound normally heard over the sternum; longer on expiration than inspiration
bronchiectasis Lung disorder characterized by chronic dilation of the bronchi
bronchitis Inflammation of the bronchial tree accompanied by hypersecretion of mucus
bronchovesicular sound Breath sound normally heard in the area of the scapula and near the sternum; medium in pitched blowing sound, with inspiratory and expiratory phases of equal length
bruxism Grinding of teeth during sleep
buffer Substance that attempts to maintain pH range, or hydrogen ion concentration, in the presence of added acids or bases
burnout State of physical and emotional exhaustion occurring when caregivers use up their adaptive energy
butterfly needle Wing-tipped needle

C

cachectic Being in a state of malnutrition and wasting
cachexia State of malnutrition and protein wasting
calculus Concentration of mineral salts in the body leading to the formation of stone
calorie Amount of heat required to raise the temperature of 1 gram of water 1 degree Celsius
cancer Disease resulting from the uncontrolled growth of cells, which causes malignant cellular tumors
capitated rate Preset fee based on membership rather than services provided; payment system used in managed care
caput succedaneum Edema of the newborn's scalp which is present at birth, may cross suture lines, and is caused by head compression against the cervix
carcinogen Substance that initiates or promotes the development of cancer
carcinoma Cancer occurring in epithelial tissue
cardiac cycle Cycle of an impulse going completely through the conduction system of the heart, and the ventricles contracting
cardiac output Volume of blood pumped per minute by the left ventricle
cardiac tamponade Collection of fluid in the pericardial sac hindering the functioning of the heart
carrier Person who harbors an infectious agent but has no symptoms of disease
caseation Process whereby the center of the primary tubercle formed in the lungs as a result of tuberculosis becomes soft and cheese-like due to decreased perfusion
catabolism Destructive process of metabolism whereby tissues or substances are broken into their component parts
cataplexy Sudden loss of muscle control
catharsis Process of talking out one's feelings; "getting things off the chest" through verbalization
cation Ion bearing a positive charge
cavitation Process whereby a cavity is created in the lung tissue through the liquefaction and rupture of a primary tubercle
ceiling effect Medication dosage beyond which no further analgesia occurs
cellular immunity Type of acquired immunity involving T-cell lymphocytes
Centers for Disease Control & Prevention (CDC) An agency of the federal government that provides for the investigation, identification, prevention, and control of diseases; it plays an important role in preparing for, and disseminating information about, possible terrorist attacks
central line Venous catheter inserted into the superior vena cava through the subclavian or internal or external jugular vein
central nervous system System of the brain and spinal cord
cephalalgia Headache; also known as cephalgia
cephalhematoma Collection of blood between the periosteum and the skull of a newborn; appears several hours to a day after birth, does not cross suture lines, and is caused by the rupturing of the periosteal bridging veins due to friction and pressure during labor and delivery
cephalopelvic disproportion Condition in which the fetal head will not fit through the mother's pelvis
certification Voluntary process that establishes and evaluates standards of care; mandatory for any health care services receiving federal funds
cerumen Earwax
cervical dilatation Enlargement of the cervical opening (os) from 0 to 10 cm (complete dilatation)
cesarean birth Birth of an infant through an incision in the abdomen and uterus
Chadwick's sign Purplish-blue color of the cervix and vagina noted about the eighth week of pregnancy
chain of custody Documentation of the transfer of evidence (of a crime) from one worker to the next in a secure fashion
chain of infection Describes the development of an infectious process
chalazion Cyst of the meibomian glands
chancre Clean, painless, syphilitic primary ulcer appearing 2 to 6 weeks after infection at the site of body contact
change Dynamic process whereby an individual's response to a stressor leads to an alteration in behavior
change agent Person who intentionally creates and implements change

chemical agent Substance that interacts with a host, causing disease
chemical name Precise description of the drug's chemical formula
chemical restraint Medication used to control client behavior
chemical warfare agents Poisonous chemicals and gases that are used to harm or kill a large number of persons; examples of chemical agents include nerve agents, blood agents, choking or vomiting agents, and blister or vesicant agents
Chemical, Biological, Radiological/Nuclear, and Explosive Enhanced Response Force Package A program of the National Guard that responds rapidly, following a call by the governor, and can be at the scene of a disaster, ready to function in 6 hours; it can also include a surgical suite, if needed
chemoreceptor Receptor that monitors the levels of carbon dioxide, oxygen, and pH in the blood
chemotherapy Use of drugs to treat illness, especially cancer
Cheyne-Stokes respirations Breathing characterized by periods of apnea alternating with periods of dyspnea
child abuse Any intentional act of physical, emotional, or sexual abuse or neglect committed by a person responsible for the care of a child
child life specialist Health care professional with extensive knowledge of psychology and early childhood development
chloasma Darkening of the skin of the forehead and around the eyes during pregnancy; also called the "mask of pregnancy"
cholecystitis Inflammation of the gallbladder
cholelithiasis Presence of gallstones or calculi in the gallbladder
cholesterol Sterol produced by the body and used in the synthesis of steroid hormones
chorea Condition characterized by abnormal, involuntary, purposeless movements of all musculature of the body
chorion Outer fetal membrane formed from the trophoblast
chronic acute pain Discomfort that occurs almost daily over a long period, months or years, and may never stop; also known as progressive pain
chronic nonmalignant pain Discomfort that occurs almost daily, has been present for at least 6 months, and ranges from mild to severe in intensity; also known as chronic benign pain
chronic pain Discomfort usually defined as long term (lasting 6 months or longer), persistent, nearly constant, or recurrent pain producing significant negative changes in a person's life
chronobiology Science of studying biorhythms
Chvostek's sign Abnormal spasm of the facial muscles in response to a light tapping of the facial nerve
chyme Acidic, semi-fluid paste found in the gastrointestinal tract
circadian rhythm Biorhythm that cycles on a daily basis
circulating nurse RN responsible and accountable for management of personnel, equipment, supplies, the environment, and communication throughout a surgical procedure
circumcision Surgical removal of the prepuce (foreskin), which covers the glans penis
circumoral cyanosis Bluish discoloration surrounding the mouth
cirrhosis Chronic degenerative changes in the liver cells and thickening of surrounding tissue
claiming process Process whereby a family identifies the infant's "likeness to" and the "differences from" family members, and the infant's unique qualities
clean object Object on which there are microorganisms that are usually not pathogenic
cleansing Removal of soil or organic material from instruments and equipment used in providing client care
client behavior accident Mishap resulting from the client's behavior or actions
clinical Observing and caring for living clients
closed reduction Repair of a fracture done without surgical intervention
coarse crackle Moist, low-pitched crackling and gurgling lung sound of long duration
codependent Description for persons who live based on what others think of them
cognition Intellectual ability to think
cognitive behavior therapy Treatment approach aimed at helping a client identify stimuli that cause the client's anxiety, develop plans to respond to those stimuli in a nonanxious manner, and problem-solve when unanticipated anxiety-provoking situations arise
cognitive domain Area of learning that involves intellectual understanding
cognitive reframing Stress-management technique whereby the individual changes a negative perception of a situation or event to a more positive, less threatening perception
coitus (copulation) Sexual act that delivers sperm to the cervix by ejaculation of the erect penis
cold stress Excessive heat loss
colic Condition of acute abdominal pain
colonization Multiplication of microorganisms on or within a host that does not result in cellular injury
colostomy Opening created anywhere along the large intestine

colostrum Antibody-rich yellow fluid secreted by the breasts during the last trimester of pregnancy and the first 2–3 days after birth; gradually changes to milk
comedone Whitehead or blackhead
command hallucination Perception by an individual of a voice or voices telling the individual to do something, usually to himself and/or someone else
communicable agent Infectious agent transmitted to a client by direct or indirect contact, via vehicle, vector, or airborne route
communicable disease Disease caused by a communicable agent
comorbidity Simultaneous existence of more than one disease process within an individual
complementary therapy Therapy used in conjunction with conventional medical therapies
complete protein Protein containing all nine essential amino acids
complicated grief Grief associated with traumatic death such as death by accident, violence, or homicide; survivors often have more intense emotions than those associated with normal grief
compound Combination of atoms of two or more elements
compromised host Person whose normal body defenses are impaired and is therefore susceptible to infection
computed tomography Radiological scanning of the body with x-ray beams and radiation detectors to transmit data to a computer that transcribes the data into quantitative measurement and multidimensional images of the internal structures
conditioning Teaching a person a behavior until it becomes an automatic response; method of conserving adaptive energy
conduction Loss of heat by direct contact with a cooler object
conductive hearing loss Condition characterized by the inability of sound waves to reach the inner ear
confabulation The making up of information to fill in memory gaps
congruence Agreement between two things
conjunctivitis Inflammation of the conjunctiva
consciousness State of awareness of self, others, and surrounding environment
constipation Condition characterized by hard, infrequent stools that are difficult or painful to pass
Contact Precautions Measures taken in addition to Standard Precautions for clients known to have or suspected of having illnesses easily spread by direct client contact or by contact with fomites
contact transmission Transfer of an agent from an infected person to a host by direct contact with that person, indirect contact with an infected person through a fomite, or close contact with contaminated secretions
contraception Measure taken to prevent pregnancy
contracture Permanent shortening of a muscle
contrast medium Radiopaque substance that facilitates roentgen (x-ray) imaging of the body's internal structures
convalescent stage Time period in which acute symptoms of an infection begin to disappear until the client returns to the previous state of health
convection Loss of heat by the movement of air
copulation Sexual act that delivers sperm to the cervix by ejaculation of the erect penis
cotyledon Subdivision of the maternal side of the placenta
couvade Development of physical symptoms by the expectant father such as fatigue, depression, headache, backache, and nausea
crackle Abnormal breath sound that resembles a popping sound, heard on inhalation and exhalation; not cleared by coughing
crenation Condition wherein cells decrease in size, shrivel and wrinkle, and are no longer functional when in a hypertonic solution
crepitus Grating or crackling sensation or sound
cretinism Congenital lack of thyroid hormones causing defective physical development and mental retardation
crisis Acute state of disorganization that occurs when usual coping mechanisms are no longer adequate; stressor that forces an individual to respond and/or adapt in some way
crisis intervention Specific technique used to help a person regain equilibrium
critical thinking The disciplined intellectual process of applying skillful reasoning, imposing intellectual standards and self-reflective thinking as a guide to a belief or action
cross-tolerance Decreased sensitivity to other substances in the same category
crowning When the largest diameter of the fetal head is past the vulva
cryotherapy Use of cold applications to reduce swelling
cryptorchidism Failure of one or both testes to descend
cultural assimilation Process whereby members of a minority group are absorbed by the dominant culture, taking on characteristics of the dominant culture
cultural diversity Differences among people resulting from ethnic, racial, and cultural variations
culture Integrated, dynamic structure of knowledge, attitudes, behaviors, beliefs, ideas, habits, customs, languages, values, symbols, rituals, and ceremonies that

are unique to a particular group of people; growing of microorganisms to identify a pathogen
curative To heal or restore health
curing Ridding one of disease
cutaneous pain Discomfort caused by stimulating the cutaneous nerve endings in the skin
cyanosis Bluish discoloration of the skin and mucous membranes observed in lips, nail beds, and earlobes
cycling Alteration in mood between depression and mania
cystitis Inflammation of the urinary bladder
cystocele Downward displacement of the bladder into the anterior vaginal wall
cytology Study of cells

D

dawn phenomenon Early morning glucose elevation produced by the release of growth hormone
death rattle Noisy respirations in the period preceding death caused by a collection of secretions in the larynx
debride To remove dead or damaged tissue or foreign material from a wound
decerebration Severing of the spinal cord
decidua The endometrium after implantation
decomposition Chemical reaction wherein the bonding between atoms in a molecule is broken and simpler products are formed
decrement Decreasing intensity of a contraction
defense mechanism Unconscious functions protecting the mind from anxiety
deglutition Swallowing of food
dehiscence Complication of wound healing wherein the wound edges separate
dehydration Condition wherein more water is lost from the body than is being replaced
delirium Cognitive changes or acute confusion of rapid onset (less than 6 months)
delusion False belief that misrepresents reality
dementia Organic brain pathology characterized by losses in intellectual functioning and a slow onset (longer than 6 months)
dental caries Cavities
dependence Reliance on a substance to such a degree that abstinence causes functional impairment, physical withdrawal symptoms, and/or psychological craving for the substance; see also addiction
depersonalization Treating an individual as an object rather than as a person
depolarization Contraction of the heart
depression State wherein an individual experiences feelings of extreme sadness, hopelessness, and helplessness
detoxification Elimination of a substance from the body
development Behavioral changes in skills and functional abilities
dialysate Solution used in dialysis, designed to approximate the normal electrolyte structure of plasma and extracellular fluid
dialysis Mechanical means of removing nitrogenous waste from the blood by imitating the function of the nephrons; involves filtration and diffusion of wastes, drugs, and excess electrolytes and/or osmosis of water across a semipermeable membrane into a dialysate solution
diarthrosis Freely movable joint
didactic Systematic presentation of information
diet therapy Treating disease or disorder with special diet
dietary prescription/order Order written by the physician for food, including liquids
differentiation Acquisition of characteristics or functions different from those of the original
diffusion Process whereby a substance moves from an area of higher concentration to an area of lower concentration
digestion Mechanical and chemical processes that convert nutrients into a physically absorbable state
diplopia Double vision
dirty object Object on which there is a high number of microorganisms, some that are potentially pathogenic
disability An individual's lack of ability to complete an activity in the normal manner
disaster A situation or event of greater magnitude than an emergency and that has unforeseen, serious, or immediate threats to public health
disciplined Trained by instruction and exercise
disenfranchised grief Grief not openly acknowledged, socially sanctioned, or publicly shared
disinfectant Chemical solution used to clean inanimate objects
disinfection Elimination of pathogens, with the exception of spores, from inanimate objects
dislocation Injury in which the articular surfaces of a joint are no longer in contact
disorientation State of mental confusion in which awareness of time, place, self, and/or situation is impaired
disseminated intravascular coagulation Abnormal stimulation of the clotting mechanism causing small clots throughout the vascular system and widespread bleeding internally, externally, or both
distraction Technique of focusing attention on stimuli other than pain
distress Subjective experience that occurs when stressors evoke an ineffective response
distribution Movement of drugs from the blood into various tissues and body fluids
diverticula Sac-like protrusion of the intestinal wall that results when the mucosa herniates through the bowel wall

diverticulitis Inflammation of one or more diverticula

diverticulosis Condition in which multiple diverticula are present in the colon

domestic violence Aggression and violence involving family members

dominant culture The group whose values prevail within a given society

Down syndrome Congenital chromosomal abnormality; also called trisomy 21

Droplet Precautions Measures taken in addition to Standard Precautions for clients known to have or suspected of having serious illnesses spread by large particle droplets

drug allergy Hypersensitivity to a drug

drug incompatibility Undesired chemical or physical reaction between a drug and a solution, between a drug and the container or tubing, or between two drugs

drug interaction Effect one drug can have on another drug

drug tolerance Reaction that occurs when the body is accustomed to a specific drug that larger doses are needed to produce the desired therapeutic effects

ductus arteriosus Fetal vessel connecting the pulmonay artery to the aorta

ductus venosus Branch of the umbilical vein that enters the inferior vena cava

duration Length of one contraction, from the beginning of the increment to the conclusion of the decrement

dysarthria Difficult and defective speech due to a dysfunction of the muscles used for speech

dysfunctional grief Persistent pattern of intense grief that does not result in reconciliation of feelings

dysfunctional labor Labor with problems of the contractions or of maternal bearing down

dysmenorrhea Painful menstruation

dyspareunia Painful intercourse

dysphagia Difficulty in swallowing

dysplasia Abnormal development

dyspnea Difficulty breathing as observed by labored or forced respirations through the use of accessory muscles in the chest and neck

dysrhythmia Irregularity in the rate, rhythm, or conduction of the electrical system of the heart

dystocia Long, difficult, or abnormal labor caused by any of the four major variables (4 Ps) that affect labor

dysuria Difficult or painful urination

E

early deceleration Reduction in fetal heart rate that begins early in the contraction and virtually mirrors the uterine contraction

ecchymosis Large, irregular hemorrhagic area on the skin; also called a bruise

eclampsia Convulsion occurring in pregnancy-induced hypertension

ectopic pregnancy Pregnancy in which the fertilized ovum is implanted outside the uterine cavity

edema Detectable accumulation of increased interstitial fluid

effacement Thinning of the cervix

efferent nerve pain pathway Descending spinal cord pathway that transmits sensory impulses from the brain

effluent Liquid output from an ileostomy

electrocardiogram Graphic recording of the heart's electrical activity

electroconvulsive therapy Procedure whereby clients are treated with pulses of electrical energy sufficient to cause brief convulsions or seizures

electroencephalogram Graphic recording of the brain's electrical activity

electrolyte Compound that, when dissolved in water or another solvent, dissociates (separates) into ions (electrically charged particles)

element Basic substance of matter

emancipated minor Child who has the legal competency of an adult because of cicumstances involving marriage, divorce, parenting of a child, living independently without parents, or enlistment in the armed services

embolus Mass, such as a blood clot or an air bubble, that circulates in the bloodstream

embryonic phase Development occuring during the first 2 to 8 weeks after fertilization of a human egg

emergency Medical or surgical condition requiring immediate or timely intervention to prevent permanent disability or death

emergency medical technician (EMT) Health care professional trained to provide basic lifesaving measures prior to arrival at the hospital

emergency nursing Care of clients who require emergency interventions

emotional lability Loss of emotional control

empathy Capacity to understand another person's feelings or perception of a situation

emphysema Lung disease wherein air accumulates in the tissues of the lungs

empowerment A process through which an individual is enabled to change situations, and uses resources, skills, and opportunities to do so

empty calories Calories that provide few nutrients

encephalitis Inflammation of the brain

encoding Laying down tracks in areas of the brain to enhance the ability to recall and use information

encopresis Passage of watery colonic contents around a hard fecal mass

endemic Occurring continuously in a particular population and having low mortality
endocrine Group of cells secreting substances directly into the blood or lymph circulation and affecting another part of the body
endometriosis Growth of endometrial tissue on structures outside of the uterus, within the pelvic cavity
endorphins Group of opiate-like substances produced naturally by the brain that raise the pain threshold, produce sedation and euphoria, and promote a sense of well-being
endoscopy Visualization of a body organ or cavity through a scope
energetic-touch therapy Technique of using the hands to direct or redirect the flow of the body's energy fields and enhance balance within those fields
engagement Condition of the widest diameter of the fetal presenting part (head) entering the inlet to the true pelvis
engorgement Distentions and swelling of the breasts in the first few days following delivery
engrossment Parents' intense interest in and preoccupation with the newborn
enriched Descriptor for food in which nutrients that were removed during processing are added back in
enteral instillation Administration of drugs through a gastrointestinal tube
enteral nutrition Feeding method meaning both the ingestion of food orally and the delivery of nutrients through a gastrointestinal tube, but generally meaning the latter
entrainment Infant's ability to move in rhythm to the parent's voice
enzyme Globular protein produced in the body that catalyzes chemical reactions within the cells
enzyme-linked immunosorbent assay Basic screening test currently used to detect antibodies to HIV
epidemic Infecting many people at the same time and in the same geographic area
epidural analgesia Analgesics administered via a catheter that terminates in the epidural space
episiotomy Incision in the perineum to facilitate passage of the baby
epispadias Placement of the urinary meatus on the top of the penis
epistaxis Hemorrhage of the nares or nostrils; also known as nosebleed
Epstein's pearls Small, whitish-yellow epithelial cysts found on the hard palate
equipment accident Accident resulting from the malfunction or improper use of medical equipment
erythema Redness of the skin due to increased blood flow to the area
erythema toxicum neonatorum Pink rash with firm, yellow-white papules or pustules found on the chest, abdomen, back, and/or buttocks of a newborn
erythematous Characterized by redness of the skin
erythrocytapheresis Procedure that removes abnormal red blood cells and replaces them with healthy ones
erythropoiesis Production of red blood cells and their release by the red bone marrow
eschar Dry, dark, leathery scab composed of denatured protein
ethnicity Cultural group's perception of itself or a group identity
ethnocentrism Assumption of cultural superiority and inability to accept another culture's ways
euglycemia Normal blood glucose level
euphoric Characterized by elation out of context to the situation
eupnea Easy respirations with a rate that is age-appropriate
eustress Stress that results in positive outcomes
evaporation Loss of heat when water is changed to a vapor
evisceration Complication of wound healing characterized by a complete separation of wound edges, accompanied by visceral protrusion
exacerbation Increase in the symptoms of a disease
exclusive provider organization Organization wherein care must be delivered by providers in the plan in order for clients to receive any reimbursement
excretion Elimination of drugs or waste products from the body
Expeditionary Medical Support A total package that includes everything necessary to screen, treat, and release clients to other facilities for longer-term care
exposure Contact with an infected person or agent
extended care facility The term refers to any facility that provides care for a long period of time. It has no concrete definition and could refer to either an intermediate or skilled nursing facility
external respiration Exchange of gases between the atmosphere and the lungs
external version Manipulation of the fetus through the mother's abdomen to a presentation facilitating birth
extracellular fluid Fluid outside of the cells; includes interstitial, intravascular, synovial, cerebrospinal, and serous fluids; aqueous and vitreous humor; and endolymph and perilymph
extravasation Escape of fluid into the surrounding tissue

F

faith Confident belief in the truth, value, or trustworthiness of a person, idea, or thing
false labor Contractions that do not cause the cervix to dilate

family-centered care A philosophy of caring recognizing the centrality of the family in the child's life and including the family's contribution and involvement in the plan of care and its delivery (Potts & Mandleco, 2000)

fasciculation Involuntary twitching of muscle fibers

fat-soluble vitamin Vitamin requiring the presence of fats for its absorption from the gastrointestinal tract into the lymphatic system and for cellular metabolism: vitamins A, D, E, and K

fee for service System in which the health care recipient directly pays the provider for services as they are provided

feedback Response from the receiver of a message so that the sender can verify the message

Ferguson's reflex Spontaneous, involuntary urge to bear down during labor

fertilization Union of an ovum and a sperm

fetal attitude Relationship of fetal body parts to one another, either flexion or extension

fetal biophysical profile Assessment of five variables: fetal breathing movement, fetal movements of body or limbs, fetal tone (flexion/extension of extremities), amniotic fluid volume, and reactive NST

fetal lie Relationship of the cephalocaudal axis of the fetus to the cephalocaudal axis of the mother, either longitudinal or transverse

fetal phase Intrauterine development from 8 weeks to birth

fetal position Relationship of the identified landmark on the presenting part to the four quadrants of the mother's pelvis

fetal presentation Determined by the fetal lie and the part of the fetus that enters the pelvis first

fibrinolysis Process of breaking fibrin apart

fight-or-flight response State wherein the body becomes physiologically ready to defend itself by either fighting or fleeing from the stressor

filtration Process of fluids and the substances dissolved in them being forced through the cell membrane by hydrostatic pressure

fine crackle Dry, high-pitched crackling and popping lung sounds of short duration

first assistant Physician or RN who assists the surgeon to retract tissue, aids in the removal of blood and fluids at the operative site, and assists with homeostasis and wound closure

first responders Persons who have been identified as the first ones to appear at the scene of a disaster or accident; designated first responders include health care workers, emergency medical personnel, police, and firepersons

flashback Rushing of blood back into intravenous tubing when a negative pressure is created on the tubing; reliving of an original trauma as if the individual were currently experiencing it

flora Microorganisms that occur or have adapted to live in a specific environment, such as intestinal, skin, vaginal, or oral flora

flow rate Volume of fluid to infuse over a set period of time

fluoroscopy Immediate, serial images of the body's structure or function

fomite Object contaminated with an infectious agent

fontanelle Membranous area where sutures meet on the fetal skull

foramen ovale Flap opening in the atrial septum that allows only right-to-left movement of blood

forceps Metal instruments used on the fetal head to provide traction or to provide a method of rotating the fetal head to an occiput-anterior position

foremilk Watery first milk from the breast, high in lactose, like skim milk, and effective in quenching thirst

formal teaching Teaching that takes place at a specific time, in a specific place, and on a specific topic

fortified Descriptor for food in which nutrients not naturally occurring in the food are added to it

fracture Break in the continuity of a bone

free radical Unstable molecule that alters genetic codes and triggers the development of cancer growth in cells

frequency Time for the beginning of one contraction to the beginning of the next contraction

friction Force of two surfaces moving against one another

fulguration Procedure to destroy tissue with long, high-frequency electric sparks

fundus Top of the uterus

funic souffle Sound of the blood pulsating through the umbilical cord; rate the same as the fetal heartbeat

G

gastric ulcer Erosion in the stomach

gastritis Inflammation of the stomach mucosa

gate control pain theory Theory that proposes that the cognitive, sensory, emotional, and physiologic components of the body can act together to block an individual's perception of pain

general adaptation syndrome Physiologic response that occurs when a person experiences a stressor

general anesthesia Method of producing unconsciousness; amnesia, motionlessness, muscle relaxation, and complete insensibility to pain

generic name Name assigned by the U.S. Adopted Names Council to the manufacturer who first develops a drug

genogram A way to visualize family members, their birth and death dates, or ages and specific health problems

genuineness Sincerity

germicide Chemical that can be applied to both animate and inanimate objects for the purpose of eliminating pathogens
germinal phase Development beginning with conception and lasting approximately 10 to 14 days
gerontological nursing Specialty within nursing that addresses and advocates for the special care needs of older adults
gerontologist Specialist in gerontology in advanced practice nursing, geriatric psychiatry, medicine, and social services
gerontology Study of the effects of normal aging and age-related diseases on human beings
gingivitis Inflammation of the gums
Glasgow Coma Scale Neurological screening test that measures a client's best verbal, motor, and eye response to stimuli
glucagon Hormone secreted by the alpha cells of the pancreas, which stimulate release of glucose by the liver
gluconeogenesis Conversion of amino acids into glucose
glycogenesis Conversion of glucose into glycogen
glycogenolysis Conversion of glycogen into glucose
glycosuria Presence of excessive glucose in the urine
goiter Enlargement of the thyroid gland
Goodell's sign Softening of the cervix noted about the 8th week of pregnancy
Gower's sign Walking the hands up the legs to get from sitting to standing position (as in Duchenne muscular dystrophy)
granulation tissue Delicate connective tissue consisting of fibroblasts, collagen, and capillaries
graphesthesia Ability to identify letters, numbers, or shapes drawn on the skin
gravida Pregnancy, regardless of duration, including present pregnancy
grief Series of intense psychological and physical responses occuring after a loss; these responses are necessary, normal, natural, and adaptive responses to the loss
growth Measurable changes in the physical size of the body and its parts
gynecomastia Abnormal enlargement of one or both breasts in males

H

half-life Time it takes the body to eliminate half of the blood concentration level of the original dose of medication
halitosis Bad breath
hallucination Sensory perception that occurs in the absence of external stimuli and that is not based on reality
hallux varus Placement of the great toe farther from the other toes
hand hygiene Rubbing together of all surfaces and crevices of the hands using a soap or chemical and water, followed by rinsing in a flowing stream of water
handicap The physical or mental inability to complete a role in one or more major ADL (U.S. Office of Personnel Management, 1987)
healing Process that activates the individual's recovery forces from within; to make whole
healing touch Energy therapy using the hands to clear, energize, and balance the energy field
health According to the World Health Organization, the state of complete physical, mental, and social well-being, not merely the absence of disease or infirmity
health care delivery system Method for providing services to meet the health needs of individuals
health care surrogate law Law enacted by some states that provides a legal means for decision making in the absence of advance directives
health continuum Range of an individual's health, from highest health potential to death
health history Review of the client's functional health patterns prior to the current contact with a health care agency
health maintenance organization Prepaid health plan that provides primary health care services for a preset fee and focuses on cost-effective treatment methods
hearing Act or power of receiving sounds
heart sound Sound heard by auscultating the heart
Heberden's nodes Enlargement and characteristic hypertrophic spurs in the terminal interphalangeal finger joints
Hegar's sign Softening of the uterine isthmus about the 6th week of pregnancy
HELLP syndrome Pregnancy-induced hypertension with liver damage characterized by hemolysis, elevated liver enzymes, and low platelet count
hemarthrosis Bleeding into the joints
hematemesis Vomiting of blood
hematocrit Percentage of red blood cells in a given volume of blood
hematopoiesis Process of blood cell production and development
hematuria Blood in the urine
hemiparesis Weakness of one side of the body
hemiplegia Paralysis of one side of the body
hemolysis Breakdown of red blood cells and the release of hemoglobin
hemopneumothorax Presence of blood and air within the pleural space
hemorrhagic exudate Discharge that has a large component of red blood cells
hemorrhoid Swollen vascular tissue in the rectal area
hemostasis Cessation of bleeding
hemothorax Condition wherein blood accumulates in the pleural space of the lungs

hepatitis Chronic or acute inflammation of the liver
hesitancy Difficulty initiating the urinary stream
hindmilk Follows foremilk, is higher in fat content, leads to weight gain, and is more satisfying
hirsutism Excessive body hair in a masculine distribution
histamine Substance released during allergic reactions
holistic Whole; includes physical, intellectual, sociocultural, psychological, and spiritual aspects as an integrated whole
Homans' sign Test to check for the presence of clots in the leg
homeostasis Balance or equilibrium among the physiologic, psychological, sociocultural, intellectual, and spiritual needs of the body; maintenance of internal environment
homonymous hemianopia Loss of vision in half of the visual field on the same side of both eyes
hope To look forward to with confidence or expectation; a resource clients can use to promote physical, psychological, and spiritual wellness
hormone Substance that initiates or regulates activity of another organ, system, or gland in another part of the body
hospice Humane, compassionate care provided to clients who can no longer benefit from curative treatment and have 6 months or less to live; allows individuals to die with dignity
host Organism that can be affected by an agent
human immunodeficiency virus (HIV) Retrovirus that causes AIDS
human leukocyte antigen Antigen present in human blood
humoral immunity Type of immunity dominated by antibodies
hydatidiform mole Abnormality of the placenta wherein the chorionic villi become fluid filled, grape-like clusters; the trophoblastic tissue proliferates; and there is no viable fetus
hydramnios (polyhydramnios) Excess amount of amniotic fluid
hydrocele Fluid around the testes in the scrotum
hydrostatic pressure Pressure that a fluid exerts against a membrane; also called filtration force
hygiene Study of health and ways of preserving health
hyperbilirubinemia Excess of bilirubin in the blood
hyperemesis gravidarum Excessive vomiting during pregnancy
hypergylcemia Condition wherein the blood glucose level becomes too high as a result of the absence of insulin
hyperopia Farsightedness
hypersensitivity Excessive reaction to a stimulus
hypersomnia Alteration in sleep pattern characterized by excessive sleep, especially in the daytime
hyperthermia Condition in which the core body temperature rises above 106°F
hypertonic solution Solution that has a higher molecular concentration than the cell; also called a hyperosmolar solution
hypertrophy Increase in muscle mass
hyperuricemia Increased uric acid blood level
hyperventilation Breathing characterized by deep, rapid respirations
hypervigilant Condition of constantly scanning the environment for potentially dangerous situations
hypervolemia Increased circulating fluid volume
hypnosis Altered state of consciousness or awareness resembling sleep and during which a person is more receptive to suggestion
hypoglycemia Condition wherein the blood glucose level is exceedingly low
hypomania Mild form of mania without significant impairment
hypospadias Placement of the urinary meatus on the underside of the penis
hypothermia Condition in which the core body temperature drops below 95°F
hypotonia Lax muscle tone
hypotonic solution Solution that has a lower molecular concentration than the cell; also called hypo-osmolar solution
hypoventilation Breathing characterized by shallow respirations
hypovolemia Abnormally low circulatory blood volume
hypoxemia Decreased oxygen level in the blood

I

iatrogenic Caused by treatment or diagnostic procedures
ideal self The person whom the individual would like to be
identity An individual's conscious description of who he or she is
idiopathic Occurring without a known cause
idiosyncratic reaction Very unpredictable response that may be an overresponse, an underresponse, or an atypical response
ileal conduit Implantation of the ureters into a piece of ileum, which is attached to the abdominal wall as a stoma so urine can be removed from the body
ileostomy Opening created in the small intestine at the ileum
illness stage Time period when the client is manifesting specific signs and symptoms of an infectious agent

illusion Inaccurate perception or misinterpretation of sensory stimuli
imagery Relaxation technique of using the imagination to visualize a pleasant, soothing image
immune response Body's reaction to substances identified as nonself
immunity Body's ability to protect itself from foreign agents or organisms
immunization Process of creating immunity or resistance to infection in an individual
immunotherapy Treatment to suppress or enhance immunologic functioning
implantable cardioverter-defibrillator (ICD) Implantable device that senses a dysrythmia and automatically sends an electrical shock directly to the heart to defibrillate it
implantable port Device made of a radiopaque silicone catheter and a plastic or stainless steel injection port with a self-sealing silicone-rubber septum
implantation Embedding of a fertilized egg into the uterine lining
impotence Inability of an adult male to have an erection firm enough or to maintain it long enough to complete sexual intercourse
incidence Frequency of disease occurrence
incompetent cervix Descriptor for when the cervix begins to dilate, usually during the second trimester
incomplete protein Protein with one or more of the essential amino acids missing
increment Increasing intensity of a contraction
incubation period Time between entry of an infectious agent in the host and the onset of symptoms
independent nursing intervention Nursing action initiated by the nurse and do not require direction or an order from another health care professional
induction of labor Stimulation of uterine contractions before contractions begin spontaneously for the purpose of birthing an infant
infancy Development from the end of the first month to the end of the first year of life
infection Invasion and multiplication of pathogenic microorganims in body tissue that results in cellular injury
infectious agent Microorganism that causes cellular injury
infertility Inability or diminished ability to produce offspring
infiltration Seepage of foreign substances into the interstitial tissue, causing swelling and discomfort at the IV site
inflammation Nonspecific cellular response to tissue injury
informal teaching Teaching that takes place anytime, anyplace, and whenever a learning need is identified
informed consent Legal form signed by a competent client and witnessed by another person that grants permission to the client's physician to perform the procedure described by the physician and that demonstrates the client's understanding of the benefits, risks, and possible complications of the procedure, as well as alternate treatment options
ingestion The taking of food into the digestive tract, generally through the mouth
initial planning Development of a preliminary plan of care by the nurse who performs the admission assessment and gathers the comprehensive admission assessment data
insensible water loss Water loss of which the person is not generally aware
insomnia Difficulty in falling asleep initially or in returning to sleep once awakened
inspection Physical examination technique that involves thorough visual observation
insulin Pancreatic hormone that aids in both the diffusion of glucose into the liver and muscle cells, and the synthesis of glycogen
intellectual wellness Ability to function as an independent person capable of making sound decisions
intensity Strength of the contraction at the acme
interdependent nursing intervention Nursing action that is implemented in a collaborative manner with other health care professionals
internal respiration Exchange of oxygen and carbon dioxide at the cellular level
interstitial fluid Fluid in tissue spaces around each cell
interval Resting period between two contractions
intoxication Reversible effect on the central nervous system soon after the use of a substance
intracath Plastic tube for insertion into a vein
intracellular fluid Fluid within the cells
intradermal Injection into the dermis
intramuscular Injection into the muscle
intraoperative phase Time during the surgical experience that begins when the client is transferred to the operating room table and ends when the client is admitted to the postanesthesia care unit
intrathecal analgesia Administration of analgesics into the subarachnoid space
intravascular fluid Fluid consisting of the plasma in the blood vessels and the lymph in the lymphatic system
intravenous Injection into a vein
intravenous therapy Administration of fluids, electrolytes, nutrients, or medications by the venous route
intravesical Within the urinary bladder
intussusception Telescoping of one part of the intestine into another

invasive Accessing the body tissues, organs, or cavities through some type of instrumentation procedure
involution Return of the reproductive organs, especially the uterus, to their pre-pregnancy size and condition
ion Atom bearing an electrical charge
ischemia Oxygen deprivation, usually due to poor perfusion
ischemic pain Discomfort resulting when the blood supply to an area is restricted or cut off completely
isolation Separation from other persons, especially those with infectious diseases
isotonic solution Solution that has the same molecular concentration as does the cell; also called an isosmolar solution
isotopes Atom of the same element that has a different atomic weight (i.e., different numbers of neutrons in the nucleus)
iv push (bolus) The administration of a large dose of medication in a relatively short time, usually 1–30 minutes

J

jaundice Yellow discoloration of the skin, sclera, mucous membranes, and body fluids that occurs when the liver is unable to fully remove bilirubin from the blood
Johnsonian intervention Confrontational approach to a client with a substance problem that lessens the chance of denial and encourages treatment before the client "hits bottom"
judgment Conclusion based on sound reasoning and supported by evidence

K

Kardex A brief worksheet with basic client care information
keloid Abnormal growth of scar tissue that is elevated, rounded, and firm with irregular, clawlike margins
keratin Tough, fibrous protein produced by cells in the epidermis called keratinocytes
keratitis Inflammation of the cornea
kernicterus Severe neurological damage resulting from a high level of bilirubin (jaundice)
Kernig's sign Diagnostic test for inflammation in the nerve roots; the inability to extend the leg when the thigh is flexed against the abdomen
ketone Acidic by-product of fat metabolism
ketonuria Presence of ketones in the urine
ketosis Condition wherein acids called ketones accumulate in the blood and urine, upsetting the acid–base balance
kilocalorie Equivalent to 1,000 calories
kinesthetic learner Person who learns by processing information through touching, feeling, and doing
kwashiorkor Condition resulting when there is a sudden or recent lack of protein-containing foods
kyphosis Increased roundness of the thoracic spinal curve

L

lanugo Fine hair covering the fetus's body
large for gestational age Infant's weight falls above the 90th percentile for gestational age
late deceleration Reduction in fetal heart rate that begins after the uterus has begun contracting and increases to the baseline level after the uterine contraction has ceased
learning Act or process of acquiring knowledge, skill, or both in a particular subject; process of assimilating knowledge resulting in behavior changes
learning disability Heterogenous group of disorders manifested by significant difficulties in the acquisition and use of listening, speaking, reading, writing, reasoning, or mathematical abilities
learning plateau Peak in the effectiveness of teaching and depth of learning
learning style Individual preference for receiving, processing, and assimilating information about a particular subject
lecithin Major component of surfactant
Leopold's maneuvers Series of specific palpations of the pregnant uterus to determine fetal position and presentation
let-down reflex Neurohormonal reflex that causes milk to be expressed from the alveoli into the lactiferous ducts
leukocytosis Increased number of white blood cells
leukopenia Decreased number of white blood cells
licensure Mandatory system of granting licenses according to specified standards
life review Form of reminiscence wherein a client attempts to come to terms with conflict or to gain meaning from life and die peacefully
ligation Application of a band or tie around a structure
lightening Descent of the fetus into the pelvis, causing the uterus to tip forward, relieving pressure on the diaphragm
linea nigra Dark line on the abdomen from umbilicus to symphysis during the pregnancy
lipid Organic compound that is insoluble in water but soluble in organic solvents such as ether and alcohol; also known as fats
lipodystrophy Atrophy or hypertrophy of subcutaneous fat
lipoma Benign tumor consisting of mature fat cells
lipoprotein Blood lipid bound to protein

liquefaction necrosis Death and subsequent change of tissue to a liquid or semi-liquid state; often descriptive of a primary tubercle

listening Interpreting the sounds heard and attaching meaning to them

litholapaxy Procedure involving crushing of a bladder stone and immediate washing out of the fragments through a catheter

lithotripsy Method of crushing a calculus anyplace in the urinary system with ultrasonic waves

liver mortis Bluish-purple discoloration of the skin that is a by-product of red blood cell destruction; it begins within 20 minutes of death

living will Legal document that allows a person to state preferences about the use of life-sustaining measures should he or she be unable to make his or her wishes known

local adaptation syndrome Physiologic response to a stressor (e.g., trauma, illness) affecting a specific part of the body

localized infection Infection limited to a defined area or single organ

lochia Uterine/vaginal discharge after childbirth; initially bright red, then changing to a pink or pinkish brown, then to a yellowish white

locomotor Pertaining to movement or the ability to move

long-term care facility Health care facility that provides services to individuals who are not acutely ill, have continuing health care needs, and cannot function independently at home

long-term care managed care Care that refers to a spectrum of services provided to individuals who have an ongoing need for health care; traditionally a community-based nursing home licensed for skilled or intermediate care

long-term goal Statement that profiles the desired resolution of the nursing diagnosis over a long period of time, usually weeks or months

lordosis Exaggeration of the curvature of the lumbar spine

loss Any situation, either potential, actual, or perceived, wherein a valued object or person is changed or is not accessible to the individual

lumbar puncture Aspiration of cerebrospinal fluid from the subarachnoid space

lung stretch receptor Receptor that monitors the patterns of breathing and prevents overexpansion of the lungs

lymphokine Chemical substance released by sensitized lymphocytes (T cells) and that assists in antigen destruction

lymphoma Tumor of the lymphatic system

M

macrosomia Excessive fetal growth characterized by a fetus weighing more than 4,000 g (8.8 lb.)

magnetic resonance imaging Imaging technique that uses radiowaves and a strong magnetic field to make continuous cross-sectional images of the body

maladaptive measure Measure used to avoid conflict or stress

malignant Becoming progessively worse and often resulting in death

malpractice Negligent acts on the part of a professional; relates to the conduct of a person who is acting in a professional capacity

managed care A cost-saving system where a case management, individual, or team control what specialists the client sees, as well as the frequency or duration of that specialty care

mania Extremely elevated mood with accompanying agitated behavior

marasmus Condition resulting from severe malnutrition; afflicts very young children who lack both energy and protein foods as well as vitamins and minerals

Maslow's hierarchy of needs Theory of behavioral motivation based on needs; includes physiologic, safety and security, love and belonging, self-esteem, and self-actualization needs

mastication Chewing food into fine particles and mixing the food with enzymes in saliva

mastitis Inflammation of the breast, generally during breastfeeding

material principle of justice Rationale for determining those times when there can be unequal allocation of scarce resources

matter Anything that occupies space and possesses mass

maturation Process of becoming fully grown and developed; involves physiologic and behavioral aspects

maturational loss Loss that occurs as a person moves from one developmental stage to another

mechanism of labor Series of movements of the fetus as it passes through the pelvis and birth canal

meconium Fecal material stored in the fetal intestines

meconium ileus Impacted feces in the newborn, causing intestinal obstruction

Medicaid Government title program (XIX) that pays for health services for people who are older, poor, or disabled, and for low-income families with dependent children

medical asepsis Practices that reduce the number, growth, and spread of microorganisms

medical diagnosis Clinical judgment by the physician that identifies or determines a specific disease, condition, or pathological state

medical model Traditional approach to health care wherein the focus is on treatment and cure of disease not prevention

Medicare Amendment (Title XVIII) to the Social Security Act that helps finance the health care of persons over 65 years old and younger persons who are permanently disabled to receive Social Security disability benefits

Medigap insurance Insurance plan for persons with Medicare that pays for health care costs not covered by Medicare

meditation An activity that brings the mind and spirit in focus on the present and provokes a sense of peace and relaxation

melanin Pigment that gives skin its color

melena Stool containing partially broken down blood usually black, sticky, and tar-like

menarche Onset of the first menstrual period

meningitis Inflammation of the meninges

meningocele Saclike protrusion along the vertebral column filled with cerebrospinal fluid and meninges

menopause Cessation of menstruation

menorrhagia Excessively heavy menstrual flow

mental disorder Clinically significant behavior or psychological syndrome or pattern that occurs in an individual and is associated with present distress or disability or with a significantly increased risk of suffering, death, pain, disability, or an important loss of freedom (APA, 1994)

mental illness Condition wherein an individual has a distorted view of self, is unable to maintain satisfying personal relationships, and is unable to adapt to the environment

mentation Ability to concentrate, remember, or think abstractly

metabolic rate Rate of energy utilization in the body

metabolism Sum total of all the biological and chemical processes in the body

metastasis Spread of cancer cells to distant areas of the body by way of the lymph system or bloodstream

metritis Inflammation of the uterus including the endometrium and parametrium

metrorrhagia Vaginal bleeding between menstrual periods

micturition Process of expelling urine from the urinary bladder; also called urination or voiding

middle adulthood Development from the ages of 40 years to 65 years

milia Pearly white cysts on the face

minimum data set An assessment tool for assessing a resident's physical, psychological, and psychosocial functioning in a Medicare and Medicaid-certified long-term care facility

minority group Group of people constituting less than a numerical majority of the population and are often labeled and treated differently from others in the society

miscarriage Spontaneous abortion

misdemeanor Offense that is less serious than a felony and may be punished by a fine or by sentence to a local prison for less than 1 year

misuse Use of a legal substance for which it was not intended, or exceeding the recommended dosage of a drug

mixed agonist-antagonist Compound that blocks opioid effects on one receptor type while producing opioid effects on a second receptor type

mixture Substances combined in no specific way

mnemonic Method to aid in association and recall; a memorable sentence created from the first letters of a list of items to be used to recall the items later

mode of transmission Process of the infectious agent moving from the reservoir or source through the portal of exit to the portal of entry of the susceptible "new" host

modulation Central nervous system pathway that selectively inhibits pain transmission by sending signals back down to the dorsal horn of the spinal cord

molding Shaping of the fetal head to adapt to the mother's pelvis during labor

molecule Atoms of the same element that unite with each other

Mongolian spots Large patches of bluish skin on the buttocks of dark-skinned infants

monounsaturated fatty acid Forms a glycerol ester with a double or triple bond; nuts, fowl, and olive oil

mood Subjective report of the way an individual is feeling

moral maturity Ability to decide for oneself what is "right"

morbidity Illness

mortality Death

morula Mass of cells resembling a mulberry

mourning Period during which grief is expressed and integration and resolution of the loss occur

multigravida Condition of being pregnant two or more times

multipara Condition of having delivered twice or more after 24 weeks' gestation

myelomeningocele Saclike protrusion along the vertebral column that is filled with spinal fluid, meninges, nerve roots, and spinal cord

myocardial infarction Necrosis (death) of the myocardium caused by an obstruction in a coronary artery; commonly known as heart attack

myocarditis Inflammation of the myocardium of the heart

myofascial pain syndrome Group of muscle disorders characterized by pain, muscle spasm, tenderness, stiffness, and limited motion
myopia Nearsightedness
myringotomy Surgical incision of the eardrum
myxedema Severe hypothyroidism in adults

N

narcolepsy Sleep alteration manifested as sudden uncontrollable urges to fall asleep during the daytime
narrative charting Chronological account written in paragraphs describes the client's status, the interventions and treatments, and the client's response to treatments
necrosis Tissue death as the result of disease or injury
neglect Situation wherein a basic need of the client is not being provided
negligence General term referring to careless acts on the part of an individual who is not exercising reasonable or prudent judgment
neonatal stage First 28 days of life following birth
neonatal transition First few hours after birth wherein the newborn makes changes to and stabilizes respiratory and circulatory functions
neonate Newborn from birth to 28 days of life
neoplasm Any abnormal growth of new tissue
nephrotoxic Quality of a substance that causes kidney tissue damage
nerve agents Powerful acetylcholinesterase inhibitors that alter cholinergic synaptic transmission at neuroeffector junctions, at skeletal myoneural junctions and autonomic ganglia, and in the central nervous system
nesting Surge of energy late in pregnancy when the pregnant woman organizes and cleans the house
neuralgia Paroxysmal pain that extends along the course of one or more nerves
neurogenic shock Hypotensive situation resulting from the loss of sympathetic control of vital functions from the brain
neuropeptide Amino acid produced in the brain and other sites in the body that acts as a chemical communicator
neurotransmitter Chemical substance produced by the body that facilitates or inhibits nerve-impulse transmission
neutral thermal environment Environment in which the newborn can maintain internal body temperature with minimal oxygen consumption and metabolism
nevi Pigmented areas in the skin; commonly known as birthmarks or moles
nevus flammeus Large, reddish-purple birthmark usually found on the face or neck and does not blanch with pressure
nevus vascularis Birthmark of enlarged superficial blood vessels, elevated and red in color
nociceptor Receptive neuron for painful sensations
nocturia Awakening at night to void
nocturnal enuresis Incontinence that occurs during sleep
noninvasive Descriptor for procedure wherein the body is not entered with any type of instrument
nonmaleficence Ethical principle based on the obligation to cause no harm to others
nonshivering thermogenesis Metabolism of brown fat; process unique to the newborn
nonverbal communication Body language or a method of sending a message without words
nosocomial infection Infection acquired in the hospital or other health care facility that was not present or incubating at the time of the client's admission
noxious stimulus Underlying pathology that causes pain
nuchal cord Condition of the umbilical cord being wrapped around the baby's neck
nuchal rigidity Pain and rigidity in the neck
nulligravida Condition of never having been pregnant
nullipara Condition of never having delivered an infant after 24 weeks' gestation
nursing The art and science of assisting individuals in learning to care for themselves whenever possible and of caring for them when they are unable to meet their own needs
nursing audit Method of evaluating the quality of care provided to clients
nursing care plan Written guide of strategies to be implemented to help the client achieve optimal health
nursing diagnosis Second step in the nursing process; a clinical judgment about individual, family, or community (aggregate) responses to actual or potential health problems/life processes
nursing intervention Action performed by a nurse that helps the client achieve the results specified by the goals and expected outcomes
nursing interventions classification Standardized language for nursing interventions
nursing minimum data set Elements that should be in clinical records and abstracted for studies on the effectiveness and costs of nursing care
nursing outcomes classification Standardized language for nursing outcomes
nursing practice act Statute that is enacted by the legislature of a state and that outlines the scope of nursing practice in that state

nursing process Systematic method for providing care to clients, consisting of five steps: assessment, diagnosis, outcome identification and planning, implementation, and evaluation

nutrition All of the processes (ingestion, digestion, absorption, metabolism, and elimination) involved in consuming and using food for energy, maintenance, and growth

nystagmus Constant, involuntary movement of the eye in various directions

O

obesity Weight that is 20% or more above the ideal body weight

objective data Observable and measurable data that are obtained through standard assessment techniques performed during the physical examination and through laboratory and diagnostic tests

occult blood Blood in the stool that can be detected only through a microscope or by chemical means

occult blood test (guaiac) Test for microscopic blood done on stool

older adulthood Development occurring from age 65 years until death

oligomenorrhea Decreased menstrual flow

oliguria Diminished production of urine

oncology Study of tumors

ongoing assessment Type of assessment that includes systematic monitoring of specific problems

ongoing planning Updates the client's plan of care

onset of action Time for the body to respond to a drug after administration

oophoritis Inflammation of the ovary

open reduction Surgical procedure that enables the surgeon to reduce (repair) a fracture under direct visualization

ophthalmia neonatorum Inflammation of a newborn's eyes that results from passing through the birth canal when a gonorrheal or chlamydial infection is present

opinion Subjective belief

opisthotonos Complete arching of the body with only the head and feet on the bed

opportunistic infection Infection in persons with a defective immune system that rarely causes harm in healthy individuals

oppression Condition wherein the rules, values, and ideals of one group are imposed on another group

orchiectomy Removal of a testis

orientation Person's awareness of self in relation to person, place, time, and in some cases, situation

orthopedics (orthopaedics) Branch of medicine that deals with the prevention or correction of the disorders and diseases of the musculoskeletal system

orthopnea Difficulty breathing while lying down

orthostatic hypotension Significant decrease in blood pressure that results when a person moves from a lying or sitting (supine) position to a standing position

osmolality Measurement of the total concentration of dissolved particles (solutes) per kilogram of water

osmolarity Concentration of solutes per liter of cellular fluid

osmosis Movement of a solvent, usually water, through a semipermeable membrane, from a region of higher concentration to a region of lower concentration

osmotic pressure Pressure exerted against the cell membrane by the water inside a cell

osteoporosis Increase in the porosity of bone

Outcomes and Assessment Information Set An outcomes measurable tool developed and implemented to determine the care given and reimbursement required; Outcomes and Assessment Information Set (OASIS) data is reported to the Centers for Medicare and Medicaid Services (CMS)

overflow incontinence Leaking of urine when the bladder becomes very full and distended

oxidation Chemical process of combining with oxygen

oxidized Joined with oxygen

P

pain Unpleasant sensory and emotional experience associated with actual or potential tissue damage or described in terms of such

pain threshold Level of intensity at which pain becomes appreciable or perceptible

pain tolerance Level of intensity or duration of pain that a person is willing to endure

palliative care Care that relieves symptoms, such as pain, but does not alter the course of disease

pallor Abnormal paleness of the skin, seen especially in the face, conjunctiva, nail beds, and oral mucous membranes

palpation Physical examination technique that uses the sense of touch to assess texture, temperature, moisture, organ location and size, vibrations and pulsations, swelling, masses, and tenderness

pancreatitis Acute or chronic inflammation of the pancreas

Papanicolaou test Smear method of examining stained exfoliative cells

paracentesis Aspiration of fluid from the abdominal cavity

paradoxical reaction Opposite effect of that which would normally be expected

paramedic Specialized health care professional trained to provide advanced life support to the client requiring emergency interventions

paraplegia Paralysis of lower extremities
parasomnia Disorders that intrude on sleep in very active ways
parenteral Any route other than the oral-gastrointestinal tract
parenteral nutrition Feeding method whereby nutrients bypass the small intestine and enter the blood directly
paresthesia Abnormal sensation such as burning, prickling, or tingling
paroxysmal Descriptor for a symptom that begins and ends abruptly
paroxysmal nocturnal dyspnea Condition of suddenly awakening, sweating, and having difficulty breathing
passive euthanasia Process of working with the client's dying process
patency Being freely opened
pathogen Microorganism that causes disease
pathogenicity Ability of a microorganism to produce disease
patient-controlled analgesia Device that allows the client to control the delivery of intravenous or subcutaneous pain medication in a safe, effective manner through a programmable pump
peak plasma level Highest blood concentration of a single dose of a drug until the elimination rate equals the rate of absorption
peer assistance program Rehabilitation program that provides an impaired nurse with referrals, professional and peer counseling support groups, and assistance and monitoring back into nursing
peptic ulcer Erosion formed in the esophagus, stomach, or duodenum resulting from acid/pepsin imbalance
perception Ability to experience, recognize, organize, and interpret sensory stimuli
percussion Physical examination technique that uses short, tapping strokes on the surface of the skin to create vibrations of underlying organs
perfectionism Overwhelming expectation of being able to get everything done in a flawless manner
perfusion Blood flow through an organ or body part
pericardial friction rub Short, high-pitched squeak heard as two inflamed pericardial surfaces rub together
pericardiocentesis Removal of fluid from the pericardial sac
pericarditis Inflammation of the membrane sac surrounding the heart
perineal care Cleansing of the external genitalia, perineum, and the surrounding area
perioperative Period of time encompassing the preoperative, intraoperative, and postoperative phases of surgery
peripheral nervous system System of the cranial nerves, spinal nerves, and the autonomic nervous system
peripheral resistance Pressure within a vessel that resists the flow of blood such as plaque buildup or vasoconstriction
peristalsis Rhythmic, coordinated, serial contraction of the smooth muscles of the gastrointestinal tract
peritonitis Inflammation of the peritoneum, the membranous covering of the abdomen
permeability Ability of a membrane to permit substances to pass through it
petechiae Pinpoint hemorrhagic spots on the skin
phantom limb pain Neuropathic pain that occurs after amputation with pain sensations referred to an area in the missing portion of the limb
pharmacokinetics Study of the absorption, distribution, metabolism, and excretion of drugs to determine the relationship between the dose of a drug and the drug's concentration in biological fluids
phimosis Condition wherein the opening in the foreskin is so small that it cannot be pulled back over the glans
phlebitis Inflammation in the wall of a vein without clot formation
phlebothrombosis Formation of a clot because of blood pooling in the vessel, trauma to the vessel's endothelial lining, or a coagulation problem with little or no inflammation in the vessel
phlebotomist Individual who performs venipuncture
phlebotomy Removal of blood from a vein
phospholipid Lipid composed of glycerol, fatty acids, and phosphorus; the structural component of cells
physical agent Factor in the environment capable of causing disease in a host
physical restraint Equipment that reduces the client's movement
physical wellness Healthy body that functions at an optimal level
physically aggressive Descriptor of an individual who threatens or actually harms someone
physiologic anemia of pregnancy Condition of having delivered after 24 weeks' gestation, whether infant is born alive or dead or number of infants born
phytochemical Physiologically active compound present in plants in very small amounts that gives plants flavor, odor, and color
pica Practice of eating substances not considered edible and that have no nutritive value, such as laundry starch, dirt, clay, and freezer frost
pie charting Documentation method using the problem, intervention, evaluation (PIE) format
piggyback Addition of an intravenous solution to infuse concurrently with another infusion

placenta Membranous vascular organ connecting the fetus to the mother, which produces hormones to sustain a pregnancy, supplies the fetus with oxygena and food, and transports waste products out of the fetal system
placenta previa Condition in which the placenta forms over or very near the internal cervical os
plague An infectious disease transmitted by a bite of a flea from a rodent (usually a rat) infected with the bacillus Yersinia pestis; plague is a potential agent of bioterrorism
planning Third step of the nursing process; includes both the establishing of guidelines for the proposed course of nursing action to resolve the nursing diagnoses and developing the client's plan of care
plateau Level at which a drug's blood concentration is maintained
pleural effusion Collection of fluid within the pleural cavity
pleural friction rub Abnormal breath sound that is creaky and grating in nature and is heard on inspiration and expiration
pleurisy Condition arising from inflammation of the pleura, or sac, that encases the lung
pneumonia Inflammation of the bronchioles and alveoli accompanied by consolidation, or solidification of exudate, in the lungs
pneumothorax Condition wherein air or gas accumulates in the pleural space of the lungs, causing the lungs to collapse
point-of-care charting Documentation system that allows health care providers to gain immediate access to client information at the bedside
poison Any substance that when taken into the body interferes with normal physiologic functioning; may be inhaled, injected, ingested, or absorbed by the body
polydipsia Excessive thirst
polymenorrhea Menstrual periods that are abnormally frequent, generally less than every 21 days
polyp Abnormal growth of tissue
polyphagia Increased hunger
polypharmacy Problem of clients taking numerous prescription and over-the-counter medications for the same or various disease processes, with unknown consequences from the resulting combinations of chemical compounds and cumulative side-effects
polyunsaturated fatty acid Forms a glycerol ester with many carbons unbonded to hydrogen atoms; fish, corn, sunflower seeds, soybeans, cotton seeds, and safflower oil
polyuria Increased urination
Port-a-Cath Port that has been implanted under the skin with a catheter inserted into the superior vena cava or right atrium through the subclavian or internal jugular vein
portal of entry Route by which an infectious agent enters the host
portal of exit Route by which an infectious agent leaves the reservoir
postictal After a seizure
post-mortem care Care given immediately after death before the body is moved to the mortuary
postoperative phase Time during the surgical experience that begins at the end of the surgical procedure and ends when the client is discharged, not just from the hospital or institution, but from medical care by the surgeon
postpartum blues Mild transient condition of emotional lability and crying for no apparent reason, which affects up to 80% of women who have just given birth, and lasts about 2 weeks
postpartum depression Condition similar to postpartum blues but is more serious, intense, and persistent
postpartum hemorrhage Blood loss of more than 500 mL after the third stage of labor or 1,000 mL following a cesarean birth
postpartum psychosis Condition more severe than postpartum depression and characterized by delusions and thoughts of self-harm or infant harm
postprandial After eating
postterm Delivery after 42 weeks' gestation
post-void residual Urine that remains in the bladder after urination
prayer A type of communication between an individual and spiritual entities
preadolescence Development from the ages of approximately 10 years to 12 years
precipitate birth Birth occurring suddenly and unexpectantly without a CNM/physician present to assist
precipitate labor Labor lasting less than 3 hours from the onset of contractions to the birth of the infant
preeclampsia Phase of pregnancy-induced hypertension prior to convulsions
preferred provider organization Type of managed care model wherein member choice is limited to providers within the system for full reimbursement and other providers for less reimbursement
prenatal care Care of a woman during pregnancy, before labor
prenatal stage Development beginning with conception and ending with birth
preoperative phase Time during the surgical experience that begins when the client decides to have surgery and ends when the client is transferred to the operating table
presbycusis Sensorineural hearing loss associated with aging

presbyopia Inability of the lens of the eye to change curvature to focus near objects
preschool stage Development from the ages of 3 years to 6 years
prescriptive authority Legal recognition of the ability to prescribe medications
presenting part Part of the fetus in contact with the cervix
pressured speech Rapid, intense style of speech
preterm Delivery after 24 weeks' gestation but before 38 weeks (full term)
preterm birth Birth that takes place before the end of the 37th week of gestation
preterm labor Onset of regular contractions of the uterus that cause cervical changes between 20 and 37 weeks' gestation
prevention Obstructing, thwarting, or hindering a disease or illness
priapism Prolonged erection that does not occur in response to sexual stimulation
primary care provider Health care provider whom a client sees first for health care, typically a family practitioner (physician/nurse), internist, or pediatrician
primary health care Client's point of entry into the health care system; includes assessment, diagnosis, treatment, coordination of care, education, prevention services, and surveillance
primary hypertension High blood pressure, the cause of which is unknown; also known as essential hypertension
primary prevention All practices designed to keep health problems from developing
primary source Major provider of information about a client
primary tubercle Nodule that contains tubercle bacilli and forms within lung tissue
primigravida Condition of being pregnant for the first time
primipara Condition of having delivered once after 24 weeks' gestation
privacy The right to be left alone, to choose care based on personal beliefs, to govern body integrity, and to choose when and how sensitive information is shared (Badzek & Gross, 1999)
problem-oriented medical record Documentation method employs a structured, logical format and focuses on the client's problem
process Series of steps or acts that leads to accomplishing some goal or purpose
procrastination Intentionally putting off or delaying something that should be done
prodromal stage Time interval from the onset of nonspecific symptoms until specific symptoms of the infectious process begin to manifest
professional boundaries Limits of the professional relationship that allow for a safe, therapeutic connection between the professional and the client
progressive muscle relaxation Stress-management strategy in which muscles are alternately tensed and relaxed
projectile vomiting Forceful ejection (up to 3 feet) of the contents of the stomach
prolapsed cord Condition in which the umbilical cord lies below the presenting part of the fetus
prolapsed uterus Downward displacement of the uterus into the vagina
prospective payment Predetermined rate paid for each episode of hospitalization based on the client's age and principal diagnosis and the presence or absence of surgery or comorbidity
protocol Series of standing orders or procedures that should be followed under certain specific conditions
proxemics Study of the space between people and its effect on interpersonal behavior
pruritus Severe itching
pseudocyesis False pregnancy
pseudomenstruation Blood-tinged mucus discharge from the vagina of a newborn caused by the withdrawal of maternal hormones
psychoanalysis Therapy focused on uncovering unconscious memories and processes
psychological wellness Enjoyment of creativity, satisfaction of the basic need to love and be loved, understanding of emotions, and ability to maintain control over emotions
psychomotor domain Area of learning that involves performance of motor skills
psychoneuroimmunology Study of the complex relationship among the physical, cognitive, and affective aspects of humans
psychoprophylaxis Mental and physical preparation for childbirth; synonymous with Lamaze
psychosis State wherein an individual has lost the ability to recognize reality
psychotherapy Treatment of mental and emotional disorders through psychological rather than physical methods
ptosis Drooping upper eyelid
puberty Emergence of secondary sex characteristics that signal the beginning of adolescence
public law Law that deals with an individual's relationship to the state
public self What the client thinks others think of him or her
pudendal block Injection of a local anesthetic into the pudendal nerve to provide perineal, external genitalia, and lower vaginal anesthesia

puerperal (postpartum) infection Infection following childbirth occurring between the birth and 6 weeks postpartum
puerperium Term for the first 6 weeks after the birth of an infant
pulse amplitude Measurement of the strength or force exerted by the ejected blood against the arterial wall with each heart contraction
pulse deficit Condition in which the apical pulse rate is greater than the radial pulse rate
pulse rate Indirect measurement of cardiac output obtained by counting the number of peripheral pulse waves over a pulse point
pulse rhythm Regularity of the heartbeat
purpura Reddish-purple patches on the skin indicative of hemorrhage
purulent exudate Discharge resulting from infection; also called pus
pyelonephritis Bacteral infection of the renal pelvis, tubules, and interstitial tissue of one or both kidneys
pyorrhea Periodontal disease
pyuria Pus in the urine

Q

quadriplegia Dysfunction or paralysis of both arms, both legs, and bowel and bladder
quickening Descriptor for when the mother first feels the fetus move, about 16 to 20 weeks' gestation

R

race A group of people with biological similarities
radiation Loss of heat by transfer to cooler near objects, but not through direct contact
radiation sickness An abnormal condition resulting from exposure to ionizing radiation, either purposefully or by accident
radiography Study of x-rays or gamma-ray-exposed film through the action of ionizing radiation
radiotherapy Treatment of cancer with high-energy radiation
rapport Mutual trust established between two people
readiness for learning Evidence of willingness to learn
real self How the individual really thinks about him- or herself
reasoning Use of the elements of thought to solve a problem or settle a question
reconstructive To rebuild or reestablish
rectocele Anterior displacement of the rectum into the posterior vaginal wall
recurrent acute pain Identified by repetitive painful episodes that recur over a prolonged period or throughout a client's lifetime
referred pain Discomfort from the internal organs that is felt in another area of the body
reframing Technique of monitoring negative thoughts and replacing them with positive ones
regional anesthesia Method of temporarily rendering a region of the body insensible to pain
rehabilitation Process or therapy designed to assist individuals to reach their optimal level of physical, mental, and psychosocial functioning
relapse Return to a previous behavior or condition
relaxation technique Method used to decrease anxiety and muscle tension
religion A system of organized beliefs, rituals, and practices with which a person identifies and wishes to be associated
religious support system Group of ministers, priests, nuns, rabbis, shamans, mullahs, or laypersons who are able to meet clients' spiritual needs
REM movement disorder Condition wherein the normal paralysis of REM sleep is absent or incomplete and the sleeper acts out the dream
remission Decrease or absence of symptoms of a disease
renal colic Severe pain in the kidney that radiates to the groin
repolarization Recovery phase of the cardiac muscle
reportable conditions Diseases or injuries that the government requires be reported to the appropriate authority or agency; include suspected abuse and/or neglect, sexually transmitted diseases (STDs), and certain other contagious illnesses that could threaten the health of the general public
reservoir Place where the agent can survive
resident flora Microorganisms that are always present, usually without altering the client's health
residual urine Urine remaining in the bladder after the individual has urinated
respect Acceptance of an individual as is and in a nonjudgmental manner
respiration Process of exchanging oxygen and carbon dioxide
respite care Care and service that provides a break to caregivers and is used for a few hours a week, for an occasional weekend, or for longer periods of time
rest State of mental and physical relaxation and calmness
restitution Rotation of the fetal head back to normal alignment with the shoulders after delivery of the fetal head
restless leg syndrome Condition characterized by uncomfortable sensations of tingling or crawling in the muscles, and twitching, burning, prickling, or deep aching in the foot, calf, or upper leg when at rest

restraint Protective device used to limit the physical activity of a client or to immobilize a client or extremity
resuscitation Support measures implemented to restore consciousness and life
reticulocyte Immature red blood cell
retroperitoneal Behind the peritoneum outside the peritoneal cavity
reverse isolation Barrier protection designed to prevent infection in clients who are severely compromised and highly susceptible to infection; also known as protective isolation
reverse tolerance Phenomenon whereby a smaller amount of substance will elicit the desired psychic effects
review of systems Brief account of any recent signs or symptoms related to any body system
rhinorrhea Watery nasal discharge
Ricin A poison made from the waste products of castor bean processing; a potential agent of bioterrorism because of its ease of dissemination
rigor mortis Natural stiffening of muscles after death; begins about 4 hours after death
risk nursing diagnosis Nursing diagnosis indicating that a problem does not yet exist but that specific risk factors are present; composed of "Risk for" followed by the diagnostic label and a list of the risk factors
role An ascribed or assumed expected behavior in a social position or group
role performance Specific behaviors a person exhibits within each role
rooming-in Practice of staying with the client 24 hours a day to provide care and comfort

S

salpingitis Inflammation of the fallopian tube
salt Product formed when an acid and a base react with each other
sanguineous Bloody drainage from a wound or surgical drain
sarcoma Cancer occurring in connective tissue
Sarin A dangerous man-made nerve agent, first developed as an insecticide that is a potential agent for bioterrorism
satiety Feeling of adequate fullness from food
school-age stage Development from the ages of 6 years to 10 years
sclerotherapy Treatment that involves injecting a chemical into the vein, causing the vein to become sclerosed (hardened) so blood no longer flows through it
sclerotic Hardened tissue
scoliosis Lateral curvature of the spine
scrub nurse RN, LP/VN, or surgical technologist who provides services under the direction of the circulating nurse and who is qualified by training or experience to prepare and maintain the integrity, safety, and efficiency of the sterile field throughout an operation
sebaceous cyst Sebaceous gland filled with sebum
sebum Oily substance secreted by the sebaceous glands of the skin
secondary care Care focused on diagnosis and treatment after the client exhibits symptoms of illness
secondary hypertension High blood pressure occurring as a sequel to a pre-existing disease or injury
secondary prevention Early detection, screening, diagnosis, and intervention, to reduce the consequences of a health problem
sedation Reduction of stress, excitement, or irritability via some central nervous system depression
self-awareness Consciously knowing how the self thinks, feels, believes, and behaves at any specific time
self-care deficit State wherein an individual is not able to perform one or more activities of daily living
self-concept Individual's perception of self; includes self-esteem, body image, and ideal self
self-efficacy Belief in one's ability to succeed in attempts to change behavior
self-esteem A personal opinion of oneself
semipermeable membrane Membrane that allows passage of only certain substances
sensation Ability to receive and process stimuli received through the sensory organs
sensible water loss Water loss of which the person is aware
sensitivity Susceptibility of a pathogen to an antibiotic
sensorineural hearing loss Condition in which the inner ear or cochlear portion of cranial nerve VIII is abnormal or diseased
sensory deficit Change in the perception of sensory stimuli; can affect any of the senses
sensory deprivation State of reduced sensory input from the internal or external environment, manifested by alterations in sensory perception
sensory overload State of excessive and sustained multisensory stimulation manifested by behavior change and perceptual distortion
sensory perception Ability to receive sensory impressions and, through cortical association, relate the stimuli to past experiences and form an impression of the nature of the stimulus
seroconversion Evidence of antibody formation in response to disease or vaccine
serosanguineous exudate Discharge that is clear with some blood tinge; seen with surgical incisions
serous exudate Discharge composed primarily of serum; is watery in appearance and has a low protein level.

serum lithium level Laboratory test done to determine whether the client's lithium level is within a therapeutic range
shaman Folk healer-priest who uses natural and supernatural forces to help others
shearing Force exerted against the skin by movement or repositioning
shift report Report about each client between shifts
shock Condition of profound hemodynamic and metabolic disturbance characterized by inadequate tissue perfusion and inadequate circulation to the vital organs
shroud Covering for the body after death
sibilant wheeze Abnormal breath sound that is high pitched and musical in nature and is heard on inhalation and exhalation
sickle When red blood cells become crescent-shaped and elongated
single point of entry Common feature of HMOs wherein the client is required to enter the health care system through a point designated by the plan
single-payer system Health care delivery model wherein the government is the only entity to reimburse health care costs
situational loss Loss that takes place in response to external events generally beyond the individual's control
slander Words that are communicated verbally to a third party and that harm or injure the personal or professional reputation of another
sleep State of altered consciousness during which a person has minimal physical activity, changes in levels of consciousness, and a slowing of physiologic processes
sleep apnea A period during sleep of not breathing; often associated with heavy snoring
sleep cycle Sequence of sleep beginning with the four stages of NREM sleep, a return to stage 3 and then stage 2 (first phase), followed by the first REM sleep (second phase)
sleep deprivation Prolonged inadequate quality and quantity of sleep
small for gestational age Infant's weight falls below the 10th percentile for gestational age
smallpox (variola) A highly contagious and frequently fatal viral disease, which is a potential agent for a bioterroristic attack; there are two varieties, known as variola major and variola minor
Snellen Chart Chart containing various-sized letters with standardized numbers at the end of each line of letters
sociocultural wellness Ability to appreciate the needs of others and to care about one's environment and the inhabitants of it
somatic nervous system Nerves that connect the central nervous system to the skin and skeletal muscles and control conscious activities
somatic pain Nonlocalized discomfort originating in tendons, ligaments, and nerves
somnambulism Sleepwalking
Somogyi phenomenon In response to hypoglycemia, the release of glucose-elevating hormones (epinephrine, cortisol, glucose), which produces a hyperglycemic state
sonorous wheeze Abnormal breath sound that is low pitched and snoring in nature and is louder on expiration
spermatogenesis Production of sperm
spina bifida occulta Failure of the vertebral arch to close
spinal shock Cessation of motor, sensory, autonomic, and reflex impulses below the level of injury; characterized by flaccid paralysis of all skeletal muscles, loss of spinal reflexes, loss of sensation, and absence of autonomic function below the level of injury
spiritual care Recognition of and assistance toward meeting spiritual needs
spiritual distress A client in this situation may have a troubled, fragmented, or possibly disintegrating spirit
spiritual needs Individual's desire to find purpose and meaning in life, pain, and death
spiritual wellness Inner strength and peace
spirituality The core of a person's being, a higher experience or transcendence of oneself
spore Bacteria in a resistant stage that can withstand unfavorable environments
sprain Injury to ligaments surrounding a joint caused by a sudden twist, wrench, or fall
stable Alert with vital signs within the client's normal range
staff development Delivery of instruction to assist nurses achieve the goals of the employer
standard Level or degree of quality
Standard Precautions Preventive practices to be used in the care of all clients in hospitals regardless of their diagnosis or presumed infection status
standards of practice Guidelines established to direct nursing care
startle response Overreaction to minor sounds or noises
stasis dermatitis Inflammation of the skin due to decreased circulation
station Relationship of the fetal presenting part to the ischial spines
status asthmaticus Persistent, intractable asthma attack
status epilepticus Acute, prolonged episode of seizure activity that lasts at least 30 minutes and may or may not involve loss of consciousness
statutory law Law enacted by legislative bodies
steatorrhea Fatty stool

stent Tiny metal tube with holes in it that prevents a vessel from collapsing and keeps the atherosclerotic plaque pressed against the vessel wall; any material used to hold tissue in place or provide support
stereognosis Ability to recognize an object by feel
stereotyping Belief that all people within the same ethnic, racial, or cultural group act the same way, sharing the same beliefs and attitudes
sterile Without microorganisms
sterile conscience Individual's personal sense of honesty and integrity with regard to adherence to the principles of aseptic technique, including prompt admission and correction of any errors and omissions
sterile field Area surrounding the client and the surgical site that is free from all microorganisms; created by draping of the work area and the client with sterile drape
sterilization Destroying all microorganisms, including spores
stock supply Medications dispensed and labeled in large quantities for storage in the medication room or nursing unit
stoma Surgical opening between a cavity and the surface of the body
stomatitis Inflammation of the oral mucosa
strabismus Inability of the eyes to focus in the same direction
strain Injury to a muscle or tendon due to overuse or overstretching
stress Nonspecific response to any demand made on the body (Selye, 1974)
stress incontinence Leakage of urine when a person does anything that strains the abdomen, such as coughing, laughing, jogging, dancing, sneezing, lifting, making a quick movement, or even walking
stress test Measure of a client's cardiovascular response to exercise
stressor Any situation, event, or agent that produces stress
striae gravidarum Reddish streaks frequently found on the abdomen, thighs, buttocks, and breasts; also called "stretch marks"
stridor High-pitched, harsh sound heard on inspiration when the trachea or larynx is obstructed
stroke volume Volume of blood pumped by the ventricle with each contraction
stye Pustular inflammation of an eyelash follicle or sebaceous gland on the eyelid margin
subacute care Short-term, aggressive care for clients who are out of the acute stage of illness but who still require skilled nursing, monitoring, and ongoing treatment
subcutaneous Injection into the subcutaneous tissue
subinvolution Incomplete return of the uterus to its prepregnant size and consistency
subluxation Partial separation of an articular surface
substance A drug, legal or illegal, that may cause physical or mental impairment
suicidal ideations Thoughts of hurting or killing oneself
supine hypotensive syndrome Lowering of blood pressure in a pregnant woman when lying supine due to compression of the vena cava by the enlarged, heavy uterus
surfactant Phospholipids that are present in the lungs and lower surface tension to prevent collapse of the airways
surgery Treatment of injury, disease, or deformity through invasive operative methods
suture Thin, fibrous, membrane-covered space between skull bones
synarthrosis Immovable joint
syndactyly Fusion of two or more fingers or toes
synergism Result of two or more agents working together to achieve a greater effect than either could produce alone
synthesiasis Hearing colors and seeing sounds
synthesis Chemical reaction when two or more atoms, called reactants, bond and form a more complex molecular product; putting data together in a new way

T

tachycardia Heart rate in excess of 100 beats per minute in an adult
tachypnea Respiratory rate greater than 24 beats per minute
talipes equinovarus A congenital deformity in which the foot and ankle are twisted inward and cannot be moved to a midline position; also known as clubfoot
teaching Active process wherein one individual shares information with another as a means to facilitate learning and thereby promote behavioral changes
teaching strategy Technique to promote learning
teaching–learning process Planned interaction that promotes a behavioral change that is not a result of maturation or coincidence
telangiectasic nevi Birthmarks of dilated capillaries that blanch with pressure; also called stork-bites
telangiestasia Permanent dilation of groups of superficial capillaries and venules; commonly known as "spider veins"
telehealth An electronic information services that offer increased client and family participation; for example, nurse and client use interactive videos, telephone

cardiac rate monitoring with EKG readout, digital subscriber lines, and Internet transmission of data

telemedicine An element of telehealth permitting physicians to provide care through a telecommunication system

teleology Ethical theory that states that the value of a situation is determined by its consequences

tenesmus Spasmodic contradiction of the anal or bladder sphincter, causing pain and a persistent urge to empty the bowel or bladder

teratogen Agent such as radiation, drugs, viruses, and other microorganisms capable of causing abnormal fetal development

teratogenic Causing abnormal development of the embryo

teratogenic substance Substance that crosses the placenta and impairs normal growth and development

term Descriptor for a pregnancy between 38 and 42 weeks' gestation

terrorism Instilling fear in large groups of persons by using any product, weapon, or the threat of using a harmful act or substance to kill or injure people

tertiary care Care focused on restoring the client to the state of health that existed before the development of an illness; if unattainable, then care is directed to attaining the optimal level of health possible

tertiary prevention Treatment of an illness or disease after symptoms have appeared, so as to prevent further progression

tetany Sharp flexion of the wrist and ankle joints, involving muscle twitching or cramps

therapeutic communication Communication that is purposeful and goal directed, creating a beneficial outcome for the client

therapeutic massage Application of hand pressure and motion to improve the recipient's well-being

therapeutic procedure accident Accident that occurs during the delivery of medical or nursing interventions

therapeutic touch Technique of assessing alterations in a person's energy fields and using the hands to direct energy to achieve a balanced state

thermogenesis Production of heat

thermoregulation Maintenance of body temperature

thoracentesis Aspiration of fluid from the pleural cavity

thrombocytopenia Decrease in the number of platelets in the blood

thrombophlebitis Formation of a clot due to an inflammation in the wall of the vessel

thrombosis Formation of a clot due to an inflammation in the wall of the vessel

thrombus Formed clot that remains at the site where it formed

time management System to help meet goals through problem solving

tinnitus Ringing sound in the ear

tocolysis Process of stopping labor with medications

tocolytic agent Medication that inhibits uterine contractions

toddler stage Development begins at approximately 12 to 18 months of age, when a child begins to walk, and ends at approximately 3 years of age

tolerance Decreased sensitivity to subsequent doses of the same substance; an increased dose of the substance is needed to produce the same desired effect

tophi Subcutaneous nodules of sodium urate crystals

tort Civil wrong committed by a person against another person or property

tort law Enforcement of duties and rights among individuals and independent of contractual agreements

touch Means of perceiving or experiencing through tactile sensation

toxic effect Reaction that occurs when the body cannot metabolize a drug and the drug accumulates in the blood

trade (brand) name Name assigned to a drug by the pharmaceutical company; always capitalized

transcendence A state of being or existence above and beyond the limits of material experience

transcutaneous electrical nerve stimulation Process of applying a low-voltage electrical current to the skin through cutaneous electrodes

transducer Instrument that converts electrical energy to sound waves

transduction Noxious stimulus that triggers electrical activity in the endings of afferent nerve fibers (nociceptors)

transmission Process whereby the pain impulse travels from the receiving nociceptors to the spinal cord

Transmission-based Precautions Practices designed for clients documented as, or suspected of, being infected with highly transmissible or epidemiologically important pathogens for which additional precautions beyond Standard Precautions are required to interrupt transmission in hospitals

trauma Wound or injury

traumatic imagery Imagining the feelings of horror felt by the victim or reliving the horror of the incident

triage Classification of clients to determine priority of need and proper place of treatment

triglyceride Lipid compound consisting of three fatty acids and a glycerol molecule

trocar Sharply pointed surgical instrument contained in a cannula
Trousseau's sign Carpal spasm caused by inflating a blood pressure cuff above the client's systolic pressure and leaving it in place for 3 minutes
trust Ability to rely on an individual's character and ability
tumor marker Substance found in the serum that indicates the possible presence of malignancy
turgor Normal resiliency of the skin
type and cross-match Laboratory test that identifies the client's blood type (e.g., A or B) and determines the compatibility of the blood between potential donor and recipient

U

ultrasound Use of high-frequency sound waves to visualize deep body structures; also called an echogram or sonogram
umbilical cord Structure that connects the fetus to the placenta
uncomplicated grief Grief reaction normally following a significant loss
unilateral neglect Failure to recognize or care for one side of the body
unit dose form System of packaging and labeling each dose of medication by the pharmacy, usually for a 24-hour period
urethrocele Downward displacement of the urethra into the vagina
urethrostomy Formation of a permanent fistula opening into the urethra
urge incontinence Inability to suppress the sudden urge or need to urinate
urgent care center A facility designed for the effective and efficient treatment of acute illnesses and injuries; clients do not require an appointment, do not see the same provider consistently, and are usually seen in the order of arrival or the order of acuity
urobilinogen Colorless derivative of bilirubin formed by the normal bacterial action of intestinal flora on bilirubin
urticaria Allergic reaction causing raised pruritic, red, nontender wheals on the skin; also called hives
uterine retraction Unique ability of the muscle fibers of the uterus to remain shortened to a small degree after each contraction
uterine souffle Sound of blood pulsating through the uterus and placenta
utility Ethical principle that states that an act must result in the greatest positive benefit for the greatest number of people involved

V

value system Individual's collection of inner beliefs that guides the way the person acts and helps determine the choices the person makes
values Influences on the development of beliefs and attitudes rather than behaviors; a principle, standard, or quality considered worthwhile or desirable
values clarification Process of analyzing one's own values to better understand those things that are truly important
variable deceleration Reduction in fetal heart rate that has no relationship to contractions of the uterus
vasectomy Surgical resection of the vas deferens
venipuncture Puncturing of a vein with a needle to aspirate blood
ventilation Movement of gases into and out of the lungs
veracity Ethical principle based on truthfulness (neither lying nor deceiving others)
verbal communication Using words, either spoken or written, to send a message
verbally aggressive Descriptor of an individual who says things in a loud and/or intimidating manner
vernix caseosa White, creamy substance covering a fetus's body
vertigo Dizziness
vesicant Agent that may produce blisters and tissue necrosis
vesicular sound Soft, breezy, low-pitched sound heard longer on inspiration than expiration resulting from air moving through the smaller airways over the lung periphery, with the exception of the scapular area
villi Finger-like projections that line the small intestine
viral load test Test that measures copies of HIV RNA
visceral pain Discomfort felt in the internal organs
visual hallucination Perception by an individual that something is present when nothing in fact is
visual learner Person who learns by processing information through seeing
vitamin Organic compounds essential to life and health
vitiligo Depigmentation of the skin caused by destruction of melanocytes; appears as milk-white patches on the skin
void Process of urine elimination
volvulus Twisting of a bowel on itself

W

water-soluble vitamin Vitamin that must be ingested daily in normal quantities because it is not stored in the body: vitamins C and B-complex

wellness State of optimal health wherein an individual maximizes human potential, moves toward integration of human functioning, has greater self-awareness and self-satisfaction, and takes responsibility for health

Western blot test Confirmatory test used to detect HIV infection

Wharton's jelly Thick substance surrounding and protecting the vessels of the umbilical cord

whistleblowing Calling public attention to unethical, illegal, or incompetent actions of others

windowing Cutting a hole in a plaster cast to relieve pressure on the skin or a bony area and to permit visualization of the underlying body part

witch's milk A whitish fluid secreted by a newborn's nipples

withdrawal Symptoms produced when a substance on which an individual has dependence is no longer used by that individual

word salad Nonsensical combination of words that is meaningless to others

wound Disruption in the integrity of body tissue

Y

yin and yang Opposing forces that yield health when in balance

young adulthood Development from the ages of 21 years through approximately 40 years

Z

zoonotic disease A disease of animals that is directly transmissible to humans from the primary animal host

zygote Fertilized ovum

INDEX

Page numbers followed by "f" denote figures, "t" denote tables, and "b" denote boxes.

B

C

D

J

K

L

M

N

O

P

Q

R

S

U

V